OXFORD MEDICAL PUBLICATION

Oxford Desk Reference

Obstetrics and Gynaecology

Oxford Desk Reference
Obstetrics and Gynaecology

Sabaratnam Arulkumaran
Professor and Head of Obstetrics & Gynaecology
St George's, University of London
Cranmer Terrace, London, UK

Lesley Regan
Professor and Head of Obstetrics & Gynaecology
Imperial College at St Mary's Hospital, London, UK

Aris T. Papageorghiou
Consultant in Obstetrics and Maternal Fetal Medicine
Honorary Senior Lecturer
St George's, University of London, Cranmer Terrace, London, UK

Ash Monga
Consultant Gynaecologist and Sub-specialist in Uro Gynaecology
Department of Obstetrics & Gynaecology
Southampton University Hospital, Southampton, UK

David I. M. Farquharson
Consultant Gynaecologist
Department of Obstetrics & Gynaecology
Simpson Centre for Reproductive Health
Royal Infirmary, Edinburgh, UK

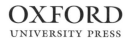
OXFORD
UNIVERSITY PRESS

OXFORD
UNIVERSITY PRESS

Great Clarendon Street, Oxford OX2 6DP

Oxford University Press is a department of the University of Oxford.
It furthers the University's objective of excellence in research, scholarship,
and education by publishing worldwide in

Oxford New York

Athens Auckland Bangkok Bogotá Buenos Aires Cape Town
Chennai Dar es Salaam Delhi Florence Hong Kong Istanbul Karachi
Kolkata Kuala Lumpur Madrid Melbourne Mexico City Mumbai Nairobi
Paris São Paulo Shanghai Singapore Taipei Tokyo Toronto Warsaw

with associated companies in Berlin Ibadan

Oxford is a registered trade mark of Oxford University Press
in the UK and in certain other countries

Published in the United States
by Oxford University Press Inc., New York

British Library Cataloguing in Publication Data

Data available

Library of Congress Cataloguing in Publication Data

Data available

ISBN 978-0-19-955221-4

10 9 8 7 6 5 4 3 2 1

Typeset in GillHandbook
by Glyph International, Bangalore, India
Printed in Great Britain
on acid-free paper by
CPI Antony Rowe, Chippenham, Wiltshire

Preface

The new training system in medicine brought about by Modernising Medical Careers (MMC) in the UK and the new European Working Time Directives (EWTD) present new challenges for the practising clinician on the ward, clinic or operating theatre. The structured training period is for seven years but s/he will be expected to know the details of each and every condition, how they present and how to manage them from Day 1. Reduction of training time is not unique to Europe and similar reductions are taking place in other countries such as America and Asia Oceania. Although there will be seniors present to train the junior doctor, they should have some baseline knowledge in order to ensure that they are in a position to have an intelligent and useful discussion with their Senior mentor. A Desk Reference that is available in every clinic, ward or theatre should be able to provide the user with enough information to understand the nature of the problem. It may even provide sufficient knowledge to solve it or at least to prompt initial investigations and management. Not all the conditions one encounters in daily working life are common problems; they will be varied and of different magnitudes. Even an experienced clinician may not remember all the detailed steps to follow to help resolve every problem. Furthermore, if they have not encountered the problem recently, the optimal investigation and management plan may have changed significantly. The Desk Reference provides information on the breadth and depth of Obstetrics & Gynaecology that will help the clinician to provide optimal care for their patients by offering appropriate investigations and treatment.

The sections and chapters in the book are organised in a way that is to easy to navigate once the major area is identified – akin to the 'Yellow Pages' Telephone Directory. Within each section the topics are displayed in alphabetical order. Not all topics in each section will fit into the same mould, but effort has been taken to prepare it in the same style, in order to make it easy for the reader. The book therefore is different from conventional books. Many practising clinicians may have good knowledge in several topics but be weak in others. This book should cater for those who like to "zoom in" straight to the problem they are trying to solve.

The Editors are internationally renowned for their expertise in the different subspecialties. The authors have been chosen based on their special expertise to cover the entire field of Obstetrics & Gynaecology. They have taken great effort to consult the latest articles in Pubmed, the Cochrane Reviews, NICE and RCOG Guidelines in constructing their chapters. Each of the editors have edited their subsection.

This book will improve knowledge and enhance high quality, safe, evidence based practice. Every book is likely to have errors and omissions. The editors and the publishers welcome constructive criticism from their reader, which will enable them to make the next edition even more comprehensive.

Contents

Detailed contents *xi*
List of contributors *xiii*

1 **Examination of the obstetric patient** 1

2 **Examination of the gynaecological patient** 7

3 **Communication: confidentiality, breaking bad news, and obtaining consent** 11

4 **Legal framework for care in obstetrics and gynaecology** 19

5 **Normal pregnancy** 31

6 **Complications of early pregnancy** 73

7 **Care of the fetus** 83

8 **Maternal medicine and infections** 175

9 **Obstetric conditions** 319

10 **Care in labour** 363

11 **Common obstetric techniques, procedures, and surgery** 429

12 **Reproduction** 463

13 **Benign and urogynaecology** 599

14 **Benign, premalignant, and malignant tumours in gynaecology** 639

15 **Common gynaecological procedures and surgery** 687

Index *713*

Detailed contents

List of contributors *xiii*

Part 1 **Introduction**

1 **Examination of the obstetric patient** *3*

Examination of the obstetric patient *4*

2 **Examination of the gynaecological patient** *7*

Examination of the gynaecological patient *8*

3 **Communication: confidentiality, breaking bad news, and obtaining consent** *11*

Communication: confidentiality, breaking bad news and obtaining consent *12*

4 **Legal framework for care in obstetrics and gynaecology** *19*

Legal framework for care in obstetrics and gynaecology *20*

Part 2 **Obstetrics**

5 **Normal pregnancy** *31*

Antenatal care *32*
Booking *38*
Breastfeeding *42*
Dating in pregnancy *48*
Diagnosis of pregnancy *50*
Minor symptoms of pregnancy *52*
Physiological changes in pregnancy *56*
Preparing for pregnancy *60*
Puerperium *64*
Routine blood tests in pregnancy *68*

6 **Complications of early pregnancy** *73*

Bleeding and pain in early pregnancy *74*
Hyperemesis gravidarum *76*
Pregnancy of unknown location *80*

7 **Care of the fetus** *83*

Biophysical profile *84*
Cardiotocography *86*

Doppler ultrasound *90*
Fetal abnormalities: cardiovascular *94*
Fetal abnormalities: central nervous system *98*
Fetal abnormalities: chromosomal anomalies *106*
Fetal abnormalities: genetic disorders *110*
Fetal abnormalities: face *116*
Fetal abnormalities: gastrointestinal system *118*
Fetal abnormalities: limbs *124*
Fetal abnormalities: head and neck *128*
Fetal abnormalities: skeletal abnormalities/dysplasias *132*
Fetal abnormalities: thorax *136*
Fetal abnormalities: urinary system *140*
Fetal movement charts *144*
Fetal nuchal translucency *146*
Fetal abnormalities: hydrops *148*
Invasive procedures *152*
Intrauterine growth restriction (IUGR) *156*
Multiple pregnancy *158*
Oligohydramnios *160*
Placental abnormalities *162*
Polyhydramnios *164*
Red blood cell isoimmunization *166*
Screening for fetal aneuploidy *168*
Symphyseal fundal height *172*

8 **Maternal medicine and infections** *175*

Adrenal disorders in pregnancy *176*
Anaemia in pregnancy *180*
Autoimmune disease *182*
Bacterial vaginosis *184*
Chicken pox/herpes zoster *186*
Chlamydia *188*
Coagulation disorders *190*
Connective tissue disorder *192*
Cytomegalovirus *196*
Dermatology *198*
Diabetes in pregnancy *200*
Drugs in pregnancy *208*
Epilepsy and other neurological conditions *214*
Gonorrhoea *218*
Perinatal group B streptococcus *220*
Haemoglobinopathies *222*
Heart disease *224*
Hepatitis B *238*
Herpes simplex infection *242*

HIV infection 244
Human papillomavirus 250
Hypertension 252
Immunization 258
Inflammatory bowel disease 262
Jaundice 266
Listeriosis 272
Liver disease 274
Measles: rubeola 278
Parvovirus 280
Pituitary disorders in pregnancy 282
Psychiatric disorders in pregnancy 286
Renal disease 290
Respiratory disease 296
Rubella 302
Substance abuse in pregnancy 304
Syphilis 306
Thromboembolic disease 310
Thyroid and parathyroid disease 312
Toxoplasmosis in pregnancy 316
Vulvovaginal candidiasis 318

9 **Obstetric conditions** 319
Abdominal pain in pregnancy 320
Amniotic fluid embolism 324
Antepartum haemorrhage 326
Cancer in pregnancy 328
Fibroids in pregnancy 330
Obstetric cholestasis 332
Ovarian cysts in pregnancy 336
Postnatal depression 338
Puerperal psychosis 342
Pre-eclampsia and eclampsia 344
Premalignant conditions of the genital tract in pregnancy 349
Preterm labour 350
Preterm prelabour rupture of membranes 354
Prolonged pregnancy 358
Puerperal sepsis 360

10 **Care in labour** 363
Analgesia and anaesthesia in obstetrics 364
Breech 368
Brow presentation 371
Cord prolapse 372
Episiotomy and obstetric perineal trauma 374
Face presentation 376
Fetal surveillance in labour 378
Home birth 384
Induction of labour 386
Labour 390

Maternal collapse 394
Meconium-stained liquor 398
Placenta praevia 402
Placental abruption 406
Postpartum haemorrhage 408
Prelabour rupture of membranes at term 412
Resuscitation of the newborn 414
Retained placenta 418
Shoulder dystocia 420
Shoulder presentation 424
Uterine inversion 426

11 **Common obstetric techniques, procedures, and surgery** 429
Balloon tamponade 430
Caesarean section 434
Forceps delivery 446
Uterine compression sutures 452
Ventouse delivery 456

Part 3 **Gynaecology**

12 **Reproduction** 463
Ambiguous genitalia 464
Anatomy of female pelvis 468
Chronic pelvic pain 476
Contraception 478
Disorders of sex development 482
Donor insemination 484
Heavy menstrual bleeding 486
Dysmenorrhoea 488
Ectopic pregnancy 490
Embryo freezing 494
Emergency contraception 498
Endometriosis 500
Female infertility 502
Fertility in survivors of childhood malignancy 508
Imaging in reproductive medicine 512
Induction of ovulation 514
Intracytoplasmic sperm injection 518
Intrauterine devices 520
In vitro fertilization 524
In vitro oocyte maturation 528
Malformations of the genital tract 532
Male subfertility 536
Menopause and hormone replacement therapy 542
Menorrhagia 550
Menstrual cycle: physiology 554
Miscarriage: early 556

Oocyte donation 560
Oligomenorrhoea and amenorrhoea 562
Ovarian hyperstimulation syndrome 566
Paediatric and adolescent problems 570
Polycystic ovary syndrome 574
Preimplantation genetic diagnosis 578
Premature ovarian failure 580
Premenstrual syndrome 582
Psychosexual problems 584
Recurrent miscarriage 590
Termination of pregnancy 594

13 **Benign and urogynaecology** 599

Endometrial polyps 600
Female genital cutting 602
Fibroids 606
Ovarian cysts 610
Pelvic inflammatory disease 612
Female urinary incontinence 614
Urinary frequency and urgency 618
Urinary retention (voiding difficulty) 620
Urinary tract injury 622
Uterovaginal prolapse 626
Urodynamic investigation 630
Vaginal discharge 632
Vesicovaginal fistulae 634
Vulval pain and pruritus 636

14 **Benign, premalignant, and malignant tumours in gynaecology** 639

Cancer screening for women 640
Cervical cancer 644
Cervical dysplasia and human papillomavirus 648
Neoplastic conditions of the endometrium 652
Gestational trophoblastic neoplasia 658
Ovarian and fallopian tube cancer 664
Palliative care 670
Vulval cancer 676
Vulval intraepithelial neoplasia 682

15 **Common gynaecological procedures and surgery** 687

Colposcopy 688
Endometrial ablation techniques 690
Hysteroscopy 694
Hysterectomy 698
Continence procedures 702
Pipelle biopsy 705
Laparoscopy 706
Pelvic floor surgery 710

Index 713

List of contributors

Dr Nihal Abdu
Clinical Fellow in Maternal Medicine
Epsom and St Helier Hospital, Surrey, UK

Mr Nigel Acheson
Consultant Gynaecological Oncologist
Centre for Women's Health
Royal Devon and Exeter NHS Foundation Trust,
Exeter, UK

Dr Rina Agrawal
Consultant and Honorary Associate
Professor in Obstetrics/Gynaecology and
Specialist in Reproductive Medicine
University College London and University Hospitals of
Warwickshire London and Warwickshire, UK

Dr Adil Akram
Academic Clinical Fellow in
Social & Community Psychiatry
St George's, University of London,
Cranmer Terrace, London, UK

Dr Sakina Ali
Specialist Registrar in Neonatology
St George's Healthcare NHS Trust
London, UK

Dr Meredith J. Alston
Department of Obstetrics and Gynecology
Denver Health Medical Center
University of Colorado School of Medicine,
Denver, CO, USA

Dr Tiziana Arcangeli
Clinical Fellow
Fetal Medicine Unit
St George's Healthcare NHS Trust
London, UK

Professor Sir Sabaratnam Arulkumaran
Professor and Head of Obstetrics & Gynaecology
St George's, University of London,
Cranmer Terrace, London, UK

Dr Baris Ata
Clinical and Research Fellow in Reproductive
Endocrinology and Infertility
McGill Reproductive Centre,
Dept of Obstetrics and Gynecology,
McGill University
Royal Victoria Hospital, Montreal, Canada

Dr Antonio Barbera
Assistant Professor of Obstetrics & Gynaecology
University of Colorado Medical Center,
Denver, CO, USA

Professor Ahmet A Baschat
Head, Section of Fetal Therapy
University of Maryland School of Medicine Baltimore,
MD, USA

Dr Amarnath Bhide
Consultant in Obstetrics and Fetal Medicine,
St George's Healthcare NHS Trust
Hon. Senior Lecturer
St George's, University of London,
Cranmer Terrace, London, UK

Professor Arijit Biswas
Associate Professor
National University of Singapore, Singapore

Dr Cecilia Bottomley
Consultant in Obstetrics & Gynaecology
Chelsea and Westminster Hospital, London, UK

Professor Peter Braude
Head of Department of Women's Health
King's College London, School of Medicine,
Guy's, King's and St Thomas' Hospitals
St Thomas' Hospital, London, UK

Professor Joanna Cain
Professor & Chair, Obstetrics and
Gynaecology Department and Julie Neupert Stott
Director,
Center for Women's Health Oregon Health & Science
University, Portland, OR, USA

Valerie Cameron
Department of Obstetrics & Gynaecology
McGill University
Montreal, Canada

Dr J. Chris Carey
Director of Obstetrics and Gynecology and
Director of Medical Education, Denver Health Professor
and Affiliate Dean,
University of Colorado School of Medicine Denver,
CO, USA

Dr Cissy Caroline
Specialist Registrar in Obstetrics & Gynaecology
St George's Healthcare NHS Trust
London, UK

Dr Julene Carvalho
Consultant in Fetal & Paediatric Cardiology,
St George's Healthcare NHS Trust, London, UK
and Royal Brompton Hospital, London, UK

Dr Charlotte Chaliha
Consultant Obstetrician & Gynaecologist and
Sub-specialist in Uro Gynaecology
Department of Obstetrics and Gynaecology,
Royal London and St Bartholomew's Hospitals,
London, UK

Mr Edwin Chandraharan
Consultant Obstetrician & Gynaecologist
Lead Consultant Labour Ward & Lead for Clinical
Governance
St George's Healthcare NHS Trust
London, UK

Dr Mahesh A Choolani
Associate Professor of Obstetrics & Gynaecology
National University of Singapore, Singapore

Professor Tony Kwok Hung Chung
Professor of Obstetrics and Gynaecology
The Chinese University of Hong Kong, Shatin,
Hong Kong

Dr Britt Clausson
Consultant Obstetrician and Gynaecologist and Honorary
Senior Lecturer
St George's University of London and
Mayday Healthcare, Department of Obstetrics and
Gynaecology, Mayday Healthcare,
Croydon, London, UK

Dr Edward Coats
Specialist Registrar Obstetrics & Gynaecology
St Michael's University Hospital, Bristol, UK

Mr Jason Cooper
Clinical Director and Consultant Gynaecologist,
University Hospital of North Staffordshire, Maternity
Centre, Stoke on Trent, UK

Miss Sarah Creighton
Consultant Gynaecologist
Department of Women's Health
University College Hospital, London, UK

Professor Hilary OD Critchley
Professor of Reproductive Medicine/Honorary
Consultant in Obstetrics and Gynaecology
University of Edinburgh, Edinburgh, UK

Dr Mary Crofton
Consultant Radiologist
Imperial College Healthcare NHS Trust
St Mary's Campus, London, UK

Dr Naomi Crouch
Specialist Registrar in Obstetrics and Gynaecology
UCL Hospitals, London, UK

Professor Howard Cuckle
Adjunct Professor
Department of Obstetrics and Gynecology
Columbia University Medical Center, New York, USA

Dr Rohan D'Souza
Clinical Fellow
Fetal Medicine Unit,
St George's Healthcare NHS Trust
London, UK

Miss Melanie Davies
Consultant Obstetrician and Gynaecologist
University College London Hospitals,
Reproductive Medicine Unit, London, UK

Miss Mandish K Dhanjal
Consultant Obstetrician and Gynaecologist
Honorary Senior Lecturer
Queen Charlotte's and Chelsea Hospital,
Imperial College Healthcare NHS Trust, London, UK

Ms Claudine Domoney
Chair of the Institute of Psychosexual Medicine,
Consultant Obstetrician and Gynaecologist
Chelsea and Westminster Hospital, London, UK

Dr Stergios K. Doumouchtsis
Senior Specialist Registrar in Obstetrics and Gynaecology
St George's Healthcare NHS Trust
London, UK

Ms Anita Dutta
Senior Registrar in Obstetrics and Gynaecology
Guy's and St. Thomas' NHS Foundation Trusts,
London, UK

Dr David I M Farquharson
Consultant Gynaecologist
Department of Obstetrics & Gynaecology
Simpson Centre for Reproductive Health,
Royal Infirmary, Edinburgh, UK

Miss Azza Fattah
Consultant Obstetrics & Gynaecology
Pontefract General Infirmary, Pontefract, UK

Dr Daniel Forton
Consultant Hepatologist and Honorary Senior Lecturer
St George's Healthcare NHS Trust
London, UK

Dr Markus Gess
Clinical Research Fellow
St George's, University of London
Cranmer Terrace, London, UK

Dr Madhusree Ghosh
Specialist Registrar
Obstetrics and Gynaecology
St George's Healthcare NHS Trust
London, UK

Professor Ronald Gibbs
Professor & Head of Obstetrics & Gynaecology
University of Colorado, USA

Dr David Gillott
Lecturer
Obstetrics & Gynaecology
St Bartholomew's Hospital London University, London, UK

Dr Catriona Hardie
Specialist Registrar
Department of Gynaecological Oncology
Oncology, Glasgow Royal Infirmary, Glasgow, UK

Dr Phillip Hay
Reader and Honorary Consultant
Genitourinary and HIV Medicine
St George's, University of London, Cranmer Terrace,
London, UK

Mr Kevin Hayes
Consultant/Senior Lecturer in Obstetrics and
Gynaecology
Department of Obstetrics and Gynaecology
St George's Healthcare NHS Trust
London, UK

Dr Gretchen Heinrichs
Assistant Professor
Obstetrics and Gynaecology
Denver Health and UCDenver SOM, Denver, CO, USA

Professor Jenny Higham
Director of Education
Faculty of Medicine, Imperial College London,
London, UK

Professor Pak Chung Ho
Chair Professor of Obstetrics and Gynaecology
Department of Obstetrics and Gynaecology, The
University of Hong Kong, Hong Kong, China

Professor G Justus Hofmeyr
Consultant/Associate Professor
Department of Obstetrics and Gynaecology,
East London Hospital Complex, London
and Walter Sisulu University, South Africa

Dr Tessa Homfray
Consultant Geneticist
St George's, University of London
Cranmer Terrace, London, UK

Mr Etienne Horner
Consultant Obstetrician and Gynaecologist
St Mary's Hospital, Imperial College Healthcare NHS
Trust, London, UK

Miss Polly Hughes
Consultant Obstetrician and Gynaecologist
St George's Healthcare NHS Trust
London, UK

Dr Jennifer Hyer
Obstetrics and Gynecology, Attending Physician,
Denver Health Medical Center
Senior Instructor, Department of Obstetrics and
Gynecology,
University of Colorado School of Medicine,
Denver, Colorado, USA

Associate Professor A Ilancheran
Senior Consultant
Division of Gynaecologic Oncology, Department of
Obstetrics & Gynaecology
National University Hospital, Singapore

Hilary Kele
Senior Registrar
Department of Obstetrics & Gynaecology
Southampton University Hospital, Southampton, UK

Dr Christos Ioannou
Clinical Research Fellow, Nuffield Department of
Obstetrics and Gynaecology
John Radcliffe Hospital, Oxford, UK

Dr Smita Jain
Consultant Obstetrician and Gynaecologist,
University Hospital of Northern British Columbia, Prince
George, British Columbia, Canada

Anna Jamil
Department of Obstetrics and Gynaecology
University College Hospital
London, UK

Dr Haider Jan
Specialist Registrar in Obstetrics & Gynaecology
St George's Healthcare NHS Trust
London, UK

Dr Swati Jha
Subspecialist in Urogynaecology,
Consultant Obstetrician and Gynaecologist,
Sheffield Teaching Hospitals NHSFT, Sheffield, UK

Miss Antoinette Johnson
Consultant Obstetrician & Gynaecologist
Epsom and St Helier Hospital, Surrey, UK

Mr Davor Jurkovic
Consultant Gynaecologist, Department of
Obstetrics and Gynaecology
University College Hospital, London, UK

Miss Vijaysri Kakumani
Consultant Obstetrician and Gynaecologist
Epsom and St Helier University Hospital NHS Trust, UK

Dr Nigel Leonard Kennea
Consultant Neonatologist
St George's Healthcare NHS Trust
London, UK

Dr Stephen Kennedy
Clinical Reader & Head of Department
Nuffield Department of Obstetrics & Gynaecology,
University of Oxford
John Radcliffe Hospital, Oxford, UK

Dr Andrew Kent
Consultant Psychiatrist and Senior Lecturer
St George's, University of London, Cranmer Terrace,
London, UK

Professor Chris Kettle
Midwife
Professor of Women's Health,
University Hospital of North Staffordshire (NHS Trust),
Stoke-on-Trent, UK

Dr Rahat Khan
Clinical Fellow in Maternal Medicine
Epsom and St Helier Hospital, Surrey, UK

Professor Mark Kilby
Professor of Fetal Medicine,
School of Clinical & Experimental Medicine,
The College of Medical & Dental Sciences
University of Birmingham,
and
Department of Fetal Medicine, Birmingham Women's
Foundation Trust, Edgbaston, Birmingham, UK

Dr Emma Kirk
Specialist Registrar
Obstetrics and Gynaecology
The Whittington Hospital, London, UK

Dr Mona B Krull
Department of Obstetrics and Gynecology
Denver Health Medical Center
Assistant Professor, University of Colorado School
of Medicine
Denver, CO, USA

Dr Ali Kubba
Consultant Community Gynaecologist,
Guy's and St Thomas' Hospital NHS Trust,
Honorary Senior Lecturer,
Department of Obstetrics and Gynaecology,
Kings College, London, UK

Dr Terence Lao
Associate Professor of Obstetrics & Gynaecology
Chinese University of Hong Kong, Hong Kong

Professor William Ledger
Professor of Obstetrics and Gynaecology
University of Sheffield, Sheffield, UK

Mr Christoph Lees
Consultant in Obstetrics and Fetal-Maternal Medicine
Lead, Fetal Medicine
Rosie Maternity-Addenbrookes Hospital, Cambridge, UK

Dr Karin Leslie
Clinical Lecturer,
St George's, University of London
Cranmer Terrace, London

Miss Jilly Lloyd
Specialist Registrar,
Obstetrics and Gynaecology,
University Hospital Lewisham, London, UK

Associate Professor Jeffrey JH Low
Head, Division of Gynaecologic Oncology
Senior Consultant, Department of Obstetrics & Gynaecology
National University Hospital, Singapore

Professor Mary Ann Lumsden
Professor of Gynaecology and Medical Education, Head of
Division of Developmental Medicine University of
Glasgow, UK

Dr Lizbeth K McCarthy
Assistant Professor of Obstetrics & Gynaecology
University of Colarado, USA

Professor Neil McClure
Professor of Obstetrics and Gynaecology
Queen's University Belfast, Belfast, UK

Dr Jane MacDougall,
Consultant in Reproductive Medicine
Addenbrooke's Hospital, Cambridge, UK

Dr Gemma Malin
Clinical Research Fellow, Department of Obstetrics and
Gynaecology, University of Birmingham
Birmingham Women's Hospital, Birmingham, UK

Dr Sahar Mansour
Consultant Geneticist
SW Thames Regional Genetics Service
St George's, University of London, Cranmer Terrace,
London, UK

Mr Isaac Manyonda
Consultant Obstetrician & Gynaecologist & Clinical
Reader in Obstetrics & Gynaecology
St George's, University of London, Cranmer Terrace,
London, UK

Dr Louise Melson
Consultant Obstetrician and Gynaecologist
Poole Hospital, Poole, Dorset, UK

Dr Lina Michala
Lead in Paediatric and Adolescent Gynaecology
Alexandras Hospital, Athens, Greece

Dr Pedro Miranda-Seijo
Clinical Instructor
University of Colorado School of Medicine, Denver
Health Hospital, Denver, CO, USA

Dr Hannah Missfelder-Lobos
Addenbrooke's Hospital
Cambridge, UK

Miss Shruti Mohan
SpR Obstetrics & Gynaecology
Imperial College Healthcare NHS Trust
St Mary's Hospital, London, UK

Mr Ash Monga
Consultant Gynaecologist and Sub-specialist in
Uro Gynaecology
Department of Obstetrics & Gynaecology,
Southampton University Hospital, Southampton, UK

Dr Judy Myles
Senior Lecturer/Consultant Psychiatrist
Division of Mental Health,
St George's University of London
Cranmer Terrace, London, UK

Dr Vivek Nama
Clinical Research Fellow
Department of Obstetrics and Gynaecology
St George's, University of London, Cranmer Terrace,
London, UK

Professor Kypros H Nicolaides
Director, Harris Birthright Research
Centre for Fetal Medicine
King's College Hospital, London, UK

Dr Rachel L O'Donnell
Specialist Trainee Obstetrics and Gynaecology
Simpson Centre for Reproductive Health, Royal Infirmary
of Edinburgh, Edinburgh, UK

Dr Tim J von Oertzen
Consultant Neurologist/Epileptologist
Epilepsy Group, Atkinson Morley Neuroscience Centre,
St. George's Hospital, London, UK

Mr Kamal Ojha
Consultant Gynaecologist
St George's Healthcare NHS Trust (St George's
Hospital), London, UK

Mrs Caroline Overton
Consultant Obstetrician & Gynaecologist
Subspecialist in Reproductive Medicine & Laparoscopic
Surgery
St Michael's University Hospital, Bristol, UK

Miss Louise M Page
SpR Obstetrics & Gynaecology
Imperial College Healthcare NHS Trust
St Mary's Hospital, London, UK

Dr Nick Panay
Consultant Gynaecologist, Subspecialist in Reproductive
Medicine & Surgery
Imperial College Healthcare NHS Trust and Chelsea &
Westminster Hospital NHS Foundation Trust, London, UK
and
Honorary Senior Clinical Lecturer, Imperial College
London, UK

Dr Aris T Papageorghiou
Consultant in Obstetrics and Maternal Fetal Medicine
Honorary Senior Lecturer
St George's, University of London
Cranmer Terrace, London, UK

Dr Leonie Penna
Consultant Obstetrician,
King's College Hospital, London, UK

Dr Nicola Persico
Clinical Research Fellow,
Harris Birthright Research Centre for Fetal Medicine,
King's College Hospital, London, UK

Mr Christian Phillips
Consultant in Obstetrics and Gynaecology
Basingstoke and North Hampshire Hospital,
Basingstoke, UK

Dr Gianluigi Pilu
Department of Obstetrics and Gynecology
University of Bologna and Policlinico S. Orsola-Malpighi,
Bologna, Italy

Ms Sheila Radhakrishnan
Consultant in Community Gynaecology
Royal Free Hospital, London, UK

Dr Kalaivani Ramalingam
Registrar- Obstetrics and Gynaecology
Princess Anne Hospital, Southampton, UK

Professor Lesley Regan
Professor and Head of Obstetrics & Gynaecology
Imperial College at St. Mary's Hospital, London, UK

Professor Wendy Reid
Royal Free Hospital, London, UK

Shauna L. Reinblatt
Clinical and Research Fellow
McGill Reproductive Centre, Dept of Obstetrics and
Gynecology,
McGill University Health Center, Montreal, Canada

Shaun Rogers
Senior Embryologist
The London Bridge Fertility, Gynaecology and Genetics
Centre, London, UK

Dr Shanthi Sairam
Associate Specialist in Fetal Medicine and Fetal Cardiology
Fetal Medicine Unit
St George's Healthcare NHS Trust
London, UK

Mr Rehan Salim
Consultant Gynaecologist
Reproductive Medicine Unit, University College London
Hospitals, London, UK

Dr Ippokratis Sarris
Specialist Registrar in Obstetrics and Gynaecology
London Deanery, London, UK

Dr Frank Schroeder
Consultant Anaesthetist
St George's Healthcare NHS Trust
London, UK

Einat Shalom-Paz
Clinical and Research Fellow
McGill Reproductive Center,
McGill University Health Center
Royal Victoria Hospital, Montreal, Canada

Mr Hassan Shehata
Consultant Obstetrician and Obstetric Physician
Maternal Medicine Unit
Epsom and St Helier University Hospital NHS Trust,
UK

Dr Nadeem Siddiqui
Consultant Gynaecological Oncologist
Dept of Gynaecological Oncology
Glasgow Royal Infirmary, Glasgow, UK

Dr Giuliane Simonazzi
Department of Obstetrics and Gynecology
University of Bologna and Policlinico S. Orsola-Malpighi,
Bologna, Italy

Dr Norma J. Stiglich
Associate Director of Obstetrics and Gynecology
Denver Health Medical Center,
and
Assistant Professor
University of Colorado School of Medicine,
Denver, CO, USA

Abdul H. Sultan
Consultant Obstetrician & Gynaecologist
Department of Obstetrics & Gynaecology
Mayday University Hospital
Croydon, UK

Dr Jo Sykes
Macmillan Consultant in Palliative Medicine
Department of Palliative Medicine
Torbay Hospital, Torqusy, Devon, UK

Dr Seang Lin Tan
James Edmund Dodds Professor and Chairman
Department of Obstetrics & Gynecology,
McGill University
and
Obstetrician & Gynecologist-in-Chief
McGill University Health Centre
and
Medical Director, McGill Reproductive Centre
Department of Obstetrics and Gynecology
McGill University, Royal Victoria Hospital,
Montreal, Quebec, Canada

Dr Alison Taylor
Consultant Gynaecologist and Subspecialist in
Reproductive Medicine
Lister Fertility Clinic
Lister Hospital, London, UK

Miss Ranee Thakar
Consultant Urogynaecologist
Mayday University Hospital, Croydon, UK

Professor Basky Thilaganathan
Director, Fetal Medicine Unit
Department of Obstetrics and Gynaecology
St George's Healthcare NHS Trust
London, UK

Dr L Chesney Thompson
Associate Professor
Vice Chair Dept. Obstetrics and Gynecology
Chief of General Obstetrics and Gynecology
University of Colorado School of Medicine,
Aurora, CO, USA

Dr Sifa Turan
Perinatal Instructor
Obstetrics, Gynecology and Reproductive Sciences
University of Maryland School of Medicine,
Baltimore, MD, USA

Mr Dhiraj Uchil
Consultant Obstetrician and Gynaecologist,
University Hospital Lewisham, London, UK

Mr Austin Ugwumadu
Consultant Obstetrician & Gynaecologist /
Senior Lecturer
Department of Obstetrics and Gynaecology
St George's Healthcare NHS Trust
London, UK

Mr Sameer Umranikar
Consultant Obstetrician & Gynaecologist
Princess Anne Hospital, Southampton, UK

Dr Catalina Valencia
Clinical Research Fellow
Harris Birthright Research Centre for Fetal Medicine
King's College Hospital, London, UK

Dr W Hamish B Wallace
Consultant Paediatric Oncologist,
Royal Hospital for Sick Children, Edinburgh, UK

Miss Lisa Webber
Consultant Gynecologist
Specialist in Reproductive Medicine, St Mary's Hospital,
Imperial College Healthcare NHS Trust, London, UK

Dr Andrew Weeks
Senior Lecturer in Obstetrics
University of Liverpool, Liverpool Women's Hospital,
Liverpool, UK

Dr Davinia White
Consultant in Reproductive Medicine
St Mary's Hospital, London, UK

Professor Catherine Williamson
Professor of Obstetric Medicine
Chelsea and Queen Charlotte's Hospital, London, UK

Dr Kathryn Witzeman
Assistant Professor, University of Colorado
Department of Obstetrics and Gynaecology
Denver Health Medical Center, Denver, CO, USA

Dr Ernest Hung Yu NG
Associate Professor
The University of Hong Kong, Department of Obstetrics
and Gynaecology
Queen Mary Hospital, Pokfulam, Hong Kong

Part 1

Introduction

Examination of the obstetric patient *3*
Examination of the gynaecological patient *7*
Communication: confidentiality, breaking
    bad news, and obtaining consent *11*
Legal framework for care in obstetrics
    and gynaecology *19*

Examination of the obstetric patient

Examination of the obstetric patient

Taking a history of the obstetric patient will vary whether it is a booking visit or presentation with a clinical problem or presentation in labour. For most women their pregnancy, labour, and delivery are normal physiological events and they will not present with serious complaints or complications. Each woman must be treated as an individual and the purpose of any consultation must be outlined to her, beginning with an appropriate introduction. In every case an account of the pregnancy to date and any background risk need to be acquired logically to allow an appropriate focused clinical examination to follow. The following template is suggested below.

Obstetric history

History of present pregnancy

Once basic biographical details (name, age, current gestation, gravidity, and parity) have been obtained enquiry will follow more in-depth questioning about the current pregnancy:

- last menstrual period (LMP) and expected date of delivery (EDD)
- ultrasound scan results (e.g. first trimester scan agreed with LMP date, nuchal translucency screening test, anomaly scan and site of placenta, any subsequent scans)
- screening and laboratory tests and results if known
- any problems or concerns during the pregnancy to date.

A detailed history of the presenting complaint should be taken.

Past obstetric history

Details of all previous pregnancies in chronological order and their outcomes (gestation, mode of delivery, birthweight, and condition of the baby). If there have been any abnormal pregnancy outcomes, e.g. second trimester miscarriages, premature deliveries or still births, then enquiry of any subsequent investigations should be sought in a compassionate manner. If the patient reports a previous termination of pregnancy then it can be prudent to ensure that she is happy for this to be documented in her hand-held maternity notes.

Past gynaecological history

Previous gynaecological conditions and operations may be relevant to the current pregnancy, in particular previous myomectomy or laparotomy, for severe endometriosis with bowel involvement might influence surgical expertise available at the time of a possible Caesarean section. Previous or current sexually transmitted infections may be relevant as this could influence the fetus or neonate if left untreated, e.g. syphyllis and chlamydia respectively. Details that should also be noted are a cervical smear and contraceptive history as these are important factors that can be addressed in the postnatal period.

Past medical and surgical history

A detailed history of any current medical condition is important and enquiry about the condition within a previous pregnancy may be useful for management or surveillance of the current pregnancy. All previous surgery should be noted, but in particular abdominal procedures should be thoroughly detailed. For example, entry into the abdomen might be affected at the time of Caesarean section by the location of a pelvic kidney in a renal transplant patient.

Drug history and allergies

Current medication should be noted and thought given to whether it is licensed in pregnancy and breast feeding and may even need to be changed due to potential teratogenesis. Specific drug allergies must be clearly marked on the notes

Social history

Whether the woman works, has support (emotional and financial) and living conditions now and for the rest of the pregnancy are important factors to ascertain. Where suitable, support agencies can be offered. Appropriate sensitive questioning of certain women about female genital mutilation (FGM) is advised to identify these women early.

Smoking, past or current recreational drug use and alcohol consumption are important for documentation and provide an opportunity for advice and offer of help if abuse is suspected. When unaccompanied by partner, family or friends, enquiry about domestic violence, both physical and verbal, may be appropriate to give the woman the opportunity to disclose any issues.

Family history

Family history should include history of multiple pregnancies, diabetes, hypertension, pre-eclampsia in a first-degree female relative, and congenital disorders. In certain ethnic minorities it may be appropriate to ask about consanguineous marriage.

Clinical examination

Explanation about the purpose of the examination must be given and it is essential that the woman be put at ease and every effort taken to ensure that the woman remains as comfortable as possible throughout the examination. Do not allow a woman in late pregnancy to lie on her back for a prolonged period of time as the reduced venous return to the heart by pressure from the gravid uterus can make her feel faint.

At the booking visit, general examination of the patient includes height and weight to calculate body mass index. Auscultation of the chest (heart sounds and lungs) is essential at the booking visit to rule out previously undetected or asymptomatic conditions. Examination of the breasts is not recommended as identification of flat or inverted nipples antenatally does not affect breast feeding rates postnatally (NICE clinical guideline 62). Subsequent visits, unless otherwise indicated will have a more specifically directed examination of the patient.

Measurement of blood pressure in all women is vital and should ideally be taken manually with a sphygnometer using Korotkoff V (value at which the sounds disappear) as the recorded diastolic blood pressure value. The correct size cuff must be used for the size of the arm. Those women with an arm circumference larger than 35 cm should have a large cuff applied to ensure that a correct reading is obtained, as a smaller cuff can result in a falsely high blood pressure.

Abdominal examination

This should follow the routine examination of any system: inspection, palpation, and auscultation. Percussion is rarely used but can illicit a fluid thrill in a case of polyhydramnios. The history and general examination will direct the specific part of the clinical examination. Where appropriate, the examination may take place concurrently with resuscitation, e.g. massive antepartum haemorrhage or eclampsia.

Inspection

Distension of the abdomen may indicate the size of the uterus and visible fetal movements can be documented.

Surgical scars must be noted. Special attention must be given to identifying a low transverse Pfannestiel incision and laparoscopic scar within the umbilicus both of which are often obscured.

Cutaneous signs of pregnancy (linea nigra and striae gravidarum and albicans) can be seen but are of no clinical significance. The umbilicus can change from being inverted to flat or everted as the pregnancy advances. Superfical veins can become evident as the pressure on the vena cava by the increasingly gravid uterus causes alternative paths of venous drainage to become more prominent.

Palpation

Uterine size

Using the ulnar border of the left hand and starting at xiphisternum, move it downwards until the fundus is identified. When the highest part of the symphyseal fundal height (SFH) is located, a tape measure (ideally paper for single use) is used to measure to the upper border of the symphysis pubis in the midline. Care should be made when palpating for this bony prominence as it is often tender in advanced pregnancy and in women with symphysis pubis dysfunction. The SFH in centimetres should equate to the gestation in weeks: 20–36 weeks ±2 cm and from 36 weeks ± 3 cm. If the patient has not presented for antenatal scans then it should be remembered that palpation may diagnose a multiple pregnancy.

Lie and presentation

Lie describes the longitudinal axis of the fetus(es) in relation to that of the uterus, and presentation describes the fetal part that overlies the pelvic brim. Prior to 28 weeks lie and presentation are not important (and often difficult to determine on palpation) unless the woman is in premature labour. After this, gestation it is of more clinical relevance and longitudinal lie with a cephalic presentation are most important from 36 weeks.

Palpation of lie is done by placing the hands over the anterolateral sides of the abdomen and moving towards the midline and feeling at the pelvic inlet for the presence or absence of a fetal pole. A fetal back will demonstrate a firm resistance and fetal limbs an irregular or less solid 'feel'. To determine presentation and engagement, towards term, palpate with two hands in the lower pole of the uterus. This can be uncomfortable for the woman and should be done cautiously. The head will feel round and hard. It can be balloted between the examining hands prior to engagement whereas the buttocks are softer and more diffuse and the breech is not ballotable. Beware of the deeply engaged head as this may in fact be a breech presentation. Reassessment of the upper pole of the fetus is advised and an ultrasound performed (or vaginal examination if appropriate) to confirm the presentation. Powlik's grip (examining the lower pole between the thumb and index finger of the right hand) can also be used for assessment of engagement of the fetal head.

Engagement

This describes the passage of the largest diameter of the presentation past the pelvic inlet and is referred to in 'fifths' palpable abdominally. The level of the head is described as engaged if the widest diameter has passed beyond the pelvic brim, i.e. only two-fifths felt abdominally.

Assessment of liquor volume

Estimating liquor volume on palpation can be difficult. If there is difficulty palpating fetal parts and particularly if the abdomen feels large, tense, and looks shiny then the suspicion of polyhydramnios should be raised. Although not a definitive indicator of polyhydramnios, a fluid thrill may be elicited in such cases. A detailed ultrasound to exclude any obvious anomaly can be undertaken and blood glucose levels checked to rule out a pathological cause. In contrast, a pregnancy with oligohydramnios may reveal fetal parts very easily without the feeling of adequate liquor and a small for dates SFH. Again referral for detailed ultrasound is appropriate as a further investigation.

Auscultation

The fetal stethoscope, Pinard, or electronic device using Doppler ultrasound can be used to hear the fetal heart by placing the device over the anterior shoulder in the third trimester. Prior to this the Doppler device can usually elicit a fetal heart rate placed anteriorly on the lower abdominal wall over the uterus from 12–14 weeks onwards. Routine auscultation for the fetal heart is not recommended at antenatal visits (NICE clinical guideline 62) although women and their partners often expect it.

Vaginal examination

A vaginal examination is performed in the obstetric patient only when indicated.

Antenatally

This is not a routine examination during the antenatal period. In the first and second trimesters a woman presenting with bleeding ± pain (e.g. miscarriage) should be fully assessed including a speculum examination to visualize the cervix, assess the quantity of bleeding and determine digitally whether the cervical os is open or closed. In the third trimester the possibility of placenta praevia should be excluded first by ultrasound examination. Speculum examinations can be done to investigate vaginal discharge, to take swabs as appropriate, and to confirm or dispute the leakage of amniotic fluid. Cervical smears can be taken during pregnancy but unless overt malignancy is suspected then this can usually be postponed until the postpartum period.

Prior to induction

A digital examination of the cervix can be offered to a woman as part of a membrane sweep at a 41-week antenatal visit (NICE clinical guideline 62) and is undertaken prior to induction of labour to determine its Bishop Score, a subjective assessment of favourability of the cervix

In labour

At term a digital vaginal examination is done in labour to assess the dilatation of the cervix and hence progress in labour.

A final summary must present a logical synopsis of the patient's current pregnancy, relevant background or risk factors followed by the salient findings of the clinical examination. This will then lead on to appropriate investigations and a plan of management.

Further reading

www.nice.org.uk NICE Reference: NICE Guidance 62. Antenatal care: Routine care for the healthy pregnant women.

Chapter 2

Examination of the gynaecological patient

Examination of the gynaecological patient

Gynaecological history

Taking a good history will go a long way towards arriving at the correct diagnosis. In order to do this it is important to develop a good rapport with the patient. Greeting the patient with a proper introduction, an explanation of the purpose of the consultation and guaranteeing privacy and confidentiality are all vital. Having a model for history taking can help to ensure that all aspects are covered but the need to be flexible and sensitive to individual patients and their problems should be appreciated. An outline is given below.

Current history

Name, age, and parity.

Presenting symptom(s). Three examples of common gynaecological complaints:

- Pelvic pain: site, onset, duration, character, radiation, exacerbating, relieving factors, any relationship to the menstrual cycle, dyspareunia, associated symptoms such as vaginal discharge, dysuria, vomiting.
- Abnormal menstrual bleeding: regular/irregular including post coital or intermenstrual, quantification of loss (does she report flooding or use of double sanitary protection?), dysmenorrhoea, dyspareunia, any previous treatments and their effects.
- Vaginal discharge: onset, colour, odour, itchiness, presence of blood, use of over-the-counter remedies, relation to the menstrual cycle, concurrent symptoms from sexual partner.

Menstrual history

First day of last menstrual period (LMP), length of cycle and days of bleeding, age of menarche/menopause as appropriate.

Contraceptive and sexual history

Current method of contraception and previous methods with any side-effects. Dyspareunia—superficial/deep/positional, libido, vaginal dryness, problems with orgasm, recent change in partner, vaginal discharge.

Past gynaecological history

Details that have not yet been covered such as details of last cervical smear, previous gynaecological conditions and relevant treatments or operations (e.g. pelvic inflammatory disease, endometriosis, use of hormone replacement therapy (HRT) and laparoscopies.)

Past obstetric history

Details of previous pregnancies and their outcomes (gestation, mode of delivery, any complicating factors e.g. haemorrhage, perforation of uterus at time of evacuation of retained products of conception (ERPC)) in chronological order.

Past medical and surgical history

This is important as accurate information may help lead to a diagnosis (e.g. thyroid disorders and menstrual disturbances, colorectal carcinoma and endometrial carcinoma), planning management with regard to anaesthetic assessment preoperatively (cardiovascular and respiratory conditions) and multidisciplinary input and follow up (e.g. haematologist involvement when managing a thrombophilic patient).

Drug history and allergies

Current medication should be noted and specific drug allergies clearly marked on the notes. Thought must always be given to any current medication to avoid drug interactions, e.g. enzyme-inducing action of antiepileptic drugs leading to higher failure rate of the combined oral contraceptive.

Social and family history

This should include how the current complaint impacts on the patient's life. Enquiry into smoking, drinking, recreational drug use and living conditions may be relevant to the condition and impact on the future management of the patient. Ascertaining a family history of conditions such as malignancies and venous thrombolic disease may also direct diagnoses or influence therapeutic options.

Clinical examination

This will start with a general examination of the patient, including blood pressure and weight to calculate body mass index. Initial inspection of the woman will include her general wellbeing, but attention to detail such as the presence of a goitre, acne and hirsuitism may be relevant before moving on to the actual gynaecological examination.

It is essential that the woman be put at ease and every effort to ensure that the woman remains as comfortable as possible throughout the examination, e.g. given a clean sheet to cover herself to protect some modesty, a female chaperone present for all patients, and curtains providing full privacy. The doctor must ensure that interruptions (e.g. pagers, mobile phones) are avoided throughout the examination.

Abdominal examination

This should follow the routine examination of any system: inspection, palpation, percussion, and auscultation. The emphasis will be guided by the patient's history but in the gynaecological patient particular attention to pubic hair distribution, striae, surgical scars including laparoscopy scars are worth noting. Palpation should allow description of any maximal site of tenderness with associated signs of peritonism and define any palpable mass in terms of site, size consistency and, importantly, mobility. Percussion can be a useful sign to differentiate between a solid mass, full bladder or distended bowel as well as the presence of fluid within the peritoneal cavity, e.g. blood from a ruptured ectopic or ascites from an ovarian malignancy. Auscultation is not routinely used in gynaecological practice but can be important for the initial assessment of a patient presenting with an acute abdomen and postoperatively to guide commencing oral intake or to rule out paralytic ileus.

Vaginal examination

Vaginal examination is normally carried out with the patient lying on her back with her knees flexed and hips abducted and includes

- inspection of the external genitalia
- speculum examination of the cervix and vagina
- bimanual examination of the uterus and adnexae.

Inspection of the external genitalia: mons pubis and pubic hair distribution. Any obvious lesions of the labia majora, minora, clitoris, urethral meatus, vaginal introitus, and perianal region should be documented. Further visualization of the perineal region and introitus may be aided by gently separating the labia further with the thumb and index finger of the examiner's left hand. This may reveal the presence of a cystourethrocoele or rectocoele. Alternatively, at this stage, asking the patient to cough or 'bear down' may unmask the presence of urinary stress incontinence or other uterovaginal prolapse. On occasion it may be necessary to ask the patient to use her own hands to localize any particular area of tenderness in this area.

Speculum examination

After explanation to the patient, the labia are parted by the examiner's finger and thumb as above and a warm lubricated Cuscoe's speculum is inserted gently in one smooth movement into the vagina directed at approximately 45° as if towards the coccyx, i.e. along the axis of the vagina. When the speculum can be advanced no further the blades are opened to visualize the cervix. If the cervix is not in view at this stage, closing the blades and drawing the instrument back before reopening them again may help. It is wise to tell the patient that you are gently going to move the speculum slightly within the vagina and the purpose of doing so. If the cervix remains out of view, occasionally it can be visualized with a Cuscoe's speculum, performed with the patient in the left lateral position.

Documentation of the appearance of the cervix and any vaginal discharge is important. Under direct vision of the cervix a cervical smear, high vaginal and endocervical swabs can be obtained as appropriate. Taking care with removal of the speculum can allow further visualization of the vagina and is essential to prevent unnecessary discomfort to the patient. The blades should be allowed to close slightly after the cervix has disappeared from view. Care should be taken not to entrap lax vaginal wall within the blades and complete the closure of the blades before final withdrawal of the instrument through the introitus is advisable.

A Sim's speculum examination, of the patient lying in the left lateral position can allow full visualization of uterovaginal prolapse and is also appropriate when suspecting vesicovaginal fistulae.

Omission of vaginal examination

It may be appropriate not to proceed with a vaginal examination during an outpatient consultation, either due to patient's request/virgo intacta/an adult unable to give consent/paediatric patient. Consideration should be given to whether examination under anaesthesia is going to add to the management of the patient. In the case of women who are virgo intacta, some are happy to be examined and a small Cuscoe's can be introduced if the patient is suitably relaxed and then proceeding to a one finger vaginal examination.

Bimanual examination

Ensure the bladder is empty prior to this examination to prevent discomfort to the patient and maximize correct identification of the pelvic organs. The index and middle fingers of the right hand are inserted into the vagina with the palmar aspect facing anteriorly until the cervix is felt. The left hand presses gently on the lower abdomen to bring the abdominal wall close to the pelvic organs, which are simultaneously being pushed upwards by the 'vaginal hand'. The uterus is palpated first between the two hands, followed by the adnexae, by moving the vaginal fingers into the lateral fornices and the abdominal hand over the respective iliac fossae. The pouch of Douglas is then felt by feeling in the posterior fornix. The size, consistency and mobility of any pelvic mass(es) detected are documented.

Rectal

This may be indicated in specific circumstances and may need to be performed simultaneously with a digital vaginal examination such as in women with suspected cervical carcinoma to asses the pelvic side walls to aid staging, severe endometriosis where involvement of the rectum is likely, urogynaecological conditions such as urinary/faecal incontinence and rectocoele where there are also defaecatory difficulties.

Chapter 3

Communication: confidentiality, breaking bad news, and obtaining consent

Communication: confidentiality, breaking bad news and obtaining consent

Communication

Communication is a core clinical skill that constitutes a main ingredient in the complex physician–patient relationship. There is strong evidence that physician–patient communication is a good predictor of patient compliance, adherence to treatment, clinical outcomes and general patient satisfaction. There are three essential communication skills that are vital to a successful patient-centred consultation.

- Rapport-building: the shaking of hands and a general introduction which transmits dynamism and expressiveness often establishes the social tone of the consultation, helping to dissipate worries.
- Partnership-building: setting the main reason for the visit and asking if the patient has any other issues or concerns paves the way for the physician to help the patient understand the course of the treatment and to legitimate the role of the woman in the process, thereby contributing to the development of an active partnership.
- Information transfer: this occurs on multiple levels:
  - the content level of communication is usually transmitted linguistically,
  - the relationship level may be transmitted either linguistically, paralinguistically (tone of voice, gestures, etc.) or may be derived from the context.

Patient–gynaecologist communication

This is characterized by several specific features placing great demand on the communication behaviour of the physician.

- The health problems presented are frequently of intimate nature and have a high emotional impact. Gynaecologists have to respond to these emotions and personal beliefs and values of their patients.
- Diagnostic and therapeutic interventions influence body image, sexuality and self-esteem.
- Reproduction and sexuality are issues that encompass the patient's whole life, involving specific life cycles and psychosocial issues. Gynaecologists have to be able to take a psychosocial, biographical and systemic perspective to understand their patients.
- Many healthy women consult with concerns regarding health maintenance, promotion and health behaviour. They are not patients in a traditional sense but partners with an interest in informed decision-making, autonomy and enhancement of their health-related interests and objectives.

Although formerly thought that patients were more satisfied with female gynaecologists regarding the relationship and consultation process, regression analyses has demonstrated that it is not gender by gender-related specific communication skills, mainly patient-centred communication, that seemed to be the crucial factor influencing patient satisfaction. Gynaecologists and obstetricians therefore need a specific competence in patient education, information exchange, behavioural change and negotiation. A recent survey on hospital care showed that, in Obstetrics and Gynaecology, women rate early postnatal care in hospital far less favourably largely based on the interaction with care-givers. It has been well documented that malpractice claims are often associated with poor communication and that effective communication could reduce these claims (Tsai et al. 2004).

The General Medical Council (GMC) emphasizes that for a relationship between a doctor and patient to be effective, it should be a partnership based on openness, trust and good communication. Good communication skills in general and knowing how to impart bad news in particular are considered central to being a good doctor (GMC 2004). Equally, good interprofessional communication is essential for effective and coordinated care.

Standards have been set by the Royal College of Obstetricians and Gynaecologists (RCOG) with regard to communication both in Obstetrics and in Gynaecology (RCOG 2008a,b). These include an emphasis on effective communication between team members and each discipline, as well as with women and their families and imparting training to all healthcare professionals on how to communicate in an effective and sensitive manner. Some of the other standards include:

1. Offering information to each patient in an accessible form, on the full range of options available, including locally available services and allowing enough time to reflect upon the information, consider options and seek additional information and advice prior to making 'informed choices'.
2. Providing interpreting services to women whose first language isn't English and making funding available for these services in the community, especially in emergency situations.
3. Making a summary of the woman's care available to her GP within 10 working days and ensuring that a local mechanism is in place to communicate urgent results to the woman and her GP.
4. Ensuring that routine appointment letters are worded appropriately and that pre-appointment letters for one-stop clinics provide clear information regarding the procedure and the investigations that might be performed.

Effective communication between doctors and children/ young people

This is essential to the provision of good care.

- You should be available to see children and young people on their own if that is what they want. The presence of a parent or chaperone can sometimes deter young people from being frank and from asking for help.
- You should talk directly and listen to children and young people who are able to take part in discussions about their care. It is preferable to 'speak to' rather than 'speak about', because the latter is often resented. The views of young people should be taken seriously and not dismissed.
- When they want or need to know about their illness or treatment, information should be provided in a manner that is easy to understand and appropriate to their age and maturity. Information should only be kept from them if they ask you to, or if it would cause them serious harm.

Confidentiality

Confidentiality is central to trust between doctors and patients (GMC 2004). Patients have a right to expect that information about them will be held in confidence by their doctors. When responsible for personal information about patients, a doctor must make sure that it is effectively protected against improper disclosure at all times. Equally, when a doctor is satisfied that information should be disclosed, one should act promptly to disclose all relevant information. This is often essential to the best interests of the patient, or to safeguard the wellbeing of others. The GMC receives more enquiries on confidentiality than any other topic and is now in the process of preparing a 'Revised Confidentiality Guidance' incorporating the views of a wide range of professional, public and patient groups as well as individual patients and doctors (GMC 2008).

The following standards have been outlined by the GMC in its current guidance on confidentiality (GMC 2004):
1. One should take reasonable steps to ensure that all consultations with patients are private.
2. Patients should not be discussed where one may be overheard; nor should records be left either on paper or on screen where they may be seen by other patients, unauthorized healthcare staff or the public.
3. One must ensure that anyone to whom personal information is disclosed understands that it is given to them in confidence, which they must respect. All staff members receiving personal information in order to provide or support care are bound by a legal duty of confidence, whether or not they have contractual or professional obligations to protect confidentiality.
4. Disclosures should be kept to the minimum necessary and patients should be informed.
5. Data should be anonymized prior to disclosure when possible, and when not patients' express consent to disclosure of information must be sought, save in the exceptional circumstances described later.
6. Doctors must keep up to date with and observe the requirements of statute and common law including data protection legislation.

Disclosure of information requires a patient's consent. Implied consent to disclosure may be sufficient in the following circumstances:
1. Within members of the healthcare team: Most people understand and accept that information must be shared within the healthcare team in order to provide their care. The wishes of any patient who objects to particular information being shared with others providing care, except where this would put others at risk of death or serious harm, must be respected. In emergency situations, where a patient cannot be informed about the sharing of information, relevant information must be passed promptly to those providing the patient's care.
2. For purposes of clinical audit: Clinical audit is essential to the provision of good care and all doctors in clinical practice have a duty to participate in clinical audit. Identifiable information may be disclosed for purposes of clinical audit provided the patients have been informed, are aware of their right to object to the disclosure and have not objected. When audits are to be undertaken by another organization, information should be anonymized wherever that is practicable. If not, express consent must be obtained prior to the disclosure of identifiable data.

Express consent must be obtained in the following circumstances:
1. Before the disclosure of identifiable information of purposes such as research, epidemiology, financial audit or administration.
2. Where doctors have contractual obligations to third parties, such as companies or organizations, they must obtain patients' consent before undertaking any examination or writing a report for that organization and should offer to show patients the report, whether or not this is required by law.

Disclosure in connection with judicial or other statutory proceedings: information must be disclosed to satisfy a specific statutory requirement, such as notification of a known or suspected communicable disease or if ordered to do so by a judge or presiding officer of a court. Patients should be informed about such disclosures, wherever practicable, but their consent is not required.

Disclosure in public interest: personal information may be disclosed in the public interest where the benefits to an individual or to society of the disclosure outweigh the public and the patient's interest in keeping the information confidential. This 'public interest' can be determined only by the courts. Similarly, disclosure to an appropriate person or authority is also justified if disclosure is deemed necessary to protect a third party from death or serious harm, such as child abuse. Such disclosures are permissible without the patient's consent and in exceptional cases also where patients have withheld consent.

Disclosure in specific circumstances
1. Children and those lacking the capacity to give consent: disclosure of information to relevant authorities is permissible if deemed essential and consent cannot be obtained despite persuasion and involvement of appropriate persons in the consultation. The discussions with the patient, views of an advocate or carer and reasons for deciding to disclose information should be documented in the patient's notes.
2. Victims of neglect or abuse: if a patient is believed to be a victim of neglect or physical, sexual or emotional abuse and the person withholds consent to disclosure, information must be given promptly to an appropriate responsible person or statutory agency in the patient's best interest. A decision not to disclose information must be discussed with an experienced colleague and would warrant justification.
3. After a patient's death: a doctor still has an obligation to keep personal information confidential after a patient dies, especially if the patient had asked for information to remain confidential. Where unaware of any directions from the patients, requests for information should be considered taking into account whether the disclosure may cause distress to or be of benefit to the patient's partner or family; whether disclosure will in effect disclose information about the patient's family or others and the purpose of the disclosure. A decision to disclose confidential information could be challenged and may warrant explanation and justification.

Breaking bad news
Any information that produces a negative alteration to a person's expectations about their present and future could be deemed 'bad news.' Bad news does of course,

have gradations, which to a certain extent are subjective (Fallowfield and Jenkins 2004). In Obstetrics and Gynaecology this could involve a pregnancy loss, the diagnosis of a structural or chromosomal fetal anomaly, the diagnosis of a malignancy or that of an uncorrectable cause of infertility. Breaking sad, bad and difficult news will always be an unpleasant but necessary part of medicine. Bad news communicated badly can cause confusion, long-lasting distress and resentment. If done well, it can assist understanding, acceptance and adjustment.

Breaking bad news in obstetrics

A planned conception is generally associated with months of excitement and anticipation, in the hope of an uneventful pregnancy, a safe delivery and a normal, healthy baby. When things do not follow the anticipated pattern, it becomes distressing to all concerned. Bereavement is extremely traumatic and the providers of maternity care need to ensure support and information for women and their families both during the acute time of the event and continuing throughout the weeks or months afterwards. The standards set by the RCOG (2008b) have been summarized below

1. Care providers should ensure there are comprehensive, culturally sensitive, multidisciplinary policies, services and facilities for the management and support of families (and staff) who have experienced a maternal loss, early or mid-pregnancy loss, stillbirth or neonatal death.
2. Information about the grieving process, support offered by local groups and other agencies as well as details about investigations (including post-mortem), birth and death registration and options for disposal of the body should be available in different languages, with particular cultural beliefs or sensitivities appropriately reflected.
3. Local guidelines must include clear communication pathways between secondary care and the primary care team with both the woman's GP and community midwife informed of any death within 1 working day
4. There must be a clear and consistent local policy about the sensitive disposal of fetal tissues after early pregnancy loss.
5. Following the death of a baby, results of all investigations, including placental and post-mortem histology should be available within 6 weeks. The woman and her partner should be given the opportunity to meet with the lead obstetrician and/or paediatrician to discuss these results.

Breaking bad news concerning fertility (Lalos 1999)

In society, the ability to conceive is closely related to self-esteem, identity, sexuality and body image. Breaking bad news to infertile couples therefore often means interference in an already vulnerable process. Involuntary childlessness is not a question of once receiving bad news but repeatedly receiving bad news during investigation and treatment. Feelings of shock, surprise, disbelief and denial generally give way to feelings of frustration, anger, loss of control and anxiety and sometimes even to guilt, embarrassment, disappointment, isolation, depression, grief and mourning. Success, in an infertility setting, stands not only for a healthy baby, but also about helping couples to cope with bad news.

Unlike in a general traumatic crisis, in which the duration of the reactive phase is usually approximately 6 weeks, in these cases, new events, new hopes and new forms of bad news result in a state of a prolonged, chronic crisis.

Although there are rituals in society to handle loss through death, there are no rituals to deal with lost dreams and future possibilities, such as the dream of a child. One way of coping during the crisis of infertility is to try to hang on to the medical system to get support and comfort. The doctor and the couple in this setting have a common goal and complementary roles and form a relational triangle—a sensitive social system, which in itself is complex and potentially unstable. Nurses and counsellors, in different capacities form new and separate relational triangles with the couple, which in turn could influence the primary doctor–couple triangle. Good teamwork is essential for effective communication with the couple. The following standards have been suggested.

1. Both partners should be involved and addressed during investigations and treatment and the man should not be allowed to feel excluded from the relationship between the doctor and the female partner.
2. Bad news should be brought to both members of the couple, rather than allowing one member to communicate results to another.
3. Specific communication skills on the part of the whole medical staff are desirable especially as the medical language itself can sometimes act as a hindrance to intellectual understanding and a relationship barrier. Doctors should attempt to listen more attentively and to stay quiet after the couple have been given a short and informative summary of the problem. The behaviour of healthcare professionals must vary and adapt according to the responses they get. It is of no use to give more information than the couple ask for or are able to handle.
4. Most couples claim that the most stressful information, the worst bad news, is that of not having a diagnosis. However, doctors must accept that arriving at a diagnosis is not always possible. Also, when medical treatment of infertility fails, it is important to terminate treatment, to avoid protracted suffering by allowing the couple to swing between hope and despair. Reducing stress by effective communication not only increases psychological, social and sexual wellbeing, but also increases fertility.

Breaking bad news in oncology (Fallowfield and Jenkins 2004)

Communication of bad news in Oncology is by far one of the most complex tasks but is frequently thwarted by the pressures of time constraints, together with political imperatives to meet targets and contain costs. Bad news in Oncology could take the form of communicating the diagnosis or recurrence, or discussion of transition from curative treatment to palliative care. It could also involve explaining the need for often complex therapeutic options and their debilitating side-effects and the eventual uncertainty about optimum treatments and dismal prognosis. Patients with cancer expect to be given the diagnosis and prognosis honestly and in simple language, by a doctor who is at the same time, encouraging, hopeful and supportive. The difficulty for most doctors is getting this balance right. Patients' perceptions of the way in which doctors deliver bad news alter understanding, decisions about treatment and later adjustment. Cancer care is frequently delivered by multidisciplinary teams and therefore demands excellent continuity of communication and awareness about what has been said within the team and between individual team members, patients and families.

The importance of clear documentation cannot be over-emphasized. A number of guidelines to this effect have been designed, one of which has been described later in this chapter.

Obtaining consent

The law relating to consent is evolving and becoming increasingly complex. Guidance on Consent has been recently issued by the GMC (2004, 2008, 2007).

Valid consent: consent is only valid if
1. it is given by a legally competent person
2. it is real (i.e. the patient has been adequately informed)
3. it is given freely.

Expressions of consent

Consent can be either 'implied' or 'express'.

Implied consent: this is generally considered acceptable for minor or routine investigations or treatments, if the doctor is satisfied that the patient understands what one proposes to do and why. An example of this would be a patient rolling up her sleeve to have her blood pressure taken.

Express consent: this could either be oral or written.

Oral consent is generally considered acceptable prior to a routine or gynaecological history taking or examination, and also prior to performing minor procedures like the suturing of an episiotomy or performing a smear test. Oral consent can also be relied on in emergency situations where it may not be possible to obtain a written consent. In these situations, a record of the fact that consent has been given must be made in the medical notes.

Written consent: this is required in cases that involve higher risk, in order that everyone involved understands what was explained and agreed. By law, written consent is required for certain treatments such as fertility treatment, and also if the primary purpose of the investigation or treatment is not to provide clinical care, but rather for research, or if there may be significant consequences for the patient's employment or social or personal life.

The basic model for obtaining consent

This applies to patients who have capacity to make decisions. It includes the following steps.
- The patient's condition is assessed taking into account the medical history, views, experience and knowledge
- The doctor uses specialist knowledge, experience, clinical judgement and the patient's views and understanding of the condition to identify the appropriate investigations and/or treatment that are likely to result in overall benefit for the patient. The doctor explains the options, setting out the potential benefits, risks, burdens and side-effects of each option, including the option to have no treatment. The doctor may recommend a particular option which they believe to be best for the patient, but they must not put pressure on the patient to accept their advice.
- The doctor provides all relevant information that a patient wants or needs in a balanced way using up-to-date written material, or visual and other aids, if required. Other sources of information and support, including patient information leaflets, advocacy services, expert patient programmes or support groups for people with special needs are sought. Patients with additional needs, such as those with disabilities, are allowed the time and support they need to make a decision. An opportunity is given to ask questions, which are then answered

honestly and fully. Patients are made aware that they can change their mind about a decision at any time.
- The patient weighs up the potential benefits, risks and burdens of the various options as well as any non-clinical issues that are relevant to them and decides whether to accept any of the options and, if so, which one. They also have the right to accept or refuse an option. Although no one else can make a decision on behalf of an adult who has capacity, one should accommodate a patient's wishes if they want another person such as a relative, partner, friend, carer or advocate to be involved in discussion or to help them make decisions. It is important to ensure that all decisions made are voluntary and not under coercion from family, employers, insurers or others.
- Once made, the patient's decisions must be respected, even if it involves refusal of an investigation or treatment or if the decision seems wrong or irrational.
- If the patient asks for a treatment that a doctor considers inappropriate, the reasons for their request should be sought and explored. If, after discussion, the doctor still considers that the treatment would not benefit the patient, he/she does not have to provide the treatment, but should explain the reasons to the patient, and explain any other available options, including the option to seek a second opinion.

Reviewing decisions

Before beginning treatment, it is important to check that the patient still wants to go ahead. Any new or repeated concerns or questions must be responded to especially if
1. significant time has passed since the initial decision was made
2. there have been material changes in the patient's condition or in any aspect of the proposed investigation or treatment
3. new information has become available, for example about the risks of treatment or about other treatment options.

Patients must be kept informed about the progress of their treatment and should be able to make decisions at all stages, not just in the initial stage.

The issue of 'capacity'

Presumption of capacity

One must work on the presumption that every adult patient has the capacity to make decisions about their care and to decide whether to agree to or refuse an examination, investigation or treatment. A patient must only be regarded as lacking capacity once it is clear that, having been given all appropriate help and support, they cannot understand, retain, use or weigh up the information needed to make that decision, or communicate their wishes. One mustn't assume that a patient lacks capacity to make a decision solely because of age, disability, appearance, behaviour, medical condition (including mental illness), beliefs, apparent inability to communicate, or they make a decision that one disagrees with.

Assessing capacity

A patient's capacity to make a particular decision must be assessed each time a decision needs to be made. Advice in this regard can be found in the 'Codes of Practice' that accompany the Mental Capacity Act 2005 and the Adults with Incapacity (Scotland) Act 2000. If the assessment leaves the patient's capacity to make a decision in doubt, advice must be sought from others involved in the patient's care, those close to the patient and colleagues with relevant specialist experience, such as psychiatrists, neurologists or speech and language therapists. If still in doubt, legal advice must be sought with a view to asking a court to determine capacity.

Obtaining consent when an adult lacks capacity

Making decisions about the treatment and care for patients who lack capacity is governed in England and Wales by the Mental Capacity Act 2005 and in Scotland by the Adults with Incapacity (Scotland) Act 2000, which set out the criteria and procedures to be followed in making decisions when patients lack capacity to make decisions. It also grants legal authority to certain people to make decisions on behalf of patients who lack capacity. In Northern Ireland, there is currently no relevant primary legislation and decision-making for patients without capacity is governed by the common law, which requires that decisions must be made in a patient's best interest. It is important for healthcare professionals to keep up to date and comply with the laws and codes of practice that apply where one works. If unsure about how the law applies in a particular situation, one should consult defence bodies or professional associations, or seek independent legal advice.

While obtaining consent from patients who lack capacity, a doctor must first establish whether this lack of capacity is temporary or permanent. It must be ensured that the care of the patient is his/her first concern, that their dignity is respected and they are not discriminated against. They should be encouraged to be involved as far as they want to and are able to. Consideration must be given to any previously expressed preferences, such as an advance statement or decision and to the views of those appointed to represent them.

Children and young people

The right to human papillomavirus (HPV) vaccination recently attracted much media attention. In the UK the principle of adolescent autonomy is recognized and logically should include the right to choose to be vaccinated (Brabin et al. 2007). However, while some parents disapproved of HPV vaccination without parental consent, some others desired to overrule their children's decision not to be vaccinated. The GMC, in its recent guidance on 0–18 year olds states the following.

- Those under the age of 18 years should be involved as much as possible in discussions about their care, even if they are not able to make their own decisions.
- A young person's ability to make decisions depends more on their ability to understand and weigh up options than on their age. At 16, a young person can be presumed to have capacity to make most decisions about their treatment and care. A young person under 16 may have capacity to make decisions, depending on their maturity and ability to understand what is involved.
- Parents cannot override the competent consent of a young person to treatment that is in their best interests. But parental consent can be relied upon when a child lacks the capacity to consent. In Scotland parents cannot authorize treatment a competent young person has refused. In England, Wales and Northern Ireland, the law is complex. Legal advice is best sought when a young person refuses treatment that is clearly in his/her best interest.

Improving communication skills

Education and training for doctors (Alder 2007; Harlak et al. 2008)

Communication is a non-predictable activity and although communication skills can be developed, they have not been shown to improve from mere experience. The recognition that these skills can be developed and/or improved through training and through continuing medical education has resulted in the development of numerous courses and programmes. The Lipkin Model used in Oncology has been shown to significantly alter and improve oncologists' communication skills while also significantly altering attitudes and beliefs about the importance of psychosocial issues and communicating well. The improvement in skills was still evident 12 months later, despite no further intervention. However, there is little evidence to suggest that most of the other available courses lead to any improvement that successfully transfer into practice, or that any measurable improvements are sustained over time. In fact, the specific communicative demands in women's healthcare have yet to be clearly defined and operationalized. The need to teach medical students to communicate clearly, sensitively and effectively through well-designed courses that are resource intensive and expensive is probably necessary and even urgent.

Patient involvement (Leite et al. 2005; Alder et al. 2007 Harlak et al. 2008)

- Patients could be previously prepared for visits so that they would come armed with information and questions.
- Clearly written educational material, illustrated aids, or even a video, all matching the patient's literacy level, could be tentative strategies to encourage the individual to have a more active role in the consultation and not to leave the office with unanswered questions.
- New technologies for education and communication could be used in the waiting room, before the visit, to provide guidance and to teach patients how to explain their problem clearly, to ask questions, seek clarification and make sure they understood what had been communicated.

Such initiatives could serve as starting points for improving physician–patient interaction.

Further reading

Alder J, Christen R, Zemp E, Bitzer J. Communication skills training in obstetrics and gynaecology: whom should we train? A randomized controlled trial. Arch Gynecol Obstet 2007;276:605–12.

Brabin L, Roberts SA, Kitchener HC. A semi-qualitative study of attitudes to vaccinating adolescents against human papillomavirus without parental consent. BMC Public Health 2007;7:20.

Brown SJ, Davey MA, Bruinsma FJ. Women's views and experiences of postnatal hospital care in the Victorian Survey of Recent Mothers 2000. Midwifery 2005;21:109–26.

Christen RN, Alder J, Bitzer J. Gender differences in physicians' communicative skills and their influence on patient satisfaction in gynaecological outpatient consultations. Soc Sci Med 2008;66:1474–83.

Fallowfield L, Jenkins V. Communicating sad, bad, and difficult news in medicine. Lancet 2004;363:312–9.

General Medical Council (GMC). Confidentiality: protecting and providing information—Frequently asked questions. London: GMC 2004.

GMC. 0–18 years: Guidance for all doctors. London: GMC 2007.

GMC. Consent: patients and doctors making decisions together. London: GMC 2008.

GMC Confidentiality guidance. GMC Today. 2008;21(Sept/Oct 2008).

Harlak H, Gemalmaz A, Gurel FS, et al. communication skills training: effects on attitudes toward communication skills and empathic tendency. Educ Health 2008;21:62.

Lalos A. Breaking bad news concerning fertility. Hum Reprod 1999;14:581–5.

Leite RC, Makuch MY, Petta CA, Morais SS. Women's satisfaction with physicians' communication skills during an infertility consultation. Patient Educ Couns 2005;59:38–45.

Royal College of Obstetricians and Gynaecologists (RCOG). Standards for gynaecology: report of a working party. London: RCOG 2008a.

RCOG. Standards for maternity care: report of a working party. London: RCOG 2008b.

Tsai WC, Kung PT, Chiang YJ. Relationship between malpractice claims and medical care quality. Int J Health Care Qual Assur Inc Leadersh Health Serv 2004;17:394–400.

Legal framework for care in obstetrics and gynaecology

Legal framework for care in obstetrics and gynaecology

Litigation is one of the health service's most pressing concerns, and obstetric litigation one of its most prominent features. The sharp increase in new claims against doctors and Obstetricians in particular has resulted in an increase in the practice of defensive medicine, a destruction of good patient–doctor relationships and a reduction in the number of new recruits to the specialty. Reference should also be made to the fact that the average retirement age for Obstetricians is 59 years, as opposed to the usual 65 years for other medical professionals. It is worthwhile emphasizing that the practice of 'good medicine' and the upholding of medical ethics would not only avoid litigation, but also result in greater job satisfaction for the doctor, better patient care and a healthier patient–doctor relationship.

Women's sexual and reproductive rights

Whereas medical ethics are protected by codes monitored primarily by the medical profession, human rights are protected by national laws and constitutions. The International Federation of Gynaecologists and Obstetricians (FIGO) constantly emphasizes the importance of the medical profession in upholding these human rights and supporting women's right to autonomy and confidentiality.

Sexual and reproductive rights are the key to the survival and health of women around the world, and understanding the relevance of respecting and promoting these rights is critical to the provision of current standards of care. Women's sexual and reproductive health is often compromised not by the lack of medical knowledge, but because of infringements of their basic human rights. These rights are often fraught with controversy, requiring the involvement of multiple stakeholders including healthcare providers, policy-makers, parliamentarians, lawyers, human rights activists, women's groups and society at large, in order to make advances. The International Planned Parenthood Federation summarized the human rights from international instruments relevant to sexual and reproductive health in a Charter document and in September 2004 at the Global Roundtable of Countdown 2015, new recommendations were made in a number of areas concerning sexual and reproductive rights.

Sexual rights

These include
- women's right to have control over and decide freely and responsibly on matters related to their sexuality, including sexual and reproductive health, free of coercion, discrimination and violence.
- the ability to enjoy mutually fulfilling sexual relationships.
- freedom from sexual abuse, coercion or harassment.
- safety from sexually transmitted diseases
- success in achieving or preventing a pregnancy.

'Reproductive health services'

These include
- family planning services
- prenatal care, safe delivery and postnatal care, especially breastfeeding and infant and women's healthcare
- prevention and treatment of infertility
- safe abortion (where it is legal), including prevention of abortion and post-abortion care

- prevention, diagnosis and treatment of reproductive tract infections and sexually transmitted infections (STIs).

Legal aspects of practice and women's rights

Although Obstetricians and Gynaecologists are natural advocates for women's health, they are often found to be limited in their understanding of the application of national laws regarding sexual and reproductive health and rights and in the limits of conscientious objection. This is probably because ethical and legal education is not yet part of the postgraduate curriculum in Obstetrics and Gynaecology. The need for this and how this may be undertaken in the UK has been discussed by Kalu and Chowdhury (2005). This chapter outlines the framework for sexual and reproductive rights, and explores the relevance of various aspects of the law to the practising clinician. Issues such as access to information and care, confidentiality and informed consent have been discussed in the previous chapter.

The principles of medical litigation

- Not every medical mishap gives the patient the right to sue for damages, as the success of a claim depends on the ability of the injured party to prove negligence.
- In law, negligence is defined as the breach of duty to practise to the standard of care that must be a proximate cause of substantial injury to a patient.
- The following elements should be established in order to document a negligent action:
  - the defendant was duty bound to take care
  - the defendant was in breach of that duty or was careless in his duty
  - the patient was injured as a direct result of the negligent action
  - a causal relationship existed between injury and breach of care.

Medical negligence in obstetrics

Dual patient-hood makes medical negligence in Obstetrics especially complex. The mother and child usually share a set of congruent interests, but when these diverge, i.e. a mother puts her interest above that of the fetus, a maternal–fetal conflict arises. When faced with competing interests, the law requires that the mother's autonomy be protected, because it is illogical to deprive the mother of her right to self-determination by virtue of her pregnancy. Therefore, although constantly mindful of fetal interests, the Obstetrician is expected to consider these as secondary when juxtaposed against maternal wishes and is required not to impose medical opinion upon his/her patient.

Establishing medical negligence in obstetrics

According to the above-mentioned principles of medical litigation, for medical negligence to be established, there must first be a doctor–patient relationship that gives rise to the duty of care which is subsequently breached. A doctor–patient relationship is generally considered as built at the time of the first consultation. A telephone advice prior to the first consultation is considered insufficient to create a duty of care before the first consultation.

In Obstetrics, this relationship is unique as there is more than one patient that could be affected by acts or omissions. In the UK, it was only firmly established that the same doctor–patient relationship between mother and the obstetrician is also present between the fetus and the doctor, when it was accepted that the factual matrix of prenatal treatment gave rise to a potential relationship between the fetus and the Obstetrician that would later manifest into a complete duty of care upon birth. This in turn implies that it is possible to sue for injuries suffered by the child before birth, because the doctor's duty crystallizes upon birth. However, as opposed to US law, which recognizes an unborn child as a distinct biological entity from the time of conception, in the UK, the child's legal personality is not recognized until birth, and a stillbirth thereby removes the possibility of such duty. In the UK therefore, the mother is the Obstetrician's primary patient and the duty to the unborn is only a secondary duty.

Establishing the standard of care expected

- The Bolam principle: The appropriate standard of care required by the above duty is one that optimizes maternal objectives. The common law standard of care is found in the Bolam principle, which establishes the criteria for competent medical practice. This states that 'A doctor is not guilty of negligence if he has acted in accordance with a practice accepted as proper by a responsible body of medical men skilled in that particular art'.
- The Bolitho qualification: The Bolam principle has been criticized enormously for effectively sanctioning any practice that is supported by a body of medical opinion, possibly 'reducing medical negligence to being determined by the lowest standard of care (accepted by the medical profession) rather than reasonable contemporary standards (expected by the community)'. This was later modified when the Court of Appeal stated that 'if in the rare case, it can be demonstrated that the professional opinion is not capable of withstanding logical analysis, the judge is entitled to hold that the body of opinion is not reasonable or responsible.' This has come to be called the Bolitho principle. It is now generally recognized that the Bolitho qualification of Bolam has become 'commonplace within the assessment of whether or not a doctor's act or omission is or is not negligent.'
- The use of clinical guidelines: The standard of care in Obstetrics should be one that optimizes maternal objectives in the labour process. However, this standard of care is unique when contrasted with other areas of medical practice because of the unpredictable nature of labour. A modification of the current adoption of Bolam with Bolitho is often required in Obstetrics in the determination of the standard of care, and there is now a growing trend in the use of clinical guidelines to determine the applicable standard of care. The UK courts have used guidance from the Royal College of Obstetricians and Gynaecologists (RCOG) in the recent past.

Consent in obstetrics

The doctrine of informed consent

Of the 500 cases involving medicolegal obstetric and gynaecological claims, studied by B-Lynch et al., 7% were the result of failure of communication. This failure to communicate, often resulting from inadequate consent, accounted for £30 million in litigation claims in the UK in 2004. Legally, patients can pursue a remedy in the civil courts for having been deliberately touched without consent (battery) or for not having received enough information about the risks of the proposed procedure (negligence). A valid consent therefore licenses what would otherwise be unlawful. Consent and the need for it, is a legal reflection of the ethical principle of respect for the patient's individual autonomy. In the UK, as opposed to Canada and Australia, the overall burden of proving lack of consent is still upon the patient. Having said that, in the light of the Chester v Afshar case, English law is now one step closer to the doctrine of informed consent.

Maternal autonomy

The Obstetrician faces a unique decision-making process because he/she is effectively providing treatment to two patients, while one is 'within and dependent upon the other', but the trite law that the mother's autonomy prevails holds true at all times. Put simply, 'A competent woman who has the capacity to decide may, for religious reasons, other reasons, for rational or irrational reasons or for no reason at all, choose not to have medical intervention, even though the consequence may be the death or serious handicap of the child she bears, or her own death.' Her competence to give an informed consent is not vitiated by her parturient state and is presumed until and unless it is rebutted. A competent woman has the absolute right to refuse or accept recommended treatment irrespective of the consequences of her choice. Society and the law are required to uphold maternal autonomy and prevent any possible interference with personal liberty.

Court-ordered Caesarean sections

If a woman in labour is considered 'competent', an emergency application made to the courts for the performance of a Caesarean section should be considered a gross violation of patient autonomy and of the woman's basic rights to bodily integrity, a fair trial and equal treatment. Such interventions are virtually never justified and have been aptly described as 'indefensible practices in the name of defensive medicine'.

Emergency obstetric procedures

In the UK, public policy would demand that it is to the public's benefit that unconscious patients who require emergency treatments should be able to receive it. If the mother had the foresight to make an advanced medical directive, the doctor has a better indication of her wishes. If not, and in an emergency situation where the doctor does not have the privilege of consulting the patient, the Obstetrician is allowed to act in the best interest of the patient, his/her first priority being the mother's interest, even without regard to the fetus.

The concept and implications of 'maternal immunity'

It may happen that an obstetrician follows the mother's instructions and that a baby is born damaged as a result. Although, it may be arguable that the mother should be liable, as against her child the action against the mother is unenforceable due to maternal immunity. It can be argued, however, that the doctor, having given advice and offered his recommendations, should then not be made to suffer for the wilful decision of the mother either. The law is unfortunately silent about whether the child in this circumstance is allowed to sue the obstetrician.

Informed consent for obstetric research

Obstetric research is now governed by the Research Governance Framework for Health and Social Care, issued by the Department of Health (DH), which states that informed consent is at the heart of ethical research. In Obstetrics the problems of gaining informed consent prior to research can be particularly difficult, because most of Obstetrics is acute and requires emergency procedures and the impact of research interventions may have major implications for the health or welfare of the fetus, an area that is highly risky from the medicolegal perspective. Besides, mothers may be unwell or in pain and some mothers may legally be children themselves. Prior to obtaining an informed consent it is vital that competence is established and that the mother understands the detailed specifics of the proposed study, including difficult concepts such as randomization and blinding, and that the study is voluntary and that failure to consent will not jeopardize her care. When research involves interventions in emergency situations, and there is no time to obtain informed consent, it may be appropriate to commence studies on the basis of an initial simplified explanation provided that the issue of information and consent is regularly revisited and the parents are free to withdraw from the study at any time. It must be understood that informed consent to research is impossible from the fetus, even though it may be benefited. In practice, the consent of the mother-to-be is held to be sufficient consent on behalf of the fetus, but there will be a natural reluctance to rely upon this when it comes to research that may carry some significant risk, even if the resultant child is a potential beneficiary. The best way forward is to think about preparing the ground long before the acute or emergency situations arrives, which is achieved by endeavouring to inform all patients about medical research, using leaflets for example, so that they are in a better position to understand if they are approached about a specific study.

Preventing damage in obstetrics

Avoiding physical harm

The doctor clearly has a duty not to cause physical harm in the care of the mother and fetus before, during or after pregnancy. This duty is particularly important in maternal–fetal conflicts, where the proposed treatment may be harmful to the mother.

Avoiding psychiatric harm

This includes not causing distress to the mother by imposing treatments on her. Psychiatric trauma is long term in nature and extends beyond the immediate temporary shock or grief in the labour ward. Nervous shock claims were first established in UK by *Dulieu* v *White*, where it was held that it was unreasonable not to recognize nervous shock where physical injury is directly produced by it.

Damages for a stillbirth

The ancient common law principle suggests that no person has an interest in the life of another. This would imply that the mother should not be compensated for the death of her child where the child was not born alive. However, the mother should be compensated for the nervous shock of having to deliver a stillborn caused by negligent acts. But for the negligent acts of the Obstetrician, the mother would have been able to experience the joy from the time and energy that she had invested for the birth of her child.

Damages in the case of stillbirth have been awarded under the following pretexts, among others:
1. deprivation of the satisfaction of carrying the baby to full term;
2. disappointment of unfulfilled family plans;
3. being deprived of the joy in raising a healthy child;
4. initial prolongation of labour; and
5. additional pain.

Economic loss

Additionally there should be compensation for economic loss arising as a consequence of injury inflicted by obstetric negligence. Infants born brain-damaged as a result of negligence should be awarded adequate compensation to cover special education and special care required for their maintenance which would not have been necessary had they been born without their disabilities. Other than the above traditional damages, consideration of wrongful birth claims is necessary as more parents are now claiming for costs of raising an unexpected child. Damages have also been awarded for the economic loss in the event that the parents would try for a larger family. This head of damages seem to be stretching the extent of the obstetrician's liability.

Medicolegal issues concerning specific obstetric conditions

Breech delivery

Medicolegal issues are increasingly rare for the singleton breech in the UK, as most that decline or fail external cephalic version choose a lower segment Caesarean section (LSCS). However, if proper delivery techniques are not employed at LSCS or vaginal birth, the resultant trauma could result in litigation.

- It is recommended that where vaginal breech delivery is to occur at any gestation, consultant or specialist input at every point in the decision process is vital. For UK-trained doctors, competence is now an issue and those with little experience or confidence at conducting a vaginal breech birth should ensure the availability of other colleagues if necessary.

- The literature is not supportive of absolute rules on oxytocin, continuous electronic fetal monitoring (EFM), fetal buttock sampling and epidural analgesia and if these are being considered, the decision and discussions should take place at the most senior level.

- Although virtually all literature to date states that breech extraction of the second twin is superior to all other options, with decreasing skills and if there is insufficient time to allow an appropriately trained practitioner to be present, external cephalic version (ECV) or LSCS may be a better risk-management option.

Shoulder dystocia

It is accepted that the majority of cases of shoulder dystocia are unpredictable and allegations that this should have been predicted and prevented by performing an LSCS have not found favour in courts. However, inappropriate manoeuvres such as fundal pressure and the lack of departmental guidelines would not be acceptable and would be difficult to defend in present-day practice. Since it is accepted that Grade A evidence will never be possible in this field, manoeuvres recommended by expert opinion will be the basis of best practice.

Perimortem LSCS

Evidence from literature and review of maternal and fetal physiology suggests that a Caesarean delivery should begin within 4 minutes of cardiac arrest and be accomplished by 5 minutes. The unanimous consensus of the literature is that a civil suit for performing perimortem Caesarean is very unlikely to succeed. The two offences involved could be 'operating without consent' and 'mutilation of corpse'. The former may be argued as 'battery' if the mother is successfully resuscitated. However, the doctrine of emergency exception would be applied because a delay in treatment could cause harm. The latter is unlikely to succeed because an operation performed to save the infant would not be wrongful since there would be no criminal intent.

Intimate partner violence

Following the Domestic Violence Crime and Victims Act 2004, a case against a perpetrator can now proceed if there is sufficient evidence even if the victim withdraws their statement. If a victim is pregnant then, healthcare workers including midwives and obstetricians will be approached for a statement if it is known that the victim was pregnant.

Medicolegal issues related to termination of pregnancy

UK Abortion Law since 1991

UK abortion legislation (ground E) states that 'A person shall not be guilty of an offence under the law relating to an abortion when a pregnancy is terminated by a registered medical practitioner if two registered medical practitioners are of an opinion formed in good faith that there is a substantial risk that if the child were born it would suffer from such physical or mental abnormalities as to be seriously handicapped'. This legislation does not apply in Northern Ireland.

Prior to the amendment of the 1967 Abortion Act by the Human Fertilisation and Embryology Act (HFEA) (1990), the law did not permit termination for any reason after viability had been reached. The Infant Life Preservation Act (1929) defined viability as 28 weeks, but a court judgement had effectively reduced that to 24 weeks. Under the HFEA amendment, that gestational limit of 24 weeks for terminations, carried out for non-medical reasons was removed when the reason for the termination was a substantial risk of serious abnormality (and also in cases when the mother's life was at risk). Thus, third trimester terminations became legally available. The emphasis on maternal welfare is clear even from statutory provisions on abortion in the UK. The UK abortion act makes provision for abortion at any stage where the pregnancy is harmful to the mother.

RCOG Guidance on termination of pregnancy

A number of guidelines have been issued from the RCOG concerning how late terminations should be managed to be within the law.

- The need for guidance arises because the law contains words and phrases that are not absolute, e.g. 'of an opinion', 'formed in good faith', 'substantial risk', 'seriously handicapped'.
- The guidance is also clear in its direction to ensure that fetuses are not born alive, listing procedures that will ensure fetal death prior to termination if the fetus might be able to breathe if delivered. That time was first defined as gestations over '21 weeks' and modified later

to 'more than 21 weeks and 6 days'. The College also made clear that a procedure that stops the fetal heart before delivery is 'part of the legal abortion and is not murder'.

- Guidance around whether to perform a termination later in pregnancy is less clear. It has been argued that if an abortion is ethical at 22 weeks, it remains ethical whenever in pregnancy the diagnosis is made. In response, the RCOG has stipulated that 'As the protection due (to the fetus) increases with embryonic development and fetal growth, reasons for termination, at no stage trivial, must be more pressing the longer the pregnancy has progressed'. The college goes on to state that there must be 'a presumption in favour of life, not absolute but rebuttable for grave reason and the rebuttal becomes harder to establish as gestation progresses'.

Medicolegal issues involving children and young people

The Sexual Offences Act 2003

In England, Wales and Scotland the age of consent to any form of sexual activity is 16 years for males and females. In Northern Ireland it is 17 years. Under the Sexual Offences Act 2003, sexual intercourse and all forms of sexual touching of a minor are illegal in England and Wales, including kissing a minor or kissing between minors. An activity is considered 'sexual' if a reasonable person would always consider it to be so, or if it may be deemed to be depending on the circumstances and intention. 'Touching' covers a wide range of behaviour: touching any part of the body with anything else, including through clothing.

- Teenagers under 13 years of age are deemed NOT to have the capacity to consent to sexual activity and any agreement to do so is not recognized in law.
- The Sexual Offences Act allows that if both partners are aged between 13 and 15 years, discretion can be exercised by the Crown Prosecution Service, provided there is no evidence of abuse or exploitation. The DH has also assured that mutually agreed sex should not be prosecuted.
- If an individual over 16 years of age has sexual activity with someone under 16, it is the older individual who commits the offence.

Contraception and the Fraser guidelines

Lord Fraser ruled in the High Court that a doctor could give contraceptive treatment or advice provided the following criteria were met:

- the girl was mature enough to understand his advice and the implications of treatment;
- the girl was likely to begin or continue to have sex with or without treatment;
- the doctor had tried to persuade the girl to inform her parents, or to allow him to inform them;
- the girl's health would suffer without treatment or advice
- the girl's best interests required him to give treatment or advice.

A young person that meets the above criteria is termed 'Fraser ruling competent'. Fraser competence can now be assessed by professionals other than a doctor. The principles of this judgement are now central to consenting minors for all health treatments. In Scotland and Northern Ireland different laws apply, although the implications are similar. The Sexual Offences Act specifically allows a professional, including teachers, nurses and youth workers to provide sexual health care to minors provided the intention is to protect the minor from STIs, pregnancy, physical harm or to promote the minor's wellbeing. Professionals providing treatment to minors must continue to assess competence within the Fraser guidelines.

Gillick competence

The parental right to determine whether or not a child below the age of 16 will or will not have medical treatment terminates if and when the child achieves sufficient understanding and intelligence to enable him to understand fully what is proposed. Note that 'Gillick competence' relates to the particular child and the particular treatment, and there have been cases where a 17-year-old has been found insufficiently competent to refuse medical treatment, whereas in other cases much younger children have been deemed sufficiently competent. In addition, where a child is 16 or 17 either parent or child can consent to treatment independently (though neither can override the other or exercise a veto). The court can, however, override the wishes of both where treatment is vital to the child's welfare. The Access to Health Records Act 1990 further complicates the picture in allowing a child under 16, deemed 'Gillick competent' by a doctor, to veto the parent's access to medical information held by that doctor, even though the parent can consent to treatment that the child cannot veto. It is for the doctor to decide whether or not an individual child is Gillick competent or not. The courts are generally reluctant to do so.

Confidentiality

About 25% of teenagers in the UK have had sexual intercourse by the age of 16 years. There is no legal obligation to report underage sex. In fact, it is enshrined in professional practice that the duty of confidentiality owed to a person under 16 years of age is the same as that owed to any other person, and breaches of it should be treated as seriously as if the person were over 16. Maintaining confidentiality also encourages young people to access the sexual health service, thereby preventing teenage pregnancies and STIs. If a girl is Fraser competent and does not want her parents to be involved, the clinician must respect her wishes. In the case of abortion, where the young woman is competent to consent but cannot be persuaded to involve a parent, every effort should be made to help them find another adult to provide support, for example another family member or specialist youth worker.

However, no one has the right to absolute confidentiality and if a professional believes there is a risk to the health, safety or welfare of a young person (or any other minor) and that the risk is serious enough to override the young person's right to privacy, then the professional must follow child protection protocols and refer to social services. The latest version of the DH document, 'Working together to safeguard children' doesn't require all partners of minors to be police-checked or all sexually active persons under the age of 13 to be reported to social services. Instead, it states that the child's best interests must be the overriding consideration in making any decision to share information. In cases where the child is under 13 there should always be a discussion with a nominated child protection lead in the organization and there should be a presumption that the case will be reported to children's social care. In addition, detailed reasons should be documented where a decision is taken not to share information. With regard to teenagers aged 13–15 it states that consideration should be given in every case of sexual activity as to whether there should be a discussion with other agencies and whether a referral should be made to children's social care.

Coercive relationships

Although most teenage sexual activity is mutually agreed, sexual abuse in childhood is common. One young person in ten is subject to abuse. The DH has issued a checklist of factors to consider in assessing the risk of coercion in relationships, and has suggested that if a request for contraception is made, doctors and health professionals should establish rapport and give a young person support and time to make an informed choice by discussing whether there may be coercion or abuse. This can be challenging, especially with vulnerable young people and it has been suggested that someone else, outside a clinic setting, who knows more about the young person be consulted, if in doubt. If, however, the professional remains concerned that the young person is involved in abusive or seriously harmful sexual activity, they should be protected by sharing relevant information with appropriate people or agencies, such as the police or social services, quickly and professionally.

Medicolegal issues and STIs

STIs are complex as they have a tremendous impact on both the physical and emotional wellbeing of the patient and those in contact with them. The healthcare provider has to tread a perilous path when dealing with issues pertaining to disclosure. In cases where disclosure becomes necessary, the healthcare provider may come up against the wishes of the patient and, at best, risk losing their trust or, at worst, end up in a courtroom. The rule of thumb should always be to seek the patient's consent before disclosing any information to a third party, but, in the event of a patient's refusal, careful adherence to the GMC guidelines will hopefully prevent any unnecessary litigation. The medical professionals' legal duty to protect confidentiality is especially relevant with regards to STIs, since personal information concerning STIs is generally regarded as sensitive and private by patients. Although confidentiality should be respected at all times, it is not absolute and paradoxically, genitourinary medicine (GUM) services are probably the main area of medicine where confidentiality may need to be broken.

Disclosure to other medical carers

Merely confirming that a patient has attended a GUM clinic amounts to a breach of confidentiality. However, it may sometimes be necessary for the treating clinician to disclose the details of a patient's sexual health to other doctors or health authorities involved in their management. The GMC's guidelines have set a code of practice for UK doctors and are invaluable in guiding any healthcare provider in these, often tricky, situations. The issue of disclosure to other medical professionals has been discussed in the previous chapter. It should be borne in mind that any information that has to be shared with other healthcare providers must be compliant with the Data Protection Act 1998 and the Caldicott Principles. These specify that the information can only be shared for a justifiable purpose, with the minimum necessary patient-identifiable information used and revealed, on a strict need-to-know basis, to a responsible individual who understands and complies with the law. GUM clinics are able to share information about their patients through the network of health advisers but it is accepted practice that a patient's GP may not be routinely informed when they attend a clinic.

GMC guidance explicitly states that, if a patient is diagnosed with a serious communicable disease, in addition to explaining the ways of protecting others from infection, the medical, social and occupational implications have to be explained to the patient. Moreover, it has to be made clear to the patient that other healthcare providers involved in their care might have to be informed of their condition, in order for them to provide adequate clinical management. If patients still refuse to allow other healthcare workers to be informed, the patients' wishes must be respected, except where that failure to disclose the information would put a healthcare worker or other patient at serious risk of death or serious harm. If in doubt about whether disclosure is appropriate, advice should be sought from an experienced colleague and one must be prepared to justify one's decision to disclose information against a patient's wishes.

The work of GUM clinics in the UK is regulated by the National Health Service (NHS) Venereal Diseases Regulation (1974), the NHS Trust and the Venereal Diseases Directive (1991), the NHS Trusts and Primary Care Trusts (Sexually Transmitted Diseases) Directions (2000) and the Venereal Diseases Act (1974) (in Scotland).

Disclosure to a partner

The English and Scottish courts have recently confirmed that the reckless transmission of human immunodeficiency virus (HIV) can amount to a criminal offence. The offence is not confined to HIV. With regards to civil liability, there is, at present, no reported decision by the UK courts to hold a doctor liable in damages for the onward transmission of HIV by one of his or her patients. Providing proper advice to the HIV-positive patient will discharge the doctor's legal duty unless the doctor has reason to believe that the patient will not follow the advice, or if the third party is also a patient of the doctor. Where there is an identifiable third party (who is not a patient of the doctor) there is a possibility that the UK courts might hold that simply giving proper advice to the patient is insufficient. The third party or the appropriate authority might need to be informed of the risk, despite the patient's wishes. Disclosure without consent must always follow prior consultation with senior colleagues and/or advice should be sought from the GMC or defence societies, as appropriate. With regards to criminal liability, both English and Scottish law establish that criminal liability will not normally be imposed for an omission to act, unless a legal duty to act is specifically recognized.

The GMC guidance on serious communicable diseases allows the disclosure of information about a patient, whether living or dead, in order to protect a person from risk of death or serious harm. This could allow the disclosure of information to a known sexual contact of a patient with HIV where there is reason to think that the patient has not informed that person, and cannot be persuaded to do so. In such circumstances, the patient should be informed before the disclosure is made, and one must be prepared to justify a decision to disclose information. It is noteworthy here that this guideline does not specify that the partner of the infected patient has to be a patient of the clinician.

Colleagues in the medical profession with serious communicable diseases

The GMC's guidance states that a doctor or other healthcare worker with a serious communicable disease is entitled to the provision of confidentiality and support like any other patient. However, if there is reason to believe that a medical colleague or healthcare worker with a serious communicable disease, is practising, or has practised, in a way which places patients at risk, an appropriate person in the healthcare worker's employing authority or the relevant regulatory body should be informed. Wherever possible, the healthcare worker should be informed of this disclosure. Similarly, the advice given by the DH for the management of HIV-infected healthcare workers has three main principles: there is a duty to protect patients; there is a duty of confidentiality towards infected healthcare workers; infected healthcare staff should avoid carrying out certain procedures where exposure of patients to HIV is possible.

Pregnant women with HIV

The issues relating to HIV in pregnant women are detailed in the British HIV Association's guidelines. Although, antenatal HIV testing of all pregnant women is recognized as an effective way of preventing mother–child transmission, the psychosocial, emotional and economic impact of routine testing is significant, especially if there is discordance between the couple. About 20–80% of couples are discordant and there are situations where a newly diagnosed HIV-positive woman refuses to disclose to a current sexual partner, or appears to want to delay disclosure indefinitely. These cases should be dealt with on an individual basis and priority should be given to finding the causes of non-disclosure. The importance of disclosure to appropriate health workers should be emphasized.

In cases of reverse discordance (where the male partner is HIV positive and the female partner HIV negative) there is an increased risk of vertical transmission associated with seroconversion in pregnancy and breastfeeding. If the male partner is reluctant to inform his partner, the issue of disclosure without consent should be based on weighing the potential harms and benefits of non-disclosure. It is of the utmost importance to consider the risk of HIV to the baby in order to determine whether breach of confidentiality is justified. There has been concern that forced disclosure can have a negative impact on HIV testing uptake. It could also mean that, by compelling doctors to disclose HIV infection to sexual contacts, they would lose the trust of their patients.

Disclosure after a patient's death

A doctor is still obliged to keep personal information confidential after a patient's death. However, GMC's guidance on serious communicable diseases, states that where a communicable disease contributed to the cause of death, this must be recorded on the death certificate and that this information should be passed to relevant for the purpose of communicable disease control and surveillance. Disclosure after a patient's death is permissible if it is done to protect other people from serious harm, or it is required by the law.

Miscellaneous legislation related to Obstetrics and Gynaecology

Making decisions when patients lack capacity

- Mental Capacity Act 2005 (England and Wales): This act provides the legal framework for making decisions in relation to people who lack capacity, and clarifies who can make decisions and how those decisions should be made. In this Act, people lack capacity in relation to a particular matter if, at the material time, they are unable to make a decision for themselves in relation to the matter because of an impairment of, or a disturbance in the functioning of, the mind or brain. Section 1 of the Act sets out five statutory principles that apply to any action taken and decisions made under the Act. The issue of 'capacity' has been discussed in the previous chapter.

- Adults with Incapacity (Scotland) Act 2000: This Act provides ways to help safeguard the welfare of people aged 16 and over who lack the capacity to take some or all decisions for themselves because of a mental disorder or inability to communicate. It also allows other people to make decisions on their behalf. The Act provides various methods of intervening on behalf of an adult who lacks capacity, and sets out the principles that must be followed when deciding whether to intervene. In this Act, incapacity means being incapable of acting on, making, communicating, understanding, or remembering decisions by reason of mental disorder or inability to communicate due to physical disorder.
- Northern Ireland: There is currently no primary legislation on capacity covering Northern Ireland and decisions about medical treatment and care when people lack capacity must be made in accordance with the common law, which requires decisions to be made in a person's best interests.

The use of human tissue

- Human Tissue Act 2005 (England, Wales and Northern Ireland): The Act requires that consent is obtained before a living person's organs and tissue can be stored or used for purposes such as research, post-mortem examination, and transplantation or a deceased person's organs and tissue can be removed for these purposes. The Act specifies whose consent is needed and in what circumstances. The Human Tissue Authority (HTA) publishes a Code of Practice, which gives detailed advice on how consent should be obtained and recorded.
- Human Tissue (Scotland) Act 2006: The Act requires that authorization is obtained before a deceased person's organs and tissue can be stored or used for purposes such as research, post-mortem examination and transplantation. It does not cover the use and storage of tissue from living people, other than organ donation for transplantation.

Fertility treatments

- Human Fertilisation and Embryology Act 1990 as amended by the Human Fertilisation (Disclosure of information) Act (1992): This Act provides a legal framework across the UK for all those involved in fertility treatments. It defines the rights of donors, patients and the children who may result from the treatment, restricts research on human embryos to specified purposes and places time limits on the storage of embryos, eggs, and sperm. HFEA was created under the Act to oversee the licensing and compliance of treatment clinics and research centres and to keep new developments under review. A number of contentious issues are constantly being debated and the even now the Parliament is considering a number of amendments to the Act. A few of these have been highlighted below
  - Children conceived with donated gametes: From April 2005, children conceived with donated gametes have the right to seek identifying information about the gamete provider when they reach the age of 18 years.

- Egg sharing: Although it is illegal within the UK, to sell or purchase eggs, egg donation is permissible and donors may receive a nominal sum, as defined by HFEA. The authority allows egg sharing, which has undoubtedly brought happiness to a select group of young infertile women able to trade their eggs for IVF treatment and to the privileged couples able to meet their costs. The concept and practice of egg trading offends the principle with respect to the trade in human cells, organs and tissues. However, it has been founded on the needs of a desperate group of vulnerable infertile women who see no other way to obtain IVF treatment, hitherto denied to them on the NHS because of inadequate funding.
- Consent in Assisted reproduction: A summary related to Consent in Assisted Conception is given in an article by Sawers and Avery (2006)

Other relevant legislation
- Data Protection Act 1998
- The Human Rights Act 1998
- Access to Health Records Act 1990
- Access to Medical Reports Act 1988
- Age of Legal Capacity (Scotland) 1991
- Age of Majority Act (Northern Ireland) 1969
- Children Acts 1989 and 2004
- NHS Regulations 1974

Further reading

B-Lynch C, Coker A, Dua KA. Clinical analysis of 500 medico-legal claims evaluating the causes and assessing the potential benefit of alternative dispute resolution. Brit J Obstet Gynaecol 1996;103: 1236–42.

General Medical Council (GMC) Consent: patients and doctors making decisions together. London: General Medical Council 2008.

FIGO Professional and Ethical Responsibilities concerning sexual and reproductive rights. International Joint Policy Statement. J Obstet Gynaecol Can 2004;26:1097–9, 1105–7.

Kalu G, Chowdhury RR. Ethical and legal education as part of structured training in obstetrics and gynaecology. Obstet Gynaecol 2005;7:44–48.

Luo LL. Medical negligence in obstetrics and maternal autonomy. Singapore J Obstet Gynaecol 2007;38:38–70.

Verschuuren M, Badeyan G, Carnicero J, et al. The European data protection legislation and its consequences for public health monitoring: a plea for action. Eur J Pub Health 2008;18:550–1.

Mavroforou A, Mavrophoros D, Koumantakis E, Michalodimitrakis E. Liability in prenatal ultrasound screening. Ultrasound Obstet Gynecol 2003;21:525–8.

Nicholas N, El Sayed M. The changing face of consent: past and present. Obstet Gynaecol 2006; 8:39–44.

FIGO. Recommendations on Ethical Issues in Obstetrics and Gynecology by the FIGO Committee for the Study of Ethical Aspects of Human Reproduction. Londonl: FIGO 2006.

Sawers R, Avery S. Risk Management: Consent in assisted conception. Obstet Gynaecol 2006;8:245–250.

Shaw D, Faundes A. What is the relevance of women's sexual and reproductive rights to the practising obstetrician/gynaecologist? Best Pract Res Clin Obstet Gynaecol 2006;20:299–309.

Spencer SA, Dawson A. Implications of informed consent for obstetric research. Obstet Gynaecol 2004;6:163–167.

Statham H, Solomou W, Green J. Late termination of pregnancy: law, policy and decision making in four English fetal medicine units. Br J Obstet Gynaecol 2006;113:1402–11.

Tillett, J. Adolescents and informed consent: ethical and legal issues. J Perinat Neonatal Nurs 2005;19:112–21.

RCOG publications and guidelines on termination of pregnancy

Law and Ethics in Relation to Court-Authorised Obstetric Intervention.

RCOG report Termination of pregnancy for fetal abnormality in England, Wales and Scotland (Jan 1996);.

Joint Report of the RCOG/RCPCH Guidelines for screening, diagnosis and management of fetal abnormalities (Dec 1997).

Report of the RCOG Ethics Committee Late termination of pregnancy for fetal abnormality: A consideration of the law and ethics (Mar 1998).

The British Association of Perinatal Medicine Memorandum, November 1999—Fetuses and Newborn Infants at the Threshold of Viability: A Framework for Practice.

Further issues relating to late abortion, fetal viability and registration of births and deaths.

Part 2

Obstetrics

Normal pregnancy *31*
Complications of early pregnancy *73*
Care of the fetus *83*
Maternal medicine and infections *175*
Obstetric conditions *319*
Care in labour *363*
Common obstetric techniques, procedures,
   and surgery *429*

Normal pregnancy

Antenatal care *32*
Booking *38*
Breastfeeding *42*
Dating in pregnancy *48*
Diagnosis of pregnancy *50*
Minor symptoms of pregnancy *52*
Physiological changes in pregnancy *56*
Preparing for pregnancy *60*
Puerperium *64*
Routine blood tests in pregnancy *68*

Antenatal care

The main principles of antenatal care in uncomplicated pregnancies are to provide advice, education, reassurance and support. It is also to address and treat the minor problems of pregnancy, to provide effective screening during the pregnancy and to identify major problems as they arise and to manage them.

Booking appointment
Refer to Chapter 5.2, Booking.

Antenatal information
- Information should be given in a form that is easy to understand and accessible to pregnant women including those with additional needs, such as physical, sensory or learning disabilities, and to pregnant women who do not speak or read English. Information can also be given in other forms such as audiovisual or touch screen technology; this should be supported by written information.
- Pregnant women should be offered information based on the current available evidence together with support to enable them to make informed decisions about their care. This information should include where they will be seen and who will undertake their care.
- At each antenatal appointment, healthcare professionals should offer consistent information and clear explanations, and should provide pregnant women with an opportunity to discuss issues and ask questions.
- Pregnant women should be offered opportunities to attend participant-led antenatal classes, including breastfeeding workshops.
- Pregnant women should be informed about the purpose of any test before it is performed. The healthcare professional should ensure the woman has understood this information and has sufficient time to make an informed decision. The right of a woman to accept or decline a test should be made clear.
- Information about antenatal screening should be provided in a setting where discussion can take place; this may be in a group setting or on a one-to-one basis. This should be done at or before the booking appointment.

Provision and organization of care
Who?
- Midwife- and GP-led models of care should be offered to women with an uncomplicated pregnancy. Routine involvement of obstetricians in the care of women with an uncomplicated pregnancy at scheduled times does not appear to improve perinatal outcomes compared with involving obstetricians when complications arise.
- Antenatal care should be provided by a small group of healthcare professionals with whom the woman feels comfortable. There should be continuity of care throughout the antenatal period.
- A system of clear referral paths should be established so that pregnant women who require additional care are managed and treated by the appropriate specialist teams when problems are identified.

Where?
- Antenatal care should be readily and easily accessible to all pregnant women and should be sensitive to the needs of individual women and the local community.

- The environment in which antenatal appointments take place should enable women to discuss sensitive issues such as domestic violence, sexual abuse, psychiatric illness and recreational drug use.

Documentation of care
- Structured maternity records should be used for antenatal care.
- Maternity services should have a system in place whereby women carry their own case notes.
- A standardized, national maternity record with an agreed minimum data set should be developed and used. This will help healthcare professionals to provide the recommended evidence-based care to pregnant women.

Frequency of antenatal appointments
A schedule of antenatal appointments should be determined based upon the needs of the individual mothers. For a woman who is nulliparous with an uncomplicated pregnancy, a schedule of 10 appointments should be adequate. For a woman who is parous with an uncomplicated pregnancy, a schedule of seven appointments should be adequate.

Gestational age assessment
Pregnant women should be offered an early ultrasound scan between 10 weeks 0 days and 13 weeks 6 days to determine gestational age and to detect multiple pregnancies. This will ensure consistency of gestational age assessment and reduce the incidence of induction of labour for prolonged pregnancy. Crown–rump length measurement should be used to determine gestational age. If the crown–rump length is above 84 mm, the gestational age should be estimated using head circumference.

Lifestyle considerations
- Working during pregnancy should be discussed.
- Pregnant women should be informed of their maternity rights and benefits.
- Nutritional supplements
  - Pregnant women (and those intending to become pregnant) should be informed that dietary supplementation with folic acid, before conception and throughout the first 12 weeks, reduces the risk of having a baby with a neural tube defect (for example, anencephaly or spina bifida). The recommended dose is 400 μg per day.
  - Iron supplementation should not be offered routinely to all pregnant women. It does not benefit the mother's or the baby's health and may have unpleasant maternal side-effects.
- Prescribed medicines: see Chapter 8.12, Drugs in pregnancy
- Complementary therapies
  - Pregnant women should be informed that few complementary therapies have been established as being safe and effective during pregnancy. Women should not assume that such therapies are safe and they should be used as little as possible during pregnancy.
- Exercise in pregnancy
  - Pregnant women should be informed that beginning or continuing a moderate course of exercise during pregnancy is not associated with adverse outcomes.

- Pregnant women should be informed of the potential dangers of certain activities during pregnancy, for example contact sports, high-impact sports and vigorous racquet sports that may involve the risk of abdominal trauma, falls or excessive joint stress, and scuba diving, which may result in fetal birth defects and fetal decompression disease.
- Sexual intercourse in pregnancy is not known to be associated with any adverse outcomes.
- Alcohol consumption in pregnancy
  - Pregnant women and women planning a pregnancy should be advised to avoid drinking alcohol in the first 3 months of pregnancy if possible because it may be associated with an increased risk of miscarriage.
  - Excess alcohol can give rise to fetal alcohol syndrome.
  - Fetal alcohol spectrum disorders are diagnosed in childhood and may present as attention disorders and inappropriate behaviour. The quantity of alcohol that causes these late problems is not known and hence avoidance is best.
- Smoking in pregnancy
  - Pregnant women should be informed about the specific risks of smoking during pregnancy (such as the risk of having a baby with low birthweight and preterm birth). The benefits of quitting at any stage should be emphasized.
  - The direct effects of cannabis on the fetus are uncertain but may be harmful. Cannabis use is associated with smoking, which is known to be harmful; therefore, women should be discouraged from using cannabis during pregnancy.
- Pregnant women should be informed that long-haul air travel is associated with an increased risk of venous thrombosis. In the general population, wearing correctly fitted compression stockings is effective at reducing the risk.

Minor ailments in pregnancy

- Women should be informed that most cases of nausea and vomiting in pregnancy will resolve spontaneously within 16–20 weeks and that nausea and vomiting are not usually associated with a poor pregnancy outcome. Information about all forms of self-help and non-pharmacological treatments should be made available for pregnant women who have nausea and vomiting.
- Women who present with symptoms of heartburn in pregnancy should be offered information regarding lifestyle and diet modification. Antacids may be offered to women whose heartburn remains troublesome despite lifestyle and diet modification.
- Women who present with constipation in pregnancy should be offered information regarding diet modification, such as bran or wheat fibre supplementation.
- Haemorrhoids: In the absence of evidence of the effectiveness of treatments for haemorrhoids in pregnancy, women should be offered information concerning diet modification. If clinical symptoms remain troublesome, standard haemorrhoid creams should be considered.
- Varicose veins are a common symptom of pregnancy that will not cause harm. Compression stockings can improve the symptoms but will not prevent varicose veins from emerging.
- An increase in vaginal discharge is a common physiological change that occurs during pregnancy. If it is associated with itch, soreness, offensive smell or pain on passing urine there may be an infective cause and investigation should be considered. A 1-week course of a topical imidazole is an effective treatment and should be considered for vaginal candidiasis infections in pregnant women. The effectiveness and safety of oral treatments for vaginal candidiasis in pregnancy are uncertain and these treatments should not be offered.

Clinical examination of pregnant women

- Maternal weight and height should be measured and body mass index (BMI) calculated at the booking appointment (BMI = weight (kg)/height (m)^2).
- Routine breast examination during antenatal care is not recommended for the promotion of postnatal breastfeeding.
- Routine antenatal pelvic examination does not accurately assess gestational age, nor does it accurately predict preterm birth or cephalopelvic disproportion. It is not recommended.
- Female genital mutilation: Pregnant women who have had female genital mutilation should be identified early in antenatal care through sensitive enquiry. Antenatal examination will then allow planning of intrapartum care.
- Healthcare professionals need to be alert to the symptoms or signs of domestic violence and women should be given the opportunity to disclose domestic violence in an environment in which they feel secure.
- In all communications (including initial referral) with maternity services, healthcare professionals should include information on any relevant history of mental disorder. At a woman's first contact with services in both the antenatal and the postnatal periods, healthcare professionals (including midwives, obstetricians, health visitors and GPs) should ask about past or present history of severe mental illness including schizophrenia, bipolar disorder or psychosis in the postnatal period. Severe depression, previous treatment by a psychiatrist/specialist mental health team, including inpatient care and a family history of perinatal mental illness should be known. After identifying a possible mental disorder in a woman during pregnancy or the postnatal period, further assessment should be considered, in consultation with colleagues if and when necessary.

Screening for haematological conditions
Anaemia
- Pregnant women should be offered screening for anaemia. Screening should take place early in pregnancy (at the booking appointment) and at 28 weeks when other blood screening tests are being performed. This allows enough time for treatment if anaemia is detected.
- Haemoglobin levels outside the normal range for pregnancy (that is 11 g/100 mL at first contact and 10.5 g/100 mL at 28 weeks) should be investigated and iron supplementation considered if indicated.

Blood grouping and red cell alloantibodies
- Women should be offered testing for blood group and rhesus D status in early pregnancy.
- It is recommended that routine antenatal anti-D prophylaxis is offered to all non-sensitized pregnant women who are rhesus D negative.
- Women should be screened for atypical red cell alloantibodies in early pregnancy and again at 28 weeks, regardless of their rhesus D status.

- In some countries, if a pregnant woman is rhesus D negative, consideration is given to partner testing to determine whether the administration of anti-D prophylaxis is necessary.

Screening for haemoglobinopathies

- Screening for sickle cell diseases and thalassaemias should be offered to all women as early as possible in pregnancy (ideally by 10 weeks). The type of screening depends upon the prevalence and can be carried out in either primary or secondary care.
- Where prevalence of sickle cell disease is high (fetal prevalence above 1.5 cases per 10 000 pregnancies), laboratory screening (preferably high-performance liquid chromatography) should be offered to all pregnant women to identify carriers of sickle cell disease and/or thalassaemia.
- Where prevalence of sickle cell disease is low (fetal prevalence 1.5 cases per 10 000 pregnancies or below), all pregnant women should be offered screening for haemoglobinopathies using the Family Origin Questionnaire.
- If the Family Origin Questionnaire indicates a high risk of sickle cell disorders, laboratory screening (preferably high-performance liquid chromatography) should be offered.
- If the mean corpuscular haemoglobin is below 27 pg, laboratory screening (preferably high-performance liquid chromatography) should be offered.
- If the woman is identified as a carrier of a clinically significant haemoglobinopathy then the father of the baby should be offered counselling and appropriate screening carried out without delay.

Screening for fetal anomalies

- Ultrasound screening for fetal anomalies should be routinely offered, normally between 18 weeks 0 days and 20 weeks 6 days.
- Women should be informed of the limitations of routine ultrasound screening and that detection rates vary by the type of fetal anomaly, the woman's BMI and the position of the unborn baby at the time of the scan.
- If an anomaly is detected during the anomaly scan pregnant women should be informed of the findings to enable them to make an informed choice of whether they wish to continue with the pregnancy or have a termination of pregnancy.
- Fetal echocardiography involving the four-chamber view of the fetal heart and outflow tracts is recommended as part of the routine anomaly scan.
- Routine screening for cardiac anomalies using nuchal translucency is not recommended.
- When routine ultrasound screening is performed to detect neural tube defects, alpha-fetoprotein testing is not required.

Screening for Down's syndrome

- All pregnant women should be offered screening for Down's syndrome. Women should understand that it is their choice to embark on screening for Down's syndrome.
- The 'combined test' (nuchal translucency, beta-human chorionic gonadotrophin, pregnancy-associated plasma protein-A) should be offered to screen for Down's syndrome between 11 weeks 0 days and 13 weeks 6 days.

- For women who book later in pregnancy, the most clinically and cost-effective serum screening test (triple or quadruple test) should be offered between 15 weeks 0 days and 20 weeks 0 days.
- When it is not possible to measure nuchal translucency, owing to fetal position or raised BMI, women should be offered serum screening (triple or quadruple test) between 15 weeks 0 days and 20 weeks 0 days.
- If a pregnant woman receives a screen positive result for Down's syndrome, she should have rapid access to appropriate counselling by trained staff.
- The routine anomaly scan (at 18 weeks 0 days to 20 weeks 6 days) should not be routinely used for Down's syndrome screening using soft markers.
- The presence of an isolated soft marker, with the exception of increased nuchal fold, on the routine anomaly scan should not be used to adjust the a priori risk for Down's syndrome.
- The presence of an increased nuchal fold (6 mm or above) or two or more soft markers on the routine anomaly scan should prompt the offer of a referral to a fetal medicine specialist or an appropriate healthcare professional with a special interest in fetal medicine.

Screening for infections

- Asymptomatic bacteriuria: women should be offered routine screening for asymptomatic bacteriuria by midstream urine culture early in pregnancy. Identification and treatment of asymptomatic bacteriuria reduces the risk of pyelonephritis.
- Asymptomatic bacterial vaginosis: pregnant women should not be offered routine screening for bacterial vaginosis because the evidence suggests that the identification and treatment of asymptomatic bacterial vaginosis does not lower the risk of preterm birth and other adverse reproductive outcomes.
- *Chlamydia trachomatis*: at the booking appointment, healthcare professionals should inform pregnant women younger than 25 years about the high prevalence of chlamydia infection in their age group, and give details of their local National Chlamydia Screening Programme.
- Cytomegalovirus: the available evidence does not support routine cytomegalovirus screening in pregnant women and it should not be offered.
- Hepatitis B virus: serological screening for hepatitis B virus should be offered to pregnant women so that effective postnatal interventions can be offered to infected women to decrease the risk of mother-to-child transmission.
- Hepatitis C virus: pregnant women should not be offered routine screening for hepatitis C virus, because there is insufficient evidence to support its clinical and cost effectiveness.
- HIV: pregnant women should be offered screening for HIV infection early in antenatal care because appropriate antenatal interventions can reduce mother-to-child transmission of HIV infection.
- Rubella: rubella susceptibility screening should be offered early in antenatal care to identify women at risk of contracting rubella infection and to enable vaccination in the postnatal period for the protection of future pregnancies.
- Group B streptococcus: pregnant women should not be offered routine antenatal screening for group B streptococcus because evidence of its clinical and cost-effectiveness remains uncertain.

- Syphilis: screening for syphilis should be offered to all pregnant women at an early stage in antenatal care because treatment of syphilis is beneficial to the mother and baby.
- Toxoplasmosis: routine antenatal serological screening for toxoplasmosis should not be offered because the risks of screening may outweigh the potential benefits.

Screening for clinical conditions

Gestational diabetes

- Screening for gestational diabetes using risk factors is recommended in a healthy population. At the booking appointment, the following risk factors for gestational diabetes should be determined:
  - body mass index above 30 kg/m^2
  - previous macrosomic baby weighing 4.5 kg or above
  - previous gestational diabetes (refer to Chapter 8.11, Diabetes in pregnancy (NICE clinical guideline 63, available from www.nice.org.uk/CG063)
  - family history of diabetes (first-degree relative with diabetes)
  - family origin with a high prevalence of diabetes.
- Women with any one of these risk factors should be offered testing for gestational diabetes.
- Screening for gestational diabetes using fasting plasma glucose, random blood glucose, glucose challenge test and urinalysis for glucose should not be undertaken.

Pre-eclampsia

- Blood pressure measurement and urinalysis for protein should be carried out at each antenatal visit to screen for pre-eclampsia.
- At the booking appointment, the following risk factors for pre-eclampsia should be determined:
  - age 40 years or older
  - nulliparity
  - pregnancy interval of more than 10 years
  - family history of pre-eclampsia
  - previous history of pre-eclampsia
  - body mass index 30 kg/m^2 or above
  - pre-existing vascular disease such as hypertension
  - pre-existing renal disease
  - multiple pregnancy.
- More frequent blood pressure measurements should be considered for pregnant women who have any of the above risk factors.
- The presence of significant hypertension and/or proteinuria should alert the healthcare professional to the need for increased surveillance.
- Hypertension in which there is a single diastolic blood pressure of 110 mmHg or two consecutive readings of 90 mmHg at least 4 hours apart and/or significant proteinuria (1+) should prompt increased surveillance.
- If the systolic blood pressure is above 160 mmHg on two consecutive readings at least 4 hours apart, treatment should be considered.
- All pregnant women should be made aware of the need to seek immediate advice from a healthcare professional if they experience symptoms of pre-eclampsia.

Preterm birth

- Routine screening for preterm labour should not be offered.

Placenta praevia

- Because most low-lying placentas detected at the routine anomaly scan will have resolved by the time the baby is born, only a woman whose placenta extends over the internal cervical os should be offered another transabdominal scan at 32 weeks. If the transabdominal scan is unclear, a transvaginal scan should be offered.

Fetal growth and wellbeing

- Symphysis–fundal height should be measured and recorded at each antenatal appointment from 24 weeks.
- Ultrasound estimation of fetal size for suspected large for gestational age unborn babies is of limited value in a low-risk population.
- Routine Doppler ultrasound should not be used in low-risk pregnancies.
- Fetal presentation should be assessed by abdominal palpation at 36 weeks or later, when presentation is likely to influence the plans for the birth. Routine assessment of presentation by abdominal palpation should not be offered before 36 weeks because it is not always accurate and may be uncomfortable. Suspected fetal malpresentation should be confirmed by an ultrasound assessment.
- Auscultation of the fetal heart may confirm that the fetus is alive but is unlikely to have any predictive value and routine listening is therefore not recommended. However, when requested by the mother, auscultation of the fetal heart may provide reassurance.
- The evidence does not support the routine use of antenatal electronic fetal heart rate monitoring (cardiotocography) for fetal assessment in women with an uncomplicated pregnancy and therefore it should not be offered.
- The evidence does not support the routine use of ultrasound scanning after 24 weeks of gestation and therefore it should not be offered.

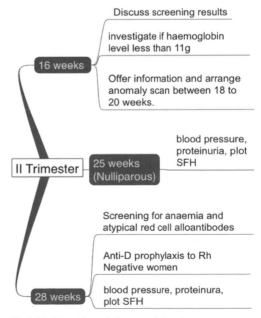

Discuss screening results

16 weeks
- investigate if haemoglobin level less than 11g
- Offer information and arrange anomaly scan between 18 to 20 weeks.

II Trimester — 25 weeks (Nulliparous)
- blood pressure, proteinuria, plot SFH

28 weeks
- Screening for anaemia and atypical red cell alloantibodes
- Anti-D prophylaxis to Rh Negative women
- blood pressure, proteinura, plot SFH

Fig. 5.1.1 Antenatal care in the second trimester.

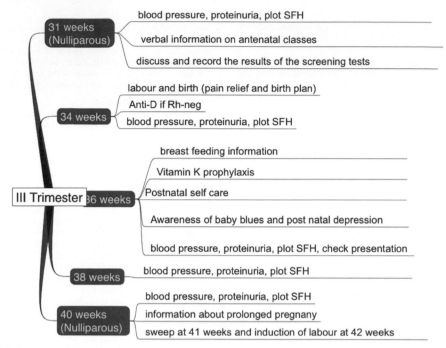

Fig 5.1.2 Antenatal care in the third trimester.

Antenatal appointments

The schedule above, which has been determined by the purpose of each appointment, presents the recommended number of antenatal care appointments for women who are healthy and whose pregnancies remain uncomplicated in the antenatal period: 10 appointments for nulliparous women and seven for parous women. These appointments follow the woman's initial contact with a healthcare professional when she first presents with the pregnancy and from where she is referred into the maternity care system.

The timing of the visits and care at each visit is summarized in Figs 5.1.1 and 5.1.2.

Further reading

NICE Guidance. Antenatal care: routine care for healthy pregnant women. Ref CG62.

Fortner KB (ed.). *The John Hopkins manual of gynecology and obstetrics.* Philadelphia: Wolters Kluwer 2008.

Steven G, Gabbe JRN, Leigh Simpson J (eds). *Obstetrics normal and problem pregnancies.* New York: Churchill Livington 1996.

Booking

Antenatal care begins when the pregnancy is registered with the midwife or GP. The vast majority of the patients would have had an ultrasound scan from the early pregnancy unit before registering with their GP. This is followed by a booking visit with the community midwife and is probably the most important visit in planning care during the pregnancy.

The booking visit is defined as the initial meeting between the pregnant woman and a professional from the maternity services.

The booking appointment or booking visit is the first official check-up in pregnancy. The term booking comes from the days when women literally had to book themselves a hospital bed for labour! It may take place in the woman's home, the GP's surgery or at the hospital antenatal clinic and usually consists of an elaborate interview with the midwife using a computerized booking form.

The aim of the booking visit is
- to introduce a woman and partner to the maternity services
- to assess the physical, social, psychological and cultural needs of the woman and family to plan future care
- to give information that allows the woman to explore the available options for care and make informed choices
- to identify risk factors and deviations from normal.

Timing of the booking visit

The National Institute for Health and Clinical Excellence (NICE) recommends that the booking appointment should take place ideally by 10 weeks of pregnancy so that the mother has the time to arrange any first trimester screening tests. The factors that affect the timing of the visit are mainly the hospital policies and the time of diagnosis of the pregnancy. Studies have shown that ethnic minority women and multigravid women who smoke usually book their pregnancies much later than primigravid Caucasian women.

Management at the booking clinic

At the booking visit a detailed history is taken, risk factors identified and appropriate referrals arranged. The details of the history include previous menstrual history, including contraception, smear tests and obstetric history to identify previous high-risk pregnancies. A detailed medical, family, social and personal history with an aim to enumerate factors that might affect the current pregnancy is taken. The first menstrual period is also confirmed and the estimated date of confinement is also confirmed or amended based on initial dating scans. Part 2 deals with the history and examination of a pregnant woman.

The visit involves examination and screening for disorders such as anaemia, haemoglobinopathies, Rhesus isoimmunization. Rubella status is checked. Screening for infections such as syphilis, hepatitis B and HIV, if recognized and treated early, makes a huge difference to the outcome. This visit also provides an ideal opportunity for the women to discuss any anxieties she may have and to provide information on maternity benefits and statutory rights (Fig. 5.2.1).

Assessment of risk

Structured maternity records with check lists and computerized data collection systems ensure that important questions are asked and risk factors identified.

The aim of risk scoring in pregnancy is to permit the classification of women into different categories for which appropriate management strategies can be implemented. Other benefits include defining populations for epidemiological purposes, allocation of resources and aid in audit and teaching. The main scores are designed to predict those who are likely to have adverse outcomes, such as perinatal death, small for gestational age, preterm labour and delivery, and perinatal asphyxia. Risk scoring tends to give a simplistic and inflexible view with the danger of 'ignoring' low-risk women. Computerized scoring systems are not widely in use to predict the likelihood of an adverse outcome, as their use has not been associated with the reduction in adverse outcomes. They also carry a risk of introducing interventions and treatments that may be of unproven value.

Lifestyle advice

The booking visit gives the opportunity to educate women regarding antenatal care, lifestyle and minor ailments. Information is given on dietary requirements, exercise during pregnancy, parent craft education programmes and antenatal classes. General advice on healthy eating, folic acid and avoidance of food that may cause infections, e.g. uncooked meat and toxoplasmosis, is reiterated.

Smoking and alcohol cessation advice should be offered as appropriate. Identifying domestic violence at this stage may help the health professional to introduce appropriate safety measures to mother and the baby.

Tests performed during the booking visit
Routine tests

Dating and a nuchal scan
A first trimester ultrasound scan, for pregnancy dating and measurement of nuchal translucency is performed between 10 and 14 weeks. With the recent guidelines for antenatal screening, nuchal translucency measurements are combined with serum markers such as human chorionic gonadotrophin (HCG) and pregnancy associated plasma protein-A (PAPP-A) as a screening test for trisomy 21. This combined test increases the sensitivity of Downs's syndrome screening to 80%, retaining the false-positive rate at 5%.

Haematological investigations
A full blood count and haemoglobin in early pregnancy help to identify those with anaemia, exclude haemoglobinopathy, and to compensate them with iron so that they can cope with the physiological dilutional anaemia which occurs in pregnancy. Many women from ethnic minorities have low booking haemoglobin and with increasing gestational age they become profoundly anaemic. Anaemic patients at booking should be investigated with assessment of ferritin, total iron binding capacity and serum B12.

Blood grouping and screening for antibodies at booking identifies women who are rhesus negative and those at risk of Rh isoimmunization. The incidence of Rh immunization has dramatically fallen over the last 30 years since the advent of anti-D. Despite screening for antibodies at 28 and 34 weeks and administration of anti-D prophylactically a small number of Rh-negative women still develop Rh antibodies. Screening for red cell antibodies should be repeated in all pregnant women and in every pregnancy as there may be other clinically significant antibodies as a consequence of previous pregnancy or blood transfusion. Antibody screening is performed to detect the presence of antibodies that may put the baby at risk of haemolytic disease.

Screening for the haemoglobinopathies

Most hospitals perform these tests routinely in all patients. Given the increasing incidence of mixed populations, routine testing for haemoglobinopathies may be justified.

Microbiological investigations

These include serum screening for evidence of immunity to rubella and screening for infections like hepatitis B or HIV. Rubella infection in early pregnancy can have serious consequences to the fetus. In an attempt to reduce the incidence of congenital rubella, vaccination for rubella was introduced. Despite vaccination, the data show that a minority of women will not be immune to rubella. And it is recommended that all women should be tested for rubella in pregnancy, and if negative postnatal vaccination is recommended.

HIV infection in the mother has implications for the mother and the fetus, and hence it is essential to test for HIV infection in pregnancy. Early recognition and treatment reduces the mother to child transmission of the HIV virus quite significantly.

Screening for hepatitis B is aimed to determine if the patient has been infected and if she is a potential risk of contracting infection to her partner or to healthcare professionals. Hepatitis B surface antibody is tested for initially and if positive, core antigen 'e' status is tested to determine the potential infectivity. Combination of active and passive immunization is undertaken in the neonate if the mother is found to be 'e' positive.

Screening for syphilis is performed as routine. Around 250 cases are detected annually in the UK. The rational is that early treatment of the disease can prevent congenital syphilis in neonates.

Screening for urinary tract infection

Urine dipstick is carried out to check for glucose, proteinuria, ketonuria, and nitrites. At the booking visit a urine specimen is sent for culture to detect and treat asymptomatic bacteriuria. Asymptomatic bacteriuria if present can lead to urinary tract infections in 15%. It also increases the risk of preterm labour. The urine dipstick is

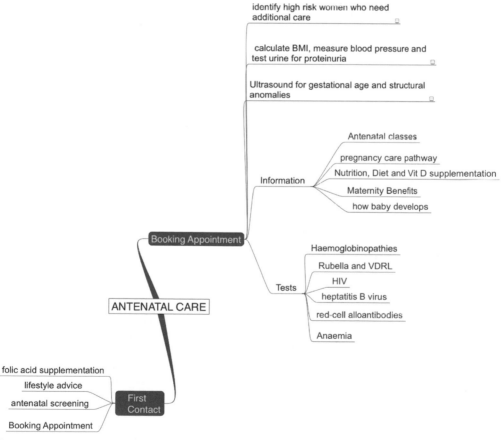

Fig. 5.2.1 Antenatal care in the first trimester in graphic presentation.

tested for glucose and protein, and if positive checking blood sugar and blood pressure and additional tests may be appropriate.

Specific tests

Specific risk-oriented tests may be done. For example, if there is a history of hypertension, a renal function test would be appropriate, and history of diabetes should prompt testing fasting blood sugar and Hb A1C.

Arrangement of appropriate referrals

Based on the history, examination and results of investigations, an individualized care plan needs to be compiled. The vast majority will be low risk and continued midwifery care is appropriate. If a medical disorder is diagnosed, appropriate referral is made to optimize the management plan.

Further reading

Fortner KB (ed.). *The John Hopkins manual of gynecology and obstetrics*, 3 edn. Philadelphia: Wolters Kluwer 2008.

Kupek E, Petrou S, Vause S, Maresh M. Clinical, provider and socio-demographic predictors of late initiation of antenatal care in England and Wales. Br J Obstet Gynaecol 2000;109:265–73.

Robson J, Boomla K, Savage W. Reducing delay in booking for antenatal care. J R Coll Gen Pract 1986;36:274–5.

Stenhouse EJ, Crossley JA, Aitken DA, *et al*. First-trimester combined ultrasound and biochemical screening for Down syndrome in routine clinical practice. Prenat Diagn 2004;24:774–80.

Steven G, Gabbe JRN, Joe Leigh Simpson (eds). *Obstetrics normal and problem pregnancies*, 3rd edn. New York: Churchill Livingston 1996.

Breastfeeding

Exclusive breastfeeding until around 6 months of age, followed by the introduction of solids with continued breastfeeding, is considered to be the optimal nutritional start for the newborn infant. It has important health benefits for both mother and baby. Breastfeeding is often accompanied by challenges, and mothers require considerable help and support from healthcare professionals.

Anatomy of breast
Each breast is divided into 15–20 lobules by fibrous tissue septae that radiate from the centre (Fig. 5.3.1). Each lobe further subdivides into lobules and consists of fibrofatty stroma, alveoli, and ductules draining the alveoli. Each alveolus is lined by columnar epithelium, where milk secretion occurs. A network of myoepithelial cells surrounds the alveoli and the smaller ducts. Contraction of these cells squeezes the alveoli and ejects the milk into the ductules. Each lobe is drained by the lactiferous duct, formed by the union of increasingly larger ductules and ducts. Each lactiferous duct dilates to form ampulla before converging onto the nipple. Milk is stored in the ampulla before release and secreted outside through nipple pores.

Physiology of lactation
For successful breastfeeding to ensue, breasts go through three stages: mammogenesis, lactogenesis, and galactopoiesis.

Mammogenesis
This takes place in two further stages: stage I around puberty and stage II during pregnancy, parturition and lactation. Normal breast tissue contains three types of lobules. Formation of type I lobules begins with puberty. Under the influence of oestrogen and progesterone they sprout new alveolar buds and evolve to more mature type 2 and 3 lobules. Further maturation does not occur until pregnancy. During pregnancy they reach their maximum branching capability and form secretory acini, which are the terminal outgrowths of the ducts. These matured lobules seen in pregnancy and lactation are called type 4 lobules. Early pregnancy is characterized by ductular proliferation and later pregnancy by secretory activity. All these processes continue during lactation, the predominant event being milk production.

Lactogenesis
Lactogenesis takes place in two stages: secretory initiation and secretory activation. Secretory initiation begins during the second half of pregnancy and is mediated by high levels of circulating progesterone. During pregnancy only minimal amounts of milk are formed in the breast, despite high levels of lactogenic hormones, prolactin, and human placental lactogen (HPL).

This is due to the inhibitory effect of oestrogen and progesterone. After delivery there is rapid decline in both these hormones and prolactin begins its milk secretory activity. This stage is known as secretory activation and occurs in women between 3 and 7 days postpartum. Secretory activation is delayed in primipara, after Caesarean and stressful vaginal deliveries, retained placental fragments and diabetes.

Galactopoiesis
This is the process of maintenance of lactation. This is regulated by the interaction of various factors, the most important being emptying of the breast by the infant's suckling. Hormones such as oxytocin, prolactin and feedback inhibitor of lactation (FIL) play their role.

Failure to empty breasts at regular intervals leads to an increase in intramammary pressure. First, this obstructs blood flow and the supply of stimulatory hormones and nutrients to the breast. Second, increased intramammary pressure disrupts the synthesis and secretion of milk components. Third, FIL is synthesized by mammary epithelial cells in response to increased intramammary pressure. This downregulates prolactin receptors and decreases milk supply. Milk production is also dependent on infant demand.

The suckling of the baby sends afferent impulses through the nerve endings in the nipple areola complex to the pituitary gland, resulting in increased secretion of prolactin and oxytocin. Prolactin acts on the alveoli and increases the production of milk proteins. This is known as the *suckling reflex*. Oxytocin acts on the myoepithelial cells aiding expulsion of milk into the ducts from the alveolar lumen and out through the nipple. At the same time the ducts expand rapidly to facilitate milk flow. This is termed the *milk ejection reflex* and is recognized by the mothers as the milk let down. The milk ejection reflex is inhibited by maternal anxiety.

Maternal benefits of breastfeeding
Breastfeeding provides both short and long-term benefits to the mother. Oxytocin released as a result of suckling accelerates uterine involution. In a randomized controlled trial, mothers who initiated frequent feedings immediately after delivery of the placenta experienced less blood loss than those who initiated later. Weight loss after pregnancy is enhanced by prolonged breastfeeding. Prolonged breastfeeding confers contraceptive benefits. The conception risk during lactational amenorrhoea is only 1–2% if three criteria apply: (1) amenorrhoea, (2) full lactation, (3) less than 6 months postpartum. It has been suggested that breastfeeding enhances maternal–infant bonding. Long-term benefits of breastfeeding include a decreased risk of developing breast cancer and ovarian cancer. It remains unclear whether lactation reduces the risk of osteoporosis, and further studies are required.

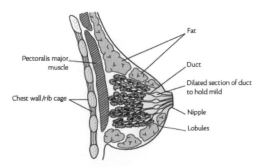

Labels: Fat; Pectoralis major muscle; Duct; Dilated section of duct to hold mild; Chest wall/rib cage; Nipple; Lobules

Fig. 5.3.1 Structure of the breast. Reproduced from *Breast cancer, the facts*, Saunders and Jassal, 2009, with permission from Oxford University Press.

Infant benefits of breastfeeding

Human milk is the ideal nutrient for term infants as it confers numerous benefits with respect to nutrition, gastrointestinal function and protection against illnesses.

Breast milk is secreted at body temperature. It generally does not need storage and is produced as and when the baby requires it. This obviates the inconveniences of warming and cooling formula, storage of milk and sterilization of bottles. Breastfeeding reduces the risk of accidental scalding or burns. Suckling helps the development of muscular coordination of the jaw and teeth of infant.

Breast milk is produced in the correct amount and is therefore not wasted. It comprises fore milk and hind milk, which vary in their fat content. The foremilk has low fat content and does not satiate baby till adequate intake is made. Hind milk occurs after the initial release of milk and contains higher levels of fat, and it is necessary for weight gain. Hind milk also retards gastric motility and aids absorption of the majority of milk lactose. Formula milk has excesses or deficiencies in substances and is prone to accidental contamination.

Breastfeeding during the first 13 weeks of life confers protection against gastrointestinal illnesses that persists beyond the period of breastfeeding itself. The risk of hospitalization for diarrhoea is reduced in infants exclusively breastfed compared with infants who never breastfed. Breastfed infants have reduced incidence of respiratory illnesses, urinary tract infections, and otitis media.

Neonatal necrotizing enterocolitis (NEC) is a major cause of morbidity in preterm infants. Human milk is known to decrease colonization of the bowel by pathogenic bacteria, promotes growth of non-pathogenic flora and maturation of the intestinal barrier. In addition it contains anti-inflammatory agents such as interleukin-10 and immunoglobulins (Ig) such as IgG and IgA. As a result it reduces inflammation-mediated ischaemic bowel injury leading to NEC.

Breastfed infants have enhanced host defence mechanisms. This is because maternal antibodies are transferred through breast milk. Enteromammary and bronchomammary immune systems have a major role to play in the protective nature of breast milk. When the mother is exposed to pathogens via her respiratory or gastrointestinal tract, protective antibodies are synthesized in the breast and secreted in the milk. Thus the infant receives passive immunity to the continuing exposure of antigens.

In addition milk proteins like lactoferrin and lysozyme have antimicrobial activity. Human milk also contains neutrophils, lymphocytes, and macrophages, which contribute to cell-mediated immunity.

Breastfeeding provides long-term benefits to infants. Meta-analysis has shown a 32% reduction in obesity in patients who were breastfed for more than 9 months. Post-breastfeeding protection appears to increase with the duration of breastfeeding. Breast-fed compared with formula-fed infants appear to have a decreased risk of developing Type 1 and Type II diabetes mellitus. A systematic review has shown that breastfeeding is associated with increased mean total cholesterol and low-density lipoprotein levels in infancy but lower levels in adulthood/adult life. This along with reduction of obesity and diabetes may have long-term benefits for cardiovascular health. Breast milk being immunologically active is thought to reduce the incidence of allergic diseases such as atopic dermatitis, allergic rhinitis, and asthma. However, most of these studies are observational and further data are required.

Combining data from the UK Childhood Cancer Study (UKCCS) with results from other published studies showed a small reduction in the odds ratios for leukaemia, Hodgkin's disease, non-haematological cancers, and all childhood cancers combined, associated with ever having been breastfed. Several studies have suggested that breastfeeding improves cognitive development in childhood and adolescence.

Economic benefits of breastfeeding

There are clear economic advantages to family and society as a whole. There is reduction in expenditure on formula as well as healthcare expenses. The cost savings from long-term benefits of breastfeeding such as reducing the incidence of chronic illnesses in children and adults and reduction in cancers in both mothers and children are substantial.

Initiation and maintenance of breastfeeding

Breastfeeding should be started within the first hour after delivery. Skin-to-skin contact immediately after delivery helps to start breastfeeding off. Subsequent feedings should be on demand. Feeding on demand means that feedings are initiated in response to behavioural changes that indicate hunger (feeding cues). Examples of feeding cues are movement of the hands towards mouth, sucking on fists and fingers, fussiness, agitation and crying. 'Rooming in' means the baby stays with mother all the time. This increases the mother's ability to understand and respond to feeding cues. Feeding the infant in response to early cues is optimal. Voluntary release of the nipple, relaxation of facial muscles and falling asleep signal satiety.

The average frequency of breastfeeding is 8–12 times per day in the first 1–2 weeks postpartum, which reduces to 7–9 times per day by 4 weeks. During the first postpartum week the duration between feeds should not be more than 4 hours. The average duration of feed on each breast is 10–15 minutes soon after birth and is dependent on efficiency of milk transfer. As efficiency improves, duration falls to 8–10 minutes by 4 weeks.

Breastfeeding mothers should have a balanced diet which is high in calories, protein, vitamins and minerals. There is an excess demand of at least 700 calories and 20 g of protein per day compared with the non-pregnant state. Daily requirements of calcium are increased by three times and vitamin A by one and a half times that of the non-pregnant state. An adequate fluid intake is important for successful breastfeeding.

Latch-on

The baby's gums should completely bypass the nipple and cover approximately 2.5 cm of the areola behind the nipple and this should form a tight seal (Fig. 5.3.2). The appearance of an adequate latch-on includes

- an angle of approximately 120 between the top and bottom lip
- the lower lip (and, to a lesser extent, the upper lip) turned outward against the breast
- the chin and nose in close proximity to the breast
- full cheeks
- the tongue extends over the lower dental ridge and is in visible contact with the breast if the lower lip is pulled away (Hopkinson and Schanler 'Breast in the perinatal period').

Colostrum is the first stage of breast milk that occurs during pregnancy and lasts for several days after the birth

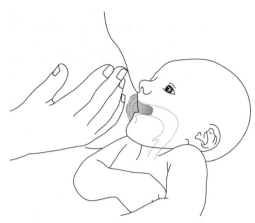

Fig. 5.3.2 Correct 'latch-on'.

of the baby. It is either yellowish or creamy in colour. It is of higher density and lower volume than the milk that is produced later in breastfeeding. Colostrum is high in protein, fat-soluble vitamins, minerals and immunoglobulins. Colostrum may be scanty in amount but is very important for passive immunity. A good amount of milk production occurs by 3–5 days. Reliable indicators of sufficient intake are weight gain, clearance of meconium and increasing urine output. Normal infants lose about 5–7% of birthweight by 5 days of age. They regain their birthweight by 1–2 weeks. Infants gain 15–40 g per day, once breastfeeding is established. Meconium is cleared by the third day and the majority of infants have four or more stools and at least six wet diapers per day. Any deviation from this should be brought to the attention of a healthcare professional.

Baby-friendly hospital

The Baby-Friendly Hospital Initiative was launched by the World Health Organization (WHO) and the United Nations Children's Fund in 1991 to improve breastfeeding rates. Hospitals can be designated baby-friendly if they comply with the following 10 steps:

- Have a written policy on breastfeeding that is communicated routinely to all staff.
- Train all healthcare staff in the skills needed to implement the policy.
- Inform all pregnant women of the benefits and management of breastfeeding.
- Help mothers start breastfeeding within 1 hour after birth.
- Show mothers how to breastfeed and maintain lactation, even if they are separated from their infants.
- Give newborns only breast milk, unless other feedings are medically indicated. Hospitals must pay a fair market price for formula and feeding supplies.
- Allow mothers and infants to remain together at all times.
- Encourage breastfeeding on demand.
- Provide no pacifiers or artificial teats to nursing infants.
- Foster the establishment of breastfeeding support groups and refer mothers to them.

A randomized controlled trial has shown that antenatal breastfeeding education and postnatal lactation support, as single interventions based in hospital, both significantly improve rates of exclusive breastfeeding up to 6 months after delivery. Postnatal support was marginally more effective than antenatal education. Hence ongoing postpartum support for patients in the form of house visits, telephone contacts with breastfeeding counsellors and peer support groups is very important in the maintenance of breastfeeding. Inadvertent promotion of artificial formula appears to reduce the number of women exclusively breastfeeding at all times.

Problems encountered during breastfeeding

Engorgement

Breast engorgement is the painful overfilling of the breasts with milk. This is usually caused by an imbalance between milk supply and infant demand. National surveys have shown that painful breasts are the second most common reason for giving up breastfeeding in the first 2 weeks after birth in the UK. One factor contributing to such pain can be breast engorgement. Early engorgement coincides with Stage II lactogenesis and typically occurs 24–72 hours postpartum. In the majority of cases, once feeding is established this resolves spontaneously. Poor latch-on interferes with the infant's ability to empty the breast and the consequent engorgement makes further latch-on difficult. Late engorgement occurs when there is inadequate emptying of the breasts due to disruption of the normal routine of breastfeeding for various reasons and the consequent accumulation of milk.

Frequent emptying of breasts is critical to prevent and treat engorgement. It is important to ensure satisfactory latch-on from the start. Breastfeeding should not be discontinued. Manual expression or breast pumps can be used if the baby is unwilling to nurse. A Cochrane database systematic review has shown that the anti-inflammatory agent serrapeptase and hand massage helps to relieve symptoms. Icepacks, cool compresses and simple analgesics are recommended for pain relief.

Galactocoeles/plugged ducts (non-infective mastitis)

A plugged duct is a sore, tender lump or knotty area in the breast. It occurs when a milk duct is not draining well and inflammation builds up. It is distinguished from mastitis by the absence of signs of systemic infection. Predisposing factors are mismatch between demand and supply and poor latching. Unrelieved plugged ducts may lead to galactocoeles, which are milk retention cysts. They are initially filled with milk and later replaced by thick, creamy or oily material. Galactocoeles can be visualized on ultrasound.

Management includes frequent emptying of breasts. Ensure that baby is properly latched on and well positioned in a way that the affected milk ducts are thoroughly drained with each feeding. Nurse as often as possible on the affected side to help drain the clogged duct. Gently massaging the lumpy area in a circular motion, starting behind the lump and working towards the nipple, can help loosen the plug. Apply warm compresses and/or stand in the shower with the spray directly on the sore area. This helps to unclog the duct. If the pain of a plugged duct or the lump does not go away within 2–3 days, appropriate advice should be sought. Galactocoeles that do not resolve are treated with needle aspiration.

Mastitis and breast abscess

Mastitis is an infection of the breast caused by bacteria. *Staphylococcus aureus*, streptococci and *Escherichia coli* are the common aetiological agents. Most studies agree that around 10% of all breastfeeding mothers are affected by mastitis. Left untreated, non-infectious mastitis can progress to infectious mastitis. This may be due to bacteria infecting the milk that remains in the breast tissue. Traumatized nipples are at risk of superficial infection that may lead to mastitis. Mastitis usually affects only one breast, causing it to become painful, red and swollen. It is associated with fever >38°C, myalgia, chills, malaise and flue-like symptoms.

Infectious mastitis requires prompt treatment to prevent more serious complications such as breast abscess. Antibiotic treatment should be started with flucloxacillin for 10–14 days. Alternatives such as cephalexin and amoxicillin are used if no response is seen in 24–48 hours. Breastfeeding should not be stopped and breasts should be emptied either manually or by pumps if the infant cannot relieve breast fullness. Supportive measures like bed rest and anti-inflammatory agents are helpful. Recurrent mastitis can result from inappropriate or incomplete antibiotic therapy or failure to resolve underlying problems in lactation management.

Breast abscess develops in 5–11% of women with mastitis and management is antibiotic therapy and drainage.

Nipple-related problems

Sore nipples are probably the most common difficulty mothers have when breastfeeding. Sore nipples can be due to nipple sensitivity, which is a normal phenomenon, or secondary to trauma. Nipple sensitivity peaks on approximately the fourth postpartum day and resolves by the seventh postpartum day. It typically subsides 30–60 seconds after suckling begins. It is due to enhanced lactational hormones like prolactin and oxytocin.

The commonest cause of trauma to nipples is poor latch-on techniques and ineffective sucking. The pain due to trauma in contrast to normal sensitivity persists throughout the nursing episode. Signs of poor latch-on include:

- contact between the upper and lower lip at the corners of the mouth;
- sunken checks;
- clicking sounds that correspond to breaking suction;
- tongue not visible below the nipple when the lower lip is pulled down;
- creased nipple following nursing (Hopkinson and Schanler 'Breast in the perinatal period').

Persistent painful latch-on should be brought to the attention of a lactation consultant. Traumatized nipples are at risk of infection predominantly by candida and staphylococci.

Sore nipples should be cleansed with clean water or saline and left to air dry after every nursing. Changing positions each time of nursing helps to avoid pressure on the same part of the nipple. Human milk has natural healing properties and emollients, and hence application of breast milk after feeding helps. Wearing a nipple shield during nursing will not relieve sore nipples. They actually can prolong soreness by making it hard for the baby to learn to nurse without the shield. Tight bras or clothes that are too tight and put pressure on the nipples should be avoided. Change Nursing pads should be changed often to avoid trapping in moisture. Application of emollients like lanolin helps to maintain moisture and facilitate healing.

A combination of antibiotic (Muciprocin), antifungal (Miconazole) and a steroid is recommended if initial steps fail.

Bloody nipple discharge is seen in some women during the first few days postpartum. This is due to vascularization of the ducts during pregnancy and resolves spontaneously. Bloody milk during lactation is often detected when the infant's stool is mixed with blood. The source of bleeding may be cracked nipples. A rare cause is intraductal papilloma and in the absence of an obvious source of bleeding this should be suspected and milk sent for cytological analysis.

Contraindications to breast feeding

Few contraindications to breastfeeding exist.

HIV and breastfeeding

The major mode of acquisition of HIV in children worldwide is through mother-to-child transmission. This happens antenatally, intrapartum and postpartum through breastfeeding. Breastfeeding alone accounts for 30–50% of mother-to-child transmission and doubles the rate of transmission. In developed countries breastfeeding is not advisable in women with HIV as the benefits of not breastfeeding outweigh the risks. The combination of antiretroviral therapy, elective Caesarean delivery, and avoidance of breastfeeding has reduced perinatal transmission to less than 2% in developed countries.

In the developing world, eliminating the risk of HIV transmission by stopping breastfeeding exposes children to different risks: increased exposure to other life-threatening infections, especially in the first year of life and malnutrition if replacement feeding is inadequate. In addition, formula may not be easily available, affordable or culturally acceptable. To date there are no proven strategies known to reduce the risk of HIV transmission during breastfeeding for those HIV-infected women who opt to breastfeed in developing countries. Breastfeeding with extended prophylaxis with antiretrovirals and vaccination of infants are currently the subject of research. The WHO recommends that women be counselled about the risk of HIV transmission through breastfeeding. When replacement feeding is affordable, feasible, acceptable, sustainable and safe, avoidance of all breastfeeding by HIV-infected mothers is recommended. When replacement feeding is not possible, then exclusive breastfeeding is recommended during the first months of life, with the time of stopping being determined by individual circumstances.

Inborn errors of metabolism

Galactosaemia is an absolute contraindication for breastfeeding as infants are unable to metabolize galactose, a component of breast milk. As a result galactose accumulates in the blood with adverse consequences. Breastfeeding is not contraindicated with other inborn errors of metabolism such as phenylketonuria. Babies suffering from phenylketonuria may be breastfed while their phenylalanine levels are monitored.

Drug abuse and other medications

Maternal drug abuse is a contraindication to breastfeeding. In the mother with an ongoing illicit drug abuse problem, drugs are secreted in breast milk. Hence the risks posed to the infant are substantial and outweigh the benefits of breastfeeding in most cases.

Most therapeutic drugs are compatible with breastfeeding. Administration of some drugs harms the infant whereas others have little effect. Toxicity to the infant can occur if the drug enters the milk in pharmacologically significant quantities. Some drugs like bromocriptine inhibit lactation. As a general rule anticancer drugs, certain anticonvulsants, ergot alkaloids, amiodarone, iodides and radiopharmaceuticals are avoided. Clinicians should consult reliable sources before prescribing drugs during breastfeeding.

In summary, exclusive breastfeeding is the ideal form of feeding infants for the first 6 months after birth as it confers invaluable benefits to mother and baby. It meets all the nutritional requirements for the infants in the first 6 months of life. The WHO advises that partial breastfeeding to be continued for at least 1 year or up to 2 years. Parental education and support is vital in initiation and maintenance of breastfeeding. It is not without its own challenges and healthcare professionals dealing with breastfeeding women should have the necessary knowledge and skills to advise and help mothers overcome these challenges. There are few contraindications to breastfeeding.

Further reading

Breastfeeding and childhood cancer. Br J Cancer 2001;85:1685–94.

Harder T, Bergmann R, Kallischnigg G, Plagemann A. Duration of breastfeeding and risk of overweight: a meta-analysis. Am J Epidemiol 2005;162:397–403.

Hopkinson J, Schanler RJ. Breastfeeding in the perinatal period. Uptodate version 16.2: www.uptodate.com

Hopkinson J, Schanler RJ. Common problems of breastfeeding in the postpartum period. Uptodate version 16.2.

Hopkinson J, Schanler RJ. Physiology of lactation. Uptodate version 16.2.

Howard C, Howard F, Lawrence R, et al. Office prenatal formula advertising and its effect on breastfeeding patterns. Obstet Gynecol 2000;95:296–303.

Howie PW, Forsyth JS, Ogston SA, et al. Protective effect of breastfeeding against infection. BMJ 1990;300:11–15.

Millennium Cohort Study. Paediatrics 2007;119:e837–42.

Owen CG, Martin RM, Whincup PH, et al. Does breastfeeding influence risk of type 2 diabetes in later life? A quantitative analysis of published evidence. Am J Clin Nutr 2006;84:1043–54.

Owen CG, Whincup PH, Odoki, K, et al. Infant feeding and blood cholesterol: a study in adolescents and a systematic review. Paediatrics 2002;110:597–608.

Quigley MA, Kelly YJ, Sacker A. Breastfeeding and hospitalization for diarrhoeal and respiratory infection in the United Kingdom.

Schanler RJ. Infant benefits of breastfeeding. Uptodate version 16.2.

Schanler RJ. Maternal and economic benefits of breastfeeding. Uptodate version 16.2.

Sobhy SI, Mohame NA. The effect of early initiation of breastfeeding on the amount of vaginal loss during the fourth stage of labour. J Egypt Public Health Assoc 2004;79:1–12.

Su LL, Chong YS, Chan YH, et al. Antenatal education and postnatal support strategies for improving rates of exclusive breastfeeding: randomised controlled trial. BMJ 2007;335:596.

Ten steps to successful breastfeeding. www.unicef.org/newsline/tenstps.htm

Dating in pregnancy

Estimation of gestational age and the expected date of delivery are valuable to the expecting couple to arrange for the arrival, but also are important in the diagnosis of intrauterine growth restriction of the fetus and for management of high-risk pregnancy.

Clinical dating

Estimation of gestational age by last menstrual period

Gestational age (GA) is about 280 days calculated from the first day of the last normal menstrual period (LMP). If the periods are regular, common practice is to calculate the expected date of delivery by Naegele's formula. Without a history of regular, predictable, cyclic, spontaneous menses that suggest ovulatory cycles, accurate dating of pregnancy by history and physical examination is difficult. Unfortunately 30% of patients do not fulfil the criteria, making estimation of expected date of delivery (EDD) based on LMP unreliable[1]. If the interval of cycles is longer, the number of extra days is added to the EDD, and if shorter, the days are subtracted from the EDD. One-quarter of patients either don't remember LMP or give it inaccurately. The last menstrual period is even more accurate if conception occurs during lactation amenorrhoea or immediately after stopping oral contraceptive pills. Estimation of EDD from last menstrual period becomes reliable if the patient remembers the date of fruitful coitus.

Estimation of GA by quickening

A crude estimate of the EDD can be derived if the woman remembers the exact date of quickening. Quickening appears in a multigravida at 16 weeks and in a primigravida at 18 weeks. Adding 24 weeks in a multigravida and 22 weeks in a primigravida from the date of quickening can estimate EDD. The reliability of EDD estimated in this way is highly inaccurate especially in primigravid mothers, as quickening is very subjective and varies with individual perception of fetal movements.

Estimation of GA by objective signs

Pelvic examination: the size of the uterus gives a rough guidance to the gestational age. At 12 weeks the uterus becomes an abdominal organ and at 24 weeks reaches the umbilicus. At 36 weeks the uterus reaches the xiphisternum and falls forwards because of lightening. Maternal obesity, observer experience, position of the uterus, amount of amniotic fluid, multiple gestation, uterine myomatosis and fetal growth disorders are variables that make assessment of gestation by uterine size unreliable.

In some patients EDD can be established by the date of the first positive pregnancy tests. It could be reliable if the pregnancy test was carried out on the fifth week of amenorrhoea. Clinical dating is inaccurate and if feasible all women should have an ultrasound in the first trimester to confirm dating.

Ultrasound estimation of GA

Sonographic measurements of fetal ultrasound parameters are the basis for accurate determination of gestational age and detection of fetal growth abnormalities. Selection of the most useful single biometric parameter depends on the timing and purpose of measurement and is influenced by specific limitations (Degani 2001).

First trimester

In the early first trimester, when no structures are visible within the gestational sac, GA may be estimated from the sac diameter. A common method is to measure the mean sac diameter (MSD) by calculating the mean of the three sac diameters. An alternative simpler method is to add 30 to the sac size in millimetres, to give GA in days. By the time the embryo becomes visible on ultrasound the sac diameter is no longer accurate in estimating gestational age. GA in the first trimester is usually calculated from fetal crown–rump length (CRL) (Fig. 5.4.1). This is the longest demonstrable length of the embryo or fetus, excluding the limbs and the yolk sac. CRL measurement is used in embryos from 20 to 60 mm as the embryo loses the extreme flexion at the neck so that its greatest length becomes the CRL measurements (Goldstein 1991). The correlation between CRL and GA is excellent until approximately 12 weeks' amenorrhea. The GA estimate has a 95% confidence interval of ±2–3 days before 11 weeks and 2–5 after 11 weeks.

Second trimester

Fetal biometry in the second trimester can yield acceptably accurate estimates of GA from 12 to approximately 22 weeks of amenorrhea. The best parameters are the biparietal diameter (BPD) and the head circumference (HC), which are virtually linearly related to GA. BPD measurements in the second trimester predict dates within a margin of ±7–11 days. BPD measurements before 20 weeks estimate GA by ±7 days. In cases where BPD may be altered because of head compression, head circumference has the advantage of being shape independent and can be used effectively as an alternative means of establishing gestational age. The femur length (FL) can also be used and is nearly as accurate as head measurements. The range of dates varies more with FL as gestation advances than with BPD. Racial differences in FL are significant, but differences in HC are not. GA estimates by the BPD or HC have a 95% confidence interval of ±8 days.

Third trimester

Fetal biometry in the third trimester is subject to much greater individual size variations than in the second trimester. Its accuracy for GA assignment is reduced considerably, and estimates may have confidence intervals of ±3 weeks. There is significant improvement in ultrasound estimation of EDD when two or more parameters were used, however the approach should be individualized excluding parameters that are suspected to be abnormal[4].

When CRL measurement is not available, gestational age should not be changed unless the discrepancy between menstrual and second trimester ultrasound dating is 9 days or more, as this policy would result in the smallest proportion of incorrect adjustments. In the majority of cases, the gestational age of the fetus and the expected date of delivery will be established with a single ultrasound examination between 18 and 24 weeks if the results agree with clinical information. If there is more than a 1-week discrepancy between the clinical dating and the results of the ultrasound examination the ultrasound should be repeated 4 weeks later. If the second set of ultrasound measurements agrees with the first examination, the gestational age and the EDD become clearly established. If the second set of measurements deviate more than 1 week from the first set, abnormality in fetal growth should be suspected and the EDD determined by the first ultrasound examination should be used.

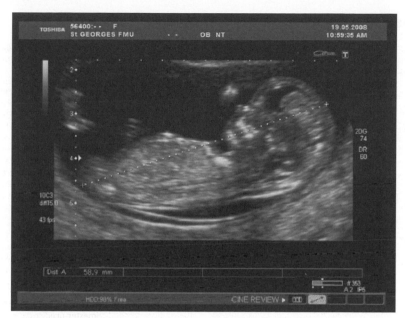

Fig. 5.4.1 Measurement of crown rump length for dating pregnancy. Reproduced from *The Oxford handbook of obstetrics and gynaecology*, Colins, Arulkumaran, Hayes, Jackson, and Impey, 2008, with permission from Oxford University Press.

Reliability of EDD

Good reliability
- Based on CRL in the first trimester is the most accurate.
- Women with adequate clinical information plus ultrasound examination between 16 and 24 weeks, indicating that the fetal measurements are in agreement with the clinical estimation of gestation.
- Women with inadequate or incomplete clinical information, but two ultrasound examinations between 16 and 24 weeks show linear fetal growth with the expected date of confinement.

Acceptable reliability
- Women who provide adequate clinical information and one confirming ultrasound examination obtained after 24 weeks of gestation.
- Women with inadequate or incomplete clinical information but two or more ultrasound examinations show adequate growth and similar expected date of confinement.

Poor reliability
Based on clinical history with none of those measurements listed above (Arias 1988).

Further reading

Cunningham G (ed.). *Williams obstetrics*, 22nd edn. New York: McGraw-Hill 2005.

Arias F. Practical guide to high-risk pregnancy and delivery, 2nd edn. Bangalore: Harcourt Brace and Company Asia 1988.

Degani S. Fetal biometry: clinical, pathological, and technical considerations. Obstet Gynecol Surv 2001;56:159–67.

Deter RL, Rossavik IK, Cortissoz C, et al. Longitudinal studies of thigh circumference growth in normal fetuses. J Clin Ultrasound 1987;15:388–93.

Goldstein SR. Embryonic ultrasonographic measurements: crown-rump length revisited. Am J Obstet Gynecol. 1991;165:497–501.

Diagnosis of pregnancy

The diagnosis of pregnancy usually begins when a woman presents with symptoms, and possibly a positive home urine pregnancy test. Most women receive confirmatory testing for human chorionic gonadotrophin (hCG) in urine or blood. There may be presumptive or diagnostic findings of pregnancy on examination. Ultrasound is often used, particularly in those cases in which there is a question about pregnancy viability or location.

Signs and symptoms
First trimester
Cessation of menstruation
Cessation of menstruation in a healthy reproductive age woman who has been experiencing normal, regular cycles before is suggestive of pregnancy. There may be a variation in the length of the follicular phase and thus date of menstruation among women. Hence the probability of pregnancy increases 10 days after the missed period.

Uterine cyclical bleeding suggestive of menstruation may occur after conception. Such bleeding episodes can occur up to 12 weeks and usually correspond with the date of the expected period. This occurs until the decidual space is obliterated by the fusion of decidua vera with decidua capsularis and is known as the placental sign. Bleeding can also occur as a consequence of blastocyst implantation.

Morning sickness
Morning sickness occurs in 50% of women and is more common in first pregnancy. It appears following a missed period and persists until 16 weeks.

Frequency of micturition
Frequency of micturition is common between 8 and 12 weeks and is due to the pressure of the enlarging uterus on the bladder and congestion of the bladder mucosa.

Breast discomfort
Breast discomfort is evident as early as 6–8 weeks and more pronounced in primigravidae.

Fatigue
Fatigue is common in early pregnancy and usually less marked by 14 weeks.

Objective signs of pregnancy
Breast changes
The anatomical changes in the breasts that accompany pregnancy are quite characteristic during the first pregnancy. These are less obvious in multiparas, whose breasts may secrete a small amount of colostrum for months after childbirth. There is vascular engorgement evidenced by the delicate veins visible under the skin. The nipple and the areola become more pigmented and Montgomery's tubercles are prominent.

Skin changes
Increased pigmentation and changes in appearance of abdominal striae are common to, but not diagnostic of, pregnancy. They may be absent during pregnancy and may be seen in women taking oestrogen–progestin contraceptives.

Discolouration of the vagina
During pregnancy, the vaginal mucosa usually appears dark-bluish or purplish-red and congested, known as the Chadwick sign. There are increased pulsations felt though the lateral fornices from 8 weeks, known as Osiander's sign.

Changes in cervical mucus
The level of sodium chloride in vaginal secretions in the presence of oestrogen causes fern-like patterns when dried on a slide. After approximately the twenty-first day in the presence of progesterone gives a beaded or cellular appearance. This beaded pattern is usually encountered during pregnancy. This concentration, and in turn the presence or absence of the fern pattern, is determined by the cervical glandular response to hormonal action. Thus, if copious thin mucus is present and if a fern pattern develops on drying, early pregnancy is unlikely.

Changes in the cervix
The cervix becomes soft as early as 6 weeks and is called 'Goodell's sign'. The softening is pronounced surrounding the external os, and on speculum examination the cervix has a bluish discoloration due to an increase in vascularity.

Changes in the uterus during pregnancy
During the first few weeks of pregnancy the uterus enlarges, mainly in the anteroposterior diameter. By 12 weeks, the body of the uterus is almost globular, and an average uterine diameter of 8 cm is attained. If there is a lateral implantation the uterus will be asymmetrically enlarged, known as Piskacek's sign. At about 6–8 weeks' menstrual age, on bimanual examination a firm cervix is felt, which contrasts with the softer body of the uterus. Because of the soft body of the uterus, on bimanual examination the abdominal and vaginal fingers seem to appose below the body of the uterus (Hegar's sign). In inexperienced hands the soft uterus may be mistaken for an adnexal mass.

Changes in the cervix
The cervix undergoes increased softening as pregnancy advances. In primigravidas, the consistency of the cervical tissue that surrounds the external os is more similar to that of the lips of the mouth than to that of nasal cartilage, characteristic of the non-pregnant cervix. Other conditions, such as oestrogen–progestin contraceptives, may cause cervical softening. As pregnancy progresses, the cervical canal may become sufficiently patulous to admit the fingertip.

Investigations
Hormonal tests of pregnancy
Presence of hCG in maternal plasma and its excretion in urine provides the basis for the endocrine test for pregnancy. hCG is produced by the syncitiotrophoblast and is a heterodimer, with the two units designated alpha and beta. Trophoblast cells produce hCG and increase exponentially from the day of implantation. The peak of hCG is at 60–70 days and the nadir is at approximately 14–16 weeks.

Immunoassay
Antibodies are developed with high specificity for the β-subunit of hCG. This specificity is the basis for detection of hCG in urine or blood. One commonly employed technique for detection and quantification of hCG is the sandwich-type immunoassay. This test uses a monoclonal antibody against the β-subunit, which is bound to a solid-phase support. The bound antibody is then exposed to

hCG in the serum or urine specimen. A second antibody is then added to 'sandwich' the bound hCG. In some assays, the second antibody is linked to an enzyme, such as alkaline phosphatase. When the test sample with hCG is added the second antibody is unbound exposing the enzyme and bringing a colour change that is proportional to the amount of the hCG present in the sample. The sensitivity for the laboratory detection of hCG in serum is as low as 1.0 mIU/mL using this technique. A false-positive hCG test occurs in women having circulating factors in their serum that may interact with the hCG antibody. The most common are heterophilic antibodies, which are human antibodies directed against animal-derived antigens used in immunoassays.

Home pregnancy tests
The immunometric/immunochromatographic method is used to detect hCG in urine. It is a rapid test and takes 2–5 minutes. Sensitivity ranges from 10 to 50 mIU/mL.

Quantitative laboratory test kits
Radioimmunoassay can be used to detect the hCG β-subunit 7–10 days after conception, even before the period is missed. Specific assays for the β-subunit are less likely to give false positives due to the binding of the β-subunit of LH.

Ultrasound
The use of transvaginal sonography has revolutionized imaging of early pregnancy and its growth and development. A gestational sac may be demonstrated by abdominal sonography after only 4–5 weeks' menstrual age. By 35 days, all normal sacs should be visible, and after 6 weeks or when the crown–rump length (CRL) is 5 mm, a heartbeat should be detectable. Up to 12 weeks, the CRL is predictive of gestational age within 4 days.

Second trimester

Perception of fetal movements or quickening
Primigravid women start feeling fetal movements between 20 and 22 weeks and multigravid women 2 weeks earlier.

Objective signs
A linear pigmented area stretching from the umbilicus to the symphysis pubis known as linea nigra may be seen. Pink and white striae may be visible to varying degrees.

Fundal height
The uterus progressively increases in size. The duration of pregnancy can be roughly estimated based on the height of the uterus in relation to different levels on the abdomen. The fundus reaches the level of the umbilicus at about 22 weeks and below the xiphisternum at 36 weeks.

Braxton–Hicks contractions
During pregnancy the uterus undergoes palpable but painless contractions at irregular intervals from the early stages of gestation. These contractions are referred to as Braxton–Hicks contractions. Close to term these contractions become more frequent, with the increase in intensity causing discomfort.

Table 5.5.1 Differential diagnosis of pregnancy

Distended urinary bladder	Associated with pain and emptying the bladder solves the confusion
Leiomyoma of uterus	Absence of early symptoms and signs of pregnancy and a negative pregnancy test
Cystic ovarian tumour	Amenorrhea is usually absent and there are no other objective signs of pregnancy
Pseudocyesis	Long history of subfertility or in women approaching menopause where menstruation becomes scanty or absent. Bimanual examination and ultrasound aid in the diagnosis

Palpation of fetal parts
Fetal parts can be distinctly palpated as early as 22–24 weeks of gestation.

Fetal heart sounds
The fetal heartbeat can be detected by auscultation with a standard non-amplified stethoscope by a mean of 17 weeks, and by 19 weeks in nearly all pregnancies in non-obese women. Because the fetus moves freely in amnionic fluid, the site on the maternal abdomen where fetal heart sounds can be heard best will vary. Instruments incorporating Doppler ultrasound are often used to easily detect fetal heart action.

Ultrasound
Ultrasound at this gestation allows prediction of gestational age with an accuracy of 2 weeks and rules out major structural anomalies. It can also be used for placental localization.

Third trimester
Distension of the abdomen, more frequent and more pronounced fetal movements, return of frequency of micturition and lightening (falling forward of the uterus with the head sinking into the pelvis resulting in the relief of pressure exerted by the gravid uterus) are some of the subjective signs of pregnancy (Table 5.5.1).

Clear palpation of fetal parts and fetal movements are objective diagnostic signs of pregnancy in the last trimester.

Ultrasound can be used to confirm the diagnosis and also to rule out multiple pregnancies.

Further reading
Arulkumaran S (ed.). *Essentials of obstetrics.* New Delhi: Jaypee Publishers 2004.

Cunningham G (ed.). *Williams obstetrics.* 22nd edn. New York: McGraw-Hill 2005.

Minor symptoms of pregnancy

Pregnancy is associated with considerable anatomical, physiological, biochemical, and immunological changes. These are adaptations for maintenance of pregnancy and preparation for delivery. However, these adaptations can give rise to minor symptoms of pregnancy. These symptoms may be trivial in some women but can cause considerable discomfort and distress in others. The adaptations of normal pregnancy can be misinterpreted as pathological and it can also unmask or worsen pre-existing disease. Hence our duty as healthcare professionals is to distinguish physiological from pathological and offer advice and reassurance.

Nausea and vomiting

These are the most common symptoms of the first trimester. It occurs in 50–75% of women and is erroneously called morning sickness. The symptoms can occur anytime throughout the day. It is commonly seen in primigravidas, with a 25% recurrence rate in subsequent pregnancies. Symptoms usually commence between 6 and 8 weeks and last until 14–16 weeks. Morning sickness is believed to be due to high levels of pregnancy hormones secreted by the placenta, particularly human chorionic gonadotrophin (hCG) and oestrogen. The time of morning sickness coincides with the rapidly rising serum levels of hCG. hCG starts rising by 6–8 weeks, reaches its peak by 10–12 weeks, starts declining and reaches its nadir by 20 weeks. Owing to higher levels of hCG in women with multiple pregnancies and molar pregnancies, these symptoms tend to be exaggerated. Psychological factors may have a role to play through their direct action at the emetic centre in the midbrain.

Normally, morning sickness does not produce any impact on health or restrict the normal activities of the woman. Hyperemesis gravidarum is defined as vomiting sufficiently to produce weight loss, dehydration, ketonuria, and electrolyte and acid–base imbalances.

Treatment

The mother should be encouraged to eat small frequent feeds that are non-fatty, dry, and of high calorific value. One should avoid dehydration by adequate fluid intake between meals and not with meals. The smell of certain foods often precipitates or aggravates the symptoms and should be avoided. If simple measures fail anti-emetics like metoclopromide, cyclizine, or promethazine are used. Heartburn-induced vomiting should be treated with antacids. Women need to be hospitalized for intravenous rehydration should it be required. It is essential to exclude other causes of vomiting such as urinary tract infections, and thyroid and liver problems. A scan is carried out to rule out multiple pregnancies and hydatiform moles if the vomiting is severe. Morning sickness is self-limiting and should diminish by the end of the first trimester.

Heartburn

Heartburn is caused by the reflux of gastric contents into the lower oesophagus. This occurs as a result of progesterone-mediated relaxation of lower oesophageal sphincter (LES) and the upward displacement and compression of the stomach by the uterus in the third trimester. The resulting reflux of acid gastric contents and bile irritates the LES and may also contribute to nausea and vomiting. The problem is aggravated by smoking and wearing tight clothing.

Treatment

Women are advised to wear loose-fitting clothes and avoid bending soon after meals. Lying in a propped up position and cessation of smoking also help to relieve heartburn. The mainstay of treatment is antacids like aluminium or magnesium hydroxides, magnesium trisilicate singly or in combination and alginate containing antacids (e.g. Gaviscon). These are given half hour after meals and at night. H2 receptor antagonists and proton pump inhibitors are safe in pregnancy and are reserved for intractable cases.

Pica and ptyalism

Pregnant women experience cravings for strange foods and at times non-foods. This desire is sometimes triggered by underlying iron deficiency, the incidence of which is twice in women with pica than those without it. Not all women with pica have iron deficiency. Pregnant women may be distressed by excessive salivation known as ptyalism. Most cases are unexplained.

Constipation and haemorrhoids

The reduced gut motility due to the smooth muscle relaxant effects of progesterone gives rise to constipation in pregnant women. This problem is further aggravated by iron supplementation and pressure from the enlarged uterus and presenting part late in pregnancy. In addition to the discomfort caused by the passage of hard faecal matter, bleeding and painful fissures may develop in the oedematous and hyperaemic rectal mucosa. Haemorrhoids are seen in 1 in 3 women in pregnancy. This may arise de novo or may represent exacerbation of pre-existing ones. This is a consequence of venous stasis in the perirectal plexus of veins, further aggravated by the increased intra-abdominal pressure caused by gravid uterus and straining at stools.

Treatment

High-fibre diet, plenty of fresh fruits and vegetables, and adequate intake of water are recommended. If laxatives are needed, bulk-forming laxatives (e.g. ispaghula husk) are preferred as they are not absorbed from the gastrointestinal tract and hence safe during pregnancy. Other alternatives are prune juice, milk of magnesia, lactulose, and senna. Haemorrhoids are best managed by avoidance of constipation, local anaesthetics, and analgesics. Haemorrhoids regress after pregnancy but may take several months. Surgery may be required in severe cases and is usually deferred until after pregnancy.

Urinary problems

Women experience increased frequency of micturition in the first trimester and at term when the head engages. In the first trimester the uterus enlarges and presses on the bladder decreasing its capacity. This eases off by the twelfth to fourteenth week when the uterus becomes an abdominal organ. Near term, particularly in nulliparas in whom the presenting part often engages before the onset of labour, the entire bladder base is pushed forwards and upwards, reducing its capacity and impairing the venous and lymphatic drainage. The resulting bladder is small, oedematous and susceptible to infection. In addition, the increased urine production due to increased glomerular filtration rate and renal plasma blood flow leads to frequency. There is increased risk of urinary tract infections (UTIs) in pregnancy because of oedematous bladder, incomplete emptying, vesicoureteral reflux and pelvicalyceal dilatation. UTIs particularly cystitis can cause increased frequency of micturition and should be ruled out. Stress incontinence occurs in the latter part of pregnancy due to increased intra-abdominal pressure from the gravid uterus.

Treatment

Mothers should be advised to have a sensible fluid intake throughout the day, avoiding caffeine and alcohol. Restricting fluids before going to bed helps with nocturia. UTIs should be treated. Stress incontinence usually resolves in the postpartum period.

Backache

About half of pregnant women experience low backache.

Previous back pain and obesity are risk factors. Back pain increases with the duration of gestation. A woman's centre of gravity shifts from its prepregnancy position, where it passes through the knees, to the gravid situation, where it moves forward and is in front of the knees. Women compensate for this by an exaggerated lumbar lordosis, otherwise known as the 'proud walk of pregnancy'. This causes strain on the vertebrae and lumbosacral joints and pressure on nerve roots, causing back pain. When it affects the sciatic nerve, it causes pain, tingling or numbness running down the buttocks, hips, and thighs, the condition being called sciatica. The relaxation effect caused by progesterone and relaxin in preparation for delivery sometimes can be excessive, resulting in undue separation of pubic bones, mobility of symphysis pubis and hip joints. This can cause back pain, pubic bone pain, and difficulty in walking and mobilization. This is called symphysis pubis diastasis. Other causes of back pain are due to muscular spasm and fibrositis from local strain injury and pregnancy-associated osteoporosis. Severe back pain not responding to conservative measures should not be attributed simply to pregnancy until a thorough orthopaedic examination has been conducted.

Treatment

Preventive measures include adopting a proper posture, having sufficient rest, avoiding lifting heavy objects, avoidance of high heels, using a back support with pillows while sitting and lying down on a firm mattress. Women should be advised to squat rather than bend over when reaching down. Muscular spasms and acute strain respond well to analgesics, anti-inflammatory agents, heat, and rest. Physiotherapy is found to be beneficial. In severe cases, a pregnancy brace girdle is used to lift the weight of the gravid uterus off the pelvis.

Aches and pains of pregnancy

- Lower abdominal and groin pain: some women experience aching or sharp pain at the lower abdomen and groin. It maybe unilateral or bilateral. This typically appears between 16 and 20 weeks and continues till about the thirty-second week. This is due to the enlarging uterus pulling on round ligaments.
- Headaches: this complaint is common in early pregnancy and most cases decrease in severity or disappear in mid-pregnancy.
- Calf pain: this is due to muscle spasm and tends to occur at night. Venous stasis due to poor circulation can also give rise to calf pain.
- Treatment: simple analgesics and reassurance is all that is required in the absence of any other pathology.

Avoidance of long periods of standing and ankle exercises to improve circulation help to relieve calf pain. Calf muscle spasm is relieved by straightening of legs and dorsiflexion of ankles. Before attributing the symptoms to pregnancy, other pathological causes that can give rise to similar symptoms should be ruled out. For instance, deep vein thrombosis in cases of calf pain, and pre-eclampsia in headaches occurring after 20 weeks should be ruled out.

Carpal tunnel syndrome

Carpal tunnel syndrome occurs when the median nerve, which runs from the forearm to the hand, becomes pressed or squeezed at the wrist. It is otherwise known as median nerve neuropathy. The carpal tunnel is a narrow, rigid passageway under the flexor retinaculum of the hand housing the median nerve and tendons. The nerve gets compressed in the carpal tunnel secondary to oedema in pregnancy. The symptoms are vague ache or pain at the wrist, radiating to hand, forearm, or arm, tingling or numbness of the fingers, excluding little finger, inability to hold or grip objects, a sense of weakness and loss of sensation in the hand. The symptoms are worse early in the morning and gets better later during the day.

Treatment

The patients should be reassured that there is no underlying sinister pathology and that it will improve after delivery. Splinting the hand in dorsiflexion to relieve pressure on the median nerve helps relieve symptoms. Surgical intervention is rarely required in pregnancy, unless there is neurological deficit. Surgery involves making an incision on the carpal tunnel to release the nerve.

Varicosities

The progressively enlarging gravid uterus causes compression of the pelvic veins and the inferior vena cava, leading to diminished venous drainage of the ileofemoral veins. As a result, there is enhanced venous pressure and exacerbation of pre-existing varicosities or the appearance of new ones. Other contributory factors are progesterone-mediated venous dilatation, congenital weakness of veins, familial tendency and prolonged standing. Varicosities are found in as high as 40% of pregnant women. They are more pronounced in the third trimester, but it has been reported as early as the first trimester. Varicosities may affect the lower limbs, vulva, abdominal wall and are also present as haemorrhoids. Varicose veins in the legs can be disfiguring and painful and secondary to phlebitis and thrombosis.

Mothers should avoid using tight-fitting elastic garters, panty girdles, and corsets that can obstruct venous return. The treatment involves periodic rest in the lateral decubitus position with elevation of legs and use of compression stockings. Exercises that improve leg circulation help to reduce venous stasis. If support stockings are to be used these should be put on while the patient is still horizontal, before getting out of bed, while the veins are relatively collapsed. Surgical correction is seldom advised, although rarely injection, ligation or stripping of the veins is necessary.

Abdominal wall varicosities rarely cause problems. Occasionally a varicocele of the round ligament can present as a groin swelling.

Vulval varicosities are seen rarely, except in pregnancy and tend to remit post partum. They may be small or large and may be seen around the introitus and extend into the vagina. They may become thrombosed, bleed, itch, and cause problems in delivery. The diagnosis is made on clinical grounds and biopsy is contraindicated as it can cause heavy bleeding. Episiotomy if required at delivery should be directed away from the varicosity. Vulvar varicosities may be aided by application of a foam rubber pad suspended across the vulva by a belt.

Skin changes in pregnancy

Hyperpigmentation occurs in as high as 90% of pregnant women. It begins early on in pregnancy and is more pronounced in naturally hyperpigmented areas such as the areolae, perineum, umbilicus, and areas prone to friction such as inner thighs. This is due to increased melanocyte-stimulating hormone secreted by the intermediary lobe of the pituitary gland, leading to increased melanin deposition into the epidermal and dermal macrophages.

The linea nigra is the line that often forms when the abdominal linea alba darkens during pregnancy. Pigmentation of the face is referred to as the mask of pregnancy, chloasma or melasma. This is present in 50–70% of pregnant women in the second half of pregnancy. The usual distribution involves the forehead, cheeks, upper lip, and chin. This is exacerbated by ultraviolet rays and hence avoidance of sun exposure and use of sun screens are protective. Pigmentation usually regresses postpartum, but persists in one-third of affected women.

Cutaneous neavi darken and enlarge during pregnancy.

There is augmented cutaneous blood flow and oestrogen-induced changes in small blood vessels. As a result, vascular changes such as spider naevi and palmar erythema appear in pregnancy. Spider naevi occur on the face, upper trunk, and arms. Twenty-five per cent may persist. Palmar erythema is present in up to 75% of women and fades within 1 week after delivery.

Similarly, because of increased blood flow in the gum capillaries, gums bleed easily and are prone to gingivitis in pregnancy. Occasionally, some pregnant women will develop a localized swelling on the gum, known as a pregnancy epulis. Typically, this will occur in the second or third trimester, sometimes even appearing for the first time in the final month of the pregnancy. A pregnancy epulis will often bleed easily, and can appear very red and inflamed; however, they are generally not painful. They are also not cancerous and do not have the potential to become cancerous. Some women who have an epulis will have it removed during pregnancy, usually because of bleeding, for cosmetic reasons or because the diagnosis is uncertain. However, if left alone, the epulis will usually regress after childbirth.

Striae gravidarum (stretch marks, striae distensae) appear as red or pink-purple lines or bands on the abdomen, breasts, thighs, and buttocks. They occur due to breakage of subdermal collagen as a result of stretching in pregnancy. Risk factors for overstretching of the abdomen are macrosomia, obesity, family history and non-Caucasian ethnic origin. Striae gravidarum regress postpartum or persist as white, atrophic lines called striae albicantes.

Rashes are common in pregnancy and are not often serious. Other pregnancy-specific dermatoses such as PUPP (pruritic urticarial papules and plaques of pregnancy) should be ruled out. Most rashes will disappear after childbirth. Pruritis without either rash or cholestasis can be a feature in up to 20% of normal pregnancies. Liver function tests should be done in pregnant women with pruritis to exclude obstetric cholestasis.

Treatment

Most of the skin changes regress in the postpartum period and rarely require treatment. Apart from the cosmetic impairment, they have no implications on the pregnancy or fetus.

Numerous creams, emollients and oils (e.g. vitamin E cream, cocoa butter, aloe vera lotion, and olive oil) are used to prevent striae; however, there is no evidence that these treatments are effective. Limited evidence suggests that two topical treatments may help prevent striae. One contains *Centella asiatica* extract plus alpha-tocopherol and collagen elastin hydrolysates. The other treatment contains tocopherol, essential fatty acids, panthenol, hyaluronic acid, elastin, and menthol. However, the safety of these medications in pregnancy needs to be confirmed with further studies before these can be recommended. Postpartum treatment involves use of retinoic acid and laser, both of which are contraindicated with breastfeeding.

Pruritis is treated with topical agents such as calamine and systemic antihistamines. Topical or systemic steroids are rarely indicated.

Palpitations

Palpitation is defined as unpleasant awareness of one's own heartbeat. It is a symptom very common in pregnancy, usually occurring due to physiological changes in the cardiovascular system rather than any identifiable underlying heart disease. The exact mechanism still remains unknown.

It is important, however, to be aware that the incidence of arrhythmias due to underlying heart disease is significantly increased during pregnancy. Other causes of palpitations such as severe anaemia, hyperthyroidism, and beriberi should be excluded. In the absence of any significant pathology, reassurance is all that is required.

Breathlessness

This is a common symptom experienced by pregnant mothers in the last trimester. There is a 40–50% increase in minute ventilation in pregnancy to accommodate for the additional oxygen demand. The expanding uterus pushes up the diaphragm reducing the lung capacity. These two factors are responsible for women experiencing breathlessness in pregnancy. Shortness of breath improves with engagement of the fetal head. Lying on the side helps to relieve breathlessness while sleeping.

Insomnia

Women complain of inability to sleep in pregnancy. This is particularly pronounced in the third trimester. Discomfort due to the increased size of the abdomen, backache, heartburn, frequent urination in the night, anxiety, and the occurrence of vivid dreams are responsible for this.

Treatment

Women are advised to adopt comfortable sleeping positions. It is helpful to exercise during the day, try relaxation techniques, and take warm baths just prior to sleeping. Women rarely require sedatives and long-term use of sedatives is certainly not advised.

Braxton–Hicks contractions

These are painless tightenings of the uterus that the pregnant women experiences after the twentieth week.

They become stronger and more frequent towards the end of pregnancy. They originate from the top of the uterus, radiate downwards, and fade after 30–60 seconds.

Tiredness

Feeling fatigued or more tired is a pregnancy symptom that can start as early as the first week after conception. This feeling will generally ease off towards the second trimester but may return towards the end of pregnancy. Stress, exhaustion, depression, the common cold or flu, or other illnesses can also leave the woman feeling tired or fatigued.

Vaginal discharge

Pregnant women commonly develop excessive vaginal discharge secondary to vaginal hyperaemia and oestrogen-mediated increased cervical glandular secretions. This is called leucorrhoea of pregnancy. The discharge is non-offensive, white in colour, clear, and mucoid. Bacterial vaginosis, candidiasis, and trichomoniasis are seen in 20–30% of pregnant women. This should be excluded in case of excessive vaginal discharge.

References

Arulkumaran S. Minor symptoms of pregnancy. In: Arulkumaran S, Symonds IM, Fowlie A. (eds) *Oxford handbook of obstetrics and gynaecology.* Oxford: University Press 2004:57–63.

Cunningham FG *et al.* (eds) Prenatal care. In: *Williams obstetrics.* McGraw-Hill 2005:200–29.

Tamizian O, Arulkumaran S. Minor disorders of pregnancy. In: Arulkumaran S, *et al.* (eds) *Essentials of obstetrics.* New Delhi: Jaypee Brothers 2004:115–17.

Physiological changes in pregnancy

Many organs undergo physiological changes in Pregnancy. Understanding these changes is important to
- determine what is abnormal in pregnancy
- explain the multitude of symptoms described in normal pregnancy
- explain the altered reference ranges in pregnancy for a laboratory investigations and their subsequent interpretation
- explain that there are different responses to some emergencies and corrective measures in pregnancy.

All the changes are best explained as individual systems that adapt to the changing needs of pregnancy.

Alimentary tract
- Most pregnant women experience an increase in appetite beginning early in the first trimester and persisting throughout pregnancy. In the absence of nausea and vomiting the increase in appetite gives 200 kcal, which is almost equal to the additional 300 kcal required per day.
- Ptyalism although uncommon occurs in women who have severe hyperemesis gravidarum.
- The tone and motility of the stomach decreases during pregnancy because of the smooth muscle relaxing effects of progesterone. A decrease in levels of motilin, a gut hormone that stimulates smooth muscle, has also been implicated. The decreased tone of the stomach contributes to the nausea of pregnancy.
- In the first and second trimester there is reduced gastric acid secretion, which decreases the symptoms of peptic ulcer disease. It increases significantly in the third trimester both during fasting and after histamine stimulation, which leads to symptoms like heart burn later on in pregnancy.
- The motility of the small bowel is reduced during pregnancy but the absorption of nutrients from the small bowel remains unchanged except for iron. The increase in iron absorption is due to the increasing demand rather than decreasing gastric motility.
- Constipation is a common problem occurring during pregnancy and is because of mechanical obstruction by the uterus, decreased motility of the bowel, and increased water absorption from the colon.
- Increase in portal venous pressure leads to the dilatation of porta systemic venous anastomosis, making haemorrhoids more common in pregnancy.

- The amount of blood supply to the liver remains unchanged, although there is a significant increase in the cardiac output. Serum albumin levels fall progressively during pregnancy. Serum cholesterol levels are increased twofold by the end of pregnancy. Fibrinogen levels rise 50% by the end of the second trimester. The levels of bilirubin, aspartate amino transferase, and alanine amino transferase fall in the third trimester.

Respiratory tract system
- The configuration of the thoracic cage changes in pregnancy with an increase in the subcostal angle and transverse diameter of the chest.
- As pregnancy progresses the level of the diaphragm is pushed up. The elevation of the diaphragm decreases the residual volume. Since there is a reduction in the expiratory reserve volume and residual volume there is a decrease in the functional residual capacity.
- The oxygen consumption increases up to 29%, which leads to higher alveolar and arterial PO2 levels. This change is important as the increase in the CO2 gradient between fetus and mother facilitates transfer of CO2 from the fetus to the mother.
- The maternal arterial pH is maintained at normal levels because of increased renal excretion of bicarbonate. Hence the serum bicarbonate concentration is significantly below non-pregnant levels (Table 5.7.1).

Urinary and renal system
Please refer to Table 5.7.2.

Anatomic changes
- The kidneys enlarge during pregnancy and the right kidney tends to enlarge more than the left. Dilatation of the ureters and renal pelvis begins by the second month of pregnancy and becomes maximal by the middle of the second trimester. The right ureter is more dilated than the left. Mechanical factors are the most important cause of this dilatation, although early onset of ureteral dilatation supports the hypothesis that smooth muscle relaxation caused by progesterone may play a role.
- The consequences of ureteral–calyceal dilatation are an increased incidence of pyelonephritis among patients with asymptomatic bacteriuria, difficulty in interpreting urinary radiographs and in diagnosing urinary tract obstruction during pregnancy, and interference with studies of renal blood flow in glomerular filtration and tubular function.

Table 5.7.1 Respiratory changes in pregnancy

Vital capacity	Maximum amount of air that can be forcibly expired after maximum inspiration	Unchanged
Inspiratory capacity	Maximum amount of air that can be inspired from resting expiratory level	Increases 5%
Tidal volume	Amount of air inspired and expired with normal breath	Increases 30–40%
Functional residual capacity	Amount of air in the lungs at resting expiratory level	Decreases by 20%
Expiratory reserve volume	Maximum amount of air that can be expired from resting expiratory level	Decreases by 20%
Inspiratory reserve volume	Maximum amount of air that can be inspired at the end of normal inspiration	Unchanged
Residual volume	Amount of air in lungs after a maximum expiration	Decreases by 20%
Total lung capacity	Total amount of air in lungs at Maximal inspiration	Decreases by 5%

Table 5.7.2 Physiological changes of the renal system in pregnancy

Increased	Frequency of micturition
	Nocturia
	Stress incontinence
	Bladder capacity
	Kidney size and weight
	Renal plasma flow and GFR
No change	Residual urine

Physiological changes

- Renal plasma flow (RPF) increases by 35–60% early in pregnancy and this increase is maintained until the late third trimester. Because the effective renal plasma flow increases up to 75% and the glomerular filtration (GFR) rate increases by 50%, the filtration fraction falls significantly. As a result of the increased GFR during pregnancy, serum urea and creatinine decrease and the blood urea nitrogen levels fall.

- Serum uric acid decreases in early pregnancy, reaching a nadir by 24 weeks. The serum uric acid levels start rising due to increased renal tubular reabsorption of urate during the third trimester and is elevated to a much higher extent in patients with pre-eclampsia. Because urate levels normally rise during late pregnancy, it is necessary to know a woman's non-pregnant urate level before third trimester values can be used in the clinical setting.

- The plasma osmolality begins to decline as early as 2 weeks after conception and is mainly due to the reduction in serum concentration of sodium and associated anions. Sodium metabolism is delicately balanced in normal pregnancy to permit a net accumulation of 900–1000 mEq of sodium in the fetus.

- Glucose excretion increases in almost all pregnant women. In the non-pregnant state the glucose loss is usually not more than 100 mg but can increase up to 10 g in pregnancy. The cause for this increase in glucose excretion is said to be due to the increased filtered load being presented to the tubules as a result of an increase in GFR. Altered tubular reabsorptive capacity may also be involved. The increase in glucose excretion raises the chance of urinary tract infection and makes monitoring of urinary glucose unreliable in pregnancy.

Cardiovascular system

Pregnancy causes marked and usually reversible changes in the cardiovascular system (Table 5.7.3). Characteristic haemodynamic changes include an increase in blood volume and cardiac output. With peripheral vasodilatation and a decrease in total vascular resistance the arterial blood pressure drops in the midtrimester.

Heart rate

Heart rate in pregnancy rises as a response to falling systemic vascular resistance. The rise is evident as early as 7 weeks and increases by up to 20% by the end of the third trimester. The rise in the heart rate leads to decreased diastolic filling and hence a decrease in the cardiac output and also a decrease in left atrial emptying, increasing the risk of pulmonary oedema.

Cardiac output

Cardiac output starts increasing as early as 5–6 weeks and increases by 30–50%. Initially there is an increase in stroke

Table 5.7.3 Cardiovascular changes in pregnancy

Cardiac output	Increases progressively, starting as early as 10 weeks until 34 weeks. Starts decreasing thereafter and is higher in multigravid pregnancy and multiple pregnancy
Plasma volume	Increases from week 10 to 25 and is maintained till term and is due to the estrogenic effect. Increases by about 50% during pregnancy and further with each contraction. It is more pronounced in lateral position.
Stroke volume	10% increase in pregnancy
Pulse rate	Increases by 15–20 beats per minute
Blood pressure	Systolic and diastolic blood pressure decrease in midtrimester. Diastolic blood pressure is lowest at 16–20 weeks' gestation
Peripheral vascular resistance	Low in early pregnancy. Allows accumulation of blood volume that acts as a reservoir to compensate for blood loss in labour

volume and later an increase in the heart rate. As pregnancy progresses, stroke volume decreases to near non-pregnant levels and the increase in heart rate is responsible for maintaining increased cardiac output. Haemodynamic measurements during labour demonstrate a rise in cardiac output of about 40% compared with late pregnancy levels.

Peripheral vascular resistance

As pregnancy advances the peripheral vascular resistance varies to change blood flow patterns. The mechanisms for vasodilatation in pregnancy are not clear, but the increase in progesterone causing smooth muscle relaxation, circulating prostaglandins, and atrial natriuretic factor may act independently or collectively in an environment of increased heat production in the fetus and an enlarged uterus with low resistance. The reduction in resistance results in a progressive fall in systemic arterial blood pressure during the first 24 weeks of pregnancy. After 24 weeks, systolic and diastolic pressures gradually rise, returning to non-pregnant levels by term. The increase in the residual blood volume in the vasculature provides a reserve in blood volume that is not haemodynamically active. These changes protect against sudden changes in blood pressure, sudden decreases in venous return, blood loss, and higher oxygen and work load demands of pregnancy, labour, and delivery.

Heart

There is an increase in left ventricular dimensions and volume during pregnancy. Despite the increase in the left ventricular dimensions, most parameters of left ventricular function remain the same as in the non-pregnant state, preserving myocardial function during pregnancy. The cardiovascular status in pregnancy resembles that seen in response to physical training. The structural changes in the heart are consistent with the effects of chronic strain put upon the heart.

Central pressures

Central haemodynamic monitoring has shown a decrease in systemic vascular resistance and pulmonary vascular resistance and colloid oncotic pressure, pulmonary capillary wedge pressure, central venous pressure, or left

Table 5.7.4 Haematological changes in pregnancy

Red cell volume	Increases in pregnancy secondary to increase in red cell mass. Since the increase in rates and mass is less than the increase in plasma volume dilutional anaemia of pregnancy occurs
White cell count	Increases in pregnancy, up to 20 000 per cubic millimetre considered as normal
Platelet count	There is a gradual decline in platelet counts in pregnancy, although it remains within the normal non-pregnant levels
ESR	Increases four- to fivefold in pregnancy mainly due to increase in fibrinogen and Immunoglobulins
Clotting factors	Increased fibrinogen, increased plasminogen, and decreased fibrinolytic activity

ventricular/work index during normal pregnancy. The pulmonary capillary wedge pressure is maintained despite the increase in stroke volume because of a marked fall in systemic vascular resistance.

Haematological changes

Please refer to Table 5.7.4.

- In normal pregnancy, maternal plasma volume begins to increase at 10 weeks' gestation and increases progressively until 30–34 weeks, after which it plateaus. The mean increase in plasma volume by 30–34 weeks is 50%, although higher increases may be found in normal pregnancies. At 34 weeks the plasma volume in a healthy pregnancy is about 3800 mL. The plasma volume will start to decline by 200–300 mL from 34 weeks, with a further drop at delivery. It will return to the non-pregnant value by 6–8 weeks postpartum. There are many reasons for increased blood volume during pregnancy. It protects the mother from the possibility of a haemorrhagic decompensation at the time of delivery. The increased plasma volume serves to dissipate fetal heat production and provide for increased excretion by glomerular filtration. The increased red blood cell mass is necessary to increase oxygen transport to meet the needs of the fetus.
- Erythrocyte mass also begins to increase at about 10 weeks. Without iron supplementation, the RBC mass increases about 18% by term. Women with dietary supplement of iron show a greater RBC mass increment, increasing about 400–450 mL or 30% by term. Because plasma volume increases by 50% and the average RBC mass increases by 18–30%, the haematocrit level drops during a normal pregnancy. This so-called physiological anaemia of pregnancy reaches its nadir at 30–34 weeks.
- The peripheral white blood cell count rises progressively during pregnancy. In the first trimester, the range is from 3000 to 15 000/mm³. During the second and third trimesters, the range is from 6000 to 16 000/mm³. In labour it may increase to 20 000–30 000/mm³, after which it gradually returns to non-pregnant levels by the end of the first week of puerperium. This causes a left shift with granulocytosis and more immature white cells.
- The platelet count gradually falls throughout pregnancy, although the counts remain within the normal range for non-pregnant subjects. The fall in platelet count could be either due to increased destruction in the periphery,

which is supported by a shorter average platelet lifespan in pregnancy or due to haemodilution.
- Pregnancy is a procoagulable state with alteration in coagulation and fibrinolysis. Fibrinolytic activity decreases due to increase in plasminogen activator inhibitors. The levels of fibrinogen increase during pregnancy to 400–500 mg/dL. Bleeding time and clotting time remain unchanged during normal pregnancy.

Endocrine and metabolic changes

Thyroid

- The normal pregnant women are euthyroid despite the alterations in thyroid function and laboratory values. However, pregnancy is a state of iodine deficiency due to inadequate intake and increased renal clearance. The change in thyroid function tests are due to an increase in oestrogen-mediated thyroid-binding globulin. Human chorionic gonadotrophin simulates the actions of thyroid-stimulating hormone (TSH). There is a decrease in the availability of iodide because of fetoplacental losses and increased renal clearance.
- TSH concentrations are decreased during the early weeks of gestation and then rise to prepregnancy levels by the end of the first trimester.
- The concentration of thyroid hormones, total T4, and total triiodothyronine rise sharply and then plateau. That is maintained until after delivery. Despite the increase in concentration of T4 and T3, the concentration of active hormones, free T4, and free T3 do not change in normal pregnancy. Determination of free T4 is the most reliable method of evaluating thyroid function in pregnancy.
- At physiological maternal blood levels, little if any transplacental passage of thyroid hormones T4 and T3 occurs. Maternal TSH does not cross the placenta, but the thyroid-stimulating immunoglobulins and TRH cross readily.

Adrenal glands

- The plasma concentration of corticosteroid-binding globulin increases because of oestrogen-induced increase in hepatic synthesis resulting in elevated plasma cortisol concentration. The cortisol concentrations show a twofold increase in the first trimester and a threefold increase in the third trimester.
- Marked elevation of maternal plasma concentration of deoxycorticosterone (DOC) is present by midgestation. Since the plasma DOC levels do not respond to adrenocorticotropic hormone (ACTH) stimulation or dexamethasone suppression the increase may be specifically arising from the fetoplacental unit.
- Dehydroepiandrosterone Sulphate levels decrease in pregnancy because of the marked rise in the metabolic clearance of this steroid.

Pancreas

During normal pregnancy an exaggerated starvation ketosis is observed with maternal hypoglycaemia and hypoinsulinaemia as a response to starvation. In response to feeding, hyperglycaemia hyperinsulinaemia, hypertriglyceridaemia, and reduced tissue sensitivity to insulin occur. The factors responsible for this diabetogenic effect are the hormones released by the placenta, mainly human placental lactogen (hPL). This hormone reduces the effectiveness of insulin by decreasing the sensitivity of peripheral tissues. Since hPL secretion is proportional to the total placental mass, the diabetogenic effect is higher in the later part of pregnancy.

Breast changes

Breast changes occur very early in pregnancy. Tenderness, tingling sensations, and a feeling of heaviness occur within 4 weeks of the last menstrual period. The breasts rapidly enlarge in the first 8 weeks, mainly because of vascular engorgement. Oestrogen stimulates ductal growth and progesterone stimulates alveolar growth.

Postural changes

The enlarging uterus shifts the centre of gravity quite anteriorly. This is compensated by progressive increased anterior convexity of the lumbar spine during pregnancy. This keeps the woman's centre of gravity over the legs. This postural change unfortunately leads to low backache. The ligaments of the pubic symphysis and sacroiliac joints loosen during pregnancy secondary to the hormone relaxin. This mobility of the pelvic joints is to facilitate delivery, but it can lead to pelvic discomfort in late pregnancy. Relaxation of the joints coupled with the increase in lordosis and protuberant abdomen lead to unsteadiness of the gait.

Further reading

Cunningham G (ed.). *Williams obstetrics*, 22nd edn. New York: McGraw-Hill;2005.

Fortner KB (ed.). *The John Hopkins manual of gynecology and obstetrics*, 3rd edn. Philadelphia: Wolters Kluwer 2008.

Steven G, Gabbe JRN, Leigh Simpson J (eds). *Obstetrics normal and problem pregnancies*, 3rd edn. New York: Churchill Livingston 1996.

Preparing for pregnancy

Preconception care and counselling are important, because they identify women who can benefit from interventions before pregnancy. Preconceptional screening and counselling offer an opportunity to identify and mitigate maternal risk factors before pregnancy begins. The preconception care can be incorporated into any visit to the GP for women of childbearing age. The chances of becoming pregnant and having a healthy pregnancy and baby are better if both partners are as fit and healthy as possible. The aim of the preconceptional clinic should be to provide a strategy to reduce or eliminate the pathological influences revealed by her family, medical, or obstetrical history, or by specific testing.

Counselling in a preconceptional clinic should begin with a thorough review of the medical, obstetrical, social, and family histories. Useful information is more likely to be obtained by asking specific questions regarding each aspect of the history. Commercially prepared questionnaires can be used in preconceptional clinics, but the answers should be reviewed with the patient to ensure appropriate follow-up. Review of an up-to-date history allows prospective parents to explore their concerns and questions. Reproductive history should include questions regarding infertility, abnormal pregnancy outcomes, including miscarriage, ectopic pregnancy, recurrent pregnancy loss, and preterm delivery, and complications such as pre-eclampsia and placental abruption. History suggestive of an incompetent cervix or uterine abnormality should warrant further investigations.

Social assessment

A social and lifestyle history should be obtained to identify potentially risky behaviours and exposures that may compromise a good productive outcome.

Specialist referral for patients with disabilities who wish to become pregnant should be offered. Referral for maternity care to the same hospital where the disability care is carried out should be provided. Addresses of support groups such as Disability Pregnancy and Parenthood international (DPPi) is provided.

Victims of domestic violence should be identified before they conceive, as they're more likely to be abused during pregnancy. Information about available community, social, and legal resources should be made available to women. They should have plans devised for dealing with the abusive partner.

Family history should include genetic risks that may help to incorporate carrier screening or prenatal diagnosis for genetic diseases.

Medical assessment should include an assessment of potential risks to the fetus and to the mother:
- diabetes or epilepsy
- heart or circulatory problems, such as high blood pressure or thrombosis
- hereditary conditions in the family, such as sickle cell anaemia, thalassaemia, cystic fibrosis, or muscular dystrophy
- gynaecological problems, such as endometriosis, polycystic ovary syndrome (PCOS), or previous ectopic pregnancy.
- genetic counselling should be discussed if either of the couple have an inherited condition.

After thorough assessment the following advice should be given to women attending the preconceptual clinic and appropriate follow-up arranged.

Infectious disease screening

- Rubella screening should be carried out in all women planning for a pregnancy. Women not immune to rubella should be vaccinated at least 1 month prior to trying for a pregnancy.
- Universal screening of pregnant women for hepatitis B virus has been recommended by the CDC. Women with social or occupational risks of exposure to hepatitis B virus should be counselled and offered vaccination.
- Cytomegalovirus screening should be offered preconceptually to women who work in neonatal ICUs, childcare facilities, or dialysis units.
- Testing for immunity against parvovirus B19 may be offered preconceptually to schoolteachers and childcare workers.
- Human immunodeficiency virus counselling and testing should be offered confidentially and voluntarily to all women.
- Toxoplasmosis is an infection caused by a parasite that can live in soil, raw meat, and cat faeces. Infection with toxoplasmosis during pregnancy can cause miscarriage, stillbirth, or damage to the baby's eyes, ears, or brain. To reduce the risk of infection patients should avoid handling cat litter, wear gloves when gardening, and wash all soil off fruit and vegetables before consumption.
- Screening for the varicella antibody should be performed if a positive history cannot be obtained. The varicella-zoster virus vaccine is now recommended for all non-immune adults.

Medicines and drugs

- Medications considered harmful to the fetus and with proven teratogenic risk should either be stopped or changed to safer alternatives preconceptually.
- If no alternatives are available the risk of congenital abnormalities should be discussed in detail with the couple and the benefit to risk ratio calculated.
- Any over-the-counter medications should be checked with the pharmacist to see whether these are safe to take while trying for a baby or when pregnant.
- Any herbal or alternative remedies or complementary therapies should be checked if they are safe to use during pregnancy, or while trying to get pregnant.
- Couples using recreational (illegal) drugs should be advised to stop all the drugs and appropriate referral arranged if required for methadone therapy. Information on street drugs and where to go for help and advice can be found on www.talktofrank.com.

Sexual health

- Patients suspected to have sexually transmitted infections should be referred to GUM clinic for confidential advice. Some sexually transmitted infections can affect the chances of getting pregnant, and if not treated they can be passed to the baby during pregnancy or birth.
- Offer cervical screening tests if not done in the last 5 years.

- If the couples have a sexual problem they should be referred to a counsellor with expertise in that field.

Stopping contraception

- Many women worry that some methods of contraception, such as the pill, injection, or IUD, will make it difficult to get pregnant when they stop using them. No method of contraception causes infertility.
- Patients should be warned that sometimes ovulation can be delayed or be irregular for a short time after stopping hormonal contraception. With implanon and depot medroxy progesterone injections menstruation and fertility take longer to return than after other methods of contraception.

Eating healthily

Eating a variety of foods, with as much fresh food as possible, helps to ensure adequate intake of vitamins and minerals.
   A healthy diet is made up of

- starchy foods, such as potatoes, sweet potatoes, bread, pasta, rice, and cereals
- at least five portions of fruit and vegetables a day (these can be fresh, dried, frozen, tinned, or juice)
- protein foods, such as meat, beans, chicken, eggs, pulses (e.g. lentils), and nuts (seek advice on foods to avoid)
- dairy foods, such as milk, yoghurt, and cheese (see 'Foods to avoid' for advice on cheese)
- fish (see 'Foods to avoid' for advice on fish).

Folic acid

- All women planning a pregnancy should take a daily supplement of folic acid: 0.4 mg (400 µg) of folic acid should be taken from the time of stopping contraception or as soon as pregnancy is confirmed until week 12 of pregnancy.
- Folic acid prevents neural tube defects and if a previous pregnancy was affected by spina bifida, or either of the partners have a neural tube defect, or suffer from epilepsy a higher dose of folic acid should be taken.
- Patients should be advised to eat foods that contain folic acid, such as green leafy vegetables, breads, and cereals with folic acid added to them.

Foods to avoid

Severe food poisoning during pregnancy can cause miscarriage, stillbirth, or damage to the developing baby. Pregnant women are advised to avoid foods that have a higher risk of causing food poisoning. The following foods can contain harmful bacteria:

- unpasteurized milk and cheese
- soft-cooked or raw eggs, for instance in homemade mayonnaise or mousse (check food labels to make sure eggs are pasteurized)
- soft cheeses with rind, such as Brie
- blue cheeses, such as Stilton
- undercooked meat, including pâté, or cold prepared meals, and cook–chill foods
- shellfish, such as mussels, prawns and clams.

   Foods containing substances that can cause harm to the unborn baby:

- vitamin A supplements (including cod liver oil)
- liver (including liver pâté) contains high levels of vitamin A, so limit this to no more than one portion a week

- fish such as swordfish, marlin and shark, which can contain high levels of mercury
- peanuts or foods containing peanuts, especially with a history of allergy.

X-rays

Patients should not have an X-ray while trying for a pregnancy unless it is essential for health.

Lifestyle issues

Exercise

- Both partners should be advised to continue exercise before planning for a pregnancy, and if not doing any exercise should be advised to start. The more active and fit the patient is the easier it is to cope with pregnancy.
- Walking and swimming are good ways to start getting fit, and a yoga or Pilates class can help with relaxation and muscle tone.
- Avoid exercise or sports where there is a risk of being hit in the abdomen, such as martial arts. Extra care should be taken during activities where there is a risk of falling or losing balance, such as cycling and horse riding.

Weight

- Being overweight or underweight can disrupt menstruation and reduce the chances of getting pregnant.
- Body mass index (BMI) more than 29 or less than 19 may make getting pregnant difficult.
- A BMI less than 18.5 is considered underweight, and a BMI above 25 is considered overweight. If you or your partner are concerned about your weight, talk to your doctor, nurse, or midwife.

Smoking

Stopping smoking may be the most important thing women can do for their health and the baby. Women who smoke during pregnancy have a greater risk of:

- miscarriage
- stillbirth
- giving birth too early (premature birth)
- complications during and after pregnancy and labour
- having low birthweight babies.

   Babies who have low birthweight or are born prematurely are more likely to have health problems and are at higher risk of sudden infant death syndrome (SIDS, or cot death). See www.gosmokefree.nhs.uk for further information.

Alcohol

- Alcohol should be limited to one or two units per week and binge drinking should be avoided.
- Alcohol can damage sperm production. Partners should be advised to avoid drinking too.
- Drinks heavily and frequently during pregnancy, or regularly binge drinking (has five or more units of alcohol on any one occasion) can harm the baby's development and health.
- Very heavy drinking can lead to fetal alcohol syndrome (FAS) and fetal alcohol spectrum disorder (FASD). These describe a range of symptoms that can be caused by alcohol in pregnancy, including damage to the facial features, brain, heart, and kidneys, and learning difficulties and behavioural problems in later life. See www.drinkaware.co.uk for further information

Work environment

There are some occupations, such as working as a radiographer or working with chemicals, or exposure to substances in some surroundings, that may be harmful for pregnancy. Further information can be obtained from the Health and Safety Executive website at www.hse.gov.uk.

Patient information and contacts

Disability Pregnancy and Parenthood international (DPPi), tel: 0800 018 4730, textphone: 0800 018 9949, www.dppi. org.uk

Further reading

Cunningham G (ed.). *Williams obstetrics*, 22nd edn. New York: McGraw-Hill 2005.

Fortner KB (ed.). *The John Hopkins manual of gynecology and obstetrics*, 3rd edn. Philadelphia: Wolters Kluwer 2008.

FPA. *Planning a pregnancy*. FPA 2006.

Puerperium

Definition
Puerperium is the period following childbirth during which the pelvic organs revert back to the prepregnant state both anatomically and physiologically. It lasts for 6 weeks after the delivery of the baby.

Normal changes of the puerperium

Involution of the uterus, cervix, and vagina
The postpartum uterus, which weighs about 1 kg, returns to its prepregnant size of 80 g. Immediately after placental expulsion, the fundus of the contracted uterus is slightly below the umbilicus. By a process called involution it shrinks, and becomes a pelvic organ in 2 weeks and regains its prepregnant size in 6 weeks. The total number of muscle cells does not decrease appreciably; instead the individual cells decrease markedly in size. Simultaneous involution of the connective tissue framework also occurs. Endometrial regeneration is complete by the third week, except at the placental site. Complete extrusion of the placental site takes up to 6 weeks. If this process is defective, late puerperal haemorrhage may ensue.

The cervical opening readily admits two fingers for a few days after labour. By a process of gradual contraction the opening narrows, the cervix thickens, and the canal reforms. By 2–3 weeks into the puerperium the internal os is closed. The lower uterine segment over a course of a few weeks is converted into the uterine isthmus.

The vagina gradually diminishes in size, but rarely returns to nulliparous dimensions. Rugae reappear by the third week. The hymen is represented by small tags of tissue known as caruncalae myrtiformis.

Lochia
Lochia is the vaginal discharge for the first 2–3 weeks during puerperium. It occurs because of the sloughing of the superficial layer of the decidua. The basal layer remains and new endometrium regenerates from it (Table 5.9.1).

Urinary tract
Puerperal diuresis occurs between the second and the fifth days. This is a reversal of the excessive extracellular water that accumulated during pregnancy. Because of the relative insensitivity to the raised intravesical pressure because of the nerve plexus trauma sustained during delivery, the bladder maybe over distended without the desire to pass urine. The paralysis effect of regional anaesthesia further compounds this. Stagnation of urine along with dilated ureters and renal pelvis predisposes to urinary tract infection (UTIs). Dilated ureters and renal pelvis return to normal size within 8 weeks.

Pelvic floor
Evidence of neuropathic injury of the pudendal nerve has been reported in up to half of the women following vaginal delivery. This leads to weakening of pelvic floor muscles and can result in incontinence of urine, faeces, or flatus and may contribute to development of prolapse later in life. Stress incontinence is known to affect one-third of women 3 months after normal delivery. Occult anal sphincter injury as identified by endoanal ultrasound is seen in one-third of primiparous women 6 weeks after normal delivery; 10–20% of women who had a normal delivery report symptoms of altered faecal incontinence 6 weeks after

Table 5.9.1 Types of lochia

Name	Colour	Duration (days)	Contents
Lochia rubra	Red	1–4	Erythrocytes, decidua, epithelial cells, bacteria
Lochia serosa	Pale	5–9	More leucocytes than erythrocytes, cervical mucus, decidua
Lochia alba	Yellowish white	10–14	Serous fluid, leucocytes, epithelial cells

delivery. Both direct trauma and pudendal nerve injury causes altered faecal or flatus incontinence.

Recovery of pudendal nerve function was observed in two-thirds of women by 2 months postpartum with evidence of persistent neuropathy in the remainder. Postnatal pelvic floor exercises are very important and help women regain tone.

Blood
Blood volume returns to normal after the first week. Although the heart rate falls, stroke volume increases and overall cardiac output rises soon after delivery and remains elevated for at least 48 hours postpartum. The rise in cardiac output is due to the rise in stroke volume from venous return. Thus, early puerperium is a time that requires close surveillance in any woman at risk of cardiac compromise. By 2 weeks, these changes return to normal non-pregnant values.

The haemoglobin concentration and haematocrit level fluctuate moderately during the first few postpartum days. Haematocrit returns to normal by the end of first week. Considerably lower haemoglobin levels than the predelivery state indicate excessive blood loss at delivery. In response to the stress of labour there is marked leucocytosis in the puerperium. The platelet count falls soon after separation of the placenta, but secondary elevation occurs by 4–5 days. Puerperium is a hypercoagulable state due to increased platelet count, platelet adhesiveness, and fibrinogen levels. Women are at high risk of developing thromboembolism in the puerperium, and appropriate anticoagulant regimens should be instituted for those at risk.

Weight loss
Average weight loss in puerperium is 7–10 kg, 5–6 kg attributed to uterine evacuation and 2–3 kg due to diuresis.

Peritoneum and abdominal wall
The laxity of broad and round ligaments requires considerable time to recover. The abdominal wall remains soft and flabby as a result of the rupture of elastic fibres in the skin caused by prolonged distention of the abdomen by the pregnant uterus. A return to normal for these structures take several weeks. Exercise helps to regain abdominal tone.

Most striae fade to pale/white (striae albicantes) lines and shrink postpartum, although they do not disappear completely.

Management of puerperium

Postnatal examination

At least for the first hour after delivery vital signs should be monitored every 15 minutes. Monitoring of the amount of vaginal bleeding and palpation of the fundal height and tone should be done to ensure that the uterus is well contracted.

In the postnatal ward women should be asked about general wellbeing, psychological wellbeing, adequacy of sleep and diet, pain control, excessive bleeding, bowel and bladder functions. Clinical examination should include monitoring of vital signs, involution of uterus, examination of perineum, and recording of colour and amount of lochia.

There may be a slight reactionary rise in temperature by 0.5° following delivery, which comes down to normal within 12 hours. The rate of involution is assessed by measuring the symphysiofundal height after emptying the bladder. The average rate of involution is 1 cm per day. The most common causes of delayed involution include full bladder, loaded rectum, uterine infection, retained products, fibroids, or broad ligament haematoma. Offensive lochia along with pyrexia and tender uterus suggest endometritis. Persistent red lochia along with subinvolution should alert the clinician to infection or retained products. Perineal examination is carried out daily to asses healing of episiotomy or tears and also to rule out vulval haematomas and infection.

General care of the mother

The mother is encouraged to get good sleep and adequate rest. Rooming in with the baby improves breastfeeding and mother–baby bonding.

The mother can be ambulant a few hours after delivery. Early ambulation decreases the risk of thromboembolism, and bladder and bowel dysfunction. Women who have had regional analgesia should delay ambulation till the muscle power of the lower limbs returns to normal. For this reason and to avoid injury due to syncopal attacks, a trained attendant should be present at least at the first ambulation.

There are no dietary restrictions for women who have delivered vaginally. If the mother does not breastfeed, her dietary requirements are the same as for non-pregnant women. Breastfeeding mothers should have a balanced diet that is high in calories, protein, vitamins, and minerals. There is an excess demand of at least 700 calories and 20 g of protein per day compared with the non-pregnant state. Daily requirements of calcium are increased three times and vitamin A by one and a half times that of the non-pregnant state. An adequate amount of fluid intake is important for successful breastfeeding.

Women should be encouraged to start exercise to tone up the abdominal and pelvic floor muscles as soon as they are able to do so. These exercises should be continued for at least 3 months.

After pain

Oxytocin liberated in response to suckling causes strong uterine contractions and is felt by the patient as spasmodic pain. Simple analgesics and antispasmodics are required occasionally to relieve the pain.

Care of the bladder

Women should be encouraged to void soon after delivery. This may not be possible for women who have undergone regional analgesia: an indwelling catheter is desirable until the patient is adequately mobile. Overdistension of the bladder is quite common in the puerperium. The infusion of intravenous fluids during labour and sudden withdrawal of the antidiuretic effect of oxytocin can lead to rapid bladder filling. This along with inadequate bladder sensation due to neuropraxia and epidural analgesia result in overdistension. Difficult instrumental deliveries, painful genital lesions such as extensive episiotomies and lacerations cause pain and periurethral oedema and prevent bladder emptying. Other sources of pain, such as prolapsed haemorrhoids, abdominal wound pain, or even faecal impaction may all contribute to voiding difficulties. In general, after Caesarean section and difficult instrumental deliveries with extensive perineal repair, an indwelling catheter for 12–24 hours is recommended.

One should look for overdistended bladder during abdominal palpation. The bladder may be palpated as a cystic mass suprapubically, or the enlarged bladder may falsely elevate fundal height. If the women has not voided within 4–6 hours of delivery, her bladder is in danger of overdistension. She should be encouraged to void. Analgesics are administered to relieve pain. If these measures fail, an indwelling catheter should be left in situ for 24–48 hours or until bladder tone is regained.

The incidence of UTI in puerperium is 3–5%. The increased incidence of UTIs may be due to bladder stasis, voiding difficulties and catheterization in labour. UTIs should be monitored, and if present should be treated with antibiotics.

Care of the bowel

Constipation is common in pregnancy and remains so in the puerperium. Fear of defaecation due to pain of prolapsed haemorrhoids, anal fissure, and perineal injuries further exacerbate the problem. The mother should be encouraged to drink plenty of fluids, consume a high-fibre diet, and be ambulant. Non-responders to conservative measures should receive bulk-forming agents or laxatives. Prophylactic stool softeners should be given to women who had third- or fourth-degree repair to avoid straining at defaecation; 20–50% of women who had primary third- and fourth-degree repairs are known to suffer faecal or flatus incontinence. This has implications on their future pregnancy management and quality of life. Hence these women should routinely be followed up in the hospital at 6 weeks to detect these problems and institute appropriate management.

Perineal care

Perineal discomfort is the most common problem encountered postnatally, occurring in 42% of women after spontaneous vaginal delivery and persisting after the first 2 months in 8–10%. The figures following assisted vaginal deliveries are 84% and 30% respectively. Perineal pain is worse following instrumental delivery, episiotomy, or spontaneous tears. A warm sitz bath helps to relieve local pain and oedema. Topical cooling measures and local anaesthetic provide short-term relief. Non-steroidal anti-inflammatory drugs (e.g. diclofenac suppositories) are the mainstay of treatment.

Women should be advised of perineal hygiene and regular changing of sanitary pads. Perineal toilet should be carried out regularly with antiseptic solutions. Any evidence of infection should be aggressively treated with antibiotics. In case of episiotomy wound dehiscence, resuturing is contraindicated in the presence of infection, and healing by secondary intention should be allowed. Any local abscess or haematomas should be drained.

Postpartum blues

As many as half of women experience 'postpartum blues' in the puerperium. This is a passing state of heightened emotions and in itself is not an illness. Levels of oestrogen, progesterone, and cortisol fall dramatically within 48 hours after delivery. This sudden fall in hormones leads to an 'emotional let down' and is thought to play a role as this state classically peaks 3–5 days after delivery and can last up to 2 weeks. Other contributory factors are discomfort, fatigue, sleep deprivation during labour and puerperium, and anxiety over parenting capabilities.

These women cry easily, are irritable, and suffer from sleep disturbances. Postpartum blues usually do not interfere with a woman's ability to care for her baby. Supportive therapy is all that is required. This condition should however be differentiated from a more serious postnatal depression.

Traumatic neuritis

This may present with foot drop, paraesthesia, sciatic pain, and muscle wasting in one or both limbs following delivery. The mechanism is thought to be herniation of lumbosacral discs at L4–5 due to exaggerated lithotomy position and instrumental delivery. Management entails bed rest, physiotherapy, and spinal/orthopaedic opinion with appropriate imaging. Peroneal neuritis may result from compression of the proneal nerve between the head of the fibula and the lithotomy pole, and presents as foot drop. Treatment is supportive with physiotherapy.

Diastasis of the symphysis pubis

Incidence is around 0.1% after spontaneous delivery. It maybe associated with a forceps delivery, a rapid second stage, or exaggerated flexion and abduction of maternal thighs such as in McRobert's manoeuvre. The symptoms are of pain over the symphysis, which is exaggerated by weight bearing. The clinical signs are a waddling gait, tenderness over the joint, and occasionally a palpable interpubic gap. Management is supportive with bed rest, physiotherapy, analgesia, and anti-inflammatory drugs and a pelvic support brace.

Immunization

Anti-D gammaglobulin is administered within 72 hours to Rh-negative mothers bearing a Rh-positive baby. Rubella-susceptible women can be vaccinated postnatally. Pregnancy should be avoided until 1 month after vaccination. Breastfeeding should not be stopped.

Return of menstruation and ovulation

The time of return of menstruation and ovulation after delivery is variable and dependent on lactation. Menstruation returns by 6–8 weeks in non-lactating mothers; 70% of women with full or nearly full breastfeeding remain amenorrheic till 6 months. Ovulation is suppressed during the greater part of lactational amenorrhoea, except for the last 4 weeks when 30% of cycles are thought to be ovulatory. The conception risk during lactational amenorrhoea is only 1–2% if all three criteria, (1) amenorrhoea (2) full lactation (3) less than 6 months postpartum, continue to apply.

Contraception

Ovulation is found to return in non-lactating mothers as early as 3 weeks. Hence they should use appropriate contraception as early as possible. The choice of contraceptives available to non-lactating mothers is the same as any other woman. Contraceptive pills containing oestrogen are not prescribed during breastfeeding as they inhibit lactation. Instead, the progesterone-only pill is used. If an intrauterine device is preferred, the insertion is performed after 6 weeks, once involution is complete.

Resumption of intercourse

Women should resume intercourse as soon as they are physically and emotionally ready for it. It is preferable to postpone it until the third week when the lochia has ceased, the cervix has closed, and the uterus has become a pelvic organ. Dyspareunia is quite common in the postpartum period due to the hypo-oestrogenic effects of breastfeeding. Topical lubricants or vaginal oestrogen creams are recommended.

Time of discharge

NICE guidelines recommend that the length of stay in a maternity unit should be discussed between the woman and the healthcare professional, taking into account the health and wellbeing of the mother and the baby. After uncomplicated deliveries, woman can be discharged from the hospital as early as 6 hours.

Postnatal visit

Postnatal examination is carried out at the end of 6 weeks. The doctor should enquire about physical, emotional and social wellbeing and that of the infant. An abdominal and pelvic examination is performed to look for tone of abdominal and pelvic musculature, uterine involution, and healing of episiotomy and tears. Contraceptive advice should be given.

Further reading

Arulkumaran S. Care in the puerperium. In: Arulkumaran S, Symonds IM, Fowlie A. (eds) *Oxford handbook of obstetrics and gynaecology.* Oxford: Oxford University Press 2004:365–72.

Fynes M, O'Herlihy C. The influence of mode of delivery on anal sphincter injury and faecal continence. Obstet Gynaecol 2001;3:120–25.

Groom KM, Paterson-Brown S. The influence of mode of delivery on anal sphincter injury and faecal continence. Obstet Gynaecol 2002;4:4–9.

Shetty J. Normal puerperium. In: Arulkumaran S, Sivanesaratnam V, Chatterjee, Kumar P. (eds) *Essentials of obstetrics.* New Delhi: Jaypee Brothers 2004:373–77.

Cunningham FG, Leveno KJ, Bloom SL, *et al.* (eds). The puerperium. In: *Williams obstetrics*, McGraw-Hill 2005:695–710.

Internet resources

Postnatal care: www.nice.org

Patient resources

Postnatal care: www.nice.org

Routine blood tests in pregnancy

It is important to screen for certain illnesses in pregnancy, as these illnesses have adverse consequences on the mother and baby. By detecting and intervening at the right time, adverse outcomes can be reduced or prevented. This chapter focuses on the reasons for undertaking such blood tests and interventions available. A detailed discussion of individual conditions is beyond the scope of this chapter and the reader is advised to consult appropriate chapters of this textbook.

Routine blood tests

- At booking: full blood count (FBC), blood group, presence of atypical antibodies, blood tests for syphilis, HIV, hepatitis B, immunity to chicken pox and rubella.
- 28 weeks: FBC, atypical antibodies
- 34 weeks: FBC, atypical antibodies.

Special blood tests

- 8–10 weeks: haemoglobin electrophoresis
- 10–13 weeks: serum markers (PAPP-A, free β-human chorionic gonadotropin (hCG)) for first trimester Down's syndrome screening
- 15–20 weeks: serum markers (α-fetoprotein (AFP), β-hCG, unconjugated oestradiol, inhibin) for second trimester down syndrome screening.
- 16-18 weeks: oral glucose tolerance test (OGTT) in women with previous history of gestational diabetes (GDM).
- 24-28 weeks: OGTT in women with risk factors for GDM.

Anaemia

The incidence of anaemia in pregnancy varies from 10–30% in the developed world and 40–80% in the developing world. Anaemia in pregnancy is due to physiological haemodilution, increased demand, nutritional deficiency, and poor reserves. The lower limit of normal for haemoglobin in pregnancy is taken as 10.5 g/dL as opposed to 11.5 g/dL in a non-pregnant individual to account for physiological haemodilution. Iron deficiency anaemia is the commonest cause of anaemia in pregnancy followed by folate deficiency. If anaemia is detected in pregnancy, it should be investigated further by assessing other indices such as ferritin, total iron binding capacity (TIBC), serum and red cell folate, and serum B12 levels.

Anaemia and pregnancy

Minor symptoms of pregnancy such as tiredness, lethargy, breathlessness, and palpitations are exacerbated due to iron deficiency anaemia. Iron deficiency adversely affects neuromuscular transmission because of the malfunction of iron-dependent tissue enzymes. Iron deficiency is associated with low birthweight, preterm delivery, and postpartum haemorrhage. There is increased incidence of childhood anaemia and impaired cognitive development in infants born to anaemic mothers. Low birthweight is in itself a risk factor for development of adult hypertension.

Treatment

Correction of iron deficiency anaemia can be achieved by iron supplementation, either oral or parenteral. The maximum rise in haemoglobin achievable with oral or parenteral iron is 0.8 g/dL/week. Hence a woman presenting with anaemia late in pregnancy is treated with blood transfusion if rapid restoration of haemoglobin is indicated. Women with low haemoglobin presenting in labour should have their blood grouped and saved should blood be needed in case of postpartum haemorrhage. Megaloblastic anaemia is treated by high-dose folate or vitamin B12 injections.

Blood grouping and screening for antibodies

Determining the blood group at booking makes it possible to identify women who are Rhesus negative and therefore at risk of Rhesus immunization. It also helps to identify other atypical antibodies acquired as a result of previous pregnancies or blood transfusions, quantify them, monitor their progress, and make appropriate management plans.

The current recommendation is to give universal Anti-D prophylaxis for pregnant women who are Rh D negative who have not already been sensitized. This is given at 28 weeks, 34 weeks, and after delivery. This is to prevent Rhesus alloimmunization and subsequent development of haemolytic disease of the newborn (HDN). Not all fetuses of sensitized mothers develop HDN. HDN can vary in severity from being detectable only in laboratory tests, through to stillbirth or birth of newborns with severe anaemia and jaundice leading to neonatal morbidity and death.

Since the implementation of post-delivery immunoprophylaxis using anti-D immunoglobulin (Ig) in the UK in 1969, deaths attributed to RhD alloimmunization have fallen from 46/100 000 births before 1969 to 1.6/100 000 in 1990.

A dose of 500 IU anti-D IgG is given at 28 and 34 weeks. After delivery, if the baby is found to be Rh negative, post-delivery prophylaxis is not indicated. Similarly, if the partner's blood group is known to be Rhesus negative from the beginning and paternity is not in doubt antenatal prophylaxis is not indicated. Studies have shown that a dose of 500 IU is sufficient to cover a fetomaternal haemorrhage (FMH) of up to 4 mL at delivery. This is the case in more than 99% of deliveries. Further dosing is required if the amount of FMH is estimated to be more than 4 mL using quantification techniques. Anti-D is also indicated after sensitizing events such as termination of pregnancy at any gestation, miscarriages before 12 weeks managed surgically, spontaneous or threatened miscarriages after 12 weeks, recurrent episodes of threatened miscarriage, after external cephalic version, and antepartum haemorrhage. A dose of 250 IU should suffice before 20 weeks and 500 IU after 20 weeks. Routine prophylaxis should be carried on irrespective of recent administration of Anti-D after a sensitizing event.

Despite routine anti-D prophylaxis a small proportion of women develop anti-D antibodies. The most important cause is unrecognized transplacental bleeds late in pregnancy. The remainder appear to be due to inadequate prophylaxis, late prophylaxis, or no prophylaxis.

Haemoglobin electrophoresis

Haemoglobin electrophoresis should be routinely performed in women of ethnic origin with a high incidence of haemoglobinopathies. These include women of Cypriot, Eastern Mediterranean, Middle Eastern, Indian and Southeast Asian origin, in whom the incidence of thalassaemia is greatest, and women of African or Afro-Caribbean origin, who are at risk of sickle cell disease. Persistent anaemia unresponsive to haematinics may be an indication for haemoglobin electrophoresis in any woman, irrespective of racial origin.

Haemoglobinopathies and pregnancy

Both sickle cell disease and thalassaemias have an autosomal recessive pattern of inheritance.

Pregnancy in women with β-thalassaemia major is very rare as this condition is usually fatal in the first or second decade. Similarly α-thalassaemia major is incompatible with life. What we routinely encounter in antenatal clinics are those women with thalassaemia traits. These women have chronic anaemia.

There are significant fetal and maternal complications in pregnancies experienced by mothers with sickle cell disease. The increased metabolic demands, hypercoagulable state, and vascular stasis associated with pregnancy predispose to these complications. Fetal complications are due to compromised placental blood flow.

There is increased incidence of miscarriage, preterm labour, intrauterine growth restriction, and stillbirths. Anaemia, infection, pre-eclampsia, thromboembolic episodes and sickling crises are increased in mothers.

Management

If the mother is known to have sickle cell or thalassaemia trait, partner testing is done to establish the carrier status of the partner. If both parents are have traits the woman should be referred for prenatal diagnosis as there is a 25% chance that the fetus is affected. Parents may opt for further invasive testing or termination of pregnancy.

Women with thalassaemia traits need iron and folate supplementation throughout pregnancy, but should not be given parenteral iron. If anaemia does not respond to haematinics, blood transfusion may be required prior to delivery.

Women with sickle cell disease should be managed in an appropriate centre with multidisciplinary input from haematologists, obstetricians, anaesthetists, and paediatricians.

Screening for gestational diabetes

GDM is defined as glucose intolerance of variable severity with onset or first identified during pregnancy. The incidence varies from 0.2–0.5% in white population to 3–6% in south Asian, Afro-Caribbean and Middle Eastern populations. GDM constitutes 90% of diabetes in pregnancy.

GDM and pregnancy

GDM occurs usually in the latter half of pregnancy and hence has no effect on organogenesis. There is increased incidence of pre-eclampsia, polyhydramnios, preterm labour, and recurrent urinary tract infections and candidiasis with uncontrolled or poorly controlled GDM; 20–30% of women with GDM have macrosomic infants. This leads to the need for early induction of labour, prolonged labour, shoulder dystocia, increased incidence of operative deliveries, and postpartum haemorrhage. Poorly controlled diabetes can lead to sudden intrauterine deaths. In the neonatal period macrosomic infants are prone to hypoglycaemia, electrolyte imbalances, hyaline membrane disease, hyperviscosity syndromes, birth injuries and birth asphyxia. Women identified as having GDM are at 50% increased risk of developing non-insulin-dependent diabetes mellitus (NIDDM) within 10–15 years.

Although management of GDM is relatively clear-cut there exists lots of controversy in the screening methods used to detect GDM, the timing of screening, and the population to be screened. Studies have shown that selective screening misses 30% of cases of GDM, but universal screening is not cost-effective, especially in populations where there is low prevalence of GDM.

The National Institute of Clinical Excellence (NICE) recommends risk factor-based screening at booking using the OGTT. The risk factors are maternal obesity (BMI above 30 kg/m^2), previous macrosomic baby weighing >4.5 kg, previous gestational diabetes, first-degree relative with diabetes, and south Asian, black Caribbean and Middle Eastern ethnic origins. The test is repeated at 16–18 weeks and 28 weeks if the previous tests are normal. If any new risk factors develop in the present pregnancy, such as persistent glycosuria, macrosomia, or polyhydramnios, the OGTT should be carried out at around 24–28 weeks. After delivery the OGTT is repeated at 6 weeks to identify those women with NIDDM.

Management

Identifying women with GDM is important as there is clear evidence that appropriate therapy can reduce both fetal and maternal morbidity. In a large randomized controlled trial, perinatal complications were 4% versus 1% and the incidence of macrosomia 21% versus 10% in the untreated and treated groups respectively. Treatment includes diet control, exercise, and use of insulin to achieve good blood sugar control. It is also possible that by diet control, regular exercises, and avoidance of obesity, these women can prevent or delay the later development of diabetes.

Screening for Down's syndrome

Down's syndrome is associated with a spectrum of physical and mental handicaps, and some couples elect to terminate an affected pregnancy. Various tests are available for Down's syndrome screening. An ideal screening test is one with maximum sensitivity and specificity. Parents may opt for further invasive tests to confirm diagnosis once they are found to be screen positive.

These invasive tests are not without complications, hence the need for a screening test with a low false-positive rate.

Studies have shown that levels of several fetoplacental products in the maternal circulation are strikingly altered in the presence of a Down's syndrome fetus. Hence blood tests are carried out to measure these markers and give a risk scoring. The screening tests available are first trimester serum screening, measurement of nuchal translucency, second trimester serum screening, and anomaly scan. Combined testing utilizes both first trimester serum markers and nuchal translucency. Triple tests and quadruple tests utilize various serum markers of the second trimester. An integrated test is one in which a combination of first and second trimester screening is used to quantify the risk. A serum integrated test is one in which only first and second trimester serum markers are used in the absence of a scan (Table 5.10.1).

The National Screening Committee recommended that by April 2004 all women should be offered a screening method with a detection rate of 60% and FPR of <5% as a minimum standard. Good standard screening requires all women who present in the first trimester to have a screening test with 75% DR and FPR <3% by April 2007. To achieve this serum markers form an integral part of Down's syndrome screening.

Table 5.10.1 Serum markers for Down's screening (DS) in the first and second trimester and the detection and false-positive rate.

First trimester markers (11–13 weeks)	Deviation in DS (MoM, multiples of median)
PAPP-A (pregnancy associated plasma protein)	0.43
Free β-hCG	1.79
Second trimester markers (15–20 weeks)	
AFP (α-fetoprotein)	0.72
μE₃ (unconjugated oestriol).	0.73
hCG, free β-hCG	2.22
Inhibin-A	1.79

Tests	Detection rate (DR) (%) for 5% FPR	False-positive rate (FPR) for 85% DR
Double test (AFP+hCG)	58	13.1
Triple test (AFP+hCG+ μE₃)	68	9.3
Quadruple test (AFP+hCG+μE₃+inhibin-A)	75	6.2
Combined test	85	6.1
Integrated test	93	1.2
Serum integrated test	88	2.7

Infections in pregnancy

Five infections routinely checked for during pregnancy are rubella, chickenpox, syphilis, hepatitis B and HIV. These tests are done at the time of booking.

Rubella

If pregnant women get primary infection with rubella there is a high risk of the fetus getting congenital rubella. The risk of fetal infection and congenital anomalies is over 80% in the first trimester and 25% in the early second trimester. Congenital rubella affects almost every organ system in the body. One-third of the infected but asymptomatic infants may develop encephalitis and type I diabetes in the second or third decade of life. If a pregnant woman gets primary infection she may wish to terminate the pregnancy after appropriate counselling.

Prevention of maternal infection is the best strategy to avoid congenital rubella. Vaccination of all children with the MMR vaccine and vaccination of susceptible individuals planning for pregnancy is recommended. It is a live attenuated vaccine and contraindicated during pregnancy. Pregnancy should be avoided for at least 3 months after vaccination. Susceptible individuals should avoid contact with other cases of rubella, although in practice this is difficult as most cases are subclinical. Susceptible individuals first detected during pregnancy should have postpartum vaccination 3 months after delivery. Vaccination is known to produce long-term immunity of 16–25 years in 95% of those who receive the vaccine.

Varicella zoster (chicken pox)

Ninety per cent of the antenatal population are seropositve to varicella zoster virus (VZV) and have the IgG antibody. This is acquired immunity due to childhood disease, as chickenpox is a common childhood infection. Primary VZV infection in pregnancy complicates 3 out of 1000 pregnancies.

Chicken pox in pregnancy is associated with increased morbidity to the mother in the form of pneumonia, hepatitis and encephalitis; 1–2% of maternal infection before 20 weeks of gestation results in fetal varicella syndrome (FVS) in the newborn. FVS is characterized by neurological abnormalities, eye defects, limb hypoplasia, and cicatrization of skin. Maternal infection between 20 weeks and up to 36 weeks may present as shingles in the infant in the first few years of life; 25% of the babies develop neonatal varicella if maternal infection occurs 1–4 weeks before delivery.

A live attenuated vaccine is available for prevention of chicken pox. Susceptible women planning a pregnancy are offered this vaccine in the USA and some European countries. Susceptible women should avoid contact with chicken pox. Varicella zoster immunoglobulin (VZIG) is used as post-exposure prophylaxis in susceptible pregnant women to prevent or reduce the clinical manifestation of the disease. Pregnant women who develop chickenpox should be given acyclovir as it is known to lessen disease severity. Intravenous acyclovir is indicated in severe maternal infections, particularly pneumonia. Neither acyclovir nor VZIG is known to reduce the incidence of FVS. Mothers should have a detailed scan in a specialist centre to detect stigmata of FVS. Delivery should be delayed at least a week after the onset of maternal infection to ensure transfer of protective antibodies to fetuses. Babies who are born in the high infectivity period are given VZIG. Acyclovir is the treatment of choice for neonatal infection.

Hepatitis B

Hepatitis B virus (HBV) infection has an acute phase and a chronic carrier state. In the healthy adults 90% of acute HBV infection resolves by 6 months, the remaining 10% develop a chronic carrier state. The risk of perinatal infection from these carriers is as high as 90% in non-immunized infants; 25% of affected children are at increased risk of developing hepatic cirrhosis and hepatocellular carcinoma later in life.

The incidence of the HBV carrier state in pregnant women is approximately 1–2%. 95% of maternal neonatal transmission occurs at delivery and the remainder due to transplacental transmission in the later weeks of gestation.

Mothers who are HBsAg positive are tested further for the presence of anti-HBs, anti-HBc, HBeAg, anti-HBe, specific IgG and IgM for hepatitis A and C. Highly infective carriers are HBeAg positive. The risk of transmission increases from 2–15% in HBeAg-negative carriers to 90% in HBeAg-positive carriers. Carrier mothers should be managed by hepatologists, and their liver function tests monitored to detect chronic active or chronic persistent hepatitis. Partner screening and appropriate counselling of family members is important. Healthcare professionals coming into contact with these mothers should take appropriate precautions during labour and delivery.

Infants born to HBsAg-positive mothers should be given hepatitis B Ig and full course of vaccination. This intervention is found to be protective against transmission in 90% of cases. Breastfeeding is not contraindicated in immunized babies.

Syphilis

Syphilis is a sexually transmitted illness caused by the spirochete *Treponema pallidum*. It has three stages: primary, secondary, and tertiary. Transplacental transmission can occur at any stage. Untreated maternal primary and secondary syphilis lead to symptomatic congenital syphilis in 50% of neonates. These figures are 40% for early latent syphilis and 10% for late latent syphilis. Infection *in utero* can lead to stillbirths, non-immune hydrops, early congenital syphilis and late congenital syphilis of the newborn. Congenital syphilis is a multisystem disorder with the involvement of skin, lymph nodes, liver, spleen, eye, bone, nerves, and heart.

Penicillin therapy in pregnancy is effective for treating maternal disease, preventing transmission to the fetus, and treating established fetal disease. Pregnant women with syphilis should be treated with the appropriate penicillin regimen according to their stage of disease. The risk of congenital infection can be reduced from 10–50% to 1–2% by maternal treatment with penicillin. Partners should be screened and treated. Patients should be screened and treated for other sexually transmitted diseases. There is no contraindication to breastfeeding.

HIV

The prevalence of HIV infection in pregnant women varies from 0.06–0.38% in the developed world to 10–15% in Africa. The National Screening Committee recommends universal screening for HIV. The aim is to increase the uptake of HIV testing to 90%.

HIV and pregnancy

Pregnancy does not accelerate disease progression or reduce the CD4 lymphocyte count. There is increased incidence of miscarriage, preterm delivery, IUGR, and low birthweight. Women on highly active antiretroviral therapy (HAART) do not seem to have an increased incidence of congenital malformations. The major mode of acquisition of HIV in children worldwide is through mother-to-child transmission. This happens antenatally, intrapartum, and postpartum through breastfeeding. Breastfeeding alone accounts for 30–50% of mother-to-child transmission and doubles the rate of transmission. The rate of vertical transmission without prophylactic treatment varies from 15–20% in the developed world to 25–40% in Africa.

Advantages of screening

Reduction of vertical transmission

The risk of perinatal transmission of 15–40% can be reduced to less than 2% with antiretroviral therapy (both antepartum and intrapartum), avoidance of labour and breastfeeding. A blanket policy of Caesarean section for all HIV-positive women is not appropriate. The viral load and CD4 count should be taken into consideration in deciding mode of delivery. It is recommended that breastfeeding should be avoided in HIV-infected women in the developed world, where there is easy access to alternatives. In the developing world the risk of stopping breastfeeding in the form of malnutrition and infections far outweighs the benefits of reducing transmission of HIV.

Appropriate medical management of the woman can be initiated

HIV-infected women should have multidisciplinary care involving an HIV specialist, obstetrician, and paediatrician. HAART in these women is known to reduce viral load, improve CD4 count, and reduce disease progression to AIDS. Women with high viral load and low CD4 count are at high risk of developing opportunistic infections. Such women receive prophylaxis for *Pneumocystis pneumonia*. Women with AIDS may make an informed decision about termination of pregnancy because of reduced life expectancy and increased risk of vertical transmission.

Partner screening and contact tracing

The antenatal period is a good time to offer partner testing and contact tracing in HIV-infected women. Studies have shown that about 30–40% of HIV-infected men and women are unaware of their HIV status.

Precautions for healthcare professionals

Healthcare professionals can take appropriate precautions to prevent risk of transmission to themselves once the HIV status is known. Post-exposure prophylaxis is available for healthcare professionals coming into accidental contact with the blood and body fluids of infected women. There should be clear departmental guidelines on the disposal and disinfection of instruments that have come into contact with infected mothers.

Further reading

Crowther CA, Hiller JE, Moss JR, *et al.* Effect of treatment of gestational diabetes mellitus on pregnancy outcomes. N Engl J Med 2005;352:2477–86.

NICE. Diabetes in pregnancy. NICE clinical guideline 63, July 2008. www.nice.org.uk

Royal College of Obstetricians and Gynaecologists (RCOG). Chickenpox in pregnancy. Guideline No. 13, July 2001. Royal College of Obstetricians and Gynaecologists. www.rcog.org.uk

RCOG. Anti-D Immunoglobulin for Rh Prophylaxis. Guideline no. 22, May 2002. Royal College of Obstetricians and Gynaecologists. www.rcog.org.uk

RCOG. Management of HIV in pregnancy. Guideline no. 39, April 2004. Royal College of Obstetricians and Gynaecologists. www.rcog.org.uk

NICE. The use of routine antenatal anti-D prophylaxis for RhD-negative women. May 2002. www.nice.org.uk

Wald NJ, Rodeck C, Hackshaw AK, *et al.* First and second trimester antenatal screening for Down's syndrome: the results of the Serum, Urine and Ultrasound Screening Study (SURRUS), Health Technology Assessments 2003: 7(11); www.hta.nhsweb.nhs.uk

Yankowitz J, Pastorek II JG. Maternal and fetal viral infections including listeriosis and toxoplasmosis. In: James DK, Steer PJ, Weiner CP, Gonik B. *High risk pregnancy management options.* W.B Saunders 1999:525–58.

Internet resources and patient information:

www.rcog.org.uk
www.nice.org.uk
www.screening.nhs.uk/an
www.arc-uk.org

Complications of early pregnancy

Bleeding and pain in early pregnancy 74
Hyperemesis gravidarum   76
Pregnancy of unknown location 80

Bleeding and pain in early pregnancy

Epidemiology
Vaginal bleeding occurs in about 25% of pregnancies with a positive pregnancy test within the first trimester. It is imperative to make an accurate diagnosis as it can cause unnecessary distress and, rarely, can be life-threatening.

Aetiology
The causes of vaginal bleeding in early pregnancy include:
- miscarriage (threatened, spontaneous, missed, complete, incomplete, or septic)
- ectopic pregnancy
- gestational trophoblastic disease
- gynaecological causes of bleeding such as ectropion
- tumours of the reproductive tract (rare).

Prognosis
In pregnancies complicated by bleeding in the first trimester, 50% will progress beyond 20 weeks, 30% will miscarry, 10% will be an ectopic pregnancy, and 0.2% will be a hydatidiform mole; about 5% will elect to terminate the pregnancy.

Clinical approach
The first step in management is to assess the blood loss and the need for resuscitation. If severe blood loss is seen or suspected, resuscitative measures must begin immediately.

If the patient is clinically stable, diagnostic measures can be undertaken.

Diagnosis
History
- Menstrual history with an accurate last menstrual period where known
- Amount of vaginal bleeding
- Associated backache or abdominal pain: central or lateral
- Shoulder-tip pain (may occur due to diaphragmatic irritation in intra-abdominal bleeding)
- Previous obstetric history.

Examination
- Vital signs, especially pulse rate and blood pressure
- Abdominal distension and tenderness (distension occurs in intra-abdominal bleeding, unilateral tenderness may denote an ectopic pregnancy)
- Speculum examination may help establish the cause of bleeding. A bleeding ectropion may be visible. An open cervical os implies an inevitable or incomplete miscarriage. Products of conception may be seen.
- Bimanual pelvic examination may help to identify an enlarged uterus consistent with an intrauterine pregnancy or reveal a tender adnexal mass in an ectopic pregnancy.

Investigations
Urinary pregnancy test
- Serial β-human chorionic gonadotrophin (hCG). A doubling rate of less than or equal to 48 hours is suggestive of a normal intrauterine pregnancy. Falling levels denote a failing pregnancy. A suboptimal rise occurs in ectopic pregnancy. Unduly high levels occur with trophoblastic disease.

Ultrasound scan
- With a transvaginal scan, an intrauterine gestational sac may be seen as early as 4 weeks. Presence of a yolk sac from 5 weeks is suggestive of an intrauterine pregnancy. A viable intrauterine pregnancy may be visualized from 5 to 6 weeks' gestation. The presence of free fluid with an adnexal mass and empty uterus are associated with an ectopic pregnancy. A snowstorm appearance in the uterus occurs with a hydatidiform mole.
- Serum progesterone levels are also used in some units.

Counselling and management
- In the presence of a viable, intrauterine gestation, the patient is reassured and advised to return if there is excessive bleeding.
- In the presence of a non-viable intrauterine pregnancy, the patient is given the options of conservative, medical, or surgical management of miscarriage considering the clinical conditions.
- A diagnostic laparoscopy may need to be considered if an ectopic pregnancy is suspected with salpingectomy if necessary.
- Ongoing counselling is very important at every step, as it is often an emotionally difficult situation for the parents.
- Use of anti-D should be considered if the patient's blood group is Rhesus negative.
- The parents must be reassured that most subsequent pregnancies will have a normal outcome.

It is important to remember that isolated abdominal pain may be due to an ectopic pregnancy in any woman of reproductive age. Other surgical causes of abdominal pain, such as ovarian accidents, appendicitis, cholecystitis, etc., must also be considered, depending on the clinical presentation.

Further reading
Royal College of Obstetricians and Gynaecologists (RCOG). *The management of early pregnancy loss.* Guideline No. 25. London: RCOG 2006.

Royal College of Obstetricians and Gynaecologists. *The management of tubal pregnancy.* Guideline No. 21. London: RCOG 2004.

Patient information and contacts
Royal College of Obstetricians and Gynaecologists. Patient information leaflet—Bleeding and pain in early pregnancy: information for you. London: RCOG 2008.

Hyperemesis gravidarum

Definition
Nausea and vomiting in pregnancy typically in the first tri-mester resulting in dehydration and ketonuria severe enough to justify hospital admission and require intrave-nous fluid therapy, after exclusion of other causes of vom-iting (Verberg 2005).

Epidemiology
Nausea or vomiting in early pregnancy affects up to 80% of women, but hyperemesis gravidarum (HG) affects only 0.3–1.5%. Typically, symptoms start between 5 and 10 weeks of gestation and resolve by 20 weeks, although up to 10% of women will continue to vomit throughout the pregnancy. The rate of admission for HG falls from 8 weeks onwards (Fell 2006).

Associations
• Ethnicity: higher incidence in Asian women in UK, Asians and Africans in USA, and Pacific Islanders in New Zealand.
• Body mass index: BMI below the normal range (and in some studies above the normal range) is associated with HG.
• Younger maternal age.
• Nulliparity.
• Female fetal sex.
• Multiple pregnancy.
• Family history of hyperemesis.
• Gestational trophoblastic disease (GTD): a recent study suggests this may not now be the case as GTD tends to be diagnosed earlier due to the prevalence of early preg-nancy transvaginal ultrasound (Kirk 2007).
• Coexistent medical disorders (hyperthyroidism, psychi-atric illness, previous molar pregnancy, pre-existing DM, gastrointestinal disorders, and asthma), though these disorders themselves may be causal factors for vomiting.
• Reduced incidence with maternal smoking.
• Psychological stress or ambivalence about pregnancy (may be a cause or effect of HG).

Aetiology
The aetiology of HG is unknown and is likely to be com-plex and multifactorial.

Anatomical
Excessive fluid secretion causing distension of upper gas-trointestinal tract and vomiting.

Infective
Several studies confirm a higher incidence of *Helicobacter pylori* in HG patients than in normal pregnant controls (Golberg 2007) with the density of colonization correlated with the severity of symptoms. This may be due to a change in the gastric pH or an altered immune system dur-ing pregnancy. Alternatively, vomiting itself may cause damage to the oesophagus, facilitating colonization of the mucosa. There is no randomized controlled trial of *H. pylori* treatment to confirm treatment benefit.

Hormonal
• Human chorionic gonadotrophin (hCG) is often thought to be a causal factor and several studies show higher hCG levels in women with HG. This is consistent with the peak incidence of HG occurring when the corpus

luteum is most active in producing hCG and with women with multiple pregnancies and molar pregnancies having a reported increased incidence of HG, but does not explain why some women have prolonged vomiting throughout pregnancy when hCG levels have declined. In addition, women with excess hCG levels (e.g. chorio-carcinoma or exogenous hCG in *in vitro* fertilization (IVF) treatment) do not generally suffer HG. There may be different isoform patterns of hCG in different women, or individual variation in responsiveness to hCG.
• Lower, higher, and similar levels of progesterone have been found in women with HG than in those without HG. Progesterone does not help symptoms, and women with exogenous progesterone support in IVF or with multiple corpora lutea do not have a high incidence of HG; progesterone is unlikely to be a true causa-tive factor.
• High levels of oestrogen have been found in some HG studies and may have a role in slowing the intestinal transit time and gastric emptying, altering gastric pH and causing increased *H. pylori* colonization. However, a causative role does not correlate with the usual resolu-tion of HG after the first trimester, when the oestrogen level continues to rise.
• Leptin, cortisol, adrenocorticotropic hormone (ACTH), growth hormone, and prolactin have been postulated to have causative roles but this is not strongly supported in the literature. In particular some studies suggest lower cortisol and ACTH levels in HG but this is not support-ed by a clear value in corticosteroid treatment.
• Vitamin B6 (pyridoxine) deficiency has been reported but no benefit has been demonstrated with replacement therapy, and the deficiency is likely to be an effect (rath-er than cause) of HG due to increased demands, poor absorption, and decreased intake.

Immunological
Altered immunological factors have been found in women with HG but it is unclear whether these associations are causal or a response to HG.

HG and thyroid disease
• Pregnancy induces physiological alterations in thyroid function (including changes in iodine metabolism, serum thyroid binding proteins and maternal goitre develop-ment) that should be taken into account in the interpre-tation of thyroid funtion test (TFT) results. Physiological stimulation of the thyroid gland is common in early preg-nancy. This is usually assumed to relate to the structural similarity between β-hCG and thyroid stimulating hor-mone (TSH), causing cross-reactivity and excessive stimulation of the thyroid. This association is supported by the mirroring of hCG rise and TSH fall in early preg-nancy and an increased incidence of thyroid overactivity in women with molar or multiple pregnancies. The TSH level has also been shown to correlate with HG symp-tom severity and electrolyte levels.
• If thyroid hormone concentrations fall outside the nor-mal range (high T4, low TSH) this is then termed gesta-tional transient thyrotoxicosis (GTT). In contrast to Grave's disease, GTT is not associated with adverse fetal outcome, and without treatment T4 usually returns to normal levels by 15 weeks and TSH by 19 weeks (Tan 2002).

Prognosis

There is a 15% recurrence rate of HG in future pregnancies (compared with 0.7% if there is no previous HG) and it may be of increased severity in subsequent pregnancies.

Clinical approach

Diagnosis

History

The history should include protracted vomiting. This can be assessed using the validated pregnancy-unique quantification of emesis and nausea (PUQE) score (Koren 2002), which quantifies symptoms over the preceding 12 hours. The history should also aim to exclude symptoms of alternative causes of vomiting such as urinary tract infection, gastrointestinal infection (e.g. diarrhoea), or preceding morbidity (e.g. diabetes). Epigastric pain and haematemesis should be specifically enquired about.

Examinations

Examination of pulse and blood pressure as well as assessment of dehydration from mucous membranes and skin turgour. Abdominal examination should include epigastric palpation, assessment for organomegaly, and lower abdominal examination.

Investigations

- Urinalysis (at least 1+ ketonuria for the diagnosis to be confirmed)
- MSU if positive urinalysis for nitrites or leucocytes.
- FBC to assess for raised haematocrit associated with dehydration as well as anaemia.
- Hypokalaemia is typical with hyponatraemia and raised urea and creatinine in severe cases.
- Elevated liver function tests (LFT) (commonly alanine transaminase or aspartate transaminase) occur in up to 67% of cases, probably from a combination of dehydration, malnutrition, and lactic acidosis. Usually resolves quickly with rehydration and establishment of oral feeding.
- Liver ultrasound and hepatitis screen should be reserved for women with significantly abnormal LFT or in whom liver function does not resolve rapidly with treatment of HG.
- Raised amylase has been reported with hyperemesis due to increased secretions of saliva rather than excessive pancreatic amylase production.

Ultrasound

Although classically twin and molar pregnancies are more common in HG, a recent study suggests that there is no increased prevalence in HG and the early pregnancy loss rate is significantly lower in the presence of HG. However, ultrasound is recommended for maternal reassurance.

Differential diagnosis

Urinary tract infection, gastrointestinal disease, hepatitis, pancreatitis, and Grave's disease.

Management

General points

- Maternal weight, ketonuria, and serum electrolytes should be assessed daily during admission.
- Dextrose-containing solutions should be avoided as they increase the body's requirements for thiamine and thus the chance of precipitating Wernicke's encephalopathy.

- Potassium supplementation should be given initially with the fluid replacement and then tailored to the serum potassium concentration.
- There is good evidence of benefit from antihistamine antiemetics and little evidence of adverse outcomes. 5-Hydroxytryptamine 3 (5HT3) antagonists have a less clear safety record and thus should not be used unless other treatments fail, and after consultation with the woman.
- The benefit of i.v. corticosteroid treatment remains equivocal (Nelson-Piercy 2001). Oral prednisolone alone has not been shown to be effective.
- Serotonin inhibitors have been described for hyperemesis but are not routine.
- Ginger (*Zingiber officinale*) 500–1500 mg orally in divided doses has been shown to be effective in reducing nausea and vomiting in four randomized controlled trials.
- Pryidoxine (B6) also has some effect at reducing symptoms.
- There is equivocal evidence of benefit from acupressure at the P6 point (wrist).
- Thiamine replacement is indicated once vomiting has been occurring for at least 3 weeks (the minimum time shown for thiamine stores to be depleted), to prevent development of Wernicke's encephalopathy.
- Treatment with antithyroid drugs or beta-adrenergic blockers is only indicated if clinical and biochemical features of hyperthyroidism are apparent.

Treatment approach

Treatment is supportive and aimed at managing the symptoms of nausea and vomiting, correcting dehydration and electrolyte imbalance, and at preventing complications such as Wernicke's encephalopathy. Admission to hospital has been recommended for any woman who is ketotic and is unable to maintain adequate hydration, but outpatient management with i.v. fluid and antiemetics is increasingly used. A suitable treatment regime is described below.

Fluids

Normal saline: 1 L with 20 mmol potassium chloride over 2 hours, 1 L with 20 mmol potassium chloride over 4 hours, 1 L over 6 hours, 1 L over 8 hours, followed by 1 L every 8 hours as maintenance regime, with appropriate electrolyte (potassium) replacement according to serum potassium result

Antiemetic

- First line: cyclizine tds i.v. until oral tolerated. An alternative (suitable for outpatient management) is prochlorperazine 3 mg buccal twice daily, increased to 6 mg twice daily if not effective.
- Second line: metoclopromide 10 mg po/i.m./i.v. tds or promethazine 25 mg at night.
- Third line: hydrocortisone 100 mg i.v. bd until able to tolerate oral prednisolone 20 mg bd, reducing weekly to 15 mg bd then continued reducing regime over a further 4 weeks. The reduction should be stopped at a dose below which symptoms recur.
- Steroids should be discontinued if there is no treatment effect within 24 hours of commencement.
- Fourth line: specific 5HT3 antagonists such as granisetron 1 mg po or i.v. or ondansetron 4 mg orally or i.v.

Vitamin supplementation
Thiamine 50 mg orally three times daily. If oral is not tolerated then one pair of Pabrinex (includes thiamine hydrochloride 250 mg) ampoules (diluted in 100 mL of normal saline and infused over 30–60 minutes) as a single i.v. dose. Repeat weekly until oral thiamine is tolerated.

Folic acid 5 mg orally per day (once tolerating oral feeding) to replace diminished stores as a result of the vomiting.

Ranitidine
For women with epigastric pain ranitidine 50 mg i.v. tds followed by 150 mg orally twice daily once tolerated

Iron therapy
Iron therapy, which is likely to exacerbate symptoms, should be stopped and restarted once nausea has settled.

Diet advice
No specific dietary advice (e.g. nil by mouth for first 24 hours) is needed as there is no evidence of benefit of withholding food or fluids.

Antithrombotic prophylaxis
Thromboembolic deterrent (TED) stockings are necessary for all women admitted and low-molecular-weight heparin prophylaxis should be considered.

Management of severe prolonged hyperemesis
In severe cases nasogastric or nasoduodenal feeding has been used. Peripherally inserted central catheters (PICC) lines are associated with an increased rate of maternal infection and venous thromboembolism (VTE) with no extra benefit. Total parenteral nutrition may be indicated in extreme situations.

Complications
Wernicke's encephalopathy, due to vitamin B1 (thiamine) deficiency, is potentially fatal. The classical presentation with the triad of confusion, ocular abnormalities and ataxia occurs in 47%. It is mostly reversible but some residual impairment remains in 60%. The fetal loss rate (excluding termination of pregnancy) with Wernicke's encephalopathy is 37%.

The earliest reported case developed 3 weeks after the onset of vomiting and it is therefore suggested that to prevent Wernike's encephalopathy thiamine is given to women with symptoms for more than 3 weeks.

Serum thiamine levels are unhelpful in making the diagnosis as little vitamin B1 is carried in serum. Magnetic resonance imaging has a high sensitivity for diagnosis, although treatment should not be delayed pending investigation. Observation of rapid improvement helps confirm the diagnosis and any woman presenting with a neurological abnormality in association with HG should be treated with intravenous thiamine (100 mg thiamine i.v. daily (or Pabrinex) then 50 mg orally until a balanced diet resumes.

Other maternal complications
- Central pontine myelinolysis, vasospasm of cerebral arteries, rhabdomyolysis, coagulopathy, acute renal failure and peripheral neuropathy, rupture of the oesophagus and pneumomediastinum have been reported.
- Social, economic, and psychological complications are common with HG, with possible job loss, depression, anxiety, and fear of future pregnancies. Such effects may last into the postpartum period. In particular there is evidence that women with HG can feel uncared for or dismissed by healthcare providers.
- Termination of pregnancy may be carried out for psychological indications (such as the woman feeling she is unable to care for self or existing children) or if the maternal condition is life threatening.

Fetal complications
Retrospective studies suggest possible low birthweight, fetal growth restriction, preterm delivery, low APGAR scores, or congenital abnormality. However, these findings seem restricted to those with poor pregnancy weight gain (less than 7 kg).

Further reading

Fell DB, Dodds L, Joseph KS, *et al*. Risk factors for hyperemesis gravidarum requiring hospital admission during pregnancy. Obstet Gynecol 2006;107:277–84.

Golberg D, Szilagyi A, Graves L Hyperemesis gravidarum and Helicobacter pylori infection: a systematic review Obstet Gynecol 2007;110:695–703.

Jewell D, Young, G. Interventions for nausea and vomiting in early pregnancy. Cochrane Database Syst Rev 2003;4:CD000145.

Kirk E, Papageorghiou AT, Condous G, *et al*. Hyperemesis gravidarum: is an ultrasound scan necessary? Hum Reprod 2006;21:2440–2.

Koren G, Boskovic R, Hard M, *et al*. Motherisk-PUQE (pregnancy-unique quantification of emesis and nausea) scoring system for nausea and vomiting of pregnancy. Am J Obstet Gynecol 2002;186:S228–31.

Nelson-Piercy C, Fayers P, de Swiet M. Randomised, double-blind, placebo-controlled trial of corticosteroids for the treatment of hyperemesis gravidarum. Br J Obstet Gynaecol 2001;108:9–15.

Tan JY, Loh KC, Yeo GS, Chee YC. Transient hyperthyroidism of hyperemesis gravidarum. Br J Obstet Gynaecol 2002;109:683–8.

Verberg MF, Gillott DJ, Al-Fardan N, Grudzinskas JG. Hyperemesis gravidarum, a literature review. Hum Reprod Update 2005;11:527–39.

Patient information and contacts
www.nhsdirect.nhs.uk/articles/article.
aspx?articleId=260&sectionId=11 (23 Sept 2008)

Pregnancy of unknown location

Definition

Pregnancy of unknown location (PUL) is a descriptive term used to classify a pregnancy in a woman who has a positive pregnancy test, but no intra- or extrauterine pregnancy is visualized on a transvaginal ultrasound scan (TVS). There is no evidence of an intrauterine gestational sac or retained products of conception and no adnexal mass suggestive of an ectopic pregnancy.

Epidemiology

It is reported that between 8% and 31% of women referred for an ultrasound in early pregnancy will be classified as having a PUL. It is thought that the higher the quality of ultrasound assessment provided, the lower the PUL rate will be, as hopefully more early intrauterine pregnancies and ectopic pregnancies will be visualized on the initial TVS assessment. It has been suggested that modern units should try to maintain a PUL rate of less than 15%.

Aetiology

PUL has four possible clinical outcomes: intrauterine pregnancy, failing PUL, ectopic pregnancy, and persistent PUL. Although the main concern for many clinicians is that a diagnosis of ectopic pregnancy has been missed, fortunately the majority of PULs are not ectopic pregnancies.

Very rarely a positive pregnancy test is not due to a pregnancy. Other causes include placental trophoblastic tumours and posterior cranial fossa germ cell tumours.

Intrauterine pregnancy

There is no doubt that performing an ultrasound assessment too early in pregnancy may lead to the finding of a PUL. A large number of women will present with intrauterine pregnancies that were just too early to be seen on the initial TVS assessment.

Failing PUL

Studies have shown that the majority of women (50–70%) will have spontaneously resolving pregnancies. However, the true location of the pregnancy may never be known. Although the majority will almost certainly be failed intrauterine pregnancies, a proportion will have failed ectopic pregnancies that were never visualized.

Ectopic pregnancy

Studies have shown that the majority of ectopic pregnancies (>90%) should be visualized on TVS prior to treatment. However, not all of these are visualized on the initial TVS assessment. One study has shown that a quarter of ectopic pregnancies are initially classified as PULs. The reason they are not seen on the initial TVS is that they are probably too small and early in the disease process to be visualized. However, only 7–20% of all women presenting with a PUL will subsequently will diagnosed with an ectopic pregnancy.

Persistent PUL

A small group of women will be diagnosed as having a persistent PUL, which tends to behave biochemically as an ectopic pregnancy. The serum human chorionic gonadotrophin (hCG) levels fail to decline and no evidence of the pregnancy is ever identified by TVS or laparoscopy.

Clinical approach: diagnosis

History

A woman can only be classified as having a PUL if she has a positive urinary pregnancy test or serum hCG level and has had a TVS performed which shows no evidence of either an intra- or an extrauterine pregnancy.

Important things to elucidate from the history include
- date of the last menstrual period
- date of the first positive pregnancy test
- history and nature of any pain
- history and nature of any bleeding: with or without clots, passage of any possible products of conception
- risk factors for ectopic pregnancy (previous ectopic pregnancy, history of pelvic inflammatory disease, history of infertility, previous tubal surgery, assisted conception, use of an intrauterine contraceptive device, or emergency contraception in this pregnancy)
- the results of any previous TVS examinations that may have already been performed.

Although the finding of an empty uterus on TVS with a history of heavy bleeding with clots is highly suggestive of a complete miscarriage, unless a previous ultrasound scan has shown an intrauterine pregnancy, such women should be classified as having a PUL. These women need to be followed up, as a proportion will have an underlying ectopic pregnancy. One study has shown that 6% of women with a history suggestive of a complete miscarriage had an ectopic pregnancy.

Examination

- Abdominal palpation may be unremarkable or confirm an acute abdomen.
- Vaginal examination may be unremarkable or confirm cervical excitation or adnexal tenderness.

Investigations

Serum hCG: Serum hCG is the most commonly used hormone in the management of PULs.

Single levels

A single serum hCG measurement is used by some as a discriminatory level to help with the detection of ectopic pregnancy within the PUL population. The concept was developed with respect to transabdominal ultrasound, when it was reported that the absence of an intrauterine sac at an hCG concentration of >6500 IU/L has a sensitivity of 100% for the detection of ectopic pregnancy. Lower discriminatory serum hCG levels of between 1000 and 2000 IU/L are often used with TVS. However, the use of a single value of serum hCG in a PUL population is of limited value. Many ectopic pregnancies in a PUL population have a low serum hCG level, well below used discriminatory zones, so the clinician may be falsely reassured. Conversely some failing PULs and intrauterine pregnancies may have an initial serum hCG level above the discriminatory zone leading to possible unnecessary intervention in this group.

Serial levels

Serial hCG levels taken 48 hours apart are more useful in the prediction of PUL outcome. Although there are suggested cut-offs for the minimal rise and minimal decrease in serum hCG levels over 48 hours for the prediction of intrauterine pregnancies and failing PULs respectively, unfortunately there is no single way to characterize the behaviour of serum hCG levels in ectopic pregnancies.

The concept of a minimal rise in serum hCG levels of 66% in 48 hours to predict an intrauterine pregnancy has been around for more than 20 years. Recently a more conservative minimal rise of 35% over 48 hours has been suggested to predict intrauterine pregnancy. However, it has been reported that 13–21% of ectopic pregnancies have an hCG rise that mimics an intrauterine pregnancy.

A decrease in serum hCG of >15% over 48 hours has been used to predict a failing PUL. Again, around 10% of ectopic pregnancies will have a fall in serum hCG similar to spontaneous miscarriages.

Serum progesterone: levels of <20 nmol/L have been shown to be highly suggestive of a failing pregnancy. Levels >25 nmol/L are 'likely to predict' and levels >60 nmol/L are 'strongly associated' with viable pregnancies. However, although progesterone levels seem to be good at predicting pregnancy viability, they are relatively poor at predicting pregnancy location.

Management

Expectant management

Expectant management has been shown to be safe for the majority of haemodynamically stable women with PULs. Intervention rates of 0.3–29% have been quoted, but at present there is no consensus as to what is an acceptable intervention rate in this group. Women should be followed up with hormone measurements and repeat TVS examinations until a diagnosis is confirmed or serum hCG levels decline to non-pregnant levels. Diagnostic laparoscopy and curettage may be needed in cases where the clinical situation remains unclear or if the woman is symptomatic or haemodynamically unstable.

Diagnostic laparoscopy

The combination of a positive pregnancy test, an empty uterus on TVS and a serum hCG level above a discriminatory level of hCG is an accepted indication for laparoscopy in many units. However, this policy may lead to a high number of unnecessary surgical interventions. Diagnostic laparoscopy should be reserved for symptomatic women or cases where a concomitant condition such as fibroids may reduce the ability to visualize a pregnancy on TVS.

Uterine curettage

Uterine curettage has been combined into various diagnostic algorithms along with serum hCG and progesterone levels for the prediction of PUL outcome. It should not be used routinely in the management of PULs. It may play a role in diagnosing the location of failing or persistent PULs, but should not be used until the possibility of a viable intrauterine pregnancy has been excluded.

Further reading

Banerjee S, Aslam N, Woelfer B, et al. Expectant management of early pregnancies if unknown location: a prospective evaluation of methods to predict spontaneous resolution of pregnancy. Br J Obstet Gynaecol 2001;108:158–63.

Condous G, Okaro E, Khalid A, Bourne T. Do we need to follow up complete miscarriages with serum human chorionic gonadotrophin levels? Br J Obstet Gynaecol 2004;111:1–3.

Condous G, Timmerman D, Goldstein S, et al. Pregnancies of unknown location: consensus statement. Ultrasound Obstet Gynecol 2006;28:121–22.

Kirk E, Daemen A, Papageorghiou, et al. Why are some ectopic pregnancies characterized as pregnancies of unknown location at the initial transvaginal ultrasound examination? Acta Obstet Gynecol Scand 2008;87:1150–4.

Kirk E, Bourne T. Predicting outcomes in pregnancies of unknown location. Women's Health 2008;4:491–9.

Sagili H, Mohamed K. Pregnancy of unknown location: an evidence-based approach to management. Obstet Gynaecol 2008;10:224–30.

Royal College of Obstetricians and Gynaecologists (RCOG). The management of tubal pregnancy. Green-top Guideline No. 21. London: RCOG 2004.

RCOG. Green-top Guideline No. 25. The management of early pregnancy loss. London: RCOG 2006.

Patient resources

The Ectopic Pregnancy Trust www.ectopic.org.uk

The Miscarriage Association www.miscarriageassociation.org.uk

Care of the fetus

Biophysical profile *84*
Cardiotocography *86*
Doppler ultrasound *90*
Fetal abnormalities: cardiovascular *94*
Fetal abnormalities: central nervous system *98*
Fetal abnormalities: chromosomal anomalies *106*
Fetal abnormalities: genetic disorders *110*
Fetal abnormalities: face *116*
Fetal abnormalities: gastrointestinal system *118*
Fetal abnormalities: limbs *124*
Fetal abnormalities: head and neck *128*
Fetal abnormalities: skeletal abnormalities/dysplasias *132*
Fetal abnormalities: thorax *136*
Fetal abnormalities: urinary system *140*
Fetal movement charts *144*
Fetal nuchal translucency *146*
Fetal abnormalities: hydrops *148*
Invasive procedures *152*
IUGR (intrauterine growth restriction) *156*
Multiple pregnancy *158*
Oligohydramnios *160*
Placental abnormalities *162*
Polyhydramnios *164*
Red blood cell isoimmunization *166*
Screening for fetal aneuploidy *168*
Symphyseal fundal height *172*

Biophysical profile

Definition

The fetal biophysical profile (BPP) score is a real-time ultrasound-based surveillance method that is used to estimate the probability of fetal hypoxaemia at the time of testing. The five variables that constitute the BPP are affected by the amount of oxygen delivery to the brain and kidney. The advantage of the BPP is its ability to evaluate for both acute and chronic fetal compromise (Manning 1984).

This score consists of five parameters: fetal tone, gross fetal movements, fetal breathing movements, amniotic fluid volume (principally related to fetal urine output), and fetal heart rate reactivity (Table 7.1.1).

Pathophysiology

The fetal dynamic variables examined in the BPP are dependent on the activity of their regulatory centres in the brain, the integrity of efferent nervous connections, and an intact effector peripheral apparatus. The activity of these connections can be modulated by physiological mechanisms and fetal disease (Manning 2002).

The most important physiological modifier of fetal activity is physiological variation of its behavioural state. During active states dynamic variables can be observed in a short observation period, while in resting states there may be long periods of inactivity. This is particularly common beyond 34 weeks as fetal rest periods become more frequent.

Pathological conditions that can modulate dynamic variables include chronic hypoxaemia, acidaemia, anatomic defects leading to disruption of neural pathways, and medications that interfere with neurotransmission.

Because individual biophysical variables may be absent due to physiological as well as pathological conditions, five variables have been combined to provide the most accurate prediction of fetal health. To account for behavioural states the BPP is scored over a 30-minute interval and may even be extended over 1 hour near term.

Fetal heart rate variables provide a record of autonomic regulation of intrinsic cardiac activity and its modulation by regulatory centres. The main regulatory centres are the vasomotor centre, reticular activating system, and autonomic nervous system. For the BPP the fetal heart rate reactivity is assessed visually by gestational age-graded criteria.

Amniotic fluid production is dependent on fetal urination and therefore renal plasma flow as well as fetal fluid balance. Since these parameters are dependent on oxygenation, placental fluid exchange and fetal cardiovascular status, the amniotic fluid volume is the only parameter in the BPP that allows longitudinal assessment for chronic fetal deterioration.

Clinical management protocol

The clinical use of the BPP also predicates the appropriate management steps for each score. These recommendations are based on the perinatal morbidity and mortality associated with each score and the accuracy of predicting prelabour acidaemia. The five-component BPP provides an accurate assessment of fetal acid–base status from 20 weeks onward. One parameter that requires special mention is fetal breathing, which is principally determined by maternal/fetal glucose levels: the absence of fetal breathing should be re-evaluated after correction of maternal fasting.

Normal BPP

- Score 10/10, 8/10 (normal AFV), and 8/8 (non stress test not done); normal test result. Fetus is not compromised at the time of testing. The risk for unexplained stillbirth in the week following is 0.9/1000. Interventions should be based on maternal/obstetric factors.

Equivocal BPP (perinatal mortality 7–10/1000)

- Score 8/10 with decreased AFV; in the absence of rupture of membranes this indicates an increased risk for chronic compensated hypoxaemia and/or acute-on chronic decompensation. Delivery is indicated in the presence of fetal lung maturity. For absent fetal lung maturity repeat testing daily.

- 6/10 with normal AFV (equivocal); indicates increased risk for acute asphyxia. In the presence of maturity delivery is indicated otherwise repeat testing in 24 hours should be performed.

Abnormal BPP (perinatal mortality 12–300/1000)

- *6/10 with decreased AFV*; fetus is at risk for chronic asphyxia with possible acute asphyxia. In this group delivery is indicated if gestational age ˘32 weeks. Repeat daily testing is warranted if gestational age is <32 weeks.

- *4/10*; fetus is at risk for acute hypoxia. <32 weeks immediate retesting with extension of the BPP to a full one hour is indicated. For a persistent score of 4/10 delivery is indicated beyond 28 weeks. Before 28 weeks the risk of fetal death versus the risk of prematurity related complications should be individualized. Daily to twice daily monitoring is indicated if delivery is deferred.

- *2/10*; fetus at risk for perinatal death and damage due to acute asphyxia. Caesarean delivery for prelabour acidaemia is indicated at viability.

- *0/10*; fetus is at risk for gross severe asphyxia. Caesarean delivery for prelabour acidaemia is indicated at viability (Manning 1999).

Table 7.1.1 Biophysical profile score (30 minutes)

Variable	For each component presence = 2 points, absence = 0 points
Tone	At least one episode of active limb, trunk or hand extension with return to flexion
Breathing	At least one episode of at least 30 seconds' duration (includes hiccups)
Movement	At least two or more limb movements in 30 minutes (active continuous considered as single movement)
Heart rate	At least two accelerations of 10 beat × 10 seconds (24–28 weeks) 15 beat × 15 seconds (28–34 weeks) 20 beat × 20 seconds (>34 weeks)
Amniotic fluid volume (AFV)	At least one single vertical pocket >2 cm

Adapted from Manning FA, Obst Gynecol Clin North 1999.

The modified biophysical profile

The modified BPP combines the non-stress test (NST, with the option of acoustic stimulation) as a short-term indicator of fetal acid–base status, and the four-quadrant amniotic fluid index (AFI) as an indicator of long-term placental function. An AFI >5 cm generally is considered to represent an adequate volume of amniotic fluid. Thus, the modified BPP is considered normal if the NST is reactive and the AFI is >5, and abnormal if either the NST is non-reactive or the AFI is 5 or less. A normal score gives similar reassurance as a normal five-component BPP. An abnormal modified BPP requires a full five-component evaluation to verify fetal compromise.

Factors that affect the biophysical profile score

There are several important factors that can affect fetal dynamic variables and therefore interpretation of the BPP.

Absence of fetal breathing can occur in the maternal fasting state, and therefore may require retesting after a meal.

A decrease in amniotic fluid volume requires exclusion of membrane rupture.

Administration of corticosteroids (dexamethasone or bethamethasone) to promote fetal lung maturity for anticipated preterm delivery cause a transitory decline in fetal breathing, heart rate reactivity, variability, and fetal movements in the 48 hours following administration. A reduction in amniotic fluid volume may be observed after 72 hours of administration.

Administration of magnesium sulphate can result in decreased fetal activity due to the neuromuscular effects.

In fetal anomalies of the central nervous system, behaviour and heart rate variables may be abnormal due to effects on the central regulatory centres or the connecting pathways.

In certain fetal conditions, such as placenta-based growth restriction or twin–twin transfusion, the rate of clinical progression cannot be anticipated by the BPP alone and other testing modalities such as fetal Doppler are required to adjust surveillance intervals.

The interpretation of the BPP and the appropriate management steps therefore always require consideration of the clinical circumstances.

Further reading

Baschat AA Integrated fetal testing in growth restriction: combining mutivessel Doppler and biophysical parameters. Ultrasound Obstet Gynecol 2003:21:1–8.

Carlan SJ, O'Brien WF. The effect of magnesium sulfate on the biophysical profile of normal term fetuses. Obstet Gynecol 1991;77:681–4.

Jackson JR, Kleeman S, Doerzbacher M, Lambers DS. The effect of glucocorticosteroid administration on fetal movements and biophysical profile score in normal pregnancies. J Matern Fetal Neonatal Med 2003;13:50–3.

Manning FA, Lange IR, Morrison I, Harman CR. Fetal biophysical profile score and non-stress test: a comparative trial. Obst Gynecol 1984;64:326–31.

Manning FA. Fetal biophysical profile. Obst Gynecol Clin North 1999;26:558.

Manning FA. Fetal biophysical profile: a critical appraisal. Clin Obst Gynecol 2002;45:975.

Cardiotocography

Definition

Cardiotocography (CTG) is a well-established and widely practised method of fetal surveillance during labour. Its use has been extended to the antenatal period, and is often also referred to as the non-stress test (NST).

The aim of antenatal CTG is to screen and identify babies with acute/chronic hypoxia or those at risk of developing hypoxia. Fetal hypoxia results in adaptations in the fetus that result in changes in heart rate patterns. Therefore CTG has become a screening tool in high-risk pregnancies (Table 7.2.1).

At present CTG is not recommended as a method of routine fetal assessment in low-risk pregnancies in the UK.

The technique

The CTG is a record of the fetal heart rate (FHR) obtained through a transducer placed on maternal abdomen, usually paired with another transducer that registers uterine activity. The registration is printed on a paper strip. Information regarding baseline fetal heart rate, variability, accelerations, and decelerations is provided.

Antenatal CTG is most commonly performed in the third trimester. But at times, can be performed early on but usually not before 26 weeks. A 20–30 minute long recording of the fetal heart rate pattern is often used on its own (the NST).

Interpretation of the test

Normal/reassuring/reactive (Fig. 7.2.1)

- Should have at least two accelerations (>15 bpm for >15 seconds) in 20 minutes, baseline heart rate 110–160 bpm, baseline variability 5–25 bpm, absence of decelerations

Table 7.2.1 Indications for antenatal fetal monitoring

Maternal conditions	Fetal conditions
Pre-eclampsia	Fetal growth restriction (FGR)
Hypertension	Reduced fetal movements
Diabetes	Multiple pregnancies
Prolonged pregnancy	Fetal anomalies
Vaginal bleeding	Infections
Prolonged rupture of membranes	Genetically inherited diseases
Maternal thyroid, renal or autoimmune disease	

- Sporadic decelerations amplitude <40 bpm are acceptable if duration <15 seconds, <30 seconds following an acceleration
- When there is moderate tachycardia (160–180 bpm) or bradycardia (100–110 bpm) a reactive trace without decelerations is reassuring.

Suspicious/equivocal/non-reactive (Fig 7.2.2)

- Absence of accelerations for >40 minutes. Baseline heart rate 160–180 bpm or 110–100 bpm
- Reduced baseline variability (5–10 bpm for >40 minutes)
- Baseline variability >25 bpm in the absence of accelerations
- Sporadic decelerations of any type unless severe as described below.

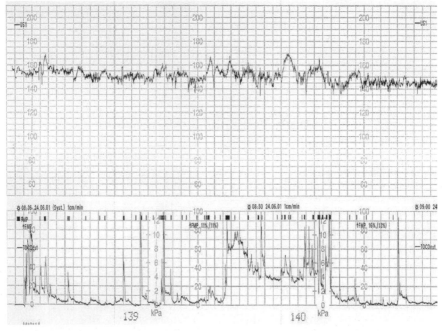

Fig 7.2.1 Normal antenatal cardiotocographs: normal rate, baseline variability, and accelerations.

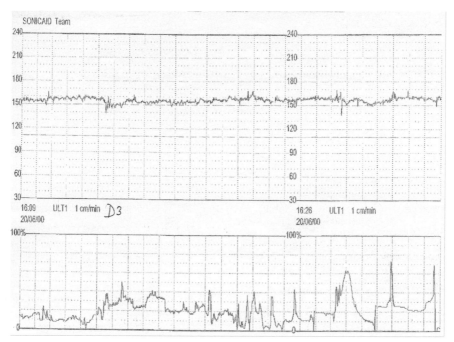

Fig 7.2.2 Equivocal antenatal cardiotocograph. There are no accelerations, the variability is reduced but no decelerations.

Pathological/ominous

- Baseline heart rate <100 or >180 bpm
- Silent pattern (baseline variability <5 bpm) for >40 minutes
- Sinusoidal pattern (oscillation frequency <2–5 cycles/minute, amplitude of >10 bpm for >40 minutes with no accelerations and no period of normal baseline variability)
- Repeated late, prolonged (>1 minute) and severe variable (>40 bpm) decelerations (Fig. 7.2.3).

The main drawback of antenatal CTG is that the analysis of the trace is visual, and there is lack of consistency even between 'experts'. Indeed, the same trace is not interpreted consistently by the same observer.

The NST has been used in combination with other antenatal assessment tools as:

- Contraction stress test (CST): it is based on the intrapartum observation that linked recurrent late FHR decelerations occur with fetal hypoxaemia. The underlying mechanism for this event is a slowing of the fetal heart rate in response to transient systemic hypertension, provoked by reduction in arterial oxygen levels. As developed by Freeman, the CST was performed with intravenous oxytocin infusion until at least three moderate or strong contractions per 10 minutes were generated in a 20-minute window.
- The test was classified as follows:
- Negative: No late or significant variable decelerations.
- Positive: Late decelerations with at least 50% of contractions.
- Suspicious: Intermittent late or variable decelerations.
- This test has shown to have very low rate of false-negative results and false-positive rates at approximately 30%. In current practice, it is used very infrequently following an abnormal NST, due to the introduction of

other non-invasive tests such as the biophysical profile (BPP), and Doppler velocimetry.

- Biophysical profile (BPP): assessment and scoring that includes fetal movements, fetal breathing movements, tone, amniotic fluid volume and assessment of FHR (Chapter 7.1). It was developed by Manning *et al.*, based on the observation that fetal responses to hypoxia are not random, but occur in a precise order. FHR and breathing are affected first, followed by fetal movements and finally tone. Amniotic fluid measurement is important component of fetal biophysical profile.
- Doppler assessment: see chapter on Doppler Ultrasound.
- Computerized CTG: Is an automated evaluation of the fetal heart rate trace. There is a system of analysis that gives criteria of normality for computerized CTG known as Dawes/Redman criteria. The main advantage of a computerized system over visual interpretation is consistency in the interpretation of the CTG trace on different occasions.

Several studies suggest that among all information provided by computerized CTG, the most valuable in predicting fetal hypoxia is short-term variability (STV). Values of STV <5 ms can predict acidaemia with high positive predictive value, which reaches 60% if STV is less than 3 ms (Fig. 7.2.4).

Frequency of testing

The frequency of antenatal surveillance with CTG varies widely in practice, depending on the indication for the CTG and the gestational age. It ranges from weekly to three times a day.

Fig. 7.2.5 shows fetal response to placental insufficiency in a growth-restricted fetus over time.

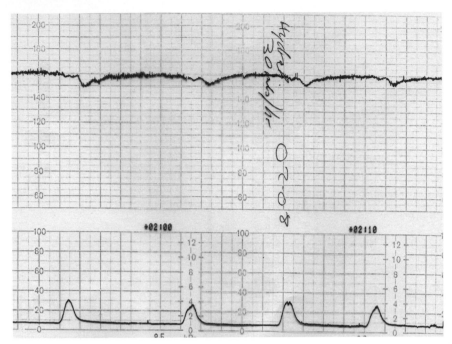

Fig 7.2.3 Pathological cardiotocograph. Poor baseline variability with repeated late decelerations.

It is clear that the changes in Doppler measurements occur well before reduction of fetal movements and intrauterine demise. They have prognostic value and therefore can be a useful tool (e.g. changes in umbilical artery PI) in antenatal surveillance. The fetal heart trace changes take place at the end of the spectrum, occurring as a preterminal event. Indeed, the CTG can be normal within hours of intrauterine demise.

Moreover, an abnormal traditionally carried out CTG is associated with a false-positive rate of up to 50%.

This could explain the lack of benefit of antenatal CTG on perinatal outcome observed in the majority of studies. Six randomized controlled trials have been reported, enrolling 2000 patients, where study groups received either traditional or computerized CTG and control groups received standard care. The meta-analysis failed to show a reduction in rates of perinatal death with CTG use (RR 2.05; 95% CI 0.95–4.42), and even a possibility of harm. In contrast, a comparison of traditional and computerized CTG showed a significant reduction in perinatal mortality with the computerized CTG (RR 0.20; 95% CI 0.04–0.88).

Interpretation and action

Whenever antenatal assessment of fetal wellbeing is performed there should be a plan of intervention/action that depends on both CTG classification and fetomaternal situation.

When CTG is classified as normal it should be repeated according to the clinical situation and the degree of fetal risk.

If a suspicious/equivocal pattern is present, the monitoring should be continued or a CTG repeated within 24 hours. Further testing could also be added (biophysical profile, amniotic fluid index, fetal Doppler flow velocity waveform analysis). If despite these assessments fetal wellbeing is uncertain, admission of the patient with intensive monitoring and betamethasone to accelerate lung maturity (if appropriate) is the most advisable action.

Evidence of a pathological CTG trace should be always followed by action, such as admission of the patient with either induction of labour or Caesarean section. The choice and timing, as previously stated, will depend on gestational age, clinical conditions, and on the health practitioner's evaluation.

Potential adverse effects of antenatal CTG

It is important to take into account the potential adverse effects of this screening test. These may include the consequences of false negative results, inappropriate interpretation and subsequent false reassurance of fetal wellbeing for the mother. On the other hand one should also remember the false-positive results with subsequent unnecessary procedures or interventions that expose both mother and fetus to potential risks. Maternal anxiety following antenatal surveillance should not be underestimated, because high-risk pregnancies are already associated with high anxiety levels that become even more pronounced before and during CTG.

Dawes / Redman criteria NOT MET by FHR1 at 46 minutes.

Signal loss (%) 1.2

Contractions.. 0

Fetal movements (per hour).. 1

    per minute in high... N/A

    per minute in low.. 0.00

Basal heart rate (bpm)... 128

Accelerations > 10bpm and <= 15bpm.. 1

Accelerations > 15 bpm 0

Minor decelerations (area <= 20 lost beats).. 1

Significant decelerations (area > 20 lost beats).. 0

    area of largest deceleration (lost beats)............................. 10

High episodes (minutes).. 0   **✶ ✶**

Low episodes (minutes)... 23

Short term variation (ms).. 4.1   **✶**

Reasons for Failure

No episodes of high variation.

ADVICE ONLY. This is NOT a diagnosis.

Fig. 7.2.4 Pathological computerized cardiotocograph analysis.

Further reading

Dawes GS, Lobb M, Moulden M, *et al.* Antenatal cardiotocogram quality and interpretation using computers. Br J Obstet Gynaecol 1992;99:791–7.

Devoe LD. Antenatal fetal assessment: contraction stress test, non-stress test, vibroacoustic stimulation, amniotic fluid volume, biophysical profile, and modified biophysical profile. An overview. Semin Perinatol 2008;32:247–52.

Grivell RM, Alfirevic Z, Gyte ML, *et al.* Antenatal cardiotocography for fetal assessment. Cochrane Database Syst Rev 2010;1:CD007863.

Lalor JG, Fawole B, Alfirevic Z, *et al.* Biophysical profile for fetal assessment in high risk pregnancies. *The* Cochrane Database Syst Rev 2008;1:CD000038.

National Institute for Health and Clinical Excellence (NICE). Antenatal care: routine care for the healthy pregnant woman. London: RCOG Press 2008.

Turan S, Miller J, Baschat AA. Integrated testing and management in fetal growth restriction. Semin Perinatol 2008;32:194–200.

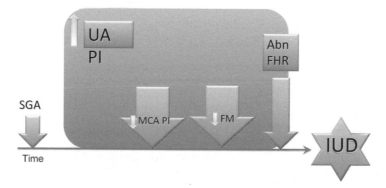

Fig. 7.2.5 Abnormal Doppler pathway. FM, fetal movements; IUD, intrauterine death; MCA, middle cerebral artery; SGA, small for gestational age; PI, pulsatility index.

Doppler ultrasound

Doppler ultrasound is now widely used to investigate the fetal circulation. 'Fetal Doppler' examination involves, in the vast majority of cases, evaluation of the umbilical and middle cerebral artery and, where indicated, the ductus venosus.

The commonest indication for fetal Doppler examination is in the context of a growth-restricted or compromised baby, where there might be fetal hypoxia or even acidaemia. In this context, fetal Doppler changes of individual vessels, using pulse wave Doppler, are highly correlated with hypoxia, and examination of the fetal circulation can give a clinically helpful assessment of the baby's state of health. A recent development of fetal Doppler, the middle cerebral artery peak systolic velocity in the assessment of fetal anaemia, has made a major impact into the fetal medicine care of these babies.

This chapter considers these most common applications of fetal Doppler, and the theory underlying the practice.

Types of Doppler and their clinical application

Most Doppler methods measure velocity in the direction of the ultrasound beam from which the colour flow and Doppler spectrum displays are produced. The requirements of colour flow imaging (including power Doppler) and pulsed wave Doppler are very different.

Colour flow imaging

Produces a colour map of flow over a region of the image. There is limited flow information—the colour shows the mean velocity vector at each point. In general, there is poor temporal resolution—because of the need to sample over a large area, flow images are usually updated at a low frame rate and only moderate spatial resolution.

Pulsed wave (spectral) Doppler

Examines flow at one point within a vessel and represents the distribution of flow velocities within the sample volume with time as the x axis. The static image allows calculation of velocity and flow waveform indices.

Power Doppler (also described as Doppler energy)

This is similar to colour flow imaging but directional information is sacrificed and temporal resolution is reduced to gain better sensitivity to low flow and low velocity situations. It is usually considered a qualitative technique, although there are methods to allow semi-quantitative analysis.

In the majority of applications for obstetric Doppler, a colour flow box is placed over the region of interest, then a specific blood vessel is visualized and then insonated using pulsed wave Doppler. These two Doppler modes will be discussed in more detail. Doppler energy/power Doppler can allow visualization of low velocity flow areas of the fetal circulation but provides mainly qualitative rather than quantitative information.

Fetal Doppler using colour flow imaging can be useful in assessing fetal anatomy; for example, intracardiac Doppler, which requires specialized Doppler settings; arteriovenous malformations; or the extent of liver displacement in diaphragmatic hernia.

Basic physics

For pulsed wave and colour flow Doppler imaging, measurement of velocity is achieved by measurement of the change in phase in the returning echoes from blood at a particular time after transmission. This produces a Doppler frequency described in the well-known equation (Eqn 7.3.1):

$$\text{Doppler frequency } f_d = \frac{2V f_t \cos\theta}{c} \text{ (Eqn 7.3.1)}$$

Where:
f_t is the transmitted ultrasound frequency,
V is the velocity of the blood
θ is the angle between the beam and the direction of flow
c is the speed of sound in tissue

The Doppler frequency determines the colour flow signal or Doppler spectrum. As the equation shows us, the Doppler frequency is dependent on
- blood velocity: as velocity increases so does the Doppler frequency;
- the angle between the Doppler pulse beam and the vessel: The Doppler frequency increases as the beam is at a narrower angle to the flow. There is very little or no signal at angles close to 90 degrees, which is often represented by no colour showing on the colour flow map at these angles.
- ultrasound frequency: higher ultrasound frequencies give increased Doppler frequencies. The 'trade off' is that lower ultrasound frequencies penetrate tissue better.

How are the waveforms assessed and measured?

Multiple indices have been described for the assessment of resistance, for example A/B ratio; S/D ratio; (resistive or Pourcelot index (RI)); (pulsatility index (PI)). Similarly, velocity is described in many different ways: time-averaged velocity (TAV); time-averaged maximum velocity (TAMX); means velocity; peak systolic velocity (PSV); minimum velocity (Vmin), etc.

The most commonly used index, for which most charts exist for fetal Doppler, is the PI, and this index will be discussed below. For velocity, excluding blood flow measurements, PSV is almost universally used in the context of assessing fetal anaemia in the middle cerebral artery (Table 7.3.1).

Fetal vessels

The umbilical artery

The umbilical artery waveform represents placental, not fetal, vascular resistance and should therefore be regarded primarily as an indicator of resistance in the fetoplacental vascular bed rather than representing the fetal circulation.

Studies from the late 1980s and early 1990s established the relationship between abnormal umbilical artery findings (absent end diastolic flow (EDF) or reversed EDF) and adverse perinatal outcome in the context of fetal growth restriction. A meta-analysis of studies of umbilical artery Doppler in a high-risk population showed improved perinatal outcomes where umbilical artery Doppler is performed, although the reason for this is not clear. More recently, it has been suggested that the risk for adverse outcome is highest in small babies with abnormal umbilical

Table 7.3.1

Flow waveform shape:	
Advantages	Does not require angle correction
	Is reproducible across different ultrasound systems
	Provides qualitative information on the circulation and changes in the circulation
	Allows qualitative assessment-'absent end diastolic flow'; reversed end diastolic flow' etc
Disadvantages	Does not provide quantified or standardized information.

Blood flow impedance/velocities:	
Advantages	A measure of quantity, increased in velocities in a vessel can imply increase in flow (for example, MCA PSV in fetal anaemia)
	Velocity can be measured reliably if angle correction is made but requires angles between beam and vessel as close to zero to be accurate
	Impedance indices (PI, RI, S/D, A/B ratio can be calculated from the waveform)
Disadvantages	Angle correction must be correct for velocity measurement
	Mean velocity measurements are subject to instrumentation errors.

Volume flow measurements:	
Advantages	Quantifies volume flow
Disadvantages	Requires measurement of vessel area/diameter, only possible in comparatively large vessels
	Requires measurement of mean velocity in the spectrum
	Difficult to get accurate results; very large errors are possible and likely.

artery Doppler, but also appreciable in those with normal umbilical artery Doppler.

How to perform umbilical artery Doppler
Umbilical artery waveforms are usually obtained from a free loop of umbilical cord, in most cases near the placental insertion where movement artefact is less. The angle of insonation should be less than 60 degrees. There is no consistent significant difference in the shape of the waveform depending upon where the cord is insonated, nor is it common for there to be a difference in waveform between the two arteries, although impedance indices are slightly higher at the fetal end of the umbilical cord, and lower at the placental insertion.

Three major abnormalities of umbilical artery flow are described:
• raised resistance (PI >95th centile)
• absent EDF
• reversed EDF.

From the sixteenth week onwards, the umbilical artery waveform should show positive end diastolic flow. Reduction in end diastolic flow, a rise in PI, absent EDF (Fig. 7.3.2), and reversed EDF represent increasing fetoplacental resistance. At 24–34 weeks, a fetus may have absent EDF in the umbilical artery for days or weeks before delivery is necessary. At very early gestations (between 24–32 weeks), even reversed EDF in the umbilical artery should not, without corroborating evidence from other fetal Doppler measurements, be the sole indication for delivery. At 32–34 weeks, delivery decisions in a growth-restricted baby may be made on the basis of amniotic fluid volume, movements, cardiotocography (CTG), and umbilical artery Doppler. After 34 weeks, absent EDF is unusual and almost always suggests severe fetoplacental pathology warranting delivery; at 32 weeks, reversed EDF would normally warrant delivery.

Key points
• Umbilical artery Doppler is not the same as 'fetal Doppler', but gives an indication about fetoplacental vascular resistance. This does not necessarily correlate Doppler findings of the fetal circulation.
• Absent or reversed umbilical artery end diastolic flow should not dictate delivery prior to 32–34 weeks. This finding normally warrants more detailed investigation in units where fetal Doppler is available, or close observation and investigation using CTG in units where it is not.

The middle cerebral artery
Examination of the fetal middle cerebral artery (MCA) relies on the physiological fetal adaptation to hypoxia called 'brainsparing' or 'cerebral redistribution'. The normal, healthy MCA waveform shows little or no EDF, or even a little reverse flow. From 28–34 weeks end diastolic flow is often seen, and after 34 weeks, the MCA PI may be reduced to its maximum from 'physiological redistribution' due to changes in flow through the heart leading to relatively deoxygenated blood being shunted to the cerebral circulation.

In hypoxia there is a progressive reduction in resistance in the MCA (brain sparing). Where severe hypoxia leads to fetal acidaemia (fetal decompensation), the fetal MCA PI may however show a paradoxical increase in resistance for 24–48 hours before irreversible fetal heart rate changes or fetal death occur. Recent work suggests that hypoxia leading to cerebral redistribution involves subtle differences in perfusion of different areas of the fetal brain. Using a semi-quantitative technique known as fractional moving blood volume (FMBV), based on colour Doppler energy/power Doppler, perfusion of the hindbrain, forebrain, and midbrain has been shown to map differently in normal versus hypoxic fetuses. The clinical importance of this finding is as yet unknown.

MCA Doppler:

Indicator of fetal redistribution-doesn't help time delivery
Difficult in interpretation beyond 36 weeks physiological
increase in cerebral flow

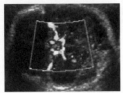

- False negative value not reliable (normal = not reassuring)
- Not all babies redistribute
- Only valuable if abnormal

Fig. 7.3.1 Key points for performance of middle cerebral artery Doppler.

How to perform MCA Doppler
The fetal head is visualized in the biparietal diameter section, and the probe tilted to allow visualization of the greater wing of the sphenoid bone. The course of the MCA follows the wing of the sphenoid bone, allowing it to be seen easily on colour flow Doppler. The anterior vessel is insonated with pulsed wave Doppler in the segment nearest the Circle of Willis (Fig. 7.3.1).

The MCA in anaemia
Measuring MCA peak systolic velocity (PSV) is useful for non-invasive monitoring of babies at risk of anaemia (for example rhesus disease) or a hyperdynamic circulation (for example sacrococcygeal teratoma). The technique is simple and reproducible; the MCA PSV correlates well with fetal anaemia: above the 1.5 multiples of the median (MoM) PSV for gestation, a baby is likely to have anaemia whereas below this level anaemia is very unlikely. Babies at risk of anaemia are frequently followed up on a weekly or 2 weekly basis in fetal medicine units, whereas previously cordocentesis was the only way to establish whether they were anaemic and required transfusion.

The thoracic aorta
The thoracic aorta (TA) is the least frequently visualized major vessel in the investigation of fetal condition. Its flow velocity waveform mirrors the umbilical artery closely, although the resistance in it is usually higher.

Key points
- *Fetal Doppler may become abnormal even in normally grown babies.* This may occur with rapid onset pre-eclampsia or poorly controlled diabetes.
- *Fetal Doppler may be normal after 34 weeks in compromised babies.* Fetal Doppler assessment is not normally considered a reliable in the assessment of post-34-week pregnancies. Umbilical artery Doppler rarely shows major changes, and the MCA PI range already shows maximum physiological dilatation.

Fetal venous Doppler
Umbilical vein
The umbilical vein can give important information especially if for technical reasons the fetal ductus venosus cannot be visualized. It normally has a low velocity continuous flow. Using pulsed wave Doppler, it may be obtained transposed on an umbilical artery waveform;

however, this is not recommended as reversed umbilical EDF may be 'lost' in the venous waveform in the opposite channel. Umbilical vein pulsations may be confused with the common physiological undulations associated with fetal breathing or even fetal movements.

Ductus venosus
The ductus venosus is a short, narrow connection between the umbilical vein and the right atrium of the heart. Early studies established the normal ranges for ductus venosus PI and characterized the changes associated with hypoxia and acidaemia. More recently, the ductus venosus waveform has been considered as the vessel most likely to differentiate between normal and abnormal outcome. 'Early' and 'late' changes in the ductus venosus waveform form the basis for the multicentre TRUFFLE randomized study (www.trufflestudy.org), a management study of severe fetal growth restriction.

How to perform ductus venosus Doppler
Oxygenated blood is directed from the umbilical vein into the fetal circulation towards the foramen ovale. The blood flow in the ductus venosus therefore reflects the pressure gradient between these two stuctures.

The ductus venosus waveform is quite distinguishable from that of the inferior vena cava and hepatic vein. The typical ductus venosus waveform has 's', 'd', and 'a' waves.

The ductus venosus abnormalities are categorized below:
- raised ductus resistance (pulsatility index for vein >95th centile)
- exaggerated a wave approaching the baseline
- reversed a wave (a wave beneath the baseline).

A reversed a wave is an ominous sign and suggests fetal decompensation in the context of uteroplacental insufficiency severe hypoxia/acidaemia. This may also occur in the recipient twin in twin-to-twin transfusion syndrome, and in end-stage fetal anaemia or viral myocarditis.

Integrating fetal Doppler into obstetric practice for the hypoxic baby
Fetal Doppler is useful tool in the management of fetal compromise, particularly in the context of placental insufficiency and hypoxia, and there is good correlation between hypoxia and impedance in individual fetal blood vessels. There are, however, few clues from the literature as to how fetal Doppler measurements should be integrated with assessment of fetal growth, amniotic fluid, movements, and cardiotocography in the management of a fetus. The Growth Restriction Intervention Trial (GRIT), which randomized 'compromised' babies into immediate or delayed delivery, did not show any significant difference in outcome between the two groups nor were there any clues in the use of Doppler. The TRUFFLE study (above) seeks to establish whether delivery of growth-restricted fetuses on the basis of abnormal CTG, 'early', or 'late' ductus venosus changes leads to an improved 2-year perinatal outcome; however, the results will not be available until 2012.

In this context, 'pragmatic' guidelines, such as those in Fig. 7.3.2, agreed by many perinatologists are reasonable to use in everyday practice until definitive evidence becomes available.

Umbilical artery Doppler, delivery if...
at 32/40 reversed EDF
at 34/40 absent EDF
at 36/40 increased PI (>95th centile)

Ductus venosus <32 weeks deliver if...
absent or reversed a wave + CTG STV
abnormal

Doubt still remains about optimal timing of delivery of IUGR fetuses: but evidence
supports waiting until delivery is definitely warranted rather then early
intervention especially in pregnancies <29 weeks

Fig. 7.3.2 Pragmatic consensus of delivery criteria in interuaterin growth restriction.

Further reading

The GRIT study group. Infant wellbeing at 2 years of age in the Growth Restriction Intervention Trial (GRIT): multicentred randomised controlled trial. Lancet 2004;364:513–20.

Figueras F, Eixarch E, Gratacos E, Gardosi J. Predictiveness of antental umbilical artery Doppler for adverse pregnancy outcome in small-for-gestational-age babies according to customised birthweight centiles: population-based study. Br J Obstet Gynaecol 2008;115:590–4.

Loughna P. Intra-uterine growth restriction: investigation and management. Curr Obstet Gynaecol 2003;13:205–11.

Baschat AA, Galan HL, Bhide A, et al. Doppler and biophysical assessment in growth restricted fetuses: distribution of test results. Ultrasound Obstet Gynecol 2006;27:41–7.

Baschat AA. Doppler application in the deliver timing of the preterm growth-restricted fetus: another step in the right direction. Ultrasound Obstet Gynecol 2004;23:111–18.

Turan OM, Turan S, Gungor S, et al. Progression of Doppler abnormalities in intrauterine growth restriction. Ultrasound Obstet Gynecol 2008;32:160–7.

Figueras F, Benavides A, Del Rio M, et al. Monitoring of fetuses with intrauterine growth restriction: longitudinal changes in ductus venosus and aortic isthmus flow. Ultrasound Obstet Gynecol 2009;33:39–43.

Baschat AA, Viscardi RM, Hussey-Gardner B, et al. Infant neurodevelopment following fetal growth restriction: relationship with antepartum surveillance parameters. Ultrasound Obstet Gynecol 2009;33:44–50.

Tchirikov M, Schräder HJ, Hecher K. Ductus venosus shunting in the fetal circulation: regulatory mechanism, diagnostic methods and medical importance. Ultrasound Obstet Gynecol 2006;27:452–61.

Figureras F, Fernandez S, Eixarch E, et al. Middle cerebral artery pulsatility index: reliability at different sampling sites. Ultrasound Obstet Gynecol 2006;28:809–13.

Figueras-Diesel H, Hernandez-Andrade E, Acosta-Rochas R, et al. Doppler changes in the main fetal brain arteries at different stages of hemodynamic adaptation in severe growth restriction. Ultrasound Obstet Gynecol 2007;30:297–302.

Hernandez-Andrade E, Figueroa-Diesel H, Janssons T, et al. Changes in the regional fetal cerebral blood flow perfusion in relation to hemodynamic deterioration in severely growth-restricted fetuses. Ultrasound Obstet Gynecol 2008;32:71–6.

Fetal abnormalities: cardiovascular

Definition
Congenital heart disease (CHD) is defined as an abnormality of the cardiovascular system that is present at birth. The heart is a complex organ, but already formed at around 8 weeks of gestation. Most CHD includes structural defects, but abnormalities with primary myocardial involvement (e.g. cardiomyopathy) or rhythm disturbances (e.g. tachycardias and heart block) may also be congenital. Major heart defects can be defined as those that are lethal or require intervention, either surgical or by cardiac catheterization, in infancy or on long-term follow-up.

Epidemiology
Structural CHD is one of the most serious forms of congenital defects and accounts for approximately 8 in 1000 live births with approximately half being considered major. The percentage of major CHD seen in fetal life is higher, as well as associated chromosomal defects, genetic syndromes, and extracardiac anomalies. Minor defects are being increasingly detected postnatally and if all minor problems are included, postnatal incidence may be as high as 5%.

Aetiology and associations
Chromosomal, genetic abnormalities and environmental agents are well-recognized factors in the aetiology of CHD. Specific genes are increasingly being linked to CHD but non-specific factors and random errors may also lead to heart defects. A non-exhaustive list of some important associations is presented below.

Chromosomal defects and genetic syndromes
- Trisomy 21: About 40–50% of these fetuses will have CHD. The most characteristic defects are atrioventricular septal defect and perimembranous ventricular septal defect (VSD).
- Trisomy 13 and 18: Approximately 90% will have CHD, from simple septal defects to complex lesions. Large perimembranous inlet VSDs are commonly seen in trisomy 18 fetuses.
- Turner syndrome (monosomy X): Left heart involvement including coarctation of the aorta and hypoplastic left heart syndrome.
- Di George sequence and velocardiofacial syndrome (microdeletion of 22q11 and 10p deletion): Typically, conotruncal malformations such as tetralogy of Fallot, truncus arteriosus and interrupted aortic arch.
- Noonan syndrome (chromosome 12q): Pulmonary valve stenosis and hypertrophic cardiomyopathy.
- William syndrome (microdeletion 7q11): Supravalvar aortic stenosis and peripheral pulmonary artery stenosis.
- Holt–Oram syndrome (chromosome 12p): atrial septal defects.
- Ellis–van Creveld syndrome (chromosome 4p).
- VACTER association.
- CHARGE association.

Environmental and maternal factors
- Maternal infection (e.g. rubella)
- Maternal use of teratogenic drugs (e.g. lithium, antiepileptic medication, retinoic acid, alcohol)

- Maternal diabetes: about 2–3% risk of structural CHD in pregestational diabetes. Fetuses may also develop diabetic (hypertrophic) cardiomyopathy later in pregnancy.
- Maternal phenylketonuria
- Maternal collagen disorders (lupus and Sjogren disease). The presence of maternal antibodies (anti-Ro/SSA and anti-La/SSB) is associated with a 2 to 7.5% risk of conduction abnormalities in the fetus (heart block), occurring from around 18 weeks of gestation with the greater risk at 22–24 weeks. Recurrence risk is increased further to 16%.

Family history
Most congenital heart defects occur in low-risk pregnancies, but if there is an affected first-degree relative, the risk of CHD is increased. Table 7.4.1 gives an overall risk estimate for these families, but the relative risk may still vary according to the type of defect present in the proband.

Nuchal translucency
There is a clear association between increased nuchal translucency (NT) in the first trimester and the presence of major CHD. In chromosomally normal fetuses, the higher the NT thickness, the higher the risk of CDH. Table 7.4.1 gives a breakdown of risks depending on NT thickness.

Natural history and antenatal prognosis
Spontaneous fetal demise due to CHD is relatively rare.

In general, most forms of structural CHD are well tolerated during pregnancy and thus do not require fetal therapy. Patency of the three natural shunts in the fetal circulation (the foramen ovale, ductus arteriosus and ductus venosus) allows the circulation to 'bypass' critical lesions and therefore ensure that most fetuses are haemodynamically stable throughout gestation, even though the neonate may require intervention in the first few days of life.

However, structural lesions which are associated with significant atrioventricular or semilunar valve regurgitation or myocardial dysfunction, have a more guarded outlook, as this often coexists with cardiomegaly and heart failure (fetal hydrops). Hydrops may also develop in a fetus with persistent tachyarrhythmia or complete heart block. In the former, hydrops is reversible if the tachycardia is controlled prenatally. In the latter, hydrops is associated with a poor prognosis.

Table 7.4.1 Groups at increased risk for CHD

Family history	Approximate risk
Affected offspring	2–3% (1 child); 10% (2 children)
Parent affected	5% (mother); 2–3% (father)
NT thickness (normal karyotype)	
>95th centile—3.4 mm	2.5%
3.5–4.4 mm	3%
4.5–6.4 mm	10%
6.5–8.5 mm	20%
>8.5 mm	60%

Fetal therapy

Maternal administration of anti-arrhythmic drugs or, less often, direct fetal therapy may be indicated in cases of persistent tachyarrhythmias or when there is circulatory compromise. A decision to treat the arrhythmia prenatally should be balanced against early delivery and postnatal treatment of the newborn.

Fetal intervention for structural CHD such as aortic stenosis was initially attempted long ago but with disappointing results. However, with recent technical advances and better ultrasound image resolution, balloon dilatation of either aortic or pulmonary valves has been performed in highly selected cases in an attempt to improve postnatal morbidity. If balloon valvuloplasty of stenotic valves or atrial septectomy is to be performed in the fetus, a multidisciplinary approach in specialist tertiary referral centres is essential. Long-term results are not available.

Clinical approach to CHD in the fetus

Screening for CHD

Most screening programmes incorporate assessment of the four-chamber view at the time of the 18–23 week scan. Antenatal detection rates based on this alone are generally low, but there is wide regional variation. Screening programmes that include assessment of the outflow tracts have higher detection rates.

In the UK, recent guidelines of the National Institute for Clinical Excellence (NICE) and the Fetal Anomaly Screening Programme (FASP) recommended that all pregnancies be screened by a combination of four-chamber and outflow tract views.

Referral to tertiary centre

Fetal echocardiography should be offered to families at risk of CHD or when an abnormality is suspected.

Suspected (structural or functional) abnormality

If a fetal cardiac abnormality is suspected at any time during pregnancy (often at the routine 18–23 week scan) referral to a specialist in fetal echocardiography should be made as soon as possible. Specialist assessment is essential for accurate diagnosis of the abnormality and to allow concomitant or subsequent counselling by the fetal and/or paediatric cardiologist. A multidisciplinary team that also includes a specialist in fetal medicine and clinical genetics is indicated to assess the presence (or not) of extracardiac malformations and to perform invasive tests, if appropriate.

High-risk pregnancies

Families considered to be at higher risk of CHD should be referred for elective fetal echocardiography, around the time of the routine obstetric scan (18–23 weeks). In selected centres where there are experts in early fetal echocardiography, cardiac scans may be performed from around 12 weeks of gestation. This may be offered to fetuses with markedly increased NT (usually NT >4 mm) or to families with previous history of CHD (usually for reassurance). Owing to the relatively high number of associated non-cardiac problems, a multidisciplinary team approach to early scans is highly desirable.

Ultrasound: diagnostic fetal echocardiography

The variable types of CHD, their wide morphological spectrum and, often, their complex nature means that accurate diagnosis requires the input of a professional who is highly familiar with congenital cardiac malformations and their manifestation both prenatally and postnatally.

There are various terminologies used to describe CHD. The sequential segmental analysis to diagnosis offers a logical approach to describing simple and most importantly, complex malformations.

Counselling and pregnancy management

Extensive consultation usually follows the diagnosis of major CHD in the fetus. Postnatal management options and timing of intervention for the neonate/child with CHD varies with each diagnosis and will be provided by the paediatric/fetal cardiologist. Associated extracardiac malformations need to be diagnosed or excluded by an experienced fetal medicine specialist.

Consideration needs to be given to the option of invasive tests (CVS, amniocentesis or cordocentesis) to assess fetal karyotype. Depending on gestational age at the time of diagnosis, the severity of the lesion and family/religious/social and legal issues, the option of termination of pregnancy will also be discussed.

Follow-up cardiac scans are usually planned at a few weeks' interval. Fetal growth may also be monitored. The importance of a multidisciplinary team approach cannot be overemphasized and a clear perinatal plan should be in place to ensure optimal clinical care of mother and baby.

Perinatal management

The various forms of CHD may be broadly divided into the following categories regarding perinatal management:

CHD requiring early neonatal treatment

Duct-dependent lesions require elective intravenous infusion of prostaglandin E to maintain patency of the ductus arteriosus. This allows early transfer to a cardiac unit where surgery/intervention will be performed prior to discharge from hospital.

Duct-dependent systemic circulation

- Coarctation of the aorta/interrupted aortic arch
- Critical aortic stenosis
- Hypoplastic left heart syndrome
- Complex lesions associated with severe systemic outflow obstruction/aortic arch obstruction.

Duct-dependent pulmonary circulation

- Pulmonary atresia with VSD
- Pulmonary atresia/critical pulmonary stenosis with intact ventricular septum
- Complex lesions associated with critical pulmonary stenosis/atresia.

Simple, complete transposition of the great arteries
Tachy- and bradyarrhythmias

Major CHD associated with neonatal stability

This group includes defects that have a balanced circulation at birth. The newborn baby is expected to be stable, albeit cyanosed in many instances. An elective postnatal assessment should be organized to plan further cardiac follow-up. Time of surgery or interventional cardiac catheterization is often beyond the first month of life.

- Septal defects without significant outflow tract obstruction.
- Tetralogy of Fallot with pulmonary stenosis and adequate forward flow.
- Complex lesions without significant/critical systemic or pulmonary outflow obstruction.

Relatively minor CHD that may not require any treatment

Follow-up can be organized for a few weeks after birth in order to document postnatal findings and plan further follow-up, if needed. Included in this group are small muscular VSDs.

Place and timing of delivery

Delivery should take place where there are good neonatal facilities to support the needs of the newborn baby with CHD, including artificial ventilation if necessary. Women whose fetuses have complete transposition should have their obstetric care transferred to deliver as close as possible to the cardiac unit as balloon atrial septostomy may be required shortly after birth.

In general, delivery will take place at term, providing there are no concerns regarding fetal growth or progression of the cardiac disease to such an extent as to impact on postnatal management.

Most fetuses can be delivered vaginally, but induction of labour may be necessary in order to plan neonatal surgery. A Caesarean section is rarely indicated for cardiac reasons. Exceptions include rhythm abnormalities (e.g. heart block and tachyarrhythmias) that may impact on fetal heart rate monitoring during labour.

Further reading

Lee W, Allan LD, Carvalho JS, et al. ISUOG Consensus Statement: What constitutes a fetal echocardiogram? Ultrasound Obstet Gynecol 2008;32:249–52.

Carvalho JS, Ho SY, Shinebourne EA. Sequential segmental analysis in complex fetal cardiac abnormalities: a logical approach to diagnosis. Ultrasound Obstet Gynecol 2005;26:105–111

Hyett JA, Perdu M, Sharland GK, et al. Increased nuchal translucency at 10–14 weeks of gestation as a marker for major cardiac defects. Ultrasound Obstet Gynecol 1997;10:242–46.

Ghi T, Huggon IC, Zosmer N, et al. Incidence of major structural cardiac defects associated with increased nuchal translucency but normal karyotype. Ultrasound Obstet Gynecol 2001;18:610–14.

Tegnander E, Eik-Nes SH, Johansen OJ, et al. Prenatal detection of heart defects at the routine fetal examination at 18 weeks in a non-selected population. Ultrasound Obstet Gynecol 1995;5:372–80.

Bull C. Current and potential impact of fetal diagnosis on prevalence and spectrum of serious congenital heart disease at term in the UK. Lancet 1999;354:1242–7.

Carvalho JS, Moscoso G, Tekay A, et al. Clinical impact of first and second trimester fetal echocardiography on high risk pregnancies. Heart 2004;90:921–6.

Bonnet D, Coltri A, Butera G, et al. Detection of transposition of the great arteries in fetuses reduces neonatal morbidity and mortality. Circulation 1999;99:916–8.

Internet resources

National Institute for Clinical Excellence: www.nice.org.uk

British Heart Foundation: www.bhf.org

Children's Heart Federation: www.childrens-heart-fed.org.uk

Fetal abnormalities: central nervous system

Neural tube defects

Definition

Neural tube defects include a group of anomalies that share failure of closure (or secondary reopening) of the neural tube: anencephaly, spina bifida and encephalocele.

Incidence

This is subject to large geographical and temporal variations; in the UK the prevalence is about 5 per 1000 births. Anencephaly and spina bifida, with an approximately equal prevalence, account for 95% of the cases, and encephalocele for the remaining 5%. About 90% of cases of spina bifida identified at birth are open.

Aetiology

Chromosomal abnormalities, single mutant genes and maternal diabetes mellitus, or ingestion of teratogens, such as antiepileptic drugs, are implicated in about 10% of the cases. However, the precise aetiology for the majority of these defects is unknown. When a parent or previous sibling has had a neural tube defect, the risk of recurrence is 5–10%. Periconceptual supplementation of the maternal diet with folate reduces by about half the risk of developing these defects.

Pathology

In anencephaly there is absence of the cranial vault (acrania) with secondary degeneration of the brain. Encephaloceles are cranial defects, usually occipital, with herniated fluid-filled or brain-filled cysts. In spina bifida the neural arch is incomplete. Spina bifida is subdivided into open and closed lesions. In open lesions the neural tube is exposed to the external environment and there is always a malformative process of the neural cord. In closed spina bifida the defect is covered by skin and the neural tube is usually intact, although it may undergo secondary damage because of adhesions or compression.

Clinical approach: diagnosis

Anencephaly is usually rapidly recognized from 11 weeks' gestation. At this time the main finding is the absence of the calvarium with exposure of the cerebrum, that usually appears severely deformed (Fig. 7.5.1). This is the first stage of anencephaly, which is also frequently referred to as acrania, or exencephaly. In the following weeks there is progressive reabsorption of the abnormal brain tissue, which is usually completely absent by the second trimester. Associated spinal lesions are found in up to 50% of cases. In the first trimester the diagnosis can be made after 11 weeks, when ossification of the skull normally occurs.

Diagnosis of open spina bifida requires the systematic examination of each neural arch from the cervical to the sacral region both transversely and longitudinally. In the transverse scan the normal neural arch appears as a closed circle with an intact skin covering, whereas in spina bifida the arch is 'U' shaped and there is an associated bulging myelomeningocele (thin-walled sometimes septated cyst). The extent of the defect and any associated kyphoscoliosis are best assessed in the longitudinal scan (Fig. 7.5.2).

The diagnosis of open spina bifida has been greatly enhanced by the recognition of associated abnormalities in the skull and brain. These abnormalities include frontal bone scalloping (lemon sign), and obliteration of the cisterna magna with either an 'absent' cerebellum or abnormal anterior curvature of the cerebellar hemispheres (banana sign) (Fig. 7.5.2). These easily recognizable alterations in skull and brain morphology are often more readily attainable than detailed spinal views. A variable degree of ventricular enlargement is present in virtually all cases of open spina bifida at birth, but in only about 70% of cases in the midtrimester. In England and in many Western countries, screening for fetal neural tube defects with maternal serum alphafetoprotein (where women with an increased concentration of alphafetoprotein (usually 2.5 MoM or more) are referred for a detailed ultrasound examination) has largely been replaced by sonographic screening.

In about 10% of cases, spina bifida is closed, that is covered by skin. In these cases, fetal intracranial anatomy is normal.

Encephaloceles are recognized as cranial defects with herniated fluid-filled or brain-filled cysts. They are most

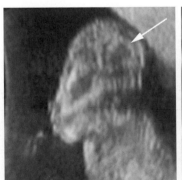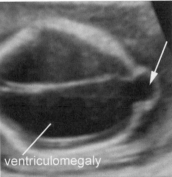

Fig. 7.5.1 (a) anencephaly in late first trimester; the calvarium is absent and distorted brain tissue (arrow) is seen arising from the skull base and floating in the amniotic fluid; (b) cephalocele: severe ventriculomegaly associated with a posterior protrusion of intracranial contents (arrow).

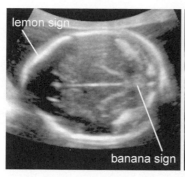
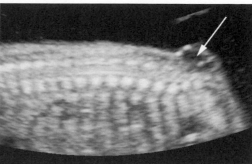

Fig. 7.5.2 (a) Arnold–Chiari malformation in a fetus with open spina bifida: there is frontal bossing (also referred to as *lemon sign*) the cerebellum is poorly delineated because of the absence of fluid in the cisterna magna (also referred to as *banana sign*); (b) myelomeningocele in a midtrimester fetus in the sacral area the neural canal is open and communicates with a septated cystic mass.

commonly found in an occipital location (75% of the cases) but alternative sites include the frontoethmoidal and parietal regions.

Prognosis

Anencephaly is fatal at or within hours of birth. In encephalocele the prognosis is inversely related to the amount of herniated cerebral tissue; overall, neonatal mortality is about 40% and more that 80% of survivors are intellectually and neurologically handicapped. In open spina bifida the surviving infants are often severely handicapped, with paralysis in the lower limbs and double incontinence; despite the associated hydrocephalus requiring surgery, intelligence may be normal. The outcome of closed spina bifida is difficult to predict. Some infants are completely asymptomatic. In other cases, neurological deficits including lower limb weakness to complete paralysis and urinary incontinence may be found.

Management

Termination of pregnancy can be offered to couples. In continuing pregnancies there is no indication to modify standard obstetric management. It has been debated whether fetuses with open spina bifida may benefit from Caesarean section, but no clear evidence exists.

Fetal therapy

There is some experimental evidence that *in utero* closure of spina bifida may reduce the risk of handicap because the amniotic fluid in the third trimester is thought to be neurotoxic. However, there are high risk from such intervention and it remains part of research.

Prevention

Periconceptual supplementation with folic acid reduces the risk of neural tube defects by as much as 50%. The recommended dosage is 400 µg daily for low-risk pregnancies and 4 mg in patients with an increased risk because of a positive familial history.

Ventriculomegaly

Definition

Enlargement of the cerebral lateral ventricles.

Prevalence

Ventriculomegaly (lateral ventricle diameter of 10 mm or more) is found in 1% of pregnancies at the 20–23 week scan.

Aetiology

This may result from chromosomal and genetic abnormalities, intrauterine haemorrhage or congenital infection, although many cases have as yet no clear-cut aetiology.

Clinical approach: diagnosis

Fetal ventriculomegaly is diagnosed sonographically by the demonstration of abnormally dilated lateral cerebral ventricles (Fig. 7.5.3). Certainly before 24 weeks and particularly in cases of associated spina bifida, the head circumference may be small rather than large for gestation. A transverse scan of the fetal head at the level of the cavum septum pellucidum will demonstrate the dilated lateral ventricles, defined by a diameter of 10 mm or more of the posterior horn. The choroid plexuses, which normally fill the lateral ventricles are surrounded by fluid.

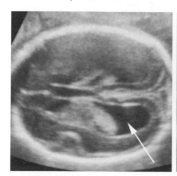
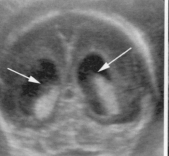
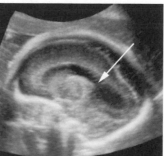

Fig. 7.5.3 Ventriculomegaly: the arrows indicate the distended lateral ventricles.

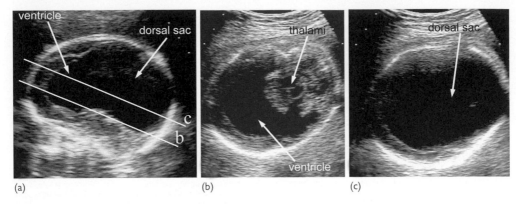

Fig. 7.5.4 Alobar holoprosencephaly in the midtrimester. (a) median plane demonstrating the single ventricular cavity, that has a rim of cortex anteriorly and amply communicates posteriorly with a dorsal sac; (b) axial scan at the level of the thalamus, demonstrating the crescent shaped single ventricle and the absence of the midline in the anterior cortex; (c) in a slightly craniad axial plane than the previous one, the communication between the ventricular cavity and the dorsal sac is demonstrated.

Ventriculomegaly is commonly subdivided into two main groups: mild ventriculomegaly (10–15 mm) and severe ventriculomegaly (15 mm or more).

Prognosis

Fetal or perinatal death and neurodevelopment in survivors are strongly related to the presence of other malformations and chromosomal defects. Although mild ventriculomegaly (atrial width of 10–15 mm) is generally associated with a good prognosis, it is also the group with the highest incidence of chromosomal abnormalities (often trisomy 21). In addition, in a few cases with apparently isolated mild ventriculomegaly there may be an underlying cerebral maldevelopment (such as lissencephaly) or destructive lesion (such as periventricular leukomalacia). Recent evidence suggests that in about 10% of cases there is mild to moderate neurodevelopmental delay. Severe ventriculomegaly is associated with a much increased risk of neurological compromise, that is some studies is in the range of 50% of cases. Fetuses with severe ventriculomegaly may develop intracranial hypertension (hydrocephalus) and require postnatal drainage.

Fetal therapy

There is some experimental evidence that *in utero* cerebrospinal fluid diversion may be beneficial. However, attempts in the 1980s to treat hydrocephalic fetuses by ventriculo-amniotic shunting have now been abandoned because of poor results, mainly because of inappropriate selection of patients.

Management

Excluding associated anomalies is critical. This requires a detailed examination of cerebral and extracerebral anatomy with ultrasound. Fetal karyotyping and work-out for cytomegalovirus and toxoplasmosis infections should be offered. The use of magnetic resonance imaging has also been advocated, although the relative value of this examination compared with ultrasound remains controversial. In continuing pregnancies no modification of standard obstetric management is required. Caesarean section is only clearly indicated in cases with associated macrocrania.

Holoprosencephaly

Definition

This is a spectrum of cerebral abnormalities resulting from incomplete separation of the forebrain. There are three types according to the degree of forebrain cleavage. The alobar type, which is the most severe, is characterized by a monoventricular cavity and fusion of the thalami. In the semilobar type there is partial segmentation of the ventricles and cerebral hemispheres posteriorly with incomplete fusion of the thalami. In lobar holoprosencephaly there is normal separation of the ventricles and thalami but absence of the septum pellucidum. The first two types are often accompanied by microcephaly and facial abnormalities.

Prevalence

Holoprosencephaly is found in about 1 in 10 000 births.

Aetiology

Although in many cases the cause is a chromosomal abnormality (usually trisomy 13) or a genetic disorder with an autosomal dominant or recessive mode of transmission, in many cases the aetiology is unknown. The risk of recurrence for sporadic, non-chromosomal holoprosencephaly, the empirical recurrence risk is 6%.

Clinical approach: diagnosis

In the standard transverse view of the fetal head for measurement of the biparietal diameter there is a single dilated midline ventricle replacing the two lateral ventricles or partial segmentation of the ventricles (Fig. 7.5.4). The alobar and semilobar types are often associated with facial defects, such as hypotelorism or cyclopia, facial cleft and nasal hypoplasia or proboscis.

Prognosis

Alobar and semilobar holoprosencephaly are lethal. Lobar holoprosencephaly is associated with mental retardation

Management

Given the poor prognosis of these defects, termination of pregnancy can be offered to the couples. In continuing pregnancies, no modification of standard obstetric management is indicated.

Agenesis of the corpus callosum

Definition
The corpus callosum is a bundle of fibres that connects the two cerebral hemispheres. It develops at 12–18 weeks of gestation. Agenesis of the corpus callosum may be either complete or partial (usually affecting the posterior part).

Prevalence
Agenesis of the corpus callosum is found in about 5 per 1000 births.

Aetiology
Agenesis of the corpus callosum may be due to maldevelopment or secondary to a destructive lesion. It is commonly associated with chromosomal abnormalities (usually trisomies 18, 13 and 8) and more than 100 genetic syndromes.

Clinical approach: diagnosis
The corpus callosum is not visible in the standard transverse views of the brain but agenesis of the corpus callosum may be suspected by the absence of the cavum septum pellucidum and the 'teardrop' configuration of the lateral ventricles (enlargement of the posterior horns). Agenesis of the corpus callosum is demonstrated in the midcoronal and midsagittal views, which may require vaginal sonography (Fig. 7.5.5).

Prognosis
This depends on the underlying cause. Prenatal studies indicate that 50–100% of fetuses with isolated agenesis of the corpus callosum will have a normal to borderline intelligence at long-term follow-up. Recent studies however suggest a progressive decline in intellectual capacity over the years.

Management
Excluding associated anomalies is critical. This requires a detailed examination of cerebral and extracerebral anatomy with ultrasound. Fetal karyotyping should be offered. The use of Magnetic resonance imaging has also been advocated, although the relative value of this examination compared with ultrasound remains controversial. In continuing pregnancies no modification of standard obstetric management is required.

Dandy–Walker complex

Definition
The Dandy–Walker complex refers to a spectrum of cystic abnormalities of the cerebellum. Most cases diagnosed *in utero* will fall into one of these categories: (a) Dandy–Walker malformation (cystic dilatation of the fourth ventricle that occupies and distend the cisterna magna associated with superior rotation of the cerebellar vermis); (b) vermian hypoplasia (absence of part of the cerebellar vermis usually associated with a cystic dilatation of the fourth ventricle that does not distend the cisterna magna); (c) Blake's pouch cyst (cystic dilatation of the fourth ventricle that causes a superior rotation of the cerebellar vermis that is intact, with a normal sized cisterna magna) and (d) mega-cisterna magna (large cisterna magna, normal vermis, and fourth ventricle).

Prevalence
Dandy–Walker malformation is found in about 1 per 30 000 births. No clear-cut epidemiological data exist with regard to the other entities.

Aetiology
The Dandy–Walker complex is a non-specific endpoint of chromosomal abnormalities (usually trisomies 18 or 13 and triploidy), genetic syndromes, congenital infection or teratogens such as warfarin, but it can also be an isolated finding.

Clinical approach: diagnosis
Enlarged cisterna magna is diagnosed if the vertical distance from the vermis to the inner border of the skull is more than 10 mm (Fig. 7.5.6). Dandy–Walker malformation, vermian hypoplasia and Blake's pouch cyst share in common a cystic dilatation of the fourth ventricle and may be difficult to differentiate. In expert hands, careful scanning with multiple views may however identify the expansion of the cisterna magna with superior elevation of the sinus confluence that is typical of Dandy–Walker malformation, the incomplete formation of the vermis in the presence of a normal cisterna magna that is typical of vermian hypoplasia and the normal appearance of both cerebellum and cisterna magna that is typical of the Blake's pouch cyst (Fig. 7.5.7).

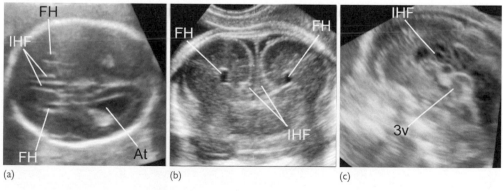

Fig. 7.5.5 Complete agenesis of the corpus callosum; (a) axial plane: the frontal horns are more distant than normal, the cavum septi pellucidi is not present and in its position only a distended interhemispheric fissure is seen; there is a slight enlargement of the atria; the increased separation between the frontal horns and the enlargement of the atria result in a tear-shaped configuration of the ventricle; (b) coronal view: the frontal horns are more distant than normal and have a typical 'comma' shaped appearance; the interhemispheric fissure is distended and the two cerebral hemispheres are separated without any intervening corpus callosum; (c) sagittal view: above the area of the third ventricle the complex formed by the corpus callosum and cavum septi pellucidi is absent and replaced by the fluid contained into the interhemispheric fissure (3v, third ventricle; At, atria; FH, frontal horns, IHF interhemispheric fissure).

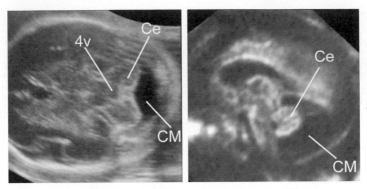

Fig. 7.5.6 Megacisterna magna in axial and sagittal views the cisterna magna is enlarged but the cerebellum appears intact (4v, fourth ventricle; Ce, cerebellum; CM, cisterna magna).

Prognosis

Prognosis depends heavily upon the presence of associated anomalies that are very frequently encountered. Blake's pouch cyst and megacisetrna magna usually have a normal outcome when isolated, and intrauterine regression is often documented. The experience with Dandy–Walker malformation and vermian hypoplasia is limited and no clear-cut figures exist. It would seem however that isolated cases may be completely asymptomatic.

Management

Excluding associated anomalies is critical. This requires a detailed examination of cerebral and extracerebral anatomy with ultrasound. Fetal karyotyping should be offered. The use of magnetic resonance imaging has also been advocated, although the relative value of this examination compared with ultrasound remains controversial. In continuing pregnancies no modification of standard obstetric management is required.

Microcephaly

Definition

Small head and brain.

Prevalence

Microcephaly is found in about 1 in 1000 births.

Aetiology

This may result from chromosomal and genetic abnormalities, fetal hypoxia, congenital infection and exposure to radiation or other teratogens, such maternal anticoagulation with warfarin. It is commonly found in the presence of other brain abnormalities, such as encephalocele or holoprosencephaly.

Clinical approach: diagnosis

The diagnosis is certain when the fetal head circumference is extremely small, 3 SD or more below the mean. However, in many cases the condition is progressive and diagnosis is not possible until late in gestation or after birth. The association with intracranial anomalies (roughly 50% of cases) greatly increases the index of suspicion.

Prognosis

This depends on the underlying cause, but in more than 50% of cases there is severe mental retardation.

Management

Fetal karyotyping and work-out of fetal infection should be offered. In continuing pregnancies no modification of standard obstetric management is required.

Destructive cerebral lesions

Definition

These lesions include hydranencephaly, porencephaly and schizencephaly. In hydranencephaly, there is absence of the cerebral hemispheres with preservation of the midbrain and cerebellum. In porencephaly, there are cystic cavities within the brain that usually communicate with the ventricular system, the subarachnoid space or both. Schizencephaly is associated with clefts in the fetal

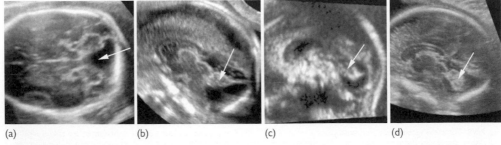

(a)   (b)   (c)   (d)

Fig. 7.5.7 Differential diagnosis of open fourth ventricle; (a) open fourth ventricle in the axial view; (b) Dandy–Walker malformation: the sagittal view (is the most useful approach for a specific diagnosis; the posterior fossa is distended by a fluid accumulation; the cerebellar vermis (arrow) is rotated superiorly; hypoplasia is inferred by the small dimensions and by the absence of the common landmarks, the triangular shape of the fourth ventricle and the main fissures. Notice the high riding tentorium; (c) vermian hypoplasia; the cerebellar vermis (arrow) is rotated superiorly, is very small and is lacking the normal anatomic landmarks; (d) Blake's pouch cyst the cerebellar vermis appears intact and is slightly rotated superiorly, with fluid interposed between it and the brain stem (arrow).

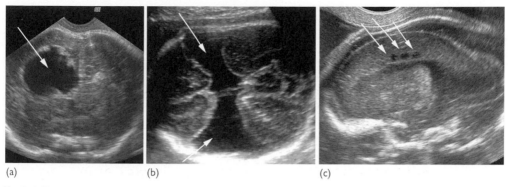

(a)   (b)   (c)

Fig. 7.5.8 Destructive lesions (arrows) of the fetal brain: (a) porencephalic cyst; (b) schizencephaly; (c) periventricular leucomalacia.

brain connecting the lateral ventricles with the subarachnoid space.

Prevalence
Destructive cerebral lesions are found in about 1 in 10 000 births.

Aetiology
Hydranencephaly is a sporadic abnormality that may result from widespread vascular occlusion in the distribution of the internal carotid arteries, prolonged severe hydrocephalus, or an overwhelming infection such as toxoplasmosis or cytomegalovirus. Porencephaly may be caused by infarction of the cerebral arteries or haemorrhage into the brain parenchyma. Schizencephaly may be a primary disorder of brain development or it may be due to early bilateral occlusion of the middle cerebral arteries.

Clinical approach: diagnosis
Differentiation between hydranencephaly and severe hydrocephalus may be difficult at times; the former condition should be suspected when no cerebral mantle can be demonstrated; even with the most severe form of hydrocephalus, a thin cortex and a midline echo are usually demonstrated. In porencephaly there is one or more cystic area in the cerebral cortex, which usually communicates with the ventricle (Fig. 7.5.8); the differential diagnosis is from intracranial cysts (arachnoid, glyoependymal) that are usually found either within the scissures or in the midline and compress the brain. In schizencephaly there are bilateral clefts extending from the lateral ventricles to the subarachnoid space, this is usually associated with absence of the cavum septum pellucidum (Fig. 7.5.8).

Prognosis
Hydranencephaly is usually incompatible with survival beyond early infancy. The prognosis in porencephaly is related to the size and location of the lesion and although there is increased risk of impaired neurodevelopment in some cases development is normal. Schizencephaly is usually associated with severe neurodevelopmental delay and seizures.

Further reading
Adamsbaum C, Moutard ML, Andre C, *et al*. MRI of the fetal posterior fossa. Pediatr Radiol 2005;35:124–40.

Bennett GL, Bromley B, Benacerraf BR. Agenesis of the corpus callosum: prenatal detection usually is not possible before 22 weeks of gestation. Radiology 1996;199:447–50.

Blaas HG, Eik-Nes SH, Vainio T, Isaksen CV. Alobar holoprosencephaly at 9 weeks gestational age visualized by two- and three-dimensional ultrasound. Ultrasound Obstet Gynecol 2000;62–5.

Blaas HG, Eriksson AG, Salvesen KA, *et al*. Brains and faces in holoprosencephaly: pre- and postnatal description of 30 cases. Ultrasound Obstet Gynecol. 2002;19:24–38.

Boddaert N, Klein O, Ferguson N, *et al*. Intellectual prognosis of the Dandy-Walker malformation in children: the importance of vermian lobulation. Neuroradiology 2003;320–4.

Boyd PA, Wellesley DG, De Walle HE, *et al*. Evaluation of the prenatal diagnosis of neural tube defects by fetal ultrasonographic examination in different centres across Europe. J Med Screen 2000;7:169–74.

Bromley B, Benacerraf BR. Difficulties in the prenatal diagnosis of microcephaly. J Ultrasound Med. 1995;303–6.

Chervenak FA, Jeanty P, Cantraine F, *et al*. Spina bifida and anencephaly before and after folic acid mandate—United States, 199 996 and 199 000. MMWR Morb Mortal Wkly Rep. 2004;53:362–5.

Chervenak FA, Rosenberg J, Brightman RC, *et al*. A prospective study of the accuracy of ultrasound in predicting fetal microcephaly. Obstet Gynecol. 1987;69:908–10.

Filly RA, Cardoza JD, Goldstein RB, Barkovich AJ. Detection of fetal central nervous system anomalies: a practical level of effort for a routine sonogram. Radiology 1989;403–8.

Pilu G. Sonographic demonstration of brain injury in fetuses with severe red blood cell alloimmunization undergoing intrauterine transfusions. Ultrasound Obstet Gynecol 2004;23:428–31.

Ghi T, Brondelli L, Simonazzi G, *et al*. Outcome of antenatally diagnosed intracranial hemorrhage: case series and review of the literature. Ultrasound Obstet Gynecol 2003;22:121–30.

Guibaud L, des Portes V. Plea for an anatomical approach to abnormalities of the posterior fossa in prenatal diagnosis. Ultrasound Obstet Gynecol 2006;27:477–81.

Gupta JK, Bryce FC, Lilford RJ. Management of apparently isolated fetal ventriculomegaly. Obstet Gynecol Surv. 1994;49:716–21.

Gupta JK, Lilford RJ. Assessment and management of fetal agenesis of the corpus callosum. Prenat Diagn 1995;15:301–12.

Hobbins JC. The diagnosis of fetal microcephaly. Am J Obstet Gynecol 1984;512–7.

Johnson SP, Sebire NJ, Snijders RJ, *et al*. Ultrasound screening for anencephaly at 11–14 weeks of gestation. Ultrasound Obstet Gynecol 1997;9:14–6.

Klein O, Pierre-Kahn A, Boddaert N, *et al*. Dandy-Walker malformation: prenatal diagnosis and prognosis. Childs Nerv Syst 2003;19:484–9.

Malinger G, Lev D, Kidron D, *et al.* Differential diagnosis in fetuses with absent septum pellucidum. Ultrasound Obstet Gynecol 2005;25:42–9.

Malinger G, Lev D, Zahalka N, *et al.* Fetal cytomegalovirus infection of the brain: the spectrum of sonographic findings. AJNR Am J Neuroradiol 2003;24:28–32.

Melchiorre K, Bhide A, Gika AD, Pilu G. Papageorghiou AT. Ultrasound Obstet Gynecol 2009; 34: 212–24.

Moutard ML, Kieffer V, Feingold J, *et al.* Agenesis of corpus callosum: prenatal diagnosis and prognosis. Childs Nerv Syst 2003; 19:471–6.

Nicolaides KH, Campbell S, Gabbe SG, Guidetti R. Ultrasound screening for spina bifida: cranial and cerebellar signs. Lancet 1986;2:72–4.

Pilu G, Falco P, Perolo A, *et al.* Differential diagnosis and outcome of fetal intracranial hypoechoic lesions: report of 21 cases. Ultrasound Obstet Gynecol 1997;9:229–36.

Pilu G, Sandri F, Perolo A, *et al.* Sonography of fetal agenesis of the corpus callosum: a survey of 35 cases. Ultrasound Obstet Gynecol 1993;3(5):318–29.

Volpe P, Paladini D, Resta M, *et al.* Characteristics, associations and outcome of partial agenesis of the corpus callosum in the fetus. Ultrasound Obstet Gynecol 2006;27:509–16.

Zalel Y, Gilboa Y, Gabis L, *et al.* Rotation of the vermis as a cause of enlarged cisterna magna on prenatal imaging. Ultrasound Obstet Gynecol 2006;27:490–3.

Fetal abnormalities: chromosomal anomalies

Definition
An abnormality in the number or structure of one or more chromosomes.

Epidemiology
The frequency of chromosomal abnormalities is dependent on the age distribution of the population in question as aneuploidies are age related.

Pathology
Abnormal chromosome results
Down's (trisomy 21), Edward's (trisomy 18) and Patau's (trisomy 13) are serious well-described abnormalities associated with severe mental handicap and multiple other congenital abnormalities. Survival even in the absence of major structural malformations in trisomies 13 and 18 is extremely limited; the median survival is 10–15 days. Expectant management during labour is appropriate following discussion with the parents in those that continue the pregnancy.

Fetal aneuploidy: autosomal aneuploidy
Down's syndrome
↑ Nuchal translucency at 11–13 + 6 weeks; also congenital heart disease especially atrioventricular septal defect (AVSD), hyperechogenic bowel, duodenal atresia, other features very subtle.

Edward's syndrome
↑ Nuchal Translucency at 11–13 + 6 weeks; also exomphalos, megacystis, strawberry-shaped head, multiple choroid plexus cysts, congenital heart disease (VSD, dysplastic valves), rocker bottom feet, renal abnormalities, intrauterine growth restriction (IUGR).

Patau syndrome
↑ Nuchal translucency at 11–13 + 6 weeks; also megacystis, exomphalos, holprosencephaly, tachycardia, cleft lip and palate, anophthalmia, polydactyly, congenital heart disease, renal cystic disease.

Triploidy 69,XXY or XXX
Severe early onset symmetrical IUGR. Redating has often occurred at the first trimester scan. Otherwise there are inconsistent ultrasound features such as ↑ nuchal translucency at 11–13 + 6 weeks; spina bifida, congenital heart disease, risk of severe early-onset preeclampsia, abnormal placenta.

Sex chromosome aneuploidies
Turner's syndrome 45,X0
- Very high NT (lethal form), increasing lethality with increasing NT.
- NT <4.5 mm; here the majority will survive. Short stature, primary infertility, coarctation of aorta/other congenital heart disease, horse shoe kidney, neck webbing, and near normal intelligence are features postnatally.

Turner's mosaic 46,XX/46X0
As above, but this tends to be milder; there are no consistent features.

Turner's Mosaic 46,XX(r)/46X0
May have significant mental retardation, particularly likely if XIST gene deleted as the second X chromosome will remain active.

46,XY/45,X0
Majority will be normal males; check genitalia on ultrasound, abnormal genitalia may suggest intersex. Further invasive prenatal diagnosis by amniocentesis is not helpful in assessing the degree of mosaicism. It is not possible to assess future fertility.

47,XXX
Phenotypically normal females, stature minimally raised, IQ 10–15 points on average below unaffected siblings, mild speech delay, introverted personalities, may undergo premature menopause.

47,XXY
Phenotypically normal at birth, one-third have undescended testis, may develop mildly abnormal body proportions, gynaecomastia in puberty, IQ 10–15 points below unaffected siblings, frequently need extra support in normal educational environment, delayed puberty, small testes, primary infertility, poor social adjustment and difficult peer relationships.

47,XYY
Phenotypically normal with a tendency to tall stature. IQ 10–15 points lower than unaffected siblings, speech delay common, impulsive behaviour with poor concentration can cause problems during schooling and antisocial behaviour in adolescence.

Chromosome deletions and duplications (microscopic)
Small chromosome deletions and duplications are more difficult to identify prenatally than postnatally as chromosomes from amniocytes and chorionic villi are shorter than from blood.

Refer for specialist advice as all are rare; there are a few that are more frequent that might be identified antenatally.

4p- (Wolff Hirchorn syndrome)
IUGR, cleft lip and palate, congenital heart disease (CHD), talipes, occasionally exomphalos, postnatally dysmorphic with severe mental retardation.

5p- (Cat Cry syndrome)
Difficult to identify antenatally, maybe IUGR, CHD, postnatally characteristic cry and severe mental retardation.

18p
Mild IUGR, talipes, holoprosencephaly postnatally dysmorphic with severe mental retardation.

Cryptic terminal deletions and duplications and well-known microdeletion syndromes can be rapidly diagnosed using multiple ligation dependent probe amplification (MLPA) but will not be identified on standard karyotype analysis. MLPA can detect up to 40 copy number variants in one reaction and can be used prenatally to look at telomere deletions and duplications when suspected.

Comparative genomic hybridization (CGH) is a powerful tool that can identify microdeletions and duplications in cohorts of previously undiagnosed patients with mental handicap. There is a large variation in copy number variants (CNVs) in the normal population and therefore it is not used in prenatal diagnosis.

Balanced translocations
Robertsonian (whole long arm translocations involving chromosomes 13, 14, 15, 21, and 22, resulting in 45 numerical chromosomes but no phenotypic abnormality as all the

important genetic material is present) (Fig. 7.6.1). Incidence 1:1000.

If it involves chromosomes 14 or 15 check that the fetus has inherited one copy of each chromosome from each parent (UPD, uniparental disomy) as these are both imprinted chromosomes with a parent of origin effect. The risk of heterodisomy is <1%. De Novo Robertsonian translocations need to be checked for UPD but do not have an associated risk of a microdeletion.

Balanced reciprocal translocation (no apparent genetic material missing on cytogenetic analysis under light microscope) (Fig 7.6.2).

Check parental chromosomes, and if the parent carries the translocation reassure that the baby will be normal (if parent is normal); refer for genetic consultation at some stage to discuss implications for future pregnancies and the affected fetus reproductive risks. If it has arisen *de novo* there is a 5% chance of a deleterious effect on the fetus, as it may be associated with a cryptic deletion or duplication or transection of an important gene. Offer a detailed anomaly scan; if this is normal reassure that the risk is lower but still above the population risk of fetal abnormality.

Chromosome mosaicism (more than one cell line with different chromosome numbers)

If this is identified on CVS, 66% will be due to confined placental mosaicism (CPM), i.e. the baby's chromosomes are normal. If there is a high percentage of CPM, placental insufficiency may develop and therefore regular growth scans and early delivery may be required. An amniocentesis will be needed to clarify whether it is true mosaicism or CPM.

If the mosaicism is identified on amniocentesis in the absence of any ultrasound abnormalities, it is not possible to advise on the degree of disability from the percentage of abnormal cells, it is only possible to say that there is a high risk of mental handicap; the presence of associated ultrasound abnormalities raises the risk enormously. Mosaic trisomy 20 in amniotic fluid maybe associated with a normal outcome. Other mosaic trisomies that are more commonly seen at amniocentesis and may have a phenotypic effect include trisomies 8, 9, 16, and 22; mosaic trisomy 1 has never been seen; trisomy 2 is reasonably frequently seen at CVS but very very rarely at amniocentesis.

Marker chromosome (extra chromosome material not identified as a whole extra chromosome)

Check for presence in parents; if present in parent outcome is excellent, there is a small risk if it is mosaic in the parent that if present in every cell that it could have a phenotypic affect.

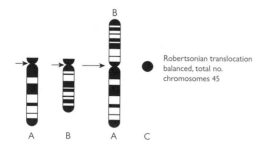

Fig. 7.6.1 Reciprocal and Robertsonian translocation.

Robertsonian translocation balanced, total no. chromosomes 45

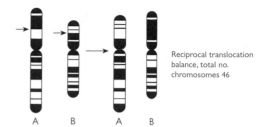

Reciprocal translocation balance, total no. chromosomes 46

Fig. 7.6.2 Reciprocal translocation.

Poor prognostic indicators for marker chromosomes:
- de novo
- large markers
- ring chromosome
- known deleterious marker
- fetal anomalies present on ultrasound
- contains euchromatin.

Approximately 30% of *de novo* markers identified prenatally will be associated with a phenotypic effect.

Common marker chromosomes

Idic(15), psudic (15)(pter-q12::q13-pter)

No ultrasound abnormalities, severe mental retardation with epilepsy and autism. Check marker chromosome by FISH using SNRPN probe; if present abnormal phenotype confirmed, if absent normal phenotype, may have some affect on fertility.

Idic (22)

In the absence of euchromatin, the normal phenotype is likely. Large markers cause variable phenotype. Cat eye syndrome idic (22) (pter-q11.2) May pick up congenital heart disease (total anomalous pulmonary venous drainage (TAPVD), Fallots tetralogy), renal abnormalities (atresia, ectopic kidneys) other features such as eye coloboma, preauricular skin tags and anal abnormalities cannot be picked up antenatally.

Iso chromosome 12p (Pallister Killian syndrome)

Diaphragmatic hernia, large birthweight, sacral teratoma, severe mental retardation; multiple other dysmorphic features are unlikely to be diagnosed antenatally.

The marker chromosome needs to be identified; a second invasive test may be required to confirm its origin as it may be present in only a small proportion of cells and the preparation of the original sample may not be appropriate for such tests.

Further reading

Crolla JA. FISH and molecular studies of autosomal supernumerary marker chromosomes excluding those derived from chromosome 15: II. Review of the literature. Am J Med Genet 1998; 75:367–81.

Crolla JA, Long F, Rivera H, Dennis NR. FISH and molecular study of autosomal supernumerary marker chromosomes excluding those derived from chromosomes 15 and 22: I. Results of 26 new cases. Am J Med Genet. 1998;75:355–66.

Gardner RJM, Sutherland GR. *Chromosome abnormalities & genetic counseling.* 2003.

Gribble SM, Prigmore E, Burford DC, *et al.* The complex nature of constitutional de novo apparently balanced translocations in patients presenting with abnormal phenotypes. J Med Genet 2005;42:8–16.

Kagan KO, Avgidou K, Molina FS, *et al*. Relation between increased fetal nuchal translucency thickness and chrom. defects. Obstet Gynecol 2006;107:6–10.

Kalousek DK, Vekemans M. Confined placental mosaicism. J Med Genet 1999;33:529–33.

Pandya PP, Kondylios A, Hilbert L, *et al*. Chromosomal defects and outcome in 1015 fetuses with increased nuchal translucency. Ultrasound Obstet Gynecol 1995;5:15–9.

Rasmussen SA, Wong LYC, Yang Q, *et al*. Population based analyses of mortality in trisomy 13 and trisomy 18. Pediatr 111:777–84.

Surerus E, Huggon IC, Allan LD. Turner's syndrome in fetal life. Ultrasound Obstet Gynecol 2003;22:264–7.

Vissers LE, de Vries BB, Osoegawa K, *et al*. Array-based comparative genomic hybridization for the genomewide detection of submicroscopic chromosomal abnormalities. Am J Hum Genet 2003;73:1261–70.

Wolstenholme J. Confined placental mosaicism for trisomies 2, 3, 7, 8, 9, 16, and 22: their incidence, likely origins, and mechanisms for cell lineage compartmentalization. Prenat Diagn 1996;16:511–24.

Internet resources

Antenatal results and choices:www.arc-uk.org

Down's syndrome association: www.downs-syndrome.org.uk

Fetal abnormalities: genetic disorders

Definition

A genetic disorder is a pathological condition caused by an absent or defective gene or by a chromosomal aberration (the latter are discussed in Section 3.6, Chromosomal anomalies).

Clinical approach

Prenatal diagnosis is available for an ever-increasing number of genetic disorders. It is important to ascertain at the beginning of a consultation a couple's expectations for prenatal diagnosis and their desired outcome. For many couples, continuation of the pregnancy is the only option they would consider and therefore invasive prenatal diagnosis will be putting the pregnancy at unnecessary risk. For others, even a low risk of abnormality is too high.

There are a number of different investigations that may confirm a diagnosis of a genetic disease. It is important to consider the gestation at which it is possible to diagnose the disorder and the accuracy and safety of the investigation being considered.

There are two different ways in which a diagnosis might be suspected:

- known genetic disorder in the family
- suspected genetic disorder from screening investigations.

The UK has a comprehensive Genetics Service and advice/appointments can be available for pregnancies at risk within a week of a request (see BSHG website).

Inheritance patterns: Mendelian inheritance patterns

Mendelian inheritance patterns are summarized in Figure 7.7.1 and consist of autosomal dominant, autosomal recessive and x-linked inheritance patterns. Some diseases become more severe as they pass from one generation to the next, a process known as anticipation. This includes fragile X syndrome, Huntington's chorea, and myotonic dystrophy. All are due to variable numbers of triplet repeats within the gene. The transmitting parent may influence the chance of expansion.

Inheritance patterns: non-Mendelian inheritance

Mitochondrial

All mitochondria are inherited maternally and they have their own genome. If a gene is transcribed from the mitochondria, all children of an affected mother are at risk, but the risk is impossible to predict, as it is likely that both normal and mutated mitochondria will both be present (heteroplasmy). Many genes that are coded for by the nuclear genome are transcribed in the mitochondria and in this case would follow Mendelian inheritance patterns.

Parent of origin affect

Uniparental disomy

Deletion from one parent having a different effect depending if of maternal or paternal origin.

Epigenetic

All cells in an individual with an altered gene expression pattern that does not affect the DNA structure and therefore will not be passed on to future generations.

Known genetic disorder within the family

Confirm the diagnosis in the affected patient within the family

Letter of confirmation needed or follow-up from clinician involved in affected patient's care.

What is the risk to the present pregnancy?

- Does this risk justify prenatal diagnosis?
- Would a termination of pregnancy be considered by the couple for this disease?
- Would a diagnosis alter the management of the pregnancy, labour or early neonatal care?

Type of prenatal diagnosis to be considered

- Invasive prenatal diagnosis
  - Molecular: confirmation of parental carrier status and affected patient's mutations essential. Check that the laboratory will undertake prenatal diagnosis and if they need extra samples. Most laboratories will require parental samples to check for maternal contamination. Some tests take longer than others and therefore prompt testing is advisable for example myotonic dystrophy and fragile X syndromes.
  - Enzyme diagnosis: confirmation of enzyme diagnosis in affected patient, parental enzyme levels may be necessary as in some diseases such as metochromatic leukodystrophy there maybe abnormally low levels of the enzyme even in carriers due to rapid metabolism of the enzyme.
  - Cytogenetic: karyotype report in affected/carrier individuals to look at chromosome breakpoints, these maybe more difficult to visualise in prenatal samples and therefore may require FISH or molecular cytogenetic techniques for accurate analysis. (see further under chromosome abnormalities)
- Non-invasive prenatal diagnosis
  - Ultrasound: what gestation is it possible to identify the abnormalities?
    The variability of the syndrome features needs to be considered.
    — Certain conditions can only be visualized later as there are no phenotypic abnormalities early on such as achondroplasia
    — Others cannot be seen due to the resolution of the ultrasound and evolving development of the normal structure such as the corpus callosum (see later for US diagnosis)
  - MRI scan: specialized investigation that normally aids rather than replaces ultrasound as the investigation of choice.
  - Non-invasive prenatal diagnosis (NIPD) by free fetal DNA (ffDNA) (see below).

Non-invasive prenatal diagnosis

ffDNA

Three per cent of free DNA in maternal blood is of fetal origin and these short segments of DNA (100–200 kb) are mainly in the form of nucleosomes. This free DNA needs to be enriched for the fetal component to be identified from the maternal ffDNA.

At the present time we can use this for fetal sexing (e.g. fetus at risk of an X-linked disorder) to avoid invasive prenatal diagnosis (PND) and for sexing in congenital adrenal hyperplasia for steroid treatment of possible affected females only. It is also used for Rhesus genotyping of the fetus in Rhesus-negative mothers.

Other uses of this technology at the time of going to press are still in the research setting. New dominant mutations suspected on ultrasound can be identified if there is a

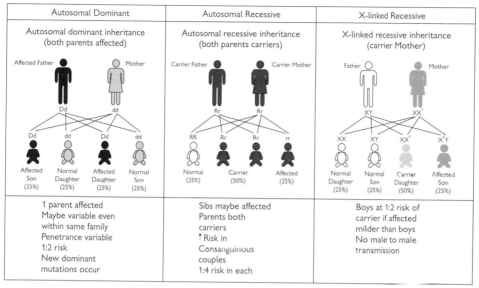

Autosomal Dominant	Autosomal Recessive	X-linked Recessive
Autosomal dominant inheritance (both parents affected)	Autosomal recessive inheritance (both parents carriers)	X-linked recessive inheritance (carrier Mother)
Affected Father — Mother Dd — dd Dd / dd / Dd / dd Affected Son (25%) / Normal Daughter (25%) / Affected Daughter (25%) / Normal Son (25%)	Carrier Father — Carrier Mother Rr — Rr RR / Rr / Rr / rr Normal (25%) / Carrier (50%) / Affected (25%)	Father — Mother XY — XX^r XX / XY / XX^r / X^{r}Y Normal Daughter (25%) / Normal Son (25%) / Carrier Daughter (50%) / Affected Son (25%)
1 parent affected Maybe variable even within same family Penetrance variable 1:2 risk New dominant mutations occur	Sibs maybe affected Parents both carriers ↑Risk in Consanguinous couples 1:4 risk in each	Boys at 1:2 risk of carrier if affected milder than boys No male to male transmission

Fig. 7.7.1 Mendelian inheritance patterns. See also colour plate section.

single mutation causing the disease, such as in achondroplasia and Apert's syndrome. Paternally inherited mutations can also be looked for in maternal blood. If a couple are at risk of having a child with an autosomal recessive disease, then providing the parents carry different mutations, i.e. an affected baby would be a compound heterozygote, it would be possible to look for the paternal allele in the maternal blood.

At the present time much work is going on to develop a test for chromosomal aneuploidy by ffDNA. Such tests may not be able to detect all trisomic fetuses, as they require heterozygosity of the markers used.

Genetic abnormality suggested from screening investigations

Increased nuchal translucency (NT)
- <3.5 mm, and normal chromosomes on chorionic villus sampling (CVS): no further extra investigations. In units only offering quantitative fluorescence polymerase chain reaction for chromosomes 13, 18, and 21 any NT >3 mm should automatically generate a full karyotype.
- >3.5 mm: a 20-week detailed cardiac scan and detailed anomaly scan by a fetal medicine specialist should be performed.
- The higher the NT the poorer the prognosis, whatever the underlying cause; congenital heart disease and diaphragmatic hernias are the most consistent associations but many rare genetic syndromes have been associated with increased NT.

Abnormal first trimester serum biochemistry
- Very low pregnancy-associated plasma protein-A (PAPP-A): pregnancy at increased risk of placentation problems
- ↓ oestriol steroid sulphatase deficiency (X-linked ichthyosis), may have microdeletion at Xp22.3 therefore need to check chromosomes and FISH analysis for this.

- ↓PAPP-A in second trimester maybe associated with Cornelia de Lange syndrome.

Second trimester ultrasound abnormalities (at the 20-week scan)
Confirmation of abnormality is strongly recommended in a fetal medicine unit.

Head
- *Microcephaly*: check parental head circumference, examine brain structure, follow growth, as frequently it is progressive. Fetal MRI in the third trimester to check for neuronal migration abnormalities, exclude congenital infection, and examine rest of the baby. Many syndromes—including chromosomal and syndromes such as Cornelia de Lange syndrome, frequently do not present until late in gestation and many are of postnatal onset. Familial recurrence is easily missed. Boys head circumference is normally bigger than girls even antenatally
- *Macrocephaly*: check parental head circumference, examine brain structure, if normal look at overall growth of baby. Generalized macrosomia in second trimester think of Simpson Golabi Behmel Syndrome; late macrosomia consider other overgrowth syndromes—Beckwith Weidemann, Soto's, isolated macrocephaly – PTEN mutations, Gorlin's syndrome:

Simpson Golabi Behmel Syndrome
X-linked recessive
- Prenatal: early-onset overgrowth, congenital heart disease (VSD/other), diaphragmatic hernia, cleft lip and palate.
- Postnatal: mental retardation, supernumerary nipples, cardiac dysrythmias, tumour risk, e.g. hepatoblastoma, sarcoma.

Beckwith Wiedemann
Complicated genetics, mostly sporadic secondary to imprinting defects. Autosomal dominant and chromosomal abnormalities around 11p15 account for a proportion.

- Prenatal: small omphalocele, macroglossia, nephromegaly, overgrowth
- Postnatal: hypoglycaemia. The majority have normal IQ, tumour risk, Wilms and hepatoblastoma depending on genetic cause of Beckwith Weidemann syndrome.

Offer full karyotyping and methylation studies of chromosome 11p15.

Soto's syndrome
Majority new dominant secondary to NSD mutations on chromosome 5q35
Unlikely to pick up prenatally as no major congenital abnormalities.
- Postnatal: mental retardation, triangular shaped head.

PTEN and Gorlin's
Both have large heads in the absence of other evidence of overgrowth. PTEN very variable presentations; can be associated with mental retardation and autism and tumour risk. Gorlin's syndrome is secondary to mutations in the PTCH gene. Shows fusion of ribs occasionally, cleft lip and palate mandibular cysts and propensity to develop basal cell carcinomas.

Abnormal skull shape: consider craniosynostosis syndromes

Apert's syndrome
The majority are due to new dominant mutations. All are caused by two mutations in FGFR2
- Prenatal: all sutures but lamboidal fused at birth but unsure at what gestation this is apparent. Prominent eyes/proptosis, flat face, cutaneous/bony syndactyly of hands and feet. 3D ultrasound may be helpful. It can be confirmed by fetal DNA studies.
- Postnatal associated with mild to moderate mental retardation.

Pfeiffer syndrome
Autosomal dominant, prenatal lethal form FGFR1 + FGFR2 mutations
- Prenatal: coronal craniosynostosis, Lethal form clover leaf skull, severe proptosis, broad halluces and thumbs, partial hands and feet syndactyly

Saethre Chotzen
Autosomal dominant very variable penetrance
- Prenatal: unlikely to identify any features in absence of family history and even then very unlikely without molecular confirmation of TWIST mutation
- Postnatal: asymmetrical coronal synostosis, ptosis, mild mental retardation, prominent ear crus, skin syndactyly.

Clover leave
Skull may be present with thanatophoric dysplasia (FGFR3 mutation). Look at long bones: telephone handle femur
- Prominent forehead maybe present in achondroplasia.

Brain abnormalities
- Ventriculomegaly: If severe, consider hydrocephalus in a male, look for aqueduct stenosis (X-Linked hydrocephalus) with severe mental retardation. Store DNA for LICAM mutational analysis
- Risk of mental handicap with isolated ventriculomegaly in absence of any other brain abnormality.
  - Mild 12–13 mm at 22 weeks ~90% normal development

- Moderate 14–15 mm at 22 weeks ~60% normal development
- Severe >15 mm at 22 weeks; very high risk of moderate to severe mental retardation
- Agenesis of the corpus callosum. If isolated, risk of mental handicap is around 50%. In the presence of associated abnormalities, it is likely to be nearly 100%
- Cerebellum
  - Agenesis of the cerebellar vermis: almost 100% risk of mental handicap. If partial risk is about 25%. Consider Joubert's syndrome
  - Cerebellar hypoplasia: bilateral is associated with poor prognosis, unilateral maybe normal if brain is otherwise normal. Chromosome abnormalities are common.

MRI is useful to look for evidence of lissencephaly in the third and LIS1 + DCX1 lissencephaly syndromes + Walker Warburg Syndrome.
  - Other syndromes associated with cerebellar hypoplasia: Smith Lemli Opitz syndrome. Prenatal: ambiguous genitalia in male, polydactyly; Postnatal: mental retardation, two or three toe syndactyly, microcephaly, ptosis. If suspected, maternal urine can be tested for seven dehydrosteroids.

Carbohydrate deficient glycoprotein syndrome (CDG): Many different types have been described. This is unlikely to be picked up prenatally in the absence of family history. Cannot screen antenatally using isoelectric focusing of transferring. Phosphomannomutase levels for CDG1 can be measured
- Encephalocele
  Small encephalocele with no apparent brain tissue good prognosis
  Other encephaloceles high risk of mental handicap
- + polycystic kidneys and polydactyly: Meckel Gruber syndrome
- + hydrocephalus and lissencephaly: Walker Warburg Syndrome.

Short Long bones
  (see Chapter 7.12 on skeletal dysplasia)

Other skeletal problems
- Talipes
  - Diastrophic dysplasia
  - Relative macrocephaly
- Flat face
  - Chondrodysplasia punctata (look for punctuate calcification particularly in knee + ankle + spine)
- Polydactyly
  - First trimester short rib polydactyly syndromes, from 15 weeks Ellis Van Creveld look for congenital eart disease), Jeunes asphyxiating thoracic dystrophy
- Late onset short limbs achondroplasia +frontal bossing.

Limb reduction defects
- Terminal transverse defect single limb good prognosis
- Radial ray defect
  - + cardiac abnormalities, Holt Oram syndrome
  - Chromosome breakage (need to contact laboratory prior to taking sample to arrange special transfer to appropriate laboratory) Fanconi syndrome,

- + vertebral + renal abnormalities consider VATER syndrome if chromosome breakage is normal.
- Limb reduction with ectrodactyly
  - Look for IUGR, low PAPP-A in mid-trimester Cornelia de Lange syndrome.

Arythrogryposis

Talipes normally isolated but need to undertake second scan 4 weeks after first to check isolated and no progression to another joints

If multiple joints:
- Joint dislocations: Larsen's syndrome, nail patella
- Fetal constraint
  - Prelabour rupture of membrane
  - Uterine abnormalities (rare)
- Fetal akinesia sequence
  - Primary muscle disorder: congenital muscular dystrophy, congenital myopathy, may have polyhydramnios.
  - Primary neurological disorder: many disorders including haemorrhage/anoxia. Check for hepatosplenomegaly (neurometabolic).
  - Maternal + fetal myotonic dystrophy. This maybe asymptomatic in the mother check for premature cataracts, shake her hand for evidence of myotonia, DNA for myotonin expansion.
  - Maternal myasthenia gravis, may be asymptomatic, ask about symptoms muscle weakness especially when tired; measure maternal anti cholinesterase antibodies. If diagnosis confirmed seek specialist advice for Rx.

Polyhydramnios is a poor prognostic sign as suggests baby is unable to swallow and baby may die soon after birth from pulmonary hypoplasia.

Fetal hydrops see Chapter 7.17
- Fetal anaemia (high middle cerebral artery Doppler)
  - Rhesus disease + other blood group incompatibility (haemolysis)
  - Parvovirus (aplastic anaemia)
  - Haemorrhage
  - Blackfan diamond syndrome (aplastic anaemia).
- Cardiac causes
  - Cardiac conduction defects
  - Long QT (maternal + paternal ECGs)
  - Anti-Rho antibodies (maternal systemic lupus erythematosis)
  - Cardiomyopathy
  - Noonan's syndrome (look for ↑ NT, pulmonary valve disease) PTPN11 mutation
  - Costello syndrome (look for ↑NT, early onset polyhydramnios) HRas mutation
- Neurometabolic, look for hepatosplenomegaly Gaucher's disease, Nieman pick type C, carbohydrate-deficient glycoprotein syndrome
- Obstructive
- Idiopathic.

Fetal renal disease

Bilateral renal agenesis

Universally lethal, associated with oligohydramnios. 25% will be secondary to a *de novo* mutation in RET. Mainly sporadic but need to undertake. Parental renal ultrasound as may have renal abnormality which will affect recurrence

risk, parents will need to be examined for evidence of branchio Oto renal syndrome (branchial clefts, ear abnormalities).

Unilateral renal agenesis

Good prognosis, look for single umbilical artery, features of VACTERL (vertebral, cardiac, tracheo-oesphageal fistula, renal defects, limb defects (radial ray) will not see anal abnormalities.

Polycystic kidneys

Bright kidneys on ultrasound if large and oligohydramnios likely diagnosis autosomal recessive polycystic kidney disease (ARPKD) but differential includes multiple acyl-CoA dehydrogenase deficiency (MADD). PM essential to differentiate different diseases.

Bright kidneys with normal amniotic fluid which may be large need to consider autosomal dominant polycystic kidney (ADPKD) look at parental kidneys, prognosis is good, renal function tends to be normal in childhood but follow up required with paediatric nephrologists for prompt management of hypertension and UTIs.

Bright kidneys with development of second trimester polyhydramnios, check maternal α-fetoprotein if ↑consider Finnish nephropathy (if parents of Finnish ancestry can undertake mutational analysis to confirm otherwise not possible).

Gastrointestinal abnormalities

Exomphalos

Thirty per cent associated with chromosome abnormalities, small exomphalos and those with other abnormalities highest risk. Need to consider Beckwith Weidemann syndrome 11p15 methylation studies can be undertaken to look for this.

Gastroschisis

Normally isolated in young mothers, incidence increasing for unknown reasons often associated with IUGR, may require early delivery. Associations:
- Hyperechogenic bowel
- Cystic fibrosis
- Trisomy 21
- Fetal infection.

Ambiguous genitalia

Discordance between fetal karyotype and ultrasound appearance, occasionally identified on ultrasound in absence of karyotypic known sex.

Check with laboratory that no error in report writing has taken place or sampling; take maternal and paternal blood to check for maternity/paternity. FISH studies for SRY gene. If necessary undertake ffDNA studies on mother.

46,XX with male genitalia
- Congenital adrenal hyperplasia
- SRY translocated to X chromosome.

46XY with female genitalia
- Campomelic dysplasia: look at long bones
- Smith Lemli Optiz syndrome
- Androgen insensitivity syndrome (AIS) (may have family history).

Further investigations during the pregnancy
- Fetal blood sample

- FBC for anaemia and platelets, can identify immunodeficiency syndromes but first trimester diagnosis by DNA diagnosis should be used if available
- Viral infections PCR for virus and immunoglobulins
- Chromosomes
- Amniocentesis
- Chromosomes if not performed
- Amniotic fluid for culture of fibroblasts.

Non-invasive
- 3D ultrasound, can see facial features more clearly may help to define a syndrome more clearly
- Fetal MRI
  - Brain abnormalities more clearly identified, most useful in third trimester, brain pathology difficult at post mortem and therefore even if termination is going to be performed it maybe useful to clarify abnormalities:
  - Lissencephaly
  - Neuronal migration defects (nodular heterotopias, polymicrogyria)
  - Tubers in tuberculus sclerosis
- Maternal blood sample
  - Viral titres: compare with booking blood samples (may not show evidence of infection). If strongly suspicious, may need invasive test
  - Maternal antibodies
  - ABO/Rh, platelets—fetal anaemia, ventriculomegaly
  - Anti-Rho: fetal Heart block
  - anticholinesterase antibodies: arythrogryposis.

Further investigations on the baby
Feticide
If a feticide is being performed and if DNA might be needed, store a sample at this stage. If a karyotype has not been undertaken, take blood. Amniotic fluid may need to be used for metabolic investigations, store at −20°C.

Delivery
Live birth
Cord blood can be used for many investigations. Planning ahead is essential with correct bottles and laboratory addresses. Discussion with neonatal unit on possible complications and interventions that can be anticipated.

After termination of pregnancy
Post mortem
Post mortem is essential to try and clarify underlying diagnosis, it may not clarify this but without a certain prenatal diagnosis recurrence risks will definitely be inaccurate. For example many syndromes cause polycystic kidneys and a ductal plate malformation needed to confirm ARPKD from ADPKD and other cystic kidney diseases. Skeletal Dysplasia need X-rays and histology for clarification of the type.

Placental histology may be useful in clarifying evidence of placental insufficiency secondary to pre-eclampsia, chronic intervillositis, or chromosome mosaicism.

Further reading
Bakalis S, Sairam S, Homfray T, et al. Outcome of antenatally diagnosed talipes equinovarus in an unselected obstetric population. Ultrasound Obstet Gynecol 2002;20:226–9.

Boltshauser E. Cerebellum-small brain but large confusion: a review of selected cerebellar malformations and disruptions Am J Med Genet A 2004;126A:376–85.

Brady AF, Pandya PP, Yuksel B, et al. Outcome of chromosomally normal livebirths with increased fetal nuchal translucency at 10–14 weeks' gestation. J Med Genet. 1998;35:222–4.

Estroff JA, Scott MR, Benacerraf BR. Dandy-Walker variant: prenatal sonographic features and clinical outcome. Radiology 1992;185:755–8.

Fratelli N, Papageorghiou AT, Prefumo F, et al. Outcome of prenatally diagnosed agenesis of the corpus callosum. Prenat Diagn 2007;27:512–7.

Has R, Ermiş H, Yüksel A, et al. Dandy-Walker malformation: a review of 78 cases diagnosed by prenatal sonography Fetal Diagn Ther 2004;19:342–7.

Joó JG, Tóth Z, Beke A, et al. Etiology, prenatal diagnostics and outcome of ventriculomegaly in 230 cases Fetal Diagn Ther 2008;24:254–63.

Mehta TS, Levine D. Imaging of fetal cerebral ventriculomegaly: a guide to management and outcome. Semin Fetal Neonatal Med 2005;10:421–8.

Niesen CE. Malformations of the posterior fossa: current perspectives Semin Pediatr Neurol. 2002;9:320–34.

Pandya PP, Kondylios A, Hilbert L, et al. Chromosomal defects and outcome in 1015 fetuses with increased nuchal translucency. Ultrasound Obstet Gynecol 1995;5:15–9.

Papageorghiou AT, Fratelli N, Leslie K, et al. Outcome of fetuses with antenatally diagnosed short femur. Ultrasound Obstet Gynecol 2008;31:507–11.

Poretti A, Wolf NI, Boltshauser E. Differential diagnosis of cerebellar atrophy in childhood. Eur J Paediatr Neurol 2008;12:155–67.

Poretti A, Prayer D, Boltshauser E. Morphological spectrum of prenatal cerebellar disruptions. Eur J Paediatr Neurol 2008 Oct 20. [Epub ahead of print]

Scott RH, Douglas J, Baskcomb L, et al. Methylation-specific multiplex ligation-dependent probe amplification (MS-MLPA) robustly detects and distinguishes 11p15 abnormalities associated with overgrowth and growth retardation. J Med Genet. 2008;45:106–13.

Shackleton CH, Marcos J, Palomaki GE, et al. Dehydrosteroid measurements in maternal urine or serum for the prenatal diagnosis of Smith-Lemli-Opitz syndrome (SLOS). Am J Med Genet A 2007;143A:2129–36.

Vissers LE, de Vries BB, Osoegawa K, et al. Array-based comparative genomic hybridization for the genomewide detection of submicroscopic chromosomal abnormalities. Am J Hum Genet 2003;73:1261–70.

Volpe P, Paladini D, Resta M, et al. Characteristics, associations and outcome of partial agenesis of the corpus callosum in the fetus. Ultrasound Obstet Gynecol 2006;27:509–16.

Wolstenholme J. Confined placental mosaicism for trisomies 2, 3, 7, 8, 9, 16, and 22: their incidence, likely origins, and mechanisms for cell lineage compartmentalization. Prenat Diagn 1996;16:511–24.

Wright CF, Burton H. The use of cell-free fetal nucleic acids in maternal blood for non-invasive prenatal diagnosis. Hum Reprod Update 2008.

Internet resources
Gene Reviews: www.geneclinics.org
OMIM: www.ncbi.nlm.nih.gov
BSHG: www.bshg.org.uk
National Metabolic Biochemical Network: www.metbio.net

Fetal abnormalities: face

Facial clefts

Definition
Facial clefts encompass a wide spectrum of defects (unilateral, bilateral and less commonly midline) usually involving the upper lip, the palate, or both. The typical cleft lip will appear as a linear defect extending from one side of the lip into the nostril. Cleft palate associated with cleft lip may extend through the alveolar ridge and hard palate, reaching the floor of the nasal cavity or even the floor of the orbit. Isolated cleft palate may include defects of the hard palate, the soft palate, or both. Cleft lip and palate is unilateral in about 75% of cases and the left side is more often involved than the right side. Cleft palate without cleft lip is a distinct disorder.

Prevalence
Facial clefting is found in about 1 per 800 births. In about 50% of cases both the lip and palate are defective, in 25% only the lip and in 25% only the palate is involved.

Aetiology
Cleft lip with or without cleft palate is usually an isolated condition, but in 20% of cases it is associated with one of many genetic syndromes. Isolated cleft palate is a different condition. All forms of inheritance have been described, including autosomal dominant, autosomal recessive, X-linked dominant and X-linked recessive. Associated anomalies are found in about 50% of patients with isolated cleft palate and in about 15% of those with cleft lip and palate. Chromosomal abnormalities (mainly trisomy 13 and 18) are found in 1–2% of cases and exposure to teratogens (such as antiepileptic drugs) in about 5% of cases. Recurrences are type specific; if the index case has cleft lip and palate there is no increased risk for isolated cleft palate, and vice versa. Median cleft lip, which accounts for about 0.5% of all cases of cleft lip, is usually associated with holoprosencephaly or the oral-facial-digital syndrome.

Clinical approach: diagnosis
The sonographic diagnosis of cleft lip depends on demonstration of a groove extending from one of the nostrils inside the lip and possibly the alveolar ridge and anterior palate. Both axial and coronal planes can be used (Fig. 7.8.1). Three-dimensional ultrasound may be useful (Fig. 7.8.2). The diagnosis of isolated cleft palate is difficult.

Prognosis
Minimal defects, such as linear indentations of the lips or submucosal cleft of the soft palate, may not require surgical correction. Larger defects cause cosmetic, swallowing, and respiratory problems. Recent advances in surgical technique have produced good cosmetic and functional results. However, prognosis depends primarily on the presence and type of associated anomalies.

Micrognathia

Definition
Mandibular hypoplasia causing a receding chin. Differentiation from cases in which the mandible is of normal size but is dislocated posteriorly (retrognathia) may be difficult.

Prevalence
Micrognathia is found in about 1 per 1000 births.

Aetiology
Micrognathia is usually associated with genetic syndromes (such as Treacher Collins, Robin and Robert syndromes), chromosomal abnormalities (mainly trisomy 18 and triploidy), and teratogenic drugs (such as methotrexate). The Robin anomalad (severe micrognathia, glossoptosis and a posterior cleft palate or an arched palate) may be a sporadic isolated finding (in about 40% of cases) or it may be associated with other anomalies or with recognized genetic and non-genetic syndromes.

Clinical approach: diagnosis
Several approaches to diagnosis have been suggested, including measurement of the mandible. However, most would use a subjective evaluation of the profile in which there is evidence of a receding chin (Fig. 7.8.3). In severe cases, glossoptosis can also be noted and increases the likelihood of the condition.

Prognosis
This depends on the presence of associated anomalies. Severe micrognathia can be a neonatal emergency due to airway obstruction by the tongue in the small oral cavity.

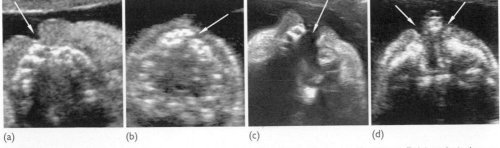

(a)   (b)   (c)   (d)

Fig. 7.8.1 Axial planes of the maxilla in fetuses with facial clefts: (a) isolated cleft lip: the alveolar ridge is intact albeit irregular in shape as frequently happens in these cases; b) unilateral cleft lip and palate: the defect only extends to the alveolar ridge; note that one toothbud is missing but that the secondary palate does look intact; these defect is frequently referred to as cleft alveolus; (c) unilateral cleft lip and palate: the defect is seen extending to the secondary palate: (d) bilateral cleft lip and palate; the anterior protrusion of the central portion of the maxilla (or premaxilla) indicates that the defect expends posteriorly to the secondary palate.

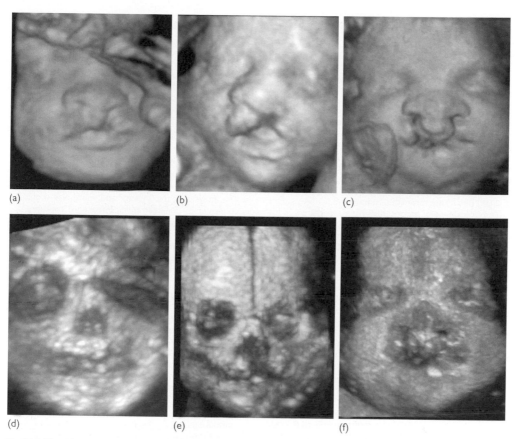

Fig. 7.8.2 Three dimensional ultrasound of cleft lip in rendering of the surface (a, b, c) and skeletal mode (d, e, f); (a, c) unilateral cleft lip; b,e) unilateral cleft lip and palate; c,f) bilateral cleft lip and palate.

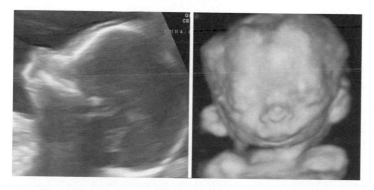

Fig. 7.8.3 Severe micrognathia in bidimensional and three-dimensional ultrasound.

If prenatal diagnosis is made, a paediatrician should be present in the delivery room and be prepared to intubate the infant.

Further reading

Berge SJ, Plath H, Van de Vondel PT, et al. Fetal cleft lip and palate: sonographic diagnosis, chromosomal abnormalities, associated anomalies and postnatal outcome in 70 fetuses. Ultrasound Obstet Gynecol 2001;18:422–31.

Bromley B, Benacerraf BR. Fetal micrognathia: associated anomalies and outcome.J Ultrasound Med. 1994 Jul;13(7):529–33.

Ghi T, Perolo A, Banzi C, et al. Two-dimensional ultrasound is accurate in the diagnosis of fetal craniofacial malformation. Ultrasound Obstet Gynecol 2002;19:543–51.

Rotten D, Levaillant JM, Martinez H, et al. The fetal mandible: a 2D and 3D sonographic approach to the diagnosis of retrognathia and micrognathia. Ultrasound Obstet Gynecol. 2002;19:122–30.

Rotten D, Levaillant JM. Two- and three-dimensional sonographic assessment of the fetal face. 2. Analysis of cleft lip, alveolus and palate. Ultrasound Obstet Gynecol 2004;24:402–11.

Fetal abnormalities: gastrointestinal system

Anterior abdominal wall defects

Definition
Defect in the anterior abdominal wall allowing herniation of intra-abdominal contents.

Epidemiology
Exomphalos (also referred to as omphalocele) prevalence of 1:4000 births; gastroschisis prevalence of 1:3000 births.

Body stalk anomaly (1:10 000 births with some studies reporting 1:14 000–42 000). Exstrophy and epispadias complex: bladder exstrophy (1 in 30 000 births) and cloacal exstrophy (which can be part of omphalocele-exstrophy-imperforate anus-spinal defects (OEIS) complex) (1 in 200 000 births) are rarer conditions.

The prevalence of gastroschisis has risen sharply in the last 20 years and is strongly associated with young maternal age. Mothers under 20 years old have a 12-fold increase in risk. Exomphalos in contrast increases with advanced maternal age.

Pathology
Exomphalos: This is a midline defect of the abdominal closure that involves the cord insertion. There is herniation of small bowel and/or liver, which are both wrapped in a two-layered sac formed by the amnion and the peritoneum. Exomphalos can also be a large defect and cases containing stomach, large bowel, bladder, and spleen have been reported. Rupture of the sac can occur and in such cases differential diagnosis with gastroschisis can be difficult. Less often there is associated failure of the cephalic or caudal embryonic folds with Pentalogy of Cantrell and bladder/cloacal exstrophy respectively.

Gastroschisis: This involves evisceration of bowel through a small abdominal wall defect, usually to the right of the umbilical cord insertion. The defect is possibly related to abnormal involution of the right umbilical vein.

Body stalk anomaly, or more appropriately, amniotic rupture sequence is characterized by a large body wall defect with fusion of the fetal peritoneum to the amniotic cavity and fetal tethering to the side wall. It is thought to occur as a result of early rupture of the amnion before the coelomic cavity is obliterated.

Bladder exstrophy results from a defect in the caudal fold of the anterior abdominal wall. These range in size from an epispadias to exposure of the posterior bladder wall.

Cloacal exstrophy is usually present as part of multiple defects present in OEIS complex that comprises exomphalos, bladder exstrophy, imperforate anus, and spinal defects.

Aetiology
Exomphalos: In the majority of cases the aetiology is sporadic. There is a strong association with chromosomal abnormalities, mainly trisomy 18 and 13 (about 50% at 12 weeks, 30% at midgestation and 15% of neonates). The risk may be highest with a small exomphalos; a large exomphalos containing the liver is more rarely associated with chromosomal abnormalities. Associated structural abnormalities are present in 60–80% of cases and in 40% of cases with normal karyotype (mainly cardiac, other gastrointestinal (GI) and urogenital malformations). The association with non chromosomal syndrome is also high and Beckwith–Wiedemann syndrome (suspect if there is fetal macrosomia) is the cause in 15–20% of cases.

Gastroschisis: usually sporadic and isolated, with no association with chromosomal abnormalities. Although in 10–30% of cases other GI tract abnormalities are found, these are mainly bowel atresias due to *in utero* strangulation and infarction. A link to an environmental teratogens and drug abuse use has been postulated but not proven.

Clinical approach
Ultrasound findings: key points
- The stomach can be visible in the left upper quadrant from 9 weeks' gestation.
- The integrity of the anterior abdominal wall should be confirmed by demonstrating normal cord insertion.
- Exstrophy can be ruled out by confirming the presence of the fetal bladder in the pelvis.
- Physiological herniation of the midgut into the umbilical sac can be present until 11 weeks' gestation and any abnormality after this should prompt careful assessment.
- Exomphalos: central, midline sac containing bowel/liver at the level of the umbilicus with the umbilical vessels traversing through the sac (Fig. 7.9.1).
- Gastroschisis: free-floating loops of bowel are seen herniating (cauliflower appearance) lateral to a normal cord insertion (Fig. 7.9.2).
- Body stalk anomaly/amniotic rupture sequence: large midline abdominal defect with severe kyphoscoliosis and a short or absent umbilical cord.
- Bladder/cloacal exstrophy: infraumbilical defect, usually large, a low protruding mass with an absent bladder and normal amniotic fluid volume. In cloacal exstrophy commonly there are lumbar sacral, lower limb and renal anomalies.

Diagnosis key points
The vast majority of anterior abdominal wall defects are now diagnosed in the first or second trimester by routine ultrasound screening (USS). Sensitivity for USS detection is ~95% (RCOG). Gastroschisis and exstrophy may still present with markedly raised AFP levels.

Investigation
The diagnosis should be confirmed by a Fetal Medicine Specialist.

Invasive testing should be considered, except in the case of isolated gastroschisis where the risk of aneuploidy is low.

Antenatal and delivery
As in all cases of fetal anomaly, multidisciplinary input including the fetal medicine team, geneticists, neonatologists, and surgeons is essential. In particular, early involvement of the paediatric surgical team is particularly important in cases of GI tract abnormalities.

Both exomphalos and gastroschisis are associated with a high risk of fetal growth restriction. Difficulty in accurately measuring abdominal circumference can make monitoring fetal growth more difficult. Therefore, regular growth scans and Doppler/biophysical assessment of fetal wellbeing should take place.

Progressive bowel dilatation has been associated with a poorer prognosis.

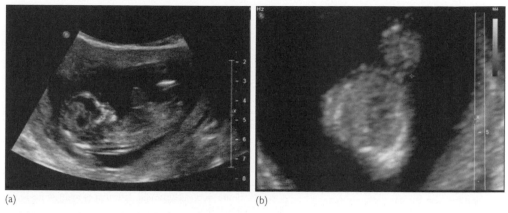

(a)   (b)

Fig. 7.9.1 (a) Sagittal and (b) axial view of a fetus with exomphalos at 12 weeks.

In particular, the occurrence of bowel obstruction has been recently demonstrated to be correlated with prenatal detection of intra-abdominal bowel dilatation.

Planned delivery in a unit with adequate neonatal care and surgical facilities is advised and fetal growth restriction often mandates induction previous to term.

The majority of cases with GI abnormality are suitable for vaginal delivery. There is no evidence of benefit of delivery by Caesarean section in gastroschisis or exomphalos unless there are other fetal or maternal indications.

Postnatal

Early management involves stabilization of the neonate and immediate covering of the affected area by clingfilm. There may be respiratory compromise with a large exomphalos due to a small chest and pulmonary hypoplasia.

Surgical management involving primary or staged closure of the wall defect can then take place in due course. The intra-abdominal contents may also be slowly reduced over time with a bag and the aid of gravity in a large number of cases.

Prognosis

Exomphalos with normal chromosomes has a survival at 1 year of over 95%.

Gastroschisis has a 90% survival at 1 year with most of the mortality relating to preterm delivery and short gut syndrome in cases with extensive bowel atresia.

Amniotic rupture sequence is almost invariably lethal due to the multiple and severe fetal anomalies.

In bladder and cloacal exstrophy, the prognosis is dependent on the site and size of the defect. Survival has been reported to be over 80% at 1 year, but a variable degree of long-term morbidity is often present. Extensive reconstructive surgery and permanent urinary diversion may be required. Male fetuses may have severely abnormal external genitalia and almost in all cases despite size, there is a certain grade of urinary continence and reproductive problems.

Termination of pregnancy

In the case of an anterior abdominal wall defect with a predictable poor prognosis a termination may be offered. The presence of a severe associated chromosomal

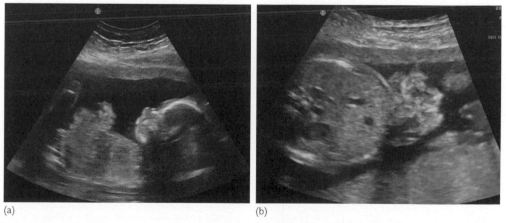

(a)   (b)

Fig 7.9.2 (a) sagittal and (b) axial view of the fetal abdomen at 21 weeks showing gastroschisis at the level of the umbilical cord insertion.

abnormality (such as trisomy 18 or 13) may influence this decision.

Owing to earlier diagnosis, usually in the first trimester, more parents may choose this option. Parents should have the opportunity to discuss their case with both a fetal medicine specialist and a paediatric surgeon prior to making this decision.

A detailed post-mortem is valuable in confirming the diagnosis and providing information for future pregnancies, although most of these cases are sporadic.

Future pregnancies

In general, the majority of these anomalies are sporadic with a low recurrence risk.

The recurrence risk for exomphalos is about 1%. When it is part of a genetic syndrome such as Beckwith–Wiedemann, a definition of the particular syndrome and a consultation with the geneticists is required to define possible increased recurrence risk.

Gastroschisis has a low recurrence risk of ~1%.

Bladder exstrophy is usually sporadic with ~1% recurrence, even though rare familial cases have been reported.

Amniotc rupture sequence and cloacal exstrophy (OEIS complex) are very rare, sporadic, and with a low recurrence risk.

GI tract abnormalities

Oesophageal atresia

Definition
Atresia of the oesophagus; this is associated with tracheo-oesophageal fistula (TEF) in about 90% of cases.

Epidemiology
1:3000–3500 births.

Pathology
Failure of the primitive foregut to divide into the trachea and oesophagus in the fourth week of gestation.

Aetiology
Usually sporadic in nature, and a clear aetiology is unknown in the majority of cases. About 20% are associated with chromosomal abnormalities (trisomy 18, 21 and 13). Other major structural defects are seen in 50% of cases, mainly cardiac and other bowel anomalies. TEF may also occur as part of VACTERL/VATER association (**v**ertebral defects–**a**nal atresia–**c**ardiac anomalies–**t**racheoesophageal fistula–**e**sophageal atresia–renal defects **l**imb defects).

Duodenal atresia

Definition
Lack of normal canalisation of the duodenal lumen leading to partial (web) or complete obstruction (atresia).

Epidemiology
1 in 5000 births.

Pathology
The lumen of the duodenum in early embryonic life is completely obliterated by proliferating epithelium and is normally canalized by the eleventh week. Failure of this process leads to duodenal atresia, which can also be caused by external compression due to an annular pancreas, or peritoneal bands.

Aetiology
Over 30% of cases are associated with trisomy 21. Other structural abnormalities are seen in up to 50% of cases and these are mainly skeletal, cardiac, renal, and other GI abnormalities.

Intestinal obstruction

Definition
Stenosis or atresia involving the distal small bowel in one or more areas of the GI tract. Equally frequent in the jejunum and ileum.

It also includes anorectal atresia or Hirschprung's disease.

Epidemiology
Intestinal obstruction occurs in about 1 in 2000 births. Many cases are not diagnosed antenatally and present in the first few days of neonatal life with abdominal distension and vomiting. The more proximal the lesion is the more likely it is to present itself antenatally with polyhydramnios and ultrasound detection of multiple fluid-filled bowel loops.

Jejunal and ileal atresia occur in 1 in 3000 births.

Hirschprung's disease is rare (1 in 5000 births) and more commonly seen in male fetuses.

Pathology
Small bowel atresias probably result from a vascular insult to the developing bowel during rotation at 6–12 weeks of embryonic life. They are frequently associated with volvulus and malrotation. There may be multiple segments involved; absence of large sections of small bowel is known as 'apple peel atresia'.

Anorectal atresia results from abnormal cloacal division in the ninth week of development.

Other causes of obstruction include meconium ileus, peritoneal bands, volvulus, and agangliosis of the colon (Hirschprung's disease). In Hirschprung's there is absence of the neural crest-derived enteric neural ganglion along a variable length of the intestine.

Aetiology
Jejunal and ileal obstructions are usually sporadic and not associated with chromosomal abnormalities; extraintestinal anomalies are uncommon. It is associated with cystic fibrosis (CF) in 10% of cases but up to 90% of cases if meconium ileus is present.

In contrast, anorectal atresias are frequently associated with chromosomal abnormalities (mostly trisomy 18 and 21) and other structural anomalies in 80% of cases. These include other GI, genitourinary, cardiac, and vertebral anomalies (VACTERL association).

Hirschprung's is associated with chromosomal abnormalities (particularly trisomy 21) in 10% of cases and other congenital anomalies or syndromes in 20% of cases. The remainder of cases are sporadic and isolated.

Echogenic bowel

Definition
Increased echogenicity (brightness) of the fetal bowel on ultrasound, with brightness similar to that of the bone (iliac crests and lumbar spine).

Epidemiology
A common finding in 1–1.8% of pregnancies in the second and third trimester.

Aetiology
In the majority of cases it is a normal variant and occasionally due to fetal ingestion of blood; however, it is also

associated with chromosomal anomalies, congenital infection, CF, and intrauterine growth restriction.

Clinical approach

Ultrasound findings key points

- Polyhydramnios due to intestinal obstruction tends not to present until 25 weeks' gestation.
- Suspect esophageal atresia in a late second and third trimester fetus with a small or absent stomach and polyhydramnios (Fig.7.9.3).
- Diagnosis can be difficult as the stomach may fill normally with an associated TEF.
- Duodenal atresia has a classic 'double bubble' appearance due to dilatation of both the stomach and proximal duodenum (Fig. 7.9.4).
- This is commonly not diagnosed until after 25 weeks, although can sometimes be seen as early as 20 weeks. Continuity of the duodenum with the stomach must be demonstrated to differentiate it from other cystic masses e.g. choledochal cyst.
- Look at the fetal heart; duodenal atresia carries a very high risk of trisomy 21 and may be associated with an atrioventricular septal defect (AVSD) or other markers for trisomy 21.
- Suspect more distal obstruction (jejunal or ileal) with hyperperistalsis in multiple loops of dilated bowel.
- It is not possible antenatally to determine the exact site and cause of the obstruction.
- Additional features such as echogenic bowel or ascites indicate the possibility of meconium peritonitis, which is more common in CF.
- With echogenic bowel assess fetal growth and uterine artery Doppler as this may be the first manifestation of subsequent fetal growth restriction.

History

- Ask about family history of genetic disorders, GI anomalies and in particular CF.
- Prior results of screening or diagnostic tests for aneuploidy should be reviewed.
- With echogenic bowel, ask about any bleeding in pregnancy or invasive testing, maternal illness or rash suggestive of congenital infection, and again family history of CF.

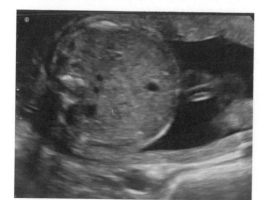

Fig 7.9.3 Axial view of the fetal abdomen showing a collapsed or small stomach.

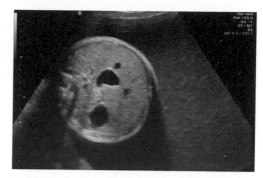

Fig 7.9.4 The appearance of a double bubble due to proximal small bowel atresia. Note the presence of polyhydramnios.

- If polyhydramnios present enquire about shortness of breath and maternal discomfort. Remember to ask about signs and symptoms of threatened preterm labour.

Investigation

- The diagnosis should be confirmed by a fetal medicine specialist with a careful search for other associated abnormalities.
- Invasive testing for karyotype and CF DNA studies should be offered depending on the findings.
- In cases of echogenic bowel send maternal serum for a congenital infection screen (CMV and toxoplasmosis), perform uterine artery and fetal Doppler studies (increased risk of IUGR) and consider parental CF carrier testing.

Management

Antenatal and delivery

- As in all cases of fetal anomaly multidisciplinary input including the fetal medicine team, neonatologists, and geneticists is essential. Early involvement of the paediatric surgical team is particularly important in these cases.
- Polyhydramnios increases the risk of preterm labour and abnormal presentation. Serial amnio reduction may be discussed and performed after a certain gestational age to reduce the risk of preterm labour and maternal discomfort.
- Systemic corticosteroids should be given to promote fetal lung maturity.
- Planned delivery in a unit with adequate neonatal care and surgical facilities is optimal. However, polyhydramnios due to upper GI obstruction will frequently result in unplanned early labour; parents should always be advised to attend the nearest hospital in an emergency.
- The majority of cases with GI abnormality are suitable for vaginal delivery, unless there are other fetal or maternal indications.

Postnatal

Early management involves stabilization of the neonate. There may be respiratory compromise due to severe abdominal distension. In cases of suspected oesophageal fistula and TEF oral feeds should be withheld until after a full assessment by the neonatal team. Surgical management of intestinal obstruction will usually involve resection of the affected bowel segment. The need for a colostomy and

Table 7.9.1 Causes of abdominal cysts

Type	Definition	Epidemiology and aetiology	Imaging key points	Clinical approach	Prognosis
Intestinal duplication cyst	Duplication of a section of GI tract	Rare. Associated with vertebral anomalies especially hemi vertebrae	Difficult to diagnose. Thick walled cyst at any point along the GI tract, peristalsis may be seen	Monitor for bowel obstruction. Postnatal surgical resection	Excellent
Choledocal cyst	Congenital cystic dilatation of the biliary tract	Rare, more common in Japan and Asia	Cystic mass in the right upper quadrant (RUQ) inferior to the liver	Neonatal work up including MRCP or ERPC. Postnatal surgical resection	Good with surgical resection. Natural history if untreated progresses to cholestasis, biliary cirrhosis and liver failure
Ovarian cyst	Benign functional cyst within the fetal ovary	Female fetuses only. Common, found in up to a third of female fetuses at autopsy. More common in diabetic pregnancies. Thought to be related to the increased placental hCG	Document sex. Most common cause of a cystic mass in a third trimester female fetus. Confirm that it is separate from urinary tract. Most are unilocular and unilateral and can be located anywhere in the abdomen	Majority are small and benign. Potential complications include torsion and haemorrhage. Large cysts can cause bowel compression and polyhydramnios. No alteration of obstetric management unless a very large cyst or polyhydramnios. Postnatal scan is required	Excellent, virtually all will spontaneously resolve, most within 6 months
Mesenteric or omental cysts	Benign cyst within the mesentery or omentum	Rare. May represent lymphatic obstruction	Midline cyst of variable size, either multiseptate or unilocular. It has a thinner wall than a duplication cyst from which it may be difficult to distinguish	Conservative. Antenatal aspiration occasionally required when a massive cyst causes thoracic compression	Usually good with conservative management. A minority will require surgical resection because of pain or bowel compression

subsequent surgery depends on the site and extent of the stenosis or atresia.

Prognosis
The prognosis for GI tract anomalies in the absence of associated chromosomal abnormalities depends largely on the gestation at delivery and the site and extent of any atresia. Large areas of atresia may lead to short gut syndrome, which has a very poor prognosis. Meconium peritonitis is associated with a poor prognosis and over 50% neonatal mortality.

Survival after surgery for isolated duodenal atresia is over 95%. TEF has a variable prognosis due to the high frequency of associated anomalies, but, in isolated cases, survival is excellent. Small bowel atresia has a good final outcome, except for the rare cases of apple peel atresia or multiple atresias.

Termination of pregnancy
These cases can be difficult as presentation is often after 24 weeks' gestation. If there is a very poor prognosis due to chromosomal abnormalities or coexisting defects, termination of pregnancy is an option in some countries, after careful counselling.

Particular ethical dilemmas are raised in cases involving a late diagnosis of trisomy 21. Many centres would not offer late termination in these circumstances.

In any case of pregnancy termination, a detailed post-mortem is valuable in confirming the diagnosis and providing information for future pregnancies.

Future pregnancies
The majority of cases are sporadic with a low recurrence risk. Rare familial cases of multiple bowel atresias have been reported. Recurrence risk is low for bowel atresia and Hirschprung's disease (respectively 1–2% and 4%).

Where the affected pregnancy involves CF, and both parents are carriers the recurrence risk is 25% for CF.

Abdominal cysts
Abdominal cystic masses are a common ultrasound finding. Renal tract anomalies or bowel dilatation are the most likely cause. Less commonly, cystic structures arise from the biliary tract or from the mesentery or from the ovary in female fetuses.

The origin is usually determined by the position of the cyst and its relation to other organs.

A definitive diagnosis may not be possible antenatally. A summary of causes of abdominal cysts's is given in Table 7.9.1; renal tract anomalies are not covered here.

Further reading

David A, Tan A, Curry J. Gastroschisis: sonographic diagnosis, associations, management and outcome. Prenatal Diagnosis 2008;28;633–44.

Fratelli N, Papageorghiou AT, Bhide A, Sharma A, Okoye B, Thilaganathan B. Outcome of antenatally diagnosed abdominal wall defects. Ultrasound Obstet Gynecol. 2007;30:266–70.

Hyett J, Intra-abdominal masses: prenatal differential diagnosis and management. Prenatal Diagnosis 2008;28;645–55.

Sparey C, Jawaheer G, Barrett AM, Robson SC. Esophageal atresia in the Northern Region Congenital Anomaly Survey, 1985–1997: prenatal diagnosis and outcome. Am J Obstet Gynecol 2000:182:427–31

Twining, McHugo, Pilling. Abdominal and abdominal wall abnormalities In: *Textbook of fetal abnormalities*, 2nd edn. Edinburgh: Churchill Livingstone Chapter 11.

Wilson RD, Johnson MP. Congenital abdominal wall defects: an update. Fetal Diagn Ther. 2004;19:385–98.

Patient resources

GEEPS (Gastroschisis, Exomphalos, Exstrophies Parents Support Group): www.geeps.co.uk

TOFS (Tracheo-Oesophageal Fistula Support): www.tofs.org.uk

Fetal abnormalities: limbs

Club foot

Definition
Malformation of the ankle joint characterized by a fixed position of the foot held in adduction, supination, and varus positions, in the classical type namely talipes equinovarus.

Incidence
Approximately 1 in a 1000.

Aetiology
May be isolated (commonest form) or complex due to an underlying chromosomal abnormality, neuromuscular and skeletal disorder or genetic syndrome.

Ultrasound features
Usually identified at the 18–23-week scan. In the normal foot, the foot is in a plane that is perpendicular to the long axis of the tibia and fibula. In talipes, the plantar aspect of the fetal foot is imaged in the same longitudinal plane as the tibia and fibula (Fig. 7.10.1).

It is important to do a full fetal survey to assess whether the talipes is a manifestation of a generalized disorder as listed in the box or an isolated condition. Additionally, serial scans need to be organized to assess if there are other joints showing progressive developmental abnormality as in neuromuscular disorders and to assess the liquor volume, as muscular disorders can impair the swallowing of the fetus.

Management
Antenatal: In isolated talipes, especially in the presence of low risk from previous first trimester screening, the pregnancy should be treated as any other low-risk pregnancy. However, in the absence of any screening or in the presence of other structural abnormalities, invasive prenatal diagnosis should be offered to rule out chromosomal associations.

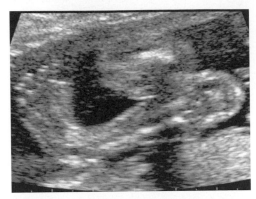

Fig. 7.10.1 Image of a fetal foot with talipes: the foot is in the same plane as the two long bones of the lower limb.

Postnatal: Mild forms of talipes may not require any treatment. More severe forms will require physiotherapy (traditional or Ponseti technique). Surgical correction is now rarely used as results from the Ponseti technique are excellent.

Prognosis
Depends on underlying aetiology. In isolated talipes, prognosis is good although surgical correction may be needed in some cases.

Ectrodactyly

Definition
Ectrodactyly, by definition describes a diverse group of hand and foot malformations that could vary from the absence of one digit to absence of all but one digit. It is also known as split hand and foot malformation and in the typical form is characterized by a median cleft of the hands and/or feet and may be associated with syndactyly, and aplasia and/or hypoplasia of the phalanges, metacarpals, and metatarsals.

Incidence
Very rare, about 1:20 000 live births.

Aetiology
It may occur as an isolated feature or as a part of a genetic syndrome (Table 7.10.1), almost all of which have a dominant mode of inheritance.

Some conditions that are associated with club foot deformity in the fetus

Chromosome abnormalities

Neuromuscular disorders

Meningomyelocele

Pena shokeir phenotype

Arthrogryposis multiplex cogenita

Skeletal dysplasias

Campomelic dysplasia

Diastrophic dysplasia

Ellis–van Creveld syndrome

Genetic syndromes

Multiple pterygium syndrome

Larsen syndrome

Smith–Lemli–Opitz syndrome

Table 7.10.1 Clinical features of some ectrodactyly syndromes

Syndromes	Additional features
EEC	Ectodermal dysplasia, cleftlip/palate, tear duct abnormality, genitourinary abnormalities, hearing loss, dysmorphic facies
EE	Ectodermal dysplasia, tear duct abnormality
ADULT	Ectodermal dysplasia, tear duct abnormality
ACFS	Cardiac defects, cleft palate, genitourinary abnormalities

EEC, ectrodactyly–ectodermal dysplasia–cleft syndrome; EE, ectrodactyly–ectodermal dysplasia; ADULT, acro-dermato-ungual-lacrimal-tooth; ACFS, acro-cardio-facial syndrome.

Ultrasound features

Typically identified at the time of the 18–23-week scan, although earlier diagnosis is reported. The findings are that of a V- or U-shaped cleft in the middle of the fetal hands and/or legs (Fig. 7.10.2). There is usually a paucity of digits, which may be due to actual absence of the digits or due to syndactyly. There may be additional features as mentioned in Table 7.10.1.

Management

Antenatal: Should include counselling for the parents in the presence of a multidisciplinary team comprising an obstetrician, fetal medicine consultant, genetics consultant and a paediatric plastic surgeon. The session should highlight the likely inheritance and any identifiable syndrome, the role of invasive prenatal diagnosis and the need for surgical correction. Some parents may opt for pregnancy termination based on the features identified.

Postnatal: The anatomical deformity will require surgical correction. For the ectrodactyly, the main aim of the surgery is to establish successful opposition of the two main digits, as complete normality of hand anatomy can usually not be restored. Owing to the possibility of associated renal tract abnormalities, prophylactic antibiotics are often advocated until normality of the renal tract can be established.

Prognosis

In the familial type of ectrodactyly, the outcome tends to be good with normal mentation and development. Morbidity caused by the associated hearing loss and ocular manifestations owing to lacrimal gland involvement in the syndromic patients should be considered.

Radial aplasia

Definition

Radial aplasia or hypoplasia is characterized by complete or partial absence of the radius and/or radial ray structures. This may manifest as a single forearm bone in the fetus with or without an absent thumb and abnormal positioning of the fetal hand. These abnormalities are collectively called radial ray defects.

Incidence

Rare: radial ray defects occur in 1 in 30 000 live births.

Aetiology

Radial ray defects and associated anomalies encompass a group of disorders with most defects being unilateral and

Table 7.10.2 Associated features of some syndromes that may present with radial ray defects

Syndromes	Additional features
Trisomy 13, 18	Growth restriction, abnormal digits, cardiac abnormality, renal abnormality, facial abnormality
Fanconi's anaemia	Growth restriction, cardiac abnormality, abnormal thumb
Cornelia de Lange	Growth restriction, abnormal digits, facial abnormality
Roberts	Growth restriction, abnormal digits, facial abnormality, renal abnormality
VACTERL	Cardiac abnormality, renal abnormality
Holt–Oram	Cardiac abnormality, abnormal thumb
Acrofacial dysostosis	Facial abnormality, abnormal thumb
TAR	Renal abnormality, normal thumb

VACTERL, Vertebral-Anal-Cardiac-TRACHEO-ESOPHAGEAL-RENAL-LIMB DEFECTS. TAR, Thrombocytopenia with Absent Radius.

sporadic while bilateral defects are more likely to be part of a multiple malformation syndrome (Table 7.10.2). It would be useful to identify any medication that the woman has been taking during the course of the pregnancy such as Valproates.

Ultrasound features

Usually identified at the 18–23-week anomaly scan. The findings are either absent or hypoplastic radius, with only bone identified in the fetal forearm (Fig. 7.10.3). This defect may be uni- or bilateral with radial deviation of the hand. There may be associated aplasia or hypoplasia of the thumb. As with any other structural abnormality, a thorough fetal survey is essential in making an assessment and a diagnosis.

Management

Antenatal management should aim for making a diagnosis if possible of the underlying syndromes as outline above. Invasive prenatal diagnosis would be required to clarify the karyotype, chromosomal breakage disorders, and fetal thrombocytopenia. Genetic counselling in these cases would be mandatory.

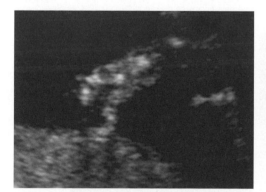

Fig. 7.10.2 Image showing ectrodactyly in the fetal hand, with a V-shaped cleft in the hand and paucity of digits.

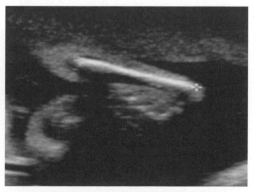

Fig. 7.10.3 Image showing single forearm bone with abnormal positioning of the fetal hand.

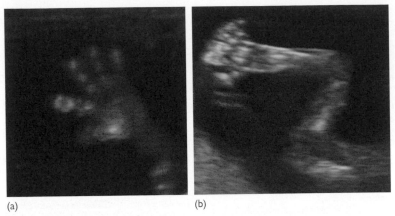

Fig. 7.10.4. Image showing normal number of fingers in (a) and postaxial polydactyly in the hand in (b).

Prognosis

Isolated unilateral radial ray defects tend to have a good prognosis as the vast majority of them are due to non-syndromic limb reduction defects. The syndromic cases have varied outcome. In the presence of other structural malformations, most parents tend to opt for termination.

Polydactyly

Definition

Polydactyly is defined as the presence of one or more extra digits in the hands (Fig. 7.10.4) or feet (Fig. 7.10.5). It is classified as pre-axial if the extra digit is on the radial or tibial side and as postaxial if it is on the ulnar or fibular aspects of the hand and foot respectively.

Incidence

Varies between 1:3000 to 10 000 with postaxial being more common.

Aetiology

The vast majority of polydactyly that are identified antenatally are isolated and familial. Polydactyly is thought to be a feature of many genetic syndromes some of which are listed in the Table 7.10.3.

Ultrasound features

Extra digits are noted on hands and/or feet (Fig. 7.10.4). These digits may either be pre- or postaxial and may or may not have bony elements in them. Occasionally, these digits are seen fused with the normal digits presenting as syndactyly.

Management

As with any other abnormality, a thorough search is mandatory to exclude other structural abnormalities. As indicated above in the table, coexisting abnormalities would point towards a genetic syndrome.

If the polydactyly is isolated, the family should be reassured and given information about postnatal surgical management that may be required. Depending on the associated anomaly pattern, invasive prenatal diagnosis will have to be considered.

Prognosis

Polydactyly, in the absence of any other abnormality is associated with an excellent prognosis. If it is not isolated, the underlying aetiology and the associated abnormalities would dictate the prognosis.

Amniotic band syndrome

Definition

Amniotic band syndrome refers to a group of congenital anomalies that are thought to be a consequence of amniotic bands that adhere to various organs, more commonly to the fetal extremities, resulting in amputations or peripheral nerve damage due to ischaemia. The amniotic bands

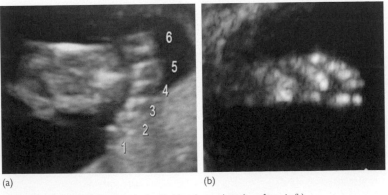

Fig. 7.10.5. Image showing postaxial polydactyly in the foot in (a) and normal number of toes in (b).

Table 7.10.3

Syndromes	Additional features
Trisomy 13	Growth restriction, holoprosencephaly, cardiac abnormality, renal abnormality, facial abnormality
Meckel–Gruber	Encephalocele, multicystic kidneys, liver cysts
Bardet–Biedl	Obesity, hypogonadism, mental retardation
Short-rib polydactyly	Skeletal dysplasia
Ellis–van Creveld	Skeletal dysplasia, cardiac anomalies
Smith–Lemli Opitz	Growth restriction, holoprosencephaly, ambiguous genitalia
Pallister Hall	Midline central nervous system anomalies
Di George	Cardiac and renal anomalies

can cause extensive disruptions in the craniofacial and truncal regions as well with the fetus presenting with bizarre clefts and abnormalities.

Incidence
Incidence varies from 1:1200 to 15000.

Aetiology
The exact underlying aetiology still remains unknown, although some authors believe that this syndrome is caused by early amnion rupture with the fetal parts being exposed to the sticky chorionic membrane. As a result, fibrous band-like adhesions are thought to be formed between the chorion and the exposed fetal parts, usually the extremities. These bands then wrap around the extremity causing ischemic changes in the distal parts, or causing transverse amputations across the limbs or digits.

Ultrasound features
The presenting feature is variable and may be an oedematous arm distal to a constriction, amputated appearance of the extremities (Fig. 7.10.6) or digits, or abnormal

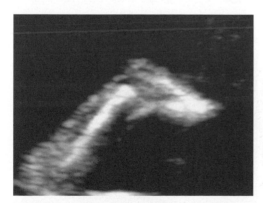

Fig. 7.10.6 Image of the fetal upper limb showing transverse amputation at the forearm.

posturing of the hands or feet that are oedematous. These may be associated with bizarre malformations of the fetal trunk, head, and neck. Amniotic bands may be noted at the line of constriction in the extremity with or without Doppler evidence of ischaemia distal to the occlusion.

Management
The presence of abnormalities as described should prompt the diagnosis of amniotic band syndrome. It is important to ascertain the extent of damage with particular reference to level of amputation and degree of ischemia in the affected limb. It may be possible to limit the damage by fetoscopic surgical release of the constricting membrane in rare cases. There are also anecdotal reports of spontaneous release of the constricting membrane with complete resolution of the changes in the limb.

Prognosis
Isolated limb abnormalities are usually non-lethal and compatible with normal life. Some abnormalities are likely to cause physical deformity and limitation of function. This may not be acceptable to some parents and they may opt for termination of the pregnancy. The prognosis depends on the severity of the abnormality and the possibility of reconstruction to near normal state with plastic surgery. Multiple malformations due to amniotic bands may be lethal or incompatible with normal life.

Further reading

Bakalis S, Sairam S, Homfray T, et al. Outcome of antenatally diagnosed talipes equinovarus in an unselected obstetric population. Ultrasound Obstet Gynecol 2002;20:226–9.

Bromley B, Shipp TD, Benacerraf B. Isolated polydactyly: prenatal diagnosis and perinatal outcome. Prenat Diagn 2000;20:905–8.

Canto MJ, Cano S, Palau J, Ojeda F. Prenatal diagnosis of clubfoot in low-risk population: associated anomalies and long-term outcome. Prenat Diagn 2008;28:343–6.

Cox H, Viljoen D, Versfeld G, Beighton P. Radial ray defects and associated anomalies. Clin Genet 1989;35:322–30.

Elliott AM, Evans JA, Chudley AE. Split hand/foot malformation (SHFM). Clin Genet 2005;68:501–5.

Kennelly MM, Moran P. A clinical algorithm of prenatal diagnosis of Radial Ray Defects with two and three dimensional ultrasound. Prenat Diagn 2007;27:730–7.

Keswani SG, Johnson MP, Adzick NS, et al. In utero limb salvage: fetoscopic release of amniotic bands for threatened limb amputation. J Pediatr Surg 2003;38:848–51.

Leung KY, MacLachlan NA, Sepulveda W. Prenatal diagnosis of ectrodactyly: the 'lobster claw' anomaly. Ultrasound Obstet Gynecol 1995;6:443–6.

Paladini D, Foglia S, Sglavo G, Martinelli P. Congenital constriction band of the upper arm: the role of three-dimensional ultrasound in diagnosis, counseling and multidisciplinary consultation. Ultrasound Obstet Gynecol 2004;23:520–2.

Pedersen TK, Thomsen SG. Spontaneous resolution of amniotic bands. Ultrasound Obstet Gynecol 2001;18:673–4.

Quintero RA, Morales WJ, Phillips J, et al. In utero lysis of amniotic bands. Ultrasound Obstet Gynecol 1997;10:316–20.

Zimmer EZ, Bronshtein M. Fetal polydactyly diagnosis during early pregnancy: clinical applications. Am J Obstet Gynecol 2000;183(3): 755–8.

Internet resources
www.steps-charity.org.uk/
www.ponseti.info

Fetal abnormalities: head and neck

Cystic hygroma

Definition

Cystic hygromas (CHs) are fluid-filled spaces that are typically noted at the back or sides of the fetal neck (Fig. 7.11.1). They may have septations within them and in the first trimester are usually manifest as increased nuchal translucency. A distinct group of cystic lesions that are sometimes identified in the third trimester tend to be fetal manifestation of lymphangiomas.

Incidence

Variable 1–3:1000.

Aetiology

The vast majority of CHs are thought to be associated with chromosomal abnormalities (>50%), most commonly Turner's syndrome. Some authors consider CHs as an independent marker for aneuploidies, whereas others have questioned this by demonstrating a strong relationship with increased nuchal translucency. In the absence of aneuploidies, CH has still a high incidence of associated malformations of the fetal heart, skeletal system, etc. (>33%). More recently the association between CH and several genetic syndromes has been described, including Noonan's syndrome, Cornelia De Lange syndrome and Roberts syndrome.

Management

The presence of CH in the first trimester should prompt a management plan as for increased nuchal translucency over the 95th centile. This should include offering invasive prenatal diagnosis, early fetal echocardiography, and a thorough search for other structural anomalies. Markers for specific genetic syndromes should be sought and the genetics team involved early in the process of counselling.

Prognosis

The outcome for CH in general is guarded and depends on the underlying diagnosis and associated abnormalities, if any. In the case of isolated CH, where no chromosomal, structural, or genetic associations have been established, the prognosis tends to be good in about 95% of cases. However, only a small proportion of CH is isolated.

Fetal goitre

Definition

Fetal goitre is a diffuse enlargement of the fetal thyroid gland.

Incidence

Fetal goitre is a very rare abnormality and can occur in the presence of a hyperthyroid, hypothyroid or euthyroid state in the fetus.

Aetiology

Maternal hyperthyroid states due to autoimmune antibodies are at risk of causing fetal goitre. The risk is increased when the mother is on antithyroid drugs, as both the antibodies and the drugs can cross the placenta and cause goitre. This risk is present when mothers are euthyroid or hypothyroid following surgical or radioisotope treatment for Graves' disease. Women in areas with endemic iodine deficiency or those with inborn errors of metabolism are similarly at risk of having fetal goitre.

Ultrasound findings

Typically, the fetal goitre is usually detected in the third trimester and is noted as a diffuse swelling in the anterior region of the fetal neck. The mass can be seen to be symmetrical on both sides of the fetal neck abutting the trachea (Fig. 7.11.2). Normograms are available for the length and width of the fetal thyroid and measurements above 2 SD are considered abnormal. The presence of goitre does not indicate hyper- or hypothyroid status in the fetus (this can only be diagnosed with fetal blood samples). In general hyperthyroid fetuses tend to have a higher fetal heart rate (over 160 bpm). If the goitre is big enough to obstruct the oesophagus, fetal swallowing may be hampered and polyhydramnios follows. Rarely, the goitre may be big enough to cause hyperextension of the fetal neck causing problems during labour.

Management

In the vast majority of cases the fetal goitre remains a chance finding, with the scan being done for other indications. Some centres have protocols to scan fetuses of mothers with thyroid abnormalities even in the euthyroid

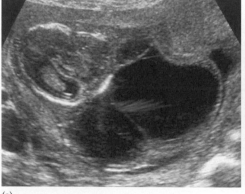

(a)

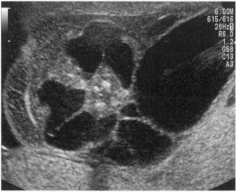

(b)

Fig. 7.11.1 Cross-section through the fetal head at the level of the occiput (a) and fetal neck (b) showing the cystic hygromas with septae.

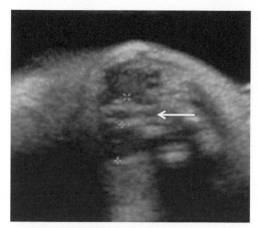

Fig. 7.11.2 Coronal section at the level of the fetal neck showing enlarged fetal thyroid gland (within callipers) on either sides of the fetal trachea (←).

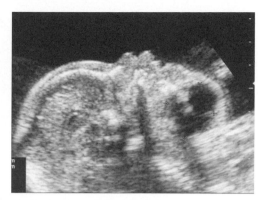

Fig. 7.11.3 Image showing cervical teratoma with mixed echogenicities.

state. As the scan does not usually give a clue to the fetal thyroid state, fetal blood sampling may be required to clarify this. Most of the available literature is on case reports due to the rarity of the fetal condition. This makes counselling difficult and is individualized for each fetus. There are several case reports suggesting successful treatment of the fetus with thyroid hormones and antithyroid drugs. Polyhydramnios may require drainage. It would be prudent to consider delivery of the fetus with a goitre in a tertiary centre in the event of there being tracheal compression. Postnatal follow up is usually organized by the neonatal team for managing the thyroid status in the baby.

Prognosis
Although there are no long-term studies, shrinkage of the goitre is the norm in the postnatal period, usually following treatment. Obviously congenital hypothyroidism is a potential problem if the condition is not appropriately treated.

Cervical teratomas
Definition
Cervical teratomas are masses noted on either side of the fetal neck, usually having a mixture of cystic and solid components and derived from any/or all of the embryonic tissues.

Incidence
These masses are extremely rare and the precise incidence is difficult to assess.

Aetiology
Cervical teratomas are not associated with underlying fetal conditions and are almost entirely sporadic.

Ultrasound findings
The vast majority of these lesions are incidental findings when identified in the second trimester. However, in the third trimester, the presenting clinical feature may actually be polyhydramnios leading to this fetal diagnosis. Invariably, the mass is unilateral on the anterolateral aspect of the fetal neck with cystic and solid components (Fig. 7.11.3) extending to the face and crossing the midline. These lesions usually do not have high vascularity as they are essentially benign. Depending on the size of the mass and

its extensions, there might be polyhydramnios and hyperextension of the fetal neck. As these are isolated conditions, the rest of the fetal anatomy is usually normal.

Management
Antenatal management of these lesions include serial scans to assess the size of the lesion, fetal growth velocity and the development of polyhydramnios. In the event of there being polyhydramnios developing, amnio drainage should be considered with a view to reducing the risk of preterm delivery. A multidisciplinary team needs to be involved in the management of the perinatal period, comprising neonatologists, neonatal anaesthetists, paediatric ENT specialist, and a paediatric surgeon along with the obstetric team. This is in the event of the baby needing an *ex utero intrapartum treatment* (EXIT) procedure at delivery and emergency tracheostomy for establishing an airway. The baby will need surgery to remove the cervical mass postnatally and plastic surgery to try and restore the anatomy.

Prognosis
The prognosis for these lesions tends to be very good as they are isolated lesions and do not tend to recur.

Further reading
Castillo F, Peiró JL, Carreras E, *et al.* The exit procedure (ex-utero intrapartum treatment): management of giant fetal cervical teratoma. J Perinat Med 2007;35:553–5.

Larsen ME, Larsen JW, Hamersley SL, *et al.* Successful management of fetal cervical teratoma using the EXIT procedure. J Matern Fetal Med 1999;8:295–7.

Martino F, Avila LF, Encinas JL, *et al.* Teratomas of the neck and mediastinum in children. Pediatr Surg Int 2006; 22:627–34.

Sayan A, Karaçay S, Bayol U, Arikan A. Management of a rare cause of neonatal airway obstruction: cervical teratoma. J Perinat Med 2007;35:255–6.

Molina FS, Avgidou K, Kagan KO, *et al.* Cystic hygromas, nuchal edema, and nuchal translucency at 11–14 weeks of gestation. Obstet Gynecol 2006;107:678–83.

Kharrat R, Yamamoto M, Roume J, *et al.* Karyotype and outcome of fetuses diagnosed with cystic hygroma in the first trimester in relation to nuchal translucency thickness. Prenat Diagn 2006;26:369–72.

Malone FD, Ball RH, Nyberg DA, *et al.* FASTER Trial Research Consortium. First-trimester septated cystic hygroma: prevalence, natural history, and pediatric outcome. Obstet Gynecol 2005;106:288–94.

Göktolga U, Karaşahin KE, Gezginç K, *et al.* Intrauterine fetal goiter: diagnosis and management. Taiwan J Obstet Gynecol 2008;47:87–90.

Miyata I, Abe-Gotyo N, Tajima A, *et al.* Successful intrauterine therapy for fetal goitrous hypothyroidism during late gestation. Endocr J 2007;54:813–7.

Hashimoto H, Hashimoto K, Suehara N. Successful in utero treatment of fetal goitrous hypothyroidism: case report and review of the literature. Fetal Diagn Ther 2006;21:360–5.

Van Loon AJ, Derksen JT, Bos AF, Rouwé CW. In utero diagnosis and treatment of fetal goitrous hypothyroidism, caused by maternal use of propylthiouracil. Prenat Diagn 1995;15:599–604.

Polak M, Legac I, Vuillard E, *et al.* Congenital hyperthyroidism: the fetus as a patient. Horm Res 2006;65:235–42.

Fetal abnormalities: skeletal abnormalities/dysplasias

Definition

The skeletal dysplasias or osteochondrodysplasias are a group of conditions affecting bone growth and development. However, they may be associated with other congenital anomalies.

There are over 370 forms that have been carefully classified into 37 groups based on the radiological and molecular abnormalities.

In addition, other genetic syndromes and chromosomal abnormalities may be associated with bone abnormalities and should be considered in the differential diagnosis.

Ultrasound findings

Some of the lethal skeletal dysplasias may present at 11–14 weeks with increased nuchal translucency and/or fetal oedema with very short long bones.

Femur length is measured routinely during the anomaly ultrasound scan at 18–24 weeks gestational age. It is compared with the biparietal diameter (BPD) and abdominal circumference (AC) to check for proportionate growth. A disproportionately short femur at this stage may indicate:

- inaccurate dating
- a small normal baby
- early intrauterine growth retardation
- chromosomal disorder
- skeletal dysplasia
- a malformation syndrome.

In a recent retrospective study it was found that 40% of fetuses with isolated short femurs had severe intrauterine growth restriction (IUGR) associated with abnormal umbilical Doppler studies. This group had a high incidence of pre-eclampsia (36%) and intrauterine death (33%).

Occasionally, non-lethal forms may be identified incidentally by measuring femur length in the third trimester.

Isolated or asymmetrical limb abnormalities may also be identified at any stage.

Approximately 5% of fetus with short long bones had no radiological abnormalities after birth. Thus, the outcome can range from lethality to normality.

Epidemiology

The skeletal dysplasias are individually rare, but as a group occur with an incidence of 1 in 5000 in the newborn period. The incidence is presumably higher antenatally as many are lethal *in utero*. They account for 5% of all genetic disorders. Of those detected in the antenatal period, approximately 70% are detected before 24 weeks and 30% after 24 weeks.

Pathology

The appendicular and axial skeleton undergo endochondral ossification of a cartilage template from early human gestation. The skull, clavicles and mandible ossify via intramembranous ossification from 8 weeks' gestation. Secondary (epiphyseal) ossification can be seen from 20 weeks' gestation. Many of the genes involved have been identified and code for collagens and proteins involved in bone development.

Aetiology

Skeletal abnormalities may be a feature of skeletal dysplasias, chromosomal disorders or malformation syndromes.

Skeletal dysplasias are a heterogeneous group. They may be inherited as autosomal dominant, autosomal recessive, or X-linked disorders. A few are associated with maternal disease or teratogens.

An accurate diagnosis is essential for accurate assessment of recurrence risks and prognosis.

The most important decision on identification of a skeletal dysplasia is whether or not the condition is likely to be lethal.

Lethal skeletal dysplasias

The three most common lethal skeletal dysplasias accounting for 40% for all the lethal dysplasias are:

- thanatophoric dysplasia (11%)
- osteogenesis imperfecta type II (20%)
- achondrogenesis type II (8%).

Thanatophoric dysplasia

This is a severe, sporadic, lethal skeletal dysplasia due to mutations in the fibroblast growth factor receptor 3 (FGFR3). Thanatophoric means 'death bringing', as the affected baby dies in the neonatal period due to the severe thoracic dystrophy. Antenatally, the fetus presents in the first or second trimester with marked shortening of all the long bones, relative macrocephaly, frontal bossing, absent nasal bone, and very short fingers. The bones are well mineralized but the femur is often curved like a telephone receiver (type 1 thanatophoric dysplasia). The vertebral bodies are small but present. Occasionally the baby is oedematous or hydropic and polyhydramnios develops in the third trimester.

The recurrence risk for this condition is very low (<1%) as it is not inherited and occurs as a new sporadic mutation.

Typically in thanatophoric dysplasia type I there are curved 'telephone receiver' femora, whereas in thanatophoric dysplasia type II there are 'cloverleaf' skull (severe craniosynostosis), and straight, short femora.

Osteogenesis imperfecta type II (brittle bone disease)

Type II is the severe, lethal form of osteogenesis imperfecta. The baby may present with short, broad, crumpled, often asymmetric, long bones in the first or second trimester. Bone mineralization is often reduced particularly in the skull. Beaded ribs may be visualized representing multiple rib fractures. The hands appear normal. The fetus may die *in utero* or shortly after birth.

Achondrogenesis type II (and type I)

Ultrasound findings include cystic hygroma or large nuchal translucency, flat facial profile with flat nose, relative macrocephaly, micrognathia, absent mineralization of the vertebral bodies, very short long bones often with metaphyseal spikes, protuberant abdomen, and short hands and feet. The fetus frequently dies *in utero*. This condition is due to new mutations in collagen II. Achondrogenesis type I is a less frequent condition with extreme shortening of the long bones and is associated with autosomal recessive inheritance. Accurate diagnosis is important as the recurrence risk associated with type II is very low (<1%) but type I is 25%.

Other less common lethal skeletal dysplasias

Short rib polydactyly

There are several types but all have an autosomal recessive mode of inheritance: small thorax with short ribs, short limbs, and polydactyly. Some forms are associated with a median cleft lip. This group can be readily confused with Ellis–van Creveld syndrome and Jeunes asphyxiating thoracic dystrophy. Differentiation is important, as the latter are not always lethal in the neonatal period. The degree of shortening of the long bones and severity of the small thorax are more marked in the short rib polydactyly syndromes.

Perinatal or infantile hypophosphatasia

The most severe forms of hypophosphatasia present prenatally—possibly as early as 12 weeks. There is reduced bone mineralization of long bones and skull. Fractures may be present. The long bones are short. Bony spurs may be seen on the tibiae—a helpful diagnostic feature. This is an autosomal recessive condition due to mutations in tissue the non-specific alkaline phosphatase gene (TNSALP). The recurrence risk is therefore 25%.

Campomelic dysplasia

This condition is characterized by disproportionate short long bones presenting in the second trimester. The scapulae, if visualized, are hypoplastic and there is often bowing (campomelia) of the long bones especially the femurs. Three-quarters of karyotypic males have ambiguous genitalia or complete sex reversal. New sporadic mutations in SOX9 are the cause of this condition, but the recurrence risk is approximately 5% because of the incidence of gonadal mosaicism.

Non-lethal skeletal dysplasias

The most common non-lethal skeletal dysplasias presenting antenatally are discussed below.

Achondroplasia

This is an autosomal dominant disorder but with an 80% new mutation rate so there is frequently no family history. The fetus may present in the third trimester with short long bones (particularly the proximal long bones) below the 5th centile in the third trimester. It is very unusual to see any reduction in bone length before 24 weeks' gestation. Other ultrasound findings include, frontal bossing, relative macrocephaly, depressed nasal bridge, and the 'trident' hands with short fingers.

This condition is due to one of two point mutations in FGFR3 in 99% of cases (this is the same gene associated with thanatophoric dysplasia, which is due to different mutations), therefore the diagnosis may be confirmed antenatally by molecular analysis of amniotic fluid, fetal blood, or chorionic villus sampling (placental biopsy). This particular genetic test is quick and cheap and therefore useful during the pregnancy.

Achondroplasia is associated with severe short stature, and complications include deafness due to recurrent otitis media, hydrocephalus, and acute onset of spinal stenosis resulting in paraplegia. Intelligence is normal.

Spondyloepiphyseal dysplasia congenita

Spondyloepiphyseal dysplasia congenita (SEDC) is a rare autosomal dominant genetic bone dysplasia due to new dominant mutations in collagen II. It may be diagnosed by antenatal ultrasound in the second or third trimester with disproportionate short long bones and normal-sized thorax. However, it is frequently missed until early childhood.

This condition is associated with normal intelligence but extreme short stature and many orthopaedic complications including progressive scoliosis, hip dysplasia and premature osteoarthritis. The baby may have micrognathia

and cleft palate. There is a significant risk of myopia and hearing loss. The recurrence risk is very low.

Osteogenesis imperfecta

There are several forms of osteogenesis imperfecta (OI). As previously mentioned, type II is the most severe, lethal form.

Type III is also severe but compatible with survival. Antenatal ultrasound scans may detect fractures of the long bones in the second or third trimester. However, although the long bones may be mildly shortened, they are not broad and crumpled as seen in type II. Again there may be reduced mineralization of the skull and some rib fractures. Some of these babies die in the neonatal period but survivors suffer from recurrent fractures due to minimal trauma and as a result are confined to a wheelchair. Intelligence is normal.

Types I and IV are the mildest forms and usually present in childhood but may present with one or two fractures in the fetus or neonate. The long bones may be slightly shortened. There is often an autosomal dominant family history of an increased frequency of fractures.

All four types of OI are due to different dominant mutations in the α-1 and α-2 chains of collagen 1. Types I and IV may be inherited from an affected parent, but types II and III are not inherited as it is unlikely for affected individuals to reproduce. There are rare autosomal recessive forms and there is a risk of gonadal mosaicism—overall the recurrence risk is 5–7%.

Others to consider

Jeunes asphyxiating thoracic dystrophy and Ellis–van Creveld syndrome

These rare autosomal recessive conditions may present in the second trimester with disproportionate long bones and narrow thorax. Polydactyly is also a feature, so they can, occasionally, be confused with the short rib polydactyly group (see above). Ellis van Creveld may be associated with congenital heart disease. Jeunes syndrome may be fatal in the neonatal period and survivors may develop chronic renal failure. Ellis–van Creveld syndrome is less frequently lethal. Recurrence risk for both is 25%.

Chondrodysplasia punctata

Chondrodysplasia punctata (CDP) is a very heterogeneous group of conditions associated with premature ossification of the epiphyses presenting as stippling, which can sometimes be seen on a careful ultrasound examination and absent nasal bone. This can be inherited in a X-linked dominant (Conradi–Hunerman–Happle syndrome, marked asymmetry, girls only), X-linked recessive (brachytelephalangic CDP, boys only, less severe), autosomal recessive (rhizomelic chondrodysplasia punctata associated with marked developmental delay), maternal illness (systemic lupus erythematosus, maternal hyperemesis) and teratogens (warfarin). Recurrence risk and prognosis depends on the specific diagnosis (Irving et al. 2008).

Prognosis/recurrence risks

The prognosis and recurrence risk depends on the type of skeletal dysplasia. The lethal skeletal dysplasias should be identifiable in the antenatal period. These fetuses frequently die in utero or in the neonatal period. In a retrospective study by Krakow et al (2008), the correct diagnosis was made in only 42%, however in the same publication, lethality was accurately predicted in 96.8%.

Correct diagnosis is essential for prediction of complications. Many of the surviving skeletal dysplasias are associated with orthopaedic complications and morbidity.

The recurrence risk is also based on the correct diagnosis as the mode of inheritance varies depending on the type of dysplasia.

Clinical approach

History

A detailed three-generation family history can be helpful in making a specific diagnosis. Parental heights should be determined.

Consanguinity suggests an autosomal recessive disorder

Increased paternal age is associated with an increased incidence of achondroplasia and Apert's syndrome.

Increased maternal age is associated with increased risk of chromosomal aneuploidy.

Pregnancy history

Disproportionate short stature may be associated with early placental insufficiency so early bleeding or the loss of a twin may be significant.

Drug exposure exposure to warfarin (CDP), sodium valproate (isolated limb defects).

Maternal illness: hyperemesis resulting in vitamin K deficiency or maternal systemic lupus erythematosis (CDP).

Maternal diabetes can be associated with sacral agenesis, vertebral anomalies and asymmetrical shortening of the long bones particularly the femurs.

Examination

Assessment of viability

Most lethal skeletal dysplasias present before the third trimester. The following should be considered indicators of lethality:

- early presentation
- very short long bones (femur length/AC ratio <0.16)
- thoracic dystrophy/high cardiothoracic ratio
- hydrops fetalis or oedema
- very poor mineralization of the long bones and/or skull.

The converse is also true, the condition is unlikely to be lethal if

- the disproportion presents in the third trimester
- the thorax looks a normal size
- there is no oedema of the fetus.

Aids for making a specific diagnosis

Long bones

Measurement of all long bones/degree of disproportion.

Pattern of shortening

- Rhizomelia: proximal part (achondroplasia/CDP)
- Mesomelia: middle part
- Acromelia: distal part.

Bone modelling

- Bowing (campomelic dysplasia/OI)
- fractures (OI/hypophophatasia)
- absence
- bone density/mineralization (decreased in OI/hypophosphatasia/achondrogenesis: increased in sclerosing bone disorders)
- epiphyseal stippling (chondrodysplasia punctata)
- asymmetry (OI/maternal diabetes/isolated limb defects)
- scapulae (small/absent in campomelic dysplasia).

Other measurements

- BPD (relatively increased achondroplasia/thanatophoric)
- Abdominal circumference (IUGR)
- Chest circumference (cardiothoracic ratio, thoracic/AC ratio for assessment of lethality, fractures of ribs—OI/hypophosphatasia).

Skull

- Mineralization (reduced in OI type II/hypophosphatasia/achondrogenesis)
- cloverleaf (thanatophoric dysplasia type II)
- craniosynostosis (see Chapter 7.7, Genetic disorders).

Vertebrae

- Absent mineralization of vertebral bodies (achondrogenesis type II/hypophosphatasia)
- scoliosis
- hemivertebrae.

Hands and feet

- Brachdactyly (short fingers)/trident hands (achondroplasia and thanatophoric dysplasia)
- extra fingers (polydactyly) (short rib polydactyly syndromes, Ellis–van Creveld and Jeunes asphyxiating thoracic dystrophy)
- hitchhiker thumb (diastrophic dysplasia)
- radial aplasia (trisomy 18, fanconi anaemia, Holt Oram syndrome, TAR syndrome)
- syndactyly: soft tissue or bony fusion (Apert's syndrome)
- talipes equinovarus (diastrophic dysplasia, campomelic dysplasia, SEDC).

Facial profile

- Micrognathia (achondrogenesis and SEDC)
- median cleft lip (short rib polydactyly)
- absent nasal bridge (chondrodysplasia punctata).

Genitalia

- Abnormalities of the genitalia or sex reversal (campomelic dysplasia, Beemer Langer syndrome (form of short rib-polydactyly))
- hypospadias (intrauterine growth retardation).

Investigations

Chromosome analysis

Chorionic villous sample, amniocentesis or fetal blood depending on gestation. Chromosomal disorders including trisomy 21 may present with short femurs, although an isolated short femur is a poor predictor for trisomy 21.

Molecular analysis

May be usefully performed for achondroplasia during the pregnancy. If there is a family history of a known skeletal dysplasia, the causative mutation can often be identified prior to the pregnancy and prenatal diagnosis can be offered at 11 weeks' gestation by CVS.

In most other skeletal dysplasia, most genetic tests take too long to be of practical use during the pregnancy, but stored DNA can be very helpful in making a specific diagnosis after birth.

Counselling

Lethal disorders

Assessment of the likelihood of lethality is essential for the further management of the pregnancy. Termination of pregnancy is an option throughout the pregnancy for a lethal disorder. Post-mortem examination and DNA storage should be encouraged, as a specific diagnosis helps to determine accurate recurrence risks. If a post-mortem is refused, the couple should be encouraged to allow a skeletal survey and external examination as it is often possible to make a diagnosis based on these alone.

Non-lethal disorders
Counselling is more difficult in non-lethal disorders. These are frequently diagnosed later in the pregnancy. Often it is difficult to make a precise diagnosis until the baby is born. Parents should be warned that it may be a few years before a specific diagnosis is made. For this reason it is helpful to involve a geneticist who can organize investigations after birth and follow up on a regular basis. Disproportionate short limbs are often easier to detect on antenatal ultrasound than plain radiographs after birth because of the availability of antenatal centile charts.

The complications also vary depending on the specific diagnosis. However, as a general rule, if chromosomal abnormalities are excluded, most of the surviving skeletal dysplasias are associated with normal intelligence.

Prognosis, final height, and recurrence risk depends on the underlying cause of the skeletal dysplasia. Orthopaedic complications are frequent in this group.

It is important to be aware that early growth retardation may present as disproportionate short long bones.

Management
- Correct assessment of viability based on ultrasound findings (as above).
- Assessment of placental function and abdominal circumference to exclude IUGR.
- Attempt at making a specific diagnosis based on history and ultrasound findings (this is only possible in less than 50% of cases).
- Exclusion of chromosomal abnormality by CVS/amniocentesis or fetal blood.
- Molecular analysis of FGFR3 if achondroplasia is suspected.
- Serial scans to assess fetal growth.
- If the baby is suspected of having osteogenesis imperfecta, a normal vaginal delivery is still the preferred mode of delivery unless there is any indication that the delivery will be difficult.

Involvement of
- Clinical geneticists for arrangement of further testing and follow-up.
- Neonatologists
- Paediatric orthopaedic surgeon.

Careful follow-up
After intrauterine death or termination of pregnancy:
- post-mortem examination
- radiology: full skeletal survery
- store DNA.

After live birth
- Careful clinical examination by neonatologist and/or geneticist
- Skeletal survey at birth with expert radiological opinion
- The baby will require follow up by paediatrician/orthopaedic surgeon/clinical geneticist
- Depending on diagnosis may require hearing and ophthalmic assessment on a regular basis
- If no specific diagnosis is made—annual follow-up by the clinical geneticist is suggested with repeat skeletal survey at the age of 3 years.

Genetic counselling
To discuss
- prognosis
- recurrence risks
- prenatal diagnosis in future pregnancies by genetic testing or detailed scans.

Further reading
Firth HV, Hurst JA. Oxford Desk reference: clinical genetics. Oxford: Oxford University Press 2003.

Irving MD, Chitty LS, Mansour S, Hall CM. Chondrodysplasia punctata: a clinical diagnostic and radiological review. Clin Dysmorphol 2008;17:229–41.

Krakow D, Alanay Y, Rimoin LP, Lin V, Wilcox WR, Lachman RS, Rimoin DL. Evaluation of prenatal-onset osteochondrodysplasias by ultrasonography: a retrospective and prospective analysis. Am J Med Genet A 2008;1(146A):1917–24.

Mansour S, Hall CM, Pembrey ME, Young ID. A clinical and genetic study of campomelic dysplasia. J Med Genet. 1995;32:415–20.

Papageorghiou AT, Fratelli N, Leslie K, et al. Outcome of fetuses with antenatally diagnosed short femur. Ultrasound Obstet Gynecol 2008;31:507–11.

Superti-Furga A, Unger S. Nosology and classification of genetic skeletal disorders: 2006 revision. Am J Med Genet A. 2007;143:1–18.

Internet resources
The skeletal dysplasia group are a UK association created for the promotion of teaching and research of the skeletal dysplasia. Their publications include summaries of the skeletal dysplasias: www.skeletaldysplasiagroup.org.uk/index.html

Some of the summaries may be accessed on the companian web site for the Oxford Desktop Reference—Clinical Genetics (Firth and Hurst): www.oup.com/uk/booksites/content/0192628968/

Further information for patients for specific disorders can be obtained on the Contact a Family website: www.cafamily.org.uk/index.html

Patient resources
Restricted Growth Association (UK), PO Box 4008, Yeovil BA20 9AW. Tel: 01935 841364 (Mon, Wed and Thur 9 am–5 pm; Tues 9 am–9 pm; Fri 9 am–12 noon); Fax: 01935 841364; e-mail: office@restrictedgrowth.co.uk: www.restrictedgrowth.co.uk

Little People of America, Inc. (USA), 250 El Camino Real, Suite 201, Tustin, CA 92780; Toll-free: (888) LPA-2001 (English and Spanish); Direct: (714) 368 3689; Fax: (714) 368 3367; E-mail: info@lpaonline.org

Antenatal Results and Choices ARC (UK), 73 Charlotte Street, London W1T 4PN; Admin: 0207 631 0280; Helpline: 0207 631 0285; E-mail: info@arc-uk.org

Fetal abnormalities: thorax

Congenital cystic adenomatous malformation

Definition
A congenital cystic adenomatous malformation (CCAM) is a benign condition characterized by an abnormal mass of lung tissue, located usually on one lobe of the fetal lung. This lesion derives its blood supply from the pulmonary vasculature. It belongs to a heterogeneous group of echogenic lesions of the fetal lung that includes CCAM, pulmonary sequestration, bronchial atresia and transient bronchial obstruction. All of them can present antenatally as an echogenic fetal lung lesion. The commonest of these is CCAM.

Incidence
CCAM is thought to occur in approximately 1 in 4000 pregnancies.

Aetiology
The exact cause for this abnormality is unknown. It is thought to occur as a consequence of arrested and abnormal growth of the terminal respiratory bronchioles. It is usually an isolated finding and does not have a genetic or chromosomal basis. It may be occasionally associated with heart or renal abnormalities.

Ultrasound features
CCAM presents as an intrathoracic cystic or solid echogenic lesion (Fig. 7.13.1) that is usually unilateral and more commonly affects the lower lobe of the fetal lung. Both sides of the fetal lung and both sexes are affected equally. As this does not function as normal lung tissue, many fetuses show obvious cystic areas, which can cause a significant mediastinal shift. Antenatally these lesions are classified as macrocystic (with obvious cysts), microcystic (cysts not visible to the naked eye, lesion appears echogenic) or mixed. A thorough fetal anatomical survey is essential to rule out coexisting anomalies. A detailed survey of the blood supply to this lesion should be sought in order to differentiate this from the even rarer pulmonary sequestration. The latter derives its blood supply from the dorsal aorta and could lead to a hyperdynamic circulatory state owing to the shunting from this lesion. This lesion can be difficult to differentiate from congenital high airway obstruction, which causes trapping of the secretions in the lung and is imaged as an echogenic lobe or the entire lung. Transient blockage of the bronchial tree with a mucus plug tends to resolve spontaneously over the course of the pregnancy, but bronchial atresia tends to persist.

Serial scans should be organized in order to monitor the fetus for signs of fetal hydrops as that would dramatically alter the outcome for the pregnancy. Additionally, progressive increase in the size of the cysts might require thoraco-amniotic shunting.

Management
Antenatal
The vast majority of fetuses with CCAM have an uneventful course. Occasionally, intervention may need to be offered as mentioned above. It is important that the prospective parents are provided with an opportunity to meet the medical and surgical team who will be looking after the baby postnatally. It is also important to make a plan for postnatal management.

Bilateral disease and hydrops fetalis are indicators of poor outcome, whereas mediastinal shift, polyhydramnios and early detection are not poor prognostic signs. Serial scans have shown spontaneous reduction of these lesions with difficulty in demonstrating these lesions as the baby may 'outgrow' these lung lesions. This should be interpreted with caution as lesions that have regressed or disappeared antenatally may still need surgery postnatally.

Postnatal
Postnatal management includes chest X-ray and CT scan to identify the site and size of the lesion. The urgency of these investigations is based on the presence of symptoms in the newborn. Most lesions are removed surgically in order to eliminate the possibility of infection and malignancy if left *in situ*. Surgery can be either through an open thoracotomy or a minimally invasive thoracotomy.

Prognosis
The outcome in general for the uncomplicated CCAMs is very good with the vast majority of infants growing and developing normally.

Congenital diaphragmatic hernia
Definition
Congenital diaphragmatic hernia is an anomaly in the diaphragm that does not develop normally allowing the abdominal contents to herniate into the thoracic cavity. This results in poor lung development.

Incidence
CDH is thought to occur in approximately 1 in 2500 pregnancies.

Aetiology
Essentially, the defect in the development of the lung is likely to be due to defective mesenchymal incorporation. Several conditions are thought to result in this maldevelopment, which includes chromosomal abnormalities (trisomies 13, 18 and 21), genetic syndromes (Fryn's syndrome), and deficiency in retinoic acid.

Ultrasound features
Left-sided CDH (Fig. 7.13.2a) is usually identified at the 18–22-week scan when the fetal stomach and bowel are noted in the chest along with a mediastinal shift to the right. Identification can be possible at the 11–14-week

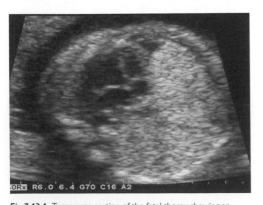

Fig.7.13.1 Transverse section of the fetal thorax showing an echogenic lesion in the right side of the fetal chest, with mediastinal shift pushing the heart to left side.

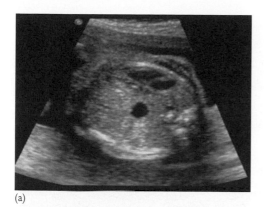

(a)

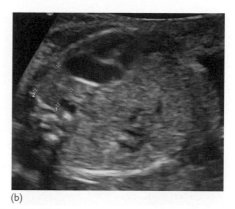

(b)

Fig. 7.13.2 (a) Transverse section through the fetal thorax showing the stomach bubble in the left side of the thorax, pushing the fetal heart to the right hemithorax: left-sided diaphragmatic hernia.

Fig. 7.13.2 (b) Transverse section through the fetal thorax showing the fetal liver in the right side of the thorax, pushing the fetal heart to the left hemithorax: Right-sided diaphragmatic hernia. Area within callipers shows normal lung tissue.

scan, when the condition is often associated with increased fetal nuchal translucency. Rarely, the liver is noted in the chest in cases of right-sided hernia (Fig. 7.13.2b) and these can be more difficult to diagnose.

CDH is an isolated finding in about 60% of cases. It can be present in association with cardiac abnormalities, other markers for chromosomal aberrations, and growth restriction. A thorough search for other abnormalities should be made and options of invasive diagnosis discussed with the parents. A proportion of CDHs may go undiagnosed, as not all hernias present at the time of the anomaly scan.

CDHs have to be differentiated from eventration of the diaphragm. This can sometimes be difficult as the thin diaphragm in the latter may not be visible and a diagnosis of CDH is made.

Management
Antenatal
The management of CDH is hinged on early inclusion of a multidisciplinary team, including neonatologists, paediatric surgeon, geneticist, and the fetal medicine team. It is important to provide as much details of outcome to the prospective parents as possible from all angles so that they are able to make an informed decision about the pregnancy. The initial management is geared towards making a diagnosis of the extent of involvement and if possible, the underlying aetiology. The pregnancy is then followed up with serial scans assessing fetal wellbeing and the development of polyhydramnios. Plans must be in place to deliver the baby in a tertiary centre that offers neonatal surgery for the CDH.

Several features have been reported as predictors of outcome in antenatally diagnosed CDH. The lung-to-head ratio (LHR), which measures the remaining area of normal lung in relation to the fetal head circumference measured on ultrasound and fetal lung volume measured with fetal MRI scan, are considered to have a role in predicting outcome in CDH. In addition, the presence of the liver in the chest confers a poor prognosis. These fetuses may be considered for *in utero* procedures such as tracheal occlusion using a balloon or plug to promote lung growth and development. This is reported to improve survival rates in some babies, but the main drawback is preterm delivery due to

the invasive intervention, and the procedure is currently a subject of a randomized trial.

Postnatal
Planned delivery in a tertiary centre is required. Once the newborn has been stabilized, surgical repair of the diaphragmatic defect is carried out. In most cases it is closed by primary repair, although some cases may require closure with a patch. Extensive respiratory support is required, including ventilation and measures to deal with the pulmonary hypertension, such as the use of nitric oxide. Pulmonary hypoplasia, abnormal pulmonary vasculature, and lung injury secondary to mechanical ventilation are the main causes of both mortality as well as long-term respiratory morbidity. A large proportion of these babies have long-term morbidity affecting gastrointestinal and neurological development as well.

Prognosis
The outcome in babies with CDH depends on the size and content of the hernia and also the associated structural chromosomal or genetic conditions. In general, for a left-sided hernia with just bowel and no liver in the fetal chest, the survival rate varies from about 40% to 60% and there is a much higher rate of other morbidity.

Fetal pleural effusion
Definition
Accumulation of fluid in the fetal pleural cavity resulting in pleural effusion can be isolated or occur with fetal hydrops.

Incidence
Pleural effusion is thought to occur in 1 in 10 000 fetuses.

Aetiology
Pleural effusion may occur as an isolated finding or in association with other conditions. Such secondary effusions occur along with diaphragmatic hernia and other lesions compressing the lungs and mediastinum such as congenital cystic adenomatoid malformation and bronchopulmonary sequestration, mediastinal tumours, and cardiac malformations. It is also noted with chromosomal abnormalities, congenital infections such as parvovirus B19, which cause fetal hydrops, and genetic syndromes such as Noonan's syndrome.

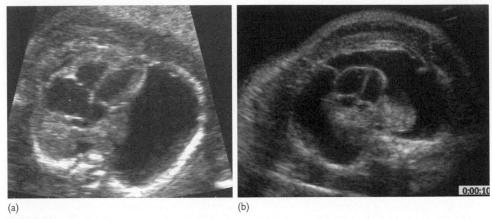

(a)   (b)

Fig. 7.13.3 (a) Transverse section through the fetal thorax showing pleural effusion (anechoeic area) in the right hemithorax with significant mediastinal shift to the left. (b) Transverse section through the fetal thorax showing bilateral pleural effusions (anechoeic area) in a fetus with hydrops (note the skin oedema). Both fetal lungs are hypoplastic.

Ultrasound features

A fluid-filled space surrounding one (Fig. 7.13.3a) or both fetal lungs (Fig. 7.13.3b) in isolation is seen and this may be associated with ascites, skin oedema, or pericardial effusion, suggesting fetal hydrops. A detailed fetal survey with specialist fetal echocardiography is essential to rule out possible associations, and the laboratory work-up should include screening for maternal viral infections, antibodies, and an invasive test for karyotyping. In the vast majority of cases with isolated effusion, no obvious cause can be identified. Accumulation of fluid in the pleural space may lead to pulmonary hypoplasia, compression of the heart, and obstruction of venous return with subsequent development of hydrops and compression of the oesophagus leading to polyhydramnios.

Management

Antenatal

Antenatal management of fetal pleural effusion should include serial scans and counselling involving the neonatal, genetics, and the fetal medicine team. The main consequence of the pleural effusion is that of pulmonary hypoplasia and pulmonary vascular hypertension. The risks of developing these depend on the time and duration of the pleural effusion. Worsening effusion indicates impaired pulmonary development and this should prompt the discussion of options to drain the effusion either by thoracocentesis or by a thoraco-amniotic shunt. Both procedures are not without risk, and this needs to be balanced against the high risk of mortality and morbidity following pulmonary hypoplasia. The delivery should be at a centre that can offer tertiary level neonatal care.

Postnatal

Postnatal care aims to stabilize the baby by promoting lung expansion (pleural drains may be needed) and by reducing the pulmonary vascular resistance. Respiratory dysfunction combined with prematurity are the main factors that contribute to neonatal death.

Prognosis

Fetal pleural effusions may regress spontaneously or show rapid deterioration with onset of fetal hydrops. There are no indicators to suggest the course of the effusion in a given fetus. The outcome is mainly determined by any underlying fetal condition/abnormality, and also depends on the trend in the fluid collection, the gestational age of occurrence, occurrence of polyhydramnios and the gestational age of delivery. Fetuses with hydrops tend to show a very high mortality of about 60% in the perinatal period. Fetuses with isolated pleural effusion that show spontaneous regression do very well. Survival for fetuses with persistent effusions following *in utero* intervention appears better for those without hydrops (around 80%) than those presenting with hydrops (around 60%).

Further reading

Cavoretto P, Molina F, Poggi S, *et al*. Prenatal diagnosis and outcome of echogenic fetal lung lesions. Ultrasound Obstet Gynecol 2008;32:769–83.

Jani JC, Nicolaides KH, Gratacós E, *et al*. Severe diaphragmatic hernia treated by fetal endoscopic tracheal occlusion. Ultrasound Obstet Gynecol 2009;34:304–10.

Lakhoo K. Management of congenital cystic adenomatous malformations of the lung Arch Dis Child Fetal Neonatal Ed 2009; 94;F73–6.

Maeda H, Shimokawa H, Yamaguchi Y, *et al*. The influence of pleural effusion on pulmonary growth in the human fetus. J Perinat Med 1989;17:231–4.

Mann S, Wilson RD, Bebbington MW, *et al*. Antenatal diagnosis and management of congenital cystic adenomatoid malformation. Semin Fetal Neonatal Med 2007;12:477–81.

Rustico MA, Lanna M, Coviello DS, *et al*. Fetal pleural effusion. Prenat Diagn 2007;27:793–9.

van den Hout L, Sluiter I, Gischler S, *et al*. Can we improve outcome of congenital diaphragmatic hernia? Pediatr Surg Int 2009;25:733–43.

Fetal abnormalities: urinary system

Definition
Abnormalities of the genitourinary tract may affect the kidney alone, including irregularities of number, structure and location. Urinary tract dilatation can result from obstruction or reflux and occur at any level, with or without associated with renal dysplasia.

Epidemiology
Genitourinary tract anomalies are relatively common, accounting for approximately 20% of all fetal malformations. The number detected antenatally varies widely, from 1 in 70 to 1 in 1200 across different centres internationally. The variation is likely to be due to gestational age at scan and definitions used rather than true population differences.

Pathology
Renal
- Renal agenesis may be unilateral or bilateral; it results from early degeneration of the ureteric bud or failed interaction between the ureteric bud and the blastema. Unilateral renal agenesis occurs in 1:3000 pregnancies. It may occur in isolation, in association with minor abnormalities such as uterine malformations, or more complicated structural abnormalities such as the VACTERL sequence:
  - Vertebral anomalies
  - Anal atresia
  - Cardiovascular anomalies
  - Tracheoesophageal fistula
  - Esophageal atresia
  - Renal (kidney) and/or radial anomalies
  - Limb defects.
- Duplex kidney is more common in females and arises from premature division of the ureteric bud resulting in two pelvicalyceal systems. The upper ureter usually enters the bladder abnormally, or may form ectopic connections to other pelvic organs. It may be associated with obstruction or reflux.
- Renal ectopy may involve one or both kidneys. It affects 1 in 1200 pregnancies and results in a caudally displaced kidney, which if located in the pelvis carries a risk of obstruction.
- A horseshoe kidney occurs due to fusion of the kidneys, usually at the lower pole. Function is usually normal but it may be associated with aneuploidy (i.e. monosomy X).
- Autosomal recessive polycystic kidney disease (infantile polycystic kidney disease) results in large kidneys which retain their shape but contain multiple cysts, often associated with other anomalies.
- Autosomal dominant polycystic kidney disease (adult polycystic kidney disease) may have an early and severe expression and therefore be detected *in utero*.
- Multicystic dysplastic kidney is an idiopathic condition in which the kidney loses its shape due to the presence of multiple cysts. The ureter is usually atretic.

Urinary tract
- Ureteric junction obstruction is the commonest abnormality of the fetal urinary tract. It may rarely be caused by external compression from an ectopic vessel.

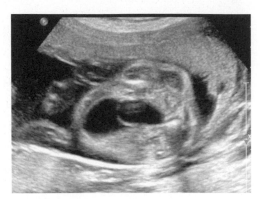

Fig 7.14.1 Ultrasound image showing ureterocele.

- Megaureter occurs as a result of dysfunction of the uterovesical junction.
- Ureterocele is a cystic dilatation of the intravesical ureter. It arises from an ectopic location of the ureter within the bladder. It may obstruct the corresponding ureter, and, if large, the bladder neck (Fig. 7.14.1).
- Obstruction of the bladder outlet (lower urinary tract obstruction) usually occurs within the urethra. This results in hypertrophy of the bladder wall and may also be associated with hydronephrosis and renal dysplasia. The commonest cause in males (1 in 5000–8000 boys) is posterior urethral valves; folds of mucosa along the posterior wall of the urethra resulting in a narrow lumen. Urethral atresia may also occur.
- Complex cloacal anomalies occur after failure of the urogenital sinus to divide normally, resulting in vesicovaginal or vesicourethral fistulae in females and urethrorectal fistulae in males.
- Urachal diverticulum results from failure of closure of the infrafunicular portion of the urachus, leading to a cystic mass within the cord wall which may persist as a vesicocutaneous fistula neonatally.
- Vesicoureteric reflux results in functional dilatation of the ureter and calyceal systems.

Ultrasound findings
The fetal bladder may be imaged from the late first trimester and the fetal kidneys by 11–14 weeks. The sonographic corticomedullary differentiation of the kidneys takes place by 24 weeks. It is not always possible to distinguish between obstruction and reflux sonographically, or to determine the underlying pathology.

Renal
- Both forms of polycystic kidney disease may appear as bilateral enlarged kidneys with a hyperechogenic cortex (Fig. 7.14.2).
- Multicystic dysplastic kidneys are easily differentiated from polycystic kidneys sonographically due to the presence of macrocysts (0.5–3 cm) (Fig. 7.14.3).

Urinary tract
- Pyelectasis is renal pelvic dilatation without calyceal involvement and is found in 2% of pregnancies. It is defined as an anteroposterior (AP) diameter greater

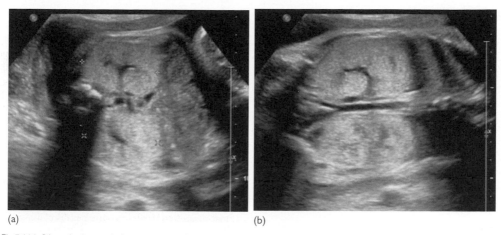

(a)   (b)

Fig 7.14.2 Bilateral echogenic kidneys in autosomal recessive (infantile) polycystic kidney disease in (a) axial and (b) coronal views.

than 6 mm in the second trimester and 8–10 mm in the third. In most cases it is physiological but it may represent reflux or obstruction.

- Fetal hydronephrosis is defined as an AP diameter greater than 15 mm and/or calyceal involvement (Fig. 7.14.4).
- Hydroureter appears as a convoluted transonic image between the kidney and bladder. A normal ureter is not visualized.
- A dilated bladder that does not empty over the course of the scan is suggestive of lower urinary tract obstruction. The bladder appears round, the wall may be hypertrophic (>3 mm). In the case of posterior urethral valves the dilated proximal urethra forms the 'keyhole' sign (Fig. 7.14.5).

Aetiology

Overall, 12% of fetal urinary tract anomalies are associated with a chromosomal abnormality. Rare familial cases of renal agenesis have been reported, with variable patterns of inheritance. Cystic kidneys may occur with several multiple malformation conditions, for example the autosomal recessive Meckel–Gruber syndrome.

Prognosis

The prognosis for isolated unilateral renal lesions is good. For bilateral lesions or obstruction, the prognosis depends on an assessment of renal function. It is not yet established whether obstructive uropathy causes renal dysplasia, or the renal abnormality arises from a simultaneous disordered embryological process.

An assessment of fetal renal function may be made via

- measurement of liquor volume: fetal urine is the main source of amniotic fluid production in the second and third trimesters. Severe oligohydramios, particularly from 16–22 weeks' gestation, results in pulmonary hypoplasia, which is invariably lethal. Anhydramnios also may result in fetal demise secondary to cord compression. Oligohydramnios is associated with a higher incidence of postnatal renal failure and perinatal mortality
- appearance of the fetal kidneys: hyperechogenicity of the cortex and the appearance of macrocysts are suggestive of renal dysplasia and poor renal function. However, the renal pelvic diameter is not a prognostic indicator; there may be gross enlargement and a thin cortex with normal renal function

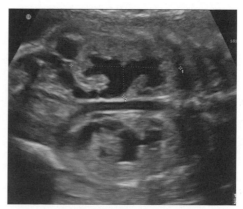

Fig 7.14.3 Multicystic dysplastic kideney.

Fig 7.14.4 severe hydronephrosis with calyceal involvement.

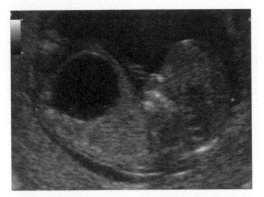

Fig 7.14.5 Fetal megacystis in the first trimester.

- fetal urinalysis: this has a controversial role in the assessment of renal function. An elevated urinary sodium and calcium show some correlation with poor postnatal renal function, but no single analyte or threshold is predictive.

No single measurement or combination of the above has been shown to accurately predict renal failure.

Clinical approach

Diagnosis

History: key points
- The majority of urinary system abnormalities will be detected by routine antenatal scanning.
- A family history of an inherited condition, chromosomal anomaly or urinary tract defect should be considered when interpreting the scan findings.

Investigations: key points
- The diagnosis should be confirmed with a detailed ultrasound performed by a fetal medicine specialist. This should include an assessment for the presence of associated anomalies.
- A fetal karyotype should be considered. In isolated pyelectasis, due to the frequency of this finding in normal pregnancy, the likelihood of aneuploidy is low and invasive testing therefore not routinely performed. If there are associated abnormalities the risk of aneuploidy increases 10- to 20-fold.

Management

Conservative: key points
- Unilateral renal lesions generally have a good prognosis and can be managed conservatively.
- In cases of bilateral hydronephrosis or features suggestive of lower urinary tract obstruction, conservative management, with regular ultrasound to monitor the condition, may be advised if the urinary tract dilatation is mild, or detected for the first time at a late gestation.
- Parents with a severe abnormality and poor prognosis may opt for conservative management.
- All parents, regardless of prognosis, should be referred to the paediatric team to discuss postnatal management, and delivery planned in a unit with appropriate neonatal care facilities.

Termination of pregnancy: key points
- In the case of a urinary tract anomaly with a poor prognosis termination of pregnancy may be offered.

- This is a difficult decision, particularly with the uncertainty in predicting renal function, and parents should be given ample time to discuss the options with the fetal medicine and paediatric teams.
- All parents who undergo termination of pregnancy or miscarry should be advised to have a post-mortem examination; this can confirm the antenatal findings and enable improved counselling for future pregnancies.

Fetal therapy: key points
- Various techniques have been proposed to relieve lower urinary tract obstruction; restoration of liquor volume allows pulmonary development and relief of the urinary pressure has been purported to allow normal renal development.
- Open fetal surgery carries a high risk of fetal and maternal morbidity and is not currently practised.
- Fetal endoscopy is difficult, is only applicable to posterior urethral valves and carries and increased risk of damage to associated organs through the use of laser in a small fetus.
- The use of a vesico-amniotic shunt, a double pigtail catheter inserted transabdominally, has been used more commonly. However, the evidence of benefit is insufficient, and there are associated risks of miscarriage, maternal, and fetal infection and injury.
- In the UK, the National Institute for Health and Clinical Excellence (NICE) therefore recommend that shunts are only used within the context of a clinical trial.
- The PLUTO trial is a multicentre randomized controlled trial to determine the effect of shunting and is now recruiting.

Follow-up
Postnatal management should involve radiological imaging of the urinary tract: further intervention will depend on the abnormality and renal function.

Future pregnancy planning
If a karyotypic abnormality or inherited disorder is present referral to a geneticist should be made.

Further reading

Twining P. Uninary tract abnormalities. In: Twining P, McHugo J, Pilling D. *Textbook of fetal abnormalities*. London: Churchill Livingstone 2000:269–314

Zaccara A, Giorlandino C, Mobili L, *et al*. Amniotic fluid index and fetal bladder outflow obstruction: do we really need more? J Urol 2005;174:1657–60.

Hutton KA, Thomas DF, Davies BW. Prenatally detected posterior urethral valves: qualitative assessment of second trimes-ter scans and prediction of outcome. J Urol 1997;158:1022–5.

Morris RK. Quinlan-Jones E, Kilby M, *et al*. Systematic review of fetal urine analysis to predict poor postnatal renal function in cases of congenital lower urinary tract obstruction. Prenat Diagn 2007;27:900–11.

Clark TJ, Martin WL, Divakaran TJ, *et al*. Prenatal bladder drainiage in the management of fetal lower urinary tract obstruction: a systematic review and meta-analysis. Obstet Gynecol 2003;102:367–82.

Dommergues M, Daikha-Dahmane F, Mueller F, *et al*. Kidney and urinary tract disorders. In: Rodeck CH, Whittle MJ (ed.) *Fetal medicine basic science and clinical practice*. London: Churchill Livingstone 2008: Ch 35.

Internet resources

PLUTO trial: www.pluto.bham.ac.uk

NICE interventional procedure guideline: www.nice.org.uk/guidance/IPG202/?c=91520

Fetal movement charts

Definition

A fetal movement chart is a record, usually kept by the mother, of her baby's movements. The objective is to monitor the baby's wellbeing, and to alert caregivers to ill-health or the risk of intrauterine death. The baby's movements may also be monitored qualitatively, without recording on a chart.

Epidemiology

Annual global stillbirths are estimated at 3.2 million (uncertainty range 2.5–4.1 million). Stillbirth rates range from 5 per 1000 in rich countries to 32 per 1000 in south Asia and sub-Saharan Africa. In South Africa, the commonest cause of perinatal loss is unexplained intrauterine death. Maternal perception of decreased fetal movements affects 5–15% of pregnancies.

Pathology

Fetuses have remarkable mechanisms for conserving oxygen and energy when deprived, including preferential circulation to essential organs and reduced breathing and body movements. Movements may also be affected by central nervous system pathology, medication and reduced amniotic fluid volume. Betamethasone administration may suppress the diurnal increase in movements in the afternoon, but not affect the morning movement pattern.

Aetiology

Risk factors for intrauterine death include maternal illness such as hypertensive disorders, diabetes mellitus, thyroid disease, and intrahepatic cholestasis; Chronic smoking, placental dysfunction with restricted fetal growth, placental abruption, amniotic fluid infection, congenital infections, fetal anaemia (from isoimmunization and other causes), fetomaternal haemorrhage, congenital anomalies and post maturity (>42 weeks for singletons, >38 weeks for twins).

Prognosis

Reduced fetal movement has poor specificity for fetal ill-health. Thus the prognosis for babies with reduced movements is in general good.

The most important question regarding the use of fetal movement assessment (as for any screening test), is whether it is likely to do more good than harm. Potential harms include anxiety induced by the screening procedure, and a cascade of unnecessary interventions, particularly when the screening test has a high false-positive rate and the population being screened is at low risk. In the case of fetal movement assessment, the matter is made worse by the fact the 'confirmatory' test usually used, cardiotocography, also has a high false-positive rate.

The evidence of effectiveness of fetal movement monitoring is not straightforward. Two prospective cohort studies found a reduction in stillbirth when fetal movement counting was used, as did one quasi-randomized trial with allocation based on initial hospital booking number.

A systematic review found no randomized trials comparing fetal movement counting with no fetal movement counting. A large cluster randomized trial (>68 000 women) compared routine formal fetal movement counting with fetal movement counting at the discretion of the caregiver. The potential effect on perinatal outcome may have been masked by contamination of the 'control' group: the rate of antepartum late fetal deaths in both groups was considerably lower than it was prior to the commencement of the study. The potential effectiveness of routine over discretionary fetal movement counting is suggested by the fact that, when fetal movements were formally counted, there were more babies with subsequent unexplained late fetal deaths who were alive when first admitted to hospital (11/59 versus 6/58). However, the warnings did not translate into fewer deaths, mainly because of falsely reassuring fetal testing, mainly cardiotocography, and clinical error. There is thus indirect evidence that fetal movement counting may be effective in screening for babies at risk of intrauterine death, but to date no direct evidence of reduced perinatal mortality.

The recommendation of the UK NICE guidelines is that formal fetal movement counting should not be used routinely.

Clinical approach to reduced fetal movements

Diagnosis

History

Fetal movements may be evaluated qualitatively by asking mothers to report their perception of reduced movements, or semiquantitatively by asking mothers to record movements on a chart. Various modifications of the 'count to 10' method developed in Cardiff, which measures the time taken for 10 movements to occur, have been found to enjoy better compliance than counting the number of movements over a specified time period. In low-risk Japanese women, the count to 10 time was almost the same from 22 weeks (10.9; 7.3–18.0 (median; interquartile range)) until 32 weeks (10.0; 6.2–15.6), then gradually increased toward 40 weeks (14.8; 9.5–24.0). Its 90th percentile was approximately 25 at 22–36 weeks and 35 minutes at 37–40 weeks.

Examination

The baby's heart is auscultated to confirm that the baby is alive. Auscultation of a regular heart rate does not confirm the baby's wellbeing. Examination of the mother is directed towards possible causes for reduced movements, and clinical assessment of the baby's growth (such as by plotting serial measurements of the symphysis–fundus distance) and volume of amniotic fluid. Evaluation of the baby's wellbeing may include clinical assessment of the baby's movement or heart rate response to vibro-acoustic stimulation. The sound produced by an electronic vibro-acoustic stimulator may be mimicked by placing the base of an empty soft drink can against the mother's abdomen, steadying it with a thumb and middle finger on the rim, depressing the ring opener with the index finger and allowing it to snap back.

Investigations

Various electronic methods of measuring fetal movements have been developed, but are not in routine clinical practice. Investigations are directed towards other methods of assessing the baby. If available, cardiotocography is often used to assess the baby's wellbeing, although systematic review of cardiotocography for antepartum fetal assessment has shown an association with a trend to increased perinatal deaths. Vibro-acoustic stimulation but not manual manipulation has been shown to evoke fetal movements and thus facilitate fetal heart rate testing. Ultrasound is used to assess growth, amniotic fluid volume, anatomy, organ blood flow and umbilical artery resistance.

Chronic placental hypoxia results in fetoplacental vasoconstriction with increased umbilical artery resistance index, a situation analogous to pulmonary hypertension in response to chronically hypoxic lungs. Observation of fetal breathing movements indicates that amniotic fluid infection is unlikely. The biophysical profile is a scoring system with 2 points each for adequate fetal body movement, tone, breathing, and amniotic fluid assessed by ultrasound, and reactive cardiotocography. There is to date inadequate evidence of effectiveness to support its use.

In some cases amniocentesis may be useful to exclude amniotic fluid infection and confirm fetal lung maturity.

Counselling

As for other methods of prenatal screening (and screening in general), even a simple recommendation to monitor the baby's movements may generate anxiety.

The perception of reduced fetal movements is a cause of considerable anxiety, particularly in women with previous pregnancy losses. Careful explanation of the implications and limitations of the test is important.

Management

The management of reduced fetal movements must take into account several parameters:

● evidence of fetal compromise, and the strength of this evidence

● any identifiable causes for fetal compromise

● the gestational age of the baby.

Where the mother's condition is contributing to fetal compromise and the baby is reasonably stable, the first priority is to optimize the mother's condition.

Very rarely, the baby may have a condition amenable to intrauterine treatment, such as transfusion for anaemia or medical treatment for a tachyarrhythmia. Equally rarely, the baby's condition may be considered irretrievable, for example severe central nervous system anomalies or extreme prematurity, and the parents may be counselled about the option of conservative care.

General measures to improve the baby's condition include ensuring that the mother avoids the supine position, and tocolysis if the uterus is contracting.

In most cases the definitive management involves deciding on the optimal timing for delivery of the baby. Here the risks of intervention and prematurity need to be weighed against the risk of intrauterine deterioration or death if managed expectantly. If delivery is considered to be in the mother and baby's best interest, the method of delivery will depend on the baby's condition and the likelihood that the baby will tolerate labour induction (as opposed to Caesarean section).

Follow-up/recurrence/future pregnancy planning

When reduced fetal movements precedes a pregnancy loss, it is most important to counsel the parents about the implications of the loss. Most parents will want to know at least three things: What was the cause of the loss? Was it our fault? Will it happen again? To address these questions, considerable attention must be paid to ascertaining the cause of the loss, including clinical examination of the baby, genetic tests if indicated, tests for maternal endocrine disorders and infections, placental histology, and post-mortem examination of the baby.

Further reading

de Heus R, Mulder EJ, Derks JB, et al. Differential effects of betamethasone on the fetus between morning and afternoon recordings. J Matern Fetal Neonatal Med 2008;21:549–54.

de Vries JI, Fong BF. Changes in fetal motility as a result of congenital disorders: an overview. Ultrasound Obstet Gynecol 2007;29:590–9.

Frøen JF, Heazell AE, Tveit JV, et al. Fetal movement assessment. Semin Perinatol 2008;32:243–6.

Gibb D, Arulkumaran S. Fetal monitoring in practice, 2nd edn. Oxford: Butterworth Heinemann 1997.

Grivell RM, Wong L, Bhatia V. Regimens of fetal surveillance for impaired fetal growth (Protocol). Cochrane Database Syst Rev 2008;2:CD007113.

Habek D. Effects of smoking and fetal hypokinesia in early pregnancy. Arch Med Res 2007;38:864–7.

Heazell AE, Green M, Wright C, et al. Midwives' and obstetricians' knowledge and management of women presenting with decreased fetal movements. Acta Obstet Gynecol Scand 2008; 87:331–9

Heazell AE, Frøen JF. Methods of fetal movement counting and the detection of fetal compromise. J Obstet Gynaecol 2008;28:147–54.

Hofmeyr GJ, Neilson JP, Alfirevic Z, et al. A Cochrane pocketbook: pregnancy and childbirth. Chichester: Wiley 2008.

Kuwata T, Matsubara S, Ohkusa T, et al. Establishing a reference value for the frequency of fetal movements using modified 'count to 10' method. J Obstet Gynaecol Res 2008;34:318–23.

Lalor JG, Fawole B, Alfirevic Z, Devane D. Biophysical profile for fetal assessment in high risk pregnancies. Cochrane Database Syst Rev 2008;1:CD000038.

Mancuso A, De Vivo A, Fanara G, et al. Effects of antepartum electronic fetal monitoring on maternal emotional state. Acta Obstet Gynecol Scand 2008;87:184–9

Martin CB Jr. Normal fetal physiology and behavior, and adaptive responses with hypoxemia. Semin Perinatol 2008;32:239–42.

Neldam S. Fetal movements as an indicator of fetal well-being. Lancet 1980;1:1222–4.

Nishihara K, Horiuchi S, Eto H, Honda M. A long-term monitoring of fetal movement at home using a newly developed sensor: An introduction of maternal micro-arousals evoked by fetal movement during maternal sleep. Early Hum Dev 2008;84:595–603.

Neilson JP, Alfirevic Z. Doppler ultrasound for fetal assessment in high risk pregnancies. Cochrane Database Syst Rev 1996;4:CD000073.

N Pattison, L McCowan. Cardiotocography for antepartum fetal assessment. Cochrane Database Syst Rev 1999;1:CD001068.

Reddy UM. Prediction and prevention of recurrent stillbirth. Obstet Gynecol 2007;110:1151–64.

Sinha D, Sharma A, Nallaswamy V, et al. Obstetric outcome in women complaining of reduced fetal movements. J Obstet Gynaecol 2007; 27:41–3.

Stanton C, Lawn JE, Rahman H, et al. Stillbirth rates: delivering estimates in 190 countries. Lancet 2006;367:1487–94.

Tan KH, Sabapathy A. Fetal manipulation for facilitating tests of fetal wellbeing. Cochrane Database Syst Rev 2001;4:CD003396.

Tan KH, Smyth R. Fetal vibroacoustic stimulation for facilitation of tests of fetal wellbeing. Cochrane Database Syst Rev 2001;1:CD002963.

Troyano Luque JM, Maeda K, et al. Fetal extremity kinetics quantified with Doppler ultrasonography. J Perinat Med 2008;36:82–6.

Westgate J, Jamieson M. Stillbirths and fetal movements. NZ Med J 1986;99:114–16.

Mangesi L, Hofmeyr GJ. Fetal movement counting for assessment of fetal wellbeing. Cochrane Database Syst Rev 2007;1:CD004909.

Internet resources

www.marchofdimes.com/professionals/14332_1198.asp

Patient resources

Stillbirth and neonatal death society: www.uk-sands.org/

Fetal nuchal translucency

Definition

Nuchal translucency (NT) is a black space seen by ultrasound behind the fetal neck and is produced by the collection of fluid under the skin.

- NT is observed in all fetuses between 11 and 13 weeks of pregnancy.
- In fetuses with trisomy 21 and other abnormalities, the size of NT tends to be higher than in normal fetuses.

Epidemiology

The median and 95th centiles of fetal NT increase with fetal crown–rump length. In a population of 100 000 fetuses 200 have trisomy 21, another 200 have other chromosomal defects and 99 600 are euploid.

- In a few (5%) of euploid fetuses the NT is above the 95th centile. Therefore, 4800 euploid fetuses (5% of 99 600) would have high NT.
- In many (75%) fetuses with trisomy 21 and other chromosomal defects the NT is above the 95th centile. Therefore, 150 fetuses with trisomy 21 (75% of 200) and 150 fetuses with other chromosomal defects (75% of 200) have high NT.
- Therefore, even when the scan shows a high NT the majority of fetuses are euploid (4800 are euploid and 300 have chromosomal defects).

Diagnosis

The diagnosis of increased fetal NT is made by ultrasound examination at 11–13 weeks of gestation.

The reasons for selecting 11 weeks as the earliest gestation are

- if after the screening test the parents choose to have CVS (chorionic villus sampling) this is not safe before 11 weeks because it can cause limb defects
- many major fetal abnormalities can be diagnosed at the NT scan, provided the minimum gestation is 11 weeks. With earlier scanning the abnormalities can be missed because the fetus is too small and the various organs are not developed enough to be visible.

The reasons for selecting 13 weeks and 6 days as the upper limit are

- to provide women with affected fetuses the option of first rather than second trimester termination
- even in fetuses with chromosomal abnormalities the high NT usually disappears after 13 weeks.

Pathophysiology

Increased fetal NT is associated with a heterogeneous group of conditions, suggesting that there may not be a single underlying mechanism for the collection of fluid under the skin of the fetal neck.

Possible mechanisms include the following:

- Cardiac defects/dysfunction: in both chromosomally abnormal and euploid fetuses there is a high association between increased NT and cardiac defects.
- Venous congestion in the head and neck: this could result from constriction of the fetal body as encountered in amnion rupture sequence and superior mediastinal compression found in diaphragmatic hernia or the narrow chest in skeletal dysplasias.
- Altered composition of the extracellular matrix: many of the component proteins of the extracellular matrix are encoded on chromosomes 21, 18, or 13. Immunohistochemical studies, examining the skin of chromosomally abnormal fetuses, have demonstrated specific alterations of the extracellular matrix which may be attributed to gene dosage effects. Altered composition of the extracellular matrix may also be the underlying mechanism for increased fetal NT in an expanding number of genetic syndromes, which are associated with alterations in collagen metabolism (such as achondrogenesis type II), abnormalities of fibroblast growth factor receptors (such as achondroplasia), or disturbed metabolism of peroxisome biogenesis factor (such as Zellweger's syndrome).
- Failure of lymphatic drainage: a possible mechanism for increased NT is dilatation of the jugular lymphatic sacs, because of developmental delay in the connection with the venous system, or a primary abnormal dilatation or proliferation of the lymphatic channels interfering with a normal flow between the lymphatic and venous systems. Immunohistochemical studies in nuchal skin tissue from fetuses with Turner syndrome have shown that the lymphatic vessels in the upper dermis are hypoplastic. In chromosomally normal fetuses with increased NT, deficient lymphatic drainage, due to hypoplastic or aplastic lymphatic vessels, is found in association with Noonan syndrome and congenital lymphoedema. In congenital neuromuscular disorders, such as fetal akinesia deformation sequence, myotonic dystrophy and spinal muscular atrophy, increased NT may be the consequence of impaired lymphatic drainage due to reduced fetal movements.
- Fetal anaemia: this is associated with a hyperdynamic circulation and fetal hydrops develops when the haemoglobin deficit is more than 7 g/dL. This is true for both immune and non-immune hydrops fetalis. However, in red blood cell isoimmunization severe fetal anaemia does not occur before 16 weeks of gestation, presumably because the fetal reticuloendothelial system is too immature to result in destruction of antibody coated erythrocytes. Consequently, red blood cell isoimmunization does not present with increased fetal NT. In contrast, genetic causes of fetal anaemia (α-thalassaemia, Blackfan–Diamond anaemia, congenital erythropoietic porphyria, dyserythropoietic anaemia, Fanconi anaemia) and possibly congenital infection-related anaemia can present with increased fetal NT.
- Fetal hypoproteinaemia: this is implicated in the pathophysiology of both immune and non-immune hydrops fetalis. In the first trimester, hypoproteinaemia due to proteinuria may be the underlying mechanism for the increased NT in fetuses with congenital nephrotic syndrome.
- Fetal infection: in about 10% of cases of 'unexplained' second- or third trimester fetal hydrops, there is evidence of recent maternal infection and, in these cases, the fetus is also infected. In contrast, in euploid pregnancies with increased NT, only 1.5% of the mothers have evidence of recent infection and the fetuses are rarely infected. Therefore, in pregnancies with increased NT the prevalence of maternal infection with the TORCH group of organisms may not be higher than in the general population. Increased NT in euploid fetuses need not stimulate the search for maternal infection unless

the NT evolves into second or third trimester nuchal oedema or generalized hydrops. The only infection that has been reported in association with increased NT is parvovirus B19. In this condition the increased NT has been attributed to myocardial dysfunction or fetal anaemia due to suppression of haemopoiesis.

Implications of increased NT

- Chromosomal defects: The prevalence of chromosomal defects increases exponentially with NT thickness from 0.2% for those with NT between the 5th and 95th centiles to 65% for NT of 6.5 mm or more. In the chromosomally abnormal group, about 50% have trisomy 21, 25% have trisomy 18 or 13, 10% have Turner's syndrome, 5% have triploidy and 10% have other chromosomal defects.
- Fetal death: In chromosomally normal fetuses, the prevalence of fetal death increases with NT thickness from about 1% for those with NT between the 95th and 99th centiles to about 20% for NT of 6.5 mm or more. The majority of fetuses that die do so by 20 weeks and they usually show progression from increased NT to severe hydrops.
- Major fetal abnormalities: These are defined as those requiring medical and/or surgical treatment or conditions associated with mental handicap. The prevalence of major fetal abnormalities in chromosomally normal fetuses increases with NT thickness, from 1.5%, in those with NT below the 95th centile, to 2.5% for NT between the 95th and 99th centiles, and exponentially thereafter to about 45% for NT of 6.5 mm or more.

Management

Although increased fetal NT thickness is associated with abnormalities and fetal death, the majority of babies survive and develop normally. After the diagnosis of increased NT the aim must be to distinguish as accurately and quickly as possible between those that are likely to have problems from those where the baby is likely to be normal.

Fetal NT between the 95th centile and 99th centile (3.5 mm)

The parents should be counselled of the possible increased risk for chromosomal defects. The decision by the parents in favour or against fetal karyotyping will depend on the patient-specific risk for chromosomal defects, which is derived from the combination of maternal age, sonographic findings and serum free β-human chorionic gonadotropin and PAPP-A.

A detailed scan should be carried out at 11–13 weeks and again at 20 weeks in search of major abnormalities. If no obvious abnormalities are seen the parents should be reassured that their baby is likely to be live born and develop normally. The chances that there would be any problems are not higher than in fetuses without increased NT.

Fetal NT above 3.5 mm

This is found in about 1% of pregnancies.

- The risk of chromosomal defects is very high and the first line of management of such pregnancies should be the offer CVS for fetal karyotyping. In patients with a family history of genetic syndromes that can be diagnosed by DNA analysis, the CVS sample can also be tested for these syndromes.
- A detailed scan should be carried out at 11–13 weeks in search of major abnormalities and genetic syndromes. A detailed scan is also carried out a couple of weeks later and again at 20 weeks.
- If no obvious abnormalities are seen and the NT has completely resolved, the parents should be reassured that their baby is likely to be live born and develop normally. The chances that the baby will have a serious abnormality or neurodevelopmental delay may not be higher than in the general population.
- If no obvious abnormalities are seen but there is persistence of increased NT at 14–16 weeks and evolution to nuchal oedema or hydrops fetalis at 20–22 weeks, it is possible that there is congenital infection or a genetic syndrome. Maternal blood should be tested for toxoplasmosis, cytomegalovirus, and parvovirus B19. Follow-up scans should be carried out every 4 weeks to define the evolution of the oedema. Consideration should be given to DNA testing for certain genetic conditions, such as Noonan syndrome, even if there is no family history for these conditions. The parents should be counselled that there is a 10% risk of perinatal death or a live birth with a genetic syndrome that could not be diagnosed prenatally. The risk of neurodevelopmental delay in the survivors is 3–5%.

Further reading

Nicolaides KH. The 11-13+6 week scan. Fetal Medicine Foundation, London, 2004. Available in pdf at www.fetalmedicine.com/

Internet resources

www.fetalmedicine.com/

Fetal abnormalities: hydrops

Definition
Hydrops is defined as an abnormal accumulation of serous fluid in at least two fetal compartments, including ascites, pleural or pericardial effusions, and skin oedema (Fig.7.17.1).

Epidemiology
Hydrops is a rare finding, affecting about 1 in 2000 pregnancies. As it can be caused by a number of recessive genetic disorders, it is more common in countries where those disorders are common. Thus, hydrops may be as common as 1 in 500 due to homozygous α-thalassaemia in South-East Asia, or glucose-6-phosphate dehydrogenase deficiency in Mediterranean countries.

Aetiology
In general terms, hydrops can be due to cardiac failure, obstructed lymphatic flow, or decreased plasma osmotic pressure.

Multiple pregnancy
The finding of hydrops in one fetus of a monochorionic pair is typical of severe twin–twin transfusion or twin reversed arterial perfusion syndromes. This is due to overload and cardiac failure of the recipient twin.

Fetal anaemia
Severe anaemia causes cardiac failure and the finding of hydrops. Hydrops will usually only result from severe anaemia, i.e. when the fetal haemoglobin deficit is more than 7 g/dL below the normal mean for gestation.
- Red cell alloimmunization: until the advent of anti-D prophylaxis, the most common cause of hydrops fetalis was blood group isoimmunization. Although usually due to Rhesus blood group antigens, other blood group antigens including C, E, and Kell antigens can cause fetal haemolytic anaemia
- parvovirus B19 infection
- homozygous α-thalassaemia
- glucose-6-phosphate dehydrogenase deficiency (X-linked, dominant)
- glucose phosphate isomerase deficiency (autosomal recessive)
- pyruvate kinase deficiency (autosomal recessive)
- Diamond–Blackfan syndrome (autosomal dominant)
- fetomaternal haemorrhage
- intrafetal haemorrhage, e.g. intracranial, into a large ovarian cyst.

Structural abnormalities of the fetus or placenta
The most common causes for hydrops in this group are due to cardiac failure due to congenital heart defects and arrhythmias. Thoracic abnormalities can cause cardiac compression, again leading to cardiac failure.

Cardiac abnormalities
- About 40% of cases in this group are due to structural cardiac defects, including left or right hypoplastic heart, large atrioventricular septal defects, or endocardial fibroelastosis.
- Cardiac arrhythmias: both tachy- and bradyarrhythmias. Causes include supraventricular tachycardia and complete heart block due to maternal anti-Ro or anti-La antibodies. Absence of a natural pacemaker (sino-atrial node) can occur in isomerism.
- Cardiomyopathies and cardiac rhabdomyoma.

Thoracic abnormalities
- Cystic lung lesions (congenital cystic adenomatoid malformation, pulmonary sequestration), or other intrathoracic neoplasms.
- Congenital diaphragmatic hernia.
- Congenital high airway obstruction syndrome (CHAOS).

Arteriovenous shunts
High output cardiac failure can be secondary to abnormal arteriovenous communications. These include:
- placental chorioangiomas
- fetal sacrococcygeal teratomas
- other placental of fetal tumours.

Fetal syndromes
- Chromosomal: most commonly trisomies 21, 18, 13, Turner's syndrome or triploidy.
- Genetic: A large number of genetic diseases can present with hydrops fetalis. The more common causes are Noonan syndrome, glycogen storage diseases, lysosome storage diseases, fetal akinesia/deformation sequence,

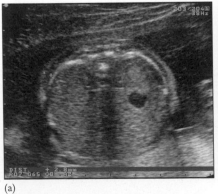
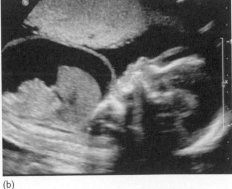

(a)   (b)

Fig. 7.17.1 Ultrasound diagnosis of (a) skin oedema and (b) fetal ascites in fetal hydrops.

achondrogenesis, Fraser syndrome, multiple pterygium syndrome and Smith–Lemli–Opitz syndrome, tuberous sclerosis (autosomal dominant).

Fetal congenital infection

These are most commonly due to early pregnancy congenital infection with cytomegalovirus or parvovirus B19 (see Anaemia, above). Other causative organisms are toxoplasmosis, coxsackie virus, listeria and syphilis.

Prognosis

The most important determinants are the underlying cause and the gestation at presentation. Estimates of mortality vary widely, but most case series report 60–90% mortality. Many cases are due to underlying congenital malformations, genetic or chromosomal abnormalities which in themselves are fatal.

Clinical approach: diagnosis

Referral to a tertiary level fetal medicine unit is indicated. This is essential not only for invasive testing to be performed, but will also allow the woman to benefit from multidisciplinary team approach. This will usually include a fetal medicine expert, cardiologist, geneticist, and other allied specialists.

History

- Previous pregnancy including previously affected pregnancies
- previous fetal congenital abnormalities or fetal death
- previous fetal or neonatal anaemia or jaundice
- previous history of rhesus or other blood group antibodies
- drug history, including recreational drug use
- haemoglobinopathy
- recent of illness or flu-like symptoms
- personal or family history of genetic or metabolic diseases.

Examination/ultrasound findings

- In monochorionic twin pregnancy the finding of hydrops is usually associated with severe twin–twin transfusion syndrome (TTTS). The hydropic twin will have polyhydramnios, a dilated heart with reduced myocardial contractility and ductus venosus Doppler will usually be abnormal. The diagnosis of TTTS is confirmed if the donor co-twin exhibits growth restriction, oligo- or anhydramnios (stuck twin), an unfilled bladder, or abnormal umbilical artery Doppler.
- Doppler measurement of the peak systolic velocity (PSV) in the middle cerebral artery (MCA) is a useful tool in predicting a hyperdynamic fetal circulation. An increased PSV is suggestive of a hyperdynamic circulation, and this is most commonly due to fetal anaemia, which can be caused by alloimmunization, parvovirus infection, congenital fetal anaemia, or fetomaternal haemorrhage. It can also be present due to a fetal or placental tumour or arteriovenous malformation.
- A detailed ultrasound examination looking for possible abnormalities outlined above, including specialist fetal echocardiography should be performed.

Investigations

These depend on the history and detailed ultrasound examination findings.

Maternal

- Blood type/blood group

- CMV, toxoplasma, and parvovirus titres
- If fetal bradyarrhythmia is suspected an antibody screen (Anti-Ro, Anti-La) should be performed
- Kleihauer test if fetomaternal haemorrhage is suspected.

Fetal

Invasive testing should be discussed with the parents. If the hydrops was diagnosed at the 11–14-week scan, chorionic villus sampling will allow fetal karyotype analysis and storage of fetal DNA. Fetal blood sampling should be considered if possible, as this allows measurement of other fetal parameters.

- Fetal karyotype.
- Full blood count.
- Coombs test.
- Metabolic tests may be indicated depending on family history.
- Serum protein may be indicated if hypoproteinaemia is suspected.
- Fetal DNA should always be stored for potential future analysis of as yet unrecognized genetic diseases.

Counselling and management

From the point of view of counselling, hydrops could be classified into treatable and untreatable causes. Treatable causes include.

Twin–twin transfusion syndrome

Left untreated, the mortality of this condition exceeds 90%, with significant neurological morbidity in 30–50% of surviving twins. Serial amnioreduction and fetoscopic laser ablation of the placental vascular anastomoses have been used for treatment of the condition. There is a significant increase in survival rates and reduction in neurological morbidity with the use of laser ablation compared with amnioreduction in severe TTTS. Overall survival rates after laser therapy range from 56% to 62%, survival of at least one twin was reported in 76–83% of cases, and neurological morbidity in about 5–10% of survivors.

Twin reversed arterial perfusion syndrome

Fetoscopic laser coagulation was assessed in a multicentre study and resulted in an overall survival rate of the pump twin of 80%. Preterm premature rupture of the membranes prior to 34 weeks' gestation occurred in 18%.

Fetal anaemia

- The procedure related fetal loss rate after fetal blood transfusion is approximately 2–3% in expert hands.
- Parvovirus infection: this has a generally good outcome if treated appropriately with fetal blood transfusion. Generally, only one or two transfusions may be necessary. One report has suggested that there is an increased incidence of neurodevelopmental delay in children born from pregnancies affected with Parvovirus infection treated with transfusion. In this series five of 16 infants (32%) exhibited some delayed psychomotor development at the age of 6–8 years. Previous reports however did not find such an association.
- Fetal anaemia secondary to immunisation: fetal blood will continue to be destroyed by maternal antibodies. The number of transfusions will depend on the gestational age at onset of the disease, the degree of anaemia, and the rate of red cell breakdown. Repeat transfusions will be necessary in the majority of cases. After 34 weeks

of gestation most practitioners would suggest delivery, as neonatal outcome is likely to be good and *ex utero* treatment removes the procedure related risks of intra-uterine transfusion.

Cardiac arrhythmias
Treatment of fetal cardiac arrhythmias has been reported. Tachyarrhythmias may respond to maternal administration of flecainide, amiodarone, or sotalol.

Chorioangiomas and other AV malformations
Successful interstitial laser therapy of placental chorioangiomas and other AV malformations have been reported. However, due to the rare nature of these conditions it is difficult to assess success rates. Such treatment is warranted in cases of severe progressive hydrops where the prognosis for the pregnancy is poor.

Non-treatable causes of hydrops
When fetal hydrops remains unexplained the prognosis for the pregnancy is very poor. In the presence of an underlying fetal structural abnormality, counselling and management will depend on the precise findings. Options for the pregnancy include monitoring, and elective pregnancy termination.

Further reading

Dembinski J, Haverkamp F, Maara H, *et al*. Neurodevelopmental outcome after intrauterine red cell transfusion for parvovirus B19-induced fetal hydrops. Br J Obstet Gynaecol 2002;109:1232–4.

Fox CD, Kilby, Khan K.S. Contemporary treatments for twin–twin transfusion syndrome. Obstet Gynecol 2005;105:1469–77.

Hecher K, Lewi L, Gratacos E, *et al*. Twin reversed arterial perfusion: fetoscopic laser coagulation of placental anastomoses or the umbilical cord. Ultrasound Obstet Gynecol. 2006;28:688–91.

Heegaard ED, Brown KE. Human parvovirus B19. Clin Microbiol Rev 2002;15:485–505.

Machin GA. Hydrops revisited: literature review of 1,414 cases published in the 1980s. Am J Med Genet 1989;34:366–90.

Nagel HT, de Haan TR, Vandenbussche FP, *et al*. Long-term outcome after fetal transfusion for hydrops associated with parvovirus B19 infection. Obstet Gynecol 2007;109:42–7.

Nicolaides KH, Fontanarosa M, Gabbe SG, Rodeck CH. Failure of ultrasonographic parameters to predict the severity of fetal anemia in rhesus isoimmunization. Am J Obstet Gynecol 1988;158:920–6.

Simpson JM. Fetal arrhythmias. Ultrasound Obstet Gynecol 2006; 27:599–606.

Van Kamp IL, Klumper FJ, Oepkes D, *et al*. Complications of intrauterine intravascular transfusion for fetal anemia due to maternal red-cell alloimmunization. Am J Obstet Gynecol 2005;192:171–7.

Useful websites

Hydrops fetalis: www.emedicine.com/ped/topic1042.htm
Parvovirus: www.hpa.org.uk/infections/topics_az/parvovirus/gen_info.htm

Patient resources

Hydrops: www.patient.co.uk/showdoc/40024818/
Rhesus disease: www.patient.co.uk/showdoc/40000464/

Invasive procedures

Prenatal diagnosis: chorionic villus sampling and amniocentesis

It is estimated that 5% of the pregnant population (30 000 women a year in the UK) are offered invasive prenatal diagnosis (RCOG), in the majority of cases this involves a choice between chorionic villous sampling (CVS) or amniocentesis.

Indications

The most common indication is for performance of fetal chromosome analysis, usually due to screen positive screening test. Other indications include analysis for genetic disease in susceptible pregnancies (for example where both parents are known to be carriers of a recessive genetic disease, or a previous history of a genetic problem).

Procedure outline

CVS is performed from 10 to 14 weeks. With transabdominal CVS a fine needle is introduced through the mother's lower abdomen into the placenta under ultrasound guidance. Transcervical CVS is used much less commonly.

Amniocentesis is performed from 15 weeks onwards. A fine needle is introduced through the mother's lower abdomen or amniotic sac under ultrasound guidance. Between 10 and 20 mL of amniotic fluid is aspirated and this contains fetal cells (from skin, lungs, and urinary tract).

Efficacy

With either technique cells are analysed for chromosomal abnormalities and DNA can be extracted for molecular analysis.

One advantage of CVS is that it is performed much earlier in gestation (between 10 and 14 weeks). As abnormalities are identified at an earlier stage, pregnancy termination may be easier, performed surgically rather than medically, and therefore may be more acceptable. A disadvantage is a small risk of confined placental mosaicism that may result in inconclusive results making additional invasive tests necessary.

Safety

Historically CVS has been thought to have higher procedure-related loss than amniocentesis (Table 7.18.1). However, evidence from meta-analysis and recent series suggest that loss rates after transabdominal CVS are similar to amniocentesis in specialized centres. This may be due to increased experience compared with the earlier studies (operator experience has been shown to have a major impact on procedure-related loss rates), taking account of the earlier gestation at which CVS is performed, and a general move towards a transabdominal approach (a transcervical approach has been associated with a higher CVS loss rate).

Table 7.18.1 Comparison between CVS and amniocentesis

	CVS	**Amniocentesis**
Gestation	10–14 weeks' gestation	15 weeks onwards
	Less than 9 weeks assoc with transverse limb defects	Early amniocentesis (less than 14 weeks) assoc with higher loss rates
Sampled	Chorion	Amniotic fluid
Approach	Transabdominal or transcervical	Transabdominal
Needle	18–22 Gauge	20–22 Gauge
Post-procedural loss rate (miscarriage risk above background)	0.5–1% (Scott *et al.* 2002; Brun *et al.* 2003)	0.5-1% (Horger *et al.* 2001; Tabor *et al.* 1986)
Complications	Vaginal bleeding 4%	Amniotic fluid leak
		Chorioamnionitis
	Severe maternal sepsis 1:1000 or less	Severe maternal sepsis 1:1000 or less
Sampling failure	3% or less	<1%
Culture Failure	0.20%	0.10%
Maternal contamination	<1% after microscopic villi selection	Very low
Mosaicism risk	2% (in the main confined to the placenta)	0.3% (50% represent true fetal mosaicism)
Timescale for results	PCR based common aneuploidy screen 2-3 days	PCR based common aneuploidy screen 2–3 days
	Routine karyotype (cultured cells) 14 days	Routine karyotype (cultured cells) 14 days
	Molecular genetic analysis 2–14 days	Molecular genetic analysis 12–28 days
	CVS procedure of choice as direct extraction of DNA from trophoblast	Amniocentesis requires amniocyte culture (10–14 days) prior to DNA extraction
Availability	Specialist centres	Most obstetric units

In utero **therapeutic interventions**

Fetal blood sampling and in utero transfusion

Fetal blood sampling (FBS) is also known as cordocentesis or percutaneous umbilical blood sampling (PUBS).

Indications

Suspected fetal anaemia or thrombocytopenia. Given the speed of results from CVS and amniocentesis, cordocentesis is rarely used for fetal chromosome analysis.

Middle cerebral artery velocity by Doppler scanning (MCA-PSV) is now the preferred method for detection of fetal anaemia and avoids the need for invasive amniocentesis or repeat fetal blood sampling. A threshold value (usually 1.5 MoM) is used to determine when FBS with possible in utero transfusion (IUT) should be performed.

Transfusion may also be needed in cases of haemolytic anaemia due to non-Rhesus antigens, non-haemolytic anaemia (e.g. fetal parvovirus infection) and fetal alloimmune thrombocytopenia when intrauterine platelet transfusions are required.

Procedure outline

A needle is introduced into the umbilical vein under ultrasound guidance. A sample of fetal blood is rapidly analysed for haematocrit and also sent to haematology. Crossmatched, irradiated, and CMV-negative blood or compatible platelet hyperconcentrates are then transfused as necessary. Rapid delivery in the event of severe fetal distress may be necessary assuming fetal viability.

Efficacy

Modern management of Rhesus disease with MCA-PSV monitoring and judicious use of FBS and IUT has successfully reduced the perinatal mortality associated with this previously devastating condition. In utero transfusion in other cases of fetal anaemia can reverse related hydrops and reduce mortality.

Weekly in utero transfusion of platelets has been shown to be effective in preventing intracranial haemorrhage in severe cases of alloimmune thrombocytopenia, although there are cumulative loss rates of up to 10% for each pregnancy as a result.

Safety

There is a fetal loss of at least 1% for each procedure. These risks include fetomaternal haemorrhage, placental abruption, acute fetal distress (bradycardia), and chorioamnionitis with maternal sepsis. These have to be balanced against the risk of preterm delivery, and in most cases delivery, rather than continuing transfusions, is undertaken beyond 34 weeks.

Laser ablation for twin–twin transfusion syndrome

Indication

Laser ablation is now the accepted best treatment for severe twin–twin transfusion syndrome (TTTS). The role of laser ablation in early TTTS is more controversial.

Outline of procedure

The aim is to divide the abnormal communicating vessels between monchorionic twins and prevent abnormal shunting of blood from the donor to recipient twin. The procedure is usually performed under regional or local anaesthesia under ultrasound guidance. A fetoscope is inserted into the amniotic sac of the recipient twin and anastomosing placental vessels are ablated using a laser.

After completion of surgery amnio drainage of the recipient twin is performed.

Efficacy

Fetoscopic laser, compared with serial amnioreduction or septostomy, both improves perinatal survival and reduces long-term neurological sequelae in survivors. A review of two randomized controlled trials showed less death of both infants per pregnancy (relative risk (RR) 0.49), less perinatal death (RR 0.59) and less neonatal death (RR 0.29) than in pregnancies treated with amnioreduction. More babies were alive without neurological abnormality at the age of six months in the laser group than the amnioreduction groups (RR 1.66) although this difference did not persist beyond six months of age. 1

In utero shunt insertion

Fetal shunts have been inserted in utero for drainage of obstructed lower urinary tracts and pleural effusions.

Outline of shunt insertion

A cannula or trocar is inserted transabdominally into the amniotic cavity under maternal local anaesthesia. This is guided through the fetal abdominal or chest wall into the bladder or pleural effusion. The entire procedure is performed under ultrasound guidance. A pigtail catheter is inserted through the cannula and positioned with one end in the target organ and the other draining into the amniotic cavity. The cannula is removed and the final position of the catheter confirmed with ultrasound

Fetal vesico-amniotic shunt

The evidence supporting shunt insertion is at present uncertain.

Indication

Fetal lower urinary tract outflow obstruction. The purpose of the shunt is to decompress the obstructed bladder and restore normal amniotic fluid dynamics with the aim of preventing the sequelae of renal dysplasia and pulmonary hypoplasia.

Efficacy

A randomized controlled trial is currently in progress (PLUTO) comparing shunt insertion with no shunt. A meta-analysis of three controlled trials comparing outcomes following shunt insertion (n = 59) with no insertion (n = 33) demonstrated an improvement in perinatal survival (OR 2.53). Overall survival rates after shunt insertion are still poor at 40%, reflecting the underlying poor prognosis. There is limited information as to the effect of shunt insertion on longer term outcomes such as need for dialysis (~25%) and long-term bladder and respiratory function.

Safety

The commonest complication is shunt displacement or blockage, occurring in 20–30% of cases, requiring a second shunt insertion. Premature labour and rupture of membranes, fetal trauma, and urinary ascites are all documented complications. Potential maternal complications include trauma to organs and infection though from the limited case series data these would appear to be rare.

Pleuro-amniotic shunt

Indication

Large pleural effusions can lead to lung compression, hypoplasia and hydrops. The aim of shunt insertion is to reverse these. Case selection is difficult as there is uncertainty about the natural history of pleural effusions, and some will resolve spontaneously. This makes it difficult to balance the risks of treatment against the natural progression of the effusion.

Efficacy

Depending on the selection of cases, pleuro-amniotic shunts are effective at draining pleural effusions and allowing lung expansion (98%) and produce resolution of hydrops in 50% of cases. Treatment outcomes vary widely across case series and probably reflect differences in underlying aetiology and case selection.

Safety

An estimated 10% of fetuses will die as a result of shunt insertion; however, in the presence of hydrops there is a high background fetal loss rate. Displacement and blockage of the shunt occur in 20–30% of cases, traumatic haemothorax has also been reported.

Balloon valvuloplasty

Indication

Severe aortic stenosis or pulmonary atresia with an intact ventricular septum. The aim is to prevent progressive damage to the ventricular muscle *in utero,* the development of hydrops and subsequent fetal death.

Careful case selection is needed given the uncertainty as to the safety and efficacy of valvuloplasty.

Procedure

Fetal positioning is critical for success. The procedure is conducted at 21–32 weeks' gestation with maternal local anaesthesia and sedation under ultrasound guidance. A needle is passed through the fetal chest into the left or right ventricle and a guidewire passed across the aortic or pulmonary valve. A balloon catheter is inserted and inflated to dilate the stenotic valve.

Efficacy

There are very limited data with the largest case series of aortic valvuloplasty including 20 fetuses. Technical success was achieved in 70% of cases with subsequent growth of the aortic and mitral valves. The data are even more limited on pulmonary valvuloplasty with only 10 cases described in the literature.

Safety

Again data are extremely limited, but fetal bradycardia, pericardial effusion, balloon rupture and fetal death are all potential complications.

An intention-to-treat registry has been developed by the Association for European Paediatric Cardiology (www.aepc.org), which it is hoped will provide much needed evidence in the future.

Further reading

Interventional procedures guidance: www.nice.org.uk/guidance

Wapner RJ. Invasive prenatal diagnostic techniques. Semin Perinatol 2005;29:401–4.

Brun JL, Mangione R, Gangbo, et al. Feasibility, accuracy and safety of chorionic villus sampling: a report of 10 741 cases. Prenat Diagn 2003;23:295–301.

Horger EO, et al. A single physician's experience with four thousand six hundred genetic amniocenteses AmJOG 2001:185:279–88.

Mujezinovic F, Alfirevic Z. Procedure-related complications of amniocentesis and chorionic villous sampling: a systematic review. Obstet Gynecol 2007;110:687–94.

Fergus S, et al. The loss rates for invasive prenatal testing in a specialised obstetric ultrasound practice Aust NZ J Obstet Gynaecol 2002;42:1:61.

Roberts et al. Cochrane Library 2008.

Tabor et al. Randomised controlled trial of genetic amniocentesis in 4606 low risk women. Lancet 1986;i:1287–93.

Patient resources

ARC (Antenatal Results and Choices): www.arc-uk.org

Intrauterine growth restriction (IUGR)

Definition
IUGR or fetal growth restriction (FGR) is slowing of expected *in utero* growth causing the fetus not to reach its genetic growth potential. This should be differentiated from small for gestational age (SGA) babies whose estimated or birthweight is below the 10th percentile for gestational age.

Epidemiology
The frequency of SGA depends on the definition used; by definition it will occur in 10% of the population if it is defined as size below the 10th percentile, 5% if defined as below the 5th percentile, etc.

The frequency of FGR is much more difficult to assess, as this also depends on the exact definition used. Owing to the wide biological variability in fetal and newborn size and uncertainties in dating/gestation, identifying a fetus that is not growing at its genetic potential is difficult. Most estimates suggest that it occurs in around 3% of pregnancies.

FGR is an important condition as it is associated with increased perinatal morbidity and mortality as well as longer term adverse health outcomes, including cardiovascular disease and metabolic syndrome.

Aetiology
In broad terms the causes are classified below.

Wrong dates
In order to plot fetal size accurately, gestational age must be known accurately. As last menstrual period dates (LMP) are either unknown or erroneous in around one-third of pregnancies the pregnancy should be dated by the first available ultrasound scan, preferably by measurement of the fetal crown–rump length (CRL) between 8 and 12 weeks of gestation. Dating in the second and third trimester is much less accurate and serial scans to assess fetal growth patterns may be needed.

Constitutionally small fetus
Estimated fetal weight (EFW) and birthweight centiles are used most commonly to diagnose FGR. This has the disadvantage of classifying a large proportion of constitutionally 'normal small' babies as being at risk. Careful examination of the fetus to differentiate between this and FGR is necessary to adequately assess risk, and this will usually involve careful assessment for abnormalities, Doppler assessment of the uteroplacental and fetoplacental circulation and serial growth assessment. It should be noted that data suggest that even when infants have SGA that is thought to be constitutional, there is an excess risk of perinatal and longer term morbidity.

Multiple pregnancy
There is an effect of fetal number on birthweight with increasing numbers of fetuses in higher order multiples being smaller at all gestations after around 24 weeks. These differences are presumed to be due to mechanical constraints of space or placental implantation, but other causes of FGR can of course affect multiple pregnancies.

Fetal abnormalities
There are a number of fetal conditions that can lead to FGR, and these can be inherent (such as a chromosomal abnormality) or acquired *in utero* (such as a congenital infection). The conditions will almost always have coexisting fetal abnormalities, and careful ultrasound examination should be mandatory in cases of severe FGR to assess for these. They include:

- fetal chromosomal abnormalities (particularly trisomy 18 and 13, and triploidy)
- rare genetic disorders (such as Silver Russell syndrome, Seckel's syndrome)
- fetal congenital infections (including cytomegalovirus and toxoplasma and, more rarely, rubella and fetal varicella syndrome)
- abnormalities of the fetal circulation, such as single umbilical artery or abnormal course of the ductus venosus.

Placental insufficiency
Once wrong dates and constitutional smallness are excluded, this is the commonest cause. The condition overlaps with pre-eclampsia and placental abruption in its pathophysiology, which has its origins in the first trimester of pregnancy—there is evidence of altered uterine artery blood flow and markers of abnormal angiogenesis at 11–13 weeks. Placental insufficiency may also be 'acquired' by heavy maternal smoking or drug abuse (especially cocaine abuse), which may affect growth through abnormal placental function. Fetuses with FGR due to placental insufficiency are often described as having 'asymmetrical' growth restriction, with the abdominal circumference falling away from the normal range before the femur length, although head measurements are generally spared. Amniotic fluid is usually reduced, uterine artery Doppler usually shows high impedance to flow and umbilical artery blood flow may be reduced, absent or reversed. The condition is progressive and management is mainly aimed at balancing the risks of intrauterine hypoxia with those of indicated preterm delivery.

Placental chorioangiomas can also be a rare cause of FGR, although in these cases a discrete placental anatomical abnormality is usually visible.

Prognosis
This depends mainly on the underlying cause and the gestational age and birthweight at delivery. When due to placental insufficiency, early-onset FGR (defined in most studies as leading to delivery before 34 weeks of gestation) has survival rates that are significantly lower than appropriately grown counterparts. There has to be a careful balance between early delivery (which carries a higher rate of neonatal complications) versus expectant management (with risks of inadvertent stillbirth or sequelae of intrauterine hypoxia). Each day *in utero* increases survival and intact survival by 1–2% and this is particularly evident at lower gestational ages.

Clinical approach: diagnosis
Referral to a fetal medicine unit with appropriate expertise in the diagnosis and management of FGR is indicated.

History
- Assess pregnancy dating. If previous dating was accurate redating of the pregnancy must not be carried out at this late gestation.
- Previous pregnancy including previous pregnancies affected by SGA, FGR, pre-eclampsia or abruption.
- Previous or family history of genetic conditions or fetal congenital abnormalities.

- Drug history, including recreational drug use.
- Recent of illness or flu-like symptoms.

Examination/ultrasound findings
- Carefully measure fetal biometry and plot in relation to previous ultrasound scans.
- Assess fetal and placental anatomy, uterine, umbilical and middle cerebral artery Doppler, amniotic fluid, and fetal biophysical profile.
- If fetal growth velocity is maintained along a centile line, with normal fetal and placental anatomy, and normal Doppler, amniotic fluid, and fetal biophysical profile, wrong dates or constitutional smallness is the most likely cause.
- In fetal conditions, Doppler, amniotic fluid, and fetal behaviour may be normal or abnormal; increased amniotic fluid in the presence of severe early-onset FGR is an ominous sign. Fetal abnormalities suggestive of the causes outlined in aetiology, above, are usually present. If uterine and fetal Dopplers are normal despite early-onset severe FGR, a fetal condition is likely. Nevertheless, abnormal Dopplers may coexist in certain fetal abnormalities (e.g. triploidy). Targeted investigations for fetal chromosomal abnormalities or congenital infections should be carried out depending on the findings.
- When the cause for the FGR is placental insufficiency the majority of pregnancies will have Doppler abnormalities in the uterine and umbilical artery. On the other hand, late-onset FGR often has few Doppler abnormalities, such as an isolated reduction in impedance to flow through the middle cerebral artery despite normal umbilical artery Doppler. Fetal heart rate abnormalities may be present.

Clinical Approach: management
Management should be targeted at the underlying cause. In early-onset FGR due to placental insufficiency there is a well-described progression of arterial to venous Doppler abnormalities which usually precedes abnormalities in biophysical profile and fetal heart rate. The sequential changes are a decrease in umbilical artery end diastolic flow (this the progresses through absent to reversed end diastolic flow); evidence of 'brain sparing', with a fall in the middle cerebral artery indices, followed by increasing ductus venosus Doppler indices. As outlined above, in late-onset FGR

Doppler changes do not typically follow this pattern. A more detailed discussion of fetal monitoring can be found in the Chapters 7.3, Doppler ultrasound, and Chapter 7.1, Biophysical profile.

Further reading
Barker DJ. Fetal growth and adult disease. Br J Obstet Gynaecol 1992;99:275–76.

Baschat AA, Cosmi E, Bilardo CM, *et al.* Predictors of neonatal outcome in early-onset placental dysfunction. Obstet Gynecol 2007; 109:253–61.

Bernstein IM, Horbar JD, Badger GJ, *et al*: Morbidity and mortality among very-low-birth-weight neonates with intrauterine growth restriction: The Vermont Oxford Network. Am J Obstet Gynecol 2000;182:198–206.

Bilardo CM, Wolf H, Stigter RH, *et al.* Relationship between monitoring parameters and perinatal outcome in severe, early intrauterine growth restriction. Ultrasound Obstet Gynecol 2004;23:119–25.

Cosmi E, Ambrosini G, D'Antona D, *et al.* Doppler, cardiotocography, and biophysical profile changes in growth-restricted fetuses. Obstet Gynecol 2005;106:1240–5.

Eixarch E, Meler E, Iraola A, *et al.* Neurodevelopmental outcome in 2-year-old infants who were small-for-gestational age term fetuses with cerebral blood flow redistribution. Ultrasound Obstet Gynecol 2008;32:894–9.

Hecher K, Bilardo CM, Stigter RH, *et al.* Monitoring of fetuses with intrauterine growth restriction: a longitudinal study. Ultrasound Obstet Gynecol 2001;18:564–70.

Manning FA. Antepartum fetal testing: a critical appraisal. Curr Opin Obstet Gynecol 2009;21:348–52.

Nyberg DA, Abuhamad A, Ville Y. Ultrasound assessment of abnormal fetal growth. Sem Perinatol 2004;28:3–22.

Thornton JG, Hornbuckle J, Vail A, *et al.* GRIT study group. Infant wellbeing at 2 years of age in the Growth Restriction Intervention Trial (GRIT): multicentred randomised controlled trial. Lancet 2004;364:513–20.

Turan OM, Turan S, Gungor S, *et al.* Progression of Doppler abnormalities in intrauterine growth restriction. Ultrasound Obstet Gynecol; 2008;32:160–7.

Turan S, Miller J. Baschat AA. Integrated testing and management in fetal growth restriction. Semin Perinatol 2008;32:194–200.

Vintzileos AM, Fleming AD, Scorza WE, *et al.* Relationship between fetal biophysical activities and umbilical cord blood gas values. Am J Obstet Gynecol 1991;165:707–13.

Patient resources
www.childgrowthfoundation.org/

Multiple pregnancy

Definition
This occurs when two or more ova are fertilized to form dizygotic (non-identical) twins or a single fertilized egg divides to form monozygotic (identical) twins.

Chorionicity
Chorionicity refers to the number of placentas in a multiple pregnancy. Dizygotic twin pregnancies always have two placentas (dichorionic). There is one placenta for each fetus and they may be fused or separate. In monozygotic multiple pregnancies, the number of placentas depends on the timing ovum division. If the embryo splits before day 4 there are two placentas. Embryos that split late (days 4–12) will have a single placenta (monochorionic). Monochorionic twins are prone to significantly more pregnancy complications than dichorionic twins.

Epidemiology
The incidence of twins is 1 in 80 and triplets 1 in 900 pregnancies. The use of assisted reproductive techniques has greatly increased the incidence of multiple pregnancies. Twinning is also slightly more common with previous multiple pregnancy, family history, increasing maternal age, and West African racial origin.

Presentation
Early symptoms include exacerbation of the usual pregnancy-related symptoms (especially hyperemesis) and a uterus that is clinically large for dates. It is possible to confirm multiple pregnancies and its chorionicity in the first trimester by ultrasound.

Complications
Vanishing twin
In a small, but significant proportion of pregnancies, one twin dies and is reabsorbed in the first trimester of pregnancy. Under these circumstances, serum screening for the risk of trisomy 21 may be unreliable.

Twin–twin transfusion syndrome
In monochorionic twin pregnancies, there can be unequal vascular sharing of the placenta with intertwin transfusion, leading to one twin developing growth restriction and the other cardiac failure.

Fetal growth restriction
Twins are usually smaller at any given gestational age than singletons. However, both mono- and dichorionic twins have a high prevalence of fetal growth restriction. The severity of the growth restriction and pregnancy outcome is often worse in monochorionic twins.

Premature delivery
The mean gestation of delivery is 37 weeks for twins and 31 weeks triplets. Multiple pregnancies have a higher incidence of preterm and severe preterm delivery.

Other complications
All maternal (anaemia, pre-eclampsia, placenta praevia) and fetal complications (cerebral palsy, perinatal mortality) of pregnancy are more common in multiple pregnancy except for prolonged pregnancy and fetal macrosomia.

Management
Prenatal screening
Fetal abnormality is more common in multiple than singleton pregnancy, as a consequence of the effects of egg splitting (monozygotic) and the number of fetuses (dizygotic).

Nuchal translucency assessment at 10–14 weeks may used to screen for risk of aneuploidy. However, invasive prenatal diagnosis is complicated by the issue of zygosity, possible sample contamination, and the ethical dilemma of managing a twin pregnancy with one abnormal fetus. Under the latter circumstances, the parents may opt for selective termination, where the miscarriage rate for the co-twin is as high as 5–8%.

Antenatal
As most pregnancy complications are seen more frequently in twin pregnancy, they should be managed by a specialist with more frequent monitoring. Ultrasound scans should be undertaken to determine chorionicity (Fig. 7.20.1), fetal growth and signs of twin–twin transfusion syndrome (TTTS).

Fetal growth restriction is managed by regular monitoring, steroids for lung maturation, and early delivery for deteriorating Doppler blood flow indices. With severe TTTS, the appropriate management is fetoscopic laser surgery to divide the monochorionic intertwin vascular placental anastomoses.

Twin pregnancies with a short cervix (<20 mm) are at significantly higher risk of preterm delivery. Cervical sutures and antibiotic prophylaxis have not shown to be of value and, in fact, may worsen pregnancy prognosis. The use of progesterone to reduce risk of preterm delivery appears promising and is being investigated currently.

Other pregnancy complications should be screened for and managed as for singleton pregnancy.

Delivery
In dichorionic twins, if the first twin presents as cephalic, vaginal delivery may be attempted. Elective Caesarean section is indicated for the same reasons as in singleton pregnancy. Monochorionic twins and triplets are usually

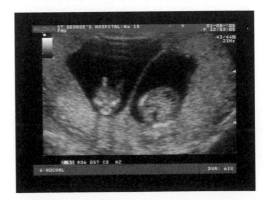

Fig. 7.20.1 The λ-sign of a dichorionic placenta.

delivered by Caesarean section because of the risks of acute intertwin transfusion in the former, and high rate of emergency Caesarean and difficulty in fetal monitoring in the latter.

Intrapartum

The main fetal risk in labour is thought to be as a result of hypoxia to the second twin during a protracted second stage and premature placental separation.

The first stage of labour can be managed as for singleton pregnancy and vaginal birth of twin 1 usually proceeds as normal. Immediately after the birth of the first twin, it is important to

- continuously monitor the fetal heart rate of twin 2 to ensure fetal wellbeing. Where there is concern, a vacuum extraction or breech extraction can be performed without resorting to Caesarean section
- determine the position of twin two. If longitudinal, normal delivery will usually result after rupture of the second amniotic sac. If transverse, internal podalic version or external version may be used to establish a longitudinal lie
- contractions usually abate after the birth of the first twin. An intravenous oxytocin infusion is usually required to help deliver the second twin. The second twin should deliver within 30 minutes of the first twin.

The third stage of labour should be actively managed.

Higher order multiple pregnancy

The outcomes of higher order multiples (three or more) are significantly worse than twin or singleton pregnancies.

Although previously a relatively common occurrence with *in vitro* fertilization (IVF) treatment, the Human Fertilization and Embryology Authority has limited the maximum number of embryos (two) transferred per cycle of IVF in order to reduce the number of multiple pregnancies.

Multifetal pregnancy reduction may be carried out, but carries a risk of miscarriage (5–8%) as well as considerable ethical problems. It is usually performed after the nuchal translucency scan at 12 weeks with ultrasound-guided injection of potassium chloride into the selected fetuses to leave a twin pregnancy.

Further reading

Taylor MJ. The management of multiple pregnancy. Early Hum Dev 2006;82:365–70.

Patient resources

www.tamba.org.uk

Oligohydramnios

Definition
Oligohydramnios is defined as reduced amniotic fluid volume (AFV) for a given gestational age. Oligohydramnios is secondary to either an excess loss of fluid, or a decrease in fetal urine production or excretion.

Epidemiology
Oligohydramnios is a complication in ~5% of all pregnancies, and severe oligohydramnios in ~1% of pregnancies. Oligohydramnios is more common in pregnancies beyond term, because the AFV normally decreases at term. It complicates as many as 12% of pregnancies that last beyond 41 weeks.

Differential diagnosis
Physiological changes in amniotic fluid volume
Amniotic fluid volume decreases with advancing gestation, especially in the third trimester. The significance of reduced amniotic fluid volume in late pregnancy is debatable.

Estimation of amniotic fluid volume
Measurement of the amniotic fluid index (AFI) or single deepest pool is only a proxy for the amniotic fluid volume. This technique has a poor specificity and sensitivity for the diagnosis of oligohydramnios.

Pathology/aetiology
Uteroplacental insufficiency
Oligohydramnios is an early feature of uteroplacental insufficiency and is associated with decreased fetal biometry particularly the abdominal circumference. Other ultrasound and Doppler features of fetal growth restriction aid in the confirmation of uteroplacental insufficiency as the cause for the reduced amniotic fluid volume.

Amniotic membrane rupture
The maternal history of persistent vaginal loss and dampness would suggest a diagnosis of prelabour membrane rupture. This is often associated with anhydramnios rather than oligohydramnios. The finding of normal amniotic fluid volume or oligohydramnios, however, does not exclude this diagnosis.

Abnormal fetal renal function
Bilateral renal agenesis, polycystic kidney disease, multicystic dysplasia and obstructive uropathy (bladder outflow obstruction) characteristically present with anhydramnios. However, early on in the process of renal impairment, transient oligohydramnios may be evident.

Post-term gestation
Although oligohydramnios may be physiological, it may be related to placental failure that is known to occur more frequently at this gestation. Oligohydramnios in the post-term patient is associated with more fetal decelerations, a higher incidence of meconium-stained fluid, and an increased risk for caesarean delivery.

Anhydramnios
Anhydramnios is defined as absent amniotic fluid at any gestation. The finding of anhydramnios in the first and second trimesters is usually associated with a poor prognosis because of the subsequent development of lethal fetal pulmonary hypoplasia. The presence of anhydramnios is also associated with joint contractures such as talipes (club foot).

Clinical approach
Assessment of amniotic fluid volume
The amniotic fluid volume increases from approximately 250 mL at 16 weeks to 1000 mL at 34 weeks, declining thereafter to approximately 800 mL at term. The amniotic fluid volume reflects both the maternal and fetal status and is altered in many physiological and pathological conditions. There are three methods for assessing amniotic fluid volume.

Subjective assessment
It is possible to classify amniotic fluid volume into broad categories such as absent, low, normal, increased, and excessive. This method has proved impossible to standardize in clinical and research terms.

Single deepest pool
The size of the deepest, cord-free pool of amniotic fluid is assessed using ultrasound. A 2–3 cm pool is considered acceptable in normal pregnancy.

Amniotic fluid index
Using the maternal umbilicus as a reference point, the abdomen is divided into four quarters. Using ultrasound, the largest vertical pool depth is recorded in each quadrant. The sum of these measurements represents the amniotic fluid index (AFI). Although the AFI is known to vary with gestational age, an AFI <5 cm is classified as oligohydramnios. This method is accepted as superior to the single deepest pool technique, but considerable intra- and interobserver variation exists.

The importance of quantification of amniotic fluid volume is of unquestionable value. However, a practical and reproducible technique for the accurate assessment of amniotic fluid volume is yet to be introduced into clinical practice.

Management
Anhydramnios as a consequence of renal pathology or early/midtrimester membrane rupture is frequently associated with a poor prognosis. If oligohydramnios is due to uteroplacental insufficiency, the management will depend on the severity of growth restriction and the gestation of the pregnancy.

Oligohydramnios of unknown aetiology on the other hand is of dubious clinical significance. Given the poor reproducibility of subjective and objective amniotic fluid estimations, one could question the value of reporting this when present as an isolated finding. The exception to this recommendation would appear to be prolonged or post-term pregnancy, where reduced amniotic fluid volume may be associated with poorer fetal and neonatal outcomes.

Amnio-infusion
Increasing the amount of fluid within the amniotic cavity can be accomplished during delivery with the use of amnio-infusion (instillation of warm sodium chloride solution into the cervix). This procedure increases the amount of fluid around the umbilical cord, which has been shown to decrease the frequency and severity of fetal heart

decelerations in labour. Unfortunately, this is not reflected in lower caesarean section rates or improved neonatal outcomes.

Vesico-amniotic shunts

Vesico-amniotic shunts may be used to divert fetal urine to the amniotic fluid cavity in patients with a fetal obstructive uropathy. Although it is effective in reversing oligohydramnios, its ability to achieve sustainable neonatal renal and pulmonary function remains to be established.

Further reading

Sherer DM, Langer O. Oligohydramnios: use and misuse in clinical management. Ultrasound Obstet Gynecol 2001;18:411–19.

Placental abnormalities

The placenta is an organ with both maternal and fetal origins. It is composed of functional units called villi, through which the mother and fetus exchange nutrients and waste products. The placenta is also implicated in the mechanism of immune avoidance by the fetus and undertakes an important endocrine role in pregnancy.

Normal variation in placental morphology

Succenturiate lobe

This refers to the presence of one or more accessory lobes of the placenta. Making the diagnosis is important as it is possible to have a fundal placenta together with a low-lying succenturiate lobe where the internal cervical os is covered by placenta (placenta praevia) or membrane with blood vessels within them (vasa praevia). These can be life-threatening conditions to the mother and baby. Succenturiate lobes may also be retained after delivery and become a cause of postpartum haemorrhage or infection.

Placental lakes

These are areas within the bulk of the placenta that are filled with slowly moving blood. There is a relationship between the presence of placental lakes and fetal growth restriction, but it is weak enough to be of little clinical significance.

Placental cysts

These are found just below the chorionic plate. They are though to represent deposition of fibrin in the intervillous space and are of no apparent significance.

Placental maturation

This is a classification of the normal changes that occur in the placenta during the course of a pregnancy; it is often known as Grannum grading. Originally it was suggested that increasing Grannum grades were associated with placental dysfunction. However, grading is no longer routinely used because of other, more accurate ways of assessing fetal wellbeing and placental function.

Placental abnormalities

Chorioangioma

This is a benign vascular tumour of the placenta (Fig. 7.22.1). Such tumours vary both in appearance and size. If the tumours have numerous feeding vessels, are large or

are close to the umbilical cord insertion, they may result in significant fetal arteriovenous shunting. This can cause fetal hyperdynamic circulation, high-output fetal cardiac failure and the development of polyhydramnios and hydrops fetalis. Occasionally they can be associated with fetal growth restriction, presumably because they reduce the effective functional capacity of the placenta.

Circumvillate placenta

In approximately 1% of cases, there is a small central chorionic area inside a paler thick ring of membranes on the fetal side of the placenta. This is associated with an increased rate of antepartum bleeding, prematurity, abruption, multiparity, and perinatal death.

Other placental problems

For information on placenta praevia, accreta, abruption, and retained placenta, see Chapter 10, Care in labour.

Umbilical cord abnormalities

Two-vessel cord

The absence of one umbilical artery is relatively common, with a reported incidence of approximately 1%. Associated malformations are thought to be present in as many as 50% of cases, with cardiac and renal being the systems most commonly affected. The risk of an underlying fetal chromosomal abnormality is unaltered in a previously screened population. The likelihood of the pregnancy being affected by intrauterine growth restriction is also thought to be increased making follow-up growth scans part of the routine management.

Marginal insertion of cord (Battledore)

Where the cord has a marginal rather than central insertion to the placenta. This has no clinical significance.

Velamentous cord insertion

The placental vessels run and divide in the membrane before reaching the cord. This is only of clinical significance if the vessels cross the lower pole of the uterus (vasa praevia, see Chapter 10, Care in Labour). With the latter finding, there is high risk of fetal haemorrhage and death at rupture of membranes. It can be diagnosed prenatally by ultrasound examination and managed by elective Caesarean section.

Coiling of the umbilical cord

Reduced coiling of the umbilical cord is associated with uteroplacental insufficiency. Hypercoiling of the cord is also associated with poorer neonatal outcomes, because of associated fetal abnormalities. There is no established, reproducible method of assessing umbilical vessel coiling reliably. Hence coiling is not used clinically to indicate the need for regular scans or detailed fetal assessment.

Umbilical cord masses

These may be primary in nature, originating from the remnants of the allantoic or vitelline duct. The use of colour Doppler will help differentiate cord masses of vascular origin and their relationship to the umbilical vessels.

Abnormal length of cord

A long cord (>100 cm) is associated with increased risk of fetal entanglement, knots and prolapse of the cord. A short cord (<40 cm) may be associated with a poorly active fetus, Down's syndrome, cord rupture, breech position, prolonged second stage, uterine inversion and abruption.

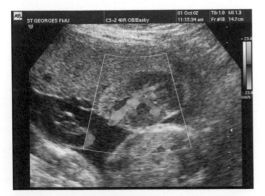

Fig. 7.22.1 Ultrasound image showing a placental chorioangioma, with colour Doppler blood flow within it. See also colour plate section.

Further reading

Benirschke K, Kaufmann P. *Pathology of the human placenta*, 2nd edn. New York: Springer-Verlag 1990.

Kaplan CG. Postpartum examination of the placenta. Clin Obstet Gynecol 1996;39:535–48.

Polyhydramnios

Definition
Subjectively assessed, or amniotic fluid index above the 95th centile for gestational age, or a maximum vertical pool length of ≥8 cm or AFI ≥24 (Fig. 7.23.1).

Epidemiology
It complicates 0.5–1% of pregnancies.

Aetiology
Excessive amniotic fluid is the result of either excessive liquor production or reduced clearance. Mild idiopathic polydramnios with no identifiable cause accounts for 55% of cases.

Diabetes in pregnancy is the commonest identifiable cause (25%).

Early onset polyhydramnios with associated structural anomalies (18%) should prompt consideration of chromosomal syndromes.

Increased liquor production
- Maternal diabetes
- Twin pregnancy (mostly monochorionic with twin–twin transfusion syndrome)
- Placental tumour i.e. chorioangioma (rare)
- Fetal macrosomia.

Decreased swallowing
- Gastrointestinal atresia
  - tracheoesophageal fistula
  - oesophageal atresia
  - duodenal atresia
- Chest malformations
  - diaphragmatic hernia
- Neuromuscular disorder
  - myotonic dystrophy
  - anencephaly
- Lethal skeletal dysplasia.

Hydrops
- Fetal anaemia (parvovirus infection, red cell alloimmunization)
- Cardiac arrhythmia
- Other causes (see Chapter 7.17).

Prognosis
In the presence of structural anomalies or chromosomal syndromes, prognosis depends on the underlying pathology.

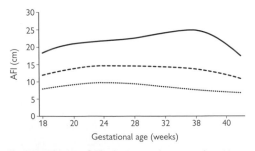

Fig. 7.23.1 Amniotic fluid index in normal pregnancy from 16 to 42 weeks' gestation (lines represent the 5th, 50th, and 95th centiles) modified from Moore TR, Cayle JE.

Idiopathic polyhydramnios is not associated with an increased rate of preterm delivery. However, perinatal mortality appears increased two- to fivefold compared with healthy control pregnancies.

Clinical approach
Diagnosis
History
- Presenting complaint
  - abdominal discomfort
  - dyspnoea
- Current pregnancy
  - gestational diabetes
  - dipstick glycosuria
  - maternal red cell antibodies
- Risk factors
  - high BMI
  - previous pregnancy affected
  - pre-existing diabetes
  - previous macrosomia
  - previous structural malformation or genetic syndrome.

Ultrasound findings
- A detailed structural survey should be performed to rule out congenital malformations:
  - markers for chromosomal defects
  - absent stomach bubble
  - 'double bubble' sign
  - diaphragmatic hernia.
- Abnormal posture or absent movements may suggest neuromuscular disorder.
- Abnormal size or shape of long bones may suggest lethal skeletal dysplasia.
- Middle cerebral artery (MCA) Doppler assessing peak systolic velocity to diagnose fetal anaemia.
- Fetal cardiac scan if there is evidence of cardiac arrhythmia or hydrops.
- Placental survey for vascular masses.

Investigations
- Glucose tolerance testing
- Red cell antibodies (if not previously done)
- Parvovirus serology, if raised MCA peak systolic velocity on Doppler
- Maternal screening for toxoplasamosis and cytomegalovirus
- In the presence of structural anomalies or hydrops consider amniocentesis for karyotyping
- In the presence of hydrops for full list of investigations see Chapter 7.17.

Counselling and management
In the presence of associated structural anomalies, counselling will be guided by the underlying condition. In mild idiopathic cases, guarded reassurance may be given. However, it should be explained that it is not possible to exclude oesophageal atresia or tracheo-oesophageal fistula if one is not seen on ultrasound: postnatal assessment of the neonate is always indicated.

Aetiological treatment

- In diabetic pregnancies presence of worsening polyhydramnios is a sign of poor glycaemic control. Frequent glucose monitoring and increased insulin requirement is indicated.
- In TTS the options of laser ablation of arteriovenous anastomoses, amnio drainage, or delivery may be considered depending on the gestational age, stage, and severity of disease.
- Fetal anaemia may be managed with cordocentesis and intrauterine fetal transfusion.

Symptomatic treatment

- Serial amnio reductions may become necessary, especially in upper gut obstructions, in order to treat maternal symptoms or prevent preterm delivery.
- Indomethacin may reduce fetal urine production through direct renal effect and may also exert a tocolytic effect. However, it is associated with premature closure of the ductus arteriosus and is therefore not recommended.
- Steroid cover should be considered in cases of severe tense polyhydramnios at less than 34 weeks gestation when the risk of preterm delivery is significant.

- In women with severe discomfort and respiratory compromise induction of labour at or beyond 37 weeks may be indicated.

Further reading

Desmedt EJ, Henry OA, Beischer NA. Polyhydramnios and associated maternal and fetal complications in singleton pregnancies. Br J Obstet Gynaecol 1990;97:1115–22.

Magann EF, Chauhan SP, Doherty DA, *et al.* A review of idiopathic hydramnios and pregnancy outcomes. Obstet Gynecol Surv 2007;62:795–802.

Williams K. Amniotic fluid assessment. Obstet Gynecol Surv 1993;48:795–800.

Further reading

Thilaganathan B, Sairam S, Papageorghiou A I, Bhide A. *Problem based obstetric ultrasound*, 1st edn. Informa Healthcare 2007.

Internet resources

www.emedicine.com (needs free registration)

Patient resources

www.babycentre.co.uk/pregnancy/complications/polyhydramnios/

Red blood cell isoimmunization

Definition

Fetomaternal blood group incompatibility may result in the development of maternal antibodies, which cross the placenta, become attached to the fetal red cells, and cause their destruction.

Epidemiology

There are at least 100 red blood cell surface antigens and the development of maternal antibodies to approximately 30 of these can lead to fetal haemolytic disease. However, the vast majority of cases are the result of either ABO or rhesus incompatibility.

ABO fetomaternal incompatibility occurs in about 20% of all pregnancies, but fetal haemolysis occurs in less than 2% of cases and this is usually mild. The antibodies are usually immunoglobulin (Ig)M, which do not cross the placenta and no special antenatal measures are necessary for the management of these pregnancies.

The commonest antibody causing severe fetal haemolysis is anti-D. Other antibodies causing fetal haemolysis are anti-C, anti-Kell and anti-E and rarely antibodies such as anti-M, anti-N, anti-S. Pregnancies complicated by the presence of these antibodies should be managed in the same way as those of Rhesus (D) incompatibility, including maternal antibody level estimations, Doppler studies, cordocentesis, fetal blood transfusion, and early delivery.

A Rhesus (D)-positive infant is born to a Rhesus (D)-negative mother in 10% of Caucasian and 3% of Black pregnancies.

Clinical management

Rh-negative women with no Rh antibodies

Anti-D administration is effective in preventing immunization in a Rhesus-negative woman but has no effect if the woman is already isoimmunized. The administration of 100 μg of anti-D IgG to a mother, will neutralize at least 4 mL of Rhesus (D)-positive fetal erythrocytes that might have entered her circulation. This is equivalent to a Kleihauer count of 80 fetal cells per 50 low-power fields. Routine antenatal anti-D prophylaxis with anti-D IgG is recommended for all pregnant women who are Rh D negative and who are not known to be sensitized, and within 72 hours of the delivery of a Rhesus-positive baby and also after termination, miscarriage, antepartum haemorrhage, amniocentesis, or other potentially immunizing episodes. Routine prophylaxis is commonly given as two doses of 500–1650 IU (one at 28 weeks and one at 34 weeks' gestation), or as a single dose of 1500 IU either at 28 or 30 weeks of gestation.

At the first antenatal visit the ABO and rhesus blood group should be determined in all patients. Furthermore, screening for other atypical antibodies should be performed. If the woman is Rhesus negative, the Rhesus status of the partner is determined. If he is also Rhesus negative then the fetus must be Rhesus negative and the mother is not at risk of Rhesus isoimmunization.

If the father is Rhesus positive then further maternal antibody screening should be undertaken at 20 weeks and at 4-week intervals thereafter until delivery.

After delivery, the blood group and rhesus status of the fetus and the direct Coombs test for the presence of antibodies on the fetal erythrocytes should be performed. If the mother has no antibodies and the baby is Rhesus D positive, anti-D IgG should be given.

Red cell isoimmunized pregnancies

In the management of red cell isoimmunized pregnancies the aims are
- to predict whether the fetus is severely affected
- to correct the fetal anaemia by intrauterine blood transfusion
- to deliver the baby at the optimal time by balancing the risks of prematurity versus intrauterine transfusion.

The only accurate method of assessing the severity of fetal anaemia is by fetal blood sampling. However, cordocentesis should only be undertaken if there is a strong suspicion that the fetus is severely affected because the procedure itself can cause miscarriage and it can also cause fetomaternal haemorrhage thereby exacerbating the severity of the disease.

The fetal haemoglobin concentration normally increases with gestation from a mean of 11 g/dL at 18 weeks to 14 g/dL at 38 weeks and 1 SD is about 1 g/dL. Mild anaemia is defined by a haemoglobin deficit of 2–4 g/dL, moderate disease by a deficit of 4–6 g/dL, and severe disease by a deficit of more than 6 g/dL. When the fetal haemoglobin concentration deficit exceeds 6 g/dL hydrops fetalis develops.

In cases where the father is homozygous for the Rhesus (D) antigen, the fetus is Rhesus positive. If the father is heterozygous the fetus could be negative, and in these cases the fetal Rhesus status can now be determined accurately by examination of the cell-free fetal DNA in maternal plasma.

Assessment of the severity of fetal haemolysis should be based on:
- the history of previous affected pregnancies
- the levels of maternal haemolytic antibodies
- ultrasonographic examination for the detection of ascites
- Doppler studies for diagnosis of a hyperdynamic circulation. Cordocentesis can safely be reserved only for those pregnancies demonstrating increased fetal middle cerebral artery peak systolic velocity (MCA-PSV); in more than 95% of the severely anaemic fetuses the MCA-PSV is more than 1.5 multiples of the median above the normal median for gestation. This high sensitivity can be achieved with a relatively low false-positive rate and therefore avoidance or delay in invasive testing in more than 80% of isoimmunized pregnancies with high maternal serum antibody concentration.

For patients with a previous red blood cell isoimmunization-affected pregnancy, it should be aimed to perform the first ultrasound scan and Doppler studies at approximately 10 weeks before the time of the earliest previous fetal or neonatal death, fetal transfusion, or birth of a severely affected baby, but not before 17–18 weeks. Fetal death or the development of hydrops do not occur before this gestation, presumably because the fetal reticuloendothelial system is too immature to result in destruction of antibody coated erythrocytes. Assessment should be carried out at intervals of 1–2 weeks and cordocentesis need only be performed if there is fetal ascites or if the fetal MCA-PSV is more than 1.5 MoM above the normal mean for gestation.

In patients that had no or mildly affected previous pregnancies the maternal haemolytic antibody levels should be measured at 2–3 weekly intervals from 17 weeks onwards. When the antibody concentrations are persistently below 15 IU/mL (equivalent to a dilution of 1 in 128), the degree of fetal haemolysis is insignificant or mild and delivery can be delayed until term. If the antibody levels are higher than 15 IU/mL the disease may be severe and the fetus should be assessed by ultrasound and Doppler examinations at 1-week intervals and cordocentesis should be considered in those that develop ascites or a high MCA-PSV.

Fetal blood transfusions

In very severe disease requiring fetal transfusions before 20 weeks the intraperitoneal approach is safer, but after 20 weeks the intravascular approach is preferred.

Intraperitoneal transfusions are performed by the ultrasound guided insertion of a 20-gauge needle into the amniotic cavity. The transducer is aligned allowing a view transverse to the fetal abdomen and perpendicular to the course of the needle, which is directed towards the anterolateral aspect of the fetal abdomen between the bladder and umbilicus and then thrust forward into the peritoneal cavity. The hub of the needle is connected to a syringe through a three-way tap. Donor blood is drawn into the syringe and infused manually at 10 mL/minute, during which time the fetal heart rate is monitored continuously by ultrasound. The total volume of blood transfused is 5 mL for 16–18 weeks, 10 mL for 19–21 weeks, and 10 mL per week of gestation after 21 weeks. This avoids over transfusion, which would cause the intraperitoneal pressure to rise above the umbilical venous pressure, obstruct the placental circulation, and result in fetal death.

Intravascular transfusions are given by cordocentesis using a 20-gauge needle. Where the placenta is anterior the needle is advanced through the placenta and into the base of the umbilical cord. When the placenta is posterior, the needle is introduced into the amniotic cavity and the cord punctured near the placental insertion. The stylet of the needle is then removed, a heparinized syringe attached to the needle hub, and pure fetal blood aspirated. The fetal haemoglobin concentration is determined and if this is below the normal range, the tip of the needle is kept in the lumen of the umbilical cord vessel and fresh, packed, Rhesus-negative blood compatible with that of the mother is infused manually into the fetal circulation. The sonographically detectable echogenicity in the umbilical cord produced by the infused blood allows identification of the punctured vessel. The fetal heart rate and the flow of the infused blood are monitored continually throughout the procedure by ultrasonography. At the end of the transfusion a blood sample is aspirated for determination of the final haemoglobin concentration. The volume of donor blood is calculated by considering the pretransfusion fetal haemoglobin concentration, the haemoglobin of the transfused blood, the desired post-transfusion haemoglobin, and the normal mean fetoplacental blood volume for that gestation.

Subsequent transfusions are given at 1–3-week intervals and the babies are delivered at 35–40 weeks.

Prognosis

The survival rate of red cell-isoimmunized pregnancies treated with cordocentesis is more than 90%.

Further reading

Hecher K, Snijders R, Campbell S, Nicolaides KH. Fetal venous, intracardiac, and arterial blood flow measurements in intrauterine growth retardation: relationship with fetal blood gases. Am J Obstet Gynecol 1995;173:10–5.

Mari G. Noninvasive diagnosis by Doppler ultrasonography of fetal anemia due to maternal red-cell alloimmunization. N Eng J Med 2000;342:9–14.

Nicolaides KH, Rodeck CH. Maternal serum anti-D antibody concentration and assessment of rhesus isoimmunisation. BMJ 1992;304:1155–6.

Nicolaides KH, Soothill PW, Clewell WH, et al. Fetal haemoglobin measurement in the assessment of red cell isoimmunisation. Lancet 1988;1:1073–5.

Nicolaides KH, Soothill PW, Rodeck CH, Clewell W. Rh disease: intravascular fetal blood transfusion by cordocentesis. Fetal Therapy 1986;1:185–92.

Rightmire DA, Nicolaides KH, Rodeck CH, Campbell S. Fetal blood velocities in Rh isoimmunization: relationship to gestational age and to fetal haematocrit. Obstet Gynecol 1986;68:233–6.

Vyas S, Nicolaides KH, Campbell S. Doppler examination of the middle cerebral artery in anemic fetuses. Am J Obstet Gynecol 1990;162:1066–8

Internet resources

www.nice.org.uk/ I A156

Patient resources

www.patient.co.uk/doctor/Haemolytic-Disease-of-the-Newborn.htm

Screening for fetal aneuploidy

There is a fundamental difference between antenatal screening and prenatal diagnosis for congenital abnormalities.

- Screening is limited to the identification of those at high enough risk to justify further investigation.
- Diagnosis is definitive but involves invasive procedures, mainly chorionic villus sampling (CVS) and amniocentesis, which carry a risk of miscarriage.

Currently, screening assesses risk of fetal aneuploidy by combining information on maternal age and multiple markers in maternal serum and ultrasound. Markers are continuous variables with a distribution of values that is, on average, higher or lower in affected pregnancies.

Aneuploidy

This is a common event in pregnancy but most affected embryos miscarry spontaneously early in the first trimester, many of them even before there are clinical signs of pregnancy. Those that survive into the second trimester also experience high late-intrauterine mortality and increased risk of infant death.

Birth prevalence in the absence of prenatal diagnosis and therapeutic abortion:

- Down's syndrome (DS): 1–2 per 1000, depending on the maternal age distribution, of which 95% are non-disjunction, 4 % translocation, 1% mosaic
- Edwards' syndrome: 1/9 less frequent
- Patau's syndrome: 1/20 less frequent
- Turner's syndrome and other sex chromosome aneuploidies are more common but relatively benign.

DS screening

This chapter is mainly concerned with DS risk assessment. Increasingly Edwards' syndrome risks are also included on DS screening reports (see below).

Natural history

The life expectancy is considerably greater than in the past, although precise estimates are difficult to derive. However, it remains the most common known cause of severe mental handicap. In addition, many adults may experience cognitive deficits due to pathological changes in the brain normally associated with Alzheimer's disease.

Prescreening risk

This can be expressed as a rate 1 in 1/p, where p is prevalence; or as an odds p:(1 − p) or 1:(1 − p)/p.

- Trimester: Most centres quote the risk at term, but some give the mid- or first trimester risks, which are respectively about one-quarter higher and double.
- Maternal age: This is the most important prescreening factor. Risk changes little from 1 in 1500 at age 20 to 1 in 900 at 30 and then increases rapidly to 1 in 30 at 45.
- Paternal age: Contributes little or no additional risk.
- Family history: Unless there is a familial translocation or mosaicism, only a previous affected pregnancy is relevant. This increases risk to 1 in 200 at 30 and 1 in 25 at 45.

Markers

Of the more than 50 maternal blood, maternal urine or ultrasound markers, currently seven are widely used: maternal serum human chorionic gonadotrophin (hCG), the free β-subunit of hCG, α-fetoprotein (AFP), unconjugated oestriol (uE3), inhibin A and pregnancy-associated plasma protein (PAPP)-A, and ultrasound measurement of fetal nuchal translucency (NT), the single most discriminatory marker, albeit limited to 11–13 weeks of gestation and optimal at 11 weeks.

Adjustments

- Gestation: all the widely used markers change with gestation. Therefore, results are expressed as multiples of the normal gestation-specific median (MoM) using a local regression equation.
- Operator: NT can be difficult to quality control and some centres use operator-specific regression equations (Logghe et al. 1995).
- Maternal weight: all serum marker levels decline with weight and MoMs are adjusted for this.
- Ethnicity: women of Afro-Caribbean origin have PAPP-A levels about 50% higher. Either ethnic-specific normal medians or a multiplication factor is needed. Other markers are altered less as are those in Oriental and Asian origin women.
- Smoking: PAPP-A levels are reduced in smokers; hCG and free β-hCG levels are also reduced but only in the second trimester. Information collected during pregnancy on daily intake is often inaccurate. Hence, although some centres adjust for smoking per se, adjustment for intake is not recommended.
- Assisted reproduction: PAPP-A, hCG and free β-hCG levels are raised in pregnancies conceived by IVF, ICSI, intrauterine insemination or following ovulation induction alone. However, there is considerable between-study heterogeneity, possibly due to the method of gestational assessment, the cause of infertility, and treatment. Hence, adjustment is not generally applied.

Frequency distributions

After log transformation each of the widely used markers, both in DS and unaffected pregnancies, follows a Gaussian distribution over most of the range. Moreover, all combinations of two or more markers follow a multivariate Gaussian distribution.

The distribution parameters are the means and standard deviations of the individual markers and the correlation coefficients between markers. They are probably best derived by meta-analysis.

Risk calculation and interpretation

The prescreening risk, expressed as odds is multiplied by a factor known as the 'likelihood ratio' (LR) derived from the marker profile. The resulting odds are then re-expressed as a rate. This posterior risk is then compared with a fixed cut-off risk. If the risk is greater than the cut-off the result is regarded as positive, otherwise it is negative.

The likelihood ratio for a single marker is calculated by the ratio of the heights of the two overlapping distributions at the specific level. For extreme results that fall beyond the point where the data fit a Gaussian distribution, it is standard practice to use the LR at the end of the acceptable range. For more than one marker the heights of multivariate log Gaussian distributions are used.

Predicting screening performance

This is determined by the detection rate (DR), the proportion of DS pregnancies referred for prenatal diagnosis and the false-positive rate (FPR).

The most robust predictions are from statistical modelling. The same Gaussian model used to calculate LR is used to generate distributions of risk in DS and unaffected pregnancies. The maternal age distribution can either be derived nationally or modelled (e.g. Gaussian, mean 27 and SD 5.5 years).

Either the DR is predicted for a fixed FPR (e.g. 1% or 5%), the FPR for a fixed DR (e.g. 75% or 85%), or DR and FPR for a given cut-off (e.g. 1 in 250 at term or 1 in 270 at midtrimester).

Principal strategies

Initially DS screening was carried out at 15–19 weeks to utilize the existing neural tube defect screening programme. Over the last decade there has been a gradual realization of the benefits of moving from the second to the first trimester. Today strategies are emerging that use both first and second trimester markers sequentially.

Second trimester (1T) tests
- Double: AFP and hCG or free β-hCG
- Triple: double plus uE3
- Quadruple: triple plus inhibin A.

First trimester (2T) tests
- NT alone
- Combined: NT, PAPP-A and free β-hCG.

Sequential tests
- Serum-integrated: first trimester PAPP-A plus second trimester quadruple markers. The first trimester result is not disclosed until the test is complete.
- Integrated: serum integrated plus NT.
- Stepwise: first trimester combined markers but using a very high cut-off; women with risks below the cut-off are offered second trimester quadruple markers and risk revision using all markers.
- Contingent: stepwise except that only women with borderline risks are offered the second stage.

Some regard non-disclosure of the two integrated tests to be unethical, or at least impractical due to the difficulty for the professional not to act on intermediate findings which would of themselves be abnormal, particularly the NT, and any increase in detection is paid for by sacrificing early diagnosis and reassurance.

Another approach, the 'independent sequential' test, albeit statistically invalid, is being practised to some degree by default, namely to carry out a combined test followed by a quadruple test and to calculate separate risks from each.

Model predicted DR for 5% FPR
Using parameters from one meta-analysis:
- double: 56% with hCG and 61% with free β-hCG
- triple: 60% and 65%
- quadruple: 67% and 71%
- NT alone: 71% at 13 weeks and 77% at 11 weeks
- combined: 81/80% and 84/87% with first trimester hCG/ free-β hCG
- serum integrated: 73% and 78%
- integrated: 89% and 93%
- stepwise: 91/91% and 94/94% with first trimester hCG/ free β-hCG
- contingent: 88/88% and 90/92% with first trimester hCG/ free β-hCG
- independent: 84% for all weeks and hCG types.

These rates are useful for health policy planning. However, for individual choice the maternal age-specific DR and FPR is needed; for a given risk cut-off, both increase with age.

Prospective intervention studies
In such studies the observed DR overestimates the actual value. This arises because some DS pregnancies terminated following a high-risk result are destined to miscarry anyway, whereas non-viable DS pregnancies with low-risk results are lost to follow-up. The DR can be corrected using trimester-specific viability factors.

Meta-analysis of published studies confirms predictions for the well established strategies:
- double: 234 000 tests, corrected DR 59%, FPR 5.0%
- triple: 612 000, 67%, 6.5%
- quadruple: 86 000, 79%, 7.4%
- NT alone: 104 000, 72%, 8.4%
- combined: 145 000, 81%, 5.9%.

So far there are insufficient published sequential test studies, but head-to-head retrospective comparison within the intervention FaSTER trial confirmed that integrated, step-wise and contingent tests had similar DR.

Possible future strategies

Contingent combined test
Where there is limited availability of quality NT, the combined test serum markers are tested on all women and NT is limited to those with high post-test DS risks. Predicted DR is 82% when one-third have NT.

Three-stage contingent test
The small loss of detection with the contingent combined test can be completely recouped by the contingent determination of second trimester serum markers just like a standard sequential contingent test.

Additional first trimester serum markers
AFP, uE3 and inhibin are weak first trimester markers but can be added to the combined test. Another marker, A disintegrin and metalloprotease (ADAM)12s, might be discriminatory prior to 9 weeks gestation.

Additional first trimester ultrasound markers
Four can be determined at the same time as NT: absence of the fetal nasal bone (NB), abnormal blood flow in the ductus venosus, tricuspid regurgitation, and the frontal-maxillary facial angle, requiring three-dimensional scanning. Few centres are sufficiently proficient to determine these routinely although NB is now becoming more available.

Based on meta-analysis the LRs for absent and present NB are 49 and 0.31, although different values are needed according to CRL, NT, and ethnicity.

Modelling predicts a substantial increase in DR:
- NT and NB: 87% and 90% at 13 and 11 weeks.
- combined with NB: 92/91% and 93/94% with hCG/free β-hCG.
- contingent with NB: 91/90% and 92/93%.

First trimester contingent test
Where there is limited availability of additional first trimester markers, refer those with borderline contingent test risks for specialist ultrasound and risk re-evaluation.

Soft markers
The results of an 18–22-week 'anomaly scan' are sometimes used in the *post hoc* modification of risk among women considering amniocentesis. Major anomalies are

risk factors as are so-called 'soft' markers: increased nuchal skinfold (NF), short femur and humerus lengths, hydrone-phrosis, echogenic intracardiac focus, and echogenic bowel.

These markers could also be formally incorporated into routine screening policies outside specialist centres. NF is most suited to this together with facial profile markers: nasal bone length (NBL) and prenasal thickness (PT). All three are all continuous variables with good Gaussian fit.

Second trimester combined test
Uses quadruple test markers together with ultrasound NF, NBL and PT. Modelling predicts the following DRs (Cuckle and Benn 2009):
- quad and NF: 78/80% with hCG/free β-hCG
- quad, NF, and NBL: 83/84%
- quad, NF, NBL, and PT: 92/93%.

Repeat measures
Markers which are more discriminatory at one gestation than another (e.g. PAPP-A) could be measured sequentially to capture a changing profile. Modelling predicts a large benefit.

Twins
Serum marker levels are approximately double those of singletons except for uE3, where they are two-thirds higher. In monozygotic twins, determined by ultrasound examination of the intertwine membrane, DR is similar to singletons, but in dizygotic twins the normal co-twin 'masks' the DS serum marker profile and DR is reduced.

If there is a 'vanishing twin the first trimester serum marker profile may be altered and some advocate delayed testing.

Other disorders
- Edwards' syndrome: four-fifths are detected through high DS risk in a combined test and one-third in second trimester tests. Explicit use of Edwards' syndrome risk changes the DR for the combined test little but increase to one-half for second trimester tests.
- Neural tube defects: about 90% of cases of anencephaly and 75% of spina bifida have raised AFP after 15 weeks. However, there is a much higher DR with the anomaly

scan where, in the BPD view, the 'lemon and banana' signs are seen.
- X-linked ichthyosis: identified with low uE3.
- Smith–Lemli–Opitz syndrome: low uE3 and other 2T markers.
- Cornelia de Lange syndrome: low PAPP-A and possibly free β-hCG and inhibin.
- Cardiac abnormalities: increased NT with normal karyotype is an indication for detailed fetal heart examination.
- Molar pregnancy or placental dysplasia: undetectable AFP and uE3 or very low PAPP-A.
- Fetal demise: low PAPP-A and low or high free β-hCG.
- Pre-eclampsia: reduced PAPP-A and increased inhibin.

References

Arbuzova S, Cuckle H, Mueller R, Sehmi I. Familial Down syndrome, evidence supporting cytoplasmic inheritance. Clin Genet 2001;60:456–62.

Cicero S, Rembouskos G, Vandecruys H, et al. Likelihood ratio for trisomy 21 in fetuses with absent nasal bone at the11–14-week scan. Ultra-sound Obstet Gynecol 2004;23:218–23.

Cuckle H. Down's syndrome screening in twins. J Me Screening 1998;5:3–4.

Cuckle H, Benn P. Multianalyte maternal serum screening for chromosomal defects. In: Genetic disorders and the fetus: diagnosis, prevention and treatment, 6th edn, Milunsky A. (ed.). Baltimore: Johns Hopkins University Press 2009.

Cuckle HS, Wald NJ, Thompson SG. Estimating a woman's risk of having a pregnancy associated with Down's syndrome using her age and serum alpha-fetoprotein level. Br J Obstet Gynaecol 1987;94:387–402.

Cuckle H, Aitken D, Goodburn S, et al. UK National Down's Syndrome Screening Programme, Laboratory Advisory Group. Age-standardisation when target setting and auditing performance of Down syndrome screening programmes. Prenat Diagn 2004;24:851–6.

Logghe H, Cuckle H, Sehmi I. Centre-specific ultrasound nuchal translucency medians needed for Down's syndrome screening. Prenat Diagn 1995;235:389–92.

Royston P, Thompson SG. Model-based screening by risk with application to Down's syndrome. Stats Med 1992;11:257–68.

Wright D, Bradbury I. Repeated measures screening for Down's syndrome. Br J Obstet Gynaecol 2005;112:80–3.

Symphyseal fundal height

Definition
The symphyseal fundal height (SFH) measurement is a measurement of the longitudinal distance of the pregnant abdomen from the symphysis pubis to the uterine fundus. It is used as a screening tool for abnormal fetal growth in late second and third trimester antenatal care, primarily to detect intrauterine growth restriction, but also as to identify macrosomia, multifetal pregnancy, and polyhydramnios.

Background
One of the main targets of antenatal care is the timely detection of abnormal fetal growth, as growth abnormalities may lead to adverse pregnancy outcomes, including perinatal death. The intrauterine growth restriction (IUGR) fetus is at increased risk in prolonged pregnancy and in labour, and may warrant intervention. The macrosomic fetus and the pregnant woman are both at increased risk of complications at the time of delivery.

Pathology
A single point measurement of SFH is at best an estimate of fetal size, rather than growth. Detection of aberrant growth requires serial measurements. The performance of SFH as a screening test for small babies has been reported to vary from 26% to 76%. This large variation in detection rate of IUGR in different studies may partly be explained by the 'Hawthorne effect': clinicians take extra care when they know they are being studied.

SFH measurements should not be seen as an isolated technique, but as part of an overall clinical assessment of the fetomaternal wellbeing.

Whereas the American College of Obstetricians and Gynecologists recommend repeated SFH measurements and ultrasound assessment of fetal growth in the presence of serial discrepancies, the Cochrane collaboration does not. The Cochrane conclusion is based on one randomized Danish trial, showing no difference in perinatal morbidity or mortality between intervention and control groups.

SFH measurement
Technique
To measure the SFH correctly a non-elastic measuring tape should be used. The pregnant woman should be semirecumbent, knees flexed, with an empty bladder, enough of the pregnant abdomen exposed to identify anatomical landmarks, and the uterus non-contracting. The uterine fundus should be identified with two hands on the abdomen. The tape-measure should be held with the centimetre marks on the underside to reduce bias.

There are several techniques described for obtaining the measurement. Westin, in the original SFH paper from 1977, describing what he called a 'gravidogram', suggested fixating the tape-measure at the symphysis pubis and identifying the fundus with the other hand, fingers extended, and the measuring tape sliding between the fingers of the fundal hand. The second method (Fig. 7.26.1), recommended by Gardosi, appears to be more common in UK practice today. The tape measure is fixed at the fundus with one hand and allowing the symphyseal hand to take the measurement. The tape measure should stay in contact with the skin along the abdomen, and the measurement should be obtained along the longitudinal axis of the uterus, without correction to the abdominal midline, if the highest fundal point is not in the midline.

Clinician bias
It is difficult and not practical to be blinded to the gestational length of the pregnant women we see in our antenatal clinics, and it is well known that awareness of gestational length at the time of measurement introduces measurement error. A variation in clinician ability to correctly identify the uterine fundus has been reported. There is also a good evidence of an interobserver variation, which, however, appears to be improving with experience and training. The consensus is that fundal height cannot

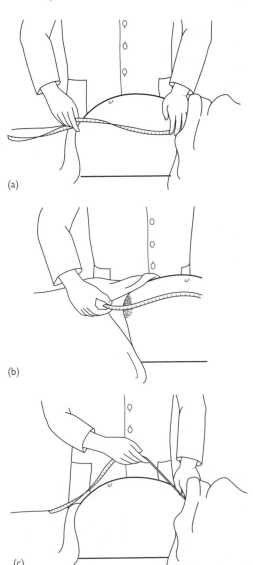

(a)

(b)

(c)

Fig. 7.26.1 (a–c) Correct technique for measuring symphyseal fundal height, courtesy of Professor Jason Gardosi, Gestation network 2010 www.gestation.net.

reliably be measured by different observers in the same pregnancy with sufficient agreement to separate small and normal or large fundal heights. This severely limits its clinical usefulness as a screening tool for both IUGR and macrosomia.

Other factors

Other fetomaternal factors that may cause variation in SHF measurement beyond the size of the fetus are

- amount of amniotic fluid
- size of placenta
- fetal presentation
- amount of abdominal fat
- thickness of myometrium
- presence of large fibroids
- relationship of uterus to the bony pelvis
- full bladder
- multifetal pregnancy
- multiparity.

Clinical management

A normal growth rate of the SFH of 1 cm per week is often assumed, based on existing SFH growth charts. When the SFH measurement appears to deviate from the standard, whether the standard is a fundal height growth curve or a simple gestational weeks ±2-cm rule (derived from observations that most pregnancies stay within this range throughout pregnancy), the recommended practice is repeat measurement by the same practitioner 1 week later. If at that stage the measurement is still the same, or smaller, referral to ultrasound for growth scan is recommended.

Similarly two consecutive measurements by the same clinician exceeding the given standard should raise the suspicion of macrosomia, and warrant investigations for macrosomia and a diabetic pregnancy. Serial ultrasound of the macrosomic fetus may not be necessary in the absence of other pathology, but an assessment of the best mode of delivery should occur at, or around term.

Previous pregnancy records often provide useful information. An otherwise low-risk woman, with what is perceived as insufficient SFH growth, which has had similar SFH growth patterns in previous pregnancies, and given birth to normal size offspring, would not need serial ultrasounds, provided that no other risk factors are identified.

Variation in SFH in different ethnic groups

The assumption that fundal height curves could be a useful adjunct to antenatal care in resource poor settings has been tested. In a small prospective study in India, a high sensitivity and specificity for both small for gestational age (SGA) and macrosomia as found using locally generated SFH curve. The authors noticed a difference of 3–4 cm compared with 'Western' fundal height curves and a corresponding birthweight difference of 500–600 g. In a larger study of Mozambican pregnant women with ultrasound-dated singleton pregnancies, locally generated charts were 0–3 cm lower in measurements at the same gestational interval as other (presumably western) charts.

It is thus likely that there are different SFH growth curves in different ethnic populations. Locally derived SFH charts will therefore perform better than more generic charts in terms of detecting abnormal growth. SFH measurements will only perform as well as the chart they are plotted on.

SFH measurement in obese women

Owing to an increasing prevalence of obesity in women of reproductive age in the Western world, the validity of SFH in obese women needs particular consideration. There is evidence that tape measurement bias increases with increasing BMI. Thus we cannot, in our clinical practice, assume that fundal height measurement have an equal validity, and will perform equally well in obese women as it has been shown to do in studies of normal weight pregnant women. On the other hand, if we do not assess SFH, considering it less useful, then ultrasound assessment of fetal growth becomes the default screening tool, and the advantage of ultrasound (often with limited vision in women with increased BMI and therefore a poorer quality assessment) in screening for fetal growth aberrations in obese women has yet to been demonstrated.

In the absence of alternative strategies, however, a low threshold for ultrasound referral for fetal growth assessment in obese women is recommended.

Customised fundal height measurements

There is thus good evidence for a significant maternal variation in fundal height and a given gestation. The often-used rule of gestational length in weeks ±2 cm has less value in a multiethnic setting, or, as we have seen, in a setting with an increasingly obese pregnant population. Serial measurements of fundal height can, however, be plotted on a 'customized' chart, controlling for physiological variables such as maternal height, weight, parity, and ethnic group, and has been shown to lead to increased antenatal detection of small and large babies. Although in a small randomized study the 'customized' chart detected 48% (compared with 29% in the control group, OR 2.2) of all SGA babies it is still disappointing to note that half the SGA infants were undiagnosed in pregnancy. However, it is reasonable to assume that in modern UK obstetric practice, with a multiethnic pregnant population and increasing contribution of obese pregnant women, the customized chart will perform better than a more generic one.

Assessment of fetal growth in the future

In current UK and European antenatal care working practice, a large proportion of pregnant women see more than one practitioner during their antenatal care, with ensuing implications for the quality of SFH measurements. The default alternative to SFH is, as we have seen, screening for growth abnormalities by serial ultrasound scans, which is expensive, time-consuming and generates false-positive results. The randomized studies of detection rates, costs, and effects of screening for abnormal growth by SFH measurement compared with ultrasound have not been done.

Self-measurement by pregnant women has been suggested as a possible future. A UK blinded pilot study recorded positive results of training in SFH measurement of pregnant women themselves. The study population performed as well as midwives in repeated, weekly measurements. Self-assessment by, we assume, interested and compliant pregnant women, would certainly address the interobserver variation problems of SFH measurement, and is simple, non-invasive, inexpensive, and well in agreement with the current ethos of patient involvement in the care they receive. SFH measurement as screening for IUGR and macrosomia should not been discarded until the comparative trial with ultrasound, using the right charts and the right techniques, has been undertaken, but in our current clinical practice it appears increasingly difficult to use SFH as a discriminating screening tool for fetal growth abnormalities.

Further reading

American College of Obstetricians and Gynecologists. *Intrauterine growth restriction.* ACOG Practise Bulletin 12. Washington: ACOG 2000.

Bailey SM, Sarmandal P, Grant JM. A comparison of three methods of assessing interobserver variation applied to measurement of the symphysis-fundal height. Br J Obstet Gynecol 1989;96:1266–71.

Boulos AN, Griffiths M, Allott H, et al. Trial of self- administered antenatal care: maternal symphysis fundal height measurements. J Obstet Gynaecol 1999;19:623.

Challis K, Osman NB, Nyström L, et al. Symphysis-fundal height growth chart of an obstetric cohort of 817 Mozambican women with ultrasound dated singleton pregnancies. Trop Med Int Health 2002;7:678–84.

Engstrom JL, McFarlin BL, Sampson MB. Fundal height measurement Part 4-Accuracy of Clinicians' identification of the uterine fundus during pregnancy J Nurse Midwifery 1993;38:318–23.

Engstrom JL, Piscioneri LA, Low LK, et al. Fundal height measurement. Part 3: The effect of maternal position on fundal height measurements. J Nurse Midwifery 1993;38:23–7.

Gardosi J, Francis A. Controlled trial of fundal height measurement plotted on customised antenatal growth charts. Br J Obstet Gynecol 1999;106;309–17.

Grover V, Usha R, Kalra S, et al. Altered fetal growth. Antenatal diagnosis by symphysis-fundal height in India and comparison with western charts. Int J Gynaecol Obstet 1991;35:231–4.

Hepburn M, Rosenberg K. An audit of the detection and management of small-for-gestational-age babies. Br J Obstet Gynaecol 1986;93:212–16.

Jelks A, Cifuentes R, Ross MG. Clinician bias in fundal height measurement. Obstet Gynecol 2007;110:892–9.

Lindhard A, Nielsen PV, Mouritzen LA, et al. The implications of introducing the symphyseal-fundal height-measurement. A prospective randomised controlled trial. Br J Obstet Gynecol 1990;97:675–80.

Neilson JP. Symphysis-fundal height measurement in pregnancy. Cochrane Database Syst Rev 1998;1:CD000944.

Parson HM. What happened at Hawthorne? Science 1974;198:922–32.

Pearce JM, Campbell S. A comparison of symphysis-fundal height and ultrasound as screening tests for light-for-gestational-age infants. Br J Obstet Gynecol 1987;94:100–4.

Petzold M, Sonesson C, Bergman E, et al. Surveillance in longitudinal models: detection of intrauterine growth restriction. Biometrics 2004;60:1025–33.

Rogers MS, Chan E, Ho A. Fundal height: does prior knowledge of gestational age influence the measurement? J Obstet Gynecol 1992;12:4–5.

Rogers MS, Needham PG. Evaluation of fundal height measurement in antenatal care. Aust NZ J Obstet Gynecol, 1985;25:87–90.

Steingrimsdottir T, Cnattingius S, Lindmark G. Symphysis-fundus height: construction of a new Swedish reference curve, based on ultrasonographically dated pregnancies. Acta Obstet Gynecol Scan 1995;74:346–51.

Westin B. Gravidogram and fetal growth. Acta Obstet Gynecol Scand 1977;56:273–82.

Internet resources

West Midlands Perinatal Institute: www.pi.nhs.uk/growth

Patient resources

Generating your own customised fetal growth and SFH chart: www.gestation.net

Maternal medicine and infections

Adrenal disorders in pregnancy 176
Anaemia in pregnancy 180
Autoimmune disease 182
Bacterial vaginosis 184
Chicken pox/herpes zoster 186
Chlamydia 188
Coagulation disorders 190
Connective tissue disorder 192
Cytomegalovirus 196
Dermatology 198
Diabetes in pregnancy 200
Drugs in pregnancy 208
Epilepsy and other neurological conditions 214
Gonorrhoea 218
Perinatal group B streptococcus 220
Haemoglobinopathies 222
Heart disease 224
Hepatitis B 238
Herpes simplex infection 242
HIV infection 244
Human papillomavirus 250
Hypertension 252
Immunization 258
Inflammatory bowel disease 262
Jaundice 266
Listeriosis 272
Liver disease 274
Measles: rubeola 278
Parvovirus 280
Pituitary disorders in pregnancy 282
Psychiatric disorders in pregnancy 286
Renal disease 290
Respiratory disease 296
Rubella 302
Substance abuse in pregnancy 304
Syphilis 306
Thromboembolic disease 310
Thyroid and parathyroid disease 312
Toxoplasmosis in pregnancy 316
Vulvovaginal candidiasis 318

Adrenal disorders in pregnancy

Addison's disease

Addison disease is adrenocortical insufficiency due to the destruction or dysfunction of the entire adrenal cortex. It affects both glucocorticoid and mineralocorticoid function. The onset of disease usually occurs when 90% or more of both adrenal cortices are dysfunctional or destroyed. Prevalence is 40–60 cases per 1 million population and so is very rarely encountered in pregnancy. Most cases (90%) are due to autoimmune destruction or tuberculosis.

Effect of Addison's disease on pregnancy

If treated, no complications are encountered.

Effect of pregnancy on Addison's disease

Pregnancy has no effect on the disease if properly treated. Steroid replacement may need to be altered at certain times during pregnancy.

Clinical approach

History

- Patients usually present with features of both glucocorticoid and mineralocorticoid deficiency and they may present with clinical features of chronic Addison's disease or in acute addisonian crisis.

Chronic presentation

- Hyperpigmentation of the skin and mucous membranes often precedes all other symptoms by months to years.
- Weakness, fatigue, poor appetite, and weight loss.
- Nausea, vomiting, and occasional diarrhoea.
- Dizziness.
- Myalgias and flaccid muscle paralysis may occur due to hyperkalaemia.
- Other reported symptoms include muscle and joint pains; a heightened sense of smell, taste, and hearing; and salt craving.

Acute presentation

- Abdominal symptoms may take on features of an acute abdomen, nausea, and vomiting. Other symptoms may include hyperpyrexia and vascular collapse.

Examination

- Increased pigmentation of the skin and mucous membranes, with or without areas of vitiligo.
- Evidence of dehydration, hypotension, and orthostasis.
- Female patients may show an absence of axillary and pubic hair and decreased body hair.

Investigations

Short synacthen test and long corticotrophin releasing hormone test.

Management

The vast majority of cases are diagnosed before conception and are well established on replacement therapy. This is usually in the form of hydrocortisone (a total of 30 mg daily in divided doses) and fludrocortisone (up to 100 mg daily).

The patients feeling of wellbeing and the lack of postural hypotension, hyponatraemia, or hyperkalaemia gauge the adequacy of replacements.

The maintenance doses are not changed by pregnancy *per se*. However, an increase in dosage is vital during periods of stress such as hyperemesis gravidarum, surgical procedures and infections, or during labour.

Hydrocortisone is administered intravenously in doses of 100 mg every 6 hour throughout the period of stress and reduced gradually over a period of days.

Congenital adrenal hyperplasia

Congenital adrenal hyperplasia (CAH) is a family of inherited disorders of adrenal steroidogenesis, resulting from a deficiency of one of several enzymes necessary for normal adrenal steroid synthesis. It occurs in 1 in 5000 and 1 in 15 000 births in most populations.

21 hydroxylase deficiency (21-OHD) is the commonest deficiency, with a particularly high frequency and carrier rates of between 1.2% and 6% of the population. The gene frequency is 1 in 200–400 and is autosomal recessive.

The risk of a subsequent child having the disorder is 1:4, if a couple have one affected child.

21-OHD deficiency leads to impaired production of glucocorticoids and mineralocorticoids. The sex steroid pathway is intact and thus provides the only option for the accumulating metabolites. The consequence is a markedly enhanced adrenal androgen production.

Affected female fetuses are at risk of masculinization. Male neonates are at risk of salt-losing crises due to mineralocorticoid deficiency as well as precocious puberty.

Effect of CAH on pregnancy

There is an increased risk of miscarriage, Caesarean section, pre-eclampsia, and intrauterine growth restriction.

Effect of pregnancy on CAH

No effect in treated patients.

Clinical approach

Key points

Aim of treatment is to ensure adequate glucocorticoid and mineralocorticoid replacement for the mother and preventing virilization of an affected female fetus.

- In women with CAH, increased antenatal surveillance should be put in place because of the increased risk of pre-eclampsia.
- Corticosteroid replacement is the mainstay of treatment. Mineralocorticoids are necessary in salt losing classical CAH.
- Monitoring with 17-hydroxyprogesterone levels is unreliable in pregnancy.
- In pregnancies with a fetus at risk of CAH, suppressing adrenocorticotrophic hormone (ACTH), the drive for the intact sex steroid production pathway, by giving dexamethasone in a dose of 250–500 µg daily is commonly used and continued throughout pregnancy.
- Fetal diagnosis should be made with sex determination, human leucocyte antigen (HLA) status and 21-hydroxylase zygosity.
- Treatment should be started preconception or before 5 weeks' gestation, prior to differentiation of the genitalia.
- All female neonates should receive corticosteroids to treat the CAH and because their adrenal glands will be suppressed following long-term high-dose maternal dexamethasone therapy.
- Male fetuses do not need to be treated *in utero*.
- Prevention of virilization is not always successful, therefore parents should be counselled regarding benefits and risks, and termination of the pregnancy should be offered if the fetus is female.

Phaeochromocytoma

These are chromaffin tumours that secrete catecholamines. It is known as the 10% tumour as approximately 10% of the disease is bilateral, malignant, located in chromaffin tissue outside of the adrenal gland, arises in childhood, familial, and recurs after being resected. They are mostly located in the adrenal medulla.

Mutations of the genes VHL, RET, NF1, SDHB, and SDHD are all known to cause familial phaeochromocytoma/extra-adrenal paraganglioma. Phaeochromocytomas may occur in certain familial syndromes, including multiple endocrine neoplasia (MEN) 2A and 2B, neurofibromatosis, and von Hippel–Lindau (VHL) disease.

Effect of phaeochromocytoma on pregnancy

These tumours are rare but dangerous if they occur in pregnancy. Fetal mortality is about 25% in undiagnosed cases and 15% in diagnosed cases. Maternal mortality most recently had decreased to about 5% in undiagnosed cases, with no maternal death when the diagnosis is made antepartum. The main causes of maternal mortality are cardiac arrythmias, cerebrovascular accidents, or pulmonary oedema.

Effect of pregnancy on phaeochromocytoma

Moribund hypertensive crisis may be precipitated by labour, delivery, general anaesthesia, or opiates. The gravid uterus may cause hypertensive attacks due to pressure on the tumour in the supine position.

Clinical approach

History
- The classic symptoms are headaches, palpitation, and excessive sweating.
- Other symptoms include tremor, nausea and vomiting, anxiety, weakness, epigastric pain, flank pain, and weight loss.

Examination
- Signs include hypertension, weight loss, pallor, fever, tremor, and tachyarrhythmias.

Investigations
- Biochemistry may reveal impaired glucose tolerance and hypercalcaemia.
- Diagnosis is from measuring plasma metanephrine and/or 24-hour urinary creatinine, total catecholamines, vanillylmandelic acid, and metanephrines
- MRI is the preferred imaging modality in pregnancy.

Management

Management of hypertension and symptoms with an alpha-blocking agent such as phenoxybenzamine is mandatory. The dose is 10–30 mg, two to four times daily. Beta-blocking agents to control tachycardia can be added if required.

Surgical removal is the only cure after control of the blood pressure is achieved by medication.

If the patient is prior to 23 weeks' gestation, then surgical resection is recommended. After 24 weeks, it is recommended that the surgery is postponed until fetal maturity is achieved and then performed either concurrently with Caesarean section or postpartum.

Adequate alpha-blockade for at least 3 days prior to surgery and expert anaesthetic care are essential.

Conn's syndrome

It is a rare disease of primary hyperaldosteroneism, caused by adrenal aldosteronomas in about 75% of cases and idiopathic bilateral adrenal hyperplasia in the remainder.

Clinical approach

History
Hypertension and hypokalaemia are sometimes the only indicators.

Examination
Symptoms and signs of hypokalaemia. Alkalosis may also be present.

Investigations

Diagnosis is by low serum potassium, suppressed renin activity and high plasma aldosterone.

Management

Treating hypertension is vital and is in the usual way. Potassium supplementation is also important. Spirinolactone, commonly used outside pregnancy, should be avoided in pregnancies with a male fetus because of its anti-androgen effects. Tumour resection is curative and laparoscopic adrenalectomy may prove to be useful during pregnancy.

Cushing's syndrome

Long-term exposure to glucocorticoids may lead to Cushing's syndrome. The most common cause is iatrogenic, from corticosteroid therapy.

Increased adrenal cortisol production causes endogenous Cushing's syndrome. Most cases are due to corticotrophin-producing pituitary adenomas leading to bilateral adrenal hyperplasia (Cushing's disease). The condition is very rare in pregnancy as most women with the disorder will have subfertility.

Effect of Cushing's syndrome on pregnancy

Maternal complications include hypertension in about 75% and gestational diabetes in about 50% of patients. Heart failure and severe pre-eclampsia are common. Buescher et al. (1992) reported a 5% maternal mortality rate among 65 pregnancies. Wound infection due to poor tissue healing is common. Perinatal morbidity, with 60% preterm delivery, and mortality (25%) are also high.

Clinical approach

History and examination
The classical clinical features can be attributed to pregnancy and include weight gain, striae, hypertension, diabetes, hirsutism, headache, and easy bruising.

Investigations
Low ACTH and high cortisol are suggestive of an adrenal cause. However, pregnancy-specific ranges for plasma and urinary cortisol must be used and the cortisol should be measured after a high-dose dexamethasone suppression test. Localization is possible with adrenal ultrasound, CT, or MRI, or pituitary CT or MRI.

Management

Long-term medical treatment is usually ineffective; however, ketoconazole blocking steroid production has been successful. Few cases during pregnancy have been successfully treated with oral ketoconazole, but there are concerns in a pregnancy with a male fetus due to blockage of testicular steroidogenesis. Surgery is the treatment of choice and it has been undertaken successfully during pregnancy.

Further reading

Nelson-Piercy C. *A Handbook of obstetric medicine*, 3rd edn. London: Informa Healthcare 2006.

Buescher MA, McClamrock HD, Adashi EY. Cushing syndrome in pregnancy. *Obstet Gynecol* 1992;79:130–7.

Burrow GN, Ferris TF. *Medical complications during pregnancy*, 4th edn. London: W.B. Saunders 1995.

Grossman A. *Clinical endocrinology*, 2nd edn. Oxford: Blackwell Scientific Publications 1997.

Shehata HA, Ahmed K. Other endocrine disorders in pregnancy. *Curr Obstet Gynaecol* 2004;14:387–94.

Internet resources

www.emedicine.com/
www.mayoclinic.com/

Anaemia in pregnancy

Definition
Anaemia is defined as a reduction in the absolute number of circulating red blood cells (RBCs), which is indirectly measured by a reduction in haemoglobin concentration, haematocrit, or RBC count. In practice, anaemia in pregnant women is said to exist when the haemoglobin level in venous blood is below 11 g/dL (WHO 1968).

Prevalence
Published rates of prevalence for developing countries range from 35% to 60% for Africa, Asia, and Latin America. This is in sharp contrast to industrialized countries where anaemia in pregnancy occurs in less than 20% of women.

Causes
- Acquired
  - nutritional : iron deficiency; folate deficiency; vitamin B12 deficiency
  - acute blood loss
  - aplastic anaemia
  - drug-induced haemolytic anaemia
  - infections: malaria, HIV
  - chronic disease: renal
  - neoplasia: leukaemia, lymphoma.
- Hereditary
  - haemoglobinopathies: thalassaemias—β, α (heterozygotes); sickle cell disease
  - congenital haemolytic anaemia.

In all of these conditions, anaemia results from one or more of three independent mechanisms: decreased RBC production, increased RBC destruction, and blood loss. Iron deficiency is the commonest cause of anaemia in the pregnant woman and is usually a result of nutritional deficiency or chronic blood loss. In both situations, the availability of iron is the rate limiting factor for RBC production by the bone marrow. Iron deficiency is relatively common in pregnancy because of the increased iron demand (500–1000 mg) and because many women start pregnancy with poor or depleted iron stores.

Effects of anaemia on mother
Suspect anaemia if mother complains of easy fatigue, pica, and appears pale. Decreased aerobic work performance in iron deficiency anaemia could result from a lack of iron-containing cellular enzymes. Anaemia is usually diagnosed on FBC, which is a part of routine antenatal screening blood tests.

Effects of anaemia on pregnancy and fetus
Fetuses of iron-deficient mothers are not anaemic at birth because of placental active transport of iron to the fetus. However, severe anaemia in the mother (Hb <6 g/dL) has been associated with reduced amniotic fluid volume, fetal cerebral vasodilation, and non-reassuring fetal heart rate patterns. Increased risks of prematurity, spontaneous abortion, low birthweight, and fetal death have also been reported.

Approach to diagnosis
The common causes are nutritional iron deficiency, folate deficiency, and haemoglobinopathies. β-Thalassaemia minor is common in Mediterranean, Arab, African and South Asian populations. α-Thalassaemia carriers are almost exclusively found in South-East Asians (1 in 25 Chinese) and Africans. Sickle cell anaemia is seen commonly in African and Afro-Caribbean populations.

Iron-deficiency anaemia
Causes of iron deficiency
The cause of iron deficiency is often multifactorial, particularly in developing countries. Iron deficiency is the most common single nutritional deficiency in women and may develop from inadequate dietary intake, impaired iron absorption, or iron loss from chronic blood loss. This is easily unmasked by the increased iron demand of pregnancy.

Diagnosis of iron-deficiency anaemia
The diagnosis is often obvious on a FBC and peripheral blood film. The FBC shows reduced haemoglobin concentration, reduced mean cell volume, reduced mean cell haemoglobin, reduced mean cell haemoglobin concentration, and mild thrombocytosis. The blood film shows microcytic hypochromic red cells with anisocytosis and poikilocytosis. Hypochromic anaemia occurs in other disorders, such as anaemia of chronic diseases and in thalassaemias. To help to differentiate the type, further haematinic assays may be necessary. Reduced serum ferritin (<15 µg/L) is the most useful indicator of iron deficiency. However, serum ferritin is an acute phase reactant, and its concentration is increased in the presence of infections, systemic inflammations, malignancies, hepatopathies, and chronic renal failure. Thus, while a low serum ferritin is diagnostic of iron deficiency, normal serum ferritin values do not exclude a deficiency state. In such a situation finding a decreased serum iron concentration and transferrin saturation is needed for diagnosis.

Management
The correction of iron deficiency involves an appropriate diet and iron supplementation. Diet modifications include more iron-rich foods and positive modification of the factors influencing iron absorption.

Oral iron replacement therapy with gradual replenishment of iron stores and restoration of haemoglobin is the preferred treatment. Foods contain iron in two forms: 'haem' iron, which is highly bioavailable (15–35% absorbed), is present in red meat, fish, and poultry. Its absorption is independent of other factors present in food. Non-haem iron, which is absorbed to a lesser extent (2–4%), is present in fruits, vegetables, cereals, and dairy products, etc. Its absorption is markedly affected by other factors. Tannins, phytates, and calcium inhibit and vitamin C, meat, and citrus juices enhance iron absorption.

Several oral iron preparations are available which vary in their degree of absorption, side-effects, and cost. Oral ferrous salts are the treatment of choice (ferric salts are less well absorbed) and should take the form of ferrous sulphate 200 mg two or three times daily (200-mg tablet provides 65 mg of elemental iron). Alternative preparations include ferrous gluconate and ferrous fumarate. Side-effects like nausea, constipation, and diarrhoea are common and may be reduced by taking the tablets after meals. Modified release preparations have been developed to reduce side-effects but in practice prove expensive and often release the iron beyond the sites of optimal absorption. Effective iron replacement therapy should result in a rise in haemoglobin concentration of around 1 g/L per day (about 20 g/L every 3 weeks) commencing after 2–3 weeks of the start of treatment.

Parenteral iron therapy may be used if oral therapy has failed or oral therapy is not tolerated. It is indicated when a pregnant woman presents with severe anaemia in the last month of pregnancy. Parenteral iron can be given by either intramuscular or intravenous route. The main drawback of intramuscular iron is the pain and staining of the skin at injection site, myalgia, arthralgia, and injection abscess. Iron-dextran and iron-polymaltose can be used by both i.m. and i.v. route. Two newer i.v. preparations, iron sucrose and ferric gluconate, are associated with lesser side-effects.

Iron can be given intravenously at one shot as total dose infusion (TDI). Utmost caution is needed for total dose iron therapy via intravenous route because of severe ana-phylactic reaction that may occur. Blood transfusion is not indicated unless the patient has decompensated due to a drop in haemoglobin concentration and needs a more rapid rise in haemoglobin. Packed red cell transfusion may be indicated for pregnant women with severe anaemia (Hb 6 g/100 mL or less) close to due date or < 8 g/d if they have an increased likelihood of blood loss at delivery.

Prophylaxis

Pregnant women need iron to cover their basic losses (0.6 mg/day for 300 days = 180 mg), the demands of the fetus (250–300 mg) and of the placenta (75 mg). In addition, 300–400 mg of iron is required for an increase in the RBC mass. Consequently, the total iron demand of pregnancy amounts to 900 mg or approximately 3 mg/day (30–40 mg of dietary iron). This requirement cannot be met by the food consumed by most pregnant women, especially from the developing world, and oral supplementation of medicinal iron is justifiable. The data from randomized trials suggest that daily antenatal iron supplementation increases haemoglobin levels in maternal blood both antenatally and postnatally (Pena-Rosas and Viteri 2006). Infant outcomes of routine supplementation have not been studied adequately.

Megaloblastic anaemias

Megaloblastic anaemias are caused by impaired DNA synthesis in the marrow secondary to either folic acid or vitamin B12 deficiency. In pregnancy it is almost always secondary to folate deficiency. Folic acid deficiency during pregnancy is usually secondary to dietary deficiency, occurring commonly in women who do not eat enough green vegetables or animal proteins. It is also commoner in multiple pregnancies, women with intestinal malapsorption and women on anticonvulsants.

Folic acid deficiency has been associated with increased risk of fetal neural tube defects, and routine supplementation periconceptually has been shown to reduce its occurrence. Although folic acid deficiency has been implicated in the occurrence of other pregnancy complications, such as placental abruption and pre-eclampsia, this has never been confirmed.

Clinical features

- Glossitis—painful red tongue with papillary flattening
- Apthous oral ulcers
- Retinal and subcutaneous haemorrhages.

Laboratory features

- Macrocytosis, megaloblasts, neutrophil hypersegmentation, anisocytosis, and Howell–Jolly bodies on peripheral smear.
- There may be associated neutropenia and thrombocytopenia:
  - serum folate levels are unreliable. Red cell folate estimate is a more accurate measure of deficiency.

Management

- A marked haematological response is seen within 7 days of starting as little as folic acid 1 mg per day orally. Treatment with folic acid should be continued throughout pregnancy.

Further reading

Pena-Rosas JP, Viteri FE, Effects of routine oral iron supplementation with or without folic acid for women during pregnancy. Cochrane Database Syst Rev 2006;3:CD004736.

WHO. Nutritional anaemias. Report of a WHO scientific group. World Health Organization Technical Report Series. 1968; 405:5–37.

Frewin R, Henson A, Provan D. ABC of clinical haematology. Iron deficiency anaemia. BMJ 1997;314:360–3.

Autoimmune disease

Multiple sclerosis

Multiple sclerosis (MS) is an inflammatory demyelinating disease of the central nervous system. It affects women more commonly than men and this often coincides with bringing up a family. It is the commonest cause of neurological disability in young adults in the UK. Pregnancy has no long-term effects on MS progression.

Aetiology

There are many causes, including viruses, autoimmune disorders, environmental and genetic factors.

Prognosis

Effect of pregnancy on multiple sclerosis
The majority of studies reported that there is a reduced frequency of relapse during pregnancy, especially during the third trimester, followed by an increase in relapse rates in the puerperium, especially in the first 3 months. There is some evidence to suggest that pregnancy may slow the rate of progression, more so in parous women than nulliparous women.

Effect of multiple sclerosis on pregnancy
There is no evidence that MS has an adverse effect on the outcome of pregnancy and delivery. Although MS is not an inherited disease, there is a slightly higher chance of the offspring developing the disease than the general population: estimated at 1–4% if one of the parents has the disease.

Clinical approach

Diagnosis
The diagnosis is one of exclusion as there is no single test that can confirm MS. Symptoms of MS vary from mild to severe and may appear in various combinations, ranging from difficulty in concentrating, poor attention, memory, and judgement. MRI can show areas of scarring and inflammation in the myelin (there are no data about safety of MRI in pregnancy). Lumbar puncture and visual evoked potentials can be helpful.

Management
There is little conclusive evidence to support a role for spinal or epidural anaesthesia precipitating exacerbations of MS postpartum. Further evidence is needed to allow a fully informed discussion about pain relief during labour for patients with multiple sclerosis. A retrospective study found the relapse rate in puerperium to be independent of breastfeeding status. Steroids are not contraindicated in pregnancy but should be used with caution after discussing the risks and benefits. Intravenous immunoglobulins have been suggested to reduce the incidence of postpartum relapse. Several new medications such as β-interferon and glatiramer acetate have demonstrated a reduction in the number and severity of MS exacerbations, but none is licensed for use in pregnancy. There are reported cases of normal pregnancies and healthy infants in women who were placed on these medications. Little is known, however, about how the use of these medications affect pregnancy and childbearing and further research is required. Planning adequate postnatal support for a family should take into account the increased risk of relapse postpartum.

Myasthenia gravis

Myasthenia gravis (MG) is a neuromuscular disease leading to fluctuating muscle weakness and fatigability. It is an autoimmune disease in women, that occurs in the second and third decades of life, caused by circulating antibodies that block the acetylcholine receptors at the postsynaptic neuromuscular junction, inhibiting the stimulative effect of acetylcholine. These antibodies are IgG and may cross the placenta causing transient neonatal MG.

Aetiology

MG is often associated with other autoimmune mediated diseases. In large series in patients with MG, 7% had diabetes mellitus, 6% had thyroid disease, 3% had non-thymic neoplasm, and more than 2% had rheumatoid arthritis. Transient MG has been observed in HIV infection and after bone marrow transplantation.

Prognosis

Effect of pregnancy on myasthenia gravis
In the long term, pregnancy does not affect MG. The course of this disease is variable and unpredictable during pregnancy and can change during subsequent pregnancies. The first trimester and the first month postpartum seem to be the most critical periods for exacerbation of the disease. Complete remission can occur in some mothers.

Effect of myasthenia gravis on pregnancy
The reported incidence of preterm delivery or low birth weight is variable. The perinatal death rate is unaffected but the death rate because of fetal anomalies is increased. About 10% of infants born to MG mothers show signs of neonatal MG, which responds well to the acetylcholine inhibitors. Very rarely, an infant can be born with arthrogryposis multiplex congenita, secondary to profound intrauterine weakness, due to maternal antibodies that target an infant's acetylcholine receptors.

Clinical approach

Diagnosis
MG can be a difficult diagnosis. Physical examination can reveal easy fatiguability, ptosis, and diplopia. If diagnosis is suspected, serology can be performed to identify acetylcholine receptor antibodies and has a sensitivity of 80–96%. Other tests are electromyography, imaging, edrophonium test, pulmonary function tests, and immunofluorescence.

Management
Acetylcholinesterase inhibitors, such as pyridostigmine and immunosuppressive therapy (corticosteroids, azathioprine, or cyclosporine A) should be continued throughout pregnancy as this reduces the chances of neonatal muscle weakness as well as controlling the mother's MG. Higher doses may be required as pregnancy advances. Serial plasmapheresis and immunosuppressive therapy have successfully been used to treat MG crisis in pregnancy. Regional anaesthesia is safe with the right choice of drugs. A Caesarean section is recommended for obstetric reasons. Large doses of acetylcholinesterase drugs may be a contraindication to breastfeeding because they can cause gastrointestinal upsets in the breastfed newborn. Corticosteroids can be safely used during lactation.

Autoimmune liver disorders

There are three different autoimmune liver disorders:
- autoimmune chronic active hepatitis (CAH)
- primary biliary cirrhosis (PBC)
- primary sclerosing cholangitis (PSC).

Autoimmune chronic active hepatitis

Autoimmune hepatitis is a chronic necroinflammatory hepatitis of unknown aetiology, caused by autoantibodies against liver-specific and non-liver-specific antigens and increased immunoglobulins IgG levels. Females make up 75% of patients with this form of chronic active hepatitis, particularly in the second and third decades of their life. It can occur by itself, but can coexist with other autoimmune diseases, such as systemic lupus erythematosus or antiphospholipid syndrome.

Clinical approach

Diagnosis

The onset is insidious with fatigue, anorexia, jaundice, but can also resemble viral hepatitis. Liver enzymes are not specifically indicative of CAH; however, elevated aminotransferases and hypergammaglobulinaemia represent another characteristic. Prothrombin time is prolonged. The presence of antinuclear, anti-smooth muscle, and anti-liver microsomal antibodies are disease specific for CAH. Liver biopsy confirms the diagnosis.

Management

Pregnancy may be uncomplicated in patients with mild treated autoimmune CAH, but there is some evidence that this group of patients has an increased risk of pre-eclampsia, prematurity, and fetal wastage. Immunosuppressive therapy with steroids or in combination with azathioprine results in remission of the disease and therapy should be continued throughout gestation to prevent relapse. Liver transplantation should be considered for end-stage cirrhosis.

Primary biliary cirrhosis

PBC is a chronic and slowly progressive cholestatic liver disease of autoimmune aetiology characterized by injury of the intrahepatic bile ducts that may eventually lead to liver failure. This disease affects predominantly women, usually in the middle age

Aetiology

PBC is associated with other autoimmune diseases such as Sjogren's syndrome, scleroderma, and Raynaud's phenomenon and is regarded as an organ-specific disease. Genetic susceptibility as a predisposing factor has been suggested. Environmental factors (e.g. infection, chemicals, and smoking) may have a causative role.

Clinical approach

Diagnosis

The majority of patients are asymptomatic, however some may present with symptoms of fatigue and pruritis. PBC may be diagnosed outside pregnancy on routine liver testing with elevated levels of alkaline phosphatase (liver isoenzyme) and γ-glutamyl transpeptidase. Diagnosis is usually confirmed by detection of antimitochondrial antibodies (AMAs). Liver biopsy may be required for those AMA-negative patients who are severely symptomatic.

Management

Maternal and fetal outcomes are variable, but the prognosis is good for well-compensated disease. Drug therapy is non-specific and aimed at relieving symptoms such as pruritis. Currently, the first line of therapy is ursodeoxycholic acid (UDCA) and an anticholestatic. Liver transplantation is an option for those with liver failure.

Primary sclerosing cholangitis

PSC is a rare, chronic, fibrosing, inflammatory disorder of unknown aetiology affecting the biliary tree. PSC often accompanies other autoimmune disorders. It is mostly observed in male patients with irritable bowel disease.

Clinical approach

Diagnosis

Patients may present with jaundice, fever, pruritis, and right upper quadrant pain. There is a hypothesis suggestive of hormonal influence which is supported by reports of patients developing the disease during or shortly after pregnancy. Patients have elevated alkaline phosphatase and γ-glutamyl transpeptidase levels and underlying bile duct abnormalities seen on ultrasound, cholangiography, magnetic resonance cholangiography, or liver biopsy.

Management

Treatment is directed at controlling symptoms with ursodeoxycholic acid to reduce itching and malabsorption and immunosupressants to reduce inflammation. In advanced cases, liver transplantation has been used successfully. In one reported series of pregnancies in women with PSC, pregnancy outcome was good. The only serious complication was severe pruritis (2 out of 13) leading to discontinuation of pregnancies. Most patients had marked disappearance or reduction of symptoms after delivery. Consequently, the cause of pruritis could have been obstetric cholestasis.

Further reading

Beth A, Mueller JZ, Critchlow C. Birth outcomes and need for hospitalisation after delivery among women with multiple sclerosis. Am J Obstet Gynecol 2002;186:446–52

Giesser B. Pregnancy and multiple sclerosis: the current view. Mult Scler Q Rep 2001;20:68.

Janczewska I, Olsson R, Hultcrantz R, *et al.* Pregnancy in patients with primary sclerosing cholangitis. Liver 1996;16:326–30.

Plauche WC. Myasthenia gravis. Clin Obstet Gynecol 1983;26:592–604.

Shehata HA, Okuson H. Neurological disorders in pregnancy. Current Opin Obstet Gynecol 2004;16:119.

Bacterial vaginosis

Definition
Bacterial vaginosis is an ecological condition of the vaginal flora characterized by variable degrees of depletion of the resident and protective, hydrogen peroxide-producing lactobacillus species and an overgrowth of vaginal anaerobes. An intermediary and less stable subtype, possibly reflecting a transitional phase between normal flora and bacterial vaginosis, is also recognized and is equally associated with adverse perinatal and gynaecological outcomes. Intermediate flora may include a range of pathological floral shifts that are unrelated to bacterial vaginosis, including aerobic vaginitis. Bacterial vaginosis has been recognized for over a hundred years albeit documented under a host of different names, including non-specific vaginitis, *Haemophilus vaginitis, Gardnerella vaginitis, Corynebacterium vaginitis* and *Anaerobic vaginosis*.

Epidemiology
The prevalence of bacterial vaginosis is population dependent. In both the USA and the UK, African American and women from African and Afro-Caribbean ethnic backgrounds have the highest prevalence of bacterial vaginosis ranging between 20% and 35% compared with their Caucasian counterparts with a prevalence rate of 10–15% (Goldenberg et al. 1996). The prevalence rates are also higher among women attending genitourinary medicine clinics, smokers, lesbians, and users of intrauterine devices.

Aetiology
The exact stimulus that initiates the transformation of the vaginal flora is unknown. The condition is polymicrobial and participating organisms include anaerobes, *Gardnerella vaginalis* and more recently *Atopobium vaginale*. Three main risk factors have emerged as possible causes of the shift from a lactobacilli-dominated flora to bacterial vaginosis, namely sexual activity, douching, and the absence of hydrogen peroxide-producing lactobacilli in the vagina. Women from African and Afro-Caribbean ethnic backgrounds practise vaginal douching more commonly than their white counterparts (Stock et al 1973; Aral et al. 1992), in the erroneous belief that douching is a health-promoting practice. Some of the antiseptic solutions used for douching may weaken the protective lactobacillus species or reduce their numbers, thereby encouraging colonization by other organisms. Douching has been independently associated with a significantly increased risk of acquisition of bacterial vaginosis. After adjusting for vaginal douching, Black race was no longer significantly associated with bacterial vaginosis (Rajamanoharan et al. 1999), suggesting that differing rates of bacterial vaginosis between racial groups may be due to cultural differences rather than genetic and socioeconomic variations.

Clinical features
Bacterial vaginosis does not elicit a cellular inflammatory response in the vagina, and up to 60% of affected women are asymptomatic. Of the minority of women with symptoms, a thin fishy smelling vaginal discharge is common, which may be accentuated by menstrual discharge or semen from unprotected sexual intercourse.

Diagnosis
Bacterial vaginosis can be diagnosed by
- amsel composite criteria: this consists of the presence of any three of the following four features: characteristic vaginal discharge, positive Whiff (10% KOH) test, pH >4.7, or the presence of clue cells
- wet mount and direct microscopy
- gram stain
- affirm VP III: this is a commercially available DNA hybridization assay for the detection of *G. vaginalis*. Since *G. vaginalis* is part of the normal flora of the vagina, it is designed to be positive only for pathological concentrations of *G. vaginalis* ($>2 \times 10^5$ bacterial cells).

Complications
- Early and late miscarriage
- Preterm labour and preterm delivery
- Preterm prelabour rupture of membranes
- Chorioamnionitis
- Postpartum endometritis
- Wound infections
- Low birthweight
- Acquisition of HIV
- Cervical dysplasias.

Management
Pregnant and non-pregnant women who have symptoms attributable to bacterial vaginosis should be treated. At present, there is insufficient evidence to recommend routine screening and treatment of all pregnant women (McDonald et al 2005). However, there is strong evidence that women with a prior history of preterm delivery or late pregnancy loss benefit significantly from screening and treatment. Treatment when indicated should be initiated early in the second trimester preferably before 20 weeks' gestation. Treatment programmes initiated after 20 weeks have not been shown to reduce adverse pregnancy outcomes. Early oral or topical clindamycin therapy eradicate bacterial vaginosis effectively, and are both associated with a reduction in the risks of late miscarriage and preterm birth (Ugwumadu et al 2003). Some authors advocate oral therapy for bacterial vaginosis in pregnancy as this is believed to eradicate subclinical endometritis, which may be important (Ugwumadu et al 2003).

Oral or topical metronidazole is also effective in the treatment of bacterial vaginosis. However, metronidazole has a narrower spectrum of activity than clindamycin acting chiefly against anaerobes, and with no activity against many aerobes and other key organisms such as mobiluncus, *Ureaplasma urealyticum* and *Mycoplasma hominis*, which are associated with bacterial vaginosis. Metronidazole has a neutral effect on the protective lactobacillus species in contrast to clindamycin, which has activity against lactobacilli. A combination of oral and intravaginal clindamycin has been suggested to ensure eradication of organisms resident in the upper genital tract through the oral component and achieve sufficient intravaginal antibiotic levels to eradicate the large burden of bacterial innoculum in the vagina, which may not be achieved easily by oral therapy. In the literature, there are no reports of embryotoxic effects attributable to clindamycin use in human pregnancy. It is well tolerated and widely used during pregnancy in the USA. Its side-effects profile compares favourably with that of other broad-spectrum antibiotics including the risk of antibiotic associated colitis.

Further reading

Aral SO, Mosher WD, Cates W, Jr. Vaginal douching among women of reproductive age in the United States: 1988. Am J Public Health 1992;82;210–14.

Goldenberg RL, Klebanoff MA, Nugent R, et al. Bacterial colonisation of the vagina during pregnancy in four ethnic groups. Vaginal Infections and Prematurity Study Group. Am J Obstet Gynecol 1996;174:1618–2161.

McDonald H, Brocklehurst P, Parsons J. Antibiotics for treating bacterial vaginosis in pregnancy. Cochrane Database Syst Rev 2005;CD000262.

Rajamanoharan S, Low N, Jones SB, Pozniak AL. Bacterial vaginosis, ethnicity, and the use of genital cleaning agents: a case control study. Sex Transm Dis 1999;26:404–9.

Stock RJ, Stock ME, Hutto JM. Vaginal douching. Current concepts and practices. Obstet Gynecol 1973;42;141–6.

Ugwumadu A, Manyonda I, Reid F, Hay P. Effect of early oral clindamycin on late miscarriage and preterm delivery in asymptomatic women with abnormal vaginal flora and bacterial vaginosis: a randomised controlled trial. Lancet 2003;361:983–8.

Chicken pox/herpes zoster

Chicken pox/herpes zoster is caused from infection with the varicella zoster virus. Varicella infection is usually seen as a childhood illness, but can occur in pregnant women and the effects vary based on the gestational age at infection. Herpes zoster is reactivation can be reactivated from latent varicella infection in a dermatomal distribution.

Epidemiology

Ninety per cent of adults in the USA demonstrate immunity to varicella zoster virus. Adult infection with varicella accounts for only about 2% of the total cases, but 25% of all varicella-related deaths. In pregnant women with varicella pneumonia, even with treatment the mortality rate is approximately 14%, with the highest rates among women infected in the third trimester of pregnancy.

Aetiology

Varicella zoster virus is a highly infectious agent that is transmitted from person to person by direct contact with respiratory droplets or aerosolization of vesicular fluid from skin lesions.

Clinical approach

Patient presentation

- The virus enters its host via the respiratory tract and has an incubation period of 14–16 days.
- The newly infected person is contagious for 1–2 days before the onset of a rash.
- Once the rash is present, it will take 4–5 days for the skin lesion to crust over
- Once the skin lesions have crusted over a person is generally considered not contagious.

Diagnosis

- Varicella infection is a clinical diagnosis and rarely requires laboratory confirmation. Patients may present with generalized symptoms of headache, fever, and malaise prior to the development of a rash.
- The classic rash will appear a few days after the generalized symptoms and begins as small pruritic macules that progress to papules and vesicles.
- Varicella pneumonia occurs in up to 20% of cases of varicella infections in pregnancy. The symptoms begin about 4 days after the initial presentation and can include cough, shortness of breath, chest pain, and haemoptysis. Characteristic radiographic findings include bilateral peribronchial nodular infiltrates.

Management

- All pregnant women diagnosed with varicella zoster infection during pregnancy should receive oral acyclovir 800 mg five times per day or valcyclovir 1 g three times a day.
- Clinicians should educate their patients about the severity of this diagnosis and encourage them to present immediately to the hospital if any respiratory symptoms develop.
- Patients diagnosed with varicella pneumonia should be hospitalized for intravenous acyclovir (10–15 mg/kg every 8 hours) and to closely monitor their respiratory status. Varicella pneumonia is considered self-limited and usually resolves within 7 days, but it can be severe enough to require mechanical ventilation.

- Intravenous acyclovir should also be used for patients with neurological symptoms, hemorrhagic rash, continued fever, or appearance of new lesions after 6 days of treatment with oral antiviral therapy.

Because pregnant women are at a higher risk for severe varicella, use of varicella zoster immune globulin (VZIG) has been previously recommended for women without evidence of immunity. According to the CDC, the only US licensed manufacturer of VZIG discontinued production in 2004. There is an investigational VZIG product known as VariZIG that is available under an investigational new drug application. This product can be requested from the sole authorized US distributor, FFF Enterprises (24-hour telephone, 800-843-7477), for patients who have been exposed to varicella who are felt to be at increased risk for severe disease. Prior to administration, patients must be counselled that this is an investigational product and should give written informed consent. Investigational VariZIG is expected to provide maximum benefit when administered as soon as possible after exposure, although it can be effective if administered as late as 96 hours after exposure. If it is not possible to administer VariZIG within 96 hours of exposure, Administration of immune globulin intravenous (IGIV) should be considered. The recommended IGIV dose for post exposure prophylaxis of varicella is 400 mg/kg administered once.

Congenital varicella syndrome

This syndrome is represented by:
- dermotomal scarring (70%)
- limb hypoplasia (68%)
- ocular abnormalities (cataracts, chorioretinitis, micropthalmos, Horner's syndrome, nystagmus; 66%)
- low birthweight (50%)
- cortical atrophy and mental retardation (46%)
- early death (28%)
- survivors can also have long-term learning defects and other developmental problems.

First trimester exposure

First trimester exposure to primary varicella zoster virus may result in stillbirth or a baby born with the stigmata of the congenital varicella syndrome at a rate of 0.55%. Maternal infection following the critical first trimester of organogenesis may be associated with reactivation zoster *in utero*, with a characteristic pattern of cicitrical skin scarring associated with the distribution of dermatomes.

Second trimester exposure

The incidence of congenital varicella syndrome is up to 2% when maternal infection occurs between 13 and 20 weeks' gestation.

Third trimester exposure

Asymptomatic infants born to women who are infected with varicella zoster virus between 25 and 36 weeks' gestation have an increased risk of zoster in the first year of life.

Peripartum exposure

Infection with primary varicella zoster virus in the peripartum period can result in neonatal varicella, which carries a significant mortality rate despite appropriate antiviral therapy. If the varicella infection is from 5 days before delivery to 2 days after delivery, an estimated 17–30% of the newborns contract severe varicella infection because of the lack of maternal antibody to protect the neonate and the relative immaturity of the neonatal immune system. If untreated, the risk of death among neonates is 31%. With varicella immunoglobulin treatment the rate of neonatal death is 7%.

Fetal outcome
- The risk to the fetus is directly dependent on when the mother was infected. Consultation with a perinatalogist should be obtained to follow the fetus by ultrasound to look for anatomic abnormalities associated with congenital varicella syndrome.
- Herpes zoster in an otherwise healthy pregnancy is not associated with intrauterine infection, even when the dermatomes innervating the uterus are involved.

Varicella screening
- Since the disease is preventable with vaccination, one should know the prior exposure status of their patient.
- If the status is negative or not known, consider serological testing to confirm prior exposure before conception.
- If the testing confirms that the patient is susceptible to varicella, she should be immunized with the vaccine on two occasions 4–8 weeks apart.

- The vaccine is a live-attenuated viral vaccine and carries a theoretical risk of causing congenital infection. Therefore, pregnancy should be deferred for at least 1 month after vaccination.

Further reading

Daley A, Thorpe S, Garland S. Varicella and the pregnant woman: Prevention and management. Austral NZ J Obstet Gynaecol 2008;48:26–33.

Gardella C, Brown Z. Managing varicella zoster infection in pregnancy. Cleveland Clin J Med 2007;74:290–6.

CDC. Varicella vaccine: questions and answers about pregnancy. 2007; www.cdc.gov/vaccines/vpd-vac/varicella/vac-faqs-clinic-preg.htm

CDC. Varicella treatment questions and answers. 2007; www.cdc.gov/vaccines/vpd-vac/varicella/dis-faqs-gen-treatment.htm

CDC. A new product (VariZIG) for post exposure prophylaxis of varicella available under an investigational new drug application expanded access protocol (ACIP). MMWR 2006; 55.

Perinatal Viral and Parasitic Infections. ACOG Practice Bulletin Number 20. American College of Obstetricians and Gynecologists. Int J Gynaecol Obstet 2002;76:95–107.

Chlamydia

Aetiology

Chlamydia is an obligate intracellular bacterium that relies on its host cells for nutrient, energy, and DNA and RNA synthesis. Of the four recognized species *Chlamydia trachomatis, psittaci, pneumoniae, and pecorium,* only the first three are known to infect man.

Epidemiology

The prevalence rate of chlamydia in the UK is approximately 10%, with higher rates among sexually active 20–24-year-old men, and 16–19-year-old women, perhaps reflecting the fact that the host immune system gradually eradicates the infection such that lower prevalence rates are observed in the older population. There were over 120 000 new cases of chlamydia reported by genitourinary medicine clinics in the UK in 2007, a 150% increase from 10 years ago. The wide spectrum of the disease presentations has hampered the epidemiological control of chlamydia infection.

Pathogenesis

C. trachomatis exists in two phases during its life cycle in man: the infective extracellular form known as the elementary body and the metabolically active and dividing intracellular form known as the reticulate body. Infection occurs with the attachment and uptake into the host cell of the elementary body. The elementary body undergoes a transformation and reorganizes itself into the active reticulate body, encapsulating itself in a cytoplasmic vacuole thus evading the activity of cellular lysosomes and most probably antibiotics too.

The reticulate body proliferates rapidly for 8–48 hours, condenses back to the elementary body and ruptures the host cell by sheer weight of numbers, resulting in the infection of neighbouring cells. The extracellular elementary bodies, the dead and dying epithelial cells activate the host's cell-mediated immunity orchestrated by interferon (IFN)-γ and interleukin (IL)-12. There is increased macrophage and natural killer cell activity with resultant tissue damage, repair, and fibrosis. The circulating IFN-γ suspends the intracellular multiplication of the of the reticulate body but does not kill or eliminate it and once the elementary bodies are cleared the stimulus for the production of IFN-γ is removed and with it the control of the reticulate body, which becomes activated, multiplies, and damages some more cells to repeat the cycle of tissue damage, repair, and fibrosis. These repeated cycles of cellular damage, immune activation, repair by fibrosis, and scarring are responsible for the tissue damage that is so characteristic of chlamydia infection.

Screening

The National Chlamydia Screening Programme (NCSP) is an opportunistic screening intervention targeted at those aged <25 years when they attend healthcare or other non-clinical venues such that asymptomatic individuals who are sexually active, but who may not otherwise seek a test, are screened. The overall aim of the NCSP is to control chlamydia through the early detection and treatment of asymptomatic infection in the under-25-year-old population to prevent the development of complications such as pelvic inflammatory disease, infertility, miscarriage, ectopic pregnancy, or infection in neonates.

Clinical features

At least 70% of women with chlamydia infection are asymptomatic and may present with complications in the long term. This is one of the most important arguments for a mass screening approach. The symptomatic minority may complain of lower abdominal or pelvic pain, intermenstrual or postcoital bleeding, dysuria, and vaginal discharge. In uncomplicated cases (approximately 70%) the infection is limited to the cervix and/or urethra, and bimanual examination is usually normal with no tenderness. In men, uncomplicated infection is limited to the urethra and also is mostly asymptomatic (approximately 52%).

Complicated chlamydia infection is associated with chronic urethritis, dysuria, inflammation of the Bartholin's glands, mucopurulent cervicitis, pelvic inflammatory disease, Fitz–Hugh Curtis syndrome, reactive arthritis, proctitis, and pharyngitis. Tubal infertility, chronic pelvic pain, and ectopic pregnancy may follow complicated infections in about 10% of affected women.

Neonatal Chlamydia trachomatis

In some series, up to 60% of infants born to women with chlamydia manifest disease including:

* inclusion conjunctivitis, affecting 15–50% of neonates of chlamydia-positive women. This presents as mucopurulent discharge, oedema of the eyelids, and erythema of the palpebral fissures, usually within the first 5–7 days of life
* pneumonia, 10–20% of cases and appears between 3 weeks and 3 months of life
* otitis media
* nasopharyngitis
* failure to thrive.

Diagnosis

Screening for and the diagnosis of chlamydia infections have become simplified and enhanced by the introduction of tests based on DNA amplification such as the polymerase and ligase chain reaction tests. Urine and self-administered low vaginal swab samples are sufficient and the sensitivity and specificities of these DNA-based tests approach 100%, a good 25–40% above previous tests based on antigen detection and cell culture.

Chlamydia is a fragile obligate intracellular organism and like viruses can only be cultured in cells, which until very recently was the sole method of diagnosis. Cell cultures were laborious, expensive, needed regional centres, live chlamydia organisms and therefore transport media, and special storage facilities.

Antigen detection tests such as the enzyme-linked immunosorbent assay (ELISA) and direct fluorescent antibody do not depend on maintaining a live organism and therefore do not require special transport or storage. They can also be automated, and therefore handle large quantities of samples with rapid turnover times.

Management

* A single oral dose of azithromycin 1 g has an excellent compliance record, is better absorbed, and achieves higher tissue concentration than erythromycin, which is maintained for up to 4 days after ingestion of the single dose. The safety profile during pregnancy has not been established.

- Alternative antibiotic regimens include oral doxycycline 100 mg once or twice daily or erythromycin 500 mg four times daily for 7 days. Emphasis should be placed on completing the course.
- Refer to GUM clinic for comprehensive screening for other sexually transmitted infections and follow up.
- Contact tracing: 65% of female and 53% of male sexual contacts are concordant for chlamydia infection.
- Provide verbal and written information.

Further reading

Chief Medical Officer's Expert Advisory Group. *Main report of the CMO's expert advisory group on Chlamydia trachomatis.* London: Department of Health, 1998.

House of Commons. Select Committee on Health. *Third report on sexual health.* Available at www.parliament. the-stationery-ffice.co.uk/pa/cm200203/cmselect/cmhealth/69/6902.htm

LaMontagne DS, Fenton KA, Randall S, *et al.* Establishing the National Chlamydia Screening Programme in England: results from the first full year of screening. Sex Transm Infect 2004;80:335–41

Department of Health. Chlamydia screening pilot: report of 1999–2000 study. London: DH 2002.

Department of Health. The national chlamydia screening programme in England, Programme overview, core requirements and data collection. London: DH 2004.

Health Protection Agency, SCIEH, ISD, National Public Health Service for Wales, CDSC Northern Ireland, the UASSG. Renewing the focus. *HIV and other sexually transmitted infections in the United Kingdom in 2002.* London: Health Protection Agency 2003.

Cates W, Wasserheit JN. Genital chlamydial infections: epidemiology and reproductive sequelae. *Am J Obstet Gynecol* 1991;164:1771–81.

Honey E, Augood C, Templeton A, *et al.* Cost effectiveness of screening for Chlamydia trachomatis: a review of published studies. Sex Transm Infect 2002;78:406–12.

Pimenta JM, Catchpole M, Rogers PA, *et al.* Opportunistic screening for genital chlamydial infection I: Acceptability of urine testing in primary and secondary healthcare settings. Sex Transm Infect 2003;79:16–21.

Pimenta JM, Catchpole M, Rogers PA, *et al.* Opportunistic screening for genital chlamydial infection II: Prevalence among health care attenders, outcome and evaluation of positive cases. Sex Transm Infect 2003;79:22–7.

Internet resources

Additional information on the epidemiology of genital chlamydia infections diagnosed in GUM clinics in the United Kingdom is available: www.hpa.org.uk/infections/topics_az/hiv_and_sti/sti-chlamydia/epidemiology/epidemiology.htm.

Coagulation disorders

The coagulation disorders are a group of disorders where there is an alteration in the coagulability of the blood. This could either result in a state of (1) bleeding disorder from coagulation defect or (2) hypercoagulable state with an increased tendency to thrombus formation in the circulation.

Coagulation defects leading to bleeding disorders

Although coagulation disorders can arise as a result of pregnancy complications (acquired defects), women with inherited coagulation defects can also become pregnant.

Inherited coagulation defects

Von Willebrand's disease: von Willebrand's disease (vWD) is the most common hereditary coagulation abnormality described in humans. It has a prevalence of approximately 1% of the population. It arises from a qualitative or quantitative deficiency of von Willebrand factor (vWF), a multimeric protein that is required for platelet adhesion. This functions as a carrier protein for Factor VIII, forming circulating vWF–Factor VIII complex. The vWF gene is located on chromosome 12. There are three main types of vWD and all, except Type 3, are inherited as autosomal dominant traits. Type 3, the most severe form, is inherited as autosomal recessive trait. Type 1 is the commonest form and is usually mild.

These patients often have a family history and/or a personal history of bleeding tendency. During pregnancy, the major haemorrhagic risk is postpartum because of the rapid decrease in Factor VIII and vWF following delivery. Laboratory diagnosis is based on assessment of vWF activity, and antigen level and Factor VIII levels.

Antenatally these patients should be managed in conjunction with the haematologists. Desmopressin (DDAVP) therapy may be useful, as some patients (Type 1) respond well with the release of vWF from endothelial cells. The majority of cases require no haemostatic support during pregnancy. In known responders, intranasal DDAVP and tranexamic acid can be used during the last few weeks to minimize the risk of postpartum bleeding.

In labour, invasive monitoring, fetal blood sampling, episiotomy, and instrumental delivery should be avoided. The third stage should be actively managed. Factor VIII replacement and i.v. DDAVP and tranexamic acid may be required for postpartum bleeding.

Haemophilias

Haemophilias are inherited deficiencies in Factor VII (haemophilia A) or Factor IX (haemophilia B). Haemophilia A is the common type. Both are X-linked conditions and hence women are usually carriers and are not usually affected.

Prenatal diagnosis is an important issue since an affected child (usually male) would require regular expensive factor replacement therapy and is at risk of significant haemorrhage.

Thrombophilia

Thrombophilia is the increased tendency to thrombosis, secondary to any hypercoagulable state. Inherited and acquired factors may determine thrombophilia. Some physiological conditions, such as pregnancy are themselves 'thrombophilic'.

Changes of coagulation system during pregnancy: Normal pregnancy is a recognized prothrombotic period.
- There is an increase in several of the coagulation factors, including fibrinogen, factors VII, VIII, X, and vWF.
- There is a decrease in the natural anticoagulant system, especially significantly lower levels of protein S and increased resistance to activated protein C (APC).
- Diminished fibrinolysis occurs as pregnancy proceeds, as evidenced by increased levels of plasminogen activator inhibitor-1 and -2 (PAI-1 and PAI-2) and increased levels of thrombin activatable fibrinolysis inhibitor (TAFI).

It has been well established that women with thrombophilic disorders are at a higher risk of venous thromboembolism (VTE) in pregnancy and puerperium. It has also been observed that those women have higher prevalence of obstetric complications in which microplacental thrombosis may play a pathogenetic role, such as placental abruption, pre-eclampsia, intrauterine growth restriction, intrauterine fetal death, and repeated spontaneous miscarriage, particularly late fetal loss.

Types of thrombophilia

Inherited thrombophilias are a heterogeneous group of conditions that have been implicated in a variety of pregnancy complications. The risk for thrombotic complications are much higher in the rarer homozygous states than in the more common heterozygous states of these inherited abnormalities.

The most common inherited thrombophilias are
- Factor V Leiden (FVL): this is the most common cause of APC resistance
- the G20210A mutation of the prothrombin gene (PGM).

Rarer causes of inherited thrombophilia include:
- antithrombin (AT) deficiency
- protein C deficiency
- protein S deficiency
- homozygosity for the thermolabile variant of methylene tetrahydrofolate reductase (MTHFR); this in conjunction with insufficient dietary intake of B vitamins, is associated with hyperhomocysteinaemia and, in turn, increased thrombotic risk
- protein Z deficiency (recently being linked to preterm delivery).

Collectively, inherited thrombophilias are present in 8–15% of Caucasian populations and they appear to be responsible for up to half of venous thromboembolism during pregnancy. Large numbers of case–control and cohort studies have now evaluated associations between thrombophilia and pregnancy loss. These studies overall suggest an association between FVL mutation, antithrombin, protein C and protein S deficiency, and recurrent and late fetal loss. The data are not consistent with regard to an association between recurrent and late fetal loss and prothrombin G20210A and MTHFR C677T homozygotes. There is no consistent evidence for an association between maternal thrombophilia and recurrent early first trimester loss (at less than 10 weeks). A recent meta-analysis, did not find an association between pre-eclampsia and FVL, prothrombin G20210A, or MTHFR C677T. When the analysis was restricted only to severe pre-eclampsia, there was a significant association with FVL and with MTHFR C677T homozygotes (Lin and August 2005).

Acquired thrombophilia

The most important cause of acquired thrombophilia is antiphospholipid antibody syndrome (APS). APS is characterized by the presence of antibodies directed against phospholipids or plasma proteins bound to anionic phospholipids. Patients may present with venous or arterial thrombosis, recurrent fetal loss, and/or thrombocytopenia. The disorder may be primary or associated with systemic lupus erythematosus and other rheumatic diseases.

The antiphospholipid antibodies in APS may be detected as

* anticardiolipin antibodies
* lupus anticoagulants
* antibodies to β2-glycoprotein-I
* other antibodies, including those to prothrombin, annexin V, phosphatidylserine, phosphatidylinositol, and others.

The mechanisms by which antiphospholipid antibodies cause thrombosis are not completely understood. The pathogenesis of the APS-associated clinical manifestations appears to result from a variety of effects of antiphospholipid antibodies upon pathways of coagulation, including the procoagulant actions of these antibodies upon protein C, annexin V, platelets, and fibrinolysis.

Adverse pregnancy outcomes attributed to the presence of antiphospholipid antibodies are

* late fetal death
* early, severe pre-eclampsia/eclampsia
* fetal growth restriction
* maternal thromboembolic disease (venous or arterial)
* recurrent pregnancy loss. Many investigators believe APS is not a cause of embryonic loss before 10 weeks.

Who should be tested for thrombophilia?

The following conditions in a pregnant woman should warrant a thrombophilia evaluation:

* previous history of thrombosis
* strong family history of thrombosis
* history of unexplained loss beyond 10 weeks
* history of severe pre-eclampsia/HELLP(haemolysis, elevated liver enzymes, low platelets)
* history of severe intrauterine growth restriction
* history of placental abruption.

Management of thrombophilias during pregnancy

* Patients with known thrombophilic defect and no prior VTE or pregnancy complication; treatment is controversial.
  * Women with antithrombin deficiency (AT) deficiency, protein C deficiency, homozygous Factor V Leiden (FVL) or prothrombin gene mutation (PGM) (high-risk thrombophilia) are at higher risk of venous thromboembolism (VTE) during pregnancy. They should receive both antepartum and postpartum thromboprophylaxis with low molecular weight heparin (LMWH).
  * Women with other heterozygous thrombophilic states with no previous history of VTE need not be

given antepartum prophylaxis. Low-dose aspirin may be used. Postpartum prophylaxis with LMWH should be considered.

* Patients with thrombophilia and previous history of VTE:
  * they should receive antepartum and postpartum prophylaxis with LMWH.
* Patients with thrombophilia and previous related pregnancy complications.
  * There is no good evidence that thromboprophylaxis improves obstetric outcome in women with inherited thrombophilia. Good randomized controlled trials are required before clear recommendations can be made.
  * In cases with acquired thrombophilia secondary to APS, a combination of low dose aspirin and LMWH is effective in reducing fetal loss rate.

Acquired coagulation defects

Disseminated intravascular coagulation

There is generalized stimulation of coagulation activity resulting in consumption of clotting factors and platelets. This results in defective clotting and stimulation of fibrinolysis. Fibrin degradation products (FDP) interfere with clot formation and myometrial activity and might contribute to further haemorrhage. Disseminated intravascular coagulation (DIVC) is never primary. In obstetrics, it usually occurs in association with

* placental abruption
* severe pre-eclampsia
* retained dead fetus *in utero* (beyond 3–4 weeks)
* sepsis
* prolonged shock from any cause
* amniotic fluid embolism.

Diagnosis

In the appropriate clinical setting, diagnosis is confirmed by a low platelet count, prolonged prothrombin time (PT), international normalization ratio (INR), and partial thromboplastin time (PTT), and high levels of circulating FDPs.

General management principles

* Treatment of the underlying triggering factor, e.g. evacuation of uterus in placental abruption and retained dead fetus.
* Component therapy:
  * fresh frozen plasma (FFP), which contains all the clotting factors
  * packed RBC (for haemorrhage)
  * platelets
  * cryoprecipitate.
* Anticoagulant therapy: controversial. It might be useful in selected cases of retained dead fetus.
* Volume replacement and maintenance of circulation.

Further reading

Brenner B, Aharon A. Thrombophilia and adverse pregnancy outcome. Clin Perinatol 2007;34:527–41.

Kujovich JL. Thrombophilia and pregnancy complications. Am J Obstet Gynecol 2004;191:412–24.

Lin J, August P. Genetic thrombophilias and preeclampsia: a meta-analysis. Obstet Gynecol 2005;105:182–92.

Connective tissue disorder

Rheumatoid arthritis

Rheumatoid arthritis (RA) is a systemic, chronic, autoimmune inflammatory disease affecting the joints mainly. There is an excessive immune response against body cells, and that leads to synovitis, pannus formation (i.e. thickening of synovium) cartilage breakdown, and bone erosion.

Epidemiology

RA affects about 1% of population, with a female to male ratio of (3:1) and approximately 1 in every 1000–2000 pregnancies is affected.

Aetiology

There is an association with the human leucocyte antigen HLA-D4 (70%). About 80–90% of patients are positive for rheumatoid factor (RhF), and 30% of cases are positive for antinuclear antibodies (ANAs).

Clinical picture

RA is characterized by periods of flares and remission. The prominent symptoms are joint pains and morning stiffness, with signs including swelling, and tenderness with limitation of movement.

The disease can affect other parts of the body causing pleuritis, pericarditis, Felty's syndrome, rheumatoid nodules, and vasculitis.

Effect of pregnancy on RA

About 70–80% of women with RA experience improvement during pregnancy. In about 25% of patients the disease is active or even worsens, requiring treatment throughout pregnancy. Of those who experience remission, 90% suffer postpartum exacerbations.

Effect of RA on pregnancy

There seems to be no adverse affect of RA on pregnancy. Rarely, limitation of hip abduction is severe enough to impede a vaginal delivery.

Management

The main concerns relate to the safety during pregnancy and lactation of the medications used to treat rheumatoid arthritis. Paracetamol, aspirin, and corticosteroids can be used safely. Non-steroidal anti-inflammatory drugs (NSAIDs) are relatively safe, but best avoided in the last 6 weeks of pregnancy to avoid their effect on the ductus arteriosus. Azathioprine, and D-penicillamine are relatively safe. Antimalarials and sulphasalazine can also be used as a second line treatment safely.

The alkylating agents cyclophosphamide and chlorambucil, and the folic acid antagonist methotrexate are all teratogenic and fetotoxic and are contraindicated in pregnancy and lactation.

Systemic lupus erythematosus

Systemic lupus erythematosus (SLE) is a chronic, multifaceted inflammatory disease that can affect every organ system of the body. It involves multisystem microvascular inflammation with the generation of autoantibodies such as ANAs, double-stranded DNA (dsDNA), extractable nuclear antigens (ENAs), including anti Ro/La antibodies and antiphospholipid antibodies (APA). There are congenital deficiencies of complement (especially C4, C2, and other early components).

Epidemiology

The prevalence of SLE is variable. It is more common in women of child bearing age (6–10-folds higher). Almost 6% of patients have other autoimmune disorders.

Clinical picture

Non-specific fatigue, fever, arthralgia, arthritis, and weight changes are the most frequent symptoms. Discoid lesions often develop in sun-exposed areas. The kidney is the most commonly involved visceral organ in SLE, which could cause hypertension, haematuria, oedema, and anasarca. Leucopenia and, more specifically, lymphopenia are common.

Effect of pregnancy on SLE

SLE flares may be difficult to diagnose during pregnancy since many features are commonly seen in pregnancy. Whether pregnancy exacerbates SLE and increases the likelihood of flare particularly postpartum is controversial. In women with lupus nephritis, pregnancy does not seem to jeopardize renal function in the long term. There is a greater risk of deterioration in patients with a higher baseline serum creatinine.

Effect of SLE on pregnancy

SLE is associated with increased risks of spontaneous miscarriage, fetal death, pre-eclampsia, preterm delivery, and intrauterine growth restriction (IUGR). These risks may be attributed to the presence of APA, lupus nephritis or hypertension, and either active disease at the time of conception or first presentation of SLE during pregnancy. Pregnancy outcome is particularly affected by renal disease. For women in remission, but without hypertension, renal involvement, or APA, the risk of pregnancy loss and pre-eclampsia is probably no higher than in the general population. Pregnancy, and especially the postpartum period, represents an additional thrombotic risk in patients with SLE who have APA.

Management

Ideally this should begin with preconception counselling. Knowledge of the anti-Ro and APA, renal and blood pressure status allows prediction of the risks to the woman and her baby. It is advised to conceive during remission. Pregnancy care is best undertaken in multidisciplinary combined clinics where physicians and obstetricians can monitor disease activity and the fetus regularly. Disease activity is monitored by appearance of symptoms, rising anti-DNA antibody titre, cellular casts in urine, and fall in the complement levels. Fetal growth should be monitored. Uterine artery and umbilical artery Doppler blood flow studies are useful.

Disease flares must be actively managed. The use of azathioprine, NSAIDs and aspirin is covered in the section on Rheumatoid arthritis. Hydroxychloroquine should be continued since stopping may precipitate flare.

Neonatal lupus syndromes

It occurs as congenital heart block or as lupus rash. It occurs in 3.5% of cases. Neonatal lupus is highly associated with maternal anti-Ro (present in about 30% of patients with SLE), although the rash may occur with anti-RNP antibodies. The risk of neonatal lupus is increased if a previous child has been affected.

There is no indication for prophylactic treatment; nevertheless, fetal four-chamber cardiac echocardiography is recommended at 16–28 weeks and if heart block is found dexamethasone 4 mg/day is given to the mother. The cutaneous form of neonatal lupus usually manifests in the first 2 weeks of life. The infant develops typical geographical skin lesions usually on the face and scalp, which appear after sun or UV light exposure. The rash disappears spontaneously within 6 months and scarring is unusual.

Antiphospholipid syndrome

Antiphospholipid syndrome (APS) is a disorder characterized by recurrent thrombosis and/or fetal loss associated with elevated levels of antibodies directed against membrane anionic phospholipids (i.e. anticardiolipin (aCL) antibody), or evidence of lupus anticoagulant.

Clinical picture

Criteria for diagnosis are
* thrombosis: venous or arterial
* pregnancy morbidity: three or more consecutive miscarriages (<10 weeks' gestation), one or more fetal death (>10 weeks' gestation with normal fetal morphology), and one or more premature birth (<34 weeks' gestation) due to pre-eclampsia or severe placental insufficiency.

Effect of pregnancy on APS

The risk of thrombosis increases because of the hypercoagulable state of pregnancy. Thrombocytopenia may worsen.

Effect of APS on pregnancy

An exceptionally high rate of pre-eclampsia has been reported in women with APS, which contributes to the high rate of preterm delivery in this condition. Recurrent pregnancy loss, typically in the second trimester, is one of the most consistent features of APS. The risk of fetal loss is directly related to the antibody titre, particularly the IgG aCL. There is also a high incidence of intrauterine IUGR and placental abruption.

Management

Women with APS and previous thromboembolism are at extremely high risk in pregnancy and the puerperium and should be given antenatal thromboprophylaxis with heparin. Many are on long-term warfarin and the change from warfarin to heparin should be achieved prior to 6 weeks' gestation to avoid warfarin embryopathy. Heparin should be continued intrapartum and postpartum until they are re-warfarinized.

The management of pregnancy in women with APS, recurrent pregnancy loss, but without a history of thromboembolism is debated. Most centres now advocate low-dose aspirin (75 mg–100 mg) for all women, often prior to conception. Any additional benefit of heparin must be balanced against the risk of heparin-induced osteoporosis. Immunosuppression with intravenous immunoglobulin (IVIG) is extremely expensive, and its use is limited to occasional salvage therapy in women who develop complications despite aspirin and heparin.

Ultrasound monitoring of fetal growth and uteroplacental blood flow is crucial. This allows for timely delivery. Assessment of uterine artery Doppler waveforms is performed in the midtrimester, and the presence of bilateral artery notches in high-risk pregnancies is associated with pre-eclampsia, IUGR, and intrapartum asphyxia. Abnormal uterine artery Doppler velocimetry is also of some value in predicting placental abruption.

Scleroderma

It is a systemic disease characterized by skin induration and thickening in addition to tissue fibrosis and chronic inflammatory infiltration in other organs, prominent fibroproliferative vasculopathy, and humoral and cellular immune alterations.

Epidemiology

The estimated incidence of systemic sclerosis is 19 cases per million population.

Clinical picture

It may be divided into a localized cutaneous form (morphoea) with areas of thickened skin usually on the forearms and hands, and systemic sclerosis associated with Raynaud's phenomenon and organ involvement. The skin in systemic sclerosis is typically bound down to produce sclerodactly, beaking of the nose, a fixed facial expression, and limitation of mouth opening. Systemic involvement usually takes the form of progressive fibrosis and includes the oesophagus most commonly (80%), the lungs (45%), the heart (40%), and the kidneys (35%).

Effect of pregnancy on scleroderma

In the localized type there is no adverse effect, but with the early diffuse type (>4 years) there is a significant risk of deterioration especially in reflux oesophagitis and renal crisis. It may be appropriate to advise women with severe organ involvement against pregnancy. Raynaud's disease improves due to vasodilatation. Postpartum deterioration occurs in cases of severe pulmonary fibrosis and pulmonary hypertension.

Effect of scleroderma on pregnancy

Pregnancy in women with systemic sclerosis is considered a high risk because of a higher risk of pregnancy loss and higher complication rates. Pregnancy risk is greatest in those who have had the disease for less than 4 years and who also have diffuse cutaneous involvement. Fetal outcome is impaired and there is an increased risk of premature delivery, pre-eclampsia, IUGR, and perinatal mortality. Venepuncture, venous access, and blood pressure measurement may be difficult because of skin or blood vessel involvement. General anaesthesia may be complicated by difficult endotracheal intubation, and regional anaesthesia may also be difficult.

Management

The management is symptomatic. Raynaud's phenomenon may be helped by heated gloves or nifedipine. Early assessment by an anaesthetist is advisable if problems with regional or general anaesthesia are anticipated.

Further reading

Chakravarty EF, Colón I, Langen ES, et al.Factors that predict prematurity and preeclampsia in pregnancies that are complicated by systemic lupus erythematosus. Am J Obstet Gynecol 2005;192:1897–904.

Shehata HA, Nelson-Piercy C, Other endocrine, connective tissue disease, and skin disorders in pregnancy. Curr Obstet Gynaecol 2001; 11:329–35.

Shehata HA, Nelson-Piercy C, Khamashta MA. Management of pregnancy in antiphospholipid syndrome. Rheum Dis Clin North Am 2001;3:643–59.

Arya R, Shehata HA, Patel RK, *et al.* Internal jugular vein thrombosis after assisted conception therapy. Br J Haematol 2001;115:153–5.

Nelson-Piercy CA. *Handbook of obstetric medicine*, 3rd edn. London: Informa Healthcare 2006.

Brennan P, Barrett J, Fiddler M, *et al.* Maternal-fetal HLA incompatibility and the course of inflammatory arthritis during pregnancy. J Rheumatol 2000;27:2843–8.

Internet resources

www.emedicine.com/
www.miscarriageclinic.co.uk

Cytomegalovirus

Definition

Cytomegalovirus (CMV) is a DNA virus of the herpesvirus group which causes cytomegalic inclusion disease. This name is derived from the characteristic large cells containing prominent intranuclear inclusion bodies that have been identified with this disease since the early twentieth century.

Epidemiology

The epidemiology of CMV infection is complex, but it is key to understanding disease manifestations. CMV is a ubiquitous virus. Overall, CMV can be cultured from the cervix or urine in 2–28% of pregnant women. In the USA and Europe, 40% of reproductive age women are susceptible to CMV. The rate of seroconversion in women in the reproductive age range is approximately 2–6% annually.

Even though CMV infection is common, serious illness occurs only in fetuses and immunodeficient or immunosuppressed individuals. Over 90% of adult infections are subclinical, with the remainder having a mononucleosis-like illness. Congenital CMV infection is acquired *in utero*, primarily from transplacental transmission. Neonates with congenital CMV are culture positive (most often in the urine) for the virus at birth. About 1% of all newborns excrete CMV at birth and are congenitally infected; an additional 3–5% of infants acquire CMV perinatally, from infected cervical secretions, infected milk, or exposure to infected transfused blood.

In utero CMV infections are the major concern, because of potentially serious adverse effects on development. On the other hand, perinatally acquired CMV infection does not result in serious complications or sequelae except in very-low-birthweight neonates. With CMV, congenital infections may occur after either primary or recurrent maternal infection, and most intrauterine infections occur in immune, rather than in susceptible, women. Symptomatic congenital CMV infection occurs mainly with primary maternal infection. Sequelae have been noted in 25–40% of the infants in the primary infection group, compared with only 8% in the recurrent CMV infection group. Common manifestations of intrauterine CMV infection are mental impairment and hearing loss.

CMV is transmitted by sexual contact or by spread within households or daycare centres.

The public health impact of congenital CMV infection is large. In the USA, for example, over 7000 infants annually either die or develop significant neurological sequelae.

The prognosis is very guarded for infants with clinically apparent disease at birth, with mortality as high as 20–30%, and with 90% having late complications. Of the 90% of congenitally infected neonates who appear normal at birth, about 15% do not develop normally, as neurological sequelae such as hearing loss, low IQ, and behaviour problems may become apparent.

Clinical approach

Diagnosis

As noted, only 10% of maternal infections with CMV are symptomatic, producing a heterophil-negative mononucleosis syndrome.

The spectrum of disease in the fetus and neonate is wide. Clinically apparent disease occurs in only 10% of infants with congenital CMV. In severely infected neonates, manifestations are hepatosplenomegaly, jaundice, thrombocytopenia, purpura, microcephaly, deafness, chorioretinitis, optic atrophy, and cerebral calcifications. A characteristic tetrad includes mental retardation, chorioretinitis, cerebral calcification, and microcephaly or hydrocephaly.

CMV infection may be documented by serological testing using one of several Ig antibody tests. Demonstration of seroconversion is the best documentation of primary infection. If infection has occurred within the previous 4–8 months, IgM-specific antibody can be detected in the serum. Avidity assays may also be helpful as low avidity indicates recent infection whereas high avidity indicates recurrent infection.

CMV infection may also be detected through culture or by PCR, but isolation does not differentiate primary and recurrent infections.

Prenatal diagnosis of CMV infection has been made by using ultrasound, amniocentesis, and cordocentesis (percutaneous umbilical cord sampling). Common ultrasound abnormalities are microcephaly (10%), hepatosplenomegaly (18%), ventriculomegaly (32%), calcifications of the brain, liver, or placenta (40%), intrauterine growth restriction/ oligohydramnios (55%), ascites, pericardial or pleural effusion, hypoechogenic bowel, and hydrops.

Detection of CMV by culture or PCR in the amniotic fluid is an excellent method for detection of *in utero* CMV infection. Amniotic fluid testing for CMV should be offered to pregnant women with documented primary CMV infection or when ultrasonography suggests CMV infection. The diagnostic sensitivity of a single amniocentesis is about 80–85%. Thus, a repeat amniocentesis may be indicated. High CMV viral load in amniotic fluid is associated with clinically evident fetal or neonatal outcomes.

Fetal blood sampling may be used to gain additional information about the fetal complications such as thrombocytopenia, anaemia, or hepatic involvement. The combination of these tests has a diagnostic sensitivity of about 80–90% in antenatal diagnosis of CMV.

Treatment

Specific treatments of CMV infection are available and include adenosine arabinoside, cytosine arabinoside, ganciclovir, and foscarnet, all of which have been used for severe clinical infection. However, these drugs are quite toxic, and their use should be undertaken in consultation with experts in perinatal infection.

Recently, one group has reported decreased symptomatic infection at birth by use of CMV-specific intravenous immunoglobulin in pregnancies complicated by documented CMV infection and abnormal ultrasound findings. In this non-randomized trial, use of the CMV-specific IVIG led to a rate of symptomatic infection at birth of 7% (1 of 15) in fetuses with abnormal ultrasounds versus a rate of 100% (7 of 7) in those not given the IVIG. Methodological problems with the study are important, however, and this approach to treatment remains to be established.

Despite the potential hypothetical advantages of a CMV vaccine in preventing congenital CMV infection, no CMV vaccine is currently available.

Routine screening for CMV infection in pregnancy is not recommended.

Further reading

Antsaklis AJ, Daskalakis GJ, Mesogitis SA, *et al.* Prenatal diagnosis of fetal primary cytomegalovirus infection. Br J Obstet Gynecol 2000;107:84–8.

Guerra B, Lazzarotto T, Quarta S, *et al.* Prenatal diagnosis of symptomatic congenital cytomegalovirus. Am J Obstet Gynecol 2000;183:476–82.

Nigro G, Adler SP, LaTorre R, Best AM. Congenital Cytomegalovirus Collaborating Group. Passive immunization during pregnancy for congenital cytomegalovirus infection. New Engl J Med 2005; 353:1350–62.

Revello MG, Gerna G. Pathogenesis and prenatal diagnosis of human cytomegalovirus infection. J Clin Virol 2004;29:71–83.

Stagno S. Cytomegalovirus. In: Remington JS, Klein JO, (eds) *Infectious diseases of the fetus and newborn*. Philadelphia: Elsevier Saunders 2006:739–81.

Dermatology

Physiological changes

Increased pigmentation
This begins in the first trimester and fades after delivery. Existing pigmented areas (e.g. areolae and axillae) become darker. Specific areas (e.g. linea nigrum, from the umbilicus to the symphysis pubis in the midline) become pigmented.

Melasma
Patches of light-brown facial pigmentation developing in about 70% of women in the second half of pregnancy. The usual distribution involves the forehead, cheeks, upper lip, and chin.

Spider naevi
Occur on the face, upper trunk and arms. They can be numerous and in some cases almost confluent. Most appear in early pregnancy and regress following delivery, although 25% may persist.

Palmar erythema
Present in up to 70% of women by the third trimester and fades within 1 week of delivery.

Hair fall
A normal feature of the postpartum period, occurring in most women at between 4 and 20 weeks after delivery. It results from the increased conversion of hairs from the anagen (growing) to telogen (resting) phase, following the increased proportion of hairs in the anagen phase during pregnancy. Hair is lost diffusely, but recovery is usual within 6 months.

Striae gravidarum
These develop in most women, but are more common in obese women and multiple pregnancy. They appear perpendicular to skin tension lines as pink linear wrinkles. They fade and become white and atrophic, although never disappear completely.

Pruritus without rash or cholestasis
This may be a feature of normal pregnancy. Liver function tests should however be checked in any pregnant woman, especially if onset occurs in the third trimester.

Pre-existing conditions

Eczema
This often, but not invariably, improves during pregnancy. Women should be reassured that if they require topical steroids to control their eczema, these are not contraindicated in pregnancy.

Psoriasis
This can improve, remain unchanged or deteriorate during pregnancy. Psoriasis may present for the first time in pregnancy. Dithranol and coal tar may be safely used in pregnancy. Methotrexate is an antimetabolite and is contraindicated in pregnancy. Rarely, a severe form of pustular psoriasis, impetigo herpetiformis, may develop. Urticated erythema, beginning in the flexures and especially the groins, is associated with sterile pustules which may become widespread and affect mucosa. This condition is associated with severe systemic upset, including fever, neutrophilia, and hypocalcaemia. An increased perinatal mortality rate is also reported and these women require intensive treatment and regular fetal surveillance.

Coincidental conditions

Acne
This may develop for the first time in pregnancy. Pre-existing acne may improve or worsen during pregnancy. Both tetracyclines and retinoids (vitamin A analogues, e.g. isotretinoin) are contraindicated in pregnancy. Erythromycin may be used safely.

Erythema nodosum
This may occur in pregnancy, without any demonstrable known underlying precipitating cause. Tuberculosis and sarcoidosis should be excluded with a chest X-ray and the woman asked about symptoms of streptococcal infection and inflammatory bowel disease, as well as any recent medications (particularly sulphonamides). If no underlying cause is discovered, the prognosis is excellent.

Erythema multiforme
This also may complicate pregnancy without any obvious underlying cause. The commoner precipitating causes should be sought (e.g. drugs and viral infections), before attributing the eruption to pregnancy alone.

Dermatoses specific to pregnancy

Polymorphic eruption of pregnancy
Occurs in about 0.5% of pregnancies, usually after 35 weeks' gestation with rapid resolution after delivery. It is more common in primiparous and twin pregnancies. The rash is pruritic in nature with urticarial papules and plaques, rarely vesicles (but not bullae) and target lesions. It is mainly distributed around the abdomen (with umbilical sparing), along striae, with spread to thighs, buttocks, and upper arms. There are no known harmful effects on the fetus.

Treatment options include 2% phenol in oily calamine or 0.5% menthol in aqueous cream, 1% hydrocortisone cream of ointment, sedative antihistamine (e.g. chlorpheniramine (Piriton) 4 mg three or four times daily or promethazine (Phenergan) 25 mg at night). Systemic steroids may occasionally be required.

Pemphigoid gestationis
It has an incidence of 1 in 10 000 to 1 in 60 000 pregnancies. It is autoimmune disorder (possibly related to exposure to fetal antigens). It is associated with bullous pemphigoid and other autoimmune conditions, e.g. Graves' disease, vitiligo, insulin-dependent diabetes, rheumatoid arthritis. The onset of rash may occur at any time (9 weeks to 1 week postpartum; usually about 20–22 weeks), with no relationship to parity. The rash is intensely pruritic with urticated erythematous papules and plaques, target lesions and annular wheals. Distribution includes abdomen (umbilicus affected), with lesions begin in periumbilical region in most patients, spreading to limbs, palms, and soles. Eruption occurs after variable delay, usually 2 weeks with vesicles and large tense bullae. If it occurs in the second trimester, there is usually an improvement at the end of the pregnancy, but a flare postpartum. Urticated plaques may persist for several months after delivery.

Diagnosis
Diagnosis is usually made by direct immunofluorescence, showing complement (C_3) deposition at the basement membrane zone. This distinguishes pemphigoid gestationis

from polymorphic eruption of pregnancy in which immunofluorescence is negative.

An increased risk to the fetus has been reported, and recent studies have shown an association with low birthweight and premature delivery. As this is an autoimmune disease, the neonate may be affected with a similar rash, but this only occurs in 10% of cases and is mild and transient.

Treatment

Treatment options include topical corticosteroid (1% hydrocortisone cream or ointment) and sedative antihistamines. Most require systemic steroids (e.g. Prednisolone 40 mg/day) and these should not be withheld in pregnancy.

It usually recurs in future pregnancies (with possibly earlier onset and more severe course). It may recur with use of combined oral contraceptive pill.

Prurigo of pregnancy

It has an incidence of 1 in 300 pregnancies. It is associated with atopy and occurs at about 25–30 weeks. The rash is pruritic with groups of red/brown excoriated papules. It affects mainly the abdomen and the extensor surfaces of limbs. The pruritus improves at delivery, but papules may persist for several months after delivery. There are no known harmful effects on the fetus.

Treatment is as polymorphic eruption of pregnancy.

Recurrence is possible.

Pruritic folliculitis of pregnancy

The incidence is not known. It occurs in the second or third trimester. The pruritic rash is widespread and acneiform in nature with erythematous, follicular papules and pustules, mainly distributed in the trunk and thighs. Resolution occurs within 2 weeks after delivery.

There are no known harmful effects on the fetus.

Treatment options are as in pruritis of pregnancy in addition to topical 10% benzoyl peroxide.

Further reading

Nelson-Piercy C. *A handbook of obstetric medicine*, 3rd edn. London: Informa Healthcare 2006.

Shehata H A, Nelson-Piercy C. Connective tissue and skin disorders in pregnancy. Curr Obstet Gynaecol 2001;11:329–35.

Diabetes in pregnancy

Prevalence of diabetes mellitus in relation to pregnancy

Of the estimated 650 000 annual births in England and Wales, 2–5% are to women with Diabetes mellitus (DM). Pre-existing type 1 and type 2 DM account for 0.27% and 0.10% of births respectively. The prevalence of both types of DM is rising, but type 2 more so, and particularly among ethnic groups, including Afro-Caribbeans, South Asians, Middle Eastern, and Chinese. The prevalence of gestational DM (GDM) is estimated as in the range 3–5% in England and Wales, with considerable regional variation depending on ethnic diversity of the populations. Approximately 87.5% of pregnancies affected by DM are thought to be due to GDM, with 7.5% due to type 1 and the remainder to type 2. However, due to a variety of factors there are immense difficulties with the accurate estimation of the prevalence of GDM.

Types of diabetes mellitus

Four types/categories of DM are described.

Type 1

Formerly type I, insulin-dependent diabetes mellitus (IDDM), or juvenile diabetes: this is characterized by β-cell destruction caused by an autoimmune process, usually leading to absolute insulin deficiency. The onset is usually acute, over a period of a few days to weeks, with the majority of patients at the onset of disease being under the age of 25.

Type 2

Formerly type II, non-insulin dependent diabetes mellitus (NIDDM), or adult-onset diabetes: This is characterized by insulin resistance in peripheral tissues and an insulin secretory defect of β-cells. This is the most common form of DM and is associated with a familial predisposition, increasing age, obesity, and lack of exercise. It is more common in women, especially those with a history of GDM.

Other specific types of diabetes mellitus

In this category are grouped types of DM of various known aetiologies, including people with genetic defects of β-cell function (formerly called maturity-onset diabetes of the young (MODY)), people with disease of the exocrine pancreas such as pancreatitis, cystic fibrosis, pancreatic dysfunction associated with other endocrinopathies such as acromegaly and also those caused by drugs, chemicals, or infection.

Gestational diabetes mellitus

This is defined as carbohydrate intolerance of variable severity with onset or first recognition during the present pregnancy. These women have normal glucose homeostasis during the first half of pregnancy and develop a relative insulin deficiency during the latter half of pregnancy leading to hyperglycaemia. This resolves after delivery in most women but increases the risk of developing type 2 DM in later life.

It should be noted that the oral glucose tolerance test (OGTT) previously recommended by the National Diabetes Data Group (NDDG) and still the criterion recommended by the World Health Organization (WHO) has been replaced with the recommendation that the diagnosis of DM be based on two fasting plasma glucose levels of 7 mmol/L (126 mg/dL) or higher.

Table 8.11.1 Diagnostic criteria for diabetes

Diabetes	Fasting plasma glucose = 7 mmol/L (126 mg/dL) or 2 hours plasma glucose* = 11.1 mmol/L (200 mg/dL)
Impaired glucose tolerance (IGT)	Fasting plasma glucose <7 mmol/L (126 mg/dL) and 2 hours plasma glucose† = 7.8 mmol/L and <11.1 mmol/L (140–200 mg/dL)
Impaired fasting glucose	Fasting plasma glucose = 7 mmol/L (126 mg/dL) and 2 hours plasma glucose (if measured) <7.8 mmol/L (140 mg/dL)

*Venous plasma glucose measured 2 hours after ingestion of 75 g of oral glucose load.
†If 2 hours plasma glucose is not measured, the status is uncertain as DM or IGT cannot be excluded.

Screening for GDM

Controversy reigns supreme on the issue of screening for GDM: who should be screened, when, and how remain unresolved questions. On one side of the debate is the assertion that evidence does not support routine screening for GDM and, therefore, it should not be offered, whereas on the other is the acknowledgement that the evidence is limited but does not conclusively support not screening for GDM. In the UK, current trends are to suggest that women with no risk factors for GDM, and therefore considered low risk, should not be screened. Similar advice is given by the American College of Obstetricians and Gynaecologists (ACOG), the American Diabetes Association (ADA), and the Joslin Diabetes Center guidelines, while the WHO and International Diabetes Centre guidelines suggest universal screening at 24–28 weeks. All guidelines advocate screening high-risk women early rather than at 24–28 weeks.

The results of recent studies may swing the debate in favour of routine/universal screening. The ACHOIS trial has provided evidence that purports to show that treatment of a screening-detected population with mild GDM reduces serious neonatal (as a composite outcome) and maternal (pre-eclamptic toxaemia (PET) or gestational hypertension) outcomes. The even more recently published HAPO study also shows a continuous relationship between glucose concentration at 28 weeks OGTT and pregnancy outcomes and makes a strong case for universal screening.

Where screening is advocated there is no universally accepted screening method, although either risk factor assessment or laboratory-based testing are the common methods. Risk factor assessment (see box Risk factors for GDM) is a common international practice and 80% of obstetric units in the UK employ this method.

Risk factors for GDM
Maternal age >37 years
Ethnicity
Prepregnancy weight >80 kg or BMI >28 kg/m^2
Family history of diabetes in first-degree relative
Previous macrosomia/polyhydramnios
Previous unexplained stillbirth
Polycystic ovarian syndrome

Other screening tests used include glycosuria, HbA1c, fructosamine, random plasma glucose, fasting glucose, the 50-g 1-hour glucose challenge test (GCT) and the OGTT. The GCT remains the most popular screening test for GDM, advocated in the USA by the ADA, the ACOG, the International Diabetes Centre, and the Joslin Diabetes Center, and is generally regarded as the yardstick for comparing all screening tests for GDM. It has a sensitivity of 79% and specificity of 87%. The fasting glucose as a screening test has the attraction of being easy to administer, well tolerated, inexpensive, reliable, and reproducible. However, it has given varied results in different populations and its use as a screening test in pregnancy remains ambiguous.

To underscore the debate surrounding screening, there is also no universal agreement on a diagnostic test for GDM. The OGTT is the gold standard diagnostic test for GDM, but its many disadvantages include the argument that it is non-physiological, that it is unpleasant for use in subjects where nausea may already be an issue, that it is not reproducible, and appears to have variable predictive values in different ethnic origin. All expert panels agree that OGTT is the confirmatory diagnostic test for GDM despite the added problem of nausea and vomiting in pregnant women. There is no agreement on the glucose load (75 g versus 100 g) or the criteria used for diagnosis of GDM. The common diagnostic tests and criteria for diagnosis of GDM are illustrated in the Table 8.11.2.

Aetiology and pathogenesis

Type 1 diabetes mellitus
This is an organ-specific autoimmune disease associated with serological evidence of autoimmune destruction of the pancreas and presence of islet cell antibodies. There is a genetic component, and the HLA region on chromosome 6 was identified very early on as a potential site of a major susceptibility gene for type 1 diabetes. Genes have been identified for rare, monogenic, or syndromic forms of diabetes. Rare variations in insulin genes result in the autosomal dominant form of diabetes. Rare syndromes like Wolfram syndrome and Wolcott Rallison syndrome with linkages to specific genes have now been described, but the discussion of these is beyond the scope of this chapter. Genes accounting for susceptibility to MODY have also been identified.

Type 2 diabetes mellitus
In contrast to type 1, there is no evidence of immune pathogenesis in type 2 DM. However, there is a much stronger genetic component. The incidence increases with age and there is a strong association with obesity. Over 25 genome-wide linkage scans for type 2 diabetes have been completed to date and the regions showing the greatest replication among studies include 1q, 12q, and 20q. An association has been reported between type 2 diabetes and a variation in the gene for transcription factor 7-like 2 (TCFL2).

Pathophysiology of GDM
Significant changes in maternal fuel metabolism occur in pregnancy: in early pregnancy fasting plasma glucose concentration decreases and there is a slight decrease in endogenous glucose production. By the end of first trimester insulin sensitivity starts to fall and by the third trimester insulin-mediated glucose utilization declines by approximately 50% in lean and 40% in obese women. There is accelerated ketosis in the fasting state and a rise in maternal fasting glucose and free fatty acids.

The cause of the insulin sensitivity in the first trimester is not known. The subsequent rise in insulin resistance is due to several factors. A rise in plasma concentration of hormones such as placental lactogen, prolactin, cortisol, and progesterone correlates with this insulin resistance in mid-pregnancy. However, a rise in the inflammatory cytokine tumour necrosis factor (TNF)-α, produced by cells of immune system, suggests the involvement of intermediate mechanisms. Compared with other potential markers such as leptin, cortisol, human placental lactogen, or prolactin, the increase in TNF-α concentration appears to be the best predictor of insulin resistance in pregnancy, independent of BMI An increase in insulin resistance in mid-pregnancy is compensated by an increase in fasting and post-meal plasma insulin concentration due to increased insulin production by the pancreatic β-cells.

Compared with normal pregnancy, there is increased insulin resistance in GDM. It has been suggested that women with GDM already have chronic underlying insulin resistance upon which pregnancy-related changes in insulin sensitivity is superimposed. The chronic insulin resistance of GDM could partly be due to increased fat mass, as GDM has a strong association with maternal obesity. Additional factors might be genetically determined defects in insulin receptor signalling.

Pancreatic β-cell dysfunction is another key feature observed in those with GDM. The exact mechanism of this is unclear. The initial response to insulin resistance is expansion of β-cell mass which is then probably followed by increased beta cell apoptosis.

Genetics of GDM
Studies have shown some links between familial clustering of GDM and type 1 and type 2 diabetes. It has been observed that the HLADR3 and DR4 antigens were uncommon overall but occur more frequently in women with GDM than in women with normal pregnancy.

Table 8.11.2 Various threshold values for diagnosis of GDM

	Fasting (mmol/L)	1 h (mmol/L)	2 h (mmol/L)	3 h (mmol/L)
100 g OGTT*	5.3	10.0	8.6	7.8
100 g OGTT†	5.8	10.6	9.2	8.0
75 g OGTT‡	5.6		7.8	
75 g OGTT¶	5.3	10.0	8.6	
75 g OGTT§	5.3	10.6	8.9	

*Carpenter & Coustan.
†National Diabetes Data Group (NDDG).
‡World Health Organization (WHO).
¶American Diabetes Association (ADA)
§Canadian Diabetes Association (CDA).
In the USA the NDDG were historically the criteria used, but in 2000 because of perceived low sensitivities with the NDDG criteria, the ADA recommended that the Carpenter and Coustan criteria should replace the NDDG. However, both are still in use, while in the UK the WHO-recommended criteria following a 75-g OGTT are mostly used. There are no randomized controlled trials comparing the one-step 75-g OGTT with the two-step 100-g OGTT, or comparing the various diagnostic criteria20. The information gained from the HAPO study may allow derivation of internationally accepted criteria for diagnosing GDM that might translate into uniform research and evidence-based clinical practice.

Effects of diabetes on pregnancy
Congenital malformation
Poorly controlled DM in women is strongly associated with an increased risk of congenital malformation. Although there is strong evidence that good glycaemic control significantly reduces this, there is still a three to five times higher incidence of congenital malformation in women with DM, suggesting that either the efforts at glycaemic control are inadequate or, more likely, that DM may have a permanent and irreversible effect on reproduction. The exact underlying mechanisms are poorly understood, but glucose metabolism is likely to be central, influencing oocyte maturation and the quality of any subsequent embryo. Poor glucose control in the mother will also be reflected in poor control in the fetus, and recent research suggests that hyperglycaemia in the fetus may predispose the offspring of a diabetic mother to develop metabolic disease later in life.

Spontaneous miscarriage
Research has that women with poorly controlled diabetes, defined as a glycosylated haemoglobin (HbA1c) value greater than 6 SD above the mean, have a spontaneous abortion rate of 28% compared with 10–17% in well-controlled diabetic women. The mechanism of miscarriage is likely to be linked to abnormal embryonic development in the early period of organogenesis, which in turn is linked to early abnormal metabolic control. It is therefore not surprising that interventions designed to decrease the rate of congenital malformation have also resulted in a decrease in the risk of spontaneous miscarriage in women with DM.

Diabetes associated stillbirth and perinatal mortality
The stillbirth, neonatal, and perinatal mortality rates for babies born to diabetic women are substantially higher than those observed in the general population, although these have improved over the last decades. This increased risk is most commonly associated with insulin requiring pregestational diabetes, but may also involve GDM. Table 8.11.3 shows the stillbirth, perinatal mortality rate, and neonatal death in type 1 and type 2 diabetes. Previous studies have reported perinatal mortality in the offspring of women with type 2 diabetes to be equivalent or higher than that seen in women with type 1 diabetes. There was no evidence from the recent CEMACH report of a difference in the mortality rates of babies born to women with type 1 compared with those from type 2 diabetic women.

Risk factors for stillbirth in diabetic women include obesity, previous Caesarean section, congenital birth defect, and intrauterine growth (restriction) IUGR. IUGR is particularly associated with vascular complications of diabetes.

The pathophysiology of fetal compromise in diabetes is poorly understood and is most likely to be multifactorial. Although at least three pathological processes have been implicated, the final common pathway leading to fatal damage or death appears to be fetal asphyxia. The three processes are fetal hypoxia, fetal acidosis, and an alteration in fetal and/or maternal metabolism, details of which are beyond the scope of his chapter.

Fetal macrosomia
Excessive fetal growth is associated with all types of DM and maternal obesity. Although different definitions have been applied to macrosomia, the conventional definition is a birthweight greater than 4.5 kg or greater than 90th or 95th percentile or the mean +2 SD for a given gestational age.

In the majority of instances it is not possible to give a convincing explanation of why macrosomia develops, but some factors appear to be contributory. It has been found that maternal glycaemia is significantly higher by the early third trimester in diabetic women destined to deliver a large baby than those destined to have a baby of average weight. There is lack of agreement however about whether the post-meal glucose and/or HbA1c or a fasting glucose taken at 29–32 weeks is a better predictor of macrosomia. Other factors having an effect on birthweight are maternal prepregnancy weight and BMI, and maternal weight gain during pregnancy, although the latter appears to have a weak correlation where GDM is concerned. Increased insulin resistance in GDM leads to increased shunting of substrate from the maternal to the fetal circulation throughout pregnancy and this excessive supply of nutrients diminishes the relative influence of maternal weight gain on birthweight. Finally the modified Pederson's hypothesis, which explains various fetal and neonatal complications, can also explain macrosomia.

Modified Pederson's hypothesis

Maternal hyperglycaemia

↓

Fetal hyperglycaemia

↓

Fetal pancreatic β-cell hyperplasia

↓

Fetal hyperinsulinaemia

↓

Macrosomia organomegaly polycythemia hypoglycaemia RDS

↓

Jaundice

Maternal considerations
There is an increased risk of pre-eclampsia, further increased if there is pre-existing hypertension or renal disease. In the presence of concomitant nephropathy or hypertension the risk is about 30%. Proteinuria significantly worsens in women with diabetic nephropathy, leading to severe oedema and hypo-albuminaemia. There is also often a normocytic normochromic anaemia which responds only to recombinant erythropoietin. There is increased risk of infection particularly urinary tract, respiratory, endometrial, and wound infections. Vaginal candidiasis is relatively more common. The Caesarean section rate is increased to about 60%, at least partly due to early induction.

Effect of pregnancy on diabetes
Diabetic nephropathy
All women with pre-existing diabetes should have a 24-hour urine collection for total protein and creatinine clearance. In women with nephropathy, changes in creatinine clearance are variable during pregnancy and most women will not exhibit a normal rise in creatinine clearance. Protein excretion will frequently rise to the nephrotic range. However, the majority of young diabetic women with overt nephropathy demonstrate only baseline proteinuria without a reduction in creatinine clearance, and in pregnancy many will have successful outcomes without renal disease progression. Angiotensin-converting enzyme (ACE) inhibitors are considered to have teratogenic potential, and therefore current standard practice

is to stop them as soon as a woman falls pregnant and substitute with a calcium channel blocker or equivalent.

Pregnancy outcomes are surprisingly good in women with diabetic nephropathy, although compared with diabetic women without vasculopathy, excess morbidity is clearly present. Preterm delivery often complicates more than 50% of pregnancies and IUGR more than 15%. Pre-eclampsia also often exceeds 50% and Caesarean section is often in excess of 70%. The outcome seems to be related to baseline renal function and women with initial serum creatinine of more than 1.5 mg/dL or urine protein excretion of more than 3 g/24 hours have an increased risk of the complications mentioned above.

Other effects of pregnancy on diabetes

Normal pregnancy is associated with increased insulin production and resistance. Therefore women with IDDM and NIDDM require increasing doses of insulin as pregnancy progresses and maximum requirements at term can be at least twofold of prepregnancy doses.

Hypoglycaemia is more common and probably related to tight control. For the same reason diabetic ketoacidosis (DKA) seems to be rare. The risk is increased in the presence of hyperemesis, infection, tocolysis or corticosteroid therapy. DKA is discussed below.

Retinopathy is a common ocular complication of diabetes with a prevalence of 17% among patients diagnosed before the age of 30 with disease duration of 5 years. After 15 years, the prevalence is over 90%. There are two well-characterized stages: non-proliferative or background retinopathy and proliferative retinopathy. Certain factors in pregnancy, such as duration of diabetes, degree of metabolic control, and hypertensive disorders influence the progression of proliferative retinopathy. It is also clearly associated with the severity of the pre-existing disease. Rapid normalization of glucose is another factor that contributes to worsening of retinopathy.

Diabetic neuropathy is a heterogeneous group of abnormalities involving both autonomic and peripheral nervous systems. Earlier studies suggested that pregnancy could enhance progression of neuropathy. This was however challenged by more recent data which concluded that parity does not influence long-term prevalence or severity of diabetic autonomic neuropathy.

Gastroparesis, which is a form of autonomic neuropathy, interferes with food absorption and is therefore associated with difficulties in blood glucose control and severe nausea and vomiting. The most worrisome aspect of diabetic autonomic neuropathy during pregnancy is the occurrence of gastroparesis diabeticorum. It may result in significant maternal complications including pulmonary oedema or aspiration, the need for parenteral nutrition, and poor glucose control. Severe fetal complications such as IUGR, preterm labour, and fetal loss have also been reported. Fortunately, severe gastroparesis in pregnancy is rare, with only a few cases being reported in the world literature.

Prognosis in GDM

Recurrence of GDM

Given that most of the risk factors for GDM persist or become worse in subsequent pregnancies, it is not surprising that the recurrence rate is high and ranges between 35% and 70%. The wide range of recurrence rate is in part due to various screening methods and different diagnostic threshold values for various GTTs. It is clear from the literature however that GDM in the index pregnancy increases both the risk of recurrence in subsequent pregnancies and also the risk of developing type 2 diabetes later in life (see box).

Risk factors for GDM and recurrence
Previous history of GDM
Previous diagnosis of GDM before 24 weeks
Insulin requirement in previous pregnancy
Previous GDM and weight gain of ≥15 lbs (6.8 kg) in between pregnancies
Previous GDM and interval between pregnancies of ≥24 months
Previous history of macrosomia (birthweight ≥9 lbs or 4.1 kg)
Previous history of adverse pregnancy outcome (not clearly attributable to a condition other than diabetes during pregnancy)
Ethnic group with an elevated risk of GDM and type 2 DM
First-degree relative with diabetes
Advanced maternal age
Obesity (BMI = 30–35 kg/m2)
Glucosuria
Conditions with insulin resistance, for example polycystic ovarian syndrome (PCOS)
Metabolic syndrome, which is defined by the presence of three or more of the following criteria:
Abdominal obesity (waist circumference >88 cm), elevated triglycerides (= 150 mg/dL), (HDL <50 mg/dL), high BP (130/85 mmHg) and elevated fasting glucose (110 mg/dL).

Long-term effects of pre-existing DM and GDM on offspring

Most research evidence indicates that intrauterine exposure to maternal diabetes or GDM increases the risks for obesity and altered glucose metabolism in the offspring. The box illustrates the chain of events in diabetic pregnancy that occurs in response to intrauterine exposure to the metabolic environment of diabetes.

Effect of intrauterine exposure to the metabolic environment of DM

Increased maternal fuel
↓
Altered fetal islet cell function
↓
Childhood obesity, pubertal impaired glucose intolerance
↓
Impaired adult islet cell function
↓
GESTATIONAL DIABETES MELLITUS
↓
Increased maternal fuel

Management of pre-existing diabetes

It is evident that in order to achieve optimal outcomes, the management of women with pregestational diabetes must start from preconception, continue throughout pregnancy and well into the puerperium.

Preconception care

Good diabetes control and normal HbA1c levels at conception lower the risk of congenital anomalies in the fetus and the risk of PET. Preconception care should ideally start 3–6 months before planned conception, thus allowing adequate time to evaluate the mother's health status and optimize glycaemic control. The main objectives of preconception counselling should therefore be as follows.

- Folic acid supplementation and adequate blood glucose control before conception to decrease the rate of major congenital anomalies. HbA1c should be monitored monthly until stable within the range 4–6% before conception. Patients should be educated regarding contraceptive use throughout this period.
- History, physical examination (including gynaecological) and laboratory investigations for presence of diabetes related complications.
- Diabetic nephropathy: 24 hours urine for protein, creatinine clearance, serum creatinine, and BUN should be determined. Urinary tract infections should be excluded by urinary cultures.
- Dilated retinal examination should be performed, and where retinopathy is found clear documentation as to its nature (background versus proliferative) is mandatory. In the presence of retinopathy sudden glycaemic changes should be avoided: rather a planned slow reduction of HbA1c should be the aim. Identification of risk factors for progression will also prompt an intensive follow-up of retinal pathology during pregnancy. Women should be counselled about the risk of progression of proliferative retinopathy. An ophthalmologist is an invaluable member of the team in this regard.
- Cardiovascular system: baseline and then regular blood pressure measurements are vital. For women with chronic hypertension antihypertensive medication should be reviewed. ACE inhibitors should be replaced by calcium channel blockers or methyldopa. An ECG should be performed in women with 10 or more years of diabetes, hypertension or other evidence of vasculopathy. An exercise stress test is indicated if there is any evidence of coronary artery disease. No maternal or fetal deaths have been reported in women who had coronary artery bypass grafts (CABGs) before pregnancy while 38% maternal or fetal mortality occurred in those who did not receive such preconception care. Thus preconception evaluation, and where indicated treatment of patients with diseased arteries with a bypass graft or angioplasty, may improve maternal and perinatal outcomes.
- Evidence of autonomic dysfunction such as lack of awareness of hypoglycaemia and orthostatic hypotension, and excessive nausea and vomiting should prompt further evaluation of these diabetic complications. As there is significant maternal and fetal morbidity in women with gastroparesis diabeticorum, these women should be counselled against pregnancy.
- Endocrine: since thyroid dysfunction is frequently associated with type 1 diabetes, thyroid function should be routinely evaluated in the preconception period.

Optimal preconception care requires a multidisciplinary team. There is a need for effective contraception until good glycaemic control is achieved. All women should be seen by diabetes educators and nutritionists for individualized counselling and instructions to reinforce self-management skills. Once the patient has achieved tight glycaemic control, she can be advised to contemplate pregnancy. If conception does not occur within 1 year, the woman's fertility should be assessed.

The preconception management outlined here is echoed by CEMACH, which also recommends that there should be clear documentation of management and counselling in a standard template.

Management during pregnancy

Medical management

Management of glycaemia

The most important goal is to achieve near normal glycaemia, which should be achieved via monitoring at least four times per day, to include a fasting level and following breakfast, midday and evening meals. The target capillary glucose levels are <6 mmol/L before breakfast, <8 mmol/L 1 hour postprandial, <7 mmol/L 2 hours postprandial. HbA1c should be measured in each trimester and the target that reflects good control is 5–6%.

The traditional basal bolus insulin regimens provide the best option for care. There are however changes in insulin requirement during pregnancy to meet maternal needs as well as to provide fuel for the growing fetus. Early in gestation maternal fasting plasma glucose levels decrease and post-prandial levels increase. As a result in the first trimester insulin may need to be reduced from prepregnancy levels and then subsequently increased in the second and third trimester as the demand for insulin rises. In the last month of pregnancy there is likely to be a decrease in insulin requirements by as much as 20–30% due to enhanced transfer of maternal glucose to the fetus. Overall there is a greater demand for mealtime insulin coupled with a need to optimize doses of intermediate acting insulin to guarantee a constant basal rate.

In an effort to simulate physiological insulin secretion basal and prandial insulin are administered in three or four injections each day or via continuous subcutaneous insulin infusion or pump therapy. Such regimens include multiple doses of short or rapid acting insulin usually before breakfast, lunch, and evening meal, the amount of each dose being dependent on the carbohydrate content of each meal, insulin sensitivity and pre-meal capillary blood glucose measurements. In the four-injection regimen most patients would take a combination of intermediate acting or at bedtime and short-acting insulin or rapid-acting insulin with breakfast, lunch, and dinner. At night, when there is a relative fasting state, placental and fetal glucose consumption continue, creating a period of accelerated starvation. Therefore, giving intermediate acting NPH at dinner can lead to nocturnal hypoglycaemia, whereas giving it at bedtime will delay its peak effect until morning.

Newer insulin analogues

Semisynthetic human insulin preparations and newer insulin analogues are now used during pregnancy. The rapid-acting insulins such as insulin lispro and insulin aspart have considerable advantages over regular insulin. They can be injected at the start of a meal, and they peak at the time of highest glucose excursion after a meal, which is approximately 90 minutes. Regular insulin must be taken 30 minutes before a meal making compliance difficult, and has its peak in 2–4 hours. It also has a long duration of action of 6–8 hours, which increases the likelihood of hypoglycaemia long after its injection.

Insulin pump therapy: open loop continuous subcutaneous insulin infusion pump (CSII) is also used by some women with type 1 diabetes, particularly those who have a hectic lifestyle and need maximum flexibility in their diet and insulin regimen. Modern pumps are small and lightweight and different basal rates can be set and boluses given as required. Potentially CSII maintains the basal rate of insulin and therefore reduces the risk of hypoglycaemia. However, patients with type 1 DM may become hyperglycaemic rapidly if there is pump failure or intercurrent infection. Of note, infection at infusion site is relatively rare. Research to date has not shown any significant difference in either maternal outcome (CS rate, mean HbA1c, hypo- or hyperglycaemia) or baby outcome (perinatal mortality rate, fetal anomaly, gestational age at delivery, and small for gestational age) between use of CSII and multiple dose injection (MDI). There was a significant increase in mean birthweight associated with CSII compared with MDI; however, there was no significant difference in macrosomia (birthweight >4000 g).

Diet therapy

A schedule consisting of three meals and several snacks is used in most patients. Diet should consist of 50–60% carbohydrate, 20% protein, and 25–30% fat with less than 10% saturated fats, up to 10% polyunsaturated fatty acid, and the remainder derived from a monounsaturated source. Caloric intake depends on prepregnancy weight and weight gain during gestation. Carbohydrate counting helps patient to determine appropriate insulin boluses for meals and snacks.

Role of oral antidiabetic agents in pregnancy

Recent research using oral antidiabetic agents (OAAs) in GDM and polycystic ovarian syndrome (PCOS) suggest that they are safe and often effective. Contrary to earlier fears, drugs such as glyburide do not increase above background the rates of major congenital malformations or neonatal deaths. Metformin has been associated with decreased rates of spontaneous miscarriage and GDM, and similar rates of pre-eclampsia, major birth defects, and similar birthweight compared with healthy controls. It has been hypothesized that type 2 women needing exceptionally high doses of insulin during pregnancy can be sensitized by using metformin, allowing a lower dose of insulin to be used. The recently published Metformin in Gestational Diabetes (MiG) trial, in which 751 women with GDM were randomly assigned at 20–33 weeks' gestation to open treatment with metformin (with supplemental insulin if required) or insulin, concluded metformin (alone or with supplemental insulin) is not associated with increased perinatal complications compared with insulin, and that women preferred metformin to insulin treatment.

Management of acute emergencies

Hypoglycaemia

Most pregnant patients with pre-existing diabetes are followed up with outpatient visits at 1–2-week intervals. However, an open-access policy should be in place, so that women should be able to call at any time with any concerns, but especially if hypoglycaemia (<60 mg/dL) or hyperglycaemia occurs (>200 mg/dL). The risk of hypoglycaemia is particularly high at 10–15 weeks because of a relative increase in oestrogen, decreased carbohydrate intake due to nausea and vomiting or overly aggressive treatment of the patient when she first presents in pregnancy. The patient and her family members should be taught to manage hypoglycaemia: mild attacks respond to drinking a glass of milk or juice, and the more severe attacks may require glucagon injections. The patients should carry candy, crackers or glucose tablets to treat themselves in an emergency when away from home.

Diabetic ketoacidosis

With the implementation of antenatal programs DKA during pregnancy has fortunately become an uncommon event, estimated at 1–2 % in women using insulin. The occurrence of DKA in GDM is extremely rare and its occurrence strongly suggests the possibility of pre-existing but undiagnosed type 1 diabetes.

The true incidence of maternal mortality in DKA is unknown although historically reported at 5–15%. Fetal loss rates are much higher and vary widely between 35% and 85%, although more recent research has reported loss rates as low as 9%.

Comprehensive details of the management of DKA are beyond the scope of this chapter. Suffice to say that this should be a multidisciplinary effort mounted on an ICU in the first instance. Although DKA represents a substantial risk to the fetus, even if late decelerations are present on cardiotocography, the aim should be to correct maternal acidosis because the fetus usually recovers with the correction of maternal acidosis.

Fetal surveillance

All women should have early booking and an early dating scan as documentation of viability is essential due to high rates of miscarriages, especially in women with poor glycaemic control. They should be offered a 11–13-week nuchal translucency scan and a detailed anomaly scan in the second trimester, as well as a cardiac scan at 22 weeks' gestation, preferably performed by a fetal cardiologist or sonoligist with appropriate expertise. Careful attention should be given to the evaluation of the great vessels.

In the third trimester evaluation of fetal growth and wellbeing are the mainstays in evaluating pregnancies complicated by diabetes. Accelerated fetal growth has been associated with a significant risk of fetal mortality. The limitations of ultrasound in consistently diagnosing and evaluating fetal macrosomia must, however, be recognized.

Other tests of fetal wellbeing include maternal monitoring of fetal movements, cardiotocography, biophysical profile, and umbilical artery Doppler flow studies. All add to the increased fetal surveillance that is required for women with DM, although efficacy is often doubtful.

Management of mother and baby around delivery

Controlling maternal blood glucose over the few hours before delivery is crucial to reduce the risk of neonatal hypoglycaemia. Blood glucose concentration of 4–8 mmol/L

Table 8.11.3 Stillbirth, perinatal mortality rate and neonatal death in type 1 and type 2 diabetes

	Type 1 (per 1000 live births)	Type 2 (per 1000 live births)	National Rate (per 1000 live births including non-diabetes)
Stillbirth	25.8	29.2	5.7
Perinatal death	31.7	32.3	8.5
Neonatal death	9.6	9.5	3.6

should be the target, and usually best achieved using glucose and insulin infusion. As soon as the cord is cut the rate of infusion should be halved as insulin sensitivity returns to normal within minutes of shut down of the uteroplacental circulation. Subcutaneous insulin administration can be resumed as soon as the mother is able to eat.

If the baby's blood glucose is checked too early in life, then it almost certainly will be low as 5% of babies of non-diabetic women have blood glucose concentrations of less than 1.7 mmol/L within 2 hours of life. If blood glucose is checked too early then the baby will unnecessarily be sent to the special care baby unit: to avoid this, early feeding should be strongly encouraged and the blood glucose checked only before the second feed. This will decrease the mother–baby separation rates as two-thirds of the separations are potentially avoidable. Blood glucose should however be checked if hypoglycaemia is suspected. These babies are also at risk of hyperbilirubinaemia, respiratory distress syndrome, asphyxia and injuries such as those associated with shoulder dystocia. It is highly recommended that all units have a written policy for care of infants of mothers with diabetes.

Timing and mode of delivery

Two arguments have been put forward for delivery of an infant of a diabetic mother 1–2 weeks before term. The first is the avoidance of unexpected fetal demise, and the second is avoidance of fetal trauma accompanying the vaginal delivery of a large infant. However, there is remarkably little hard research on the issue of the mode and timing of delivery in pregnancies complicated by DM. NICE have recommended the following with regard to timing and mode of delivery: (i) pregnant women with diabetes who have a normally grown fetus should be offered elective birth through induction of labour, or by elective Caesarean section if indicated, after 38 completed weeks; (ii) diabetes should not in itself be considered a contraindication to attempting vaginal birth after a previous Caesarean section; (iii) pregnant women with diabetes who have an ultrasound-diagnosed macrosomic fetus should be informed of the risks and benefits of vaginal birth, induction of labour and caesarean section.

Management of GDM

The management goals in GDM are similar to those of pre-existing diabetes. The first step is usually dietary and exercise advice. If diet and exercise fail to achieve the target levels of glucose, insulin therapy should be commenced. Therapy should also be considered if there is ultrasound evidence of fetal macrosomia.

With regard to OAAs, metformin is the logical choice in GDM where insulin resistance seems to be the main problem. The findings of the MiG trial have provided an evidence base for the use of metformin in GDM.

If there is satisfactory glycaemic control, pregnancy can be allowed to progress until 40 weeks. Women who need insulin/metformin are usually induced at 40 weeks, ostensibly to reduce the risk of macrosomia and/or unexplained stillbirth, but the evidence for either is at best tenuous. Women who do not need any medical intervention and are controlled by diet alone can be safely managed as other low-risk non-GDM women. Following delivery insulin or metformin can be stopped immediately, and glucose monitoring can stop after the establishment of normal fasting glucose levels. All women with GDM should be followed up with an OGTT (usually 75 g, but centres in the USA mostly use 100 g) performed 6 weeks postpartum.

Postpartum care and education

Women with type 1 diabetes often require very little insulin during the first 24–72 hours after delivery, and insulin dosing is best achieved by continuation of the sliding scale. Women with type 2 diabetes often have adequate glycaemic control following delivery and may not require any medical intervention for a while. If resumption of OAAs is necessary, glyburide, glipizide, or metformin have been shown to have little or no transfer into the breast milk and can be prescribed to breast feeding women.

Dietary counselling should also take place and the general guideline for caloric intake are about 25 kcal/kg/day in non-breastfeeding and 27–30 kcal/kg/day in breastfeeding women.

Exclusive breastfeeding is strongly recommended for the first 6 months of life, although this is not always achievable. The offspring of diabetic mothers are at increased risk of childhood obesity and type 2 diabetes later in life. Breastfed infants appear to be at lower risk of both. A delayed introduction of formula milk also appears to be protective of β-cell autoimmunity and later risk of type 1 diabetes. In GDM, evidence also suggests that women who breastfeed are themselves protected against the later development of type 2 diabetes.

In women with pre-existing diabetes the ABCs of diabetes should be stressed: A1c (controlling glucose), B (blood pressure), C (cholesterol). All these go a long way in preventing long-term complications of diabetes, especially the microvascular complications. Use of ACE inhibitors in these women is thought to be renoprotective.

Reproductive health and contraception during the postpartum period

Exclusive breastfeeding provides contraception via lactational amenorrhoea, and this can be enhanced with the use of condoms. For those desiring hormonal contraception, reassurance should be given that less than 1% of the dose is transferred in breast milk. Progestin-only methods, which can be started on day 21 postpartum, are preferred as there is no demonstrable effect on the volume of milk secretion. The use of combined oral contraceptives (COCs) should be withheld until 6 weeks postpartum because of the risk of thromboembolism, and then only in non-breastfeeding women. The short-term use of low-dose COCs and progestin-only OCs seem to have minimal metabolic effects, but data on long-term effects are lacking. In women with GDM COCs do not seem to have either short-term or long-term adverse metabolic effects or increase the risk of developing diabetes. Progestin-only OCs however appear to increase the risk of developing diabetes almost by threefold. It is therefore recommended that the lowest dose and potency progestin and oestrogen combination OC be selected to minimize glucose intolerance and adverse effect on lipid metabolism and blood pressure. Intrauterine devices can be used safely in women with diabetes without increasing the risk of pelvic inflammatory diseases. When used, the insertion should be delayed by at least 4 weeks postpartum, although copper medicated devices can be inserted 48 hours postpartum.

Further reading

Crowther CA, Hiller JE, Moss JR, et al. Australian Carbohydrate Intolerance Study in Pregnant Women (ACHOIS) Trial Group. Effect of treatment of gestational diabetes mellitus on pregnancy outcomes. N Engl J Med. 2005; 352:2477–86.

Hillier TA, Vesco KK, Pedula KL, et al. Screening for gestational diabetes mellitus: a systematic review for the U.S. Preventive Services Task Force. Ann Intern Med 2008;148:766–75.

Hunt K, Schuller K. The increasing prevalence of diabetes in pregnancy. Obstet Gynecol Clin N Am 2007;34:173–99.

Metzer BE, Lowel LP, Dyer AR, *et al.* The HAPO Study Cooperative Research Group. Hyperglycemia and adverse pregnancy outcomes. N Engl J Med 2008;358:1991–2002.

Nice Clinical Guideline 8. Diabetes in pregnancy: management of diabetes and its complications from the preconception to the postnatal period; March 2008. http://www.nice.org.uk

Reece EA, Eriksson UJ. Congenital malformations: epidemiology, pathogenesis and experimental methods of induction and prevention. In: Reece EA, Coustan DR, Gabbe SG (eds) Diabetes in women: adolescence, pregnancy and menopause, 3rd edn. Philadelphia: Lippincott Williams & Wilkins Philadelphia 2004: 169–204.

Rowan JA, Hague WM, Gao W, *et al*, for the MiG Trial Investigators. Metformin versus insulin for the treatment of gestational diabetes. N Engl J Med 2008;358:2003–15.

World Health Organization. Definition and diagnosis of Diabetes Mellitus and intermediate Hyperglycemia. Report of a WHO/IDF consultation. Geneva: WHO 2006.

Drugs in pregnancy

Pharmacological agents are not necessary during pregnancy; however, some women go through pregnancy with medical conditions that need continuing or episodic treatment (e.g. asthma, epilepsy, and hypertension). During pregnancy new medical problems may develop or the old ones can aggravate (e.g. migraine headaches), requiring pharmacological therapy. Drugs given in pregnancy can adversely affect the fetus in many ways. Studies have shown that many pregnant women use either prescribed or over-the-counter medications during pregnancy (Bonati et al. 1990; Lacroix 2000). A comparison of therapeutic drug use in pregnancy across Europe showed that 64% of women used at least one drug during pregnancy (De Vigan 1999), while in France, pregnant women were prescribed an average of five drugs during the first trimester (Lacroix 2000). In the UK about a third of women take pharmacological agents at least once in pregnancy, but only 6% take these agents in the first trimester (Moore 1988). In puerperium, the use of drugs increases substantially, with no difference in the pattern of prescribing between mothers who breastfeed and those who bottlefeed. Although most doctors are cautious with medication use in their pregnant patients, it is estimated that at least 10% of birth defects are attributed to maternal drug exposure in pregnancy.

Drug metabolism in pregnancy

The safety and efficacy of drugs for a dosage regimen is established by Phase 3 clinical trials, involving typical representatives from the target patient population. Pregnant women and those who fall pregnant during the trial are excluded from these studies. Thus, at a drug's first marketing, except for products developed to treat conditions specific to pregnancy (e.g. oxytocics, cervical ripening agents), there are seldom human data on the proper dosage and frequency of administration during pregnancy. The placenta is a relative lipid barrier between the maternal and fetal circulation and most drugs cross the placenta by passive diffusion. The practical view to take on prescribing drugs in pregnancy is that transfer of drugs to the fetus is unavoidable. Low-molecular-weight, lipid-soluble, and un-ionized drugs cross the placenta more readily than polar drugs. There are several physiological changes during pregnancy that have a marked impact on pharmacokinetics and hence some of the established therapeutic ranges might be inappropriate.

Based on all the evidence available about congenital abnormalities and its association with the drugs, the FDA has divided the drugs into different categories (Table 8.12.1).

In this section we aim to provide a quick reference guide for drug use in pregnancy. The drugs here listed here are in groups according to how they appear in the WHO 11th model list of essential drugs.

General anaesthetics

Intravenous anaesthetics induce anaesthesia rapidly and commonly used drugs are thiopentone and Propofol (risk factor B). Propofol has not been used during the first and second trimesters in humans. Reproduction studies in rats and rabbits at doses six times the recommended human induction dose revealed no evidence of impaired fertility or fetal harm.

Inhalational anaesthetics commonly used are halothane and nitric oxide. A collaborative perinatal project showed no embryonic or fetal effects of nitric oxide. Its use during

Table 8.12.1 US FDA pregnancy category definitions

Cat	Description
A	Controlled studies in women fail to show a risk to the fetus in the first trimester, and the possibility of fetal harm appears remote
B	Animal studies do not indicate a risk to the fetus and there are no controlled human studies, or animal studies do show an adverse effect on the fetus but well-controlled studies in pregnant women have failed to demonstrate a risk to the fetus
C	Studies have shown the drug exerts animal teratogenic or embryocidal effects, but there are no controlled studies in women, or no studies are available in either animals or women
D	Positive evidence of human fetal risk exists, but benefits in certain (e.g. life-threatening or serious diseases for which safer drugs cannot be used or are ineffective) may make use of the drug acceptable despite its risks
X	Studies in animals or humans have demonstrated fetal abnormalities or there is evidence of fetal risk based on human experience, or both, and the risk clearly outweighs any possible benefit

delivery will lead to neonatal depression and fetal accumulation of nitric oxide, which increases over time; therefore, it is safer to keep the induction to delivery time as short as possible.

Neuromuscular blocking agents

These agents are used in adjunct to anaesthetics to provide muscle relaxation. Succinyl choline (risk factor C) is the only depolarizing agent used. The Collaborative Perinatal Project recorded 50 282 mother–child pairs, 26 of whom had first trimester exposure to succinylcholine. No congenital malformations were observed in any of the newborns.

Non-opioid analgesics and antipyretics and non-steroidal anti-inflammatory drugs

Aspirin (Risk Factor C) and non-steroidal anti-inflammatory drugs (NSAIDs) do not produce structural defects. Salicylates (in analgesic doses) and NSAIDs may increase the risk of neonatal haemorrhage by inhibition of platelet function. NSAIDs may also lead to oligohydramnios by its effect on the fetal kidney. The use of NSAIDs in the last trimester causes premature closure of the ductus arteriosus, leading to neonatal primary hypertension. Both premature closure of the ductus and the oligohydramnios are reversible. If used during pregnancy, they should be discontinued at least 6–8 weeks before delivery.

Opioid analgesics

In a surveillance study of Michigan Medicaid recipients 375 (4.9%) major birth defects were noted (325 expected). Specific data were available for six defect categories, including (observed/expected) 74/76 cardiovascular defects, 14/13 oral clefts, 4/4 spina bifida, 25/22 polydactyly, 15/13 limb reduction defects, and 14/18 hypospadias. Only with the total number of defects is there a suggestion of an association between codeine and congenital defects, but other reasons, including the mother's disease, concurrent drug use, and chance may be involved. In an investigation of 1427 malformed newborns compared with 3001 controls, first trimester use of narcotic analgesics (codeine (risk factor C) most common) is associated with inguinal hernias, cardiac and circulatory defects, cleft lip and palate, dislocated hip, and other musculoskeletal defects. Alimentary tract defects occur when used in the second trimester. The data serve as a possible warning that indiscriminate use of codeine may present a risk to the fetus. Use of codeine during labour produces neonatal respiratory depression to the same degree as other narcotic analgesics. Neonatal codeine withdrawal has also been reported.

Disease modifying agents of rheumatic disorders

- Sulphasalazine (risk factor B): no increase in human congenital defects or newborn toxicity has been observed from its use in pregnancy. Milk concentrations were roughly 40–60% of maternal serum levels. Bloody diarrhoea in an infant only breastfed was attributed to the mother's sulphasalazine therapy (3 g/day), Cautious use of sulphasalazine in nursing women because of significant adverse effects in some nursing infants is recommended.
- Cyclophosphamide (risk factor D): various abnormalities ranging from karyotyping abnormalities to multiple structural anomalies have been described with the use of cyclophosphamide in first trimester. Use of cyclophosphamide in the second and third trimesters does not place the fetus at risk for congenital defects. Except in a few individual cases, long-term studies of growth and mental development in offspring exposed to cyclophosphamide during the second trimester, the period of neuroblast multiplication, have not been conducted. Cyclophosphamide is contraindicated during breastfeeding because of the reported case of neutropenia and because of the potential adverse effects of immune suppression, growth, and carcinogenesis.

Anticonvulsants/antiepileptics (risk factor D)

Phenytoin, primidone, phenobarbitone, carbamazepine, and sodium valproate all cross the placenta and are teratogenic. The major abnormalities produced by anticonvulsants are neural tube, orofacial, and congenital heart defects. The neural tube defects are mainly caused by sodium valproate (1–2%) and carbamazepine (0.5–1%). Orofacial defects are mainly from phenytoin, which also produces the fetal hydantoin syndrome.

The risk for any single drug is about 6–7% (i.e. double to three times the background level). The risk increases with the multiple drugs. Patients on two or more anticonvulsants the risk is 15%, and for those taking combinations of valproate, carbamazepine, and phenytoin the risk is as high as 50%. The risk of neural tube defects may be decreased with preconceptual and first trimester folic acid (5 mg). The newer anticonvulsant drugs vigabatrin, lamotrogine, topiramate, and gabapentin are often prescribed in combination with other anticonvulsants and it is therefore difficult to ascertain the teratogenic risk of these drugs in isolation. Monotherapy should be used wherever possible and special care should be taken to keep the dose as low as is compatible with seizure prophylaxis. The traditional anticonvulsants, such as phenytoin, carbamazepine, and valproic acid are considered safe for use during breastfeeding; however, observation for adverse effects such as drowsiness is recommended for women receiving high doses.

Anti-helminthic—intestinal, anti-filarials, anti-schistosmals, anti-trematode drugs

- Mebendazole(risk factor C): it has been found to be embryotoxic and teratogenic in rats and is therefore not recommended for use during pregnancy.
- Albendazole (risk factor C): observation of limb reduction defects at all doses in one animal study and limited human pregnancy data suggest that Albendazole during pregnancy is not recommended. There is no data on the safety of albendazole in breastfeeding.

Antibacterials

- Tetracycline (risk factor D): tetracycline is contraindicated during pregnancy. This broad-spectrum antibiotic crosses the placenta, chelates with calcium and is deposited in the developing teeth and bones of the fetus. Staining of the permanent teeth is most likely when tetracyclines are administered after 24 weeks' gestation.
- Ciprofloxacin (risk factor C): quinolone treatment in developing adolescents of several animal species is associated with acute arthropathy of the weight-bearing joints. A recent study examining the effect of intrauterine exposure to quinolones on the fetus inferred that the use of the ciprofloxacin during the first trimester of pregnancy is not associated with an increased risk of malformations or musculoskeletal problems. Long-term follow up is required to exclude subtle cartilage and bone damage.
- Aminoglycosides: except for eighth cranial nerve damage, no reports of congenital defects caused by streptomycin have been found. The Collaborative Perinatal Project monitored 50 282 mother–child pairs, 135 of whom had first trimester exposure to streptomycin (risk factor D). For use any time during pregnancy, 355 exposures were recorded. In neither group was evidence found to suggest a relationship to large categories of major or minor malformations or to individual defects. Aminoglycoside antibiotics have no detectable teratogenic risk for structural defects. They also concluded that the risk of deafness after in utero aminoglycoside exposure was small. Streptomycin is compatible with breastfeeding.
- Chloramphenicol (risk factor C): it should be avoided in late pregnancy and during labour because of the potential for the 'grey baby syndrome' in the newborn infant. Therefore, it should only be used in pregnancy in life-threatening conditions, when no alternative is available.
- Nitrofurantoin (risk factor B): nitrofurantoin may be administered in pregnancy, but should be avoided near term. Low levels of glutathione may predispose the foetus to haemolytic anaemia if it is exposed to nitrofurantoin shortly before birth.
- Vancomycin (risk factor B): vancomycin is a bactericidal antibiotic with a fetal ototoxic effect. It should be avoided unless benefit outweighs potential risk.
- Trimethoprim (risk factor C): the use of trimethoprim in pregnancy was associated with an approximate quadrupling the risk of cardiovascular defects and/or an oral cleft. The risk was increased with use during the second and third months after the last menstrual period but not before or after this period. It is therefore advisable to avoid trimethoprim in the first trimester unless benefit outweighs potential risk and is always used with folic acid.

Antiprotozoal drugs (anti-amoebic and anti-malarial drugs)

- Metronidazole (risk factor B): most of the published evidence now suggest that metronidazole does not present a significant risk to the fetus. A possible small risk for cleft lip with or without palate has been reported, but the validity and the clinical significance of this finding is questionable. It is also not possible to assess the risk to the fetus from the potential carcinogenic potential of metronidazole. Metronidazole is contraindicated during the first trimester in patients with trichomoniasis or bacterial vaginosis.

- Chloroquine: chloroquine is not a major teratogen, but a small increase in birth defects cannot be excluded. The amount of chloroquine excreted into milk is not considered to be harmful to a nursing infant.

- Quinine (risk factor D): quinine has effectively been replaced by newer agents to treat malaria. Although no increased teratogenic risk can be documented, its use during pregnancy should be avoided. Quinine is compatible with breastfeeding.

Adrenocortical steroids

The adrenal cortex synthesizes two classes of steroids: the corticosteroids (glucocorticoids and mineralocorticoids) having 21 carbon atoms and the androgens, which have 19. Cortisone is the main glucocorticoid and aldosterone is the main mineralocorticoid. Glucocorticoids are administered in multiple formulations for disorders that share an inflammatory or immunological basis. Except in patients receiving replacement therapy for adrenal insufficiency, glucocorticoids are neither specific nor curative, but rather are palliative because of their anti-inflammatory and immunosuppressive actions.

- Prednisolone (risk factor C) is the biologically active form of prednisone. The placenta can oxidize prednisolone to inactive prednisone or even less active cortisone. The Michigan Medicaid surveillance study looked at 229 101 patients exposed to prednisolone, prednisone and methyl-prednisolone during the first trimester. These data do not support an association between the drugs and congenital defects. There are isolated reports of cataracts in the newborn if prednisolone was used throughout the pregnancy. At maternal doses of 20 mg the infant would be exposed to minimal amounts of steroid. At higher doses (>20 mg), it is recommended to wait at least 4 hours after a dose before nursing the baby.

- Betamethazone (risk factor C) use in preterm labour is associated with a decrease in respiratory distress syndrome, periventricular leucomalacia, and IVH in preterm infants. It can precipitate myasthaenic crisis in patients with myasthaenia gravis, induce hyperglycaemia, and, rarely, a hypertensive crisis. Single courses of betamethasone have no effects on the fetus but multiple courses of betamethasone have been associated with lower birthweights and reduced head circumference at birth. Follow-up studies have not shown any differences in cognitive and pscychosocial development when compared with controls.

- Hydrocortisone (risk factor C) and its inactive precursor, cortisone, present a small risk to the human fetus. These corticosteroids produce dose-related teratogenic and toxic effects in genetically susceptible experimental animals consist of cleft palate, cataracts, spontaneous abortion, IUGR, and polycystic kidney disease.

Although the large numbers of data support no effects in much of human pregnancies, adverse outcomes have been observed and may have been caused by corticosteroids. Moreover, the decrease in birthweight and a small increase in the incidence of cleft lip with or without cleft palate are supported by large epidemiological studies. Because the benefits of corticosteroids far outweigh the fetal risks, these agents should not be withheld if the mother's condition requires their use. The mother, however, should be informed of the risks so she can actively participate in the decision on whether to use these agents during her pregnancy.

Immunosuppressive drugs

- Azathioprine (risk factor D): azathioprine is a 6-mercaptopurine derivative, which acts as a 'steroid-sparing' agent. Current evidence indicates that maternal use of azathioprine is not associated with an increased risk of impaired fetal immunity, growth restriction, and prematurity. There is no increase in congenital abnormalities or subsequent problems such as childhood malignancy in children followed for up to 20 years. There has been conflicting information on breastfeeding while taking azathioprine. Despite little or no drug being found in breast milk most rheumatologists advise avoidance of azathioprine if possible, or would counsel against breastfeeding because of theoretical risks of immune suppression of the neonate.

- Cyclosporin (risk factor C): based on relatively small numbers, the use of cyclosporine during pregnancy apparently does not pose a major risk to the fetus. No pattern of defects has emerged in the few newborns with anomalies. Skeletal defects, other than the single case of osseous malformation, have not been observed. Cyclosporine is contraindicated during breastfeeding due to the potential for immune suppression and neutropenia, an unknown effect on growth, and a possible association with carcinogenesis.

Anti-angina drugs

Nitroglycerin (risk factor B): the use of nitroglycerine during pregnancy does not seem to present a risk to the fetus. However, the number of women treated during pregnancy is limited, especially during the first trimester. With the smaller doses reported, transient decreases in the mother's blood pressure may occur, but these do not appear to be sufficient to jeopardize placental perfusion. Nitroglycerin appears to be a safe, effective, rapid-onset, short-acting tocolytic agent. The use of transdermal nitroglycerine patches is also effective when longer periods of tocolysis are required.

Anti-arrhythmic drugs

Amiodarone (risk factor D) is an iodine-rich anti-arrhythmic drug with proven benefit in the treatment of patients with ventricular and atrial arrhythmias. It can reach the fetus by transplacental passage and induce fetal hypothyroidism. It inhibits the conversion of thyroxine to triiodothyronine in most tissues. It may also inhibit thyroid hormone synthesis and secretion, causing hypothyroidism in 5–25% of patients. There may be neurotoxicity associated with transplacental exposure to amiodarone. Amiodarone-exposed toddlers showed expressive language skills that were relatively poorer than verbal skills when compared with controls. One amiodarone-exposed toddler exhibited global developmental delay.

Amiodarone exposed older children had well-developed social competence, favourable global IQ scores but had problems with reading comprehension, written language, and arithmetic. This picture is reminiscent of non-verbal learning disability syndrome. In another report, a normal psychomotor development was observed in two patients with full-scale IQ score, verbal, and performance IQ scores within normal range. These data need to be validated by larger studies. In conclusion, drug therapy with amiodarone should be avoided during the first trimester of pregnancy if possible and drugs with the longest record of safety should be used as first-line therapy. Conservative therapies should be used when appropriate.

Anti-hypertensive drugs

β-Adrenergic antagonists

β-Adrenergic antagonists have fewer side-effects than most antihypertensives, but their safety in pregnancy is not so well established. Some studies have found no adverse effects on the outcome of pregnancy while others have described a variety of foetal and neonatal complications. The concern is that if these drugs are used before 28 weeks' gestation, they may increase the risk of intrauterine growth restriction. Later complications include bradycardia, hypotension, hypoglycaemia, and respiratory distress. However, many studies suggest that they are safe antihypertensives for use in the third trimester. If treatment of hypertension is required before 28 weeks, methyldopa should be the first drug of choice. Guidelines of the International Society for the Study of Hypertension in Pregnancy (ISSHP) do not recommend the use of oral β-adrenergic antagonists for mild hypertension in pregnancy.

Angiotensin converting enzyme inhibitors

These drugs have been associated with prolonged renal failure and hypotension in the newborn, decreased skull ossification, hypocalvaria, and renal tubular dysgenesis. In addition, there are several case reports of intrauterine growth restriction, oligohydramnios, patent ductus arteriosus, and neonatal hypotension. The use of these drugs in the first trimester is not thought to produce structural malformations, so it is acceptable to cease treatment early in pregnancy and not necessarily preconception.

Antithrombotic drugs

Warfarin (risk factor D)

Warfarin is a form of coumarin with vitamin K antagonist action. Its use in pregnancy is associated with a high incidence of fetal loss, congenital malformations, and physical disability. Exposure to the drug between the sixth and ninth weeks of gestation is associated with defective ossification of bone resulting in nasal hypoplasia and chondrodysplasia punctata. On a molecular level, vitamin K inhibitors may alter calcium binding for several proteins, affecting bone ossification causing the characteristic bony abnormalities of the 'fetal warfarin' syndrome. The use of warfarin in the second and third trimester is not without serious complications. The effects are mainly CNS abnormalities and are thought to be due to microhaemorrhages in the brain. The defects include dorsal midline dysplasia (agenesis of corpus callosum and Dandy-Walker malformations) or ventral midline dysplasia (optic atrophy), mental retardation, delayed development, seizures, and microcephaly. The risk of teratogenicity with warfarin has led to the recommendation that heparin should be substituted for the treatment and prophylaxis of venous

thromboembolism. However, heparin is not as effective as warfarin in preventing arterial thromboembolism in women with artificial heart valves or mitral disease with atrial fibrillation. In these situations, the risk of thrombosis may exceed the risks of warfarin use, and warfarin therefore may be indicated. It should be used with great caution and close monitoring of both the mother and fetus.

Heparin (risk factor C)

This is the anticoagulant of choice from the fetal perspective, as it does not cross the placenta.

Thyroid hormone and other antithyroid drugs

- Propylthiouracil (risk factor D): in a surveillance study of Michigan Medicaid recipients involving 229 101 completed pregnancies conducted between 1985 and 1992, 35 newborns had been exposed to propylthiouracil (PTU) during the first trimester. One (2.9%) major birth defect was observed (one expected), a case of hypospadias (none expected). A 1992 abstract and a later full report described a retrospective evaluation of hyperthyroid pregnancy outcomes treated with either PTU (N = 99) or methimazole (N = 36). Three (3.0%) defects were observed in those exposed to PTU (ventricular septal defect, pulmonary stenosis, patent ductus arteriosus in a term infant), whereas one newborn (2.8%) had a defect (inguinal hernia) in the methimazole group. No scalp defects were observed. In comparison with other antithyroid drugs, propylthiouracil is considered the drug of choice for the medical treatment of hyperthyroidism during pregnancy. PTU is compatible with breastfeeding.

- Methimazole (risk factor D) and carbimazole (risk factor D): a specific pattern of rare congenital malformations secondary to exposure to methimazole during the first 7 weeks of gestation that consists of some or all of the following: scalp or patchy hair defects, choanal atresia, oesophageal atresia with tracheoesophageal fistula, minor facial anomalies, hypoplastic or absent nipples, and psychomotor delay is reported. These defects may indicate a phenotype for methimazole embryopathy. Because of the possible association with aplasia cutis and other malformations, and the passage of methimazole into breast milk, PTU is the drug of choice for the medical treatment of hyperthyroidism during pregnancy. Methimazole and carbimazole are compatible with breastfeeding.

Psychotherapeutic drugs

Drugs used in psychotic disorders

Antipsychotic drugs: lithium (risk factor D)

It is estimated that 7.8% of lithium-exposed embryos develop abnormalities. Early data showed that the cardiovascular system is the most affected, with Ebstein anomaly affecting a third of the malformed babies. Although initial information regarding the teratogenic risk of lithium treatment was derived from biased retrospective reports, more recent epidemiological data indicate that the teratogenic risk of first trimester lithium exposure is lower than previously suggested. The clinical management of women with bipolar disorder who have childbearing potential should be modified with this revised risk estimate. If lithium is used for prophylaxis, it is advisable to discontinue it during the first trimester, unless its withdrawal would jeopardize the woman or the pregnancy. During pregnancy, the smallest dose possible for acceptable therapeutic effects should be used. Frequent small dosages should be used to avoid larger fluctuations in maternal plasma concentrations, and each dosage should not exceed 300 mg, with even spacing throughout the 24-hour period.

Drugs used in depressive disorders

Maternal depression in pregnancy can have deleterious effects on the neonate because of the potential for poor maternal weight gain or malnutrition. If supportive counselling is not adequate, tricyclic antidepressants and fluoxetine are the first-line choices in the management of depression. Tricyclic antidepressants have a long history of use without increasing teratogenic risk in pregnant women. Fluoxetine has been studied in prospective trials and no evidence for a higher incidence of malformations or other teratogenecity was found. Doses of tricyclic antidepressants may need to be higher in pregnancy due to increased hepatic metabolism. Where appropriate, to avoid withdrawal symptoms in the neonate, antidepressants should be slowly withdrawn or reduced to the minimum dose prior to delivery.

Further reading

Banks BA, Cnaan A, Morgan MA, et al. Multiple courses of antenatal corticosteroids and outcome of premature neonates. North American Thyrotropin-Releasing Hormone Study Group. Am J Obstet Gynecol 1999;181:709–17.

Bonati M, Bortolus R, Marchetti F, et al. Drug use in pregnancy: an overview of epidemiological (drug utilization) studies. Eur J Clin Pharmacol. 1990;38:325–8.

De Vigan C, De Walle HE, Cordier S, et al. Therapeutic drug use during pregnancy: a comparison in four European countries. OECM Working Group. Occupational Exposures and Congenital Anomalies. J Clin Epidemiol 1999;52:977–82.

French NP, Hagan R, Evans SF, et al. Repeated antenatal corticosteroids: size at birth and subsequent development. Am J Obstet Gynecol 1999;180:114–21.

Lacroix I, Damase-Michel C, Lapeyre-Mestre M, Montastruc JL. Prescription of drugs during pregnancy in France. Lancet 2000;356:1735–6.

MacArthur BA, Howie RN, Dezoete JA, Elkins J. Cognitive and psychosocial development of 4-year-old children whose mothers were treated antenatally with betamethasone. Pediatrics 1981;68:638–43.

MacArthur BA, Howie RN, Dezoete JA, Elkins J. School progress and cognitive development of 6-year-old children whose mothers were treated antenatally with betamethasone. Pediatrics 1982;70:99–105.

Moore K. The developing human: clinically oriented embryology, 4th edn. Philadelphia: WB Saunders 1988.

Schmand B, Neuvel J, Smolders-de Haas H, et al. Psychological development of children who were treated antenatally with corticosteroids to prevent respiratory distress syndrome. Pediatrics 1990;86:58–64.

Terrone DA, Rinehart BK, Rhodes PG, et al. Multiple courses of betamethasone to enhance fetal lung maturation do not suppress neonatal adrenal response. Am J Obstet Gynecol 1999;180:1349–53.

Epilepsy and other neurological conditions

Epilepsy

Epilepsy is the most common chronic neurological disorder affecting 0.8% of the general population. Similar prevalence is given in pregnant women. The incidence of epilepsy is 0.05% and will be certainly lower in pregnancy as peaks of incidence are in childhood/adolescents and in older age.

Classification of epilepsy includes idiopathic generalized epilepsies (e.g. juvenile myoclonic epilepsy, juvenile absence epilepsy, epilepsy with grand mal at awakening), partial or focal epilepsies (e.g. malformations of cortical development, posttraumatic epilepsies), epilepsies with generalized and focal features and specific syndromes (e.g. reflex epilepsies, febrile convulsions, isolated seizures). Treatment of people with epilepsy should be tailored according to seizure type and epilepsy syndrome. A neurologist or epilepsy specialist should manage diagnosis and treatment of epilepsy.

Epilepsy and preconception advice

- All women in childbearing age on AEDs (anti-epileptic drugs) and with active sex life should be on folic acid 5 mg once daily to prevent folic acid-deficient induced spina bifida.
- Woman with epilepsy should consult their neurologist/epilepsy specialist for preconceptional advice.
- Women with epilepsy on AEDs should avoid falling pregnant unplanned.

Risks in pregnancy

- Teratogenic risk of AEDs
- Uncontrolled generalized tonic clonic seizures (GTCS) can induce fetal hypoxia/acidosis and five or more GTCS can reduce verbal IQ of fetus.
- Risk of traumatic fetal injury with maternal seizures
- Slightly increased maternal death rate in woman with epilepsy (3.8% of all maternal death).
- Risk of seizures during the 48 hours around delivery is 2%, indicating a 10-fold increase compared with any other 48-hour period in pregnancy.

Teratogenic effect of AEDs

AEDs have a teratogenic risk. Monotherapy with AEDs will have a lower risk then polytherapy. But uncontrolled generalized tonic clonic seizures are more hazardous to mother and fetus than AEDs.

Teratogenic risk for MCMs (major congenital malformations) for

- carbamazepine does not significantly differ from baseline
- lamotrigine is around 2.9% in low dose (<400 mg/day), but up to 5.5% in high dose (>400 mg/day). Within this figure is a particular risk of open cleft palates
- sodium valproate has a dose-dependent risk from 5.5% (<600 mg/day) up to 8.3% (>1000 mg/day). Additionally, the risk for fetal valproate syndrome (abnormalities in face, developmental delay, occasionally major organ abnormalities and autistic traits). Recent studies suggest risk of reduced verbal IQ in children with maternal valproate exposure
- figures for other AEDs in pregnancy registers are statistically less valuable because of small patient groups.

However, most AEDs seem to have a slightly increased risk for MCM. Some of the newer AEDs might be associated with a lower risk (levetiracetam) but sample sizes are still too small.

Although risks for MCMs with AEDs are thought to be an effect of exposure in the first trimester additional effects with valproate suggest vulnerability of fetus in all trimesters of pregnancy.

Peaks of AED serum levels will increase the risk for MCMs. To avoid serum level peaks, slow-release AED preparations in two or even three divided dosages should be suggested. It should be kept in mind that non-compliance (i.e. forgetting lunch time dose frequently) might increase the serum level oscillations and risk for seizures.

Genetic aspects

Children of mothers with epilepsy have a slight increased risk to develop epilepsy. This depends on the seizure syndrome and its aetiology. In maternal focal epilepsy the risk is about 3% compared with approximately 0.8% in the normal population. Idiopathic generalized epilepsies may have a higher risk for genetic predisposition (approximately 10%), in particular with positive family history.

Management

Most women with epilepsy will have no change of seizure frequency during pregnancy. Approximately 15% will have a reduction of seizure frequency and a similar percentage will have an increase in seizure frequency.

- Antenatal screening includes detailed high resolution ultrasound scanning to detect neural tube, cardiac and skeletal abnormalities.
- Serum levels of antiepileptic drugs might decrease during pregnancy with the increased liver and renal clearance. This is applicable in particular for Lamotrigine but might apply for other AEDs as well. AED dosages should be adjusted accordingly. Trough serum level control before pregnancy or during the first trimester might be helpful to ascertain a base line figure for further reference (regular serum level controls in e.g. lamotrigine and oxcarbazepine). This is of particular importance in women whose epilepsy is fully controlled.
- Folic acid 5 mg od during the first trimester at least.
- Inform/involve neurologist/epilepsy specialist.
- Advise women with epilepsy to continue AEDs regularly. In case of increased vomiting, AEDs should be taken again if vomiting occurs within 45 minutes after drug intake. Recurrent vomiting may reduce serum levels of AEDs.
- In case of hospital admission ensure that AEDs are continued without gap!
- In case of enzyme-inducing AED risk of haemorrhagic disease during delivery might be increased. Vitamin K prophylaxis 10 mg od should be given to mother for 4 weeks prior to delivery. (Enzyme inducing AEDs: carbamazepine, phenytoin, phenobarbital, primidone; to lesser extent: oxcarbazepine, topiramate, lamotrigine.)
- Home delivery is not recommended, but spontaneous delivery in the hospital environment is regarded as safe unless there are very frequent seizures.
- Pain relief during delivery can include epidurals, gas and air, TENS machine, which are regarded as safe for

women with epilepsy. Pethidine and other opioids should be avoided if possible as they may trigger seizures in some patients.
- In case of seizure during delivery: Administer magnesium *and* 1–2 mg of lorazepam i.v. (2 mg with GTCS).

Postpartum management

All newborns should receive vitamin K prophylaxis postpartum to reduce the risk of haemorrhagic disease.

In case of AED dose increase during pregnancy, dosage of AED should be reduced to previous dosage within 3–4 weeks postpartum. However, should side-effects occur after delivery (particularly in women who had increase in lamotrigine dose) dosage should be readjusted more quickly, sometimes within a few days.

Advice for breastfeeding should be discussed prior to delivery with epilepsy nurse specialist or neurologist/epilepsy specialist. Concentration of some AEDs is higher in breast milk then in serum but in general breastfeeding in mother with AEDs is not restricted unless the newborn presents with side-effects, i.e. sedation and related feeding difficulties.

Contraception

Contraception should be discussed postpartum.
- Depot injections (Depo-provera) should be repeated every 10 weeks instead of 12.
- Standard strength combined oral contraceptive pill (COCP) will be safe with non-enzyme-inducing drugs (sodium valproate, levetiracetam, benzodiazepines, pregabaline, zonisamide, gabapentin, tiagabine, vigabatrin). Enzyme-inducing AEDs including carbamazepine, phenytoin, phenobarbital, and primidone require a higher dose COCP (50 μg or more of oestradiol) and/or tricyclic might be necessary. The safety might be still compromised. Breakthough bleeds would indicate reduced effectiveness of COCP. AEDs with lesser extent of enzyme induction (oxcarbazepine, topiramate particular >200 mg/day, and lamotrigine) are likely to affect the effectiveness of COCP as well. The same rules apply.
- COCP will reduce the plasma concentration of lamotrigine. Lamotrigine serum levels pre and post COCP are recommended. The lamotrigine dose should be increased by 50% when COCP is started. This is particularly important in women with full seizure control to avoid breakthrough seizures.
- Intrauterine devices (IUDs) with local hormone release (Mirena coil) have no interaction with AEDs.
- Progesterone-only pills and contraceptive implants are not recommended for women with epilepsy on AEDs.
- Other neurological conditions.

Most frequent other neurological conditions in pregnancy include migraine, peripheral nerve compression syndromes (e.g. carpal tunnel syndrome), reversible posterior leucoencephalopathy, sinus venous thrombosis, and multiple sclerosis. Eclampsia and pre-eclampsia are discussed in section 9.10.

Migraine

Migraine without aura tends to reduce in frequency during pregnancy, particularly after the first trimester. Migraine with aura is more likely to continue during pregnancy and it rarely gets worse. Some patients might present with aura only, and do not develop the typical headaches. Aura would usually present with the same symptoms as previously. New onset migraine presenting during pregnancy is rare but it is more likely to be with aura. Caution is advised as symptoms can be similar to eclampsia.

Postpartum headache occurs in 34% of women 3–6 days postpartum. It is more common in women with migraine. The headache usually presents slightly differently, bifrontal, less severe than migraine with nausea and vomiting. If the headache is disabling and there are no contraindications (e.g. coronary or cerebrovascular disease), subcutaneous sumatriptan injection is the treatment of choice even for breastfeeding women.

Management
- Migraine attacks should be treated with paracetamol 1000 mg orally. If necessary some antiemetic should be added (e.g. chlorpromazine or prochlorperazine).
- Sumatriptan has not shown to cause a significant increase of birth defects in more then 500 patients suggesting that it does not carry a risk for mother or fetus.
- Prophylactic medication should be avoided but if necessary, low dose propanolol might be helpful.

Peripheral nerve compression syndromes

Peripheral nerves might be compressed due to changes of connective tissue in pregnancy. Most commonly this presents with a carpal tunnel syndrome (CTS) causing tingling and pains (often nocturnal) in hand/wrist or even in the upper arm. Referral to neurology clinic for nerve conduction studies is advised. Treatment of CTS during pregnancy includes splint at night in neutral position or in severe cases decompressive surgery. However, it should be kept in mind that most CTS reverse spontaneously after delivery.

Reversible posterior leucoencephalopathy

This is a rare condition presenting late in pregnancy or puerperium. It is often associated with high blood pressure, although this might be a very moderate increase.

Clinically it presents with headaches and frequently visual symptoms including visual field defects up to hemianopia or anopia, possibly also agitation, dys- or aphasia, hallucinations and other cognitive disturbance.

Management
- Urgent neurology review
- Urgent MRI brain with DWI and MRV
- Control blood pressure!
- Symptomatic treatment of headache and other symptoms (e.g. hallucinations) if necessary.

Diagnosis is made by clinical picture and MRI result (posterior vasogenic oedema). Prognosis is good and syndrome is usually fully reversible.

Sinus venous thrombosis

This is a rare condition but slightly more prone to occur in women in pregnancy or puerperium due to activation of coagulation.

Clinical symptoms might present in an acute (within hours), subacute (within days or weeks) or rarely in a hyperacute fashion (thunderclap headache). Symptoms might include headaches, seizures, nausea and vomiting, alteration in consciousness level, paresis, aphasia, ataxia, and potentially other neurological signs depending on its location.

Management
- Urgent neurological review

- Urgent MRI with DWI and MRV (contrast CT brain: delta sign, i.e. rim of contrast around thrombus in posterior sagittal sinus only in 20% of cases positive)
- If diagnosis is confirmed, anticoagulation with heparin (aPTT twice the baseline but >120 seconds) even if haemorrhage on scan. Anticoagulation to be continued on warfarin for 6 months.
- AED during the acute phase of disease (e.g. clobazam) for up to 6 months maximum. *No* phenytoin (increases thrombophlebitis risk).
- Symptomatic treatment of headache.

No clear figures are at hand but prognosis seems to be better in women in pregnancy or puerperium than other aetiologies of sinus venous thrombosis. In one study 80% showed good outcome, but mortality was 9% in the pregnant patient group compared with up to 33% in all other cases.

Multiple sclerosis

Pregnancy in MS is safe. Particularly during the third trimester relapse rate will reduce but might rise in the first 3 months postpartum. However, only 28% of women with MS will suffer a relapse in this period. Higher the prepregnancy relapse rate and relapse during pregnancy might increase the risk for postpartum relapse. In the long-term pregnancy will have no impact on disability outcome.

Management

- Disease-modifying treatment should be stopped at least 3 months prior to conceiving.
- During pregnancy MS symptoms such as fatigue or incontinence might increase. Patients should seek advice from neurology or urology services.
- Spontaneous delivery is most often appropriate.
- Epidural or anaesthesia for Caesarean section is safe.

Further reading

Cantu C and Barinagarrementeria F. Cerebral venous thrombosis associated with pregnancy and puerperium. Review of 67 cases. Stroke 1993;24:1880–4.

EURAP Study Group. Seizure control and treatment in pregnancy: observations from the EURAP epilepsy pregnancy registry. Neurology 2006;66:354–560.

Goadsby PJ, Goldberg J, Silberstein SD. Migraine in pregnancy. BMJ 2008;336:1502–4.

Hinchey J, Chaves C, et al. A reversible posterior leukoencephalopathy syndrome. N Engl J Med 1996;334: 494–500.

Kimber J. Cerebral venous sinus thrombosis. QJM 2002:95: 137–42.

Morrow J, Russell A, et al. Malformation risks of antiepileptic drugs in pregnancy: a prospective study from the UK Epilepsy and Pregnancy Register. J Neurol Neurosurg Psychiatry 2006;77:193–8.

NICE guidelines CG20: The epilepsies: the diagnosis and management of the epilepsies in adults and children in primary and secondary care. October 2004. www.nice.org.uk/Guidance/CG20

Vukusic S, Hutchinson M, et al. Pregnancy and multiple sclerosis (the PRIMS study): clinical predictors of post-partum relapse. Brain 2004;127:1353–60.

Useful websites

www.epilepsynse.org.uk
www.epilepsyandpregnancy.co.uk
www.migrainetrust.org
www.mssociety.org.uk

Gonorrhoea

Definition

Gonorrhoea is a sexually transmitted infection caused by *Neisseria gonorrhoeae*, a gram-negative diplococcus.

Epidemiology

Gonorrhoea is spread by contact with the penis, vagina, mouth, or anus. In the USA, approximately 700 000 new cases occur each year. In 2006, the rate of reported gonorrhoeal infections was 120.9 per 100 000 persons in the USA, but only half of cases are reported. In the UK, there were 18 710 new cases in 2007; cases of uncomplicated gonorrhoea increased by 42% between 1998 and 2007. Approximately one-third of UK cases are in women. In the USA, slightly more cases are reported in women than in men. In women attending selected prenatal clinics in 20 states, Puerto Rico, and the Virgin Islands, the median gonorrhoea positivity was 1.0% (range 0.0–3.2%)

Risk factors

- Younger age (<25)
- Previous gonorrhoea infection
- Other sexually transmitted infections
- New or multiple sex partners
- Inconsistent condom use
- Commercial sex work
- Drug use
- Black race.

Pathology

N. gonorrhoeae infects mucous membranes that are lined with columnar epithelium cells. The urethra, cervix, rectum, pharynx, and conjunctiva of the eye are common sites. Spreading to the upper tract can cause pelvic inflammatory disease (PID). In pregnancy, untreated cervical gonorrhoea can cause intra-amniotic infection, premature rupture of membranes, and preterm birth. Perinatal transmission can lead to neonatal conjunctivitis and blindness if untreated. Disseminated infections may cause septic arthritis, endocarditis, and meningitis. Pregnant women are at greater risk for disseminated infection than non-pregnant women. Co-infection with gonorrhoea increases the risk of transmission of HIV.

Clinical approach

Diagnosis

Because gonorrhoea is usually asymptomatic, the essential component of gonorrhoea control is the screening of women at high risk for STDs. Pregnant women should be screened at the first prenatal visit if they are at risk or if there is a high rate of gonorrhoea in the population. Patients at continued risk should be screened again in the third trimester.

Pregnant adolescents should be screened for gonorrhoea at the first prenatal visit.

History

Most cases are asymptomatic. Women may complain of a discharge or urethritis.

Examination

Mucopurulent cervicitis may be seen, but the diagnostic value is low, especially in pregnancy.

Investigations

Gram stain of the endocervix has a high positive predictive value, but is not sensitive enough to be useful as a screening tool. Specific diagnosis of infection with *N. gonorrhoeae* is made by culture, nucleic acid hybridization tests, or nucleic acid amplification tests (NAATs) of endocervical, vaginal, male urethral, or urine specimens. NAATs offer the widest range of testing specimen types. They are FDA cleared for use with endocervical swabs, vaginal swabs, male urethral swabs, and female and male urine. Non-culture tests are not FDA-cleared for use in the rectum and pharynx. Some NAATs may cross-react with non-gonococcal *Neisseria* and related organisms that are commonly found in the throat.

Non-culture techniques cannot determine antibiotic sensitivity. In cases of persistent gonococcal infection after treatment, clinicians should perform both culture and antimicrobial susceptibility testing; 25.6% of isolates collected in 2006 in 28 Gonococcal Isolate Surveillance Project sites were resistant to penicillin, tetracycline, ciprofloxacin, or some combination of these antibiotics.

All patients tested for gonorrhoea should be tested for other STDs, including chlamydia, syphilis, and HIV.

Counselling

Patients with gonorrhoea should be counselled about the nature of transmission and the risk of other sexually transmitted diseases, including HIV, syphilis, and chlamydia.

All sexual partners should be identified and treatment offered. Patients should be instructed on the effectiveness of latex condoms in preventing sexually transmitted diseases.

Management

Fluoroquinolone-resistant gonorrhoea continues to spread worldwide. Resistance to recommended doses of ciprofloxacin and ofloxacin exceeds 40% in some Asian countries. As a result, this class of antibiotics is no longer recommended for the treatment of gonorrhoea.

Recommended regimens for uncomplicated urogenital and anorectal gonorrhoea

Ceftriaxone 125 mg i.m. in a single dose
    or
    Cefixime 400 mg orally in a single dose or 400 mg by suspension (200 mg/5 mL)
    plus
    treatment for chlamydia if chlamydial infection is not ruled out
    Patients infected with *N. gonorrhoeae* frequently are co-infected with *C. trachomatis*; this finding has led to the recommendation that patients treated for gonococcal infection also be treated routinely with a regimen that is effective against uncomplicated genital *C. trachomatis* infection.

Alternative regimens

Spectinomycin 2 g in a single i.m. dose (spectinomycin is currently not available in the USA) or single-dose cephalosporin regimens.

Other single-dose cephalosporin therapies that are considered alternative treatment regimens for uncomplicated urogenital, and anorectal gonococcal infections include ceftizoxime 500 mg i.m.; or cefoxitin 2 g i.m., administered with probenecid 1 g orally; or cefotaxime 500 mg i.m. Some evidence indicates that cefpodoxime 400 mg and cefuroxime axetil 1 g might be oral alternatives.

Pharyngeal infection should be treated with ceftriaxone 125 mg i.m.

For disseminated infection, ceftriaxone 1 g i.m. or i.v. every 24 hours is recommended; alternative regimens include cefotaxime 1 g i.v. every 8 hours; ceftizoxime 1 g i.v. every 8 hours or spectinomycin 2 g i.m. every 12 hours. Treatment should be continued for 24–48 hours after clinical improvement, and then cefixime 400 mg orally twice daily or cefpodoxime 400 mg orally twice daily should be continued to complete one week of therapy.

Allergy, intolerance, or adverse reactions

Culture and antibiotic sensitivity testing can help guide the choice of antibiotic therapy in patients with allergy or intolerance. Women who cannot tolerate cephalosporins or quinolones should be treated with spectinomycin. A single dose of azithromycin 2 g is active against uncomplicated gonorrhoea, but nausea and vomiting limits the use of the drug in that dose.

Special consideration in pregnancy

Pregnant women should not be treated with quinolones or tetracyclines. Those infected with *N. gonorrhoeae* should be treated with a recommended or alternative cephalosporin. Women who cannot tolerate a cephalosporin should be administered a single 2-g dose of spectinomycin i.m. Either azithromycin or amoxicillin is recommended for treatment of presumptive or diagnosed *C. trachomatis* infection during pregnancy

Management of sex partners

Treatment of sex partners is an essential component of the control of STDs. Treatment of partners prevents morbidity in partners and reduces the risk of reinfection.

Expedited partner therapy

Expedited partner therapy (EPT) is the practice of treating the sex partners of people with STDs without an intervening medical evaluation or professional prevention counselling. The usual implementation of EPT is through patient-delivered partner therapy (PDPT). The Centers for Disease Control has funded four randomized trials of EPT by PDPT. Both clinical and behavioural outcomes of the available studies indicate that EPT is a useful option to facilitate partner management among heterosexual men and women with gonorrhoea or chlamydia. Pregnant women were not separately analysed in these trials, but because of the potential adverse effects of gonococcal or chlamydial infection on the course of pregnancy and neonatal health, preventing reinfection may have a higher priority than in non-pregnant women. Thus it is reasonable to use EPT by PDPT in a population of pregnant women.

In some jurisdictions, EPT by PDPT may not be legal. Some jurisdictions require an examination of a patient before any treatment can be given, thus making EPT by PDPT illegal. Other jurisdictions specifically allow the practice.

Further reading

Centers for Disease Control and Prevention (CDCP). Sexually Transmitted Disease Surveillance 2006 Supplement, Gonococcal Isolate Surveillance Project (GISP) Annual Report 2006. Atlanta: US Department of Health and Human Services, CDCP 2008.

Centers for Disease Control and Prevention. Sexually transmitted diseases. Treatment Guidelines 2006. MMWR, 2006;55 (No.RR-11).

Centers for Disease Control and Prevention. *Expedited partner therapy in the management of sexually transmitted diseases.* Atlanta: US Department of Health and Human Services 2006.

Centers for Disease Control and Prevention. Update to CDC's sexually transmitted diseases treatment guidelines, 2006: fluoroquinolones no longer recommended for treatment of gonococcal infections. MMWR, 2007;56:332–6.

Health Protection Agency. All new episodes seen at GUM clinics: 1998-2007. United Kingdom and country specific tables. London: Health Protection Agency 2008.

Internet resources

Centers for Disease Control: www.cdc.gov; www.cdc.gov/STD/treatment/

Planned Parenthood Federation of America: www.plannedparenthood.org

National Institute of Allergy and Infectious Diseases www.niaid.nih.gov/publications/stds.htm

Patient resources

CDC-INFO Contact Center, 1-800-CDC-INFO (1-800-232-4636), Email: cdcinfo@cdc.gov

American Social Health Association (ASHA), 1-800-783-9877: www.ashastd.org

National Women's Health Information Center, 1-800-994-9662

Perinatal group B streptococcus

Background

Group B streptococcus (GBS) emerged in the 1970s as the leading cause of neonatal sepsis, and also as an important cause of maternal septicaemia and uterine infection. Approximately 20–30% of pregnant women are GBS carriers, with higher rates of colonization in Black than in White or Asian women (Regan et al. 1991). Early clinical trials showed that intravenous penicillin or ampicillin administered during labour was effective in preventing neonatal disease (Boyer and Gotoff 1986), in contrast to antenatal treatment to eradicate GBS genital colonization before labour (Hall et al. 1976; Gardner 1979). There are no efficacy data to assess oral or intramuscular antibiotic prophylaxis during labour. Available data on oral penicillin, ampicillin (Merenstein et al. 1980), erythromycin (Klebanoff et al. 19995), and long-acting benzathine penicillin (Weeks et al. 1997; Bland et al. 2000), administered for 1 or more weeks in pregnancy, show that 20–30% of women were still colonized at the time of delivery.

Prevention of early onset neonatal GBS disease

There are two competing strategies for the prevention of early-onset neonatal GBS infection, namely a cheaper and relatively less effective monitoring of women for known obstetric risk factors (intrapartum fever (20% of GBS positive women), preterm labour, prolonged rupture of membranes (˜18 hours), GBS bacteriuria, previously affected infant and isolation of GBS at any other time), and a culture-based screening of all women before labour (35–37 weeks in practice) to identify those colonized with GBS. The first national consensus guidelines in the USA in 1996 presented both approaches as equally acceptable, and their implementation resulted in a 70% reduction in the incidence of invasive neonatal GBS disease (from 1.5–2 cases/1000 live births to 0.5 cases/1000 live births) (MMWR 2000). A subsequent large retrospective cohort study showed that late antenatal culture-based screening was over 50% more effective in reducing the GBS attack rate than the alternative risk-based approach (Schrag et al. 2002a), leading to the adoption of a single prevention strategy, namely universal antenatal culture-based screening at 35–37 weeks of gestation (Schrag et al. 2002b). This improvement may be related to the detection on culture and intrapartum treatment of the 20% of colonized women who do not display any risk factors. For optimal detection rates (up to 27%) a rectovaginal or vaginal/perianal swab inoculated into a selective medium was recommended. In addition, women who have had a previously affected infant, GBS bacteriuria, or unknown GBS status were also eligible to receive intrapartum antibiotic prophylaxis.

Intrapartum antibiotic prophylaxis

The recommended regimens for intrapartum antibiotic prophylaxis included Penicillin G, 5 million units i.v. initially, then 2.5 million units i.v. every 4 hours until delivery or alternatively Ampicillin 2 g i.v. initially, then 1 g i.v. every 4 hours until delivery. Patients who are allergic to penicillin but not at risk of anaphylaxis should receive cefazolin 2 g i.v. initially, then 1 g i.v. every 4 hours until delivery, or either clindamycin 900 mg i.v. every 8 hours or erythromycin 500 mg i.v. every 6 hours until delivery, if they were at risk of anaphylaxis. If the GBS was found to be resistant to clindamycin or erythromycin or the susceptibility was unknown, vancomycin 1 g i.v. every 12 hours until delivery should be given.

In the UK, the risk-based approach is adopted by most units with approximately 55% reduction in the incidence of invasive neonatal GBS disease. It is important to recognize that the baseline incidence of early-onset GBS disease in the UK is estimated at 0.5–1.15/1000 live births (Beardsall et al. 2000) in contrast to the 1.5–2.5/1000 rate in the USA prior to the introduction of mass screening in late pregnancy. Introduction of US-style mass screening for the prevention of early-onset disease in the UK may not be appropriate or cost-effective. The current UK NICE guidelines on intrapartum care do not recommend intrapartum antibiotic prophylaxis for women with prolonged rupture of membranes ˜24 hours or their babies, if there is no evidence of infection such as pyrexia in labour (http://www.nice.org.uk/CG55). This deviates significantly from current understanding of the risk factor-based approach to prevention of neonatal GBS sepsis, particularly as 20% of colonized women do not display any risk factors.

Emergence of resistant organisms

At present, GBS remain universally sensitive to penicillin and the narrow spectrum of activity exhibited by penicillin G (preferred over ampicillin for intrapartum antibiotic prophylaxis) drive the continuing belief that there is less selective pressure for the emergence of resistant organisms. However, recent studies have shown that both intrapartum benzylpenicillin and ampicillin were associated with a 35% increase in vaginal colonization with ampicillin-resistant Enterobacteria species, 36 hours postpartum (Moore et al. 2003). One large study found a significant increase in the rate of early-onset Escherichia coli sepsis, although this was restricted to low-birthweight neonates (Stoll et al. 2002), and the total gram-negative bacterial sepsis declined despite the increase in E. coli infections. Other studies report stable or declining rates of non-GBS sepsis.

The risk of life-threatening maternal anaphylactic reactions to penicillin or cephalosporin is very low but increased use of intrapartum antibiotics is expected to lead to more neonatal testing. Some clinicians assume that clindamycin or erythromycin is automatically effective as prophylaxis for GBS in women who are sensitive to penicillin. This is not necessarily so as some 4% and 11% of GBS are resistant to clindamycin and erythromycin respectively. Clinicians should request sensitivity studies when taking samples for possible GBS colonization from women that volunteer a history of penicillin allergy.

Late-onset neonatal disease

Intrapartum antibiotic prophylaxis to prevent early-onset neonatal GBS disease does not modify the risk of acquisition of late-onset disease. This is because at least 50% of late-onset disease is due to nosocomial spread from other infants, hospital staff, or other adults. Not surprisingly, the dramatic reduction in the incidence of early-onset disease in the USA has at least in some parts, led to the emergence of the late-onset disease as the more common variant. At present, no preventive intervention has been identified, mostly because of the low baseline incidence rate of late-onset disease (0.5/1000 live births) and the much longer period of acquisition required in comparison to the early-onset disease.

Group B streptococci and preterm birth or low birthweight

There is some evidence those women who have heavy lower genital tract colonization with GBS have a significant, albeit small, risk of delivery of a low birthweight infant (OR 1.2, 95% CI 1.01–1.5) (Regan *et al.* 1996) but do not have an increased risk of other adverse outcomes including preterm birth. Other studies have not confirmed these findings. The 2002 CDC guidelines therefore recommend not treating GBS-colonized women antepartum, because it has no benefit and will expose a large number of women to unnecessary antibiotics.

Further reading

Beardsall K, Thompson MH, Mulla RJ. Neonatal group B streptococcal infection in South Bedfordshire, 1993–1998. Arch Dis Child Fetal Neonatal Ed 2000;82:F205–7.

Bland ML, Vermillion ST, Soper DE. Late third-trimester treatment of rectovaginal group B streptococci with benzathine penicillin G. Am J Obstet Gynecol 2000;183:372–6.

Boyer KM, Gotoff SP. Prevention of early-onset neonatal group B streptococcal disease with selective intrapartum chemoprophylaxis. N Engl J Med 1986;314:1665–9.

Gardner SE, Yow MD, Leeds LJ, et al. Failure of penicillin to eradicate group B streptococcal colonisation in the pregnant woman. A couple study. Am J Obstet Gynecol 1979;135:1062–5.

Hall RT, Barnes W, Krishnan L, et al. Antibiotic treatment of parturient women colonized with group B streptococci. Am J Obstet Gynecol 1976;124:630–4.

Klebanoff MA, Regan JA, Rao AV, et al. Outcome of the Vaginal Infections and Prematurity Study: results of a clinical trial of erythromycin among pregnant women colonised with group B streptococci. Am J Obstet Gynecol 1995;172:1540–5.

Merenstein GB, Todd WA, Brown G, et al. Group B beta-hemolytic streptococcus: randomised controlled treatment study at term. Obstet Gynecol 1980;55:315–18.

MMWR Early onset group B streptococcal disease, US 1998–1999. MMWR 2000;49:793–6.

Moore MR, Schrag SJ, Schuchat A. Effects of intrapartum antimicrobial prophylaxis for prevention of group-B-streptococcal disease on the incidence and ecology of early-onset neonatal sepsis. Lancet Infect Dis 2003;3:201–13.

Regan JA, Klebanoff MA, Nugent RP. The epidemiology of group B streptococcal colonization in pregnancy. Vaginal Infections and Prematurity Study Group. Obstet Gynecol 1991;77:604–10.

Regan JA, Klebanoff MA, Nugent RP, et al. Colonisation with group B streptococci in pregnancy and adverse outcome. VIP Study Group. Am J Obstet Gynecol 1996;174:1354–60.

Schrag SJ, Zell ER, Lynfield R, Roome A, Arnold KE, Craig AS et al. A population-based comparison of strategies to prevent early-onset group B streptococcal disease in neonates. N Engl J Med 2002a;347:233–239.

Schrag S, Gorwitz R, Fultz-Butts K, Schuchat A. Prevention of perinatal group B streptococcal disease. Revised guidelines from CDC. MMWR Recomm Rep 2002b;51:1–22.

Stoll BJ, Hansen N, Fanaroff AA, et al. Changes in pathogens causing early-onset sepsis in very-low-birth-weight infants. N Engl J Med 2002;347:240–7.

Weeks JW, Myers SR, Lasher L, et al. Persistence of penicillin G benzathine in pregnant group B streptococcus carriers. Obstet Gynecol 1997;90:240–3.

Haemoglobinopathies

Definition
A group of inherited disorders of haemoglobin synthesis or haemoglobin structure that have highly variable but significant clinical manifestations.

Epidemiology
About 5% of the world's population are carriers of a potentially pathological haemoglobin gene. Each year, about 300 000 infants are born (worldwide) with sickle cell anaemia (70%) and thalassaemia syndromes (30%) (WHO 2006).

There are ethnic differences in the prevalence of sickle cell disease and the thalassaemias. Sickle cell trait/anaemia is more common in individuals of African, Greek, Turkish, and Middle-Eastern descent. Sickle cell trait (HbAS) is much more common than Sickle cell disease/anaemia (HbSS). The thalassaemias, especially α-thalassaemia, are common among the Asian population. β-Thalassaemia is also prevalent in the Mediterranean islands and Southern Italy. But the demographics are slowly changing; with more interracial marriages and population migrations, these conditions are not uncommonly seen in the UK and most major cities.

Pathology
The α-globin cluster is located on the human chromosome 16, and the β-globin cluster is located on chromosome 11. Each individual normally has two paired α-globin genes, one pair on the maternal chromosome and the other pair on the paternal chromosome. The γ, δ-, and β-globin genes are encoded on chromosome 11.

Each haemoglobin (Hb) molecule has two pairs of globin chains. The usual adult haemoglobins are HbA, HbA2, and HbF. The production of normal haemoglobins require an intact gene, intact promoters, enhancers, and silencers, and an intact locus control region (LCR).

In sickle cell disease, an abnormal form of globin chains is synthesized. An A-to-T point mutation in the sixth codon of the β-globin chain gene leads to a glutamine-to-valine substitution on position six of the β-globin chain. In deoxy conditions, the resultant Hb has decreased solubility, increased viscosity, and forms tactoids. These phenomena alter the shape of the red blood cell into the characteristic sickle shape.

In thalassaemias, production of functional haemoglobin is impaired. In general, but not always, α-thalassaemia is due to partial/total deletions of the α-globin genes, whereas β-thalassaemia arises from missense/nonsense mutations within the β-globin gene.

The phenotypic expression of α-thalassaemia is extremely varied, but generally depends on the number of functional α-globin genes present. Patients who inherit three normal α-globin genes are phenotypically normal and may be haematologically normal as well, but are silent carriers of α-thalassaemia. Patients who inherit two normal α-globin genes are phenotypically normal, but have a mild anaemia, low mean corpuscular volume (MCV) and low mean corpuscular haemoglobin (MCH) levels. Cis-type double gene deletions are common in the Asian population, and can lead to haemoglobin Bart's hydrops fetalis (below). Patients who inherit only one normal α-globin gene have HbH disease, with haemolytic anaemia, defective erythropoiesis, and splenomegaly. Functional deletion of all four α-globin genes leads to an inability to produce any HbA, HbA2, or HbF. In utero, this leads to hydrops fetalis and intrauterine/early neonatal demise. In the Asian population, Hb Bart's hydrops fetalis occurs because of fetal inheritance of two defective parental chromosomes, each with a cis double gene deletion of both α-globin genes on chromosome 16.

In β-thalassaemia minor (heterozygous/carrier state/trait), one of the β-globin genes is defective. In β-thalassaemia major (homozygous), both genes are affected so the production of β-globin chains is severely impaired.

Clinical approach
Screening and diagnosis
The implications of the major haemoglobinopathies are significant in pregnancy, especially for the fetus and newborn child. All pregnant women in the UK are offered a screening test for thalassaemia, and sickle cell disease forms part of the antenatal and newborn screening programme.

History
- Sickle cell disease is usually diagnosed in childhood, so it is unusual to diagnose this condition in pregnancy. Moderately severe anaemia (Hb <7 g/dL), leucocytosis, and dactylitis in early life are known predictors of prognosis. Vaso-occlusive crises are relatively common in adult life. Other symptoms would include joint pains, chronic haemolytic anaemia, acute chest syndrome, bony avascular necrosis, hyposplenism, infections, and cerebrovascular accidents.
- The presenting history in the thalassaemias varies widely depending on the extent of the genetic alteration and the amount of globin chains produced. Silent thalassaemia carriers may only be identified after having given birth to an affected child with α- or β-thalassaemia, or presenting with a bad obstetric history due to Hb Bart's hydrops fetalis.

Examination
Examination will usually reveal the effects of anaemia, haemolytic anaemia, and blood transfusions on the body. There may be pallor, jaundice, systolic murmurs, hepatosplenomegaly, malleolar ulcers, bony deformities from bone marrow expansion, premature closure of epiphyses, fractures, and hyperpigmentation.

Laboratory investigations
These are important to make the diagnosis of the haemoglobinopathy, and also to distinguish between the different types of haemoglobinopathies.
- Full blood counts would reveal the severity of any anaemia, microcytosis, a low MCH, reticulocytosis, and leucocytosis.
- Peripheral blood smears would demonstrate the presence of sickled erythrocytes or target cells.
- Haemoglobin electrophoresis on cellulose acetate/citrate agar is a standard method of separating the haemoglobin bands. Relative quantitation of the different forms of haemoglobins give some indication of type of haemoglobinopathy present, but confirmatory tests are helpful.

- Thin-layer isoelectric focusing and high-performance liquid chromatography are also effective in studying haemoglobin variants.
- A solubility test such as Sickledex can be used to confirm sickle cell disease as HbS precipitates in this test.
- Iron studies are useful in excluding iron deficiency anaemia as a cause of the microcytic anaemia.
- Polymerase chain reaction-based molecular diagnostic tests now play an important part in the specific diagnoses of all haemoglobinopathies. These tests allow the exact characterization of the genetic change, and allow for genetic counselling and for accurate fetal prenatal diagnosis.

Counselling and management

Sickle cell disease

- Increased metabolic requirements, hypercoagulability, and the vascular stasis associated with pregnancy particularly predispose the pregnant mother with sickle cell disease to more frequent sickling crises, infections, and thromboembolic events. Pregnant women with sickle cell disease are at a higher risk of miscarriage, fetal growth restriction, pre-eclampsia, prematurity, placental abruption, stillbirth, and perinatal and maternal mortality.
- Ideally, patients with sickle cell disease should present for prepregnancy counselling, and partner screening and prenatal diagnosis should be discussed with her then. Her care through pregnancy should be jointly managed with a haematologist experienced in haemoglobinopathies.
- Some medications used in the management of sickle cell disease such as iron-chelating agents, anti-inflammatory agents, hydroxyurea, and 5-azacytidine are contraindicated in pregnancy or should be used with great caution. In the first trimester and also in labour, hydration should be diligently maintained. Iron supplementation should be used only in the presence of low iron stores, but all women should receive adequate folic acid supplementation (5 mg/day).
- If her partner also carries the defective gene, the couple should be offered prenatal diagnosis. Fetal cells and fetal DNA necessary for carrying out the fetal genetic diagnosis can be obtained using invasive procedures such as chorionic villus biopsy, amniocentesis and fetal blood sampling. In special circumstances, preimplantation genetic diagnosis could be offered.
- In view of a higher risk of fetal complications, regular assessment of fetal growth and placental function by ultrasound and Doppler is indicated. Continuous electronic fetal monitoring is recommended during labour. Caesarean section should be performed for obstetric indications, but general anaesthesia should be avoided. Peripartum thromboprophylaxis should be considered, but the role of prophylactic antibiotics and prophylactic blood transfusions remains controversial.

Thalassaemia

- It is unusual for transfusion-dependent thalassaemic patients to present with pregnancy. Those that do get pregnant are usually mild–moderately anaemic, or not at all. Whether α- or β-thalassaemia, the principle of management of the pregnant mother is the same. Most of these patients are not iron depleted, so oral iron supplementation should follow biochemical evidence of low iron stores. In contrast, folic acid supplementation (5 mg/day) should be routine throughout the pregnancy. Blood transfusions may be necessary when clinically indicated, and all such patients should be jointly managed with a haematologist.
- Ideally, patients with thalassaemia should present for prepregnancy counselling, and partner screening and prenatal diagnosis should be discussed. If her partner is also a carrier, the couple should be offered prenatal diagnosis. Fetal cells and fetal DNA necessary for carrying out the fetal genetic diagnosis can be obtained using invasive procedures such as chorionic villus biopsy, amniocentesis, and fetal blood sampling. Preimplantation genetic diagnosis involves the need for *in vitro* fertilization and is therefore relatively expensive, but has begun playing an important role in the management of thalassaemias.
- Hb Bart's hydrops fetalis is usually lethal *in utero*, or soon after birth. Only a few rare infants have survived the perinatal period, but requiring chronic intensive transfusion regimens, iron chelation, and haemopoietic stem cell transplantation (Singer *et al* 2000). Mothers carrying affected hydropic fetuses are at an increased risk of early-onset severe pre-eclampsia, intrapartum difficulties, and postpartum haemorrhage. In view of possible maternal and fetal compromise, the option of therapeutic termination of pregnancy should be discussed with the couple.

Further reading

Chui DH. Alpha-thalassemia: Hb H disease and Hb Barts hydrops fetalis. Ann N Y Acad Sci 2005;1054:25–32

Frewin R, Henson A, Provan D. ABC of clinical haematology. Iron deficiency anaemia. BMJ 1997;314:360–3.

Gillham JC. Haematological conditions. In: Luesley DM, Baker PN (eds) *Obstetrics and gynaecology. An evidence-based text for MRCOG*. Arnold 2004.

National Institutes of Health. *The management of sickle cell disease*, 4th edn. 2002 www.nhlbi.nih.gov/health/prof/blood/sickle/index.htm

Old JM. Haemoglobinopathies. In: Rodeck CH, Whittle MJ (eds) *Fetal medicine: basic science and clinical practice*. Churchill Livingstone 1999.

Singer ST et al. Changing outcome of homozygous alpha-thalassemia: cautious optimism. J Pediatr Hematol Oncol 2000;22:539–42.

Sun PM, Wilburn W, Raynor BD, Jamieson D. Sickle cell disease in pregnancy: twenty years of experience at Grady Memorial Hospital, Atlanta, Georgia. Am J Obstet Gynecol 2001;178:1127–30.

World Health Organization. 118th Session Executive Board. Geneva: WHO 2006.

Internet resources

Hematology articles: www.emedicine.medscape.com/hematology#red

Patient resources

Antenatal and Newborn Screening Programmes: www.screening.nhs.uk/sicklecellandthalassaemia/index.htm

Thalassaemia: www.patient.co.uk/DisplayConcepts.asp?f=1&maxresults=&WordId=thalassaemia

Heart disease

Definition
Heart disease in pregnancy refers to any pre-existing or pregnancy-related heart disorder that became symptomatic or detected during pregnancy, for which treatment may or may not be required. The condition or its residual effects may persist after pregnancy.

Epidemiology
Heart disease is one of the leading causes of maternal death in developed countries such as the UK. Heart disease complicates about 1% of all deliveries, but the reported figures can vary depending on the extent and type of investigations performed to confirm or exclude the diagnosis, and whether the denominator includes miscarriages and therapeutic abortions in addition to deliveries, and whether it is the number of mothers or total pregnancies that are counted. In general there is a progressive decline in the prevalence of chronic rheumatic heart disease (RHD) but an increase in congenital heart disease (CHD), especially in women after corrective surgery, so that the proportion of pregnant women with CHD had increased from 5% to 80%. The improvement in medical care, and delayed child-bearing, also mean that conditions in women who are previously advised against pregnancy, as well as age-related conditions, will be encountered more and more often in the future.

Pathology
In normal pregnancy, cardiac output is increased by 50%, which peaks between the mid-second and third trimesters. This is achieved by increase in stroke volume and heart rate, and is in response to the increase in blood volume of 50%. There is a concomitant fall in peripheral vascular resistance with a disproportionately greater lowering of diastolic blood pressure and a wide pulse pressure. The decrease in blood pressure lasts up to 34 weeks' gestation, when the peripheral resistance begins to rise again. There is increased pulmonary blood flow, which is balanced by a reduction in pulmonary vascular resistance. Myocardial hypertrophy and chamber enlargement are demonstrable by the third trimester, and mild multivalvular regurgitation is often found. Inferior vena caval and aortic compression by the gravid uterus in the supine position can result in a marked decrease in the blood pressure and uterine perfusion, especially during labour, and results in maternal hypotension, weakness, lightheadedness and may reduce placental perfusion. During labour, cardiac output is increased further by 10–14%, so that any conditions that restrict cardiac output can easily lead to cardiac decompensation in labour.

Pregnancy is also associated with a hypercoagulable state. Increased circulating oestrogens can interfere with collagen in the media of the muscular arteries, whereas elastase can weaken the aortic media, and relaxin can decrease collagen synthesis. Thus pregnancy is a predisposing factor to dissection of blood vessels, even in the absence of an underlying connective tissue disorder.

The severity of cardiac symptoms is classified by the New York heart Association (NYHA) classification as follows.
- Class I—no limitation of activity, no symptoms from ordinary activity.
- Class II—slight or mild limitation of activity, comfortable with mild exertion.
- Class III—marked limitation of activity, comfortable only at rest.
- Class IV—confined to rest in bed/chair; any physical activity leads to discomfort and symptoms occur at rest.

Heart diseases constitute a big heterogeneous group and are traditionally categorized into congenital, rheumatic, arrhythmias, and other acquired conditions. However, to facilitate discussion on pathology, the conditions can be categorized as follows.

Valvular diseases
Valvular heart diseases constitute the largest group and include congenital and acquired conditions, as well as native and prosthetic valves. In general, women tolerate valvular regurgitation better than stenosis, because the reduction in systemic vascular resistance limits the effect of regurgitation and accentuates the effect of stenosis.

Native valves
The valves involved in descending frequency are mitral, aortic, pulmonary, and tricuspid. There may be multiple valvular involvement in RHD.

Mitral valve
Mitral stenosis, which is almost always due to RHD, is more common than mitral regurgitation, which often accompanies mitral stenosis but is more commonly due to mitral valve prolapse (MVP). In cases of mixed mitral stenosis and mitral regurgitation, the clinical problem is predominantly due to mitral stenosis. Mitral stenosis is regarded as severe when the valve area is <1.0 cm^2 and mean gradient >10 mmHg, and mild when the valve area is >1.5 cm^2 and gradient <5 mmHg. The increased left atrial pressure associated with pregnancy predisposes towards arrhythmias and atrial fibrillation, and the increased heart rate then leads to heart failure. Although maternal and perinatal outcome is correlated with the NYHA classification, 74% of patients in class I/II deteriorate in pregnancy, and those with moderate to severe stenosis have increased risk of morbidity, including the need for commencement or increase in medications and hospitalization. In one series, the complication rates from mild to severe cases were 26%, 38%, and 67% respectively. Mitral regurgitation is regarded as severe when the regurgitant fraction is ≥50% or regurgitant orifice ≥0.4 cm^2, and mild if the fraction is <30% or orifice <0.20 cm^2. Surgical repair may occasionally be required due to ruptured chordae and acute deterioration in regurgitation.

The important complications (overall rate 35%) include
- atrial fibrillation and arrhythmias—up to 11%
- pulmonary oedema—up to 31%, with 60% of the cases occurring antepartum at the mean gestation of 30 weeks. Tachycardia, of which the majority (70%) were due to atrial fibrillation, can be found in 20% of the patients with pulmonary oedema
- atrial thrombosis and embolization—left atrial thrombus formation has also been reported in patients with sinus rhythm in addition to those with atrial fibrillation, so that anticoagulant treatment is now recommended for all patients with dilated left atrium irrespective of the rhythm
- fetal growth restriction—the mean birthweight is decreased to 2706 g and 2558 g, and the incidence of

growth restriction was 27% and 33%, in the moderate and severe cases respectively

- preterm labour and birth—the incidence was as high as 14%, 28%, and 33–44% from the mild to the severe cases respectively
- maternal mortality is uncommon but it can be as high as 5% in severe stenosis, and most of the patients were in NYHA class III/IV.

Aortic valve

Aortic stenosis (AS), which is most commonly due to congenital aortic valve disease, is more frequently encountered than aortic regurgitation (AR), which is usually associated with or secondary to other aortic/cardiac lesions. AS is severe if the valve area is <1.0 cm^2 or gradient >40 mmHg, and mild when valve area is >1.5 cm^2 or gradient <25 mmHg. In severe AS, if conservative management fails to relieve symptoms and pregnancy termination at the time is not an option, percutaneous aortic balloon valvotomy or surgery should be considered. Cardiac output is affected in AS, and there is increased risk of fetal growth restriction and preterm birth. For AR, severe regurgitation refers to a regurgitant fraction of ≥50% or regurgitant orifice area ≥0.30 cm^2, and mild if the fraction is <30% or orifice <0.10 cm^2. Conservative management is usually sufficient but patients with symptomatic left ventricular failure should be monitored closely, especially during the peripartum period, and surgery may have to be considered for patients refractory to medical treatment and pregnancy termination at the time is not an option.

Pulmonary valve

Pulmonary stenosis (PS) is the main lesion, which can occur alone but more frequently with other CHDs. Isolated PS rarely causes any significant effect on pregnancy outcome. For PS associated with other CHDs, the outcome is related mainly to the presence or absence of cyanosis and the type of CHD. Severe PS refers to a maximum gradient of 60 mmHg while severe regurgitation refers to a dense continuous wave Doppler signal with a steep deceleration slope.

Tricuspid valve

Tricuspid valvular lesions are rare and may be congenital in association with other lesions (Ebstein's anomaly, tricuspid atresia) or acquired (endocarditis). Regurgitation (TR) is the more common pathology, in which case connective tissue disorders such as Marfan's syndrome, and other structural heart abnormalities should be looked for. Isolated TR usually has little impact on pregnancy outcome. Severe stenosis refers to a valve area of <1.0 cm^2, while severe regurgitation refers to a vena contracta width of >0.7 cm and systolic flow reversal in hepatic veins.

Prosthetic valves

Prosthetic valve replacement is used to treat rheumatic heart disease as well as congenital valvular stenosis, most commonly involving the mitral followed by the aortic valve, and not infrequently more than one valve is involved. There are two types of prosthetic heart valves, the mechanical and the biological valves. There are two main concerns that are related to the type of valves. For mechanical valves, it is the increased risk of thromboembolism and problems associated with the use of anticoagulants. For the biological valves, these can be heterografts (porcine) or homografts (limited data in pregnant women). There is a substantial risk of structural valve deterioration

(SVD) with both types. At 10 years, the risk of SVD is between 55% and 77%. Hence the interval between valve replacement and pregnancy and the age at prosthetic valve implantation are important factors to consider. The rate of SVD is 24% on average, which can be threefold higher than non-pregnant patients. Mitral bioprosthesis has a higher rate of SVD than aortic bioprosthesis. The mortality of reoperation during pregnancy is 3.8% to 8.7%. Other complications include prosthetic valve endocarditis, thromboembolism, and sudden death.

The best approach is probably autografts, based on the Ross principle, using pulmonary autograft for aortic valve replacement. When inserted in children, the valve increases in size with growth of the children. The limited available data suggest that the autograft is associated with lower risks of thromboembolism, infective endocarditis, and need for reoperation. An early series of 14 pregnancies in eight women reported no valve-related complications during pregnancy, and no pregnancy-induced effect on the function of the pulmonary valve autograft or right-sided homograft. Rheumatic valvulitis can occur in the autograft in patients with rheumatic heart disease, and other reported complications included peripartum cardiomyopathy (PPCM) and valvular obstruction.

Complex and surgically corrected CHDs

These patients, especially those who have undergone surgery, are particularly prone to have arrhythmias, which can lead to functional deterioration. Those with atrial surgery, such as the Mustard or Fontan procedure, and those with right ventricular impairment, are vulnerable to atrial flutter. Surgical correction for tetralogy of Fallot (TOF) may increase the risk of atrial flutter or ventricular tachycardia arising from the right ventricular outflow tract.

For TOF, there is increased fetal loss, the majority of which are in the form of miscarriages (27%), and a 6% incidence of cardiac and other congenital anomalies. In women with unrepaired TOF, the incidence of miscarriage and small-for-gestational age infants were 20% and 30% respectively. Unrepaired TOF and morphological pulmonary artery abnormality impact on birthweight. Even in women with surgically corrected TOF, there was a 21% spontaneous miscarriage rate, and among the successful pregnancies, cardiac complications occurred in 12%, but there was no clear relationship between cardiac characteristics of the mother with perinatal complications, but there was a 2.2% risk of recurrence for CHD. Other exceptional causes reported included coronary artery spasm, Kawasaki disease, and aortic prosthetic valve thrombosis. Coronary artery spasm may be induced with drugs such as methylergometrine, ergonovine, and even bromocriptine. Acute myocardial infarction (AMI) in the presence of morphologically normal coronary arteries might be due to transient thrombus and emboli that had undergone resorption, with or without preceding coronary vasoconstriction. The hypercoagulation state of pregnancy, aggravated by the release of tissue-plasminogen activator inhibitor at the time of placental separation, could be a contributing factor. Anecdotal reports of myocardial ischaemia and infarction has been reported with the use of betasympathomimetics, with/without the addition of nifedipine, for the treatment of preterm labour. This potential complication must be borne in mind in treating preterm labour even in patients without known heart diseases.

Pulmonary hypertension can arise from CHD with a left to right shunt as in ventricular septal defect, which can result in the Eisenmenger syndrome, or as an idiopathic primary event. Maternal mortality is 30–50%, usually due to further increase in pulmonary vascular resistance consequent to thrombosis or fibrinoid necrosis, which can develop rapidly in the peripartum and postpartum period with little forewarning. In Eisenmenger syndrome, right to left shunting is increased during pregnancy due to the decrease in systemic vascular resistance and right ventricular overload.

For all types of cyanotic CHD, the overall maternal mortality is 2%, and there is high risk of complications such as infective endocarditis, arrhythmias, congestive heart failure, and thromboembolism. Adverse pregnancy outcomes include spontaneous miscarriage (50%), preterm delivery, fetal growth restriction, and pre-eclampsia (up to 50%).

Dextrocardia is uncommon, with an incidence of 1 per 5000–20 000 live births. The condition includes isolated dextrocardia as well as situs inversus. There is apparently no maternal cardiac deterioration or obstetric complications, and all cases of fetal growth restriction belonged to the patients with situs inversus (67%).

Cardiomyopathies and myocarditis
There are three main categories of cardiomyopathy. The commonest is PPCM, followed by cardiomyopathies due to other conditions (hypertrophic, dilated, hypertensive, endocrine related, such as thyroid and diabetic, infection, and connective diseases), and cardiomyopathy of unknown type.

Peripartum cardiomyopathy
This condition is diagnosed mainly by exclusion, and the diagnostic criteria are
* cardiac failure developing in the last month of pregnancy or within 5 months of delivery
* absence of an identifiable cause for the cardiac failure
* absence of recognizable heart disease prior to the last month of pregnancy
* left ventricular systolic dysfunction on echocardiography, such as depressed shortening fraction or ejection fraction.

Recently, it was reported that among patients with a history of cardiomyopathy diagnosed during pregnancy that fulfilled the traditional diagnostic criteria for PPCM, one-fifth were diagnosed earlier than the last month of pregnancy, and that there was no difference between patients diagnosed earlier versus those diagnosed within the last month of pregnancy with respect to maternal demographics, associated conditions, left ventricular ejection fraction, rate and time of recovery, and outcome. Therefore, some of the cases categorized as cardiomyopathy of unknown cause might have represented the continuum of a spectrum of the same disease. The actual incidence of PPCM could therefore be higher than the reported incidence of between 1 per 1485 to 1 per 15 000 pregnancies, and a reasonable estimate is 1 per 3000–4000 live births. The classical risk factors are multiparity, advanced age, multifetal pregnancy, pre-eclampsia/gestational hypertension, and Black women. Endomyocardial biopsies have consistently revealed features of myocarditis with the highest incidence of 100%, which could be due to an underlying viral infection, or autoimmune response. Coincident with clinical improvement was the resolution of the myocarditis. The finding of myocarditis is dependent on the interval from onset of symptoms, and the focal nature of the inflammatory infiltrates may give rise to false-negative results.

Evidence of a maternal inflammatory reaction and associated cell death in PPCM is suggested by the significantly elevated plasma levels of C-reactive protein (CRP), tumour necrosis factor (TNF)-α, and Fas/Apo-1 (an apoptosis-signalling surface receptor that triggers cell death) at diagnosis. In fact, baseline CRP was correlated positively with baseline left ventricular end-diastolic and end-systolic diameters and inversely with left ventricular ejection fraction. Normalization of left ventricular ejection fraction occurred in 54% and was more likely in patients with left ventricular ejection fraction ˇ30% at diagnosis, and maternal mortality was 9%.

Hypertrophic cardiomyopathy
These women tolerated pregnancy well, and no complications were reported with either general or regional anaesthesia.

Lymphocytic myocarditis
This is extremely rare but case fatality has been reported. The case presented with nausea, vomiting, and hepatic dysfunction in the first trimester, and deteriorated rapidly with cardiopulmonary arrest.

Cardiac arrhythmias
In the general population, arrhythmias can be found on Holter recordings in up to 60% of normal individuals up to the age of 40 years, and symptomatic atrial re-entrant and atrioventricular nodal re-entry tachycardias are more common in females. Furthermore, in pregnancy, the heart rate increases by 25%, especially in the third trimester, and ectopic beats and non-sustained arrhythmias can be encountered in >50% of women. Therefore, palpitations and arrhythmias are often encountered in pregnancy, but the physiological adaptation of the cardiovascular and endocrine systems to pregnancy may render sustained arrhythmias more likely to develop. However, sustained tachycardias are found in 0.2–0.3%, whereas pathological bradycardias, usually due to congenital heart block, are found in <0.01% of pregnant women. The types of arrhythmias are listed below.

Bradycardia
Often due to vagal effects, especially in the second trimester when maximum vasodilation and hypotension occur, or is consequent to the supine hypotension syndrome. Rare causes include unrecognized hypothyroidism, medication effect, and congenital heart block. Spinal anaesthesia can be associated with a 13% incidence of bradycardia.

Supraventricular tachycardia (SVT)
Transient episodes may be due to an inability to adapt to pregnancy, especially in women lacking physical activities. Apart from structural abnormalities in the heart, other underlying conditions include anaemia, thyrotoxicosis, hypovolaemia, infection, and inflammation.

Atrial fibrillation and flutter
These are uncommon in pregnancy, and mostly associated with congenital and valvular heart disease, and metabolic and electrolyte disturbance. It is usually well tolerated, except in the case of mitral stenosis,

Restoration of sinus rhythm is required. The heart rate should be controlled with medications together with anticoagulation therapy.

Idiopathic ventricular tachycardia
This originates from the right ventricular outflow tract below the pulmonary valve, and usually manifests as

ectopic beats, bigemini, or short non-sustained runs of ventricular tachycardia (VT). On the ECG, the QRS complex can be a left (more frequent) or right bundle branch block pattern. There are two types of VT. Monomorphic ventricular tachycardia in the structurally abnormal heart, presenting as rapid VT, can degenerate into ventricular fibrillation and risk of sudden death. Urgent treatment is required. Polymorphic ventricular tachycardia can lead to rapid collapse and a high risk of ventricular fibrillation. Causes include electrolyte disturbance such as high magnesium level, class I and III anti-arrhythmic drugs, macrolide antibiotics, non-sedating antihistamines, antidepressants, and antipsychotics.

Cardiac arrest

This occurs in 1:30 000 deliveries, and apart from known heart diseases, other acute causes include amniotic fluid embolism, pulmonary embolism, PPCM, and acute coronary or aortic dissection. Relief of aortocaval compression often contributes to successful resuscitation.

Ischaemic heart disease/acute myocardial infarction

In the USA, a population study revealed that the rate of AMI was 6.2 per 100 000 deliveries, with a case fatality rate of 5.1%. AMI had occurred from ages 16 to 45 years and in all trimesters, but the risk is greater in older multigravidae and in the third trimester. The maternal mortality was 21%, with the highest rates in the peripartum or early postpartum period. Cardiac catheterization was performed in 45% and 37% underwent angioplasty, stent placement, or bypass surgery.

Location of infarct

- Subendocardial (37%)
- Anterior/anterolateral (25%)
- Inferior/inferolateral/inferoposterior (20%)
- Other sites (the remainder).

Underlying pathology on coronary angiographic studies

- Stenosis due to atherosclerotic disease (43%)
- Thrombus without atherosclerosis (21%)
- Dissection (16%)
- Aneurysm (4%)
- Normal findings (29%), mostly in those with peripartum AMI.

Risk factors

- Hypertension (OR 21.7)
- Thrombophilia (OR 25.6)
- Diabetes mellitus (OR 3.6)
- Smoking (OR 8.4)
- Transfusion (OR 5.1)
- Postpartum infection (OR 3.2)
- Age ˃30 years (OR increasing from 6.7, 16.0, to 15.2 for each 5-year increment above 29 years. One study revealed a 30-fold higher risk for women ˃40 years compared with <20 years).
- Drug effects: AMI has been reported with the use of ergot derivatives in the third stage and nifedipine for tocolysis.

Aortic dissection/aneurysm

Aortic dissection can occur in patients with the following conditions:
- severe hypertension
- underlying thoracic aortic aneurismal disease
- family history of aortic dissection or thoracic aneurysm
- connective tissue disorders.

In women in the reproductive age group, aortic dissection is mostly related to hereditary conditions and familial forms of aortic dissection. All ascending aortic aneurysms have similar histological changes, including four almost universal characteristics, elastolysis, non-inflammatory smooth muscle cell loss and dedifferentiation, mucoid degeneration, and medial degeneration, which are collectively known as cystic medial degeneration. The integrity and structure of the extracellular matrix within the wall of the aortic root or thoracic aorta are changed and these features are often found before the development of the dissection or aneurysm. There is altered expression of matrix metalloproteinases (MMPs) and tissue inhibitors of metalloproteinases (TIMPs) with an increased ratio of expression of MMP-1 to TIMP-1, MMP-2 to TIMP-2, and MMP-9 to TIMP-2, all of which reflect the relative degree of proteolysis. The heritable conditions are described below.

Marfan's syndrome

This is an autosomal dominant condition with variable penetrance affecting 1 in 3000–5000 live births, and is independent of race and sex. There are mutations (>100) in the fibrillin-1 gene in chromosome 15q21, but addition mutations in fibrillin-1 and the related fibrillin-2 have been reported in patients who do not fulfil the clinical diagnostic criteria. There are also overlapping manifestations with other types of if inherited connective tissue disorders. There are major and minor criteria of the musculoskeletal, ocular, cardiovascular, pulmonary, integument, and dural systems, and criteria of family or genetic history (85%). For diagnosis of an index case, major criteria in at least two different organ systems with involvement of a third system are required. For cases of mutation, one major criterion and involvement of a second organ system must be present. The cardiac features include mitral and tricuspid valve prolapse and regurgitation, aortic dilatation, regurgitation, and dissection.

The average age of presentation is 35 years. The mortality can be as high as 30% in the older patients. The prognosis is better if there is minimal cardiovascular involvement and the aortic root diameter is <4 cm.

For aortic involvement, the diagnosis can be suspected by the typical radiological appearance of the aortic root before aneurismal changes. The patients are usually normotensive, with larger sinus segment of the aortic root, and aortic regurgitation. There are several uniform characteristics in the Marfan aortic roots, including sinus segment dilation, elongated aortic cusps often with stress fenestrations over the leading edge by their respective commissures, a triangular valvular orifice at late systole, and markedly increased non-laminar flow within the aortic root space.

Ehlers–Danlos syndrome

The incidence is 1 in 5000–20 000 live births. There are at least six major types, type IV being the vascular type that is commonly associated with thoracic aortic disease, including rupture or dissection of first order branch arteries and aortic dissection and rupture. This condition is due to a mutation in the gene encoding type III procollagen (COL3A1) mapped to chromosome 2q24.3-q31. Clinical criteria include hyperextensibility of the skin, easy bruisability, characteristic facial features, hypermobility of joints, and rupture of arteries, intestines, and the uterus. The median survival is the fifth decade, most deaths resulting from arterial dissection or rupture in the thoracic or abdominal medium-sized to large vessels.

Familial forms of aortic dissection, aneurysm, or annuloaortic ectasia

There are multiple familial forms with autosomal dominant inheritance patterns and 20% of patients with aortic dissection have a first-degree relative with a similar history. The management is similar to that of Marfan's syndrome.

Biscuspid aortic valve with/without coarctation of the aorta

This is one of the most common congenital heart malformations, affecting 1–2% of the population, and features include aortic dilation, aneurysm, dissection, and coarctation of the aorta. There were data suggesting significantly increased expression of MMP-2 and MMP-9, which probably play a role in the pathogenesis. As aortic valve replacement for stenosis or regurgitation did not appear to impact on subsequent aortic dilation, the underlying problem is related to abnormalities of the media of aortic walls rather than the valves per se. The adverse outcomes are dissection, rupture, and sudden death. The histological changes are similar to those of Marfan syndrome, and similarly aortic root enlargement >4 cm, or an increase in aortic root size during pregnancy, is associated with high risk of type A dissection.

Pulmonary vascular disease

This group is rarely encountered, as pregnancy is contraindicated in view of the high maternal mortality, which peaks on days 2–9 postpartum from refractory heart failure.

The precipitating factors for deterioration include increase in pulmonary vascular resistance and volume overload. Echocardiography is not as accurate as pulmonary artery catheterization in assessing pulmonary arterial pressure as it tended to overestimate the value, leading to misclassification in 30% of patients with normal pulmonary arterial pressure.

Primary pulmonary hypertension

This condition refers to the finding of persistently increased pulmonary arterial pressure without an aetiology. It is rare but more commonly encountered in women. In general, pregnancy is contraindicated as the maternal mortality is as high as 50% but more recent data have suggested a rate of 30%. Preterm birth and fetal growth restriction are common.

Secondary pulmonary hypertension and Eisenmenger's syndrome

This is secondary to congenital and acquired disorders, and Eisenmenger's syndrome is the final stage where reversal of the left-to-right shunt, or bidirectional shunting, occurs thus resulting in cyanosis. Maternal mortality rate is 20–52%.

Aetiology

Rheumatic heart disease occurs following rheumatic fever in childhood, and with the control and prevention of rheumatic fever, its incidence has been on the decline.

The aetiology of PPCM remains uncertain, but the following have been suggested: myocarditis, abnormal immune response to pregnancy, maladaptive response to the haemodynamic stresses of pregnancy, stress-activated cytokines, prolonged tocolysis, familial, abnormalities of

relaxin, and deficiency of selenium. A recent series reported that the common associated factors were gestational hypertension (43%), tocolytic therapy (19%), and twin pregnancy (13%).

Cardiac arrhythmias can be related to a structurally normal or abnormal heart in relation to the following conditions

- CHDs: acyanotic, e.g. ASD, VSD; cyanotic, e.g. TOF; valvular, e.g. bicuspid aortic valve
- acquired heart disease: valvular heart disease, e.g. RHD, endocarditis; cardiomyopathy; degenerative disease of conducting system; acquired long QT syndrome, e.g. drugs, metabolic conditions
- congenital 'electrical-only' disease: dual AV nodal pathways causing AV nodal re-entry
- Wolf Parkinson White (WPW)/accessory pathways
- channelopathy.

Prognosis

In the literature, the incidences of various complications and adverse outcomes vary according to the period of study, the nature/combination of the lesions and functional classification, and the degree of objective assessment with imaging studies. Adverse neonatal outcome is increased overall, including birth before 37 weeks, fetal growth restriction, respiratory distress syndrome, and perinatal death.

The prognosis of some of the uncommon conditions is described here.

For cardiomyopathies, the mortality rate is related to the type of cardiomyopathy. Overall, PPCM accounted for up to 70%, whereas other cardiomyopathies and cardiomyopathy of unknown type accounted for 20% and 10% respectively. Of the deaths, 50% occurred between 43 days and 1 year postpartum, and 2% occurred before delivery. The rate was 0.88 per 100 000 live births.

For PPCM, adverse prognostic factors for maternal mortality include symptoms at >2 weeks postpartum, Black women, age >30 years, multiparity, significantly lower mean left ventricular ejection fraction and smaller LV end-diastolic diameter at diagnosis, and persistent cardiomegaly. The reported incidences of persistent cardiomegaly and progressive cardiomyopathy varied from 50% to >90%, and mean survival was <5 years. Recently it was shown that maternal mortality is associated with significantly higher Fas/Apo-1 level, which can be predicted from the NYHA functional classification and the baseline plasma level of Fas/Apo-1.

The measurement of cardiac troponin T (cTnT) within 2 weeks of the onset of PPCM was shown to correlate inversely with left ventricular failure (LVF) at follow-up, and a serum cTnT concentration of >0.04 ng/mL predicted persistent LV dysfunction with a sensitivity of 54.9% and a specificity of 90.9%.

In general, persistent LV dysfunction is found in about half of the survivors (59%). On echocardiography performed at diagnosis, a LV end-diastolic dimension of ˜6 cm and a fractional shortening value of <20% were both associated with a threefold higher risk of persistent LV dysfunction.

In general, patients with apparent full clinical recovery can still have recurrent cardiomyopathy and congestive symptoms in the subsequent pregnancies, and even normal resting LV size and function cannot preclude the possibility of reduced contractile reserve under haemodynamic stress. It was shown that in the first subsequent pregnancy among the survivors, left ventricular ejection fraction was significantly decreased in those whose LV function had returned to normal (Group 1, from 56% to 49%) as well as those with persistent LV dysfunction (Group 2, from 36% to 32%). Symptoms of heart failure and maternal mortality were 21% and 0% respectively in Group 1, and 44% and 19% respectively in Group 2. Group 2 also had higher incidences of preterm delivery (37% versus 11%) and therapeutic abortion (25% versus 4%). Women with persistent LV dysfunction should therefore avoid subsequent pregnancies due to the increased risk of morbidity and mortality.

For hypertrophic cardiomyopathy, cardiac symptoms during pregnancy were reported in 28%, mostly (90%) among women who were symptomatic before pregnancy. Symptoms deteriorated in <10% during pregnancy, and recurred in the subsequent pregnancy in 60%. Heart failure occurred in 1.6% after delivery. In general, the mothers tolerated pregnancy well, although unexplained intrauterine death had occurred in 1%.

For Marfan's syndrome, the mortality rate for type A dissection is 25%.

CARPREG risk index

For practical purposes, the following approach, which can be applied to different type of lesions, irrespective of treatment, is recommended.

Complications arising from the heart condition during and after pregnancy can be categorized into cardiac, neonatal, and obstetric events.

- Primary cardiac event is defined as pulmonary oedema, sustained symptomatic tachyarrhythmia or bradyarrhythmia requiring treatment, stroke, cardiac arrest, or cardiac death.
- Secondary cardiac event is defined as a decline in NYHA class (~2 classes) compared with baseline, and the need for urgent invasive cardiac procedures during pregnancy or within 6 months after delivery.
- Neonatal event includes any of the following: premature birth (<37 weeks' gestation), small-for-gestational age (SGA, birthweight <10th percentile), respiratory distress syndrome, intraventricular haemorrhage, fetal death (~20 weeks gestation), or neonatal death.
- Obstetric event include the following: non-cardiac death, pregnancy-induced hypertension/pre-eclampsia, and postpartum haemorrhage.

The incidence of cardiac events varied from 13% to 19.4%, most of which occurred in the antepartum period and the commonest were pulmonary oedema and/or cardiac arrhythmia. Maternal death was 1%. The incidence of neonatal events was 20% to 27.8%, with premature births and SGA infants being the commonest complications. The recurrence of CHD overall was 7%. The fetal or neonatal death rate was 2% without and 4% with one or more predictors (see below). The effect of the predictors are further aggravated by obstetric risk factors, extremes of maternal age (<20 or >35 years), smoking, multifetal pregnancy, and anticoagulant therapy. For obstetric events, pregnancy-induced hypertension and postpartum haemorrhage complicated 4% and 3% of the pregnancies.

Application of the CARPREG risk index

A number of predictors or risk indices (CARPREG risk index) have been established, and each of these is assigned a score of 1. Good correlation has been shown between actual and predicted rates. The actual primary cardiac events rates with 0, 1, and ~2 of the original predictors were shown to be 5%, 27%, and 75%. It has been estimated that a 1-point increase in the CARPREG index was associated with a fivefold increase in the risk of maternal cardiac complications. For cardiac event rates, the original and additional predictors are listed below:

Original CARPREG predictors

- Prior cardiac event (including transient ischaemic attack or stroke before pregnancy) or arrhythmia
- NYHA functional class >2 or cyanosis
- Left heart obstruction (mitral valve area <2 cm^2, aortic area <1.5 cm^2, or peak left ventricular outflow tract gradient >30 mmHg by echocardiography)
- Reduced systemic ventricular systolic function (ejection fraction <40%).

Additional predictors

- Smoking history
- Subpulmonary ventricular dysfunction and/or severe pulmonary regurgitation.
  For neonatal events, the predictors are
- NYHA functional class >2 or cyanosis
- heparin/warfarin during pregnancy
- smoking
- multiple gestation
- left heart obstruction.
  For pregnancy-induced hypetension/pre-eclampsia, the predictors are
- nulliparity
- systemic lupus erythematosus
- coarctation of the aorta.
  For postpartum haemorrhage, the predictors are
- peripartum heparin or warfarin
- cyanosis.

Clinical approach
Pre-pregnancy/conception counselling
Basic knowledge and understanding

- Clarify patient's wishes for pregnancy
- Check their knowledge on their treatment, occupational issues, dental hygiene, exercise tolerance, smoking.

Risk assessment

- NYHA classification
- Repeat echocardiography, assess severity of lesion
- History of complications e.g. thromboembolism
- Other health issues, e.g. anaemia, smoking
- Relevant complications in previous pregnancies.

Optimise treatment

- Determine effect of current treatment
- Assess potential teratogenicity and other risks of current medications
- Arrange early surgical treatment, e.g. balloon valvotomy or valvular replacement before conception if current medical treatment is inadequate
- Appropriate supplementation, e.g. folic acid before conception.

Obstetric assessment

- Past obstetric history

- Impact of previous obstetric complications and outcome on future pregnancies.

Genetic counselling
- Assess likelihood of inheritance of maternal cardiac condition by offspring.
- Look for other familial genetic and hereditary conditions that might impact on fetal outcome.
- Identify current risk factors, e.g. advanced maternal age.
- Review previous pregnancy losses/outcome, e.g. fetal hydrops due to Hb Bart's disease.

Assessment of family and social support
- Check socioeconomic condition
- Assess occupational environment
- Assess marital relationship
- Assess relationship with family/relatives, likelihood of support for own family and children from relatives and friends, especially if prolonged hospitalization is necessary
- Help in childcare after delivery.

In the management of women in the reproductive age group who are affected with heart disease, the cardiologist should document clearly and in regular intervals in the medical notes the patients' desire and plan for pregnancy, since their plans as well as their cardiac status can change with time. If pregnancy is considered to be acceptable, their cardiac status should be optimized and any medications prescribed are changed to those with the lowest likelihood of teratogenicity and fetal complications when pregnancy is contemplated. If pregnancy is contraindicated, this should be made clear to the patients and documented. In either case, the patients should be referred to a prepregnancy counselling clinic managed by, preferably, a maternal–fetal medicine specialist who would be able to assess the patients' conditions, and give appropriate advice and treatment, including those on contraception. Subsequent follow-up assessment in the obstetric clinic must be individualized, and an early appointment at the first sign of pregnancy should be provided as appropriate, especially in patients on warfarin for whom a changeover to heparin is contemplated. Early appointment allows accurate dating of the pregnancy and provides the opportunity for baseline investigations and assessment, and arrangement for prenatal diagnosis.

Antenatal care

Clinical assessment and management
In the first antenatal visit the family history of heart disease and significant past history should be obtained, if these were not taken before. The family history and symptoms associated with previous pregnancies (if present) should be rechecked when symptoms of heart disease appear or worsen. Many of the symptoms of heart disease are physiological features of normal pregnancy, such as ankle oedema, a slight tachycardia, and a soft systolic murmur especially at the pulmonary area. In patients without a history of heart disease, further assessment and investigations are warranted when unusual symptoms are reported. These include chest pain, dyspnoea on exertion (especially if progressive), orthopnoea, paroxysmal nocturnal dyspnoea, persistent cough, anorexia, extensive oedema, and easy fatigability. For patients with history of heart disease, these specific symptoms should be elicited in each visit and the relevant physical examination performed when necessary. On examination, auscultation of the heart and chest

should always be performed in addition to counting the peripheral pulse. General features such as jugular venous congestion, tachycardia, and peripheral oedema may be normal features of pregnancy. Abnormal features include tachypnoea, hepatomegaly, hepatojugular reflux, ascites, oedema of 3-plus or more, mental status changes, and thromboemboli phenomena, and a gallop rhythm, diastolic murmur or systolic murmur of grade 3 and above, loud P2, and rales, on auscultation.

Patients with a history of heart disease should be seen in the antenatal clinic at 4-weekly intervals initially till 24–28 weeks, then fortnightly afterwards till 32–34 weeks, and then weekly thereafter. Apart from features of cardiac deterioration, one should watch out for fetal growth restriction, preterm labour, pregnancy-induced hypertension, and other conditions that can lead to cardiac deterioration such as anaemia and infection. When features suggestive of deterioration in cardiac function appear, or at the first signs of obstetric complications, the patient should be admitted for assessment and further investigations. Following discharge from hospital, the subsequent antenatal and postnatal visits of the patient should be arranged at a conjoined medical–obstetric clinic in a tertiary centre.

Antenatal inpatient assessment should be arranged in case of suspicion of deterioration or complications. In addition to the standard examination and investigations, further assessment include daily bodyweight, temperature, blood pressure and pulse rate monitoring (screen for arrhythmias), charting fluid intake and output, pulse oximetry recording, spirometry, repeat ECG, chest X-ray, blood tests, and screening for infection. Cardiac consultation and echocardiography will be performed both in patients with and without a history of symptoms of heart disease for prognostication. A 24-hour rhythm tape should be arranged if arrhythmia is suspected. After assessment, a management plan should be drawn up, and the appropriate management team be formed under the coordination of the obstetrician in charge or preferably under a maternal–fetal medicine specialist. The team may include a neonatologist, anaesthetist, haematologist, physiotherapist, and a clinical psychologist or psychiatrist if necessary. The points to be laid down in documentation include the use of medications and monitoring of the therapeutic effects, especially drugs that can affect the fetus like anticoagulants, the frequency, methods, and venue of the follow-up assessment, predicted complications and adverse outcomes with the appropriate response plans, fetal monitoring and assessment, timing and mode of delivery, anaesthetic concerns and treatment, preventive measures such as for thromboembolic complications, and maternal psychological wellbeing. The patient and her partner should be fully informed, and, if possible, be involved in the decision-making process. The wishes of the patient should be respected. Both the maternal and fetal status should be regularly reviewed so that the management plan can be revised when necessary.

Investigations
- General aspects: chest X-ray with shielding of the abdomen can help to reveal abnormal heart size or contour, and pulmonary congestion or other lesions. Baseline blood tests include complete blood count, renal and liver function, and blood gas and acid–base measurement. Urine, sputum, and blood culture should be performed according to clinical suspicion.
- Electrocardiogram (ECG): a baseline ECG is helpful for future comparisons, and help in documenting arrhythmias.

In normal women, the ECG usually shows a normal sinus or sinus tachycardia rhythm. Normal changes include decreased PR, QRS, and QT intervals, left axis deviation, Q wave and inverted T wave in the inferior leads, ectopics and non-sustained atrial arrhythmias. Abnormal features include left ventricular hypertrophy, inverted T waves, Q waves, and non-specific ST-T changes, and delta waves of the Wolff–Parkinson–White (WPW) syndrome. A 12-lead ECG should be recorded during symptoms, and 24/48-hour Holter monitor may be necessary, but the documentation may be difficult owing to the frequency of the attacks and the presence of precipitating events, and whether the patients are taking normal activities or resting. For outpatients, a diary and patient-activated event recorder may help to establish the diagnosis.

- Echocardiography: in normal pregnancy, there is mild ventricular enlargement with physiological regurgitation in most of the valves in the absence of valvular disease. Serial echocardiographic examination is warranted in conditions where structural changes and functional deterioration cannot be easily determined from physical signs and symptoms alone. Echocardiography allows the serial assessment of the dimensions of the chambers, particularly the LV at different stages of the cardiac cycle and to document LV function and dysfunction, measuring valvular area, flow gradient, and measurement of the aortic root to exclude aneurysm.

Arrhythmias are frequently encountered in pregnancy. The following approach can be arranged in the clinic:
- confirm the diagnosis, using 24-hour (Holter) recordings if necessary;
- rule out underlying heart disease with echocardiography
- exclude systemic disorders including thyroid dysfunction, haemorrhage, pulmonary embolism, infection, and inflammatory state, through appropriate examination and investigations.

Fetal assessment

There are two aspects. In general, women with heart disease are at increased risk of fetal growth restriction and preterm labour. Fetal growth should be monitored with serial ultrasound scanning. Fetal wellbeing should be assessed and monitored if there is maternal functional deterioration, and/or the presence of obstetric complications. In patients with CHD, there is a variable risk of recurrence. While the overall incidence is usually cited as 3–5%, more recent findings suggested much higher risks in relation to the type of maternal lesion as follows:
- Marfan's syndrome: 50%
- aortic stenosis: 15–17.9%
- pulmonary stenosis: 6.5%
- ventricular septal defect: 9.5–15.6%
- atrial septal defect: 4.6–11.0%
- patent ductus arteriosus: 4.1%
- coarctation of the aorta: 14.1%
- tetralogy of Fallot: 2.6%.

Therefore, appropriate referral for detailed ultrasound scanning and prenatal diagnosis is warranted. The availability of first trimester screening for fetal aneuploidy using nuchal translucency measurement can also help to screen out fetuses with CHD, 90% of which are associated with increased nuchal translucency. First trimester ultrasound scan may identify some of the significant heart malformations, but a detailed ultrasound scan for fetal cardiac and other anomalies should always be arranged for all patients with heart disease. The option of therapeutic abortion should be made available for the parents before 24 weeks gestation should significant cardiac and/or other anomalies be found. There is little point in jeopardizing the safety of the mother by continuing the pregnancy in the presence of significant fetal anomalies, even if these are compatible with neonatal survival, because looking after such a child, as well as caring for the rest of the family or coping with employment, would be too demanding especially for the mother whose health is already affected by the underlying heart disease. If therapeutic abortion is indicated, medical termination with prostaglandin analogues such as misoprostol would be preferable.

Treatment

Since the same groups of medications are used to treat different conditions, medical treatments are grouped together for discussion. Owing to increased plasma volume, protein binding, and drug metabolism, in pregnancy, the dose of medications may need to be regularly adjusted to maintain therapeutic level for adequate treatment.

General measures

- Bed rest with non-medication prophylaxis for deep vein thrombosis (DVT) such as physiotherapy and pressure stocking
- Salt and fluid restriction, ensuring a balanced intake and output but avoid dehydration and haemoconcentration which may be detrimental to placental perfusion and increase the risk of DVT
- Adequate nutrition, including iron and vitamin supplements to prevent anaemia
- Antenatal exercise, which can be performed on the bed, and is important in minimizing muscle wasting in the lower body following bed rest, so that the ability for vaginal delivery would not be seriously compromised
- Prevention of constipation by increasing fibre intake and avoiding dehydration, as the Valsalva manoeuvre increases the risk of bradycardia and syncope
- Sleeping in the lateral position helps to avoid the supine hypotension syndrome
- Vagotonic manoeuvres such as carotid sinus massage can terminate episodes of tachycardias
- Oxygen may be necessary in symptomatic patients, especially those with functional deterioration, and during labour and delivery
- Resuscitation of cardiac arrest may be necessary and the cardiac arrest team should be called. Relief of aortocaval compression using a 'Cardiff wedge' on the right side, raising the right hip, or manual displacement of the uterus to the left side, may contribute to a successful resuscitation. Early intubation reduces the risk of aspiration. Peri-arrest Caesarean section also aids resuscitation and facilitates external cardiac massage, in addition to possibly saving the fetus.

Medical treatment

Diuretics
Furosemide
This is used to decrease congestion and blood volume in valvular heart disease and heart failure in cardiomyopathy. Excessive or prolonged use can deplete maternal

intravascular volume and decrease placental perfusion. Maternal potassium level should be monitored and supplement may be needed. For the fetus there is risk of hypoglycaemia, hyponatraemia, hypokalaemia, and thrombocytopenia. The usual dose is 20–40 mg daily by mouth. For acute treatment, intravenous boluses of 10–40 mg can be given.

Antihypertensives
Methyldopa
This is considered to be the safest antihypertensive agent in pregnancy, well tolerated by the mother and with no major adverse effects in the fetus. The usual dose is from 500 mg to 4 g daily orally in divided doses.

Beta-blockers
This lowers blood pressure and controls heart rate in case of supraventricular tachycardia, and atrial fibrillation in clinically significant mitral stenosis. It is also indicated in Marfan's syndrome, aortic aneurysm, myocardial ischaemia, and hypertrophic cardiomyopathy. It is the drug of choice for the WPW syndrome, as digoxin and calcium channel blockers may accelerate conduction through the accessory pathway leading to deterioration of the maternal condition. It is effective for VT with a left bundle branch block pattern. It has been associated with fetal growth restriction, bradycardia, apnoea, hypoglycaemia, and hyperbilirubinaemia in the newborn. This group is safe for breast feeding. Examples include propranolol, acebutolol, labetolol, metoprolol, and atenolol. Metoprolol is preferred to atenolol, which is associated with a higher incidence of fetal growth restriction. The dose may need to be titrated to achieve heart rate control, usually 100–200 mg daily in one or two divided doses. Selective beta-1-blockers are preferred since they are less likely to interfere with beta-2-mediated uterine relaxation. .

Vasodilators
Hydralazine
This is indicated in aortic regurgitation and LV dysfunction, usually in a dose of 75–150 mg daily in divided doses. There are no major adverse fetal effects.

Nitrates
This can be used in myocardial ischaemia and infarction, hypertension, and pulmonary oedema, but in pregnant women it is used to decrease venous congestion. There are minimal fetal effects.

Angiotensin-converting-enzyme inhibitors
This group of agents is contraindicated in pregnancy because of the well-documented effect of fetal urogenital defects, renal failure, anaemia, growth restriction, and death.

Antiarrhythmics
Digoxin
This is used for suppression of supraventricular tachycardia (SVT) and control of the ventricular rate in atrial fibrillation associated with severe mitral stenosis. There are no major fetal adverse effects and is safe for breastfeeding. The usual dose is 0.25 mg daily, and one or two rest days per week may be necessary since it can accumulate with long-term use. Maternal serum potassium level should be monitored especially if a diuretic is given, and potassium supplement may be required. There is no evidence of significant fetal side-effects.

Adenosine
This is used for immediate conversion of SVT, using escalating IV boluses up to a maximum of 18–24 mg until the target is achieved. Most women respond to 6–12 mg due to a reduction in adenosine deaminase. It is possible that an arrhythmia may be accelerated due to enhanced conduction down an accessory pathway, so that treatment should be monitored and resuscitation equipment is available during its administration. Owing to its very short half-life, there are no adverse fetal effects and is safe for breastfeeding.

Quinidine
This is used occasionally for the suppression of atrial or ventricular arrhythmias. It can have oxytocic effect at high dose and may lead to premature labour. Rare complications include fetal eighth nerve damage and neonatal thrombocytopenia, but is safe for breastfeeding.

Procainamide
This is used occasionally for the suppression of atrial or ventricular arrhythmias like atrial fibrillation. It is safe for short-term use, but lupus-like syndrome, gastrointestinal disturbance, hypotension, and agranulocytosis may be associated with long-term use. It is safe for the fetus and breastfeeding.

Amiodarone
This is used to suppress atrial or ventricular arrhythmias in high-risk patients but is seldom used in pregnancy because it can be associated with fetal hypo- and hyperthyroidism, goitre, growth restriction, and preterm birth.

Lignocain
This is indicated for VT with IV administration. It is safe for pregnancy and breast feeding.

Sotalol
It is a preferred drug for treating atrial fibrillation. Transient fetal bradycardia may occur but it is generally safe for pregnancy and breastfeeding.

Verapamil
This is now the second-line IV medication for SVT, using doses up to 10 mg without effect on fetal heart rate. It can also control ventricular rate in atrial fibrillation, and is effective in VT with a right bundle branch block pattern. It may cause maternal hypotension and fetal distress with rapid injection, but no other adverse fetal side-effects have been reported. It is safe for breastfeeding.

DC cardioversion
This is indicated in VT. It is safe in all stages of pregnancy, with only a small risk of inducing fetal arrhythmia due to the small amount of current reaching the fetus, but the fetus should be monitored before and during the procedure. In the third trimester, general anaesthesia and intubation may be preferred to avoid problems with the airway and aspiration of gastric contents.

Implantable cardioverter defibrillators
Good maternal and fetal outcomes have been reported in pregnant women with this device. Fetal monitoring is advisable after each therapy, but fetal distress is usually related to the hypotension associated with the arrhythmias. This is an option for women who failed pharmacological treatment, and the leads can be positioned using ECG guidance, thus avoiding fetal radiation exposure.

Cardiac pacing

This is indicated in bradycardia due to heart block to ensure an adequate heart response to the demands of pregnancy. Temporary overdrive pacing may be life saving in polymorphic VT.

Anticoagulant and antithrombotic agents

Unlike in the case of prevention of DVT and pulmonary embolism, anticoagulant therapy for cardiac indications has to be more aggressive in the sense that an adequate therapeutic level must be achieved in order to minimize the chance of thromboembolic complications, especially for patients with prosthetic heart valves. The indications for anticoagulant therapy are

• mechanical prosthetic heart valves
• atrial fibrillation
• tight mitral stenosis with dilated right atrium
• cardiomyopathies.

Warfarin

The dose of warfarin is adjusted to maintain an international normalized ratio (INR) of between 2.5 and 3.5. Warfarin crosses the placenta, and its use, especially if it is given between the sixth and twelfth weeks of gestation, may lead to 'warfarin embryopathy' in the offspring, with an overall incidence of 3.9% among the total exposed pregnancies and 6.4% to 7.4% among the total live births. This is characterized by nasal hypoplasia and stippled epiphyses. Other features include central nervous system (hydrocephalus, microcephaly, mental retardation), cleft lip and cleft palate, and eye and other miscellaneous abnormalities, some of which are attributable to warfarin exposure in later gestation. There is also increased risk of other fetal complications that include spontaneous miscarriage (24.7%) and fetal wastage (33.6%). The overall incidence of fetal complications is apparently dose related, being 15% and 88% among pregnancies in women taking a daily dose of 5 mg versus >5 mg, and the probability of fetal complications is correlated with the dose (Vitale *et al* 1999). To minimize the fetal risk, including that of haemorrhage during and after birth, the use of heparin in the first trimester and in the last 2–3 weeks before delivery is generally recommended. The combined warfarin–heparin regimen is associated with a spontaneous abortion rate of 14.7–42.2%, a fetal wastage rate of 16.3–44.4%, and a congenital anomalies rate of 0–11.1%. Despite achieving the therapeutic target as assessed by the INR, warfarin cannot prevent maternal valve thrombosis (3.9%), while the use of heparin from the sixth to the twelfth weeks' gestation was associated with a risk of 9.2%), while the corresponding incidence of maternal death were 1.8% and 4.2% respectively. Major bleeding events occurred in 2.5% of all pregnancies, usually in the peripartum period.

Heparin

Given subcutaneously, it is usually considered to be less effective than warfarin in patients with prosthetic heart valves, as the incidence of thromboembolism in pregnant patients with mechanical prosthesis is fourfold higher, with a higher maternal mortality and no improvement in fetal outcome. In general unfractionated heparin is used, either in an adjusted-dose regimen (to maintain the activated partial thromboplastin time at 2.0–2.5 times control) or low-dose regimen (15 000 units per day). The spontaneous abortion and fetal wastage rates were 25.0% and 43.8%, and 20.0% and 40.0%, for the adjusted-dose and low-dose regimens respectively. The congenital anomalies rate was 0% for both regimens. The incidence of thromboembolic

complications was 25% and 60% for the adjusted-dose and low-dose regimens respectively, respectively, while that of maternal death was 6.7% and 40% respectively.

Recently the use of LMWH, including nadroparin 0.1 mL/10 kg twice daily, enoxaparin 40 mg daily to 80 mg twice daily, tinzaparin 175 units/kg daily, and dalteparin 100 units/kg twice daily, with or without monitoring with the peak anti-Xa level 3 hours after injection to keep it between 0.4–1.0 units/mL, has been reported for this purpose. There were both successful cases and cases of thromboembolic complications, but the numbers are too small for any meaningful conclusion. The advantages of LMWH are reduced incidence of heparin-induced thrombocytopenia, allergy, osteoporosis, ease of administration, and monitoring of anticoagulant effect is usually not required. However, each LMWH is unique with different bioavailability, half life, and safety profile, so that this group of agents must be used with caution and on an individual basis until data from randomized controlled trials of adequate size are available.

Antiplatelet agents

Aspirin and dipyridamole have also been reported as the only treatment for patients with prosthetic heart valves. Although the incidences of thromboembolic complications and maternal death were 29% and 4.3% respectively, those for spontaneous abortion, congenital fetal anomalies, and fetal wastage were lower than the aforementioned regimens. Nevertheless, the use of these agents alone should not be recommended as a reasonable alternative to the above regimens and more data from prospective studies are required. Aspirin is more often given as adjunct to heparin and LMWH, prescribed in a low dose that varies between 60 and 100 mg daily in different regimens. High doses are not given as the therapeutic effect is not proven, and this approach is associated with fetal complications including haemorrhage, prolonged labour, and growth restriction.

The recommendation from the American College of Chest Physicians (ACCP) is shown in Table 8.17.1.

Surgical treatment

Balloon valvuloplasty/valvotomy can be considered in tight mitral/aortic stenosis with symptomatic deterioration and refractory to medical treatment. The optimal timing for the procedure is the second trimester.

Valvular repair/replacement should be avoided in pregnancy. If such surgery is indicated before delivery, there is a high chance of fetal death or hypoxic damage, miscarriage, or premature labour. Since fetal prognosis is poor, other options such as therapeutic termination or elective preterm delivery before the cardiac surgery should be considered, and a management plan involving all the relevant specialties be made following thorough discussion. The plan is then recommended to the patient who should be involved in the final decision.

Surgical repair for special conditions

Surgical repair is necessary in Marfan's syndrome, but the aorta is inherently fragile and difficult to work with. Replacement of the aortic root and ascending aorta, with composite mechanical valved-conduits using the modified Bentall approach, is associated with a mortality rate of 0–2.6% and 5.6–11.7% for elective and emergent replacement. Therefore this should be arranged before pregnancy is contemplated. The conduits are at risk of endocarditis and thromboembolic disease, and are less ideal than the

Table 8.17.1 Recommendations from the American College of Chest Physicians (ACCP)

Condition	Anticoagulation	Therapeutic aim
Rheumatic mitral disease and atrial fibrillation, history of systemic embolism	Long-term oral anticoagulant (OAC)	INR 2.5
Rheumatic mitral disease and atrial fibrillation, history of systemic embolism, has systemic embolism while on OAC achieving therapeutic aim	OAC plus aspirin 75–100 mg daily or dipyridamole 400 mg daily	
Mitral valve prolapse (MVP) without complications	Nil recommended	
MVP with documented transient ischaemic attacks	Aspirin 50–162 mg daily	
Mechanical prosthetic aortic valve	OAC	INR 2.5
Mechanical prosthetic mitral valve: tilting disc/bileaflet valves	OAC	INR 3.0
Mechanical prosthetic mitral valve: caged ball/caged disk valves	OAC plus aspirin 75–100 mg	INR 3.0
Bioprosthetic valve (mitral or aortic) within 3 months of insertion	OAC	INR 2.5
Bioprosthetic valve (mitral or aortic) in sinus rhythm	Long-term aspirin 75–100 mg	

newer approach using valve-sparing aortic root replacement techniques involving remodelling or reimplantation which has a survival rate of 90–92%. In a series of four patients with acute type A aortic dissection during pregnancy, three underwent composite graft replacement combined with reimplantation of the coronary artery and aortic valve replacement and the other had aortic valve replacement with coronary bypass grafting of the right coronary artery. Three patients had aortic arch repair utilizing antegrade cerebral perfusion and deep hypothermia with total circulatory arrest. The three patients with cardiac surgery performed either combined with Caesarean section (n=2) or after vaginal delivery (n=1) survived and were discharged with their babies in good condition, although the remaining patient with the fetus *in situ* during cardiac surgery had fetal demise just after surgery and then died 4 days later with disseminated intravascular coagulation and multi-organ failure. Therefore, Caesarean section with concomitant cardiac surgery appears to give better results in this situation.

Operative intervention in Ehlers–Danlos syndrome should be avoided because the vessels tear easily.

Management of labour and delivery
Two issues have to be considered separately, that is the timing and the mode of delivery. As the safe delivery of the infant with minimal maternal consequences is the penultimate objective, labour and delivery should be an event that is planned or anticipated well beforehand, and the necessary precautions must be undertaken accordingly.

Timing of delivery
For well-controlled and asymptomatic women, the pregnancy is likely to be carried to 37 weeks or later. In the absence of any obstetric complications, it is preferable to allow spontaneous labour at term. In case of obstetric indications for early delivery, the date of delivery should be decided ahead of time and appropriate consultation (with anaesthetist and cardiologist) and arrangement for peri- and postpartum care, such as the setting up of invasive monitoring and an ICU bed, must be organized beforehand. The delivery should be conducted in the daytime under the charge of the MFM team and not left to the on-call team to deal with a complicated patient having what is to them unfamiliar problems.

Mode of delivery
In the absence of obstetric or medical contraindications, vaginal delivery is preferred to Caesarean section, and a planned induction of labour can be safely conducted as for any high-risk patients with close maternal and fetal monitoring. However, if after careful assessment the mother or fetus is thought to be unable to withstand the stress of labour, or that the duration of labour may be uncertain due to an unfavourable cervix, or that the delivery could be difficult due to cephalopelvic disproportion, an elective Caesarean section to minimize the time required for the delivery may be in the best interest of the mother and infant. The most important concern is to avoid having to perform an emergency or crash caesarean section for maternal or fetal distress in a mother with significant underlying cardiac disorder, as there would be considerable maternal and fetal risks. Another concern is the difficulty in timing the administration of medications which are necessary for the mother but which would increase the risk of complications, such as anticoagulants. An elective caesarean section would be preferred under such circumstance.

Intrapartum management
Invasive monitoring: the decision for the use of invasive maternal monitoring during labour and the early postpartum period should be left to the cardiologist and ICU specialist, but this is unnecessary for most of the women. Monitoring of blood pressure, pulse rate, SaO_2, and respiratory rate is often sufficient for the mother, and cardiotocography is necessary for the fetus. If internal monitoring of the mother or fetus is indicated, watch out and cover for potential problems such as bleeding and infection.

Fluid balance: fluid restriction in the intrapartum and postpartum period is important to avoid fluid overload and iatrogenic pulmonary oedema. Diuresis induced with intravenous furosemide may be necessary after delivery if fluid intake significantly exceeds output, in order to prevent pulmonary oedema. An indwelling Foley catheter is preferred especially if epidural analgesia is given. The catheter should be removed in the second stage to avoid trauma inflicted by the balloon on the bladder sphincter and urethra.

Antibiotic cover: although routine antibiotic cover for the prophylaxis of bacterial endocarditis is considered unnecessary, the use of antibiotic cover should be individualized, taking into consideration the duration of rupture of membranes, internal monitoring, e.g. fetal scalp electrode or intrauterine pressure cannula, operative delivery, and vaginal/perineal lacerations or abdominal wound haematoma. Clinical suspicion of chorioamnionitis and previous positive vaginal culture are other indications. Intravenous antibiotic administration is necessary since anticoagulant therapy is often required in these patients.

Analgesia: adequate analgesia is necessary for labour management in cardiac patients, and epidural analgesia is the preferred option except for patients on anticoagulant treatment, in which case all intramuscular injections should also be avoided.

Prevention of postpartum haemorrhage: the usual prophylaxis for postpartum haemorrhage should be given. Oxytocin infusion should be given in a higher concentration with reduced volume of infusion fluid. Any ergot-containing medications should be avoided. Careful repair of episiotomy or caesarean section wound with good haemostasis is necessary, and additional measures like pressure dressing for the abdominal wound and packing for the vaginal wound may be necessary for the first day to avoid haematoma collection, especially in patients who has been or will be on anticoagulant therapy.

Postnatal management and breastfeeding

The management in the postpartum period follows the principle for all high-risk patients who require specific medications such as anticoagulants, antihypertensives, and antibiotics, etc. The complications to watch out for are

- infections
- wound complications
- cardiac decompensation or related complications
- thromboembolic complications
- postpartum depression.

The postpartum stay in the hospital should be flexible and premature discharge from the hospital should be avoided. Breastfeeding is not contraindicated but this should not be enforced either. One should ensure that the mother can look after herself and is coping with her baby before discharge, and assessment for depression using instruments such as the Edinburgh Postpartum Depression Scale should be performed before discharge. Early postnatal follow-up is essential, not only for patients requiring adjustment of warfarin dose, but also for patients requiring other medications. Again a flexible approach with assessment at a special clinic run by MFM specialist would ensure the optimal care for these patients.

Further reading

Adamson DL, Nelson-Piercy C. Managing palpitations and arrhythmias during pregnancy. Postgrad Med J 2008;84:66–72.

Ayhan A, Yucel A, Bildirici I, Dogan R. Fetomaternal morbidity and mortality after cardiac valve replacement. Acta Obstet Gynecol Scand 2001;80:713–18.

Bédard E, Shore DF, Gatzoulis MA. Adult CHD: a 2008 overview. Br Med Bulletin 2008;85:151–80.

Ben Farhat M, Gamra H, Betbout F, et al. Percutaneous balloon mitral commissurotomy during pregnancy. Heart 1997;77:564–7.

Bhatla N, Lal S, Behera G, et al. Cardiac disease in pregnancy. Int J Gynecol Obstet 2003;82:153–9.

Boggess KA, Watts DH, Hillier SL, Krohn NA, Benedetti TJ, Eschenbach DA. Bacteremia shortly after placenta separation during cesarean delivery. Obstet Gynecol 1996;87:77–984.

Burn J, Brennan P, Little J, et al. Recurrence risks in offspring of adults with major heart defects: results from first cohort of British collaborative study. Lancet 1998;351:311–16.

Campuzans K, Rogue H, Bolwick A, Leo MV, Campbell WA. Bacterial endocarditis complicating pregnancy: case report and systematic review of the literature. Arch Gynecol Obstet 2003;268:251–5.

Carvalho JS. Early prenatal diagnosis of major congenital heart defects. Curr Opin Obstet Gynecol 2001;13:155–9.

Chan WS, Anand S, Ginsberg JS. Anticoagulation of pregnant women with mechanical heart valves. Arch Intern Med 2000;160:191–6.

Chapa JB, Heiberger HB, Weinert L, et al. Prognostic value of echocardiography in peripartum cardiomyopathy. Obstet Gynecol 2005;105:1303–8.

Dore A, Somerville J. Pregnancy in patients with pulmonary autograft valve replacement. Eur Heart J 1997;18:1659–62.

Drenthen W, Pieper PG, Roos-Hesselink JW, et al. Pregnancy and delivery in women after Fontan palliation. Heart 2006;92:1290–4.

Elkayam U, Akhter MW, Singh H, et al. Pregnancy-associated cardiomyopathy. Clinical characteristics and a comparison between early and late presentation. Circulation 2005;111:2050–5.

Elkayam U, Bitar F. Valvular heart disease and pregnancy. Part I: native valves. JACC 2005;46:223–30.

Elkayam U, Ostrzega E, Shotan A, Mehra A. Cardiovascular problems in pregnant women with the Marfan syndrome. Ann Intern Med 1995;123:117–22.

Elkayam U, Tummala PP, Rao K, et al. Maternal and fetal outcomes of subsequent pregnancies in women with peripartum cardiomyopathy. N Engl J Med 2001;344:1567–71.

Elkayam U. Pregnancy through a prosthetic heart valve. JACC 1999;33:1642–5.

Ellison J, Thomson AJ, Walker ID, Greer IA. Use of enoxaparin in a pregnant woman with a mechanical heart valve prosthesis. Br J Obstet Gynaecol 2001;108:757–9.

Fawzi ME, Kinsara AJ, Stefadouros M, et al. Long-term outcome of mitral balloon valvotomy in pregnant women. J Heart valve Dis 2001;10:153–7.

Felker GM, Thompson RE, Hare JM, et al. Underlying causes and long-term survival in patients with initially unexplained cardiomyopathy. N Engl J Med 2000;342:1077–84.

Fung TY, Chan DLW, Leung TN, Leung TY, Lau TK. Dextrocardia in pregnancy. 20 years' experience. J Reprod Med 2006;51:573–7.

Furman B, Shohan-Vardi I, Bashire A, et al. Clinical significance and outcomes of preterm pre-labor rupture of membranes: population-based study. Eur J Obstet Gynecol Reprod Biol 2000;92:209–16.

Gei AF, Hankins GD. Cardiac disease and pregnancy. Obstet Gynecol Clin North Am 2001;28:465–512.

Gleason TG. Heritable disorders predisposing to aortic dissection. Thorac cardiovasc Surg 2005;17:274–81.

Hameed A, Akhter MW, Bitar F, et al. Left atrial thrombosis in pregnant women with mitral stenosis and sinus rhythm. Am J Obstet Gynecol 2005;

Hameed A, Karaalp IS, Tummala PP, et al. The effect of valvular heart disease on maternal and fetal outcome of pregnancy. JACC 2001;37:893–9.

Hu CL. Li YB, Zou YG, et al. Troponin T measurement can predict persistent left ventricular dysfunction in peripartum cardiomyopathy. Heart 2007;93:488–90.

Hung L, Rahimtoola SH. Prosthetic heart valves and pregnancy. Circulation 2003;107:1240–6.

Hyett J, Perdu M, Sharland G, et al. Using fetal nuchal translucency to screen for major congenital heart defects at 10–14 weeks of gestation: population based cohort study. BMJ 1999;318:81–5.

Immer FF, Bansi AG, Immer-Bansi AS, et al. Aortic dissection in pregnancy: analysis of risk factors and outcome. Ann Thorac Surg 2003;76:309–14.

James AH, Jamison MG, Biswas MS, et al. Acute myocardial infarction in pregnancy. A United States population-based study. Circulation 2006;113:1564–71.

Khairy P, Ouyang DW, Fernandes SM, *et al.* Pregnancy outcomes in women with CHD. Circulation 2006;113:517–24.

Lind J, Wallenberg HC. The Marfan syndrome and pregnancy: a retrospective study in a Dutch population. Eur J Obstet Gynecol Reprod Biol 2001;98:28–35.

Lupton M, Oteng-Ntim E, Ayida G, Steer PJ. Cardiac disease in pregnancy. Curr Opin Obstet Gynaecol 2002;14:137–43.

Malhotra M, Sharma JB, Tripathii R, *et al.* Maternal and fetal outcome in valvular heart disease. Int J Gynecol Obstet 2004;84:11–16.

Moore RC, Briery CM, Rose CH, *et al.* Lymphocytic myocarditis presenting as nausea, vomiting, and hepatic dysfunction in the first trimester of pregnancy. Obstet Gynecol 2006;108:815–17.

Nabhan A. Peripartum cardiomyopathy. ASJOG 2005;2:231–7.

Oei SG, Oei SK, Brölmann HAM. Myocardial infarction during nifedipine therapy for preterm labor. N Engl J Med 1999;340:154.

Pearson GD, Veille J-C, Rahimtoola S, *et al.* Peripartum cardiomyopathy. National Heart, Lung, and Blood Institute and Office of Rare Diseases (National Institutes of Health) Workshop Recommendations and Review. JAMA 2000;283:1183–8.

Penning S, Robinson KD, Major CA, Garite TJ. A comparison of echocardiography and pulmonary artery catheterization for evaluation of pulmonary artery pressures in pregnant patients with suspected pulmonary hypertension. Am J Obstet Gynecol 2001;184:1568–70.

Petanovic M, Zagar Z. The significance of asymptomatic bacteremia for the newborn. Acta Obstet Gynecol Scand 2001;80:813–17.

Roberts N, Ross D, Flint SK, Arya R, Blott M. Thromboembolism in pregnant women with mechanical prosthetic heart valves anticoagulated with low molecular weight heparin. Br J Obstet Gynaecol 2001;108:327–29.

Romano-Zelekha O, Hirsh R, Blieden L, *et al.* The risk for congenital heart defects in offsprings of individuals with congenital heart defects. Clin Genet 2001;59:325–9.

Roth A, Elkayam U. Acute myocardial infarction associated with pregnancy. JACC 2008;52:171–80.

Rowan JA, McCowan LM, Raudkivi PJ, North RA. Enoxaparin treatment in women with mechanical heart valve during pregnancy. Am J Obstet Gynecol 2001;185:633–7.

Sakaguchi M, Kitahara H, Seto T, *et al.* Surgery for acute type A aortic dissection in pregnant patients with Marfan syndrome. Eur J Cardiol Thorac Surg 2005;28:280–5.

Salem DN, Stein PD, Al-Ahmad A, *et al.* Antithrombotic therapy in valvular heart disease—native and prosthetic. The Seventh ACCP Conference on Antithrombotic and Thrombolytic Therapy. Chest 2004;126:457S–482S.

Salem DN, Stein PD, Al-Almad A, *et al.* Antithrombotic therapy in valvular heart disease—native and prosthetic. The Seventh ACCP Conference on Antithrombotic and Thrombolytic Therapy. Chest 2004;126:457S–482S.

Silversides CK, Colman JM, Sermer M, Siu SC. Cardiac risk in pregnant women with rheumatic mitral stenosis. Am J Cardiol 2003;91:1382–5.

Siu SC, Colman JM, Sorensen S, *et al.* Adverse neonatal and cardiac outcomes are more common in pregnant women with cardiac disease. Circulation 2002;105:2179–84.

Siu SC, Sermer M, Colman JM, *et al.* Prospective multicenter study of pregnancy outcomes in women with heart disease. Circulation 2001;104:515–21.

Sliwa K, Förster O, Libhaber E, *et al.* Peripartum cardiomyopathy: inflammatory markers as predictors of outcome in 100 prospectively studied patients. Eur Heart J 2006;27:441–6.

Thaman R, VarnavaA, Hamid MS, Firoozi S, Sachdev B, Condon M, *et al.* Pregnancy related complications in women with hypertrophic cardiomyopathy. Heart 2003;89:752–6.

The Task Force on the Management of Cardiovascular Diseases During Pregnancy of the European Society of Cardiology. Expert consensus document on management of cardiovascular diseases during pregnancy. Eur Heart J 2003;24:761–81.

Thorne SA. Pregnancy in heart disease. Heart 2004;90:450–6.

Tsui BCH, Stewart B, Fitzmaurice A, Williams R. Cardiac arrest and myocardial infarction induced by postpartum intravenous ergonovine administration. Anesthesiology 2001;94:363–4.

Uebing A, Steer PJ, Yentis SM, Gatzoulis MA. Pregnancy and CHD. BMJ 2006;332:401–6.

Veldtman GR, Connolly HM, Grogan M, *et al.* Outcomes of pregnancy in women with tetralogy of Fallot. JACC 2004;44:174–80.

Vitale N, De Feo M, De Santo LS, *et al.* Dose-dependent fetal complications of Warfarin in pregnant women with mechanical heart valves. JACC 1999;33:1637–41.

Weiss BM, Hess OM. Pulmonary vascular disease and pregnancy: current controversies, management strategies, and perspectives. Eur Heart J 2000;21:104–15.

Yentis SM, Steer PJ, Plaat F. Eisenmenger's syndrome in pregnancy: maternal and fetal mortality in the 1990s. Br J Obstet Gynaecol 1998;105:921–2.

Internet resources

www.clevelandclinicmeded.com

Hepatitis B

The hepatitis B virus (HBV) is a 3.2-kb, partially double-stranded DNA virus, which predominantly infects hepatocytes. HBV infection is a global health problem with a wide spectrum of clinical manifestations, ranging from acute hepatitis, through asymptomatic carriage to liver cirrhosis and hepatocellular carcinoma (HCC). Although antiviral treatments are increasingly effective, the prevention of transmission by vaccination, particularly from mother to child, remains the main route to reducing global morbidity and mortality.

Epidemiology

The World Health Organization (WHO) has estimated that there are over 350 million people worldwide with chronic HBV infection, defined as persistence of HBV surface antigen (HBsAg) for more than 6 months. The prevalence of chronic infection varies from high prevalence regions (>8%, such as sub-Saharan Africa, Asia, and the Pacific islands), through intermediate regions (2–8%, southern and eastern Europe, the Middle East, and the Indian subcontinent) to low prevalence regions (<2%, most of Western Europe and north America). In the UK, the prevalence of HbsAg positivity in antenatal women is 0.14% overall, but increases to 1% or more in inner-city areas with a high proportion of women born in high prevalence countries. The geographical variation is largely due to significant differences in the age of infection in different countries, which plays a crucial role in the risk of developing chronicity. Chronic infection is estimated to occur in 90% of infants who are infected in the perinatal period, in 20–50% of infections that occur between the ages of 1 and 5 years and in less than 5% in acute adult infections. Perinatal or vertical infection and childhood transmission are the major routes of infection in high and intermediate prevalence countries. Adult transmission has been the main route of transmission in low prevalence countries, although this pattern is changing with increasing migration.

Modes of transmission

HBV is transmitted by percutaneous or mucous membrane exposure to infectious blood and serum-derived bodily fluids. Only serum, semen, and saliva have been demonstrated to be infectious. No infections have been demonstrated in people who were orally exposed to HBsAg-positive saliva, and transmission has only been shown in animal experiments after subcutaneous injection of saliva. The main modes of transmission are perinatal transmission from mother to child, transmission through vaginal or anal intercourse, and as a result of blood to blood contact, e.g. sharing of needles by drug users. HBV is stable on surfaces for up to 7 days or more. Therefore, indirect inoculation from, for example shared jewellery, is possible. Higher viral loads are associated with a greater risk of transmission, particularly in the context of vertical transmission.

Acute hepatitis B

The incubation period ranges from 40 to 160 days. Acute infections (695 reported cases in England and Wales in 2003, Health Protection Agency website) may be clinically asymptomatic or present with acute hepatic inflammation leading to serious illness, including fulminant hepatic failure (in approximately 0.5% of cases). Most symptomatic cases occur in adults and are very rare in infants. Symptoms are non-specific and include general malaise, anorexia, arthritis, nausea and vomiting, pyrexia, right upper quadrant pain, or an urticarial rash due to immune complex deposition. Anicteric infections are common but some patients may develop overt jaundice. The majority of infected adults recover and develop long-lasting immunity, defined as loss of HBsAg and development of antibodies against the surface protein (anti-HBs Ab). In contrast, vertical transmission at birth or infection in early childhood carries a high risk of chronicity.

Chronic hepatitis B

Chronic infection is defined as persistence of HBsAg for more than 6 months and occurs in individuals, where the immune response is not sufficiently strong to clear the virus. These individuals are sometimes referred to as chronic carriers, but approximately 25% will develop progressive liver disease over time. The development of chronic liver inflammation, fibrosis, and cirrhosis occurs over a variable period, depending again on the age of infection. It is useful to consider four phases of chronic infection (Fig. 8.18.1), defined according to serum HBV e antigen (HBeAg) status and viral DNA levels. HBeAg is a viral protein, which historically has been measured as a marker of viral replication. However, it is now known that, over time, viral mutants may develop which replicate efficiently but do not synthesize HBeAg (termed pre-core mutants due to mutations in the HBV genome pre-core or core promoter region, which render such HBV variants unable to express HBeAg). The level of viral replication is more accurately measured using serum levels of HBV DNA, which range from just detectable up to 10^9 copies/mL or more.

In children and young adults there may an early HBeAg seropositive phase with high HBV DNA levels and normal ALT levels, characterized by very little liver inflammation due to a weak or absent immune response (immune-tolerant phase). This phase may last a variable period, even into adulthood, before the second immune clearance phase ensues, characterized by elevated liver transaminase levels and a risk of liver fibrosis. The length of this phase is short in acute infections that result in long-lasting immunity. In individuals with a suboptimal immune response, this phase may last many years and is associated with liver fibrosis and cirrhosis. This phase may be followed by a low or non-replicative third phase, when HBeAg is lost with the development of anti-HBe Ab (known as e seroconversion). The liver transaminases usually normalize and HBV DNA is undetectable or measured at $<10^3$–10^4 copies/mL. This phase may last for many years or indeed a lifetime. Each year 0.5% of individuals in this phase will develop anti-HBs Ab and lose anti-HBsAg, which is considered to represent viral clearance. However, a proportion will develop pre-core mutants and move into the fourth phase of HBeAg-negative chronic hepatitis, which again is associated with progressive liver fibrosis and cirrhosis.

Chronic infection may be completely asymptomatic or lead to the clinical manifestations of cirrhosis or HCC. Usually, progression to cirrhosis takes many years, but this is variable and may be accelerated by other risk factors such as alcohol, which should be avoided by patients with chronic HBV infection, and immunosuppression. In HbeAg-positive patients, progression to cirrhosis occurs at 2–5.5%

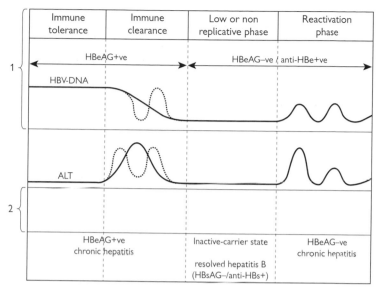

Fig. 8.18.1 Four phases of chronic infection.

per annum with an estimated yearly incidence of hepatic decompensation of 3%. Population-based studies in Taiwan have demonstrated that patients who remain HBeAg-positive with continued HBV replication are more likely to develop cirrhosis and HCC than any other HBsAg-positive group. A European longitudinal study of HBsAg positive patients with compensated cirrhosis showed a cumulative survival of 84% at 5 years and 68% at 10 years. HBV infection is the single most frequent cause of HCC, the sixth most common cancer globally.

Prevention

Hepatitis B infection is preventable by immunization. The main objective of HBV vaccination programmes is the prevention of chronic infection and chronic liver disease; the prevention of acute hepatitis B is a secondary goal. Immunization is the most effective measure and, in 1992, the WHO recommended infant immunization programmes for all countries. By 2005 immunization for HBV had been integrated into the Expanded Program of Immunization (EPI) in 155 countries, with an overall average coverage of only 50% of the global infant population.

It is now well established that HBV infection and its complications can be prevented by active and passive vaccination. Universal immunization of neonates has dramatically reduced the prevalence of chronic HBV infection in children and adolescents in parts of Africa and Asia as well as the incidence of HCC in children in Taiwan. Safe vaccines have been available since 1982. The efficacy of HBV vaccination in children and newborns has been shown to be over 90% in most countries.

Different methods of immune-prophylaxis have been used worldwide, depending on financial resources and the population prevalence of HBV infection. Taiwan instituted the first universal HBV vaccination in 1984. Pregnant women were screened for HBsAg and HBeAg. All infants received HBV vaccination. Those infants at high risk (mothers positive for HBsAg and HBeAg) also received passive immunization with hepatitis B immunoglobulin (HBIg) within 24 hours of birth. The vaccination programme was gradually extended to preschool and school children and adults. This programme has demonstrated that HBV infection rates, the incidence of HCC, and fulminant hepatitis in childhood can be reduced successfully. In the USA, antenatal screening includes HBsAg but not HBeAg. Every infant is recommended to receive HBV vaccination, while those born to HbsAg-positive mothers also receive HBIg within 24 hours of birth, regardless of HBeAg status (passive–active immunization). This strategy is considerably more expensive as HBIg is used more frequently. Some countries with intermediate or low prevalence of chronic HBV infection or insufficient resources perform no antenatal screening and vaccinate all infants (without using HBIg). This approach (used for example in Thailand) is less efficacious than the first two. In the UK, there is not a policy of universal infant vaccination. Infants of seropositive mothers receive vaccination with or without HBIg (see below). Vaccination is also recommended for other high risk categories such as injection drug users and health workers.

Treatment of chronic HBV infection

There have been major advances in the treatment of chronic HBV infection in recent years. There are two main therapeutic strategies: the use of α-IFN, which enhances T-cell-mediated viral clearance through immunomodulatory activities and the use of oral antiviral agent to suppress HBV replication. The aims of antiviral treatment are to achieve suppression of viral replication and to prevent progression to cirrhosis, end stage liver disease and HCC. Antiviral therapy should be considered in patients with active HBV replication, raised ALT levels and/or liver histology showing active inflammation, necrosis, or fibrosis. In the absence of elevated transaminases, the response to treatment is often poor. Pregnant women with high levels of viral replication may have a lower risk of vertical transmission if oral antiviral therapy is used. However, there remain concerns regarding the safety of such treatments and only limited data are available at present (see below). α-IFN is given in injectable form, often conjugated to a polyethelene glycol (PEG) moiety. In HBeAg-positive patients, seroconversion to anti-HBe or loss of HBV DNA occurs in 30–40% but HBsAg clearance occurs in less than 10%. Its use is limited by significant side-effects and reduced efficacy in HBeAg-negative patients. The oral antiviral agents include lamivudine, adefovir, entecavir, tenofovir, and telbivudine. They reduce HBV DNA levels and may induce seroconversion to anti-HBe. The loss of HBsAg occurs rarely and treatment is often long term. Their use is limited by the development of antiviral resistance. Lamivudine was the first nucleoside analogue to be used in HBV infection. Monotherapy with this agent results in resistance rates of up to 70% at 5 years due to mutations in the HBV DNA polymerase. The newer antivirals appear to have significantly lower risks of resistance and are being licensed for routine use in chronic HBV infection.

Hepatitis B in pregnancy

Risk during pregnancy and at delivery
Acute HBV infection in pregnancy does not increase maternal morbidity or mortality and does not increase the risk of fetal complications such as death or congenital abnormalitites. An increased risk of preterm labour has been reported. The risk of perinatal transmission, in the absence of appropriate immunoprophylaxis, is very high in acute infection (>70–90%).

In chronic HBV infection the risk of perinatal infection depends on the HbeAg status of the mother: 90% of babies born to HBeAg-positive mothers and approximately 10% of babies born to HBeAg-negative mothers become infected in the absence of immunoprophylaxis. This risk is also related to maternal serum HBV DNA levels. Although passive–active immunization is highly effective in the prevention of vertical transmission, high maternal serum HBV DNA levels have been associated with the failure of immunoprophylaxis. In a Dutch meta-analysis, the efficacy of passive–active immunization was 100% in infants born to HBeAg-negative mothers and 92% in those born to HBeAg-positive mothers. If the maternal HBV DNA level was greater than 10^7 IU/mL, transmission was only prevented in 68%. This may be related, in part at least, to intrauterine infection, which is thought to occur via transplacental leakage of maternal blood. There is ongoing debate about whether such patients should commence antiviral therapy in the third trimester of pregnancy (see below).

Acute or fulminant infection in infancy occurs very rarely, predominantly as a result of transmission of HbeAg-negative strains. It does not cause early neonatal viral hepatitis, occurring only after 6 weeks of age.

Clinical approach
Diagnosis: history, examination, investigations
The evaluation of pregnant women who have been identified to have HBV infection (seropositive for HBsAg) should encompass a thorough history including alcohol consumption, risk assessment for co-infection with hepatitis C or HIV and family history of HBV infection and hepatocellular carcinoma. Full clinical examination should be performed with particular attention to stigmata of chronic liver disease (e.g. evidence of ascites, asterixis, spider naevi, etc.).

Table 8.18.1 US FDA categories for antiviral drugs

	US FDA category
Lamivudine	C
Adefovir	C
Entecavir	C
Telbivudine	B
Tenofovir	B

Laboratory tests should include routine liver function tests, standard tests for other forms of potentially coexisting liver disease (e.g. testing for diabetes mellitus, dyslipidaemias, iron storage disorders, autoimmune hepatitis, etc.) and tests for potential co-infection in those at risk (hepatitis A, C, D, E, and HIV). Once the diagnosis of chronic HBV infection has been made, it is important to further define the virological status, i.e. HBeAg status and HBV DNA levels need to be established. HBV levels are measured by the polymerase chain reaction (PCR). A liver ultrasound should be performed to look for evidence of progressive fibrosis and cirrhosis. Where advanced liver disease is suspected, the serum levels of α-fetoprotein (AFP), a marker of HCC, should be determined. All women should be referred to a hepatology specialist for an assessment of liver disease to determine the need for antiviral therapy before or after delivery.

Counselling
Every patient with chronic HBV infection should be counselled regarding lifestyle changes to prevent transmission to sexual partners and household contacts. The need for disease monitoring in specialist clinics and the importance of alcohol, a risk factor for the development of cirrhosis, should be discussed. Robust systems should be in place to ensure that maternity services for pregnant HBsAg-positive women are informed to ensure immunoprophylaxis of the newborn.

Management
Acute HBV infection during pregnancy
Treatment of acute HBV infection is supportive only as currently no specific treatments are available. Fetal infection after an acute self-limiting maternal HBV infection in early pregnancy is rare. In contrast, if acute infection occurs in the third trimester or in the immediate postpartum period, the maternal–infant transmission rates are very high. Passive–active immunization is required.

Management of chronic HBV infection in pregnancy
Management decisions regarding women with chronic HBV infection who become pregnant while on oral antiviral therapy need to be made on an individualized basis. The drugs that are currently used in antiviral therapy have been allocated to categories B (no evidence of risk in humans) and C (risk cannot be ruled out) by the United States Food and Drug Administration (Table 8.18.1).

The benefit of the treatment must be weighed against the potential small risk of the antiviral drugs to the fetus. Surveys have not demonstrated substantial increases in birth defect rates in first trimester exposures to Lamivudine over rates in the general population (Antiretroviral Pregnancy Registry Steering Committee report). Early in the first trimester it may be appropriate to stop treatment with careful monitoring through pregnancy. Alternatively, depending on the stage of liver disease and treatment history, it may be optimal to continue treatment or switch drugs (Liaw 2005).

The current UK guidance recommends passive–active immunization at birth (HBIg plus vaccination; injection at different sites if given simultaneously) for infants who
- are born to HBeAg-positive mothers
- are born to mothers who are HbeAg negative but have no anti-HBe Ab
- are born to mothers where the e-markers are not known
- are born to mothers who had acute HBV infection during pregnancy
- weigh less than 1500 g at birth.

It is recommended that newborns to mothers who are anti-HBe positive (HBsAg-positive, HBeAg-negative) receive active immunization only, starting at birth. The accelerated immunization schedule is preferable, i.e. the first dose at birth and further doses at 1 and 2 months of age and a fourth dose at 12 months. HBsAg testing should take place at the same time as the last dose of vaccine to identify those babies for whom immunoprophylaxis was not successful and to ensure further specialist management.

A number of strategies have been tested to reduce the rate of failure of immunoprophylaxis in mothers with high viral loads. Studies have shown that administration of Lamivudine in the last trimester of pregnancy results in lower rates of perinatal transmission. A small study published in 2003 treated eight highly viraemic mothers (HBV DNA >1.2×10^9 IU/mL) with 150 mg of Lamivudine daily during the last month of pregnancy. Twenty-four children born to untreated HBsAg-positive mothers with similarly high HBV DNA levels served as controls. All newborns received passive–active immunization at birth and were followed-up for 12 months. Seven of the eight Lamivudine-treated mothers had a significant decrease in HBV DNA. One of the eight children (12.5%) remained HBsAg and HBV DNA positive at 12 months while all others seroconverted to anti-HBs. In the untreated control group perinatal transmission occurred in 28% of children (van Zonnveld 2003). Li and colleagues compared the use of antenatal HBIg with Lamivudine in mothers who were HBsAg positive (56 women received 200 IU of HBIg intramuscularly every 4 weeks from 28 weeks of gestation, 43 women were given 100 mg of Lamivudine daily from week 28 until day 30 after delivery and these were compared to 52 women (controls) who received no specific treatment): neonatal infection was significantly lower in those receiving HBIg (16%) or Lamivudine (16%) than in controls (33%; p<0.05). No side-effects occurred in the mothers or their newborns.

Although failure of immunoprophylaxis occurs more frequently when the maternal HBV DNA level is >10^7 IU/mL, there are no clinical trial data to inform optimal management of this group of women and further studies are required. At present, women with viral loads greater than

10^7 IU/mL may be considered for antiviral therapy during the third trimester of pregnancy. Clinicians caring for pregnant patients with chronic HBV infection should liaise with a viral hepatitis specialist to optimise treatment in individual cases.

Vaccination of preterm babies

There is evidence that preterm, low-birthweight babies have a suboptimal response to HBV vaccination. Therefore, the recommendations suggest the full paediatric dose of HBV vaccine on schedule. Babies weighing 1500 g or less should be given HBIg together with the vaccine (independent of the eAg-status of the mother).

Further reading

Alter MJ. Epidemiology of hepatitis B in Europe and worldwide. J Hepatol 2003;39:S64–S69.

Chang MH, Chen CJ, Lai MS, et al. Universal hepatitis B vaccination in Taiwan and the incidence of hepatocellular carcinoma in children. N Engl J Med 1997;336:1855–9.

Chang MH. Hepatitis B virus infection. Semin Fetal Neonatal Med. 2007;12:160–7.

Chen HL, Chang CJ, Kong MS et al. Fulminant hepatic failure in children in endemic area of hepatitis B virus infection:15 years after universal hepatitis B vaccination, Hepatology 2004;39: 58–63.

del Canho R, Grosheide PM, Mazel JA, et al. Ten-year neonatal hepatitis B vaccination program, The Netherlands, 1982–1992:protective efficacy and long-term immunogenicity. Vaccine 1991 5:1624–1630

Dusheiko G, Antonakopoulos N. Current treatment of hepatitis B. Gut 2008;57:105–124.

Liaw YF, Leung N, Guan R, et al. Asian-Pacific consensus statement on the management of chronic hepatitis B: a 2005 update. Liver Int 2005;25:472–89.

Lin HH, Lee TY, Chen DS et al. Transplacental leakage of HbeAg-positive maternal blood as the most likely route in causing intrauterine infection with hepatitis B virus. J Pediatr 1987;111:877–81.

Realdi G, Fattovich G, Hadziyannis S, et al. Survival and prognostic factors in 366 patients with compensated cirrhosis type B: a multicenter study. The Investigators of the European Concerted Action on Viral Hepatitis (EUROHEP). J Hepatol 1994;21: 656–66.

Terrault NA, Jacobson IM (). Treating chronic hepatitis B infection in patients who are pregnant or are undergoing immunosuppressive chemotherapy. Semin Liver Dis 2007;27(Suppl 1):18–24.

van Zonneveld M, van Nunen AB, Niesters HG, et al . Lamivudine treatment during pregnancy to prevent perinatal transmission of hepatitis B virus infection. J Viral Hepat 2003;10:294–7.

Internet resources

Antiretroviral Pregnancy Registry Steering Committee report: www.apregistry.com/forms/apr_report_106.pdf
Department of Health. Immunization against infectious disease—the Green Book: www.dh.gov.uk
Health Protection Agency: www.hpa.org.uk

Patient resources

British Liver Trust: www.britishlivertrust.org.uk
The Hepatitis B Foundation: www.hepb.org.uk

Herpes simplex infection

Definition
Genital herpes is a sexually transmitted infection that is caused by the herpes simplex virus (HSV). This infection is typically characterized with recurrent ulcerative lesions on the genital mucosa. During pregnancy, genital herpes causes concern for morbidity and mortality associated with neonatal infection.

Epidemiology
Genital herpes is one of the most common ulcerating diseases of the genital mucosa. The WHO estimates that 40–60 million people in the USA are HSV-2 infected, with an incidence of 1–2 million infections and 600 000–800 000 clinical cases per year. HSV-2 causes most of the genital infections whereas HSV-1 is primarily responsible for herpes labialis ('cold sores') gingivostomatitis, and keratoconjunctivitis. Given changing sexual practices, genital HSV-1 infections are becoming increasingly common, responsible for up to 80% of new genital HSV infections.

Pathology
HSV belongs to the family Herpesviridae. The virus enters the skin and travels to the sensory neurons, and then the infection becomes latent in the sensory ganglia. This plays an important role in the clinical presentation of HSV.

Aetiology
HSV is a double-stranded DNA virus that can be subdivided into HSV type 1 and HSV type 2. HSV is transmitted from person to person through direct contact. Infection is initiated when the virus contacts mucosa or abraded skin. The incubation period of HSV ranges from 2 days to 12 days. HSV then replicates, with resulting cellular destruction and inflammation. During the initial infection, vesicles appear on the vulva, which soon break to leave shallow, painful ulcers. The ulcers heal in 2–3 weeks. This primary infection is then followed by reactivation. Reactivation of viral replication usually presents as recurrent ulcerative lesions or as asymptomatic viral shedding.

Risk factors
- Female gender
- Duration of sexual activity
- Minority ethnicity
- Family income
- Number of sexual partners.

Types of infection
There are three main clinical types to HSV: primary, non-primary first episode, and recurrent. Distinguishing what type a woman presents with can have consequences on perinatal transmission rates. Serological testing and viral isolation would be required to establish type of infection. Each of the presentations can be symptomatic or asymptomatic.
- Primary infection refers to infection in a patient without preexisting antibodies to HSV-1 or HSV-2. This typically presents with systemic symptoms, including fever and malaise.
- Non-primary first episode infection refers to the acquisition of genital HSV-1 in a patient with pre-existing antibodies to HSV-2 or the acquisition of genital HSV-2 in a patient with pre-existing antibodies to HSV-1.

- Recurrent infection refers to reactivation of genital HSV in which the HSV type recovered in the lesion is the same type as antibodies in the serum.

Maternal–fetal transmission
The maternal–fetal or vertical transmission rate is dependent on clinical type and timing of episode. The mode of transmission most commonly occurs via direct contact of the fetus with infected vaginal secretions during delivery. Less commonly, ascending intrauterine infection or postnatal infection may be the cause.

Neonatal clinical manifestations
Acquisition of primary herpes in the first trimester has been associated with neonatal chorioretinitis, microcephly, and skin lesions in rare cases. HSV infection acquired in the late third trimester is associated with one of three patterns in the newborn. Initial symptoms usually occur within the first 4 weeks of newborn life. The three patterns are:
- localized to the skin, eyes, and mouth
- localized central nervous system (CNS) disease
- disseminated disease involving multiple organs.

Prognosis
The most important determinants of prognosis of neonatal infection are type and timing of the episode. Primary infections acquired during pregnancy yield a greater risk of perinatal transmission than recurrent episodes. Of those who acquire a primary HSV infection during pregnancy, the risk of vertical transmission is greatest around the time of labour. This risk is approximately 30–60%. For the newborn, mortality can be up to 4% with CNS disease and up to 30% with disseminated disease. Approximately 20% of survivors of neonatal herpes have long-term neurological problems.

Clinical approach
Diagnosis
It is not possible to distinguish primary from non-primary herpes simplex virus infection on clinical findings alone. Diagnosis is based on the combination of positive viral detection and negative serological test results or evidence of seroconversion. Even with our diagnostic tools, approximately 80% of infected infants are born to mothers with no reported history of HSV infection.

History
- Personal history of genital herpes
- If personal history of genital HSV: date of diagnosis, medications used, numbers of outbreaks per year
- Sexual history, including partners' HSV status.

Examination
- Multiple painful vesicles or shallow ulcers on the genitals
- Normal examination findings may be present in a HSV carrier.

Investigations
- Isolation of virus through viral culture or PCR
- Direct fluorescent antibody testing
- Tzank test (microscopic identification)
- Serological testing for type-specific antibodies.

Counselling

For pregnant patients with no known history of genital HSV, counselling should emphasize prevention habits. Avoiding or decreasing exposure to HSV-infected partners when active lesions are present will decrease risk of acquistion. It is important to know that acquistion can still occur with asymptomatic partners. For women with serological test results that indicate susceptibility to HSV infection, the incidence of new HSV infection during pregnancy is about 2%. The most critical time to avoid acquistion is during late pregnancy.

For pregnant patients with a primary outbreak during pregnancy, counselling should include risks and transmission rates as described above.

For pregnant patients with a history of genital HSV, counselling should include awareness of a decreased vertical transmission rate of less than 2%. For patients with multiple outbreaks, suppressive therapy may be initiated at 36 weeks of gestation.

If active lesions are present at the time of labour (preferably prior to rupture of membranes), a Caesarean section should be performed to decrease the vertical transmission risk. The neonatal risks as described above should be explained.

Management

The most common antiviral agents used during pregnancy are Category B medications. They are approved for the treatment of primary and recurrent genital herpes, and the daily treatment for outbreak suppression. There are no documented increases in adverse fetal effects secondary to medication exposure. Topical therapy offers limited benefit and should not be used.

Primary outbreak during pregnancy

Oral antiviral therapy can be initiated to reduce the duration and severity of symptoms and reduce duration of viral shedding. Intravenous antiviral therapy can be initiated in severe disseminated cases of HSV. HSV suppression may be indicated at 36 weeks to decrease recurrence. There is no evidence to support Caesarean delivery before labour to prevent vertical transmission.

Recurrent outbreak during pregnancy

Oral antiviral therapy can also be initiated to reduce number of outbreaks. Women with active recurrent genital herpes should be offered suppressive viral therapy at 36 weeks. Women with recurrent lesions at the time of delivery have a low rate of transmission at about 3%. The transmission rate decreases considerably to 2/10 000 in women with no visible lesions at the time of delivery. There is no indication for Caesarean delivery in women with a history of HSV and no active lesions or prodromal symptoms at time of delivery.

Active outbreak at the time of delivery

Cesarean delivery is indicated with active lesions or prodromal symptoms, which may indicate an impending outbreak, during labour or with ruptured membranes at or near term. This significantly decreases vertical transmission in a primary outbreak. The transmission rate is low in a recurrent outbreak, but Caesarean delivery is still recommended because of the potentially serious nature of the disease. Caesarean delivery does not eliminate the transmission risk. There is no timeframe after rupture of membranes at which a Caesarean delivery is not indicated.

Further reading

ACOG Committee on Practice Bulletins. ACOG Practice Bulletin: Management of Herpes in Pregnancy No. 82. Obstet Gynecol 2007;109:1489–98.

Brown ZA, Selke S, Zeh J, et al. The acquisition of herpes simplex virus during pregnancy. N Engl J Med 1997;337:509–15.

Brown ZA, Wald A, Morrow RA, Selke S, Zeh J, Corey L. Effect of serologic status and cesarean delivery on transmission rates of herpes simplex virus from mother to infant. JAMA 2003;289:203–9.

Paz-Bailey G, Ramaswamy M, Hawkes SJ, Geretti AM. Herpes simplex virus type 2: epidemiology and management options in developing countries. Postgrad Med J. 2008 Jun;84:299–306.

Roberts CM, Pfister JR, Spear SJ. Increasing proportion of herpes simplex virus type 1 as a cause of genital herpes infection in college students. Sex Transm Dis 2003;30:797–800.

Sauerbrei A, Wutzler P. Herpes simplex and varicella-zoster virus infections during pregnancy: current concepts of prevention, diagnosis and therapy. Part 1: herpes simplex virus infections. Med Microbiol Immunol 2007;196:89–94.

Sexually transmitted diseases treatment guidelines, 2006 [published in MMWR Recomm Rep 2006;55:997]. Centers for Disease Control and Prevention. MMWR Recomm Rep 2006;55 (RR-11):1–94.

Internet resources

World Health Organization: www.who.int

Centers for Disease Control and Prevention: www.cdc.gov/std/herpes

UptoDate: Genital Herpes Simplex Virus Infection in Pregnancy: www.utdol.com

HIV infection

Definition

Acquired immunodeficiency syndrome (AIDS) was first described in San Francisco in 1981. It is caused by infection with a retrovirus human immunodeficiency virus (HIV). Following infection cell-mediated immunity, in particular, becomes impaired as the level of CD4 (T-helper cells) cells declines. A normal CD4 count is between 500 and 1500 cells/mm^3. Four-fifths of people with AIDS present with a CD4 count <200 cells/mm^3. In some countries such as the USA a CD4 count below 200 is itself regarded as AIDS defining. AIDS-defining illnesses are essentially life-threatening opportunistic infections,- or cancers associated with immunodeficiency. The commonest AIDS presentations are listed in Table 8.20.1.

The onset of immunodeficiency can be manifest in any organ system so that a high index of suspicion is required to recognize the way in which other disease processes are altered. This section will focus on the gynaecological and obstetric aspects of HIV infection.

With effective antiretroviral therapy life expectancy is now near normal for those diagnosed with HIV infection.

Epidemiology

More than 30 million individuals are infected worldwide, and in countries with a high prevalence it is the leading cause of death in young adults. It is a particularly devastating disease because of the stigma of sexual transmission and the risk of vertical transmission to children. Even if a child is not infected, the death of one or both parents threatens his/her development and survival in many parts of the world.

As shown in Fig. 8.20.1, the prevalence is greatest in Sub-Saharan Africa, where in several cities as many as a third of pregnant women are infected. A resurgence in tuberculosis has occurred hand in hand with the AIDS epidemic.

The initial epidemic in developed countries was concentrated among men who have sex with men (MSM) and intravenous drug users. Heterosexual spread, however, is increasing worldwide. The risk factors are the same as for all sexually transmitted infections (STIs): rate of partner change; young age at sexual debut; unprotected sex. The risk of transmission is related to the viral load in the genital tract which is increased by co-infection with STIs or even bacterial vaginosis. Seroconvertors and those with AIDS have high viral loads and are most likely to transmit.

HIV-1 is responsible for the AIDS pandemic. There are three groups of HIV-1 in humans, thought to represent different transmission events: group M with multiple subtypes (A–H) is the commonest worldwide, with groups O and N originating from Central and West Africa. Subtype B is the commonest in Europe and the USA. HIV-2 infection has a more benign course but can cause AIDS after prolonged infection, and can be transmitted vertically. Its geographical distribution is more restricted to West Africa, but has spread to European countries with historical links.

Natural history

The initial infection is usually silent, although 20% develop a seroconversion illness manifest as fever, lymphadenopathy, skin rash, and malaise lasting for up to a few weeks. The virus becomes detectable after about 3–4 weeks, rising to a high level, usually >10^6 copies/mL. After 12 weeks the viral load drops to a lower level, which is usually stable for a number of years before rising again with the onset of AIDS. During seroconversion the CD4 count also falls from the normal level: >500 cells/mm^3 and can drop below 200, which is the threshold for the onset of AIDS in chronic infection. It usually recovers to a normal level before progressively declining.

A steady decline in immune function over the first few years may be manifest by non-life-threatening opportunistic conditions such as

- recurrent oral and vaginal candidiasis
- single dermatome herpes zoster (shingles)
- frequent and prolonged episodes of oral or genital herpes
- persistent genital warts (Fig. 8.20.2), CIN, VIN and AIN
- hairy oral leukoplakia (HOL) (Fig. 8.20.3)
- persistent generalized lymphadenopathy (PGL)
- skin problems, including seborrhoeic dermatitis, folliculitis, dry skin, tinea pedis, and a high frequency of allergic reactions.

Without antiretroviral treatment the median time to the development of AIDS is 10 years. Essentially AIDS is defined by the onset of life-threatening opportunistic infections, or malignancies associated with immunodeficiency. The commonest presentations are listed in Table 8.20.1.

A few individuals are resistant to infection through genetic polymorphisms such as those with a Δ32 mutation in the chemokine receptor CCR-5, which is a coreceptor for viral entry into cells. If they become infected they become immunosuppressed only slowly, if at all. 'Elite controllers' have undetectable viral loads, but can still develop immunosuppression associated with the inflammatory response to the virus.

History

Assessing risk of infection if undiagnosed

In Europe where the epidemic has been linked with particular risk factors they can be used to identify those at

Table 8.20.1 Common AIDS presenting illnesses

Pulmonary	*Pneumocystis carinii* pneumonia
	Tuberculosis: pulmonary or extrapulmonary
Neurological	Cerebral toxoplasmosis
	Cryptococcal meningitis
	Tuberculous meningitis
	AIDS dementia
Gastrointestinal	Diarrhoea and wasting syndrome which may be due to infection with Cryptosporidium, Microsporidium, Isospora
	Oesophageal candidiasis
Ophthalmic	Cytomegalovirus retinitis
Malignancy	Kaposi's sarcoma (Fig. 8.20.4a,b)
	Non-Hodgkin's Lymphoma
Systemic	Mycobacterium avium intracellulare complex (MAC) infection

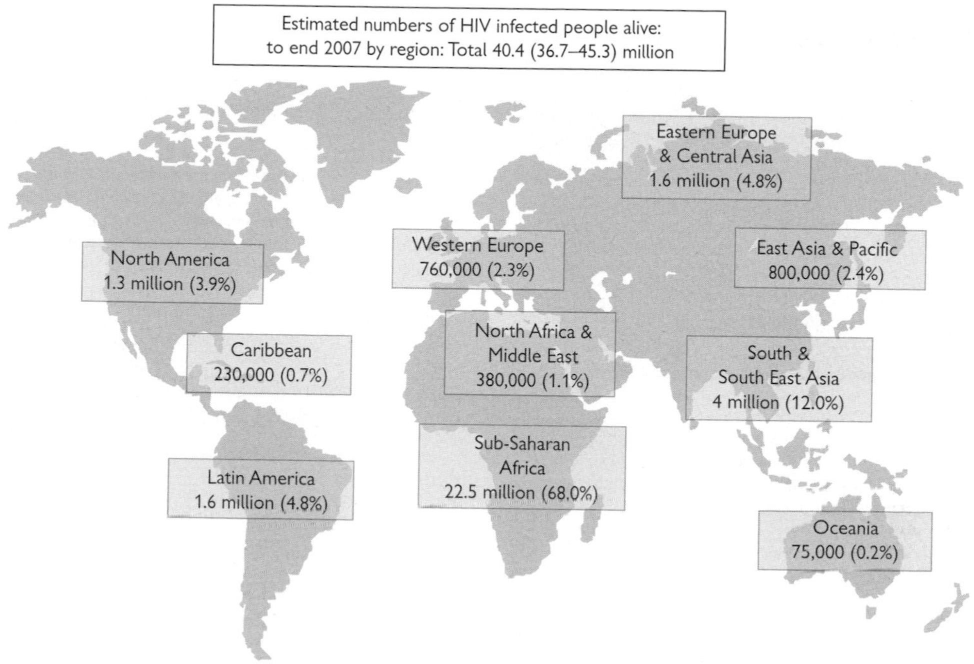

Estimated numbers of HIV infected people alive:
to end 2007 by region: Total 40.4 (36.7–45.3) million

Eastern Europe
& Central Asia
1.6 million (4.8%)

North America
1.3 million (3.9%)

Western Europe
760,000 (2.3%)

East Asia & Pacific
800,000 (2.4%)

Caribbean
230,000 (0.7%)

North Africa &
Middle East
380,000 (1.1%)

South &
South East Asia
4 million (12.0%)

Latin America
1.6 million (4.8%)

Sub-Saharan
Africa
22.5 million (68.0%)

Oceania
75,000 (0.2%)

Fig. 8.20.1 Summary of estimated worldwide epidemic 2007 from UNAIDS.

greatest risk. However, risk may be undisclosed by a patient or her partner, occasionally vertical infection stays asymptomatic until adulthood, and HIV is spreading in apparently low risk people so the safest course is to test all patients. The main risk factors are:

- injecting drug use in patient or partner
- bisexual male partner
- partner originating from a country of high prevalence (mostly sub-Saharan Africa and South East Asia)

- commercial sex
- blood products that have not been screened
- partner known to be HIV positive.

A sexual history (qv) and travel history should also be obtained.

Person known to be HIV positive

Liaison with the appropriate specialist team is essential, particularly in pregnancy. Obtain the following information:

- when diagnosed, and where
- any AIDS diagnoses or other clinical manifestations of HIV
- current treatment
- current CD4 count and viral load.

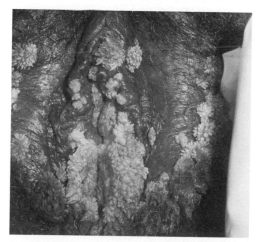

Fig. 8.20.2 Extensive genital warts in a pregnant woman presenting with a CD count of 170 cells/mm³. See also colour plate section.

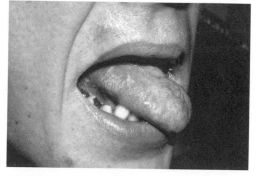

Fig. 8.20.3 Hairy oral leukoplakia is seen as white patches on the side of the tongue in HIV infection with often only moderate immunosuppression. The brown discolouration is related to smoking. See also colour plate section.

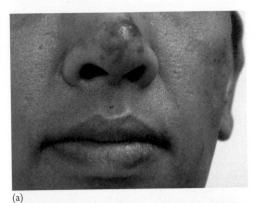

(a)

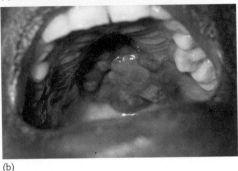

(b)

Fig. 8.20.4 Kaposi's sarcoma on the face (a) and large lesion on the palate (b). When this occurs multiple lesions are usually present in the gut and lungs as well. See also colour plate section.

If the CD4 count is >200 a new AIDS-defining illness is unlikely to develop. If on antiretroviral treatment for 6 months or more the viral load should be undetectable.

Examination and investigations

In an untested individual in whom the diagnosis of HIV is suspected look for the features of opportunistic conditions described above. HOL, oral candidiasis, and evidence of weight loss should all raise suspicion. A full description of the protean manifestation of HIV is outside the scope of this chapter.

Additional features of laboratory tests should raise suspicion of HIV infection. There is usually a polyclonal hyperimmunoglobulinaemia due to the immune dysregulation that occurs, so total protein is elevated in serum. In the blood count, autoimmune thrombocytopenia may occur; total lymphopenia and anaemia of chronic disease are seen in advanced infection.

HIV testing

The diagnosis of HIV is confirmed by identifying HIV antibody. Ideally tests should be done for antibody to both HIV-1 and HIV-2. This is often carried out using 'fingerprick' enzyme-liked immunosorbent assays (ELISAs) in developing countries, with a second one for confirmation of positive tests. In the UK we use tests combining ELISA for antibodies and viral p24 antigen detection. The latter allows earlier diagnosis of seroconvertors in the 'window period' before antibody develops. The window period is traditionally quoted as 3 months, but current tests usually become positive 4–6 weeks after exposure. If seroconversion is suspected clinically, a viral load assay may provide earlier confirmation of diagnosis, but the difference from p24 antigen detection is a few days.

CD4 count

This is a proxy measurement of the degree of immunosuppression. A normal level is between 500 and 1500 cells/mm^3. In the absence of intervention there is a 10% risk of AIDS in the year after the level reaches 200 cells/mm^3. This is usually monitored every 3–6 months.

HIV viral load

In untreated individuals the viral load may vary from <50 (undetectable) to >10^7 copies/mL. Some of the assays underquantify non-B subtypes. If there is a mismatch between the CD4 count and viral load a test should be repeated using a different assay. This is usually monitored every 3–6 months.

Management

Treatment guidelines are regularly updated from the USA, UK and WHO. There are two strategies used in treatment: antiretroviral therapy and prophylaxis against opportunistic infections in the immunosuppressed.

Combinations of antiretroviral drugs are prescribed. Treatment is recommended for those with a CD4 count below 350 cells/mm^3, or with clinical features of disease or cofactors such as hepatitis co-infection when earlier treatment improves prognosis. Currently, where there are resources to pay for the drugs, first line regimens are usually two nucleoside or nucleotide analogues reverse transcriptase inhibitors, such as lamivudine, tenofovir or emtricitabine with a non-nucleoside reverse transcriptase inhibitor (NNRTI) such as efavirenz or nevirapine. Protease inhibitors such as lopinavir/ritonavir or atazanavir with ritonavir are used instead of the NNRTI if there is resistance or other reasons not to use an NNRTI. Newer drug classes include viral entry inhibitors: enfurtide and maraviroc, and integrase inhibitors such as raltegravir.

Adverse reactions to antiretroviral drugs

There are many potential adverse reactions associated with antiretroviral therapy. A potentially fatal hypersensitivity reaction occurs with abacavir in HLA-B5701 positive individuals (rare in Sub-Saharan African populations). Allergic rashes occur commonly with NNRTIs: nevirapine more often than efavirenz. Nevirapine is particularly associated with Stevens-Johnson syndrome and severe hepatotoxicity. It should not be started in women with CD4 counts >250 cells/mm^3 when these reactions are more likely. Tenofovir should be avoided in those with renal impairment as it can cause renal tubular acidosis and exacerbate renal failure.

Protease inhibitors are associated principally with gastrointestinal toxicity: nausea and diarrhoea. Additionally they cause elevations in lipids and increased insulin resistance. They are often used in women starting antiretroviral therapy in pregnancy when efavirenz is contraindicated and nevirapine cannot be used if the CD4 count >250 cells/mm^3. Concomitant antiemetics and antidiarrhoeal medication are usually provided with the first prescription.

The newer classes of antiretroviral drugs have only been used in a limited number of pregnant women but are generally well tolerated and not known to be teratogenic (Table 8.20.2).

Table 8.20.2 FDA classification of antiretroviral drugs for safety in pregnancy

NRTIs		Protease inhibtors	
Abacavir	C	Amprenavir	C
Didanosine	B	Atazanavir	B
Emtricitabine	B	Darunavir	B
Lamivudine	C	Fosamprenavir	C
Stavudine	C	Indinavir	C
Zalcitabine	C	Lopinavir	C
Zidovudine	C	Nelfinavir	B
Tenofovir	B	Ritonavir	B
		Saquinavir	B
NNRTIs		Tipranavir	C
Efavirenz	D	Etravirine	B
Nevirapine	B		
Other			
Enfuvirtide	B		
Maraviroc	B		
Raltegravir	C		

American food and drug administration categories.
A, controlled studies show no risk; B, no evidence of risk in humans; C, risk cannot be ruled out; D, positive evidence of risk; X, contraindicated.

Drug interactions

Ritonavir is used with protease inhibitor drugs because it is a potent inhibitor of cytochrome P-450, which greatly increases the half life of other protease inhibitors allowing once or twice a day administration. Protease inhibitors and NNRTIs can inhibit and induce different enzymes making interactions complex and difficult to predict. NRTIs have fewer interactions. The most important ones for a gynaecologist to be aware of include

- rifampicin: contraindicated (rifabutin at reduced dose sometimes used with protease inhibitors)
- sex hormones: levels reduced so oral contraception unreliable. Give double dose of levonorgestrol (3 g) for post-coital contraception
- warfarin levels increased
- proton pump inhibitors decrease levels of atazanavir which can lead to virological failure.

Prognosis

If successful the viral load is usually <50 copies/mL within 24 weeks of starting treatment, and the immune system recovers at least partially with a rise in the CD4 count and decreased risk of opportunistic infection. As long as the patient continues to take the treatment carefully prolonged viral suppression and immune recovery can occur. The virus has a high mutation rate, so if replication is allowed to occur in the presence of drug, resistance arises inevitably.

Late presentation

If immunodeficiency has already occurred treatment and prevention of opportunistic infections is needed. This may include cotrimoxazole to prevent *Pneumocystis carinii* pneumonia (PCP), and in severely immunosuppressed individuals with CD4 counts <50 cells/mm^3, azithromycin to prevent disseminated *Mycobacterium avium intracellulare* complex (MAC) infection, and valganciclovir to prevent cytomegalovirus (CMV) infection. Regular administration of antifungal agents may be necessary to control oral and vaginal candidiasis. An immune restitution inflammatory syndrome (IRIS) is increasingly recognised in those presenting with advance immunosuppression. An occult condition such as tuberculosis may become symptomatic, and manifestations of a diagnosed condition such as cryptococcal meningitis become more severe leading to increased death rates if antiretroviral therapy is started before the infection is controlled.

With longer survival we are now recognising increased rates of many non-AIDS related cancers, particularly HPV related ones. Therapy is also associated with increased risk of cardiovascular disease and diabetes mellitus. Patients should be monitored for these regularly.

Counselling

All healthcare workers should be competent in discussing HIV testing. The approach is different depending on the presence or absence of risk factors described in history taking.

If no risk factors are identified and there are no clinical reasons for suspecting infection a brief discussion to assess the individuals concerns about being tested is usually sufficient. This should cover:

- The benefits of testing for the individual.
- Details of how the result will be communicated.

If there are reasons to suspect that the test may be positive, or when communicating a positive result it is important to discuss the implications.

- Who else knows that a test is being done/will the patient tell.
- Particularly the need to inform partners now that knowingly putting a partner at risk is a criminal offence in many countries.
- Treatment is now highly successful, with near normal life expectancy.
- HIV does not preclude future pregnancies as vertical transmission is rare when appropriate interventions are used.
- Support is available from many organizations.

If one of a couple is HIV-positive advocate barrier contraception to protect against infections, and an additional more reliable form of contraception if pregnancy is not wanted. If a condom splits post exposure prophylaxis after sexual intercourse (PEPSI) may be indicated and should be started within 48 hours.

Specific conditions for obstetrics and gynaecology

HIV in pregnancy

Pregnancy is a vulnerable time for a woman to be diagnosed with HIV. Disclosure of diagnosis to partners may lead to domestic violence or abandonment. However the benefits of treatment in reducing vertical transmission and prolonging the mother's life mean that all women should be encouraged to test. Those that decline should be re-offered testing and reasons for declining explored in depth.

Because the rates of vertical transmission are now so low in Europe and the USA, one of the commonest reasons for it occurring are that the mother seroconverts after her initial test, whilst pregnant or breast feeding. The potential benefits of retesting in the third trimester are being evaluated, with testing of male partners as an alternative strategy.

The CD4 count falls in pregnancy and rises after delivery, so women may present with opportunistic infections in pregnancy. This is best managed in conjunction with the HIV specialist. Where effective antiretroviral therapy is available few vertical transmissions should occur.

Vertical transmission

Without intervention vertical transmission occurs in 25–40% pregnancies. It is thought that a minority of fetuses is infected during gestation. These babies can present with AIDS in the neonatal period. The majority is infected during parturition. Breastfeeding accounts for transmission in up to 15% of pregnancies, corresponding to 37% of infected infants. Transmission by this route may occur even after several months. The risk of vertical transmission is increased if there is a high HIV viral load or a preterm delivery. The role of genital infections in vertical transmission is still being assessed. Many children infected with HIV will survive into adolescence.

Three interventions have been shown to reduce the risk of vertical transmission of HIV.
- Avoiding breast feeding
- Elective Caesarean section
- Antiviral medication prescribed during the latter half of pregnancy, and to the neonate for 4 weeks.

With combination antiretroviral therapy with a viral load of <50 copies/ml at the time of delivery the risk of vertical transmission is <1% even with a vaginal delivery so this option is becoming increasingly taken up. If the baseline viral load is <10 000 copies/mL use of zidovudine monotherapy and elective Caesarean section has a similar risk and remains an option. However Caesarean section may limit the choice in future pregnancies now that many women with HIV are choosing to have several children.

Choice of therapy

In general if a woman falls pregnant on antiretroviral therapy it is easiest to continue the current regimen. If a woman presents having fallen pregnant on efavirenz current guidelines recommend continuing it with close monitoring for fetal abnormalities. Neural tube defects such as spina bifida occur at around 2 weeks' gestation, so it is pointless to stop the drug when a woman presents at a later stage of pregnancy. If she is not yet receiving antiretroviral treatment she should plan to start in pregnancy with the timing and choice of agent dependent on the viral load and choice of triple or monotherapy.

If a pregnant woman is not on treatment, but fulfils standard criteria for treatment, e.g. CD4 count below 350 cells/mm^3 treatment should be started as soon as possible. If treatment is not indicated for the mother a short course of antiretroviral therapy (START) should be initiated to reduce the risk of vertical transmission. Ideally this should be around 20 weeks' gestation so that the viral load is reduced by 24 weeks' gestation when a premature infant is potentially viable.

In many developing countries resources for triple therapy are lacking so regimens using short course monotherapy with nevirapine for mother and infant may be used. Although this reduces perinatal infection rates to about 6% there is a risk of viral resistance for both mother and infant

if infected. Alternative short course dual therapy or triple therapy combinations have been developed.

Caesarean section is not routinely available in many developing countries, and bottle feeding or early weaning without a clean water supply is associated with a greater excess risk of death from gastroenteritis than of HIV from breastfeeding. Current approaches being studied are to support 100% breastfeeding rather than any mixed feeding, and the use of antiretroviral therapy for mother and/or infant.

Currently efavirenz is avoided in women planning pregnancy because its use was associated with teratogenicity in Rhesus macaque monkeys. The dose and frequency of dosing of nevirapine and some protease inhibitors may need to be modified with altered pharmacokinetics in the second and third trimesters of pregnancy.

HIV in gynaecology

HIV testing

Current British HIV Association (BHIVA) guidelines on HIV testing recommend exploring HIV testing in colposcopy and termination of pregnancy clinics. These may be the first point of access of healthcare for women with HIV, and the prevalence in such settings is likely to be higher than in the general community.

HPV related conditions

HPV infection flourishes in immunosuppressed individuals. Genital warts often persist despite aggressive surgical treatment. Chronic HPV infection can result in the development of carcinomas, CIN, anal and vulval intraepithelial neoplasia (AIN and VIN) and Bowen's disease. Because of this most Physicians perform cervical cytology annually in women with HIV infection. High rates of AIN are now reported in heterosexual women with chronic HIV infection, and squamous cell carcinoma of the anus is now demonstrably more common in men and women with HIV. Persistent atypical warty lesions of the skin or vulva should be biopsied.

Other infections

Other infections can also be more persistent in HIV infected individuals. There is limited evidence that PID requires longer courses of antibiotics in women with HIV. Careful follow-up is certainly indicated. Postpartum endometritis is common in this group of women. Eruptions of secondary genital herpes may become widespread, severe and persist for weeks if not diagnosed and treated. It often presents as deep, painful ulceration. If lasting more than 4 weeks it is AIDS defining in an HIV-positive individual.

Contraception

Although all HIV infected women are urged to use condoms to prevent them transmitting the infection to others, they should also be advised to use a more reliable form of contraception if they do not wish to become pregnant. Because many antiretroviral drugs induce the cytochrome P-450 enzymes that metabolise sex hormones, only Depoprovera and IUCDs are known to work reliably in women receiving antiretroviral drugs. It is important to plan future contraception during pregnancy to avoid early unwanted pregnancy in women who will not be breastfeeding.

Preconceptional planning

Preconceptional advice is important for women with HIV. With rates of vertical transmission now <1% where triple therapy is available, HIV is not a contraindication to IVF although only some centres offer it.

HIV-positive woman

If on treatment her antiretroviral medication may need modifying. Currently all antiretroviral agents are category B or C in the FDA (American food and drug administration) with the exception of efavirenz which is category D. Efavirenz, which is a favoured first line treatment in current USA, BHIVA and European guidelines, caused skeletal abnormalities in Rhesus Macaques, and four cases of spina bifida reported retrospectively led to its current classification. In prospectively reported pregnancies in the registry there is currently no excess risk of abnormalities for efavirenz and the classification may be changed in future. Current practice is to change to an alternative agent if planning pregnancy.

Use of condoms and artificial insemination is recommended to protect the male partner from infection. Even if the partner is HIV-positive there is a theoretical risk of transmission of virus which may be more pathogenic for one partner, or carry resistance mutations.

This advice is now less clear following a statement by Swiss Physicians that if a man or woman is on treatment with an undetectable viral load the risk of transmission through vaginal intercourse is less than that of couples using condoms where the index patient is not receiving treatment. It is good practice to discuss this with couples and allow them to make their own risk assessment.

Also discuss the management of HIV in pregnancy to reduce vertical transmission. Even with an undetectable viral load caesarean section offers a reduced risk of infection but when the risk is already so low it is not clear that the benefit outweighs the risks associated with caesarean section. In a resource poor setting discuss the pros and cons of bottle feeding versus exclusive breastfeeding.

HIV-positive man

If an HIV-negative woman has a positive partner sperm washing has been shown to be safe, albeit expensive. It is more difficult when this is not available locally or there is no funding for it. A retrospective study of 70 (approx) pregnancies in HIV discordant couples from Spain reported no infections if the index patient had an undetectable viral load. The Swiss statement (above) similarly supports a low risk in this scenario. If a discordant couple choose to conceive naturally the risk of transmission can be minimised by targeting unprotected intercourse to the fertile time of the menstrual cycle, and checking for and treating genital tract infections in both of them.

Internet resources

British HIV association (BHIVA) links to current guidelines: bhiva.org

United Nations UNAIDS latest worldwide statistics on the epidemic: www.unaids.org/en

World Health Organization guidelines for resource constrained settings and reports on treatment roll out programmes: www.who.int/hiv/pub/guidelines/en

US Centers for Disease Control links to current guidelines: www.cdc.gov/hiv/resources/guidelines

Antiretroviral pregnancy registry prospective reporting of pregnancies exposed to antiretroviral therapy: www.apregistry.com for

Antiretroviral drug interactions: www.hiv-druginteractions.org

Patient resources

Patient support groups generally available locally. National AIDS Manual (NAM): www.aidsmap.com

Positively Women: www.positivelywomen.org.uk

Terence Higgins Trust: www.tht.org.uk

The Swiss Statement: Vernazza P, *et al.* Les personnes séropositives ne souffrant d'aucune autre MST et suivant un traitement antirétroviral efficace ne transmettent pas le VIH par voie sexuelle. Bulletin des médecins suisses 89 (5), 2008. summarised at www.aidsmap.com/en/news/4E9D555B-18FB-4D56-B912-2C28AFCCD36B.asp

Safety and Toxicity of Individual Antiretroviral Agents in Pregnancy: www.aidsinfo.nih.gov/contentfiles/PerinatalGL-SafetyTox_Sup.pdf

Human papillomavirus

Definition

Human papillomavirus (HPV) is a non-enveloped double-stranded DNA virus that infects the epithelium, such as skin, or mucus membranes. In this case the virus is specific to humans, although there are different species-specific papillomaviruses which infect other animals. There are at least 130 different strains of HPV which can infect any part of the human integument. The consequences of infection range from warts to dysplasia, and cancer. The different strains are identified by number and tend to be associated with specific anatomic infections. There are 30–40 types that infect the genital tract in both men and women and largely transmitted by intimate sexual contact.

Epidemiology

It is likely that HPV is the most common sexually transmitted infection. Because it is not reportable and not necessarily specifically screened, the true prevalence is uncertain. However epidemiological data suggest that it is well established in younger women such as adolescents and those in their early twenties; rates for HPV infection in women younger than 25 in North America and Northern Europe are 10-fold higher than in women older than 45 (Franceschi et al. 2006). In the USA the CDC estimates that 80% of women will have been infected with at least one strain of HPV by 50 years of age (CDCP 2004). Although it is fair to say that worldwide this is a common infection, there are data from the International Agency for Research on Cancer (IARC) that suggest these trends may not be universal. Their surveys have shown overall low rates of infection in certain populations of Thailand and Vietnam, and flat or rates that increase with age in India, China, Mexico, and South America(1). It is not clear if this reflects different rates of infection or differences in the natural history of HPV among various populations.

Pathology

Some of these HPV types, such as 6, 11, 42, 43, and 44, are considered 'low risk' and rarely if ever cause cancer but do cause warts and some cases of mild dysplasia. The 'high-risk' types, such as 16, 18, 31, 33, 35, 39, 45, 51, 52, 56, 58, 59, and 68, are associated with dysplasia and cancer. This latter group is responsible for the development of cervical intraepithelial neoplasia (CIN) and cancer as well as vaginal (VaIN), vulvar (VIN), penile (PIN), and anal (AIN) neoplasia and cancer. It appears that the majority of genital tract cancers are caused by types 16 and 18 worldwide and may represent a more virulent type of infection (Munoz 2004). Although more than half of cervical cancer is caused by type 16 and approximately two-thirds by 16 and 18, over 90% of vulvar carcinoma is caused by type 16 alone (Srodon et al. 2006). At the same time relative rates for HPV 18 suggest it is more common in the aetiology of glandular pathology.

As for the actual infection process, it appears that the virus must find its way to the basal cell layer of the epithelium, where an interaction between virus and cell allows for some endocytotic event and subsequent transport to the nucleus. In the nucleus the virus usually remains separate from the host genome, as an episome. While the basal cell matures and differentiates becoming part of the superficial epithelial cells the virus genome multiplies and ultimately replicates copies of itself, which are then shed with the superficial desquamating cells. In higher degrees of dysplasia and invasive cancer the viral genome actually integrates into the host DNA suggesting this step is at the root of malignant transformation. The virus ultimately destabilizes the cell cycle with transcription products from the E6 and E7 oncogenes, which interrupt tumour suppressor proteins p53 and pRb respectfully in the host cell. Thus, length of time for harboring the infection correlates with severity of disease, probably by increasing the opportunity for genetic integration.

Prognosis

There are multiple studies demonstrating significant clearance rates of HPV infection, particularly in younger patients. The clearance of HPV has also been correlated with the clearance of clinical disease. This premise has been challenged by the notion that perhaps there are long-term latent infections that remain clinically insignificant and are missed because the current screening tools are not sensitive enough or unable to access the virus. Perhaps the greater concern is the development of pathology from latent infection in the future, if the host's immune status weakens. It is likely that both of these scenarios occur; however, this has little impact on current clinical management which includes continued screening.

Clinical approach

The role of HPV has been defined in the development of cervical cancer thanks to the efforts of the recent Nobel laureate and molecular biologist Harald ZurHausen. He established that HPV is involved in the pathogenesis of cervical cancer. His findings along with epidemiological evidence from Munoz et al. (2006) has verified the causal relationship between HPV infection and development of cancer (Srodon et al. 2006). Given this relationship, HPV has become a tool for diagnostic modalities and a target for prophylactic vaccines and therapeutic approaches.

Diagnosis

Although the pap smear alone has single-handedly reduced the mortality rate from cervical cancer by more than 70% over the last five decades, the addition of HPV typing increases the sensitivity of finding pathology. The use of HPV typing for high-risk HPV by itself has a sensitivity of greater than 89% for detecting high-grade cervical lesions. This compares favourably to the liquid-based cytology which is probably less than 80%. However, the positive predictive value of HPV typing is not robust because most women with HPV do not have cytological abnormalities. The liquid-based pap smear has a superior positive predictive value as it detects cytological abnormalities which is really the endpoint for clinical screening objectives. Liquid-based cytology is the current screening standard in Europe and was universally implemented in the UK by the end of 2008. Combining the two techniques not only improves the sensitivity but also improves the negative predictive value to nearly 100% (Arbyn et al. 2006). The latter point being that if a patient has a normal pap smear and does not harbour a high-risk HPV her chances of developing severe cervical dysplasia or cervical cancer are less than 0.1% over the next 5 years. Given this, the FDA in the USA approved clinical testing for high-risk HPV as a screening tool when combined with cervical cytology in women 30 years of age or older using the hybrid-capture test marketed by Digene to screen for 13 high-risk types of HPV. In this algorithm patients who have normal cytology and negative HPV testing are not screened for 3 years as a cost-containing measure. Thirty years of age has been selected as a slightly arbitrary age yet does reflect most epidemiological trends in screening a population with a lower prevalence of HPV and greater incidence of pathology which increases the positive predictive value for finding dysplasia. This strategy is less helpful in younger populations where the likelihood of finding HPV is very high without identifying significant neoplasia. The other scenario where High-Risk HPV typing has been approved for clinical use in the USA is as an adjunct to pap smear screening when the cytology is atypical squamous cells of undetermined significance (ASCUS). In this case approximately 50% of the patients do not have a high-risk HPV and are allowed the more conservative recommendation of a pap smear in 12 months. If they have a high-risk HPV they are referred for colposcopic evaluation (ALTS 2003). The role of HPV screening as a diagnostic tool is being evaluated in the UK. There are two major studies which should yield answers in the near future. The first is A Randomized Trial of Human Papilloma Virus Testing in Primary Cervical Screening (ARTISTIC), in which more than 24 000 attendees age 20–64 at Specific NHS Cervical Screening Programme sites are screened with liquid-based cytology and high-risk HPV typing. The HPV results are either revealed or concealed based on randomization. Outcomes will include the test characteristics for HPV typing as well as cost and efficiency. Further outcomes include insight into psychological and psychosexual differences when HPV status is known. Although publication is expected in the spring of 2009, preliminary data support previous findings where HPV prevalence is prohibitively high in younger women, which would only serve to increase the demand for follow-up measures. A second study is a Trial of Management of Borderline and other Low-grade Abnormal smears (TOMBOLA) funded by the Medical Research Council. Results should be forthcoming and will include information on the potential for HPV to be used as triage in patients with borderline or mild dyskaryosis.

Management

As for preventive and therapeutic uses, HPV technology has been employed in the production of vaccines. Within the applications of vaccines there are two approaches with one being to prevent infection as a passive vaccine and the other as an active vaccine to treat infected individuals and induce regression of disease. Presently the latter approach is still being developed and is in clinical trials. There appears to be some potential in this, but certainly no consistent and compelling data at this time.

Reproducible data have been published in multiple studies disclosing the efficacy of the prophylactic vaccines in preventing HPV-related disease. This vaccine development grew out of the discovery that the outer protein capsule would essentially self-assemble into an empty viral shell, absent the DNA contents, if the correct capsid proteins

were put together in the laboratory. The concept is that the body recognizes these empty viral coats and will produce antibodies that recognize and block future infection from the real virus. As it turns out, the surface proteins are unique to each strain of HPV and thus the vaccine is type specific. Gardasil, produced by Merck pharmaceuticals, one of two prophylactic vaccines, was approved in Europe in 2006 and Cervarix, GlaxoSmithKline, was approved in 2007. Gardasil provides protection against HPV types 6 and 11, which are low-risk types and responsible for 90% of genital warts, as well as high-risk types 16 and 18. Cervarix contains only capsid proteins from high-risk HPV types 16 and 18. Gardasil was approved in the USA in June 2006 for the prevention of cervical cancer and genital warts in females aged 9–26, whereas cervarix has not yet been approved in the USA. Most of the national health plans in Europe have implemented HPV vaccine programmes. The UK recently launched an HPV vaccine programme, using Cervarix, which initially will focus on 12–13-year-old girls. A 'catch up programme' will follow whereby 17–18-year-old girls will be vaccinated the following year and then 16–18 and 15–17-year-old girls will be vaccinated the following 2 years respectively.

Further reading

Arbyn M, Sasieni P, Meijer C, et al. Clinical applications of HPV testing: a summary of meta-analyses. Vaccine 2006;24;S3/78–89.

ASCUS-LSIL Triage Study (ALTS) Group. Results of a randomized trial on the management of cytology interpretations of atypical squamous cells of undetermined significance. Am J Obstet Gynecol 2003;188:1383–92.

Centers for Disease Control and Prevention (CDCP). Genital HPV infection fact sheet. Rockville: CDC National Prevention Information Network 2004.

Franceschi S, Herrero R, Clifford GM, et al. Variations in the age-specific curves of human papillomavirus prevalence in women worldwide. Int J Cancer 2006;119:2677–84.

HPV vaccines and screening in the prevention of cervical cancer. Vaccine 2006;24(Suppl. 3).

Munoz N, Bosch FX, Castellsaque X, et al. Against which human papillomavirus types shall we vaccinate and screen? The international perspective. Int J Cancer 2004;111:278–85.

Srodon M, Stoler M, Baber G, Kurman R. The distribution of low and high-risk HPV types in vulvar and vaginal intraepithelial neoplasia (VIN and VaIN). Am J Surg Pathol 2006;30,12;1513–18.

Stanley M, Immunobiology of HPV and HPV vaccines. Gynecol Oncol 2008;109:S15–21.

World Health Organization (WHO) Human papillomavirus and HPV vaccines: technical information for policy-makers and health professionals. WHO 2007: http://who.int/reproductive-health/publications/hpvvaccines_techinfo/index.html

Internet resources

www.asccp.org
www.hpa.org.uk

Patient information and contacts

www.asccp.org
www.cancerresearchuk.org
www.patient.co.uk

Hypertension

Definition

Hypertension is established in a pregnant woman if the blood pressure (BP) measurement is ≥140/90 mmHg for two or more occasions at least 4 hours apart using the same arm. If hypertension pre-dates pregnancy or is found before 20 weeks' gestation, the individual is considered to have chronic hypertension. Hypertension first detected after 20 weeks' gestation is gestational hypertension (GH) in the absence of significant proteinuria, and pre-eclampsia in the presence of proteinuria. Normotensive women with only an increase in systolic and/or diastolic pressure of 30 mmHg and 15 mmHg respectively are not associated with complications and should not be considered as having GH. Severe hypertension is defined as systolic BP ≥160 mmHg or diastolic BP ≥110 mmHg.

This chapter will be confined to discussion of chronic and gestational hypertension only.

Epidemiology

- Chronic hypertension is found in 1–5% of all pregnancies. It includes both essential hypertension and hypertension secondary to underlying medical conditions. The incidences of the various underlying conditions are quite variable depending on location and population.
- Gestational hypertension (GH), found in 3–10% of all pregnancies, may represent the early phase/presentation of pre-eclampsia, which can manifest as late as the time of labour or early postpartum period. It has been shown that the great majority of women presenting with GH in the early third trimester eventually progressed to pre-eclampsia with time.

Pathology

In normal pregnancy, cardiac output shows an early increase with a subsequent plateau after 20–24 weeks gestation, and a small decrease closer to term. Total peripheral resistance shows a similar but inversed pattern with an early decrease and a nadir is reached at 20–24 weeks' gestation, followed by a plateau and non-significant increase closer to term. Women with GH have significantly elevated cardiac output before and during the clinical course of the condition, reflecting a hyperdynamic circulation throughout pregnancy. The increased cardiac output is demonstrable as early as 11–14 weeks' gestation and is at a rate well in excess of that of the normal population throughout pregnancy and after the diagnosis of GH. Total peripheral resistance is generally normal throughout most of the pregnancy except towards term when it is reduced. The increased vasodilated state remained despite a clinical diagnosis of GH.

Echocardiographic Doppler studies 2–4 days postpartum revealed that women with GH had significant left ventricular dysfunction, with depressed systolic function and altered diastolic function, left atrial dysfunction, and high total vascular resistance (TVR). The most significant differences shown in the higher isovolumetric relaxation time and the Tei index (sum of both contraction and relaxation isovolumetric periods divided by the ejection time). Furthermore, the left ventricular mass index is increased due to an increase in the septal and posterior wall thickness, whereas the dimensions of the left ventricle, left atrium and aortic root do not change. There is an altered cardiac geometric pattern of concentric hypertrophy.

With respect to adverse maternal and fetal pregnancy outcomes, a stepwise increase is found from GH to pre-eclampsia, for severe maternal disease (26.5% and 63.4% respectively) as well as for preterm birth and small-for-gestational age (SGA) infants.

Aetiology

Chronic hypertension

This may be due to the following conditions:

- essential hypertension, often with a familial history of hypertension
- secondary to chronic renal diseases, including chronic glomerulonephritis and pyelonephritis
- secondary to endocrine conditions including hyper- and hypothyroidism, Cushing's syndrome/disease, Conn's syndrome, phaeochromocytoma, adrenal hyperplasia, acromegaly, hyperparathyroidism, and pre-existing type I and type II diabetes mellitus.
- cardiovascular conditions including coarctation of the aorta, renal artery stenosis
- autoimmune conditions such as systemic lupus erythematosus and antiphospholipid syndrome.

Gestational hypertension

Clinically GH may evolve into pre-eclampsia, or reveals itself as the unmasking of chronic hypertension when reassessed after delivery. However, echocardiographic studies suggested different cardiac anatomical and functional changes and adaptation that are distinct from pre-eclampsia and fetal growth restriction, or from normotensive subjects. Furthermore, mild to moderate increase in BP alone is poorly predictive of adverse maternal and fetal outcome. It is therefore possible that GH is a feature of maternal physiological adaptation to the demands of pregnancy, rather than of a pathological process, in a significant proportion of women diagnosed with GH.

Prognosis

BP alone is limited in its predictability for adverse outcome, and mild hypertension in isolation or appearing for the first time in labour are generally not associated with adverse outcomes. An increase in the diastolic pressure by 15 mmHg but short of 90 mmHg does not predict adverse outcome. On the other hand, GH may represent the early presentation of pre-eclampsia, and pre-eclampsia may be superimposed on chronic hypertension of all categories. Therefore, all hypertensive patients should be managed as high risk and monitored for the development of multisystem involvement and fetal compromise by clinical and laboratory means.

One new approach is to assess the aforementioned maternal cardiac adaptation to the development of hypertension. Adverse maternal and fetal outcomes can be better predicted from the total vascular resistance (TVR) and left ventricular concentric geometry, both of which are independent predictors. The TVR is calculated from maternal echocardiographic examination and measurement of BP at the brachial artery with a manual cuff, and using the formula:

$$TVR = (MBP(mmHg)/CO \ (L/minutes)) \times 80$$

where MBP is the mean arterial pressure. Applying a cut-off value of 1340 dyn seconds/cm^5, the sensitivity and specificity are 90% and 91% respectively. Concentric geometry is defined as a left ventricular mass index >50 g/m and a relative wall thickness >0.44 ((interventricular septum diameter + posterior wall diastolic thickness)(left ventricular end-diastolic diameter)) on echocardiography.

Clinical approach

Blood pressure measurement

The systolic blood pressure (SBP) reading is defined by phase I and diastolic blood pressure (DBP) reading by phase V of the Korotkoff sounds. The BP readings should be obtained using a mercury sphygmomanometer with an appropriate-sized cuff (length of 1.5 times the circumference of the arm) placed at the level of the heart with the patient in a sitting position. Any aneroid or automated BP device used should have been calibrated beforehand or validated, since automated devices may underestimate the BP. In case of consistently higher readings from one arm, this arm should be used for all BP measurement.

Conceptual understanding

In practice GH often merges into pre-eclampsia with progressive multisystem involvement and fetal compromise, and reliance on the presence of proteinuria to differentiate between the two conditions is also dependent on the methods of determining proteinuria (spot urine measurement or dipsticks, protein–creatinine ratio, 24-hour collection). Therefore it has been recommended that the appearance of multisystem involvement and/or fetal complications be used instead to define the appearance of pre-eclampsia. Indeed, the management should be dictated by the clinical features and complications, rather than an arbitrary definition of the condition, be it GH, pre-eclampsia, or pre-eclampsia superimposed on chronic hypertension.

Prepregnancy counselling and assessment for chronic hypertension

Women diagnosed with chronic hypertension due to whatever cause in the reproductive age group should be asked about their desire and plan for pregnancy at regular intervals in the medical clinic, and the information be clearly documented in the medical notes, since their condition and their desire might change with time. Except for severe secondary hypertension or the presence of end organ damage, pregnancy is generally not contraindicated. However, the control of hypertension should be optimized, and the types of medication be changed to ones that are safe for the fetus, when pregnancy is contemplated. For secondary hypertension, the severity and status of the underlying condition should also be assessed and the treatment optimized similarly. Referral to a prepregnancy counselling clinic managed by maternal–fetal medicine specialists is desirable, as all patients with chronic medical diseases should have a realistic picture of the likely course and outcome of pregnancy in relation to their individual condition. There is also the opportunity to discuss and adopt the most appropriate means of contraception until conception is decided. Subsequent follow-up management must be individualized, and the principle is to ensure early confirmation and dating of the pregnancy for subsequent arrangement for prenatal diagnosis and baseline clinical assessment and investigations. It will also be early enough for any change of medications to take place where necessary.

Clinical assessment

First presentation of hypertension

- For a pregnant woman found incidentally to have transient hypertension which settles after a variable period of rest in the clinic, more frequent follow-up assessment should be arranged, the interval being dependent on the gestation. At/after 28 weeks' gestation, the patient should be seen at least weekly once before spacing out the interval, if the subsequent BP readings are normal.

- For a patient with persistently elevated BP, the fluctuation in the readings should be documented in hourly to 2-hourly measurements in the day centre/day hospital, or if this is not available, then a short stay in the ward. If the BP settles after rest, then she could be seen again the following week. If the BP remains elevated, she may be warded for workup. If only the SBP is elevated, these patients should be closely followed up for the development of diastolic hypertension.

- A comprehensive physical examination should be performed for any woman with hypertension, including auscultation of the heart and chest, looking out for radial-femoral delay, and listening for bruit in the renal area. Fundoscopy should also be carried out if the instrument is available. Even if the BP reading returns to normal subsequently, any abnormal finding should call for assessment especially in the third trimester.

Known chronic hypertension

- For patients with a known history of hypertension, particularly those who are already on antihypertensive medications, symptoms and signs of deteriorating hypertension control should be elicited. The dose of medications can be adjusted in the clinic, but the frequency of follow-up may need to be increased, and the patients should be instructed to return to the clinic or admit herself should adverse effects of either the medication or the hypertension be experienced at home or at work. Sick leave for rest at home may be necessary.

- In case of uncertainty, the patients can be seen daily in the day centre/hospital, or they can measure their BP regularly at home using a sphygmomanometer that has been previously calibrated in the clinic, and to test their urine daily using dipsticks for protein. More frequent follow-up should be arranged if the BP is persistently elevated or proteinuria is significant.

Obstetric examination

- The abdominal examination should include symphysial-fundal height measurement, careful palpation for fetal parts, fetal lie and presentation, and a rough estimate of the fetal size and amount of amniotic fluid. In addition, an ultrasound scan should be carried out if available.

- Any suspected fetal growth restriction, oligohydramnios, or unexplained uterine size much larger than date (whether due to polyhydramnios or large fetus or both) would warrant admission.

- All multifetal pregnancies, and pregnancies complicated by fetal or maternal complications such as gestational diabetes mellitus, should be further assessed if hypertension is found in the clinic.

Inpatient monitoring/day-care assessment

- The women should be admitted for assessment and monitoring of maternal and fetal conditions if necessary.

- The BP should be monitored 4-hourly, watching out for the loss of the diurnal rhythm that may suggest the development of pre-eclampsia.

- Maternal symptoms should be documented daily.

- Further investigations should be arranged as indicated.

- Fetal assessment should be organized.

Investigations

Standard investigations

Serial monitoring is required to determine the progression of the condition and timing of intervention.

- Urinalysis: this should be done in the clinic at every visit. A mid-stream urine specimen for culture should always be collected if proteinuria is found. If proteinuria is 2 plus or more, a random specimen for the estimation of the protein–creatinine ratio should be sent. Confirmation of significant proteinuria calls for a 24-hour collection for quantification, which needs to be done carefully to ensure complete collection. Proteinuria is defined as a 24-hour urine protein excretion of ˇ300 mg or a protein–creatinine ratio of ˇ30 mg/mmol.
- Renal function test: this should include the measurement of serum electrolytes, urea, creatinine, and uric acid concentrations. Electrolyte disturbance, especially in the form of a low potassium concentration, should alert one to the possibility of Cushing's or Conn's syndrome. If the creatinine concentration is normal, there is no need to calculate the creatinine clearance, which can be done without resorting to a 24-hour urine collection nowadays.
- Liver function test: this should include serum albumen, globulin, bilirubin, alkaline phosphatase, transaminases, and γ-glutamyl transferase. An underlying liver disease may be present.
- Oral glucose tolerance test: this should be carried out if not done before, as there is an association between glucose intolerance and hypertension.

Additional investigations

These depend on the initial findings and clinical suspicion.

- Blood tests to assess and monitor the progression of the condition, including evidence of haemolysis (serum bilirubin, lactate dehydrogenase, serum iron).
- Blood test to monitor disturbance in coagulation, including prothrombin (PT) and activated partial thromboplastin time (APTT), D-dimer, and fibrin-fibrinogen degradation products (FDP), and platelet count and blood smear.
- Blood test for myocardial damage such as creatinine kinase (MB) and troponin-t.
- Test for possible underlying conditions, including blood tests for thyroid function, autoimmune markers, anticardiolipin antibodies and the lupus anticoagulant, calcium level and the calcium–phosphate ratio, other hormones such as growth hormone, cortisol, parathormone, and serum and urine catecholamines, after consultation with physicians.
- Imaging studies, including ultrasound, Doppler and echocardiographic studies, and magnetic resonance imaging and CT scan if necessary, to rule out lesions of the heart and major arteries, and endocrine tumours such as phaeochromocytoma, adrenal tumour, etc.

Fetal assessment and monitoring

For patients with chronic hypertension, screening for fetal anomalies should be organized as for any high-risk pregnancies. Serial monitoring for fetal growth and wellbeing should be commenced in the last 2 months of pregnancy, and earlier if complications or deterioration in BP control occur. For women with GH, the fetal condition should be assessed at diagnosis.

- Fetal anomalies should be excluded with a detailed ultrasound scan if this is not done before. The information helps the obstetrician and parents to decide the best course of action for the remainder of the pregnancy.
- Fetal size should be assessed with ultrasound scan to detect the fetus with unsuspected growth restriction. The information is especially helpful in multifetal pregnancies.
- Fetal wellbeing should be assessed with the biophysical profile (BPP), amniotic fluid index (AFI), especially in fetuses suspected of being growth restricted. The parameters provide a baseline for future comparison. Regular reassessment with the BPP is indicated if there is fetal growth restriction, if the initial BPP score is reduced, or if the antihypertensive medication has rendered the CTG difficult to interpret. A complete profile may not be necessary each time if the AFI is normal and not decreasing, and fetal growth is not slowing down.
- Doppler studies of the uterine and umbilical arteries may be helpful. A placental origin of the hypertension may be suggested from the uterine artery waveform. The umbilical artery indices provide early warning of placental deterioration.
- A fetal kick count to monitor fetal movements at home is helpful for the majority of patients, especially those on medications. They should be instructed to report to the clinic or ward for further assessment should there be sustained or progressive decrease in fetal movements noticed over a 48-hour period.

Antihypertensive medications

Principles

- Initial trial of rest and observation before prescription is useful. Mild hypertension does not require antihypertensive medication.
- Commence treatment promptly for severe hypertension with the aim to keep SBP <160 mmHg and DBP <110 mmHg. It should ideally be carried out in hospital to allow close monitoring of the response and avoid the problems related to excessive hypotension.
- For non-severe hypertension, commence treatment if presentation is before 28 weeks' gestation or with comorbid conditions, aiming to keep SBP at 130–139 mmHg and DBP at 80–89 mmHg.
- The choice of medication depends on the obstetrician's experience with the medication, safety for the fetus and breastfeeding, and the patient's preference. It may be necessary to change the medication for patients with chronic hypertension once pregnancy is confirmed, or when pregnancy is contemplated.
- For outpatients, arrange more frequent follow-up visits to monitor BP response and adjust the dose if necessary so as to avoid inducing hypotension. Patients should keep a diary. Home monitoring is preferable but the patients must be given adequate and appropriate instructions and prior calibration is necessary for the various devices available commercially for home use.

Types of medications and regimens

Methyldopa

- Dosage: 250–500 mg orally bid qid, maximum 3 g/day.
- Remarks: loading dose has been suggested but not universally recommended.

Labetolol

- Dosage: in cases of severe hypertension 20 mg i.v. repeat 20–80 mg q30 minute, or 1–2 mg/minute, maximum 300 mg. Oral 100–400 mg bid qid, maximum 1200 mg/day
- Remarks: decreases the risk of severe hypertension and the need for additional antihypertensives, maternal hospital admission, neonatal respiratory distress syndrome. Avoid in asthma. Increased risk of neonatal bradycardia, small-for-gestational age (SGA) infants. Insufficient data on perinatal mortality or preterm birth. Similar effectiveness with methyldopa.

Nifedipine

- Dosage: 5–10-mg capsule orally q30 minutes, then slow release form 10–20 mg bid qid.
- Remarks: can be used together with magnesium sulphate. Check the form of preparation available in the hospital pharmacy.

Hydralazine

- Dosage: 5 mg i.v. and repeat q 30 minutes, or 0.5–10 mg/h infusion, to a maximum of 20 mg i.v.
- Remarks: for the control of severe hypertension, it appears to be more effective than labetolol and less effective than nifedipine. Compared with other agents, there is more maternal hypotension and side-effects, Caesarean section, placental abruption, oliguria, adverse effects on fetal heart rate and low first minute Apgar score. Less fetal bradycardia compared with labetolol.

Angiotensin-converting enzyme inhibitors (ACEI)

- Remarks: serious fetal effects including renal failure, renal dysplasia, hypotension, hypocalvaria, oligohydramnios, and pulmonary hypoplasia. The effect is greatest during the second and third trimesters. Avoid in pregnancy.

Angiotensin receptor blockers

- Remarks: similar adverse fetal effects as ACEI.
  Medications for severe hypertension: labetolol, nifedipine (capsules and slow-release preparation), hydralazine.
  Medications for non-severe hypertension: methyldopa, labetolol, metoprolol (or other beta-blockers, including pindolol, acebutolol, propranolol), nifedipine.

Labour and delivery

- If labour or delivery is anticipated before 34 weeks' gestation, corticosteroid therapy should be given. On the other hand, tocolytic therapy for spontaneous preterm labour is not warranted since fetal compromise or maternal complication is very likely under the circumstance, so that tocolysis will increase the maternal and fetal risks with little benefit to the fetus.
- If the presentation/diagnosis is after 34 weeks' gestation, delivery is indicated if there is clinical deterioration or features of maternal or fetal compromise. For presentation after 37 completed weeks, there is little point in waiting for events to happen. Vaginal delivery is indicated for the majority of cases. Cervical priming should be attempted if the cervix is unfavourable but there is no maternal or fetal compromise. For an unfavourable cervix that fails to respond to priming, or evidence of maternal/fetal compromise appears, a semi-elective Caesarean delivery is preferable to an emergency Caesarean delivery for failed induction or fetal distress.

- The stress of labour and delivery often leads to an increase in the BP despite satisfactory control before. Features of pre-eclampsia may also appear for the first time. Severe or uncontrolled hypertension may be associated with fetal distress and placental abruption. Therefore, close maternal and fetal monitoring should be organized with preparation for emergency Caesarean delivery made for women with any category of hypertension during labour. However, Caesarean delivery should be reserved for obstetric indications except for the following underlying or associated conditions:
  - coarctation of the aorta
  - aortic dissection or aneurysm, or other related cardiovascular complications
  - history of stroke or the presence of cerebral aneurysm
  - unsatisfactory control of hypertension in the presence of a low likelihood of successful vaginal delivery.
- The following steps should be taken:
  - set up and maintain an intravenous access with normal saline
  - send blood for cross-match and reserve at least 2 units to cover the peripartum period
  - keep patient nil by mouth
  - prophylaxis for aspiration with antacid (sodium citrate) and ranitidine
  - monitor and document maternal vital signs and oxygen saturation
  - continuous cardiotocography
  - keep intake and output chart, follow the 'dry regime' as for the management of pre-eclampsia
  - place patient in left lateral tilt position throughout
  - provide adequate analgesia. Epidural analgesia is preferred, but caution with fluid loading while avoiding hypotension especially for patients receiving antihypertensive medication
  - assess the progress of labour regularly and use a partogram with alert and action lines; set up management plan beforehand and avoid prolonged labour; augmentation with oxytocin infusion if necessary but may need to restrict fluid infusion by using a more concentrated solution
  - maintain BP control with intravenous medication, using infusion regimens with hydralazine or labetolol. Avoid bolus doses. Absorption from oral administration is unreliable and there is a risk of aspiration. Sublingual nifedipine may result in a sudden and marked drop in BP leading to fetal distress; therefore, this should be used with caution
  - invasive cardiac monitoring with pulmonary artery catheterization or central venous access is not recommended except for specific indications and in a high-dependency setting.

Points to note for delivery

- If BP control is unsatisfactory or deteriorated during labour, avoid the Valsalva manoeuvre in the mother and assist delivery with forceps.
- A sudden increase in BP may lead to complications and intravenous medications may be necessary to stabilize BP.
- Magnesium sulphate should be given if features of impending eclampsia are found, but this should not be relied upon as the only or main form of antihypertensive therapy.

- Postpartum induction of diuresis with a diuretic may help to minimize the effect of the sudden expansion of blood volume from the return of blood from the utero-placental circulation.
- Frequent monitoring of BP (e.g. quarter- or half-hourly) may be necessary postpartum, especially in women previously on antihypertensives. The combined effects of changing/stopping the previously prescribed medications before/during labour, fluid dynamics, blood loss, and response to the stress and pain of labour and delivery, often lead to increased fluctuations of BP.
- Prophylaxis for postpartum haemorrhage should be undertaken for all cases with small boluses (5–10 units) of oxytocin, followed by an infusion of 40 units in 500 mL of normal saline given over 4–6 hours. Do not use ergot-containing preparations, which may lead to a sudden increase in BP and myocardial ischaemia
- Postpartum shock may be mistaken initially as the BP returning to normal postpartum. In this context care must be exercised with the peripartum use of nifedipine to control hypertension, since cases of postpartum haemorrhage associated with peripartum use of nifedipine in hypertensive women has been encountered.

Postnatal management and breastfeeding

- Postpartum monitoring of BP: a postpartum increase in BP commencing on day 3 and reaching a peak on days 5–6 is not uncommon, especially in patients whose antihypertensive medications have been stopped. This is attributed to fluid shift back into the circulation and the rapid decline in serum progesterone level. A significant rise in BP may be dangerous. Resumption of the original antihypertensive medication, or using a new medication and adjusting the dose according to maternal response may be required. The patient should be discharged with treatment only after the BP has been stabilized and she is asymptomatic. Early postnatal follow-up, e.g. 2–3 weeks postpartum may be necessary. The medication may be tailed off gradually over the next 3–12 weeks. Persistent hypertension after 3 months of delivery warrants referral to physicians for assessment.
- Analgesia should be given in adequate amounts since pain from whatever cause can aggravate hypertension. If an abdominal or episiotomy wound is present, persistent and unrelenting pain calls for careful inspection of the wound to exclude infection and other problems.
- For hypertension secondary to an underlying medical disorder, this should be reassessed by the appropriate specialists, especially when a change of the dose or type of treatment may be indicated, such as for endocrine and autoimmune conditions.
- Breastfeeding: hypertension or its treatment are usually not contraindications for breastfeeding, but the maternal condition should be reviewed to ensure that the mother is fit for breastfeeding.
- Hospital stay: prolonged hospital stay is not necessary provided that the mother can have easy access to the clinic or day centre for prearranged or emergent review. The patient may be discharged on day 3 in the absence of complications and rebound hypertension.

Prevention of hypertension

A number of measures, including medications/supplements, have been studied for the prevention of hypertensive disorders or the adverse effects.

Calcium
Supplementation with at least 1 g daily reduces the risk of hypertension and pre-eclampsia, maternal death, or serious morbidity. The effect is greater for high-risk women and those with low calcium intake. There is no effect on preterm birth or stillbirth.

Antioxidants
Supplementation with vitamins C and E does not appear to be effective, but may even be harmful. The data are insufficient to be conclusive.

Aspirin
Low dose (75–100 g) from prepregnancy or given after the first trimester can reduce the risk of hypertension and pre-eclampsia, and fetal or neonatal death.

Magnesium
Effect of supplementation not proven.

Salt restriction
Effect not proven.

Folic acid
Apart from the prevention of neural tube defects, 5 mg daily helps to minimize the effect of hyperhomocysteinaemia.

Rest/bed rest, stress reduction
May be useful but effect is small.

Further reading

Abalos E, Duley L, Steyn DW, Henderson-Smart DJ. Antihypertensive drug therapy for mild to moderate hypertension during pregnancy. Cochrane Database Syst Rev 2007;4:CD002252.

Blanco MV, Grosso O, Bellido CA, et al. Dimensions of the left ventricle, atrium, and aortic root in pregnancy-induced hypertension. AJH 2001;14:390–2.

Blanco MV, Roisinblit J, Grosso O, et al. Left ventricular function impairment in pregnancy-induced hypertension. AJH 2001;14:271–5.

Bosio PM, McKenna PJ, Conroy R, O'Herlihy C. Maternal central hemodynamics in hypertensive disorders of pregnancy. Obstet Gynecol 1999;94:978–84.

De Champlain J, Wu R, Girouard H, et al. Oxidative stress in hypertension. Clin Exp Hyperten 2004;26:593–601.

De Paco C, Kametas N, Rencoret G, Strobl I, Nicolaides KH. Maternal cardiac output between 11 and 13 weeks of gestation in the prediction of preeclampsia and small for gestational age. Obstet gynecol 2008;111:292–300.

Duley L, Henderson-Smart D, Knight M, King J. Antiplatelet drugs for prevention of pre-eclampsia and its consequences: systematic review. BMJ 2001;322:329–33.

Higgins JR, de Swiet M. Blood pressure measurement and classification in pregnancy. Lancet 2001;357:131–5.

Hofmeyr GJ, Atallah AN, Duley L. Calcium supplementation during pregnancy for preventing hypertensive disorders and related problems. Cochrane Database Syst Rev 2006;3:CD001059.

Magee LA, Cham C, Waterman EJ, Ohlsson A, von Dadelszen P. Hydralazine for treatment of severe hypertension in pregnancy: meta-analysis. BMJ 2003;327:955–64.

Magee LA, Duley L. Oral beta-blockers for mild to moderate hypertension during pregnancy. Cochrane Database Syst Rev 2003;3CD002863.

Magee LA, Sadeghi S. Prevention and treatment of postpartum hypertension. Cochrane Database Syst Rev 2005;1:CD004351.

North RA, Taylor RS, Schellenberg JC. Evaluation of a definition of pre-eclampsia. Br J Obstet Gynaecol 1999;106:767–3.

Novelli GP, Valensise H, Vasapollo B, et al. Left ventricular concentric geometry as a risk factor in gestational hypertension. Hypertension 2003;41: 469–75.

Quan A. Fetopathy associated with exposure to angiotensin converting enzyme inhibitors and angiotensin receptor antagonists. Early Hum Dev 2006;82:23-8.

Rumbold A, Duley L, Crowther CA, Haslam RR. Antioxidants for preventing pre-eclampsia. Cochrane Database Syst Rev 2007;4:CD004227.

SOGC Clinical Practice Guideline. Diagnosis, evaluation, and management of the hypertensive disorders of pregnancy. JOGC 2008;30(Suppl 1):S1–S48.

Valensise H, Novelli GP, Vasapollo B, et al. Maternal diastolic dysfunction and left ventricular geometry in gestational hypertension. Hypertension 2001;37:1209–15.

Valensise H, Vasapollo B, Novelli GP, et al. Maternal total vascular resistance and concentric geometry: a key to identify uncomplicated gestational hypertension. Br J Obstet Gynaecol 2006;113:1044–52.

Zhang J, Klebanoff MA, Roberts JM. Prediction of adverse outcomes by common definitions of hypertension in pregnancy. Obstet Gynecol 2001;97:261–7.

Internet resources

http://highbloodpressure.about.com

Patient resources

www.rcog.org.hk

Immunization

Definition
- Active immunization: protective immunity is obtained exposing a patient's immune system to the key antigen of a pathogen so that protective antibodies are produced.
- Passive immunization: protective immunity is obtained providing the patient antibodies preformed in human or animals.

Clinical approach
One of the greatest accomplishments of twentieth-century medicine has been the development of effective vaccines for immunoprophylaxis and one of the saddest failures of twentieth-century medicine has been the erratic and incomplete delivery of vaccines to populations at risk.

Pregnancy and breastfeeding are specific conditions that require attention in the administration of a specific vaccine.

Ideally preconceptional immunization to prevent disease in offspring would be preferred to vaccination during pregnancy. Unfortunately, the routine of fully immunizing women entering their reproductive age against common infection, is often unpracticable.

To date there is no evidence that vaccinating pregnant women with an inactivated virus or bacterial vaccine or toxoids poses a risk. In contrast, live vaccines pose a theoretical risk to the fetus of transmission of the virus used. So, if a woman becomes pregnant within 4 weeks after vaccination or if a live virus vaccine is given inadvertently to a pregnant woman, she should be counselled about the potential effects on the fetus.

In the decision of whether to immunize a pregnant woman using ether live or inactivated vaccines, the risk of exposure to disease and its adverse effect on mother and fetus must be balanced against the efficacy of the vaccine and any beneficial effect resulting from it.

Different issues are related to immunization during pregnancy and breastfeeding (Tables 8.23.1 and 8.23.2).

Vulnerable population
- Pregnant women have an altered immune response
- They are at increased risk of some infections
- There is an increased risk of severe outcomes (maternal, fetal, or both) of some infections
- Fetuses and newborns have immature immune system.

Theoretical concerns about efficacy
- the altered immune status of pregnant women may reduce the response to a vaccine
- the quantity of antibodies transferred to the fetus to confer protection may not be adequate
- the half-life of maternal antibodies may not be sufficient to protect fetus/newborn during relevant period of vulnerability.

Theoretical concerns about safety
- Live attenuated virus vaccines
- Use of additives/adjuvants/preservatives with limited or no safety data on exposure.

Timing of vaccination
- Safety risks may vary with time period of vaccination during pregnancy (early pregnancy versus. late pregnancy; immediately postpartum versus later).

Breastfeeding
Neither inactivated nor live vaccine administered to lactating women affect the safety of breastfeeding for mothers or infants. Breastfeeding does not adversely affect immunization and is not a contraindication for any vaccine, with the exception of smallpox vaccine.

The following applies to varicella vaccine, which was licensed after the ACIP General Recommendations were published: 'Whether attenuated vaccine VZV is excreted in human milk and, if so, whether the infant could be infected are not known. Most live vaccines have not been demonstrated to be secreted in breast milk. Attenuated rubella vaccine virus has been detected in beast milk but has produced only asymptomatic infection in the nursing infant. Therefore, varicella vaccine may be considered for a nursing mother'.

Further reading
ACOG, Immunization During Pregnancy, Committee Opinion, Number 282, January 2003.

Barss VA. Immunizations in pregnant women. Uptodate, October, 2008.

General recommendation on immunization. Recommendation of the Advisory Committee on Immunization Practices (ACIP) and the American Academy of Family Physicians (AAFP). CDC. MMWR 2002; Recomm Rep; 51(RR-2):1–35.

Guidelines for Vaccinating Pregnant Women, from recommendations of the Advisory Committee on Immunization Practices (ACIP), October 1998 (Updated May 2007), Centers for Disease Control and Prevention (CDC), Department of Health and Human Services (DHHS).

Guidelines Principles for Development of ACIP Recommendations for Vaccination during Pregnancy and Breastfeeding, April 2008.

Lee EV. Infectious disease. In: *Medical Care of pregnant patient.* ACP Women's Health Series. Philadelphia: American College Of Physicians 2000 Chapter 13

Prevention of varicella: recommendations of the Advisory Committee on Immunization Practices (ACIP). CDC. MMWR 1996; 45 (No. RR-15): 11.

Internet resources
www.cdc.gov/mmwr/preview/mmwrhtml/rr5102a1.htm.
www.ACOG.org
www.cdc.gov/vaccines/pubs/downloads/f_preg_chart.pdf
www.cdc.gov/vaccines/pubs/preg-guide.htm

Table 8.23.1 Active immunization during pregnancy

Vaccine	Virus	Maternal risk from disease	Fetal risk from disease	Fetal risk from vaccine	Immunization in pregnancy	Dose schedule	Comment
Measles	Live attenuated	high morbidity, low mortality	high miscarriage rate, may cause malformations	none confirmed	contraindicated	single dose SC	performed post partum
Mumps	Live attenuated	low morbidity, low mortality	possible high miscarriage rate	none confirmed	contraindicated	single dose SC	performed post partum
Rubella	Live attenuated	low morbidity, low mortality	high miscarriage rate, congenital rubella syndrome	none confirmed	contraindicated	single dose SC	performed post partum theoretic. teratogenicity not confirmed
Poliomyelitis	Live attenuated	high morbidity	anoxic fetal damage reported	none confirmed	not routinely recommended in USA, except women at increased risk of exposure	two dose SC at 4-8 weeks interval and third dose 6-12 months from second dose	indicated for susceptible pregnant women traveling in endemic areas
Yellow Fever	Live attenuated	high morbidity, high mortality	unknown	unknown	contraindicated	single dose SC	
Varicella	Live attenuated	possible increase in severe pneumonia	congenital varicella 2% if infected during 2nd trimester	none confirmed	contraindicated	2 doses needed 4-8 weeks apart	performed post partum
Influenza	inactivated	increase in morbidity and mortality during epidemic of new antigenic strain	possible increased miscarriage rate	none confirmed	any time	single dose IM	
Rabies	killed	100% fatality	determined by maternal disease	unknown	indication for prophylaxis considered individually		public health authorities consulted for indications, dosage and route
Hepatitis B	Purified surface antigen	possible increased severity in 3rd trimester	possible increased miscarriage rate and preterm birth	none reported	pre-exposure and post exposure for women at risk of infection	three-doses series IM at 0,1, and 6 months	used with hepatitis B immunoglobulin for some exposure
Hepatitis A	inactivated	no increased risk during pregnancy		none reported	pre-exposure and post exposure for women at risk of infection	two doses 6 month apart	
Pneumococcus	Polyvalent polysaccharide	no increased risk	unknown, but depends on maternal illness	none reported	recommended in case of: asplenia; metabolic, renal, cardiac, pulmonary diseases; smokers; immunosuppressed.	single dose SC or IM	consider repeat dose in 6 years in high risk women
Meningococcus	Quadrivalent polysaccharide	high morbidity, high mortality	unknown, but depends on maternal illness	none reported	recommended in unusual outbreak situations	single dose SC	public health authorities consulted

Table 8.23.1 Active immunization during pregnancy (*Contd.*)

Vaccine	Virus	Maternal risk from disease	Fetal risk from disease	Fetal risk from vaccine	Immunization in pregnancy	Dose schedule	Comment
Typhoid	killed or live attenuated	high morbidity	unknown	none confirmed	recommended for close, continued exposure or travel in endemic areas	killed: - primary: two injection SC - booster: single dose SC	oral vaccine preferred
Anthrax	preparation from cell-free filtrate of B anthracis	high morbidity, high mortality	unknown, but depends on maternal illness	none confirmed	not routinely recommended	six-dose primary vaccination SC, then annual booster	teratogenicity of vaccine theoretical
Tetanus / Diptheria	combined toxoids	tetanus mortality 30% diphtheria mortality 10%	neonatal tetanus mortality 60%	none confirmed	lack of primary series or no booster within past 10 years		updating immune status during antepartum care

SC, subcutaneously; IM, intramuscularly.

Table 8.23.2 Passive immunization during pregnancy

Vaccine	Virus	Maternal risk from disease	Fetal/Neonatal risk from disease	Fatal risk from vaccine	Immunization in pregnancy	Dose schedule	Comment
Hepatitis B	hepatitis B immune globulin	possible increased severity in 3rd trimester	possible increase in miscarriage and preterm birth, neonatal hepatitis may occur	none reported	post exposure prophylaxis	consult Practice Advisory Committee recommendation	usually given with hepatitis B vaccine
Rabies	rabies immune globulin	100% fatality	determined by maternal disease	none reported	post exposure prophylaxis	half dose at injurysite and half in deltoid	used in conjunction with rabies killed virus vaccine
Tetanus	tetanus immune globulin	high morbidity, mortality 60%	neonatal tetanus with 60% mortality	none reported	post exposure prophylaxis	single dose IM	used in conjunction with tetanus toxoid
Varicella	varicella-zoster immune globulin	possible increase in severe varicella pneumonia	can cause congenital varicella with increased mortality in neonatal period	none reported	considered for healthy pregnant women exposed to varicella to protect against maternal, not congenital infection	single dose IM within 96 hours of exposure	indicated in newborn of women who developed varicella within 4 days before delivery or 2 days following delivery, not indicated for prevention of congenital varicella
Hepatitis A	Standard immune globulin	possible increased severity during third trimester	possible increase in miscarriage and preterm birth,	none reported	post exposure prophylaxis, but the vaccine should be used with immune globulin	single dose IM	immune globulin should be given as soon as possible and within 2 weeks of exposure

IM, intramuscularly.

Inflammatory bowel disease

Definition
Inflammatory bowel disease (IBD) is divided into Crohn's disease and ulcerative colitis (UC). These are chronic inflammatory diseases of the gastrointestinal tract.

Epidemiology
- IBD is more common in the Western World than Africa or Asia. It usually presents in young adults.
- Crohn's affects women and men equally with incidence of 5 in 100 000 and prevalence of 0.5 in 1000.
- UC is more common in women, with an incidence of 5–10 in 100 000 and prevalence of 0.8–1 in 1000.
- The incidence and prevalence of IBD has increased over the last 50 years, but the reasons are unknown.

Pathology
- Crohn's disease: granulomatous inflammation extending beyond the submucosa, affecting any part of the gastrointestinal tract from the mouth to anus, in a patchy distribution (skip lesions).
- UC: mucosal and submucosal inflammation with crypt abscesses. It Always affects the rectum and extends proximally continuously to affect a variable proportion of the colon.

Causes
The causes are unknown, although 5–20% have an affected family member. Susceptibility genes have been located. Genetics, infection, autoimmunity, and environmental toxins are all likely to play a part. Crohn's is more common in smokers, whereas UC is more common in non-smokers.

Clinical features
- Crohn's disease affects both the ileum and the colon in half of cases. The terminal ileum and colon may also be commonly involved in isolation. Symptoms will depend on the site of the bowel affected.
- UC affects only the colon.

General symptoms
- Malaise
- Tiredness
- Anorexia.

Symptoms related to ileitis
- Cramping mid-abdominal pain
- Diarrhoea
- Weight loss.

Symptoms related to colitis
- Liquid diarrhoea
- Urgency of defaecation and tenesmus
- Rectal bleeding (mixed in with stool)
- Passage of mucus per rectum
- Lower abdominal pain (less frequent).

Symptoms related to proctitis
- Fresh blood passed per rectum.

Signs
- Fever, dehydration, anaemia, weight loss, abdominal distension and tenderness, perianal disease (Crohn's).

Exra-intestinal manifestations (especially with colonitis)
- Clubbing
- Mouth ulcers
- Arthritis: large joints, sacroiliitis, ankylosing spondylitis
- Eyes: conjunctivitis, iritis, episcleritis
- Biliary tract: gallstones, ascending/sclerosing cholangitis
- Skin: erythema nodosum, pyoderma gangrenosum.

Investigations
- Sigmoidoscopy ± colonoscopy and mucosal biopsy to confirm mucosal inflammation. Histology will distinguish between Crohn's disease and UC.
- ↑ WCC, ↑ C-reactive protein (CRP) (inflammation)
- ↓Ca^{2+}, vitamin D, iron, folate, B12 (terminal ileal disease)
- Blood cultures (if febrile)
- AXR: if suspecting colonic dilatation/toxic megacolon (fetal risks minimal)
- MRI: if suspecting colonic dilatation/toxic megacolon/perforation
- Avoid barium enema and small bowel contrast studies in pregnancy

Effect of pregnancy on IBD
Pregnancy does not affect IBD, but limits the ability to perform some investigations and use some treatments.

> Predictors of active IBD in pregnancy
> Active IBD/flare at conception: likely to stay active during pregnancy
> New-onset IBD in pregnancy (usually occurs in first or second trimester)

- IBD quiescent at conception: similar frequency of exacerbations in pregnancy as when not pregnant.
- Exacerbations in inactive Crohn's disease usually occur in the first trimester and in inactive UC are usually in the first two trimesters.
- Postpartum flare is more common in Crohn's disease, but not in UC.

Effect of IBD on pregnancy
Fertility: reduced in active Crohn's disease
  If disease quiescent at conception, rates of miscarriage, stillbirth, fetal anomaly, and live births are unaltered
  Active disease is associated with worse pregnancy outcome. Flares
- at conception: increased miscarriage rates
- in pregnancy: increased prematurity.
  Low birthweight babies more common irrespective of disease activity.
  Previous surgery:
- tolerated well if disease inactive
- stomas and inactive disease: most women have normal deliveries at term
- ileostomy: dysfunction can occur in the second trimester with peristomal cracking and bleeding from an enlarging abdomen. Intermittent intestinal obstruction can occur and is serious.

- Ileoanal anastomosis: good outcomes and vaginal births reported.

Management
Prepregnancy counselling
- Determine disease activity and optimize control.
- Recommend postponing pregnancy if IBD is active, and conceiving when IBD is in remission.
- Replace methotrexate with a more suitable drug (see below).
- Establish nutritional status and supplement with calcium, Vitamin D, iron, folic acid, and Vitamin B12 if deficient.
- If using an aminosalicylate (folate antagonist) add 5 mg of folic acid preconceptionally and during pregnancy.
- Encourage cessation of smoking.

During pregnancy
Management of chronic disease and acute attacks is similar to outside pregnancy. Multidisciplinary care with gastroenterologists and obstetricians is important with input from colorectal surgeons in severe cases.
- Continue with maintenance medications to reduce relapse rate
- Continue 5-mg folic acid if on an aminosalicylate
- Distinguish a flare of IBD from other conditions, e.g. abdominal pain
  - normal pregnancy: constipation or gastro-oesophageal reflux
  - unrelated to pregnancy: appendicitis, cholelithiasis, pancreatitis, pre-eclampsia
- Fetal growth scans.

If flare of IBD suspected, perform
  full blood count, urea and electrolytes, liver function tests, CRP, amylase, albumin, and stool culture
  flexible sigmoidoscopy or rigid proctoscopy to assess disease activity
  If complications suspected, imaging may be required

Drug treatment
- Aminosalicylates (sulfasalazine, mesalazine, balsalazine): safe throughout pregnancy and breastfeeding. Sulfasalazine splits into sulfapyridine and the active compound 5-aminosalicylic acid (5-ASA) in the colon. Continue as maintenance or to induce remission in colonic Crohn's disease or UC. Available orally or as rectal enemas.
- Oral and rectal corticosteroids can be used in pregnancy. There is a very slight increase in facial clefts with high-dose prednisolone used in the first trimester, but in a disease flare the benefits outweigh the risks.
- Azathioprine has extensive safety data from use in pregnant women with renal transplants and SLE. Azathioprine should be continued in women who require this to remain in remission. It can also be used as a steroid-sparing drug. It takes several weeks to take effect if started in pregnancy.
- Metronidazole and ciprofloxacin are not associated with adverse fetal effects with short-term use.
- Methotrexate results in miscarriage and is a teratogen and should not be used in pregnancy. Pregnancy should be avoided for at least 3 months following its discontinuation.
- Ciclosporin has good safety data from use in pregnant women with renal transplants. It is associated with intra-uterine growth restriction. Its use is reserved to severe flares of IBD in pregnancy.
- Infliximab (anti-tumour necrosis factor-α): there are reports of successful use of this in severe flares of IBD. Reassuring safety data are emerging from its use in pregnant women.

Medical treatment of a flare of IBD in pregnancy

Colonic disease

Start with topical corticosteroid enemas and a topical or oral aminosalicylate.
Second-line treatment is with oral steroids (20-40mg). Hydrocortisone can be used if oral treatments are not tolerated.
Poor response to steroids demands the use of third-line treatments such as ciclosporin or infliximab.

Ileal disease

Start with oral steroids and aminosalicylates.
Cyclosporin or infliximab are rarely required.

Surgery
Surgery should never be delayed because of pregnancy. For indications similar to non-pregnant state:
- IBD not responsive to medical treatment
- obstruction
- haemorrhage
- perforation
- toxic megacolon.

Delivery
- Vaginal delivery is usually preferable, particularly in the presence of previous abdominal surgery which may have resulted in extensive intraperitoneal adhesions. Women with stomas can deliver vaginally.
- Caesarean section should be performed for
  - obstetric indications
  - severe active or chronic peri-anal Crohn's disease with a scarred or deformed rectum and perineum (delayed healing of episiotomies and risks of fistula formation).
- Caesarean section can be considered in those with impaired anal continence.
- Total proctocolectomy and ileal pouch anal anastomosis: successful vaginal deliveries have been reported despite theoretical concerns regarding anal sphincter integrity at delivery.

Complications
Crohn's disease
- Perforation
- Stricture formation
- Peri-anal disease
- Fistulae
- Abscess formation.

Ulcerative Colitis
- Dilatation of colon/toxic megacolon
- Malignancy.

Contraception
- Absorption of oral hormonal contraceptives may be reduced by small bowel involvement/malabsorption.
- If on antibiotics, reduced efficacy of oestrogen containing contraceptives
  - Recommend:
  - Copper IUCD
  - Non-oral progestogen-based methods e.g. levonogestrel intrauterine system or implanon.

Further reading

Ferguson CB, Mahsud-Dornan S, Patterson RN. Inflammatory bowel disease in pregnancy. BMJ 2008;337:a427.

Alstead EA, Nelson-Piercy C. Inflammatory bowel disease in pregnancy. Gut 2003;52:159–61.

Cornish J, Tan E, Teare J, *et al*. A meta-analysis on the influence of inflammatory bowel disease on pregnancy. Gut 2007;56:830–7.

Caprilli R, Gassull MA, Escher JC, *et al*. European evidence based consensus on the diagnosis and management of Crohn's disease: special situations. Gut 2006;55(Suppl 1):i36–58.

Faculty of Family Planning and Reproductive Healthcare Clinical Effectiveness Unit. FFPRHC Guidance (July 2003). Contraceptive choices for women with inflammatory bowel disease. JFFPRHC 2003;29:127–135. www.ffprhc.org.uk

Jaundice

Definition
Jaundice is a yellow discolouration of the skin and sclera due to an increase in the level of serum bilirubin. Unconjugated bilirubin is produced from the breakdown of haem and is conjugated in the liver.

Causes
Prehepatic
- Increased production of unconjugated bilirubin:
  - haemolysis, e.g. HELLP (haemolysis, elevated liver enzymes, low platelets) syndrome, haemolytic uraemic syndrome (HUS), thrombotic thrombocytopenic purpura (TTP), malaria
  - haemoglobinopathies (e.g. sickle cell disease, thalassaemia).
- Reduced hepatic uptake of unconjugated bilirubin:
  - Severe congestive heart failure.

Hepatic
- Reduced hepatic conjugation of bilirubin
  - Gilbert's syndrome
  - Crigler–Najjar syndrome.
- Reduced excretion of conjugated bilirubin
  - hepatocellular injury, e.g. viral hepatitis, drugs (e.g. paracetamol overdose), chronic active hepatitis, sepsis
  - infiltration of liver, e.g. acute fatty liver of pregnancy (AFLP), malignancy
  - obstetric cholestasis (OC)
  - congenital defects, e.g. Dubin–Johnson and Rotor syndromes.

Cholestatic (obstructive)
- Extrahepatic bile duct obstruction
  - gallstones (choledocholithiasis)
  - ascending cholangitis
  - acute pancreatitis
  - primary biliary crrhosis.

History
- Duration of jaundice, malaise, anorexia, nausea, vomiting, fever, rash, weight loss
- Other symptoms of liver disease: Itching, abdominal pain, dark urine, pale stools, bruising, bleeding
- Recent travel abroad
- Drug treatment/abuse/overdose, amount of alcohol
- Recent tattoos or piercings
- Previous jaundice, gallstones.

Signs
- Signs of chronic liver disease are common in normal pregnancy, e.g. spider naevi, palmar erythema
- Upper abdominal tenderness
- Palpable gall bladder, hepatomegaly, splenomegaly.

> Worrying signs: call ITU ± liver unit
> Drowsiness, confusion, slurred speech, tachycardia, hypotension, severe hypertension, bleeding, tremor/flap, poor coordination, hypoxia

Initial investigations
- Urine: dipstick for protein, blood, urobilinogen (prehepatic/hepatic jaundice), bilirubin (hepatic/obstructive jaundice)
- Bloods: full blood count, reticulocytes, blood film, clotting, U+E, LFT, amylase ± paracetamol levels, hepatitis serology (A, B, C ± E), EBV, CMV, blood cultures
- USS abdomen: gallstones, dilated common bile duct.

Further investigations
As depicted by initial results and differential diagnoses: see individual diseases. Also refer to chapter on Liver Diseases which covers other conditions that can present with jaundice including acute fatty liver of pregnancy and obstetric cholestasis.

Gilbert's syndrome
Benign disease: develops as unconjugated hyperbilirubinaemia with an acute illness. Usually incidental finding of slightly raised bilirubin. No concerns in pregnancy.

Gall bladder disease
Incidence
- Gallstones: 2–8% of pregnant women: ↑ with parity
- Biliary sludge: in 30% women by the end of pregnancy
- Acute cholecystitis in 0.1% of pregnancies.

Causes
Gall bladder stasis and lithogenic bile (from an increase in bile cholesterol and a reduction of bile acids) leads to increased formation of sludge and gallstones in pregnancy

Clinical features
- Asymptomatic
- Biliary pain in right upper quadrant
- Acute cholecystitis
- Associated with obstetric cholestasis.

Acute cholecystitis
Definition
Impacted gallstone in neck of gallbladder with inflammation

Clinical
- Severe continuous right upper quadrant pain (can radiate in a band round to back)
- nausea, vomiting
- pyrexia
- tender over gall bladder (Murphy's sign +ve)
- peritonitis
- jaundice if stones in common bile duct (CBD).

Diagnosis
- ↑ WCC, ↑ CRP
- Abnormal LFT
- Amylase can double. If higher consider pancreatitis or stones in CBD
- USS gallbladder: pericholecystic fluid, gallbladder distension and thickening of wall
- Endoscopic retrograde cholangiopancreatography (ERCP) if impacted stone suspected

- Technecium-99 HIDA scan for CBD stones (minimal fetal radiation).

Differential diagnosis
- Acute pancreatitis
- Pneumonia
- Cholangitis
- AFLP
- Peptic ulcer disease
- HELLP
- Appendicitis
- Viral hepatitis.

Management
- Similar to non-pregnant
- Conservative management resolves symptoms in 75% but increased incidence of preterm delivery and relapse in pregnancy compared with surgery. Usually defer definitive surgery until postpartum:
  - Keep nil by mouth and administer i.v. fluids
  - Antibiotics
  - Analgesia (avoid NSAIDs)
- Surgery required if
  - Non-resolution of symptoms
  - Recurrent symptoms
  - CBD obstruction
- Perform surgery in second trimester if necessary
  - Laparoscopic cholecystectomy (difficult with later gestations)
  - Open cholecystectomy
  - Endoscopic removal of CBD stones.

Complications
- Pancreatitis
- Cholangitis.

Acute and chronic viral hepatitis
This is the commonest cause of jaundice worldwide

Causes
- Hepatitis A, B, C, D, E (Table 8.25.1)
- Cytomegalovirus (CMV)
- Ebstein–Barr Virus (EBV)
- Herpes simplex virus (HSV)

Hepatitis E (HEV) and herpes simplex hepatitis can cause adverse pregnancy outcome. The other viral hepatitis run a similar cause outside pregnancy (Table 8.25.1).

Hepatitis D (HDV) is dependent on hepatitis B (HBV) for transmission.
- Co-infection of HBV and HDV leads to a more severe form of acute hepatitis than HBV alone.
- Superimposed infection of a chronic carrier of HBV with HDV can lead to another episode of clinical hepatitis and can hasten the course of chronic liver disease.

Herpes simplex hepatitis
Incidence
Very rare.

Pathology
- Usually primary infection with HSV type 2.
- Liver focal haemorrhagic necrosis and intranuclear inclusion bodies.

Clinical
- Initial non-specific symptoms, e.g. fatigue, pyrexia
- Abdominal pain
- Herpetic vesicles may be absent
- ± jaundice
- Fulminant liver failure
- Disseminated infection.

Diagnosis
- Very high liver transaminases
- Mildly raised bilirubin
- Prolonged prothrombin time
- Serology: IgM HSV+
- Liver biopsy: histology and viral culture.

Treatment
Intravenous acyclovir

Prognosis
Poor without treatment in pregnant women

Acute pancreatitis
Incidence
- Same as non-pregnant 1 in 10 000
- Attacks are usually mild and occur in the third trimester.

Causes
- Gallstones
- Alcohol
- Hypercalcaemia (primary hyperparathyroidism)
- Hypertriglyceridaemia (from underlying disorder).

Clinical features
Symptoms
- Constant severe epigastric pain radiating straight through to back, improved with sitting forward
- Nausea, vomiting, anorexia.

Signs
- Tachycardia, ±, ↑RR, ↓BP, low-grade pyrexia
- Mild jaundice
- Epigastric tenderness with peritonitis
- Reduced or absent bowel sounds (paralytic ileus)
- Cullen's sign (bruised umbilicus), Grey–Turner's sign (bruised flanks)
- Pleural effusions, ascites.

Diagnosis
- serum amylase four times normal (can be >1000 U/L): rise may be masked by high lipids

> Severe disease: liaise with ITU
> Hypoxic, pyrexial, hypotensive, marked tachypnoea, prolonged paralytic ileus, ascites, pleural effusions

- ↑serum lipase more specific
- ↑ WCC, ↑CRP, ↑glucose, ↓corrected Ca^{2+}
- Abnormal LFTs
- ± Deranged clotting
- ABG
- USS upper abdomen: gallstones
- CT abdo: pancreatic swelling.

Table 8.25.1 Viral hepatitis in pregnancy

	Hepatitis A	Hepatitis B	Hepatitis B	Hepatitis C	Hepatitis E
		Acute infection	Carrier	Acute/carrier	
Epidemiology in pregnancy	Endemic areas: Asia, Africa, South America	Endemic areas: Asia, sub-Saharan Africa (seropositivity up to 50%) Western world <1% HBsAg+ve		Acute: uncommon in pregnancy Chronic carriers: 0.5–1% West 3% worldwide 30% if also HIV+	Epidemics: Asia, Africa, Mexico
Spread	Faecal–oral	Blood	Blood	Blood (i.v. drug abuse, post transfusion)	Faecal-oral (esp. water)
Incubation period	2–7 weeks	1–5 months		2 weeks to 5 months	2–6 weeks
History	Recent travel to endemic area			↑risk obstetric cholestasis (OC)	↑infection in pregnancy
Clinical	Acute: anorexia, nausea. jaundice, fever Self limited	Mild symptoms 30%: anorexia, nausea, jaundice, fever/ abdominal pain	Asymptomatic	Acute: three-quarters asymptomatic; anorexia, nausea; jaundice (rare); fever If OC, symptoms worse and ↑ premature delivery	Severity and progression of symptoms worse
Transaminases	Raised	Up to >1000 IU/L	Normal/mildly↑	Normal/mildly↑	Raised
Bilirubin	Raised	Raised	Normal	↑ in 20% of acute infections	Raised
Serology	IgM anti-HAV antibodies +	HBsAg+ HBcAb+ (IgM)	HBsAg+ HBeAg+ (high infectivity) or HBeAb+ (low infectivity)	HCV Ab+ +/- HCV RNA +	IgM anti-HEV antibodies +
Carrier Status	No	10% (esp if mild illness with no jaundice)		80%	No
Fulminant liver failure	Rare	1%	Rare	Rare	32–69%
Other maternal complications	As for non-pregnant	As for non-pregnant	Cirrhosis Chronic active hepatitis Primary liver Ca	Cirrhosis (20% in 10 years) Primary liver Ca (1–5%)	Maternal death 27–41% esp. if infection in third trimester
Vertical transmission method	If virus in faeces at delivery	Transplacental at delivery	Transplacental at delivery	Transplacental at delivery	If virus in faeces at delivery
Vertical transmission rates	Rare	First trimester 10% Third trimester 90%	HBeAg+ 70-90% HBeAb+ 2–15%	HCV RNA+ 11% f also HIV+ 16% Female fetus ↑2x	33%

	Hepatitis A	Hepatitis B	Hepatitis B carrier	Hepatitis C	Hepatitis E
Fetal complications	Preterm labour	Preterm birth / Fetal loss / 90% of infected fetuses become chronic carriers	No	No	% Preterm delivery / Fetal loss 30–62%
Delivery	Vaginal	Vaginal	Vaginal	Vaginal*	Vaginal
Maternal vaccination or immunoglobulin	Inactivated virus in vaccine	Can use HBIG and hepatitis vaccine in pregnancy and breast feeding†	N/A	None available	None available
Neonatal vaccination or immunoglobulin	Mother infectious at delivery: give baby normal immunoglobulin	Mother low infectivity: hepatitis vaccine / Mother high infectivity: HBIG and hepatitis vaccine (transmission reduced by >90%)		None available	None available
Breastfeeding	Safe	Safe if neonate immunized		Does not affect transmission*	Safe
Treatment	None	Interferon-α‡ / Lamivudine (occas. used in pregnancy)		Interferon-α‡ / Ribavarin‡	None

† HBIG within 72 hours of exposure + hepatitis vaccine within 7 days of exposure (repeat vaccine after 1 and 6 months).

* Caesarean section and breastfeeding does not affect transmission of hepatitis C.

‡ Not in pregnancy.

Differential diagnosis

Mildly raised amylase also occurs in
- cholecystitis
- peptic ulcer perforation
- bowel obstruction
- ectopic pregnancy.

Management

Making the correct diagnosis is very important to avoid an unnecessary laparotomy.

Supportive NOT surgical (unless CBD obstruction: biliary pancreatitis):
- Keep nil by mouth
- Resuscitate with intravenous fluids
- Facial O_2
- Analgesia: pethidine, NOT morphine (contraindicated as causes spasm of sphincter of Oddi)
- Urinary catheter and monitor fluid balance
- Nasogastric tube (usually have) paralytic ileus
- Prophylactic thromboprophylaxis with LMWH.

Regular monitoring of
Pulse, BP, Hb, WCC, U+E, LFT, amylase, prothrombin time, glucose, calcium.

Complications

Requires liaising with ITU
- DIC
- Renal failure
- Respiratory failure : liaise with ITU
- Thrombosis
- Pseudocyst/abscess
- Sepsis
- Chronic pancreatitis
- Fetal loss.

Further reading

Beasley RP, Hwang LY, Lee GC, et al. Prevention of perinatally transmitted hepatitis B virus infections with hepatitis B virus infections with hepatitis B immune globulin and hepatitis B vaccine. Lancet 1983;2:1099–102.

Elinav E, Ben-Dov IZ, Shapira Y, et al. Acute hepatitis A infection in pregnancy is associated with high rates of gestational complications and preterm labour.

European Paediatric Hepatitis C Virus Network. Effects of mode of delivery and infant feeding on the risk of mother-to-child transmission of hepatitis C virus. Br J Obstet Gynaecol 2001;108:371–7.

Hernandez A, Petrov MS, Brooks DC, Banks PA, et al. Acute pancreatitis and pregnancy: a 10-year single center experience. J Gastrointest Surg 2007;11:1623–7.

Kumar A, Beniwal M, Kar P, et al. Hepatitis E in pregnancy. Int J Gynaecol Obstet 2004;85:240–4.

Mendez-Sanchez N, Chavez-Tapia NC, Uribe M. Pregnancy and gallbladder disease. Ann Hepatol 2006;5:227–30.

Patra S, Kumar A, Trivedi SS, et al. Maternal and fetal outcomes in pregnant women with acute hepatitis E virus infection. Ann Intern Med 2007;147:28–33.

Yeung LT, King SM, Roberts EA. Mother-to-infant transmission of hepatitis C virus. Hepatology 2001;34:223–9.

Listeriosis

Definition
Listeriosis refers to infection by the organism *Listeria monocytogenes* and its manifestations are host dependent.

Epidemiology
- In the USA, surveillance data from 1997 showed that 2500 people become seriously ill each year as a result of listeriosis and 500 die (CDC).
- Neonatal infection is the most common clinical form of the disease
- Listeriosis is 20 times more likely in pregnancy and 300 times more likely in AIDS
- Age >65 years is associated with increased rates of Listeriosis.

Aetiology
Listeria monocytogenes is a gram-positive rod-shaped bacterium that contaminates raw food such as soft cheeses, cured meats, and prepackaged raw items such as smoked fish, sandwiches, or salads. Infection occurs when contaminated food is consumed by an at-risk individual.

The bacterium grows well at refrigeration temperatures (4–10°C)

Neonatal infection
- Caused predominantly by maternal infection in pregnancy, listeria is transmitted to the fetus via ascending or transplacental means.
- Nosocomial infection has been reported.

Pregnancy
- Pregnant women are particularly at risk in the second and third trimester due to decreased cell-mediated immunity.

Immunocompromised states and elderly people
- Immunocompromised states increase the risk of invasive infection due to decreased cell-mediated immunity.
- Ageing causes anatomic and functional changes and immune changes such as decreased macrophage efficiency Increasing the risk of complicated infection.

Prognosis
- Immunocompetent hosts may be asymptomatic or have acute febrile gastroenteritis, and nearly all make a full recovery within 2 days
- Among pregnant women, however, 22% of cases result in stillbirth or neonatal death, and spontaneous abortion is common.
- Seventy per cent of pregnancies with listeriosis result in preterm delivery at <35 weeks
- 66% of infants surviving a pregnancy complicated by listeriosis will have a clinical diagnosis of neonatal listeriosis
- Mortality in the infected neonate is 30–50%
- Early treatment of listeria sepsis can prevent invasive infection and improve outcomes.

Clinical approach
Diagnosis: history
- Recent ingestion of raw milk products, soft cheeses, cured or smoked meats, or raw packaged food

- Maternal influenza-like illness preceding delivery by 2–14 days, including the following symptoms: headache, myalgias, fever, nausea, diarrhoea, stiff neck, confusion, vertigo, or seizures
- Immunocompromise (corticosteroid use, HIV/AIDS, cancer, chemotherapy, diabetes, immune-modulating medications).

Examination
Neonates
- Early onset: Apparent in less than 7 days, and in most cases less than 2 days. Characterized by overwhelming sepsis, respiratory distress, and hepatosplenomegaly
- Late onset: More insidious, characterized by fever, meningitis, lethargy, irritability, and feeding problems, associated with nosocomial transmission.

Pregnant women and adults
- Signs of chorioamnionitis: uterine fundal tenderness, contractions, fever, vaginal discharge, ruptured membranes
- Febrile Gastroenteritis
- Meningeal signs: fever, stiff neck, confusion.

Special investigations
- Cultures of blood, cerebral spinal fluid, sputum, placenta, vagina, and rectum should be taken
- Amniocentesis with culture of the fluid may be obtained to diagnose amnionitis in pregnant patients
- If membranes have ruptured, and sample is contaminated, diagnosis may still be possible using selective media
- During a food-borne outbreak, strains of Listeria isolated from clinical specimens should be forwarded to a reference laboratory for typing.

Management
General: key points.
- Infection control precautions with gowning, gloves, and careful hand washing will prevent nosocomial infection
- During an outbreak, high-risk groups of pregnant or immunocompromised individuals with flu-like illnesses should be empirically treated with ampicillin and an aminoglycoside after cultures are obtained
- Decrease immunosuppressive drug doses if no evidence of rapid clinical response to antibiotic therapy.

Supportive therapy
- Adequate hydration and nutrition
- Intravenous fluids for blood pressure support in setting of sepsis.

Medical therapy
Listeria is sensitive to antimicrobial therapies and resistance is rare
- Ampicillin (2 g i.v. every 4 hours) or penicillin G (4 million units i.v. every 4 hours) is the drug of choice
- Gentamicin or another aminoglycoside should be used in combination with ampicillin or penicillin to treat complicated infections in the CNS, neonates, endocarditis, and immunocompromised patients. CNS infection is rare in pregnant patients. Consider monitoring renal function for prolonged use.

- Other antibiotic choices that have shown efficacy are trimethoprim-sulfamethoxazole, imepenem, or meropenem.
- Pregnant patients with isolated bacteraemia can be treated with ampicillin or penicillin alone, or trimethoprim-sulfamethoxazole, although this drug should be avoided in the first and third trimesters due to risks of affected folic acid metabolism or kernicterus, respectively, in the neonate.
- Pregnant patients with chorioamnionitis should be treated as complicated infections.
- Treatment failures have been reported with vancomycin, erythromycin, tetracyclines, cephalosporins, and chloramphenicol and therefore should be avoided in listeriosis.
- Penicillin desensitization is an option for those who are allergic
- Treatment must be continued for 2 weeks in immunocompetent patients with bacteraemia and 2–4 weeks for CNS infection, longer treatment intervals are needed in immunocompromised individuals.

Prognosis
- Highly variable based on underlying host conditions (Mortality ranges from 0–32%)
- Mortality in CNS infection is high (13–43%) in immunocompetent patients and higher among immunocompromised individuals
- After CNS infection, neurological sequelae may persist in a majority of patients.

Prevention
Prevention measures are focused on food safety, and include cooking all raw food, avoiding unpasteurized products, and preventing cross-contamination of cooking surfaces by thorough washing of hands, cutting boards or cooking surfaces.

Recommendations for pregnant women and immunocompromised patients
- Do not eat delicatessen meats or hotdogs unless heated to steaming
- Do not eat soft cheeses such as feta, Brie, or Camembert, or Mexican-style cheeses unless they are labelled as pasteurized
- Do not eat refrigerated pâtés, meat spreads, packaged salads containing meat, or smoked seafood. Canned items are safe to eat, or smoked items may be eaten if they are cooked.
- Thoroughly wash raw vegetables before consuming
- Do not drink raw milk or other foods containing unpasteurized milk.
- Keep refrigerator at 40°F (4.4°C) or lower and freezer at 0°F (−17.8°C) or lower.

Further reading

Ault K Faro S. Bacteria and protozoans in pregnancy: a sample of each. Clin Obstet Gynecol 1993;36:878–85.

Bortolussi R, Mailman TL. Aerobic gram-positive bacilli, clinical manifestations. In: Cohen and Powderly (eds) *Infectious diseases*, 2nd edn. St Louis: Mosby Elsevier 2004: Chapter 226.

Eckburg PB, Montoya JG, Vosti KL. Brain abscess due to Listeria monocytogenes: five cases and a review of the literature. Medicine 2001;80:223.

Heymann D. (ed.). *Control of communicable diseases manual*, 18th edn. Washington, DC: American Public Health Association 2004.

Lorber B. Listeriosis. Clin Infect Disease 1997;24:1.

Lorber B. Listeria monocytogenes. In: Mandell, Bennet, and Dolin (eds) *Principles and practice of infectious diseases*, 6th edn. Philadelphia: Churchill Livingstone 2005: Chapter 204.

Louria D. Sen P. Sherer C, Farrer W. Infections in older patients: a systematic clinical approach. Geriatrics 1993;48:28–34.

Mylonakis E. Hohmann EL, Calderwood SB. Central nervous system infection with Listeria monocytogenes: 33 years' experience at a general hospital and review of 776 episodes from the literature. Medicine 1998,77:313.

Internet resources

Listeriosis: Center for Disease Control and Prevention: National Center for Zoonotic, Vector-Borne, and Enteric Diseases www.cdc.gov/nczved/dfbmd/disease_listing/listeriosis_g.html

Liver disease

It is important to use pregnancy-specific ranges when interpreting liver function tests (LFT) in pregnancy (Table 8.27.1).

Obstetric cholestasis (OC)

Definition
Intrahepatic cholestasis occurring in the second and third trimesters of pregnancy and resolving postnatally.

Incidence
- In Europeans 0.5–1.5% of pregnancies.
- More common in South Americans and South Asians.

Causes
- Genetic predisposition to cholestatic effects of elevated oestrogen ± progesterone levels
- Mutations of MDR3 gene identified.

Clinical features
Specific points in history
- Prepregnancy pruritis on oral contraceptive pill or in luteal phase of menstrual cycle
- Personal or family history of pruritis in pregnancy
- Personal or family history of previous unexplained still-birth
- Onset usually in third trimester, but may be earlier.

Symptoms
- Pruritis generalized, but typically includes palms of hands and soles of feet. Disappears postnatally.
- No rash
- Dark urine, pale stools

Signs
- Excoriation of skin following scratching
- Jaundice 10%.

Diagnosis (of exclusion)
- Abnormal liver enzymes* (use normal ranges for pregnancy): moderately raised
- Raised bile acids (BAs)*
- Exclude other causes if LFT or BAs abnormal:
  - Serology: hepatitis A, B, C† –ve
  - Serology: CMV IgM –ve, EBV IgM –ve
  - Occasionally need to exclude hepatitis E
  - Antimitochondrial and anti-smooth muscle Ab –ve
  - Liver USS normal (may have gallstones†).

Table 8.27.1. Normal pregnancy values of liver function tests

Trimester	Non-pregnant	First	Second	Third
ALT	0.40	6–32		
AST	7–40	10–28	11–29	11–30
ALP	30–130	32–100	43–135	133–418
GGT	11–50	5–37	5–43	3–41

Girling JC, Dow E, Smith JH. Liver function tests in pre-eclampsia: importance of comparison with a reference range derived for normal pregnancy. Br J Obstet Gynaecol 1997;104:246–50.

*May be normal initially
†OC can occur in association

Differential diagnosis
- Hepatitis due to hepatitis A, B, or C, CMV, or EBV
- Chronic active hepatitis (antismooth muscle Ab +ve)
- Primary biliary cirrhosis (antimitochondrial Ab +ve)

Effect of OC on pregnancy
- Spontaneous preterm labour and delivery‡
- Meconium-stained liquor‡
- Fetal distress‡
- Stillbirth‡ 2% (when delivered <38 weeks)
- Vitamin K deficiency (malabsorption fat-soluble vitamins)
- Postpartum haemorrhage.

‡Fetal complications only occurred if BA ³40 μmol/L in a Swedish population and increased with increasing BA levels.

Fetal risk related to level of bile acids, not to severity of symptoms or degree of derangement of LFT.

Management
Prepregnancy counselling
If previous OC, the recurrence is 90%
- Check that baseline LFT and BA are normal
- If these are abnormal, and above extended tests are normal, refer to hepatologist
- Check hepatitis C (develop OC earlier if HCV Ab+).

During pregnancy
- If had previous OC check LFT and BA at booking
- Development of itching in pregnancy: check LFT and BA. If normal, repeat after 1–2 weeks if itching persists. If abnormal exclude other causes.
- Chlorpheniramine unhelpful (may help sleep)
- Antenatal surveillance (by USS, umbilical Doppler or cardiotocography) has not been shown to predict or prevent stillbirth
- Monitor LFT, prothrombin time and BA weekly.

Treatment of OC
- Aqueous cream and menthol: soothing
- Ursodeoxycholic acid (UDCA) start 500 mg bd. Maximum dose 2 g/day. Stop postnatally.
- Second-line drug treatment: rifampicin/dexamethasone
- Vitamin K 10 mg od (water soluble) for a few days before delivery (to prevent maternal/fetal bleeding).
  UDCA: hydrophilic bile acid which alters the bile acid pool reducing the amount of hydrophobic (hepatoxic) bile acids. Itching, LFT and BA usually improve. No reported adverse effects. Not known if reduces frequency of fetal complications.
  Rifampicin: useful in combination with UDCA in non-responders. Occasionally causes worsening of LFT.
  Dexamethasone: 12 mg po daily. Serious concerns of neurodevelopmental delay with repeated use.

Delivery
Risk of fetal death increases >37 weeks; therefore, deliver by 37–38 weeks. Continuous fetal monitoring in labour.

Postnatal
- Neonate should be given i.m. vitamin K.

- LFT and BA normalize within days or a few weeks.
- Contraception: avoid hormonal contraception particularly oestrogen-containing methods. If used, monitor LFT and BA and discontinue if deranged.
- Hormone replacement therapy can be used.

Referral to hepatologist
- If LFT/BA remain abnormal postnatally
- Anyone diagnosed with hepatitis B or C

Acute fatty liver of pregnancy (AFLP)

Definition
Reversible peripartum liver and renal impairment usually occurring in the third trimester, can be lethal

Incidence
1 in 20 000 pregnancies

Causes
- On same disease spectrum as pre-eclampsia
- Twenty per cent with AFLP are heterozygous for long-chain 3-hydroxy-acyl-coenzyme A dehydrogenase (LCHAD) deficiency (a disorder of mitochondrial fatty acid oxidation). The Fetus is homozygous.

Pathology
Microvesicular fatty infiltration of hepatocytes.

Risk factors
- Primigravidae
- Multiple pregnancies (14-fold increased risk)
- Male fetus.

Clinical features
Presentation varies from asymptomatic to fulminant liver failure, but usually gradual onset.

Symptoms
- Gradual onset nausea, anorexia, malaise (early)
- Vomiting, abdominal discomfort (later)
- Polyuria, polydipsia (transient diabetes insipidus).

Signs
- Jaundice
- Mild hypertension and mild proteinuria
- Ascites
- Hepatic encephalopathy in fulminant hepatic failure
  - Confusion
  - Liver flap.

Diagnosis
- ↑ liver transaminases (AST up to 3000), ↑ALP
- ↑bilirubin
- ↓albumin
- hypoglycaemia
- deranged clotting (initially ↓antithrombin levels, then prolonged prothrombin time)
- ↑WCC
- renal impairment (↑urea, ↑creatinine)
- ↑ urate
- ABG: metabolic acidosis
- Liver biopsy and fat stains (not done in practise due to coaglopathy)
- Imaging of liver with USS, CT or MRI is not discriminatory.

Important markers of severity of AFLP
- Hypoglycaemia
- Coagulopathy
- Falling albumin.

Differential diagnosis
- HELLP syndrome
- Fulminant viral hepatitis.

Management
- Multidisciplinary involvement of obstetricians, hepatologists, nephrologists, haematologists and intensivists is essential, usually in ITU unless mild disease
- Early discussion with specialist liver unit
- Degree of abnormality of LFT not prognostic.

Supportive management
- Adequate fluid balance (to maintain renal perfusion)
- Correct coagulopathy: FFP, ± antithrombin concentrate, platelets, cryoprecipitate
- Hypoglycaemia: 50% dextrose initially then 10% dextrose infusion
- Renal failure: dialysis
- Liver dysfunction: N-acetyl cysteine infusion.

Rapid delivery of baby (after correcting glucose and clotting)
- Remember bleeding risks with caesarean section
- Cover delivery with antibiotics

Fulminant hepatic failure and encephalopathy
- Transfer to specialist liver unit
- May need liver transplant

Postnatal
- Most women improve 1–4 weeks after prompt delivery and treatment
- Cholestatic phase with ↑bilirubin and ALP may persist longer
- Postpartum haemorrhage requiring repeated surgery not uncommon
- Avoid NSAIDs
- Screen baby for defects of fatty acid oxidation.

Table 8.27.2 differentiating features between AFLP and HELLP

Feature	AFLP	HELLP
Epigastric pain	+	++
Vomiting	++	±
Hypertension	+	++
Proteinuria	+	++
Elevated liver enzymes	moderately	mildly
Hypoglycaemia	++	±
Hyperuricaemia	++	+
DIC and coagulopathy	++	+
Low platelets (i.e. <100) without DIC	±	++
Elevated white blood count	++	+

Complications
- Maternal mortality varies from 1.8% (based on a UK population study) up to 19% (based on hospital studies)
- Perinatal mortality 10%.

Recurrence
More likely if heterozygous for LCHAD deficiency

HELLP syndrome
Definition
Part of the spectrum of pre-eclampsia. Acronym **HELLP**: **H**aemolysis, **E**levated **L**iver enzymes, **L**ow **P**latelets

Incidence
Twenty per cent of severe pre-eclamptics.

Pathology
Endothelial dysfunction (as for pre-eclampsia)
Microangiopathic platelet activation and consumption.

Clinical features
Twenty-five per cent occur postnatally.

Symptoms
- Malaise
- Nausea
- Epigastric or right upper quadrant pain
- Vaginal bleeding from placental abruption.

Signs
- Hypertension (might not be severe) ± proteinuria
- Tender right upper quadrant
- Haematuria/coke-coloured urine
- Jaundice (occasionally).

Diagnosis
- Haemolysis (infrequent):
  - peripheral blood film: red cell fragments
  - ↑lactose dehydrogenase (LDH >600 U/l)
  - ↑ unconjugated bilirubin
  - falling haemoglobin
- LFT: ↑ transaminases (AST >70 U/l)
- Platelets < 100×10^9/L
- Liver USS/CT: if suspect subcapsular haematoma or intrahepatic haemorrhage.

Differential diagnosis
- Acute fatty liver of pregnancy (Table 8.27.2)
- Haemolytic uraemic syndrome (HUS)
- Thrombotic thrombocytopenic purpura (TTP)
  In HUS/TTP thrombocytopenia is usually profound.

Management
As for severe pre-eclampsia:
- Fluid restriction
- Antihypertensives (keep BP <160/110 mmHg)
- Prophylaxis against eclampsia with MgSO4
- Steroids for fetal lung maturity
- Delivery
  - mode of delivery depends on gestation and obstetric factors
  - urgent delivery if severe upper abdominal pain, abruption, fetal distress
  - aim for vaginal delivery if possible as less morbidity

- if platelets <80×10^9/L, regional analgesia unlikely, use other methods instead, e.g. diamorphine or fentanyl patient controlled analgesia (PCA).

Specific points
- Caution with dose of MgSO4 if renal impairment
- Check blood glucose with pre-eclampsia bloods
- Steroid treatment does not improve prognosis
- Platelet transfusion if platelet count <50×10^9/L and
  - actively bleeding or
  - requiring surgery
- Correct coagulopathy with FFP.

Postnatal
Abnormal blood parameters may deteriorate initially, but resolve completely
  HELLP can occur postpartum.

Complications
- Massive hepatic necrosis
- Hepatic haemorrhage without rupture
- Liver rupture (requires immediate laparotomy ± embolization)
- Maternal mortality 1%
- Perinatal mortality 7–60%
  Recurrence of pre-eclampsia high
  Recurrence of HELLP 3–5%.

Primary biliary cirrhosis
Definition
Chronic cholestatic presumed autoimmune liver disease.

Incidence
Rare. Nine times commoner in women than men.

Clinical features
Pruritis: can become very severe and intractable in pregnancy.

Diagnosis
- raised ALP and GGT
- antimitochondrial antibodies.

Differential diagnosis
- Obstetric cholestasis
- Sclerosing cholangitis.

Treatment
- Ursodeoxycholic acid
- Plasmapharesis if intractable pruritis
- Liver transplantation.

Sclerosing cholangitis
Definition
Rare chronic fibrosing inflammation of biliary tree.

Clinical features
- Pruritis can worsen in pregnancy
- Abdominal pain
- Associated with inflammatory bowel disease
- Good outcome in pregnancy.

Complications
  Cholangiocarcinoma and other hepatic tumours.

Wilson's disease

Definition
Autosomal recessive disorder resulting in copper deposition in liver initially, then in central nervous system and other organs.

Clinical features
- Hepatic impairment
- Neurological impairment especially movement disorders
- Behavioural abnormalities.

Diagnosis:
- ↓ serum copper and caeruloplasmin
- ↑ urinary copper.

Management
- Maternal and fetal outcomes good if adequately treated
- Treatment: d-penicillamine, trientine and zinc
- Teratogenicity reported with drug treatment but continue in pregnancy as discontinuation can result in severe deterioration.

Cirrhosis
Often infertile

Clinical features in pregnancy
- Pregnancy associated with decompensation of liver disease
- ↑risk of miscarriage, preterm delivery and stillbirth
- ↑risk of bleeding from oesophageal varices if have portal hypertension (usually in second trimester).

Management
- Multidisciplinary care essential with hepatologists
- Continue beta-blockers in those with portal hypertension and oesophageal varices
- Commence beta-blockers in women not already on them with portal hypertension in second trimester of pregnancy.

Liver transplants
- Delay pregnancy for 18 months following transplant surgery when allograft is functioning well, risk of rejection low, immunosupressive drugs at lower dose and viral prophylaxis completed
- Continue immunosuppressive drugs throughout pregnancy under joint care with hepatologist to avoid graft rejection and infection
- Tacrolimus, and azathioprine are commonly used with no associated fetal malformations

- Prednisolone carries a small risk of fetal cleft lip/palate with first trimester use, but should be continued
- Delivery may be preterm, but outcomes are usually good.

Hepatitis
See Chapter 8.25, Jaundice.

Further reading

Bellig LL. Maternal acute fatty liver of pregnancy and the associated risk for long-chain-3 hydroxyacyl co-enzyme A dehydrogenase deficiency (LCHAD) in infants. Adv Neonatal Care 2004;4:26–32.

Ch'ng CL, Morgan M, Hainsworth I, et al. Prospective study of liver dysfunction in Southwest Wales. Gut 2002;51:876–80.

Christopher V, Al-Chalabi T, Richardson PD, et al. Pregnancy outcome after liver transplantation: a single-centre experience of 71 pregnancies in 45 recipients. Liver Transpl 2006;12:1138–43.

Glanz A, Marschall HU, Lammert F, Mattsson LA. Intrahepatic cholestasis of pregnancy: a randomised controlled trial comparing dexamethasone and ursodeoxycholic acid. Hepatology 2005;42:1399–405.

Glanz A, Marschall HU, Mattsson LA. Intrahepatic cholestasis of pregnancy. Relationships between bile acid levels and fetal complication rates. Hepatology 2004;40:467–74.

Janczewska I, Olsson R, Hultcrantz, et al. Pregnancy in patients with primary sclerosing cholangitis. Liver 1996;16:326–30.

Katz L, de Amorim MM, Figueiroa JN, et al. Postpartum dexamethasone for women with hemolysis, elevated liver enzymes, and low platelets (HELLP) syndrome: a double-blind, placebo-controlled, randomized clinical trail. Am J Obstet Gynecol 2008;198:283.e1–8.

Knight M, Nelson-Piercy C, Kurinczuk JJ, et al. UK Obstetric Surveillance System. A prospective national study of acute fatty liver of pregnancy in the UK. Gut 2008;57:951–6.

Royal College of Obstetricians and Gynaecologists. Obstetric Cholestasis. Guideline No. 13. London: RCOG 2006. Available on-line: www.rcog.org.uk/resources/Public/pdf/obstetric_cholestasis43.pdf

Sibai BM, Ramadan MK, Usta I, et al. Maternal morbidity and mortality in 442 pregnancies with haemolysis, elevated liver enzymes and low platelets (HELLP syndrome). Am J Obstet Gynecol 1993;169:1000–6.

Sternlieb I. Wilson's disease and pregnancy. Hepatology 2000;31:531–2.

Tan J, Surti B, Saab S. Pregnancy and cirrhosis. Liver Transpl 2008;14:1081–91.

Internet resources

The Obstetric Cholestasis Support website: www.ocsupport.org.uk

Measles: rubeola

Definition
Rubeola, measles, is an acute, highly infectious illness caused by the rubeola virus that is characterized by cough, coryza, fever, and a maculopapular rash.

Epidemiology
Although rubeola is highly contagious, the infection is uncommon in industrialized nations because of a safe and effective vaccine; it has not been considered endemic in the USA since 2000. In developing countries, there are over 20 000 000 cases per year with an estimated 242 000 deaths, mainly children, in 2006. The majority of the deaths occurred in South-East Asia.

Most epidemics occur in the spring and summer of alternate years. Since maternally derived immunity is effective up to 6–9 months of age, the peak age of infection is about 4 years.

Aetiology
The rubeola virus belongs to the Paramyxoviridae family, which are enveloped, negative single-stranded RNA viruses. Although the virion is very labile, it remains infective in droplet form in air for several hours. Spread is by direct contact with droplets from respiratory secretions of infected persons.

Clinical features
Incubation period
The incubation following exposure lasts 10–14 days. Exposure to the virus results in entry via the respiratory mucosa and/or conjuctiva. The virus replicates locally before dissemination into regional lymphatics and eventually the bloodstream. Although it is typically asymptomatic during this period, there may be transient respiratory symptoms, fever, or a morbilliform rash.

Prodromal illness
A second viraemia occurs several days after the first and is associated with the appearance of symptoms that include high, spiking fevers, irritability, nasal and conjunctival discharge, a cough, and loose stools. Koplik's spots, white, irregular lesions that appear on the buccal mucosa typically opposite the upper premolars on day 2 of the fever, are pathognomonic of prodromal measles.

Rash
On days 3–4, the erythematous maculopapular rash appears, initially at the hairline involving the forehead, behind the earlobes, and upper part of the neck. It spreads downwards to the face, neck, upper extremities, and trunk; it reaches the feet by the third day. The early lesions become confluent, although peripherally, the lesions remain discrete. It begins to fade by the third day in the order of its appearance. With disappearance, a fine branny desquamation may be noted in heavily affected areas excepting the hands and feet, a feature which distinguishes it from scarlet fever.

Convalescence
The rash appears as the temperature reaches its peak. Koplik's spots begin to slough. The coryza and conjunctivitis become profuse and the cough is persistent. Within the next 24–36 hours, the temperature falls and the remainder of the symptoms begin to clear, although the cough may last for weeks. Fever lasting beyond the third day of the rash is probably caused by secondary infection.

Diagnosis
Although the clinical course is often typical, the WHO recommends that the diagnosis be confirmed by laboratory tests. In the USA, the infection is reportable to the local health department. A serodiagnosis can be made with an IgM enzyme-linked immonosorbent assay using serum or saliva samples. Virtually 100% will be positive by the end of the first week.

Differential diagnosis
This varies with the stage of the illness. The prodromal phase symptoms are typical of a common cold except for the presence of fever. Other considerations are influenza, adenovirus, dengue virus, or respiratory syncytial virus infection.

During the exanthem phase, *Mycoplasma pneunomiae*, rubella, Rocky Mountain spotted fever, infectious mononucleosis, scarlet fever, Kawasaki disease, toxic shock syndrome, dengue, roseola, erythema infectiosum, and drug eruptions are in the differential. The intensity of the rash followed by its brownish discolouration and the associated symptoms of coryza and conjunctivitis are distinguishing features of rubeola.

Management
Vitamin A
Since measles mortality is inversely related to serum retinol levels, children from countries where health care and nutrition are compromised should receive vitamin A at the time of diagnosis. An oral dose of 10 000 IU is recommended for children up to 1 year of age; those over 1 year should receive 20 000 IU. Children with keratoconjunctivitis should receive a second dose 1 month later.

Antibiotics
Measles will generally run a fairly typical, self-limiting course, resulting in full recovery with supportive therapy such as hydration and antipyretics. Since secondary bacterial infections are frequent, however, these should be treated appropriately as soon as a diagnosis is made.

Complications
- Secondary bacterial infections, including suppurative otitis media and bronchopneumonia, are common and often severe.
- With dissemination of the virus, there can be involvement of other organ systems with manifestations that include myocarditis, pericarditis, hepatitis, mesenteric lymphadenopathy, and corneal ulceration.
- Post-infectious encephalitis occurs in 1 in 800–1600 cases and has a mortality of up to 15%. Fifty per cent of survivors have neurological sequelae.
- Subacute sclerosing panencephalitis is a rare (1 in 1 000 000 cases), late-appearing complication occurring most often in children who became infected under the age of 2 years. The onset is 3–10 years after the original illness and results in death within 2 years.
- Measles inclusion body encephalitis is seen most often in children who are immunosuppressed; the usual onset is 1–7 months after the original illness. Fever, neurological

dysfunction and seizures progress over 3 or more weeks, resulting in a 75% fatality rate and severe neurological sequelae in survivors.

Prevention

Pre-exposure prophylaxis
Live-attenuated measles vaccines introduced in the 1960s and 1970s have been highly effective in controlling epidemic disease as well as the rare neurological sequelae. Since immunization prior to age 9–12 months produces a short-lasting immunity and immunization after age 1 year leaves a window of susceptibility due to the loss of maternally derived antibodies, a two-step immunization programme is recommended. The first dose is given between the ages of 12 and 15 months and a second booster dose is given between the ages of 3 and 5 years. The first dose is recommended between the ages of 6 and 9 months in developing countries. A 96% seroconversion rate can be expected.

Common adverse effects from the immunization can occur and include:
- a mild febrile illness with a transient rash at 7 days following the first immunization
- mild allergic reactions such as urticaria or other, non-anaphylactic, reactions.

Although generally contraindicated in immunosuppressed patients, the measles live vaccine has been safely given to patients with asymptomatic and symptomatic HIV infection as long as the CD4 cell count is greater than 500.

Post-exposure prophylaxis
When given within 3 days of exposure, human immunoglobulin is effective in preventing measles as all commercially available immunoglobulin preparations contain high levels of antibodies. The recommended doses are as follows:
- less than 1 year of age: 250 mg of immunoglobulin
- ages 1– 2 years: 500 mg of immunoglobulin
- age 3 or greater: 750 mg of immunoglobulin.

Public health initiatives
The WHO and UNICEF have developed a comprehensive strategy to sustainably reduce measles deaths. The strategy was endorsed by the World Health Assembly in 2003. The strategy includes
- strong routine immunization: vaccination of at least 90% of children at the age of 9 months
- a second opportunity for measles immunization: vaccination provided to all children aged 9 months to 15 years who did not previously receive a dose as well as those who did not develop immunity
- surveillance: confirmation of suspected cases of measles through blood collection and testing in accredited laboratories
- improved clinical management: vitamin A supplementation and antibiotic treatment of secondary infections.

Further reading
Katz S. Measles (Rubeola). In: Gershon AA, Hotez PJ, Katz SL, (eds) *Krugman's infectious diseases of children*, 11th edn. Philadelphia: Mosby 2004.

World Health Organization. *Progress in global measles control and mortality reduction, 2000-2006*. Weekly Epidemiological Record 2007;48:418–24.

Baringa JL, Skolnik PR. Clinical presentation and diagnosis of measles. UpToDate May 2008. Version 16.2.

Maldonado YA, et al. Early loss of passive measles antibody in infants of mothers with vaccine-induced immunity. Pediatrics 1995;96:447–50.

Butler JC, Havens PL, Sowel AL, et al. Measles severity and serum retinol (vitamin A) concentration among children in the United States. Pediatrics 1993;91:1176–81.

Bannister BA. *Measles (Rubeola)*. In: Cohen J, Powderly WG, et al. (eds) *Infectious diseases*, 2nd edn. Philadelphia: Mosby 2004.

Strebel P, Cochi S, et al. The unfinished measles immunization agenda. J Infect Dis 2003;187(Suppl 1):S1–7.

Internet resources
www.who.int/mediacentre/factsheets/fs286/en/index.html
www.measlesinitiative.org/index3.asp

Parvovirus

Parvovirus B19 is the cause of erythema infectiosum or 'fifth disease'. These are among the smallest DNA viruses; humans are their only known hosts. It is composed of an icosahedral protein capsule without an envelope that contains a single strand of DNA.

The cellular receptor for B19 parvovirus is the erythrocyte P antigen, thus explaining their propensity to infect erythrocytes and precursors.

Epidemiology

The prevalence of parvovirus B19 infection is common and it is spread worldwide. Infections are more common in schoolchildren, with 70% of cases occurring between 5 and 15 years of age. Seasonal peaks occur in the late winter and spring, with sporadic cases throughout the year. Transmission is via the respiratory route; the transmission rate is 15–30% among susceptible household contacts. In school outbreaks, secondary attack rates range from 10% to 60%. Nosocomial outbreaks show an attack rate of 30% among susceptible healthcare workers. It is also transmissible via blood or blood products; indeed the virus was first identified in blood bank specimens in the 1970s.

Sixty-five per cent of pregnant women have serological evidence of seroconversion and are thus immune. Daycare workers, teachers, and parents are at increased risk of seroconversion.

Clinical approach

Clinical manifestations

The most common manifestation is erythema infectiosum, characterized by a malar rash with the characteristic 'slapped cheeks' appearance and a lace-like rash in the extremities. The rash may reappear for several weeks following stimulus, including changes in temperature, sunlight exposure, or emotional stress. Fever, malaise, and lymphadenopathy may accompany the infection. A symmetric arthropathy affecting most commonly the hands may also appear. Symptoms are self-limiting but may last for several months. Infection may be asymptomatic 20% of the time. Persistent infection, in patients unable to mount an appropriate immune response, is rare, and presents as pure red cell aplasia.

Fetal infection can be asymptomatic or instead an aplastic anaemia of varying severity may appear. Severe anaemia may cause high-output heart failure and non-immune hydrops.

Diagnosis

Serological testing can detect IgG and IgM antibodies to B19 Parvovirus through an enzyme-linked immunosorbent assay. Susceptible individuals will have both antibodies negative. Positive IgG and negative IgM signals immunity or infection more than 120 days prior. Recently infected patients will have positive IgM and negative IgG, and, finally, those who have had an infection more than 7 days but less than 120 days prior will show seropositivity to both G and M immunoglobulin.

Management during pregnancy

Transplacental transmission rates have been reported to be as high as 33% and fetal infection has been associated with spontaneous abortion, hydrops fetalis, and stillbirth. The rate of fetal loss is between 2% and 9%. *In utero* parvovirus B19 infection is responsible for up to 18 % of cases of non-immune hydrops.

For women exposed between the first and twelfth week of gestation, the risk of severe fetal involvement is 19%. This decreases to 15% for exposure between 13 and 20 weeks and drops down to 6% for infection occurring after 20 weeks.

Women who are exposed to Parvovirus should have their antibodies, both IgG and IgM, tested. Positive reaction to IgG shows old infection and no further workup is warranted. Susceptible women should have repeat serology in 3 weeks. In case of confirmed infection, maternal treatment is just supportive care since the infection is self-limited. Serial ultrasound examinations to evaluate the fetus for hydrops should be performed for 8–10 weeks after maternal illness; measurement of the middle cerebral artery peak systolic velocity can be useful to document fetal anaemia before hydrops ensues. It should be noted that although 33% of fetal hydrops resolves without treatment there are no reliable predictors for resolution versus fetal death, so cordocentesis and intrauterine transfusion are recommended when hydrops is present. If hydrops has not occurred by 8 weeks after maternal infection, it is unlikely to occur. Long-term developments of these fetuses appear to be normal (ACOG 2008).

Preventative measures

Options for prevention are limited during outbreaks in which prolonged, close contact exposure occurs, such as schools, homes, or childcare settings. Exposure cannot be prevented by identifying and isolating affected persons since 20% of infections are asymptomatic and those who do become symptomatic are infectious before they develop symptoms. Exclusion of pregnant women from the workplace during an endemic period is controversial and excluding members of high-risk groups from work during an outbreak is not recommended (ACOG 2000).

References

ACOGCompendium of selected publicationsPractice Bulletin #20. September 2008;651:654–5.

Bernstein H. *Gabbe obstetrics*, 5th edn. 2007: 1213–14.

Cosmi E, Mari G, Delle Chiae L, et al. Noninvasive diagnosis by Doppler ultrasonography of fetal anemia resulting from parvovirus infection. Am J Obstet Gynecol 2002;187:1290.

Hernandez-Andrade E, Scheier M, Dezerega V, et al. Fetal middle cerebral artery peak systolic velocity in the investigation of non immune hydrops. Ultrasound Obstet Gynecol 2004;23:442.

Koch CW. *Kliegman: Nelson textbook of pediatrics*, 18th edn. Ch 248.

Pituitary disorders in pregnancy

Physiological changes

The volume of the anterior pituitary increases progressively during pregnancy by up to 35%. This is mainly due to an increase in the number and size of the lactotrophic cells. Postpartum involution is slower if the woman breastfeeds. Prolactin levels increase up to 10-fold during pregnancy and return to normal by 2 weeks after delivery, unless the woman breastfeeds. This increase is thought to be mediated via increases in oestrogen and progesterone and is related to the initiation and maintenance of lactation.

Levels of luteinizing hormone (LH) and follicle-stimulating hormone (FSH) are suppressed by the concentrations of oestrogen and progesterone. Basal growth hormone (GH), antidiuretic hormone (ADH), and pituitary adrenocorticotrophic hormone (ACTH) are unaltered in pregnancy.

Hyperprolactinaemia

Prolactinomas

Epidemiology
Prolactin-producing pituitary adenomas are the commonest pituitary adenomas encountered in pregnancy.

Pathology
They are classified according to size into microprolactinomas (<10 mm in diameter) or macroprolactinoma (>10 mm in diameter).

Aetiology
Hyperprolactinaemia has multiple potential causes apart from prolactinomas:
- normal pregnancy
- hypothalamic and pituitary stalk lesions (leading to removal of dopaminergic suppression of prolactin secretion)
- empty sella syndrome
- hypothyroidism (thyroid-stimulating hormone stimulates lactotrophs)
- chronic renal failure
- seizures
- drugs, e.g. metoclopramide.

Prognosis
Effect of pregnancy on prolactinomas
The main risks are those posed by the potential expansion of the pituitary space-occupying lesion. This could potentially lead to visual field defects by impinging on the optic chiasma or to pituitary apoplexy with panhypopituitarism. This risk of symptomatic tumour expansion is 15% in untreated and 4.4% in treated patients with macroprolactinomas. The risk for symptomatic expansion of a microprolactinoma during pregnancy is minimal (1.6%).

Effect of prolactinomas on pregnancy
Hyperprolactinaemia is associated with amenorrhoea, reduced fertility and hypo-oestrogenaemia. Therefore, the majority are diagnosed preconceptually and the pregnancy would have been the result of treatment with dopamine-receptor agonists. There are no known adverse effects to the fetus and women with prolactinomas can breastfeed.

Clinical approach
Diagnosis

History
Prolactinomas may present with amenorrhoea, reduced fertility, galactorrhoea, frontal headache, visual field defects, or diabetes insipidus. In pregnancy, only the last three symptoms are discriminatory.

Examination and investigations
Formal visual field testing should be performed to confirm any symptoms of visual fields to confrontation.

Prolactin levels are of no value in the diagnosis of these patients as they are elevated during pregnancy. If a pituitary tumour is suspected, other pituitary function tests (thyroid function tests) should be performed.

Diagnosis in pregnancy largely relies on findings of pituitary magnetic resonance imaging (MRI) or computed tomography (CT).

Management
- Prolactin levels are unhelpful to monitor tumour activity in pregnancy as they are elevated in pregnancy.
- Women should be reviewed once in every trimester.
- Most physicians discontinue dopamine receptor agonists (bromocriptine/cabergoline) in cases of micropolactinomas once pregnancy is confirmed. Treatment with dopamine receptor agonists is electively continued by many endocrinologists in cases of macroprolactinomas.
- Regular follow up with formal visual field testing is mandatory for symptomatic women or those with macroprolactinomas.
- There should be a low threshold for performing pituitary images (MRI) in the presence of headaches or symptoms suggestive of visual field defects or diabetes insipidus.
- Dopamine receptor agonists are safe during pregnancy and breastfeeding. They should be reintroduced if there is concern about tumour expansion. Cabergoline has a more favourable side-effect profile than bromocriptine (causes less nausea).
- Hypophysectomy or radiotherapy is rarely necessary and is usually deferred to after delivery.

Hypopituitarism

Hypopituitarism may precede pregnancy or present for the first time during pregnancy. The usual causes are pituitary or hypothalamic tumours, pituitary surgery, or cranial radiotherapy. Causes more specific to pregnancy include lymphocytic hypophysitis and postpartum pituitary infarction (Sheehan's syndrome).

Pathogenesis

Sheehan's syndrome
This usually presents postpartum following postpartum haemorrhage and hypotension and may lead to partial or complete pituitary failure. This is because the anterior pituitary is more vulnerable to hypotension in pregnancy due to its increased size.

Lymphocytic hypophysitis
This is a condition unique to pregnancy, presenting either late in the pregnancy or in the puerperium. It is characterized

by autoimmune infiltration of the anterior pituitary, predominantly lymphocytes, causing pituitary expansion and hypopituitarism. Antipituitary antibodies have been described and this condition is associated with autoimmune thyroiditis or adrenalitis in 20% of cases.

Prognosis

Effect of pregnancy on hypopituitarism
Subsequent pregnancies after Sheehan's syndrome and lymphocytic hypophysitis have been reported. Conception may require gonadotrophic stimulation of ovulation.

Effect of hypopituitarism on pregnancy
Maternal and fetal outcome is normal, if the condition is diagnosed and treated with adequate hormone replacement therapy prior to pregnancy. Poorly treated or undiagnosed hypopituitarism is associated with an increased risk of miscarriage, stillbirth, and maternal morbidity and mortality, resulting from hypoglycaemia and hypotension.

Clinical approach

Clinical features
- Sheehan's syndrome: presenting features are due to deficiency of the relevant hormones. They include persistent amenorrhoea, failure of lactation, secondary hypothyroidism and secondary adrenocortical insufficiency.
- Lymphocytic hypophysitis: the features are those of expanding pituitary tumour with headaches, visual field defects, secondary hypothyroidism and secondary hypoadrenalism.

Diagnosis of hypopituitarism
- Investigations reveal reduced levels of thyroxine (T4), TSH, cortisol, ACTH, FSH, LH, and GH. The insulin stress test is impaired.
- Any patient with hypopituitarism should undergo pituitary imaging with MRI or CT to exclude a pituitary tumour.
- Definitive diagnosis of lymphocytic hypophysitis can only be made by histological examination of pituitary tissue.

Management
- The treatment is with replacement of deficient hormones. The vital hormone replacements are those of thyroxine and glucocorticoids.
- Requirements of the latter may change during periods of stress, and doses and route of administration may need to be changed based on the severity of the stress.
- There is a need for vigorous regular follow-up of these patients throughout pregnancy.
- The management of acute pituitary insufficiency includes intravenous fluids, dextrose and corticosteroids.
- Cases of Sheehan's syndrome and lymphocytic hypophysitis have resolved spontaneously.

Future pregnancy
Lymphocytic hypophysitis may recur in subsequent pregnancies.

During subsequent pregnancies, requirements for thyroxine do not change, but additional parenteral corticosteroids may be required.

Diabetes insipidus

Epidemiology
This is approximately the same as in the non-pregnant population, i.e. 1 in 15 000.

Pathology
Diabetes insipidus (DI) is caused by a relative deficiency of vasopressin (ADH). There are four types:
- Central: (cranial) due to decreased production of ADH by the paraventricular nuclei of the hypothalamus. Causes include prolactinomas, craniopharyngeomas, skull trauma, post-neurosurgery, rarely Sheehan's syndrome or it may be idiopathic.
- Nephrogenic: associated with chronic renal disease, or more rarely hypercalcaemia or lithium therapy.
- Transient: increased ADH production by the placenta or decreased breakdown by the liver, usually associated with pre-eclampsia or acute fatty liver of pregnancy (AFLP).
- Psychogenic: caused by compulsive water drinking.

Prognosis

Effect of DI on pregnancy
No known adverse effects in treated cases and there is no contraindication to breastfeeding. Maternal seizures and oligohydramnios can complicate pregnancies in untreated or undiagnosed cases because of electrolyte imbalance and severe dehydration.

Effect of pregnancy on DI
Established central DI worsens in pregnancy and subclinical central DI may be unmasked for the first time during pregnancy because of increased clearance of endogenous ADH by vasopressinase. It is estimated that 60% of established cases of central DI worsen, but 25% improve, and 15% remain unchanged.

Clinical approach

Clinical features
These include excessive thirst, polyuria, or seizures (more common with transient DI).

Diagnosis
Other causes of polyuria such as diuretics, hyperglycaemia, hypercalcaemia, and hypokalaemia should be excluded.

The conventional 15–22 hours fluid deprivation test is hazardous in pregnancy. Close observation with paired urine and plasma osmolality measurements may be sufficient to exclude DI. A short deprivation test, e.g. overnight, may be all that is required to demonstrate an increasing urine osmolality with normal plasma osmolality and thus exclude cranial and nephrogenic DI.

Diagnosis is confirmed by a raised plasma osmolality (>295 mOsm/kg) or raised serum sodium (>145 mmol/L) in the presence of polyuria and a low urine osmolality (<300 mOsm/kg). This excludes psychogenic DI.

Administration of DDAVP (synthetic analogue of vasopressin) 10–20 µg intranasally may be used to facilitate diagnosis. It will result in concentration of urine in cranial DI but not in nephrogenic DI.

Those with central DI have low ADH levels, but those with nephrogenic DI have high levels.

Management
- In pregnancy, central DI is best treated by 2–20 µg of DDAVP intranasally, twice daily. DDAVP is not degraded by vasopressinase.
- DDAVP is safe for use in pregnancy for diagnosis and treatment of DI. Breastfeeding is not contraindicated.
- Newly onset DI should prompt a search for pre-eclampsia and AFLP.

- Serum osmolality and electrolytes should be checked regularly to ensure adequate treatment and to avoid overtreatment and water intoxication.
- For nephrogenic DI, carbamazepine is safer than chlorpropamide, as the latter may cause fetal hypoglycaemia.

Acromegaly

Epidemiology
Acromegaly is a rare condition with an incidence of five new cases per million of population per year. It affects both sexes equally and peaks at the age of 40–60 years.

Pathology
It is characterized by excess GH secretion. In over 9% of cases, it is due to a benign pituitary adenoma. Rarely, it is due to excess growth hormone-releasing hormone (GHRH) secretion from hypothalamic pituitary somatotroph hyperplasia, carcinoid tumour, or a pancreatic tumour.

Prognosis
Effect of pregnancy on acromegaly
There is an increased risk of enlargement of GH secreting pituitary adenomas in pregnancy, with the possibility of optic chiasma encroachment and visual field defects.

Effect of acromegaly on pregnancy
Fertility is markedly reduced in acromegaly. This is due to hyperprolactinaemia as well as disturbed gonadotrophin secretion. There is an increased risk of maternal diabetes mellitus and hypertension, with their associated risks to mother and fetus.

Maternal growth hormone does not cross the placenta and has no effect on fetal growth. Macrosomia is the result of maternal GH-induced diabetes mellitus.

Clinical approach
Clinical features
Many patients are infertile and 40% of women with acromegaly have associated hyperprolactinaemia.

The main clinical features are those of growth hormone excess, of which altered facial appearance, large hands and feet, and macroglossia may be the most obvious.

Excess growth hormone can result in hypertension, left ventricular hypertrophy, diabetes mellitus, and increased risk of colonic neoplasia.

Diagnosis
Growth hormone levels using conventional radioimmunoassays can be misleading, as they cannot differentiate between pituitary and placental growth hormone. The latter peaks during the later stages of pregnancy.

Insulin growth factor (IGF)-I is used outside pregnancy as a diagnostic tool but not during pregnancy as it increases in normal pregnancy.

Management
- Acromegaly is best treated prior to conception, preferably by surgery or adjuvant radiotherapy if surgical cure is not complete. Robust contraception is therefore strongly advised.
- Regular surveillance is vital throughout pregnancy. Macroadenomas require monthly visual field perimetry and MRI confirmation in cases of suspected enlargement.
- Dopamine agonists (bromocriptine or cabergoline) are effective in reducing growth hormone in less than 50% of cases, especially when associated with high prolactin. They have no effect on tumour size and are therefore of limited value in pregnancy.
- Octreotide (long-acting somatostatin analogue) by deep intramuscular injection is the medical treatment of choice. There are reports of safe and successful use during pregnancy but data are limited. Therefore, use is best avoided in pregnancy.

Cushing's syndrome

Epidemiology
The condition is very rare in pregnancy as most women with the disorder will have subfertility.

Pathology
Eight per cent of the cases outside pregnancy are due to corticotrophin-producing pituitary adenomas leading to bilateral adrenal hyperplasia (Cushing's disease). In pregnancy, less than 50% of cases are due to pituitary disease and most are caused by adrenal adenomas (44%) or adrenal carcinomas (12%).

Prognosis
Effect of Cushing's syndrome on pregnancy
Women with previously treated Cushing's do well in pregnancy.

There is an increased rate of fetal loss and perinatal morbidity, with 60% preterm delivery, and mortality (25%) is also high.

High maternal cortisol levels lead to suppression of fetal/neonatal corticosteroid secretion and the neonate is at a risk of adrenal insufficiency.

Maternal morbidity and mortality are increased. Maternal complications include hypertension in about 75% and gestational diabetes in about 50% of patients. Heart failure and severe pre-eclampsia are common. Wound infection due to poor tissue healing is common.

Clinical approach
Clinical features
Most women with this disorder will have subfertility. The classical clinical features can be attributed to pregnancy and include weight gain, striae, hypertension, diabetes, headaches, hirsutism, acne, and easy bruising.

Diagnosis
Pregnancy-specific ranges for plasma and urinary cortisol must be used. Low ACTH, with a high cortisol level that fails to suppress with a high-dose dexamethasone suppression test is suggestive of an adrenal cause.

Localization is with ultrasound, CT, or MRI of the pituitary or adrenals.

Management
- Surgery is the treatment of choice and has been undertaken successfully during pregnancy.
- Experience with cyproheptadine, metyrapone and ketoconazole in pregnancy is very limited. Metyrapone has been associated with severe hypertension. Ketoconazole should be avoided as it is teratogenic in animal studies due to blockage of testicular steroidogenesis.

Further reading
Nelson-Piercy C. *A handbook of obstetric medicine*, 3rd edn. London: Informa health care 2006:125–35.

Shehata HA, Ahmed K. Other endocrine disorders in pregnancy. Curr Obstet Gynaecol 2004;14:387–94.

Cauley K, Dalal A, Olson B, Onyiuke H. Lymphocytic hypophysitis. Conn Med 2005;69:143–6.

Hanson RS, Powrie RO, Larson L. Diabetes insipidus in pregnancy: a treatable cause of oligohydramnios. Obstet Gynecol 1997;89:816–17.

Herman-Bonert V, Seliverstov M, Melmed S. Pregnancy in acromgaly, successful therapeutic outcome. J Clin Endocrinol Metab 1998;83:727–31.

Landolt AM, Schmid J, Wimpfheimer C, et al. Successful pregnancy in a previously infertile woman treated with SMS 201-995 for Acromegaly N Eng J Med 1989;320:671.

Beressi N, Beressir J-P, Cohen R, Modigliani E. Lymphocytic hypophysitis. Ann Med Intern 1999;150:327–34.

Psychiatric disorders in pregnancy

Subsyndromal emotional disturbances are very common in pregnancy and psychiatric disorders much more common than previously recognized. Around one in two women experience significant symptoms of anxiety and around 1 in 10 will suffer with a diagnosable anxiety disorder. These are usually pre-existing disorders that have continued into pregnancy. One in three women experience significant symptoms of depression at some stage of pregnancy and at least 1 in 10 pregnant women will develop a depressive episode. Antenatal depression is probably more common than postnatal depression.

Conception rates among women with severe and enduring psychiatric disorders appear to be increasing, probably as a consequence of more community-based care and newer treatments. Around 1 in 500 pregnant women will be suffering with schizophrenia or bipolar affective disorder. These disorders are associated with relatively high risks of perinatal relapse, treatment with potentially teratogenic medications, and higher rates of miscarriage and other obstetric complications.

Obstetricians, midwives, and general practitioners need to be aware of the risks associated with psychiatric disorders in pregnancy and will frequently need to balance the risks to the unborn child of starting or continuing any psychiatric treatment with the risks to both mother and child of stopping or changing treatment.

Screening for psychiatric disorders in pregnancy

Psychiatric disorders are associated with high rates of morbidity in pregnancy and can have longer lasting effects on maternal health and child development (Oates 2003). They also are one of the leading causes of maternal mortality. It is therefore important to identify women who have a psychiatric disorder or who are at high risk of developing a psychiatric disorder as early on in pregnancy as possible. Early identification reduces risk and facilitates timely intervention.

At booking all women should be asked about
- past or present mental illness
- previous treatment by a psychiatrist or mental health team
- family history of perinatal mental illness.

Certain factors may increase the risk of developing mental illness in pregnancy or the puerperium including
- young age of mother
- family/partner conflicts
- lack of social network
- substance misuse
- unwanted pregnancy
- pre-existing mental illness.

As the risk of perinatal depression is particularly high, NICE (2007) recommends that all women are asked the following questions at booking, during pregnancy, and at 1 and 3–4 months postpartum:
- During the past month, have you often been bothered by feeling down, depressed or hopeless?
- During the past month, have you often been bothered by having little interest or pleasure in doing things?

If a woman says yes to either of these questions, a third is suggested:
- Is this something you feel you need or want help with?

More detailed clinical assessment

History: key points
- Current presenting symptoms: Screen for affective symptoms (low or elated mood, tearfulness, low or increased energy, sleep disturbance, anhedonia, amotivation) and psychotic symptoms (auditory hallucinations, delusions, thought disorder).
- Past psychiatric history: Ask about first contact with psychiatric services, any history of medications taken before or during pregnancy, any history of self harm or suicide attempts, admissions to hospital with a mental health problem, particularly if under a section of the Mental Health Act (2007).
- Family history: Ask about any family history of serious psychiatric illness, particularly in the perinatal period.
- Medication history: What medications are they currently taking? What medications have they been on prior to the pregnancy and when did these stop? This is important if medications taken are contraindicated in pregnancy, e.g. sodium valproate.
- Enquire about past or current substance misuse and alcohol use.

Examination: key points
- Ensure a thorough physical examination has been done to rule out physical causes for psychiatric symptoms, such as anaemia, gestational diabetes, thyroid disease, or iatrogenic causes such as steroids.
- Perinatal psychiatric liaison opinion to confirm diagnosis by detailed mental state examination.
- Appearance and behaviour: any evidence of poor eye contact and rapport, poor self-care?
- Speech: increased/reduced rate, rhythm, volume, content?
- Mood changes: how does the patient describe their mood? How do they rate severity out of 10?
- Thoughts: any self-harm or suicidal ideas, plans or intention? Any thoughts of harm to the baby? Any distressing guilty ideas or paranoid thoughts, especially concerning the baby?
- Perceptions: any experiences of seeing or hearing things when alone that others cannot see or accept?
- Cognition: orientation to time, place, person? Impaired concentration or memory?
- Insight: Does the patient feel they are physically or mentally unwell? Do they wish to accept treatment and if required come into hospital?
- Special investigations
- Consider blood tests to exclude physical conditions (FBC, WBC, U&E, LFTs, TFTs, glucose)
- Consider blood serum levels of medication to check if levels are therapeutic, e.g. lithium level.

Specific disorders

Anxiety disorders
- Anxiety disorders include phobias, panic disorder, generalized anxiety disorder, obsessive compulsive disorder, and post-traumatic stress disorder.
- Around 1 in 10 women will suffer with an anxiety disorder in any one year.

- Generic symptoms include pervasive or episodic fearfulness, avoidance, and autonomic arousal.
- Pregnant women with an anxiety disorder may present with excessive reassurance seeking and an over-preoccupation with fetal wellbeing.
- The possibility of agoraphobia, blood injury phobia, and needle phobia should be considered in women who are too fearful to attend antenatal clinic appointments.
- Depression can present with anxiety and is an important differential diagnosis to consider, as it will require treatment in its own right.
- Although invariably distressing to the pregnant woman, there is conflicting evidence that marked anxiety has an adverse effect on fetal outcome.
- High antenatal anxiety is a predictive factor for postnatal depression independently of antenatal depression.
- A relatively short-term, structured psychological treatment like cognitive behaviour therapy is the treatment of choice.
- Long-term benzodiazepine use should be avoided in pregnancy.

Bipolar affective disorder
- This affects 1 in 100 women of childbearing age.
- It is characterized by severe episodes of depression, mania (elevated mood, excitability, irritability, and over-activity) or a mixture of the two (mixed affective state) often associated with psychotic symptoms that can pose a significant risk to mother and fetus.
- It is associated with high rates of subsyndromal depression between acute episodes
- It is associated with high rates of relapse if mood-stabilizing medication is stopped precipitately in early pregnancy
- It predicts a high risk of postpartum relapse, approaching 1 in 2 without preventative treatment. Most episodes of postpartum psychosis are bipolar in nature, and most present within a week of delivery.
- It is associated with a high suicide rate.

Requires careful management by a psychiatrist familiar with the risks and benefits of psychiatric medication in pregnancy

Is best managed by a combined approach between maternity services, specialist mental health services and primary care with a formal perinatal care plan.

Depression
- This is characterized by low mood, lack of energy, or increased fatigability and loss of enjoyment or interest in association with a range of other symptoms including low self-esteem, feelings of guilt, worthlessness or hopelessness, poor concentration, poor appetite, and suicidal ideation
- It is associated with an increased risk of suicide
- It can be effectively treated with pharmacological and psychological therapy, although psychological treatments such as cognitive behavior therapy are preferred in pregnancy.

Eating disorders
- Bulimia nervosa affects 1 in 100 women of child-bearing age and anorexia nervosa around 1 in 500
- Bulimia nervosa and anorexia nervosa are characterized by disturbances in eating behaviour and abnormalities in body image

- Eating disorders tend to improve during pregnancy. Deterioration in pregnancy is predicted by more severe symptoms, younger age, and lower educational attainment.
- Pregnancy complications include poor maternal weight gain resulting in intrauterine growth retardation and small for date babies, electrolyte disturbances (hypokalaemia and hyponatraemia), metabolic alkalosis as a consequence of self-induced vomiting, laxatives or diuretic misuse, and higher rates of miscarriage, premature or instrumental delivery.
- The combination of hyperemesis gravidarum and eating disorder can be particularly problematic.
- Treatment is predominantly psychological.

Schizophrenia
- Schizophrenia affects 1 in 100 women of child-bearing age
- It is characterized by a range of cognitive, emotional, and volitional symptoms including delusions, hallucinations, and abnormalities of affect, speech, and motivation
- It is associated with a wide range of outcomes, from complete remission to long term enduring illness.
- It usually requires maintenance medication throughout and after pregnancy under the supervision of a psychiatrist familiar with the risks and benefits of psychotic medication in pregnancy.

Principles of treatment
If there is evidence of mild to moderate mental illness often psychological intervention alone or regular outpatient appointments for support can be helpful. Advice can be obtained from a perinatal psychiatrist. If medication is required, then the following treatment principles should apply (NICE 2007):
- use drugs with low-risk profiles for both the mother and fetus
- start at the lowest effective dose and increase slowly if required
- aim for monotherapy
- consider increased screening of the fetus, e.g. ultrasound
- breastfeeding should always be encouraged if the woman wishes and treatment that allows the woman to do this are preferred whenever possible.

Specific treatments
Anticonvulsants
- These are widely used in the treatment of bipolar disorder
- They are associated with relatively high teratogenicity, including neural tube defects. NICE (2007) recommends that valproate is not used to treat bipolar disorder in women of childbearing age unless clinically justified on the balance of risks, the woman has been carefully counselled about potential teratogenicity, and she is using adequate contraception.
- If taken during early pregnancy, the addition of high-dose folic acid is required (5 mg a day for women taking carbamazepine and valproate), although there is no evidence that this reduces the risk of neural tube defects.
- They are associated with a risk of vitamin K deficiency bleeding if taken in late pregnancy.

Antidepressants

- Antidepressants are relatively safe in pregnancy with notable exceptions. Venlafaxine may be associated with high blood pressure if taken at high doses; paroxetine should be avoided because of its reported association with cardiac anomalies, and all other selective serotonin reuptake inhibitors (SSRIs) should be used with caution after 20 weeks' gestation because of their reported association with persistent pulmonary hypertension of the newborn.

Antipsychotics

- These are relatively safe in pregnancy they but should be used at the lowest possible dose and polypharmacy avoided.
- Newer 'atypical' drugs may be associated with maternal weight gain predisposing to gestational diabetes, and 'large for date' and heavier birth weight babies.

Electroconvulsive therapy

- This is safe in pregnancy subject to the standard precautions associated with short-term anaesthesia.

Lithium

- Lithium has an important role in the management of bipolar disorder and stopping it precipitately in early pregnancy is associated with high rates of relapse.
- It has also been associated with elevated rates of congenital heart disease if used in the first trimester of pregnancy, but estimates of risk vary between 1% and 8%.
- High-resolution fetal ultrasound and echocardiography are recommended for the assessment of lithium exposed pregnancies.

- Lithium levels should be monitored every month until 36 weeks' gestation, then every week.
- Dehydration during prolonged labour may result in increased blood levels and intrapartum levels should be taken as required.
- Occasionally reported neonatal complications of lithium exposure include hypotonia, nephrogenic diabetes insipidus, hypothyroidism, and cardiac rhythm disturbances.

The pregnant woman in the psychiatric hospital

- She requires careful multiprofessional management and a clearly formulated birth plan that considers capacity to consent to, as well as capacity to cooperate with, obstetric care
- She may require increasingly frequent midwifery assessment as term approaches if her capacity to recognize the onset of labour is compromised.

References

Confidential Enquiry into Maternal and Child Health (CEMACH). Saving Mothers Lives: reviewing maternal deaths to make motherhood safer (2003–2007). Dec 2007.

Davies A, McIvor R, et al. Impact of childbirth on a series of schizophrenic mothers. Schizophrenia Res 1995;16:25–31.

NICE Clinical guideline 45. Antenatal and postnatal mental health National Institute of Clinical Excellence. Feb 2007.

Oates M. Perinatal psychiatric disorders: a leading cause of maternal morbidity and mortality. Br Med Bull 2003;67:219–29

Patient resources

The Royal College of Psychiatrists website has a useful information leaflet:www.rcpsych.ac.uk/pnd

Mind www.mind.org.uk and www.pni.org.uk.

Renal disease

Asymptomatic bacteriuria

Definition
Significant growth of a uropathogen in the absence of symptoms.

Incidence
Incidence of 2–10% of pregnant women.

Causes
As for urinary tract infections (see below).

Clinical features
- Asymptomatic, usually infected in early pregnancy
- Associated with preterm delivery and low birthweight babies in some studies if untreated.

Diagnosis
- Urine dipstick: leucocytes, nitrites
- Midstream specimen of urine (MSU): >10^5 colony forming units of pathogen (CFC)/mL.

Management
During pregnancy
- Empirically treat with antibiotics if leucocytes and nitrites on urine dipstick. Adjust treatment according to sensitivities
- 4–6 weekly MSU (as 30% have a relapse of bacteriuria)

Complications
Development of acute pyelonephritis in
- <1% of treated women
- up to 30% of untreated women.

Urinary tract infection

Incidence
In pregnancy 1%

Causes
Escherichia coli (70–80%), *Klebsiella, Proteus, Enterobacter, Staphylococcus saprophyticus.*

Clinical features
- Dysuria
- Offensive smelling urine
- Suprapubic pain
- Symptoms common in healthy pregnant women: frequency, nocturia, strangury (urge to pass urine when already done so)

Diagnosis
As for asymptomatic bacteriuria (see above)

Management
Antibiotic treatment: normally for 3 days. If recurrent infection, or infection in a woman with renal disease, diabetes, sickle cell trait or disease treat for 7–10 days
- *E. coli* is the commonest organism and usually sensitive to:
  - nitrofurantoin 100 mg bd (avoid in late third trimester due to risk of neonatal haemolysis)
  - trimethoprim 200 mg b.d. (avoid in first trimester as it is a folate antagonist)
  - amoxicillin and cephalosporin
  - ciprofloxacin causes arthropathy in animal studies
- Increase fluid intake

- Check MSU 1 week following completion of treatment and then after every 4–6 weeks
- If ≥2 episodes of asymptomatic bacteriuria or urinary tract infections (UTIs)
  - renal USS for structural abnormalities or renal stones
  - prophylactic low-dose antibiotics given at night for the rest of pregnancy and 6 weeks postpartum.

Complications
Acute pyelonephritis.

Acute pyelonephritis

Definition
Infection of kidney(s).

Causes
As for UTIs.

Clinical features
- Fever, rigors
- Back or loin pain
- Symptoms of UTI
- Nausea, vomiting
- Sepsis if severe.

Effect of acute pyelonephritis on pregnancy
- Uterine contractions
- Preterm labour
- Sepsis.

Diagnosis
- As for UTI plus
  - FBC, U+E, CRP
  - blood culture (if febrile).

Management
- Admit for empirical IV broad-spectrum antibiotics (usually a cephalosporin). Change to oral treatment for 10 days once afebrile for 24 hours.
- Aminoglycoside may be necessary (measure drug levels as theoretical risk of fetal ototoxicity).
- Intravenous fluid rehydration.
- If sepsis suspected, perform lactate level, check for haemolysis (blood film and LDH), consider CVP line and liaise with ITU.
- Renal USS.
- Following discharge, screen for bacteriuria as in UTIs (see above).
- Prophylactic antibiotics reduce risk of recurrent acute pyelonephritis.

Complications
Chronic pyelonephritis.

Acute renal failure (ARF)

Incidence
<0.005%

Causes
- Prerenal: intravascular fluid depletion, e.g. hyperemesis gravidarum, ovarian hyperstimulation syndrome, preeclampsia, placental abruption, postpartum haemorrhage, sepsis.

- Renal: haemolytic uraemic syndrome, thrombotic thrombocytopenic purpura, acute fatty liver of pregnancy, drugs (e.g. NSAIDs, gentamicin).
- Post-renal: acute obstruction of renal tracts e.g. ureteric damage or obstruction.

> Principles of management;
> Identify and treat cause
> Fluid resuscitation (monitor CVP)
> Renal replacement therapy if other measures do not help

Clinical features
- Oliguria (but common intrapartum and postpartum especially with pre-eclampsia)
- Anuria uncommon
- Features associated with possible cause of ARF
- Bleeding, hypotension, and low CVP
- Hypertension and proteinuria (pre-eclampsia):
  - BP often remains high even if bleeding.

Diagnosis
- Raised urea and creatinine
- Low sodium
- High potassium
- Metabolic acidosis.

> Differential diagnosis of ARF + thrombocytopenia +; microangiopathic haemolytic anaemia:
> Pre-eclampsia (see Chapter 9.10)
> HELLP syndrome (see Chapter 8.27)
> Haemolytic uraemic syndrome (see below)
> Thrombotic thrombocytopenic purpura (see below)
> Acute fatty liver of pregnancy (see Chapter 8.27)

Management
Senior obstetric and anaesthetic involvement essential
- Treat underlying cause
- Insert CVP and urinary catheter
- Monitor hourly fluid balance, CVP, pulse, BP, and RR
- Treat coagulopathy.

Fluid management
- If loss of blood or dehydration, replace blood and/or fluids intravenously until normal haemoglobin and CVP between 5–10 cm H2O. Avoid giving diuretics with blood until volume replete
- If remains oliguric with a normal or high CVP, do not give fluid challenge as will develop pulmonary oedema
- When euvolaemic and if no longer bleeding, administer IV fluids: previous hour's urine output plus 20 mL/hour for insensible losses. If still bleeding treat this and replace blood loss
- Pre-eclamptics are particularly vulnerable to fluid overload especially iatrogenically if they are bleeding.

> Indications for renal replacement therapy (dialysis);
> Hyperkalaemia refractory to medical treatment
> Uraemia (usually urea >25 mmol/L)
> Acidosis
> Pulmonary oedema refractory to diuretics

Recovery
- Dialysis is required in the short-term as most causes of ARF in pregnancy are reversible
- Acute tubular necrosis is reversible
- Acute cortical necrosis is irreversible.

Haemolytic uraemic syndrome (HUS) and thrombotic thrombocytopenic purpura (TTP)
Definition
Part of the same spectrum of microangiopathic haemolytic anaemia and thrombocytopenia

Incidence
More common in women and increased incidence in late pregnancy and postpartum

Causes
- Congenital HUS/TTP: absence of ADAMTS13 (a plasma metalloprotease)
- Acquired HUS/TTP: reduction of ADAMTS13 by anti-ADAMST13 antibodies.

Pathology
- ADAMTS13 cleaves von Willebrand factor (vWF) multimers, which prevents platelets adhering to the multimers and forming microthrombi that can block end organ arterioles and capillaries (as occurs in HUS/TTP).
- ADAMST13 normally falls in pregnancy.

Clinical features
- HUS: haematuria, renal failure
- TTP: neurological or behavioural abnormalities ± symptoms of gastrointestinal vessel ischaemia.

Diagnosis
- Severe thrombocytopenia
- Severe haemolysis
  - peripheral blood film (usually diagnostic): red cell fragments
  - ↑lactose dehydrogenase (LDH >600 U/L)
  - ↑ unconjugated bilirubin
  - falling haemoglobin
- Renal impairment: severe in HUS
- DIC is rare (prothrombin time and APTT usually normal).

Differential diagnosis
Pre-eclampsia: discriminating features include abnormal LFT, ± coagulopathy, lower grade haemolysis.

Management
- Plasmapharesis
- Steroids in addition if acquired HUS/TTP
- Do not administer platelets as this can lead to rapid decline.

Chronic renal disease
Definition
- Normal glomerular filtration rate (GFR) plus structural kidney damage, or persistent proteinuria or
- Estimated GFR <60 mL/minute 1.73 m².

Use Cockcroft–Gault formula to calculate GFR in pregnancy: www.renal.org/resources/resources.html

All pregnancy studies use creatinine level rather than GFR. Creatinine varies with sex, age, weight and ethnicity. Creatinine only becomes abnormal when GFR falls <40 mL/minute 1.73m².

Causes
- Reflux nephropathy
- Chronic pyelonephritis
- Diabetic nephropathy
- Glomerulonephritis
- Vasculitic nephropathy, e.g. systemic lupus erythematosus (SLE)
- Adult polycystic kidney disease (APKD).

Clinical
- ±hypertension
- ±haematuria, proteinuria.

Effect of chronic renal disease on pregnancy
- Subfertility (with previous use of cytotoxics, e.g. cyclophosphamide, renal disease itself, degree of renal impairment)
- Genetic inheritance affecting offspring, e.g. APKD and some cases of reflux nephropathy are autosomal dominant
- Miscarriage and fetal loss
- Pre-eclampsia (may be difficult to diagnose if already hytpertensive and proteinuric (Table 8.32.1)
- IUGR (Table 8.32.1)
- Prematurity (Table 8.32.1)
- Polyhydramnios (if urea >10 mmol/L).

Effect of pregnancy on chronic renal disease
- Variable risk of progression of decline in renal function (see box): may reduce time to requiring renal replacement therapy. If creatinine >180 μmol/L have a 1 in 3 chance of requiring renal replacement therapy within a year of pregnancy (Table 8.32.1).
- If relapsing and remitting disease, e.g. SLE, pregnancy during a flare results in a worse prognosis, for the fetus, disease activity in pregnancy and progression of renal disease.
- Escalating hypertension
- Worsening proteinuria.

Pregnancy outcome in chronic renal disease depends on:
Level of kidney dysfunction (GFR/creatinine)
Hypertension
Proteinuria
Specific disease

Best outcome for those prepregnancy without significant renal impairment, hypertension or proteinuria.

Diagnosis
- U+E, FBC, LFT, clotting, urine dipstick
- Renal screen to identify cause:
  - urine microscopy (casts, rbc, wbc), culture
  - protein/creatinine ratio (PCR)

Table 8.32.1 Risks of pregnancy in chronic renal disease

Creatinine (μmol/L)	Successful obstetric outcome (%)	PET(%)	IUGR or preterm (%)	Long-term renal problems (%)
<125	96	10–20	↑	<3
125–250	89	40	30–50	25
>250	46	80	57–73	53

- ANA, anti-dsDNA Ab, ACA, ANCA, immunoglobulin subclasses, complement (C3, C4), anti-GBM Ab
- renal USS.

Management
Prepregnancy counselling
Counsel regarding maternal and fetal risks (Table 8.32.1) Advise against pregnancy if severe renal impairment (creatinine >250 μmol/L)
Genetic counselling if heritable component to the disease, e.g. APKD, reflux nephropathy.

Drugs
- Women should not conceive while on cytotoxic drugs (e.g. cyclophosphamide, methotrexate). Use effective contraception while on these drugs. Wait 3–6 months before conceiving once use discontinued.
- Mycophenolate mofetil (MMF) is teratogenic. Consider changing to another drug, e.g. azathioprine prepregnancy.
- Reassure about safety of hydroxychloroquine, azathioprine, ciclosporin A, and tacrolimus.
- ACE inhibitors (ACEI) and the closely related angiotensin 2 receptor blockers (ARB) protect kidneys from progressive renal impairment particularly when patient has proteinuria. ACEI are teratogenic in the first trimester increasing the risk of congenital anomalies from 3% to 8%. In the second and third trimesters they prevent nephrogenesis and result in oligohydramnios. As women with chronic renal disease may be subfertile stopping ACEI/ARB prepregnancy may result in loss of renal function preservation. In a planned pregnancy can consider stopping them as soon as positive pregnancy test.

During pregnancy
Multidisciplinary care involving both obstetricians and nephrologists
- If on cytotoxic agents, consider termination of pregnancy
- Stop statins (teratogenic).
- Hypertension
  - Stop ACEI and ARB if still on them. If on these for hypertension, change to methyldopa or long acting nifedipine. Second line agents include labetolol, hydralazine and doxazocin.
  - Maintain BP at ‚135/80 mmHg to protect kidneys from further damage
  - Start aspirin 75 mg daily as prophylaxis against pre-eclampsia
  - If develops pre-eclampsia reduce dose of MgSO4 for eclampsia prophylaxis if creatinine >180–200 μmol/L, and check MgSO4 levels
- Proteinuria: if nephrotic syndrome with proteinuria (>3 g/day) and albumin <25 mmol/L, give low molecular weight heparin (LMWH) for thromboprophylaxis. Consider reducing dose of LMWH if creatinine >180–200 μmol/L as heparin is renally cleared.
- Anaemia
  - iron deficiency (due to pregnancy): replace with iron
  - Erythropoietin (EPO) deficiency (due to chronic renal disease). Ensure iron replete (ferritin >200: use IV iron) prior to giving EPO to prevent blood transfusion.
- Regularly monitor, FBC, U+E, albumin, PCR (or 24 hour urinary protein).
- Regular fetal growth scans
- Women with reflux nephropathy
  - MSU each visit

- prophylactic antibiotics if recurrent UTIs or very dilated renal tracts
- Serial renal USS to check for progression or obstruction if previous ureteric surgery or dilated renal tracts
- Women with diabetic nephropathy
  - Worse pregnancy outcome compared to diabetics without nephropathy
  - Increased risks UTIs, pre-eclampsia, proteinuria and nephrotic syndrome
- Women with APKD
  - Increased risks of pre-eclampsia and UTIs in pregnancy
  - Can bleed into a cyst causing loin pain and haematuria
  - Associated with polycystic liver disease and Berry anuerysms.

Delivery
- Aim for a vaginal delivery: spontaneous or by induction of labour if clinical circumstances necessitate earlier delivery and no obstetric contraindications
- Caesarean section for obstetric indications only
- Delivery may need to be expedited if deteriorating renal function, pre-eclampsia or fetal compromise.

Postnatal
- Recommence ACEI (safe in breastfeeding)
- Avoid NSAIDs
- Consider thromboprophylaxis
- Screen offspring for inherited kidney disease.

Dialysis
Haemodialysis
  Chronic ambulatory peritoneal dialysis (CAPD)

Effect of dialysis on pregnancy
Overall successful pregnancy outcome only 30%
- Subfertility: improved with treatment of anaemia with erythropoietin
- Miscarriage and fetal loss 50–60%
- Polyhydramnios
- IUGR
- Prematurity in almost all: spontaneous or iatrogenic
- Severe pre-eclampsia
- Bleeding due to heparinization (in haemodialysis)
- Peritonitis (in CAPD)
- Maternal mortality.

Effect of pregnancy on dialysis
- More frequent dialysis required: often daily to maintain pre-dialysis urea <15 mmol/L
- Worsening anaemia
- Pregnancy is prothrombotic: may need higher doses of heparin required during dialysis
- Large fluctuations in fluid balance and blood pressure.

Poor prognostic indicators in women on dialysis
Age >35 years:
On dialysis for >5 years
Late booker (dialysis frequency increased later in pregnancy)

Management
Prepregnancy counselling
Counsel regarding severe fetal and maternal risks of pregnancy
  Advise effective contraception if decides against pregnancy

During pregnancy
Pregnancy should be managed in a tertiary centre with a specialised renal unit with multidisciplinary care involving both obstetricians and nephrologists
  Caution with fluid balance: avoid interdialysis weight gain
  Hypertension: can be severe and chaotic in pregnancy
- Stop ACEI and ARB as soon as positive pregnancy test
- Start aspirin 75 mg daily as prophylaxis against pre-eclampsia
- First trimester fall in BP does not occur
- Pre-eclampsia is more common but very difficult to diagnose as patients are usually hypertensive and anuric. If urine is produced, there is usually baseline proteinuria and haematuria. Do not give MgSO4, as will quickly accumulate to toxic levels
  Anaemia: will become more severe in pregnancy
- Increased requirements for erythropoietin and IV iron
- Monitor FBC and iron stores regularly.
  Regular fetal growth scans
  Do not perform CTG during dialysis
  A delivery pack should be kept in dialysis suite due to risk of preterm delivery

Contraception
Mirena IUS
  Copper coil (not in CAPD)

Renal transplant recipient
Successful outcome in 95% who remain pregnant after 12 weeks gestation

Effect of renal transplant on pregnancy
- Fertility restored quickly when renal function normalises
- If pregnancy >1 year after surgery, and good graft function, generally good outcomes
- Increased risk of
  - infection
  - hypertension and pre-eclampsia
  - IUGR and prematurity.

Effect of drugs (see below)

Pregnancy outcome dependent the following parameters at conception:
Renal function (better if creatinine <125 µmol/L)
Hypertension
Proteinuria
Recurrent graft rejection

Effect of pregnancy on renal transplant
- If creatinine <100 µmol/L, usually no long-term effect on renal graft function
- Renal function may deteriorate during and after pregnancy
- Obstruction of renal graft by enlarging uterus (rare).

Management

Prepregnancy counselling
Recommend pregnancy is delayed for at least 1 year following renal transplant surgery. Risks of earlier pregnancy:
- Graft rejection
- Immunosuppressive agents used in higher doses and multiple therapies, some of which may be harmful to fetus
- Viral infections e.g. CMV.

Use effective contraception until then as fertility rapidly returns after surgery

During pregnancy
Pregnancy should be managed in a tertiary centre with a specialized renal unit with multidisciplinary care involving both obstetricians and nephrologists
- careful control of blood pressure
- regularly monitor creatinine, U+E, PCR (or 24 hour urinary protein), FBC, LFT, calcium, MSU
- Fetal growth scans.

Drugs commonly used in combination for immunosuppression include:
- Azathioprine relatively safe and not teratogenic
- Ciclosporin relatively safe, not teratogenic, associated with IUGR
- Prednisolone associated with a small increased risk of fetal cleft lip and or palate if used in first trimester but benefit of use outweighs risk
- Tacrolimus appears safe with the limited available data
- Mycophenolate mofetil (MMF) teratogenic and generally avoided, but may need to be continued if this is the only drug that prevents graft rejection
- Sirolimus is an alternative to MMF but few data are available.

Continue immunosuppressive drugs at prepregnancy levels to avoid graft rejection

Monitor tacrolimus and ciclosporin levels in pregnancy

If renal function deteriorates in pregnancy
MSU to exclude infection
PET bloods
Ciclosporin levels
Renal graft USS to exclude obstruction
Renal biopsy: consider in early pregnancy if graft rejection suspected
Expedite delivery in late pregnancy if graft rejection suspected

---

Delivery
- Aim for vaginal delivery: the renal graft does not obstruct labour
- Caesarean section only for obstetric reasons
- Prophylactic antibiotics if surgery necessary
- If on prednisolone ˅7.5 mg daily, cover delivery with hydrocortisone (see Section 8.33 asthma).

Further reading

Armenti VT, Radomski JS, Moritz MJ, *et al.* Report from the National Transplantation Pregnancy Registry (NTPR): outcomes of pregnancy after transplantation. In: Cecka JM, Terasaki PI (eds) Clinical transplants 2003. UCLA Immunogenetics Centre, Los Angeles, California 131–41.

George JN. The association of pregnancy with thrombotic thrombocytopenic purpura-haemolytic uraemic syndrome. Curr Opin Hematol 2003;10:339–44.

Haase M, Morgera S, Bamberg C, *et al.* A systematic approach to managing pregnant dialysis patients: the importance of an intensified haemodiafiltration protocol. Nephrol Dial Transplant 2005;20:2537–42.

Hou SH. Pregnancy in women with chronic renal insufficiency and end stage renal disease, Am J Kid Dis 1999;33:235–52.

Jones DC, Hayslett JP. Outcome of pregnancy in women with moderate or severe renal insufficiency. N Engl J Med 1996;335:226–32.

Jungers P, Chauveau D, Choukroun G, *et al.* Pregnancy in women with impaired renal function. Clin Nephrol 1997;47: 281–8.

Lightstone L. Chronic renal disease, dialysis and transplant. In: Gree IA, Nelson-Piercy C, Walters B (eds) *Maternal medicine.* 2007 Elsevier.

Pertuiset N, Grunfeld JP. Acute renal failure in pregnancy. Ballière's Clin Obstet Gynaecol 1994;8:333–51.

Smaill F. Antibiotics for asymptomatic bacteriuria in pregnancy. Cochrane Database Syst Rev 2001;2:CD000490.

Vazquez JC, Villar J. Treatments for symptomatic urinary tract infections in pregnancy. Cochrane Database Syst Rev 2003;4:CD002256.

Respiratory disease

Asthma

Definition
Reversible airways obstruction.

Epidemiology
Respiratory disease affects 4–8% of pregnant women.

Precipitants
Pollen, dust, animals, exercise, emotion, change in weather, upper respiratory tract infections.

Pathology
Inflammatory disorder of airways mucosa with bronchial obstruction due to:
- bronchial hyper-responsiveness
- bronchial mucosal inflammation
- sticky mucus secretions blocking airways.

Specific points in history
- Onset: childhood/adult; identify precipitants
- Assess severity: current medication and frequency of use of ventolin inhaler, previous use of nebulizers, oral steroids, frequency of hospital admissions, any ITU admissions for ventilation.
- Ask if asthma worsens with non-steroidal anti-inflammatory drugs (NSAIDs).

Symptoms (usually diurnal)
- Wheeze
- Cough especially nocturnal and morning
- Shortness of breath
- Tight chest.

Signs
- Polyphonic wheeze
- Tachypnoea
- Tachycardia
- Accessory muscle use.

Diagnosis
- Variability of bronchial obstruction with reversibility
- PEFR (peak expiratory flow rate): <80% predicted, ≥20% improvement with inhaled β2-agonist
- Morning dips in PEFR: >20% diurnal variation in PEFR for ≥3 days in a 2-week period
- Severity see Table 8.33.1.

Investigations
- PEFR: reduced compared with their best
- ABG: mild hypoxia, reduced PCO_2 (hyperventilating). Beware a high PCO_2
- CXR: to exclude pneumothorax and pneumonia
- Sputum: culture
- Spirometry: low forced expiratory volume in 1 second (FEV)1; low FEV1:FVC (forced vital capacity).

Effect of pregnancy on asthma
Rule of thirds: may improve, deteriorate, or remain unchanged
    More likely to worsen if
- medications are stopped
- asthma is severe (worsens in third trimester)
- there is gastro-oesophageal reflux

Table 8.33.1 Severity of asthma

Severity of asthma	Features
Severe	Incomplete sentences PEFR <50% best HR >110, RR >25
Life-threatening	As for severe plus any of: SpO_2 <92% Silent chest, cyanosis, poor respiratory effort Bradycardia, hypotension, arrhythmia Exhaustion (normal $PaCO_2$), confusion, coma
Near fatal	Any CO_2 retention – call anaesthetist

- there is postnasal drip from pregnancy rhinitis.
    Asthma attacks after 36 weeks' gestation are unusual. Attacks in labour are rare (↑ endogenous steroids). The course of asthma is similar in successive pregnancies.

Effect of on asthma on pregnancy
- Well-controlled asthma has no adverse effects on pregnancy.
- Severe, poorly controlled asthma (regular or chronic maternal hypoxia) has a small increase in adverse pregnancy outcome (pregnancy induced hypertension, pre-eclampsia, pre-term birth, IUGR, neonatal hypoxia)
- Asthma in mother doubles risk of asthma in offspring.

Management
Preconception
- Asthma control should be optimized with medications.
- Specifically tell women not to stop or reduce asthma treatment when pregnancy is diagnosed.

During pregnancy
- This is an excellent opportunity to improve asthma control: monitor and adjust treatment (see box)
- Emphasize the importance and safety of continuing asthma medications during pregnancy to ensure good asthma control, avoid triggers, stop smoking
- Check inhaler technique: may need spacer/breath-activated inhaler
- Treat gastro-oesophageal reflux and rhinitis
- Explain to patient indications to increase inhaled steroid dose at home.

Treatment of an acute asthma attack
Please refer to Fig. 8.33.1.

Medications
Inhaled drugs: β2-agonists (short and long acting), steroids, cromoglycates, and anticholinergics (ipratropium):
- Safe in pregnancy. No adverse fetal effects. Minute proportions are systemically absorbed
- Inhaled β2-agonists do not impair uterine contractility or delay labour.
Oral/i.v. β2-agonists: may reduce uterine contractility and cause tachycardia

Stepwise treatment of asthma

Step 1 mild intermittent asthma: short-acting inhaled β2-agonist as required, e.g. salbutamol, terbutaline

Step 2 regular preventer therapy: add an inhaled steroid 'preventer', e.g. beclomethasone 200-800 µg/day (divide into two doses) if: symptomatic ≥3 times/week, or using short-acting inhaled β2-agonist ≥3 times/week, or waking up one night/week.

Step 3 Initial add-on therapy: add long-acting inhaled β2-agonist (LABA), e.g. salmeterol. Can use a combination inhaler containing a steroid and LABA. If inadequate/no response to LABA, continue/stop it and increase inhaled steroid to 800 µg/day

Step 4 persistent poor control: Additional treatments, e.g. slow-release oral theophylline, oral β2-agonist, increase inhaled steroid dose up to 2000 µg/day or consider leukotriene receptor antagonist.

Step 5 continuous or frequent use of oral steroids: use lowest effective dose of prednisolone and continue inhaled steroid at 2000 µg/day.

Prednisolone: 90% metabolized by placenta (only 10% crosses to fetus).
- Slight increased incidence of cleft lip/palate with first trimester use (benefit exceeds risk in asthma)
- Steroid-induced gestational diabetes (GDM): test if on regular steroids; treat GDM with diet, then insulin, not by reducing steroid dose
- Increased risk of infections
- Preterm rupture of membranes: risk increased with long-term high-dose steroids

Theophylline: if dependent on therapeutic theophylline levels for asthma control, check plasma level and increase dose accordingly. No adverse fetal effects.

Leucotriene receptor antagonists: continue in brittle asthmatics who depend on them for stability. Emerging good safety data for montelukast and zafirlukast. Avoid zileuton. Low-dose aspirin and NSAIDs: avoid in women who have had worsening asthma with these agents.

Intrapartum
- Continue asthma medications
- If on prednisolone >7.5 mg for >2 weeks, cover with IV hydrocortisone 50 mg tds over labour until oral drugs recommenced.
- Prostglandin E1 (e.g. prostin) is safe

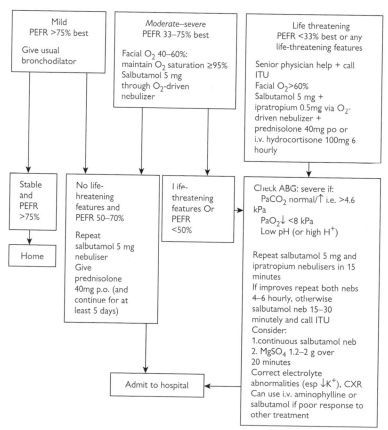

Fig. 8.33.1 Management of an acute asthma attack: treat as non-pregnant.

- Prostaglandin F2α (e.g. carbeprost) can cause bronchospasm
- Ergometrine reported to cause bronchospasm when used with general anaesthesia. No real concerns reported with syntometrine
- All forms analgesia for labour (including entonox and epidural) are safe. Avoid opiates in an asthma attack.

Postpartum
- Continue all medications: all safe with breastfeeding
- Encourage breastfeeding which is protective against the child developing atopy and asthma.

Pneumonia

Epidemiology
Similar incidence to non-pregnant
  More severe in pregnancy with atypical infections especially viral

Aetiology
- Bacterial pneumonia, e.g. *Streptococcus pneumoniae* (>50% cases), *Haemophilus influenzae*, *Staphylococcus aureus* (especially with influenza and IV drug abusers)
- Viral pneumonia, e.g. influenza, varicella (10–20% with chicken pox)
- Other, e.g *Mycoplasma pneumoniae* (atypical pneumonia), *Pneumocystis carinii* (PCP with HIV).

Symptoms
- Cough productive of coloured sputum
- Fever ± rigors
- Shortness of breath
- Pleuritic chest pain.

Signs
- Fever, tachycardia, tachypnoea
- Consolidation (dull to percussion, increased tactile vocal fremitus, bronchial breathing)
- Coarse crackles on auscultation
- Unilateral signs in lobar pneumonia, bilateral signs in community acquired/viral pneumonia).

Diagnosis
- Sputum culture ± blood culture
- Raised inflammatory markers (↑WCC, ↑CRP)
- Chest X-ray: never withhold due to pregnancy
  - *S. pneumoniae* lobar pneumonia
  - Mycoplasma pneumoniae often clear
  - *PCP* ground glass appearance
- Pneumococcal and legionella urine antigen tests, influenza testing (in severe pneumonia)
- Test for PCP if HIV positive
- ABG if O2 saturation <95% on air
- Serology for *Mycoplasma* if poor response to treatment.

Differential diagnosis
- Pulmonary embolus
- Pulmonary oedema
- Amniotic fluid embolism.

Maternal and fetal risks
- Pre-term labour
- Pulmonary oedema
- Acute respiratory distress syndrome (ARDS)

- Varicella pneumonia: increased maternal, fetal and neonatal morbidity and mortality.

Prepregnancy counselling
- Influenza vaccine during influenza season if asthmatic/ chronic cardiac or pulmonary disease/immunosuppressed/ on steroids
- Pneumococcal vaccine: sickle cell disease, post-splenectomy
- If HIV positive with CD4 count <200 cells/μL: continue PCP prophylaxis with cotrimoxazole (Septrin).

Treatment
- Sit up and give facial O2 (maintain O2 sat ˜95%)
- Intravenous fluids
- Antibiotics as for the non-pregnant woman (follow hospital protocol) and treat for 7 days:
  - community-acquired pneumonia amoxicillin and clarithromycin (for atypicals)
  - severe community acquired/hospital-acquired i.v. cephalosporin and clarithromycin
  - avoid tetracyclines >20 weeks (teeth discolouration)
- Varicella pneumonia: i.v. acyclovir
- PCP: high-dose trimethoprim-sulphamethoxazole (cotrimoxazole) ± pentamidine
- Discuss with ITU if adverse clinical features:
  - RR >30/minute
  - O2 sat <92%, pO2 <8 kPa
  - Hypotension SBP <90 mmHg
  - CXR: bilateral or multilobe involvement.

Complications
- Empyema
- Respiratory failure
- Sepsis.

Tuberculosis

Epidemiology
- Increasing rates across world especially with HIV infection.
- In the UK it is more prevalent in Asian and African immigrants.
- In pregnancy 50% of Asian and African immigrants have extrapulmonary TB.

Aetiology
- Mycobacterium tuberculosis
- Mycobacterium avium-intracellulare especially with HIV.

Pathology
Caseating granulomata

Symptoms
- Cough
- Haemoptysis
- Fever
- Night sweats
- Weight loss/ failure to gain weight in pregnancy.

Signs
- Typically affects upper lobes in lungs
- Lymphadenopathy
- Erythema nodosum

- Extrapulmonary sites: lymph nodes, liver and spleen, bone, bowel, peritoneal, CNS, eyes.

Diagnosis
- CXR: upper lobe infiltrates, cavities, hilar lymph nodes
- Microbiology from sputum, bronchiolar lavage, early morning urine or lymph node biopsy:
  - Ziehl–Neelsen stain: acid fast bacilli
  - Culture for *Mycobacterium* (6 weeks)
- Tuberculin skin test (Mantoux test) not affected by pregnancy: >10 mm induration.

Management
Treat as in the non-pregnant state in collaboration with respiratory physicians

Drugs
Treat without delay before sensitivities available with triple/quadruple therapy:
- Rifampicin (6 months minimum)
- Isoniazid (6 months minimum): add pyridoxine to reduce risk of peripheral neuritis
- Pyrazinamide and/or ethambutol (2 months).

  All non-teratogenic and safe in breastfeeding
  Monitor liver function tests monthly as risk of isoniazid/rifampicin-induced hepatotoxicity
  Avoid streptomycin (fetal ototoxicity)
  Reserve drugs for multidrug resistant TB (MDR-TB) include kanamycin, capreomycin (reassuring safety data), ethionamide (CNS defects)

Infectivity
Only pulmonary TB is infectious: non-infectious after 2 weeks of treatment.

Postnatal
- Vaccinate baby with BCG
- If mother still infectious give baby prophylactic isoniazid
- Only separate baby from mother if she is infectious with MDR-TB.

Pulmonary oedema
Epidemiology
More common in pregnancy than in non-pregnant women.

Aetiology
- Cardiac, e.g. mitral stenosis, myocardial infarction, peripartum cardiomyopathy (PPCM), arrhythmia
- Respiratory, e.g. massive pulmonary embolus, severe pneumonia
- Pre-eclampsia especially with injudicious fluid use
- Tocolysis with β2-agonists
- Sepsis
- Amniotic fluid embolus.

Symptoms
- Shortness of breath, orthopnoea
- Cough
- Haemoptysis
- Wheeze.

Signs
- Tachycardia, tachypnoea
- ↑JVP

- Bilateral inspiratory crackles
- Dull lung bases (pleural effusions)
- Dependent oedema.

Investigations
- CXR: pulmonary infiltrates, upper lobe blood diversion, Kerly B lines, pleural effusions
- ABG: initially ↓PaO2 and ↓PaCO2 (rises with tiredness)
- FBC, U+E, LFTs, clotting
- ECG for arrhythmia
- Echocardiogram: valve abnormalities, PPCM
- CT-PA if pulmonary embolus suspected.

Management
- Sit up and give facial O2 (maintain O2 sat >95%)
- Fluid restrict and monitor fluid balance
- Diuretics: frusemide 10–40 mg initially (lower dose in pre-eclampsia)
- Diamorphine 2.5 mg i.v. (+ antiemetic)
- Treat underlying cause, e.g. antibiotics if sepsis or pneumonia, low molecular weight heparin if pulmonary embolus, replace β2-agonists with atosiban or nifedipine for tocolysis.

Sarcoidosis

Definition
Epidemiology
0.05% of pregnancies.

Pathology
Multisystem disorder with non-caseating granuloma.

Clinical features
- Often asymptomatic
- Chest symptoms, e.g. shortness of breath, cough
- Extrapulmonary features:
  - Erythema nodosum
  - Anterior uveitis
  - Hypercalcaemia
  - Arthropathy
  - Fever
  - CNS involvement.

Diagnosis
- CXR: bilateral hilar lymphadenopathy, pulmonary infiltration, fibrosis
- Bronchioalveolar lavage and transbronchial biopsy
- Lung function tests: reduced transfer factor (KCO)
- Serum ACE unhelpful as altered in pregnancy.

Effect of pregnancy on sarcoidosis
Disease may be unaffected or improve with pregnancy, and relapse postnatally.

Management
Continue maintenance steroids.
  Initiate or increase steroid treatment if:
- Extrapulmonary disease
- Functional respiratory impairment.
If on >7.5 mg prednisolone for >2 weeks, cover labour with hydrocortisone i.v. 50 mg tds
  Avoid vitamin D, which can precipitate hypercalcaemia.

Cystic fibrosis

Definition
Autosomal recessive condition combining pancreatic insufficiency and repeated respiratory tract infections

Epidemiology
1:2000 Caucasians affected. 1:25 Caucasians are carriers

Pathology
- Mutations of the cystic fibrosis transmembrane conductance regulator (CFTR) gene on chromosome 7 affecting chloride channels
- All exocrine glands affected: thick mucus production (blocks ducts) and high sweat sodium.

Clinical features
- Bronchiectasis and repeated respiratory infections
- Malnutrition (loss of pancreatic digestive enzymes in >90% with CF)
- Diabetes 20%, impaired glucose tolerance 15% (loss of islet cell function).

Effect of pregnancy on CF
Most people with cystic fibrosis die in early adult life. The death rate is not increased by pregnancy, but is more likely if moderate to severe lung disease with FEV1 <50% predicted at booking

Effect of CF on pregnancy
- Reduced fertility
- Good outcomes in most women.

Maternal risks
- Poor weight gain in pregnancy
- Temporary reduction in lung function in pregnancy, reversible postnatally
- Repeated chest infections
- Congestive cardiac failure.

Predictors of poor pregnancy outcome in CF
- Pre-pregnancy FEV1 <50% predicted
- Pulmonary hypertension
- Cyanosis and O2 sat <90%
- Colonization with Burkholderia cepacia
- Pancreatic insufficiency.

Fetal risks
Hypoxia, malnutrition, infections can cause:
- IUGR
- Preterm labour and delivery (up to 50%)
- Pregnancy loss.

Management
Pre-pregnancy counselling
- Screen for diabetes and if already diabetic aim for normal HbA1c preconception
- Check partner's carrier status: risk of CF in offspring 50% if partner is a carrier.

Pregnancy not recommended in CF if
- Pulmonary hypertension/cor pulmonale
- FEV1 <30–40% predicted

- *Burkholderia cepacia:* declining lung function/recent colonisation with this organism.

During pregnancy
- Multidisciplinary care with CF centre and maternal medicine specialist.
- Offer antenatal diagnosis if father carrier of CF mutation (CVS/amniocentesis).
- Pancreatic insufficiency: give enzyme supplements (Creon) and high-calorie dietary supplements.
- Screen for GDM.
- Continue chest physiotherapy: do not reduce frequency.
- Chest infections: Send sputum for culture and treat aggressively. Most antibiotics safe; less data with newer drugs but benefits outweigh risks. Avoid tetracyclines.
- Use inhaled bronchodilators if reversibility demonstrated. May require inhaled steroids.
- Admit for bed rest and oxygen if resting hypoxia (O2 sat <92%).
- Regular growth scans.

Delivery
- May be early if symptom deterioration or fetal growth concerns.
- Aim for vaginal delivery. Instrumental delivery may be necessary for maternal exhaustion and to prevent pneumothorax from prolonged pushing.
- Breastfeeding encouraged if mother not very malnourished.

Restrictive lung disease

Generally good pregnancy outcomes.
May require bed rest and/or home oxygen to maintain O_2 saturation ≥95%.
Avoid pregnancy if associated with:
- pulmonary hypertension/cor pulmonale
- FEV1 <50%
- FVC <1 L.

Further reading

King TE Jr. Restrictive lung disease in pregnancy. Clin Chest Med 1992;13:607–22.

Laibl VR, Sheffield JS. Influenza and pneumonia in pregnancy. Clin Perinatol 2005;32:727–38.

Laibl VR, Sheffield JS. Tuberculosis in pregnancy. Clin Perinatol 2005;32:739–47.

Kothari A, Mahadevan N, Girling J. Tuberculosis and pregnancy-results of a study in a high prevalence are in London. Eur J Obstet Gynecol Reprod Biol 2006;126:48–55.

Edenborough FP, Mackenzie WE, Stableforth DE. The outcome of 72 pregnancies in 55 women with cystic fibrosis in the United Kingdom 1977–1996. Br J Obstet Gynaecol 2000;107:254–61.

Gilljam M, Antoniou M, Shin J et al. pregnancy in cystic fibrosis. Fetal and maternal outcome. Chest 2000;118:85–91.

Baughman RB, Lower EE, du Bois RM. Sarcoidosis. Lancet 2003; 361:1111–18.

British Thoracic Society Scottish Intercollegiate Guidelines Network. British Guideline on the Management of Asthma. Thorax. 2008; 63(Suppl 4):iv1–121. www.brit-thoracic.org.uk

Rubella

Definition
Rubella, also commonly known as German measles, is historically a viral illness of childhood. The rubella virus is a member of the togavirus family and is infectious only to humans. The congenital rubella syndrome (CRS) can result when rubella infection occurs during pregnancy.

Epidemiology
Prior to the rubella vaccine, rubella infection was primarily seen in school age children. Since the initiation of vaccination, rubella infection and CRS incidence have decreased dramatically. Currently, rubella infections in the developed world have become extremely rare. In the USA, the incidence of rubella decreased from 0.45 cases per 100 000 in 1990 to 0.1 cases per 100 000 in 1999. However, the number of susceptible women of reproductive age varies tremendously between countries. Vaccines are not universally available, and even where they are available, vaccination may not be accessible. Susceptibility must be considered in women living in or immigrating from developing countries.

Pathology
Rubella typically presents as an exanthematous illness associated with transient rash, arthralgias, lymphadenopathy, and fever. The classic rash is erythematous with pinpoint, puritic papules. The rash often migrates from the face to the rest of the body. The incubation period is typically 12–24 days. Rare complications from rubella infection include encephalitis, myocarditis, pericarditis, hepatitis, and thrombotic thrombocytopenic purpura/haemolytic uraemic syndrome (TTP/HUS). Conversely, up to 50% of infections may be asymptomatic. Rubella infection during pregnancy can be associated with spontaneous abortions, intrauterine fetal demise, intrauterine growth restriction, and CRS.

The definition for CRS is the presence of congenital defects with evidence of maternal rubella infection during gestation. Common congenital anomalies associated with CRS include:

- auditory defects: sensorineural deafness
- ophthalmologic defects: cataracts, glaucoma, chorioretinitis, and microphthalmia
- cardiac anomalies: patent ductus arteriosus, peripheral pulmonary artery stenosis, atrial or ventricular septal defects
- neurological abnormalities: microcephaly, meningoencephalitis, mental retardation
- other defects include hepatosplenomegaly, thrombocytopenia, bone defects, and purpuric skin lesions resulting in the classic 'blueberry muffin' presentation.

Aetiology
Neonates with CRS are born to mothers who are exposed to the rubella virus during pregnancy and do not carry immunity either by vaccination or prior infection.

Perinatal transmission of the virus varies with gestational age. Risk of fetal infection is high in the first trimester (up to 80%), decreases in the second trimester, and rises again in the third trimester. However, sequelae of infection, such as CRS, are essentially limited to infection occurring during the first 16 weeks of gestation.

The defects associated with CRS are felt to be the result of viral damage to blood vessels with resultant ischaemia to the involved organ systems.

Prognosis
Rubella infection is typically a self-limited infection for the mother. The prognosis for neonates affected with CRS is variable based on the organ systems involved and the associated complications.

Clinical approach
Diagnosis
Evaluation for rubella infection should be performed in pregnant women with known susceptibility to the virus and clinical manifestations consistent with infection or concern for exposure.

Serology is typically the method used for diagnosis of rubella infection. Testing should be performed within 10 days of the onset of the rash and repeated 2-3 weeks later. Rubella infection can be diagnosed with the presence of rubella-specific immunoglobulin (Ig)M or a significant rise in the IgG titre between acute and convalescent phases. Cultures can also be performed as the rubella virus can be isolated from nasal, blood, throat, urine, and CSF specimens. Additionally, some advocate performing PCR on chorionic villous samples or amniotic fluid. Generally, ultrasound diagnosis of rubella infection in the fetus is difficult given the nature of abnormalities seen with CRS. However, in fetuses with growth restriction, congenital rubella infection should be a component of the differential diagnosis.

Treatment
Unfortunately, treatment for acute rubella infection during pregnancy, as well as outside pregnancy, is primarily limited to supportive measures. Some advocate the use of immune globin in the setting of acute infection; however, this remains controversial. There are currently no *in utero* treatments for fetuses at risk of developing CRS.

Given the limited treatment options for CRS, focus has been placed on prevention. As mentioned previously, the overall incidence of rubella infections, and thus CRS, has decreased dramatically with the implementation of vaccination.

The rubella vaccine is a live attenuated vaccine and now commonly administered as a part of the measles, mumps, and rubella (MMR) vaccine. In the USA, vaccination is recommended via two injections, separated by 1 month, after the first year of life. Vaccination results in measurable antibody in 95% of immunized individuals. The second dose is designed to foster immunity in the small percentage of individuals who do not immunilogically respond to the first dose. Booster injections may be required.

Ideally, all women of reproductive age would be screened for immunity prior to pregnancy and immunized as needed. It is recommended by the Centers for Disease Control that pregnancy be delayed by 1 month following administration of the vaccine given a theoretical risk to the fetus with the live attenuated vaccine.

All pregnant women should be screened for rubella immunity. If immunity is not identified, vaccination should be performed postpartum, again, given a theoretical risk to the fetus with live attenuated vaccines. Given an often concomitant lack of immunity in those women found to be susceptible to rubella infection for risk of mumps and measles, the American College of Obstetricians and Gynecologists recommends administration of the MMR vaccine in the postpartum period if needed. There is no contraindication to breastfeeding with the vaccine.

References

Marret H, Golfier F, Di Maio M, et al. Rubella in Pregnancy. Management and prevention. Presse Med 1999;28:2117–22.

Miller E, Cradock-Watson JE, Pollock TM. Consequences of confirmed rubella at successive stages of pregnancy. Lancet 1982;2:781–4.

Reef SE, Redd SB, Abernathy E, zimmerman L, Icenogle JP. The epidemiological profile of rubella and congenital rubella syndrome in the United States 1998–2004: the evidence for absence of endemic transmission. Clin Infect Dis 2006;43(Suppl 3):126–32.

Rubella Prevention. Recommendations of the Advisory Committee on Immunization Practices (ACIP). MMWR Recommendations and reports 1998;47(RR-8):1–57.

Rubella Vaccination. American College of Obstetricians and Gynecologists Committee Opinion, #281 Dec 2002.

Substance abuse in pregnancy

Definition
Substance abuse covers a wide range of behaviours from use of drugs and alcohol to dependence on the drug of choice. Both the International Classification of Disease ICD-10 (WHO 1992) and the Diagnostic and Statistical Manual for Mental Disorders DSM-IV (ASA 1994) include dependence and harmful use for alcohol, drugs, and nicotine. Harmful use is defined by the negative social consequences of the behaviour and the physical and psychological consequences, dependence as the presence of withdrawal signs and symptoms on cessation. Addiction is the term used to describe the overwhelming urge to continue use despite the harmful consequence to the individual or others and usually, but not always, includes physical dependence.

Epidemiology
Drug use among 16–29-year-olds in England (General Household Survey 2002), found 25% had experienced "any drug" use, 22.7% had used cannabis and 4.9% opiates. Nicotine use was found to have declined, however 26% were nicotine users. A survey conducted in 2008 (NHS Information Centre National Centre for Social Research), of 11–15-year-olds found that 25% had tried drugs previously, 17% in the previous year, 10% in the previous month. However, smoking had decreased from 52% in 1982 to 33% in 2007. Girls were more likely to smoke regularly. Alcohol had been consumed by 3% of 11 year olds and 41% of 15 year olds. In 2004 (NHS Information Centre, 2006) 15% of men and 59% of women drank daily and 39% men and 22% women were drinking over the recommended levels per week. However, in 2000 30% of women who drank alcohol before a pregnancy reported giving up when pregnant.

It should be noted therefore that the age of exposure to drugs and alcohol is becoming lower and the proportion of using women to men in the fertile age range is increasing, that pregnancy itself has been shown to change behaviour, and that the numbers of drug users in treatment has increased significantly over the past 5 years. However, it should also be noted that patterns of drug and alcohol use have changed with polysubstance use, particularly opiates, crack cocaine, and alcohol, being more common and carrying greater risk. The baby born to the opiate-dependent mother is at risk of opiate withdrawal in the neonatal period; to the cocaine/crack using mother to neurological instability in the neonatal period and the potential for cognitive delay in infancy; to the alcohol-dependent mother to fetal alcohol syndrome and to the injecting drug using mother to infection with HIV, hepatitis B, and hepatitis C.

Injecting drug use carries the risk of infection, particularly with hepatitis B and C, and HIV. Rates of immunization against hepatitis B have increased encouragingly. The rate of HIV infection in England remains between 1% and 2% in the drug-using population but hepatitis C infection is estimated to be between 50% and 70%.

Engagement in antenatal services remains problematic for a proportion of drug and alcohol users with 'late booking'. This is, in part, due to fear of social service involvement and also due to the irregularity of menstrual cycles, particularly in opiate users. The Hidden Harm report (ACMD 2003) estimated that there are 250 000–350 000 children of drug misusers in the UK, that drug misuse causes harm to children, and that effective treatment of the parent can have major benefits for children.

Aetiology
It is noteworthy that some of the effects of exposure to drugs in utero are common across classes of drugs. Social deprivation, nicotine consumption, poor nutrition, poor compliance with healthcare, and high levels of blood-borne viral infections compound the fetal state. These common problems are those of intrauterine growth restriction, preterm deliveries, and increased rates of low birthweight and perinatal deaths.

Heroin use has a higher rate of small for date babies and preterm deliveries. There is evidence that the level of methadone exposure in utero correlates with the incidence of neonatal abstinence, although more recent evidence contests this finding.

Cocaine-exposed pregnancies have a higher rate of third trimester abruption, stillbirth, and neonatal death.

Fetal alcohol syndrome rates range from 0.5% to 1.3% of deliveries. Women who drink more than 7 units/week or 5 units/24 hours are at increased risk.

Nicotine predisposes to preterm birth and low birthweight babies.

Prognosis
Engagement in drug/alcohol treatment services, with the aim of achieving stability across parameters of behaviour, improves outcomes in terms of substance misuse and also engagement with antenatal and medical services. Cessation of illicit drug consumption with the aid of substitute opioid for the opiate-dependent woman, detoxification from alcohol, psychological interventions to reduce or cease stimulant use, medical assessment, and social interventions all improve outcomes for the neonate. All pregnant women should be screened for drug and alcohol use as early intervention and treatment reduces length of exposure by the fetus. As exemplified in the Confidential Enquiry into Maternal and Child Health (2007) 'all women should be routinely asked in early pregnancy about current and previous mental health problems including their use of prescribed and non prescribed medicine and legal and illegal substances including tobacco and alcohol'.

Clinical approach
Education about the risks to the fetus and neonate of drug and alcohol use should be routinely available to women of fertile age, in education services, in primary and in secondary care.

All drug and alcohol services in the UK now prioritize the treatment of pregnant women in recognition of the advantages of early engagement. Such services are ideally placed to assist the woman in accessing and attending antenatal services. Integrated services, although seldom available, are recommended, as these women have multiple social, psychological, medical, and psychiatric needs. There is a need for better communication about past history and present state between services and for improved assessment of drug and alcohol consumption across services.

Drug and alcohol abusers have a high comorbidity with mental illness, particularly mood disorders, and therefore assessment of mental state should be undertaken to enable early identification and treatment.

Opiate detoxification is not recommended during the first trimester; it should be undertaken at a slow rate during the second trimester and continued, with caution, during the third trimester. Detoxification should only proceed if stability is maintained as a neonate exposed to higher doses of methadone has a better prognosis than if exposed to illegal heroin.

Cocaine users should be offered psychosocial interventions as substitute prescribing is not available.

Alcohol-dependent pregnant women should be offered detoxification with benzodiazepines, the dose of benzodiazepine being kept as low as is possible to achieve abstinence.

All pregnant women should be encouraged to stop smoking and offered access to smoking cessation groups.

Services should make efforts to retain this group of women in treatment after delivery as it is evident that the families and children of drug and alcohol parents have significant need of continued help.

Further reading

ACMD Hidden Harm: responding to the needs of children of problem drug users. London: Advisory Council for the misuse of drugs 2003.

Addis A, Moretti ME, Ahmed SF, Einarson TR, Koren G. Fetal Effects of cocaine: an updated meta analysis. Reprod Toxicol 2001;15:341–367.

American Psychiatric Association (ASA). Diagnostic and Statistics Manual for Mental Disorders (DSM) American Psychiatric Association. ASA 1994.

Confidential Enquiry into Maternal and Child Health 'Saving Mothers' Lives'. The Seventh Report into Maternal Deaths in the UK 2007.

Confidential Enquiry into Maternal and Child Health Saving Mothers' Lives . The seventh report into maternal deaths in the UK. London: CEMACH 2007.

Drug misuse and dependence: UK guidelines on clinical management. DH England, the Scottish Government, Welsh Assembly Government, and Northern Ireland Executive 2007.

Evidence Based Guidelines for the pharmacological management of substance misuse, addiction and comorbidity: recommendations from the British Association for Psychopharmacology 2004. J Psychopharm 18:293–335.

General Household Survey ONS 2002.

Kaltenbach K, Finnegan L. Children of maternal substance misusers. Curr Opin Psychiat 1997;10:220–4.

Lumley J, Oliver S, Waters E. Interventions for promoting smoking prevention during pregnancy. Cochrane Database Syst Rev 2000;2:CD001055.

NHS Information Centre Statistics on Alcohol England 2006.

Stratton K, Howe C, Battaglia F. Fetal alcohol syndrome: diagnosis, epidemiology, prevention and treatment. Washington DC: National Academy Press 1996.

Survey by NHS Information Centre, National Centre for Social Research, National Foundation for Educational Research; The Health and Social Care Information Centre 2008.

World Health Organization (WHO). International Classification of Diseases (ICD) WHO 1992.

Syphilis

Definition

Syphilis is generally considered a sexually transmitted infection caused by the spirochete *Treponema pallidum*. It develops through different stages over time if undiagnosed and untreated. Syphilis is of particular concern during pregnancy secondary to the risk of transplacental transmission resulting in congenital syphilis infection in the fetus.

Clinical features

The stages of syphilis are defined below.

- Primary syphilis is the first manifestation characterized by a painless papule at the site of inoculation which ulcerates into the classic chancre. The chancre will resolve spontaneously within 3–6 weeks even without treatment. Horizontal transmission is about 30%.
- Secondary syphilis is a systemic process involving widespread dissemination of spirochetes beginning approximately 6 weeks to 6 months after initial infection, and occurs in about 25% of untreated individuals. Clinical signs include lymphadenopathy, genital condyloma lata, and an extensive maculopapular rash, particularly involving the palms and soles. Horizontal transmission is about 30%.
- Latent syphilis is the diagnosis of asymptomatic infection documented with positive serology but absent manifestation on physical examination. If this occurs within 1 year of inoculation it is called early latent; if the diagnosis occurs after 1 year or cannot be determined it is defined as late latent syphilis. Congenital transmission is extremely high during the first 4 years after inoculation when spirochetaemia is common.
- Tertiary (late) syphilis occurs after the first stages of syphilis defined above, and can arise as early as 1 year after inoculation but more frequently occurs late, 20–30 years afterwards. It is slow and progressive and can involve the central nervous system, cardiovascular system, or skin and subcutaneous tissues.
- Congenital syphilis occurs via transplacental transmission of *T. pallidum* to the fetus and can occur at any time during pregnancy and at any stage of the maternal disease. It can result in intrauterine growth restriction, intrauterine fetal demise, neonatal death, preterm birth, and congenital infection and anomalies. Fetal effects depend on stage of development at time of infection.

Epidemiology

The first well-documented outbreak of syphilis was in Naples in 1494, and subsequently spread throughout Europe. In 2001, the WHO estimated 12 million new cases per year globally in adults. Since 1998, there has been a dramatic increase in the diagnosis of syphilis in both heterosexual and homosexual populations, which has been attributed to an increase in intravenous drug abuse and human immunodeficiency virus (HIV) infection. The incidence of congenital syphilis correlates directly with the rate of syphilis in women of childbearing age. Today, most cases occur in women who did not receive prenatal care or who were inadequately treated. Global estimates of congenital syphilis range from approximately 750 000 to 1.5 million cases annually.

The risk of vertical transmission in an infected, untreated mother is significant but diminishes as maternal disease progresses. During primary syphilis perinatal transmission ranges from 70% to 100%, during secondary syphilis about 50%, during early latent disease about 40%, and during late latent and tertiary syphilis there is about 10% vertical transmission.

Treatment of maternal syphilis is the most important factor in the eradication of congenital syphilis. Vertical transmission is decreased to 1–2% in women who are adequately treated during pregnancy. Therefore, maternal screening with subsequent antenatal surveillance and adequate treatment are imperative to reducing the global impact of congenital syphilis.

Implications

Congenital syphilis and its morbidity have significant economic and social implications. Numerous economic analyses of the value of universal screening of pregnant women for syphilis have indicated it is a cost-effective approach. Most industrialized countries recommend universal screening of pregnant women. In developing countries, screening of pregnant women for syphilis is a public health bargain. When using traditional screening methods for syphilis, it is about 25 times more cost-effective in preventing one disability-adjusted life year among infants compared with those born to women who are HIV positive.

Societal and emotional implications of congenital syphilis are important as well. The loss of an infant or birth of an afflicted infant with congenital syphilis could lead to feelings of guilt, blame, and depression.

Clinical approach

Risk factors

- Poor socioeconomic status
- Sexual promiscuity
- Prostitution
- Use of illicit drugs
- HIV infection
- Lack of prenatal care
- Unmarried
- Black race
- Hispanic ethnicity
- Age less than 25 years
- Multiparity.

Screening and diagnosis

Although diagnosis of primary or secondary syphilis is quickest and most direct with darkfield microscopy and direct visualization of spirochetes, this requires the proper equipment and trained clinicians. In practice, darkfield microscopy is usually limited to clinics that specialize in the diagnosis of sexually transmitted infections. Alternatively, the predominance of clinical sites utilize serological testing, both non-treponemal and treponemal tests are available.

Non-treponemal tests, also known as reagin antibodies, test the patient's serum for reactivity to cardiolipin-cholesterol-lecithin antigen. They include the venereal disease research laboratory (VDRL) test and rapid plasma reagin (RPR) test, and are inexpensive and used primarily for screening or following treatment response. Positive tests are usually reported as a titre.

Treponemal tests are more complicated and are usually used as confirmatory tests. These tests include fluorescent treponemal antibody absorption (FTA-ABS), the micro-haemagglutination test for antibodies to *T. pallidum* (MHA-TP), and the *T. pallidum* particle agglutination assay (TPPA) and are based on detection of antibodies against treponemal cellular antigens. These tests are qualitative and reported as either reactive or non-reactive. Acute and chronic false positive results can occur with both non-treponemal and treponemal methods; therefore, use of a single test to diagnose syphilis is inadequate. False-positive results can be associated with febrile illnesses, immunizations, autoimmune conditions particularly systemic lupus erythematosus (SLE), intravenous drug use, and chronic liver disease, and HIV infections.

Other tests for detecting syphilis include direct fluorescence antibody testing (DFA-TP) and multiplex polymerase chain reaction (M-PCR); however, these test require specialized equipment and personnel and are not widely available in most outpatient settings.

The current Centers for Disease Control (CDC) guidelines recommend syphilis screening at the first prenatal visit, and for patients at high risk again during the third trimester and at delivery.

Patients with reactive serological tests for syphilis should be assessed for the stage of progression. Major morbidity occurs in the tertiary phase, including neurosyphilis. Identifying asymptomatic neurosyphilis in the latent phase is important in the optimal management of any patient with reactive syphilis serologies. Cerebrospinal fluid analysis via lumbar puncture is essential in anyone with latent syphilis, who has ophthalmic or neurological signs or symptoms, treatment failure or coexistent HIV infection, or is thought to have active tertiary syphilis.

Management

Antepartum syphilis management must consider that both maternal and likely fetal infections are present. Ultrasound can be used as a tool to determine the extent of fetal disease during the second half of pregnancy, after 20 weeks. This will assist in maternal counselling about the efficacy and potential complications associated with treatment. In the latter part of pregnancy, if there are ultrasonographic signs of fetal disease, for example, hepatosplenomegaly or hydrops fetalis, a perinatologist and neonatologist should be consulted. An abnormal ultrasound indicates antepartum fetal heart rate monitoring prior to instituting antibiotic treatment. Sonographic signs of fetal syphilis combined with abnormal fetal heart rate pattern may indicate a severely affected fetus with possible impending fetal demise.

Penicillin continues to be the *gold standard* in the treatment of syphilis, both in pregnancy and outside pregnancy. Treatment should be pursued in pregnancy when there is
- evidence of spirochetes on darkfield microscopy
- positive serologies with confirmation by specific treponemal test
- history of sexual contact with someone who has confirmed syphilis
- prior history of syphilis with treatment but continues to have persistently elevated or rising titres $\geq 1:4$.

Adequate treatment is effective in preventing maternal vertical transmission to the fetus, treating maternal disease, and treating established early fetal disease.

Primary syphilis, if there are documented negative serologies in the past year or adequate documentation of a recent chancre, can be treated with a single dose of penicillin G benzathine 2.4 millions units intramuscularly.

In all other cases, the disease should be considered latent syphilis of unknown duration and treated with a course of *three* intramuscular injections of penicillin G benzathine 2.4 million units spaced a week apart. However, neurosyphilis requires aqueous crystalline penicillin G between 12–24 million units daily in divided intravenous doses for 10–14 days.

Treatment of maternal syphilis is more complicated when the pregnant woman has a penicillin allergy, about 5–10% of cases. Confirmation of the penicillin allergy with skin testing is recommended, unless there is a documented anaphylactic reaction. The only well-studied and established treatment of women diagnosed with syphilis in pregnancy who have a true penicillin allergy is penicillin desensitization followed by penicillin treatment. Oral penicillin desensitization is given in small, gradually increasing doses with inpatient monitoring over approximately 4 hours, followed by the administration of the therapeutic dose intramuscularly 30 minutes after completion. Most adverse reactions can be managed supportively without discontinuation of the desensitization protocol.

Complications

The Jarisch–Herxheimer reaction is a common systemic reaction to the treatment of syphilis occurring in approximately 45% of pregnant women, during the first course of penicillin. It is thought to result from an endotoxin-like substance released when a large number of *T. pallidum* are killed by the antibiotics, although the true mechanism has not been elucidated. It is characterized by headache, malaise, rash, and hypotension with onset usually one to 12 hours after the initial administration of antibiotic. Symptoms can last from several hours to a few days and should be managed supportively. The reaction is not seen with subsequent antibiotic doses. The Jarisch–Herxheimer reaction can precipitate preterm contractions and preterm labour, and fetal heart tracing changes that can be concerning, therefore fetal monitoring should be considered.

Follow-up and future pregnancy

The same non-treponemal antibody serological titre used for diagnosis should be utilized to follow therapeutic response at 1-, 3-, 6-, 12-, and 24-month intervals. Patients with primary or secondary syphilis should have a fourfold decrease in their titre by 6 months and eightfold by 1 year. Those with early latent syphilis may only decline by fourfold over a 1-year period. If titres do not decline appropriately, at least fourfold, or show an increase, this probably represents either treatment failure or reinfection and the treatment regimen should be repeated. Consideration of testing for neurosyphilis is also recommended.

Women diagnosed with syphilis should be offered testing for other sexually transmitted infections, including HIV infection. Their sexual contacts should also be identified and offered treatment. Syphilis infection should be reported as indicated by local authorities. The infant's paediatrician should be notified at the time of delivery if not done previously, so they can pursue a thorough evaluation of the newborn for congenital syphilis.

Further reading

Ray, JG, Lues-Lues. Maternal and fetal considerations of syphilis. Obstet Gynecol Surv 1995;50:845.

Fiumara N, Fleming W, Downing J, Good F. The incidence of prenatal syphilis at the Boston City Hospital. N Engl J Med 1952;247:48–52.

Schmid GP, Stoner, BP. The need and plan for global elimination of congenital syphilis. Sexually Transmitted Dis 2007;34:S5–S10.

Chakraborty, R Luck, S. Managing congenital syphilis again? The more things change… Curr Opin Infect Dis 2007;20:247–52.

Walker DG, Walker GJ. Forgotten but not gone: the continuing scourge of congenital syphilis. Lancet Infect Dis 2002; 2:432–6.

Wiwanitkit V. Screening for syphilis in pregnancy: which is the proper method? Arch Gynecol Obstet 2007;276:629–31.

Wendel GD Jr, Sheffield JS, Hollier LM, et al. Treatment of syphilis in pregnancy and prevention of congenital syphilis. Clin Infec Dis 2002;35(Suppl 2):S200–9.

Wendel GD Jr, Stark BJ, Jamison RB, et al. Penicillin allergy and desensitization in serious infections during pregnancy. N Eng J Med. 1985;312:1229–32.

Myles TD, Elam G, Park-Hwang E, et al. The Jarisch-Herxheimer reaction and fetal monitoring changes in pregnant women treated for syphilis. Obstet Gynecol 1998; 92:859–64.

#MMWR Sexually transmitted diseased treatment guidelines. MMWR Recomm Rep (RR-11) 2006;55:1–95.

Thromboembolic disease

Definition
Pregnancy is a hypercoagulable, thrombogenic state. This has a synergistic effect with inherited and acquired thrombophilias: a predisposition to thrombosis. The three clinical conditions that arise from abnormal clotting mechanisms in pregnancy are deep vein thrombosis (DVT), pulmonary embolism (PE), and adverse obstetric outcomes.

Epidemiology
The risk of venous thromboembolism in pregnancy lies between 1 and 2 per 1000 pregnancies. The relative risk for venous thromboembolism in pregnancy and the puerperium is 4.3 compared to non-pregnant women, being five times higher in the postpartum period compared with during pregnancy. PE was also many-fold more common after than before birth. Inherited thrombophilias comprise about 15% of the population, but are responsible for up to 50% of venous thromboembolism in the pregnant and postpartum period.

Pathophysiology
The classical Virchow's triad includes venous stasis, endothelial injury and activation of coagulation status. Pregnancy is a thrombogenic physiological state. There is an increase in the circulating levels of fibrinogen and most clotting factors. Fibrinolytic activity is decreased with increased levels of fibrinolytic inhibitors. Levels and activity of protein S decrease in pregnancy, and resistance to activated protein C increases in later pregnancy.

Patients with acquired or inherited thrombophilias are at an even higher risk of thromboembolic complications during pregnancy. Patients with antiphospholipid antibody syndrome are at a greater risk of thrombosis. This is paradoxical to the *in vitro* prolonged partial thromboplastin time. Antiphospholipid autoantibodies, directed against plasma proteins bound to anionic phospholipids include lupus anticoagulants, anticardiolipin antibodies, and β2-glycoprotein-I antibodies.

Among the inherited thrombophilias, the guanine-to-adenine mutation at nucleotide 1691 (G1691A, factor V Leiden, FVL) is the most common abnormality in patients with thromboembolic disease. A similar autosomal dominant heterozygous G-to-A mutation in the prothrombin gene (G20210A, PGM) is associated with an elevated plasma prothrombin level and a fivefold increased risk of venous thrombosis. Other causes of inherited thrombophilias include antithrombin deficiency, protein C deficiency, and protein S deficiency. The role of the C-to-T mutation in the 5,10-methylenetetrahydrofolate reductase (C677T) causing elevated plasma homocysteine levels is uncertain, but probably not significant in pregnancy.

Maternal thrombophilias are associated with poor pregnancy outcomes, causing recurrent miscarriages, fetal growth restriction, pre-eclampsia, placental abruption, and intrauterine fetal demise.

Clinical approach
Diagnosis
History
- Only half of the patients with DVT have symptoms. These include pain and swelling of the calf/leg. Symptoms of PE include dyspnoea, chest pain, cough, and haemoptysis.

- Antiphospholipid antibody syndrome (APS) should be suspected if (1) there has been at least one unexplained thrombotic/thromboembolic event, (2) at least one specific adverse pregnancy outcome, or (3) unexplained thrombocytopenia/prolonged prothrombin time/activated partial thromboplastin time (PT/aPTT).
- Inherited thrombophilias should be suspected in patients with a history of venous thromboembolism or recurrent unexplained fetal losses after 10 weeks of amenorrhoea.

Examination
- In DVT, there may be fever, and swelling, warmth, and erythema of the affected leg; Homan's sign is not reliable.
- In PE, pyrexia, dyspnoea, tachypnoea, tachycardia, cyanosis, pleural effusion, pleural rub, raised jugular venous pressure, and right ventricular failure may be observed.
- There may be few clinical signs in acquired/inherited thrombophilias. Often, these are diagnosed on investigations. Patients with secondary APS may have physical findings such as joint swelling and tenderness that are more likely to be related to other autoimmune disorders.

Laboratory investigations
These tests are important to make the diagnosis of thromboembolic diseases, and their underlying thrombophilias.
- Compression duplex ultrasonography to detect the thrombus in the leg vein.
- Contrast venography is the gold-standard test for DVT, but may not be suitable as a first line investigation due to patient discomfort.
- Impedence plethysmography, computed tomography (CT) and magnetic resonance venography diagnosis of DVT may be available in specialised centres.
- Pulse oximetry readings in room air may be less than 95% in PE.
- Arterial blood gases in PE would usually show hypoxaemia, hypercapnia, and respiratory alkalosis.
- Serum troponin levels may be elevated in patients with a large PE.
- Electrocardiogram (ECG) changes may be typical in PE (e.g. S1Q3T3), especially in patients with massive PE and cor pulmonale.
- Chest X-ray may show cardiomegaly, atelectasis, mediastinal changes, pulmonary parenchymal abnormalities, and pleural effusion.
- Echocardiography reveals evidence of right heart strain in less than half the cases with PE.
- Ventilation-perfusion (V/Q) scan can be diagnostic.
- Spiral CT with intravenous contrast is now commonly used to diagnose PE.
- Pulmonary angiography is the gold standard in the definitive diagnosis of acute PE.
- Full blood counts could reveal leucocytosis in DVT/PE, and thrombocytopenia in acquired thrombophilias.
- D-dimers have a high negative predictive value in the diagnosis of PE, but these should be used in conjunction with other imaging techniques described above.
- Lupus anticoagulant activity by a prolonged aPTT.

- Anticardiolipin and β2-glycoprotein I antibodies, enzyme-linked immunosorbent assays for IgG and IgM.
- Protein C and Protein S activity
- Factor V Leiden activity
- Antithrombin activity.

Management

Deep vein thrombosis

When suspected, treatment with low molecular weight heparin (LMWH) should be initiated until diagnostic investigations are complete. The leg should be elevated and a graduated elastic compression (thromboembolic deterrent, TED) stocking used to reduce oedema. Intermittent pneumatic leg compression is now being used more frequently perioperatively to reduce the likelihood of DVT. LMWH is a safe and effective alternative to unfractionated heparin as an anticoagulant in pregnancy. It should be given daily in two divided doses titrated against the woman's most recent weight. Peak anti-Xa activity need be measured in underweight or overweight women only. Treatment should be continued for 6 months from the initial episode, or up to 3 months after delivery, whichever is longer.

Low dose subcutaneous unfractionated heparin and warfarin are alternatives to LMWH, but used less frequently now.

Pulmonary embolism

Upon diagnosis, or suspicion of diagnosis, respiratory and haemodynamic support needs to be initiated immediately. Intravenous unfractionated heparin is the initial treatment of choice. This condition needs to be jointly managed by senior physicians, obstetricians and radiologists. In life-threatening cases, thrombolysis with streptokinase and surgical embolectomy can be considered. In special circumstances such as recurrent PE, temporary inferior vena caval filters can be used. Warfarin can be used in the postpartum period as maintenance therapy.

Antiphospholipid antibody syndrome

These patients should be comanaged with a physician, and any underlying autoimmune diseases treated as may be necessary. In early pregnancy, normally rising titres of human chorionic gonadotrophin (hCG) indicate a good prognosis in most cases; the corollary is also true. The patients should be counselled and examined regularly for the symptoms and signs of thromboembolic disease. They should be assessed for pre-eclampsia, fetal growth restriction, and evidence of intrauterine fetal demise at frequent intervals, and counselled to observe for contractions, bleeding, and decreased fetal movements. LMWH can be used during pregnancy in these patients, and warfarin may be used in the postpartum period. Timing and mode of delivery would depend on antenatal progress.

Inherited thrombophilias

Anticoagulant therapy in inherited thrombophilias depends on past history of thrombotic events, pre-pregnancy use of anticoagulants and history of recurrent miscarriages. The evidence for use of aspirin and low-dose heparin in patients with recurrent miscarriages is clear, but clear evidence that these are beneficial in inherited thrombophilias in those with no previous complications is still lacking. In contrast, it is generally accepted that these patients need anticoagulant therapy with prophylactic/intermediate dose unfractionated heparin or LMWH if they are homozygous for FVL or PGM mutations, compound heterzygotes for FVL/PGM, or have protein C/antithrombin deficiency. A past history of venous thromboembolism may require therapeutic doses of anticoagulation with heparin ante and postpartum.

Patients with a lower risk of thromboembolic disease such as heterozygotes for FVL/PGM and protein S deficiency may benefit from low-dose aspirin antepartum, and postpartum thromboprophylaxis.

Further reading

Bertina RM et al. Mutation in blood coagulation factor V associated with resistance to activated protein C. Nature 1994;369.64–7.

Gillham JC. Haematological conditions. Obstetrics and Gynaecology. An evidence-based text for MRCOG. Luesley DM, Baker PN (ed). Arnold, 2004.

Greer IA. The challenge of thrombophilia in maternal-fetal medicine. New Engl J Med 2000;342:424–5.

Helt JA et al. Trends in the incidence of venous throm-boembolism during pregnancy or postpartum: a 30-year population-based study. Ann Intern Med 2005;143:697–06.

Marik, Plante. Venous thromboembolic disease and pregnancy. New Engl J Med 2008;359:2025–33.

McColl MD et al. Risk factors for pregnancy associated venous thromboembolism. Thromb Haemost 1997;78:1183–8.

Miyakis S et al. International consensus statement on an update of the classification criteria for definite antiphospholipid syndrome (APS). J Thromb Haemost. 2006;4:295–306.

Rai R et al. Randomised controlled trial of aspirin and aspirin plus heparin in pregnant women with recurrent miscarriage associated with phospholipid antibodies (or antiphospholipid antibodies). BMJ 1997;314:253–7.

Ray JG et al. Common C677T polymorphism of the methyl-enetetrahydrofolate reductase gene and the risk of venous thromboembolism: meta-analysis of 31 studies. Pathophysiol Haemost Thromb. 2002;32:51–8.

Thomson AJ, Walker ID, Greer IA. Low molecular weight heparin for the immediate management of thromboembolic disease in pregnancy. Lancet 1998;352:1904.

Thromboembolic disease in pregnancy and the puerperium: acute management. RCOG Green-top Guideline No. 28, Feb 2007.

Thromboembolism in pregnancy. ACOG practice bulletin #19. American College of Obstetricians and Gynecologists, Washington, DC, 2000.

Patient resources

Venous thrombosis in pregnancy and after birth: information for you: www.rcog.org.uk/index.asp?pageID=2516

Thyroid and parathyroid disease

Hypothyroidism

Definition
Thyroid hormone deficiency.

Epidemiology
More common in women. Affects 1% of pregnancies.

Causes
- Autoimmune lymphocytic thyroiditis (thyroid peroxidase autoantibodies):
  - atrophic thyroiditis (no goitre)
  - Hashimoto's thyroiditis (goitre)
- Following treatment for hyperthyroidism with radioiodine (^{131}I), partial thyroidectomy, or antithyroid drugs
- Other drugs, e.g. amiodarone, lithium, iodine
- Transient hypothyroidism: subacute/postpartum

Symptoms (*good discriminators)
- Similar to pregnancy: tiredness, lethargy, weight gain, constipation, fluid retention, muscle cramps
- Cold intolerance*
- Slowness of thought

Signs
- ± goitre
- Slow pulse rate*
- Slowly relaxing reflexes (especially ankle)*
- Dry skin
- Carpel tunnel syndrome.

Associated autoimmune diseases
Type 1 diabetes, pernicious anaemia, vitiligo

Diagnosis
↓free T4 (fT4) and ↑TSH: use pregnancy ranges (Table 8.38.1)

Effect of pregnancy on hypothyroidism
Requirements for increased dosage usually related to previous under-replacement

Effect of hypothyroidism on pregnancy
Fetus produces its own thyroxine >12 weeks. Before this time, it is dependent on maternal thyroxine. Maternal thyroxine replacement does not cause fetal hyperthyroidism as only small amounts cross placenta.
- Adequately treated, euthyroid in first trimester:
  - no risks.
- Untreated and overt hypothyroidism risks:
  - subfertility
  - miscarriage and fetal loss
  - Pre-eclampsia, abruption
  - IUGR, prematurity.

Table 8.38.1 Normal pregnancy ranges of thyroid function tests (TFTs)

Trimester	Non-pregnant	First	Second	Third
Free T4	11–23	11–22	11–19	7–15
Free T3	4–9	4–8	4–7	3–5
TSH	0–4	0–1.6	0.1–1.8	0.7–7.3

- Untreated or undertreated (subclinical) hypothyroidism in *first trimester*: risks in offspring:
  - reduction in IQ (small if subclinical)
  - neurodevelopmental delay.

Management
Prepregnancy counselling
Ensure adequate replacement of thyroxine

During pregnancy
Check thyroid-stimulating hormone (TSH) and fT4 (free thyroxine) at booking, second, and third trimesters. Adjust thyroxine dose according to pregnancy range.
  If euthyroid at booking, it is unusual to have to adjust dose
  If dose is amended:
- repeat thyroid function tests (TFTs) after 4–6 weeks
- check TFTs postpartum: most women maintain higher dose postpartum (as adjustment reflects previous under-replacement)

Complications
Fetal/neonatal hypothyroidism is very rare; the maternal TSH receptor-blocking antibodies (in a few patients with atrophic thyroiditis) cross the placenta and affect the fetal thyroid (usually has goitre).

Hyperthyroidism

Definition
Thyroid hormone excess.

Epidemiology
It occurs more often in women and affects 1 in 800 pregnancies; 50% have a family history of thyroid disease.

Causes
- Graves' disease (95%): TSH receptor stimulating antibodies (TSHR Ab) and specific antibodies against eye (occur in 50%). Both are present even when the disease is inactive.
- Toxic nodule: in a multinodular goitre/toxic solitary adenoma.
- Subacute thyroiditis (de Quervain's): usually following URTI. Fever and painful thyroid.
- Drugs: amiodarone, iodine, lithium, or inappropriate use of thyroxine.
- Hydatidiform mole, choriocarcinoma (high hCG).

Symptoms (*good discriminators)
- Similar to pregnancy: sweating, palpitations, heat intolerance, emotional lability, vomiting
- Weight loss*.

Signs
- Goitre- check for retrosternal extension
- Palmar erythema
- Persistent tachycardia*
- Tremor*
- Eye signs (with Graves' disease)*: proptosis, lid lag, lid retraction.

Diagnosis
- ↑free T3 and or ↑free T4 and suppressed TSH (use pregnancy ranges)

- TSHR Ab (helps distinguish from hyperemesis).

Differential diagnosis
- fT4 and clinically euthyroid
- Hyperemesis gravidarum
- Non-thyroid illness: sick euthyroid.

Effect of pregnancy on hyperthyroidism
- Improvement especially second and third trimesters
- Worsening in first trimester (related to ↑hCG) and in puerperium.

Effect of hyperthyroidism on pregnancy
- Adequately treated, euthyroid patient:
  - transplacental transfer of antithyroid drugs and TSHR Ab can affect fetus.
- Untreated and overt hyperthyroidism—risks:
  - subfertility
  - miscarriage, fetal loss
  - IUGR, prematurity
  - thyroid storm (see Complications).

Management
Women should not conceive for 4 months following [131]I.

During pregnancy
Check fT3, fT4 and TSH in each trimester.
Antithyroid drugs: propylthiouracil (PTU), carbimazole
- Continue in pregnancy. Don't switch drugs. Can often reduce dose maintaining free T4 at higher end of normal range for pregnancy
- Transplacental transfer: PTU less than carbimazole. They counteract stimulatory effect of TSHR Ab on fetal thyroid
- Carbimazole rarely causes aplasia cutis (scalp skin defect).

Newly diagnosed thyrotoxicosis in pregnancy
- Start PTU 200–300 mg bd/carbimazole 40–60 mg.
- Add propranolol 10 mg bd tds if significant palpitations, tremor or sweating (usually for 2–3 weeks)
- Check FBC 1 week later (agranulomatosis and neutropenia rare: must report sore throat)
- Check fT3, fT4 and TSH 2–4 weekly initially
- Usually can start to reduce dose after 4–6 weeks
- Aim to control thyrotoxicosis with smallest dose of drugs possible.

Thyroidectomy: rare in pregnancy:
- Retrosternal goitre causing stridor/ dysphagia
- Thyroid cancer
- Allergies to both PTU and carbimazole.

Radioiodine (^{131}I)
- Contraindicated in pregnancy and breastfeeding
- Avoid pregnancy for a minimum of 4 months.

Fetal wellbeing
- USS for fetal growth, goitre and heart rate if high titre of TSHR Ab, poorly controlled or newly diagnosed Graves' disease.

Postpartum
Breastfeeding safe with PTU ≤150 mg/day and carbimazole ≤15 mg/day.

Complications
Thyroid storm (thyroid crisis)
Medical emergency: urgently liaise with endocrinologists
- Rare: can be precipitated by delivery in a patient with undiagnosed Grave's disease
- Clinical: hypermetabolic with fever, sweating, marked tachycardia; can develop congestive cardiac failure, delirium/psychosis
- Treat with large doses of PTU, dexamethasone, hydration and paracetamol for pyrexia
- Fatal without treatment.

Fetal/neonatal thyrotoxicosis
- One per cent of babies whose mothers have current or previous Graves' disease (even if now hypothyroid following surgery/ radioactive iodine).
- Fetal tachycardia, IUGR, goitre, accelerated bone maturation.
- Without treatment fetal mortality up to 50%, neonatal mortality up to 15%.
- If fetus affected, treat mother with antithyroid drugs (maintain maternal euthyroidism with thyroxine).
- Neonate becomes symptomatic after maternal antithyroid drugs cleared.

Postpartum thyroiditis
Prevalence
- Variable: 2–17%
- 25% family history autoimmune thyroid disease
- 50–70% with thyroid peroxidise antibodies
- More common in type 1 diabetics.

Pathology
Autoimmune lymphocytic destruction of thyroid gland initially causing release of pre-formed thyroxine (hyperthyroid phase) and subsequently causing hypothyroidism as stores used up.

Clinical
Vague symptoms occur 3–4 months postpartum. Variable progression often resolving spontaneously:
- Only hyperthyroidism (40%)
- Only hypothyroidism (40%)
- Hyperthyroidism initially, then hypothyroidism for several months (20%).

Diagnosis
- TFTs: identifies hypothyroidism/hyperthyroidism
- Antithyroid antibodies (in 80–85%)
- Distinguish from flare of Graves': postpartum thyroiditis has no TSHR Ab and poor uptake on radioactive iodine/ technetium scans.

Management
- Treat only if symptomatic (course unaltered):
- Hyperthyroidism: beta-blockers not antithyroid drugs
- Hypothyroidism: thyroxine—stop after 6–8 months to see if resolved
- Annual TFTs if thyroid peroxidise Ab positive as 20% develop permanent hypothyroidism in 4 years.

Prognosis
- Remain hypothyroid: 3–4%
- Recurrence after future pregnancy: 70%.

Thyroid nodules/thyroid cancer

Incidence
1% (up to 40% diagnosed in pregnancy are malignant).

Cause
- Multinodular goitre
- Cyst (usually benign)
- Adenoma
- Malignancy.

Clinical
Suspect malignancy if
- Nodule is hard and fixed
- Rapid growth
- lymphadenopathy.

Diagnosis
Urgent referral to endocrine surgeon:
- TFTs and thyroid antibodies
- Thyroglobulin (can also be raised with goitre, Hashimoto's and Grave's disease). Level >100 μg/L suspicious of malignancy
- USS thyroid: cyst/solid
- Aspiration of cyst: fluid to cytology
- Fine needle biopsy
- Iodine scanning contraindicated in pregnancy.

Management
Malignancy:
- Pregnancy does not affect the course of differentiated thyroid cancer
- Surgery safest in second trimester (can perform in third trimester if necessary)
- postoperative thyroxine to suppress TSH (residual tumour dependent on TSH for growth)
- future pregnancies: check thyroglobulin level (should be low/ undetectable) and keep TSH suppressed with thyroxine.

Hyperparathyroidism

Incidence
Rare: 8 in 100 000 women of childbearing age.

Pathology
- Primary hyperparathyroidism
  - hyperplasia
  - adenoma
  - malignancy (very rare)
- Secondary hyperparathyroidism (prolonged hypocalcaemia)
  - vitamin D deficiency
  - renal insufficiency
- Tertiary hyperparathyroidism.

Clinical
- Asymptomatic
- Features of hypercalcaemia: thirst, vomiting, malaise, bone pain, abdominal discomfort (pancreatitis, renal stones, constipation), depression, hypertension.

Diagnosis
- ↑corrected calcium, ↑PTH
- ↑calcium excretion in 24-hour urine collection
- USS/MRI neck: may detect parathyroid adenoma
- Isotope studies contraindicated in pregnancy

- Surgical exploration of neck.

Differential diagnosis (of hypercalcaemia)
- Sarcoidosis
- Malignant disease with bone secondaries
- Vitamin D toxicity
- Excess antacids use (contain calcium)
- Familial hypocalciuric hypercalcaemia.

Effect of pregnancy on hyperparathyroidism
↓level of calcium in pregnancy (↑GFR, fetal demands); may rebound back up postnatally

Effect of hyperparathyroidism on pregnancy
- Miscarriage and fetal loss
- Preterm labour.

Management.
Multidisciplinary care with endocrine surgeons
  Aim to reduce corrected calcium level to upper limit of normal
- ↑fluids (orally, may need intravenously)
- Low calcium diet +/– oral phosphate
- Symptomatic cases/conservative measures ineffective:
- Surgical excision of abnormal parathyroid gland(s)
- Post-surgery daily bloods initially to detect low calcium.

Complications
- Acute pancreatitis: especially postpartum
- Neonatal hypocalcaemia:
- Fetal PTH suppressed by high maternal calcium
- Postnatally: neonatal seizures and tetany from neonatal hypocalcaemia as calcium no longer supplied from mother. Occurs within 2 weeks of delivery, or up to 2 months if baby breast fed.

Hypoparathyroidism

Incidence
Rare.

Causes
- Inadvertent removal parathyroid glands following thyroidectomy (3%)
- Autoimmunity.

Diagnosis
↓ corrected calcium, ↓PTH.

Effect of pregnancy on hypoparathyroidism
Further ↓level of calcium in pregnancy (↑GFR, fetal demands).

Effect of hypoparathyroidism on pregnancy
- Miscarriage and fetal loss
- Fetal hypocalcaemia, bone demineralisation
- Neonatal hypocalcaemia and rickets.

Management
- Vitamin D (alfacalcidol or calcitriol) and calcium supplementation
  - increased requirement in pregnancy
  - reduce dose postnatally
- Measure corrected calcium monthly.

Complications
- Neonatal hypocalcaemia seizures and tetany
- Maternal osteoporosis.

Further reading

Feldt-Rasmussen U, Hoier-Madsen M, Rasmussen NG, *et al.* Antithyroid peroxidise antibodies during pregnancy and postpartum. Relation to postpartum thyroiditis. Autoimmunity 1990; 6:211–4.

Girling J. Thyroid disease and pregnancy. In: de Swiet M (ed.). *Medical disorders in obstetric practice.* Oxford: Blackwell Science 2002:415–38.

Haddow JE, Palomaki GE, Allen WC, *et al.* Maternal thyroid deficiency during pregnancy and subsequent neuropsychological development in the child. N Eng J Med 1999;341:549–55.

Leung AS, *et al.* Perinatal outcome in hypothyroid pregnancies. Obstet Gynecol 1993;81:349–53.

Mestman JH. Parathyroid disorders of pregnancy. Semin Perinatol 1998;22:485–96.

O'Doherty MJ, McElhatton PR, Thomas SHL. Treating thyrotoxicosis in pregnant or potentially pregnant women. BMJ 1999;318;5–6.

Pop VJ, Kuijpens JL, van Baar AL, *et al.* Low maternal free thyroxine concentrations during early pregnancy are associated with impaired psychomotor development in infancy. Clin Endocrinol 1999;50:149–55.

Tan GH, Gharib H, Goeller JR, *et al.* Management of thyroid nodules in pregnancy. Arch Intern Med 1996;156:2317–20.

Wolfberg AJ, Lee-Parritz A, Peller AJ, Lieberman ES. Obstetric and neonatal outcomes associated with maternal hypothyroid disease. J Matern Fetal Neonatal Med 2005;17:35–8.

Toxoplasmosis in pregnancy

Definition
Toxoplasmosis is an infection caused by the intracellular parasite *Toxoplasma gondii*. It can be passed transplacentally from an infected mother to her unborn embryo/fetus causing congenital toxoplasmosis.

Epidemiology
Toxoplasmosis is the most common parasitic infection worldwide. Toxoplasmosis is the third leading cause of food-borne illness death. In the USA it is estimated that 22.5% of the population has been infected with toxoplasmosis and approximately 15% of reproductive age women. Serological data indicate much higher rates of infection in France and South America. In the USA approximately 400–4000 infants are born each year with toxoplasmosis. The worldwide incidence of congenital toxoplasmosis is estimated to be 1–10/10 000 live births.

Aetiology
Toxoplasma gondii exists in three stages: the oocyst, tachyozoite, and bradyzoite. The cat is the definitive host. When a cat ingests cysts of *T. gondii*, which are contained in the tissues of infected prey or raw meat, the parasite is released into the cat's digestive tract. The organisms then multiply in the wall of the small intestine and produce oocysts. These oocysts are then excreted in great numbers in the cat's faeces. Intermediate hosts, including humans, become infected when coming into contact with oocysts or ingesting other infected intermediate hosts. Oocysts and tissue cysts transform rapidly into tachyzoites upon ingestion. Tachyzoites represent an acute infection stage and localize to neural and muscle tissue. After the acute infection the tachyzoites develop into bradyzoites and they remain dormant for the remainder of the intermediate host's life. In the tachyzoite form the parasite can be passed to an unborn child from its mother. Reproductive age women are at risk of acquiring an infection if they live in a high prevalence area (South America), eat undercooked/raw meat, have contact with contaminated soil, drink contaminated water, and/or own a cat.

Prognosis
Toxoplasmosis infection, in an immunocompetent pregnant woman, is usually asymptomatic. Rarely can she develop a mononucleosis type illness including fever, fatigue, and lymphadenopathy. The risk to her unborn child is dependent on timing of seroconversion during gestation, with an approximate 10–15% transmission rate in the first trimester to a 60–70% transmission rate in the third trimester. Congenital infection tends to be more severe the earlier in gestation it is acquired, and can consist of fetal demise (rare), intracranial calcifications, hydrocephalus, and retinochoroiditis.

Clinical approach
History
- Lives in or recent travel to endemic area
- Exposure to contaminated soil/water
- Cat owner
- Mononucleosis type illness with a cervical lymphadenopathy.

Examination/ultrasound findings
- Maternal vital signs/cervical lymph node palpation
- Fetus with hydrocephalus, intracranial calcifications, increased placental thickness, intrahepatic calcifications, hepatomegaly, ascites, pericardial effusion and/or pleural effusion.

Investigations
Maternal
- the difficulty in diagnosis lies in determining if the infection is active or chronic. The primary diagnostic tool is serological studies. An acute infection in pregnancy is most accurately diagnosed when at least two blood samples drawn at least 2 weeks apart show seroconversion from negative to positive, IgG or IgM. The sensitivity/specificity varies widely between laboratories; using a reference laboratory is recommended.
- Toxoplasmosis can also be isolated from infected fluids and/or tissues using special stains or PCR.

Fetal
- When primary maternal infection is suspected an amniocentesis should be performed and the fluid sent for PCR and/or mouse inoculation.

Counselling
- In proven fetal infection with ultrasound abnormalities the outcome can be poor including fetal demise, neonatal death, neurological impairment (mental retardation, seizures, need for ventricular shunt placement), and/or chorioretinitis.
- In documented fetal infection with no ultrasound findings fetal demise/neonatal death is rare. Approximately 80% of newborns show no clinical evidence of infection. Of those that do intracranial lesions and chorioretinitis are most common. A small percentage, 1–5%, will develop severe neurological impairment (as above) and up to 30% will develop retinochoroidal lesions, leading to blindness in rare cases.

Management
- Pregnancy termination
- Maternal infection: treatment with spiramycin, a macrolide antibiotic (not available in the USA), 1 g three times a day, may reduce the risk of fetal infection by up to 60%.
- Fetal infection: treatment with pyrimethamine and sulfadiazine, two drugs that act synergistically to inhibit the synthesis of folic acid, may decrease the severity of fetal manifestations. Various dosing regimes exist. Leucovorin, folinic acid, needs to be used as add back to prevent bone marrow suppression.
- Neonatal infection: treatment with pyrimethamine and sulfadiazine has been proven to decrease the rate of clinical manifestations. Various dosing regimes exist.
- Prevention is the best strategy, thorough cooking of meats, thorough washing/peeling of fruits and vegetables, thorough washing of cutting boards, dishes, counters, utensils and hands, pregnant women should wear gloves when gardening and pregnant women should avoid changing a cats litter box.

Further reading

ACOG. Perinatal viral and parasitic infections. Practice Bulletin 2000, #20.

CDC. Preventing Congenital Toxoplasmosis. MMWR 2000, 49(RR02);57–75.

Foulon W, Pinon JM, *et al.* Prenantal diagnosis of congenital toxoplasmosis: a multicenter evaluation of different diagnostic parameters. Am J Obstet Gynecol 1999;181:843.

Foulon W, Villena I, *et al.* Treatment of toxoplasmosis during pregnancy: a multicenter study of the impact on foetal transmission and children's sequelae at age 1 year. Am J Obstet Gynecol 1999;180:410.

Jones J, Lopez A, Wilson M. Congenital Toxoplasmosis: A Review. Ob Gyn Survey 2001:56:296–305.

Wallon M, Liou C, Garner P. Congenital toxoplasmosis: systematic review of evidence of efficacy of treatment in pregnancy. BMJ 199:318:1571–4.

Internet resources

www.cdc.gov

www.ACOG.org

Vulvovaginal candidiasis

Definition
This is a superficial fungal infection of the vulva and vagina by candidal species characterized by local inflammation, pruritus, and discomfort. There are more than 100 species of *Candida* but *Candida albicans* is responsible for more than 95% of human disease. Some of the other non-albicans *Candida* species that cause diseases in man include *C. tropicalis*, *C. glabrata*, *C. krusei*, and *C. parapsilosis*.

Epidemiology
Candida may be detected in the vagina of 5–10% of non-pregnant women and in up to 40% of pregnant women. The overwhelming majority of these women are completely asymptomatic.

Pathogenesis
- The *Candida* detected in the vagina of asymptomatic women usually exists in the spore or yeast format as commensals unless their numbers increase rapidly due to alteration in the local or systemic cell-mediated immunity. The characteristic symptoms associated with thrush are caused by the transformation of the *Candida* from the spore phase into the invasive hyphae phase. It is the cell-mediated immunity through interferon-gamma (IFN-γ) that controls and inhibits this transformation and therefore the germination, growth, and proliferation of *Candida* in the vagina. Almost all women have antibodies to *Candida* but these antibodies are not protective and do not prevent the growth of *Candida*. Therefore, women with genetic or acquired alteration of cell-mediated immune function are predisposed to recurrent vulvovaginal candidal infections.
- About 20% of recurrent vulvovaginal candidiasis are due to allergic reactions to seminal components, fabrics of under clothing, douches, contraceptive spermicides, condoms, hygienic products, including soaps, and even candidal antigens. The histamine release associated with the immediate hypersensitivity response stimulates the release of prostaglandin from macrophages, which in turn inhibits the production of interleukin (IL)-2 by T-lymphocytes, thereby temporarily paralysing the cell-mediated immune response. This results in diminished inhibition and regulation of the growth of candida.

Risk factors
- Diabetes mellitus: the hyperglycaemia associated with diabetes enhances the adherence of yeast to the vaginal epithelial cells, impairs phagocytosis and supplies the *Candida* with essential nutrients for growth.
- Pregnancy and combined oral contraceptive: pregnancy and the pill suppress T-cell immunity and generate sugar substrates in the vagina by increasing mucosal glycogen stores.
- Broad-spectrum antibiotics: these decrease the number of organisms competing for resources in the vagina. Some antibiotics such as tetracycline impair host immune response by altering phagocytosis.
- Corticosteroid: this acts by attenuating the immune system and down regulating the inflammatory response.
- Tight under clothing: these create a warm, damp and moist environment in the vulva and vaginal area, which encourages the growth and multiplication of *Candida*.
- Other risk factors: obesity and intrauterine device.

Clinical features
- Vulval and vaginal itching, soreness and irritation are the commonest symptoms associated with female genital candidiasis. This may be associated with the characteristic thick, curdy white, and adherent discharge. In severe cases there may be erythematous rashes involving the inner thighs and most active at the periphery. The vulva may be oedematous, and dysuria and dyspareunia may be present. There is usually no associated malodour unless there is comorbidity with bacterial vaginosis or trichomoniasis.
- About 2–3 in 1000 women may have recurrent vulvovaginal candidiasis, defined as ≥4 attacks in a year. These women need specialist care to identify and address the underlying predisposing and precipitating factors.

Diagnosis
- Typical thick, cheesy, and adherent discharge
- Wet mount or gram stain looking for mycelia/hyphae or spores. If candidal spores only are present in a symptomatic woman consider *C. glabrata*
- Culture in Sabouraud's cornmeal media, to identify candidal species and to obtain sensitivity studies. Non-albicans candidal species are implicated in cases of recurrent vulvovaginal candidiasis and they are commonly resistant to over the counter azole agents.

Treatment
- Sporadic and single episode of vulvovaginal candidiasis may be treated with a single stat dose of intravaginal clotrimazole 500 mg + cream 1–2% applied topical for symptom relief.
- Women with recurrent vulvovaginal candidiasis should be discouraged from the use of scented soaps or similar products in the genital area, wearing tight fitting underclothing, nylon tights, and excessive consumption of sweets and refined sugars.
- In addition to eliminating the predisposing and precipitating factors, women with recurrent attacks may benefit from a 6-month course of weekly Fluconazole 100 mg. At the end of the course approximately 25% of women may relapse within 6 months. The course may be repeated. Resistant cases may respond to boric acid.
- Screen sexual partners for drugs such as penicillin to which the woman may be allergic, and which may be deposited in the vagina with the seminal plasma thus provoking an allergic reaction.

Further reading
Sobel JD. Vulvovaginal candidosis. Lancet 2007;369:1961–71.

Witkin SS, Linhares I, Giraldo P, *et al.* Individual immunity and susceptibility to female genital tract infection. Am J Obstet Gynecol 2000;183:252–6.

Witkin SS. Immunology of recurrent vaginitis. Am J Reprod Immunol Microbiol 1987;15:347.

Obstetric conditions

Abdominal pain in pregnancy *320*
Amniotic fluid embolism *324*
Antepartum haemorrhage *326*
Cancer in pregnancy *328*
Fibroids in pregnancy *330*
Obstetric cholestasis *332*
Ovarian cysts in pregnancy *336*
Postnatal depression *338*
Puerperal psychosis *342*
Pre-eclampsia and eclampsia *344*
Premalignant conditions of the genital tract in pregnancy *349*
Preterm Labour *350*
Preterm prelabour rupture of membranes *354*
Prolonged pregnancy *358*
Puerperal sepsis *360*

Abdominal pain in pregnancy

Epidemiology

This is an extremely common condition in pregnancy. Non-specific and musculoskeletal pain (or round ligament pain) are diagnoses of exclusion and can usually be managed with reassurance, rest, and outpatient care.

The commonest obstetric complications manifesting with abdominal pain are spontaneous preterm labour, placental abruption, and severe pre-eclampsia. Pyelonephritis occurs in 1–2% of pregnancies.

Acute abdomen of non-obstetric aetiology requiring surgery has an incidence of 1 in 500–635 pregnancies. The leading cause in this group is acute appendicitis.

Aetiology

Although obstetricians and gynaecologists are trained in the recognition and management of the majority of the following conditions, some of the less common causes will require multidisciplinary input.

Physiological
- Labour.
- Musculoskeletal pain from ligament stretching affects about 30% of pregnancies, and is more common in early and late gestation.
- Constipation can be physiological due to decreased bowel motility and increased water absorption of water; if severe, it can become pathological. This is usually amenable to conservative treatment and dietary advice, although bulking agents and in some cases stool softeners or laxatives are needed.

Early pregnancy
- Ectopic pregnancy
- Corpus luteum haemorrhage
- Miscarriage
- Acute urinary retention
- Urinary tract infection.

Second trimester onwards
- Preterm labour
- Chorioamnionitis
- Placental abruption
- Severe pre-eclampsia and HELLP syndrome
- Acute fatty liver of pregnancy
- Uterine rupture/scar dehiscence
- Degenerating fibroid
- Musculoskeletal.

Non obstetric causes
- Ovarian torsion
- Acute pyelonephritis or hydronephrosis
- Urolithiasis
- Gastroenteritis
- Appendicitis
- Bowel obstruction
- Inflammatory bowel disease (ulcerative colitis and Crohn's disease)
- Biliary colic or cholecystitis
- Pancreatitis
- Pleurisy

- Sickle cell crisis
- Malaria.

Postpartum
- Endometritis
- Postoperative wound infection or haematoma
- Pseudo-obstruction (Ogilvie syndrome)

Clinical approach

Interpretation of clinical findings should always take into account anatomic, physiological, and biochemical considerations that are unique to the pregnant woman.

Diagnosis

History

Any type of abdominal pain prior to ultrasound confirmation of pregnancy location should prompt consideration of an ectopic gestation. Acute epigastric pain in mid to late gestation should be interpreted in association with any other symptoms and signs of pre-eclampsia (headache, visual disturbance, hyper-reflexia). It is important to remember that HELLP syndrome may also manifest postpartum. Painful uterine contraction is the cardinal symptom in spontaneous preterm labour (intermittent) and placental abruption (continuous). Specific symptoms of non-obstetric abdominal pathology should also be sought.

Examination

The presence of a gravid uterus may alter considerably the findings of abdominal examination. The adnexa remain in proximity to the uterus, lateral and posterior to the fundus and are progressively pulled out of the pelvis and into the maternal abdomen. The appendix is usually displaced upwards to the level of the iliac crest. Abdominal guarding and rigidity may not be a reliable sign of intra-abdominal inflammation because of interposition of the growing uterus.

The presence of uterine activity is best assessed with direct palpation for several minutes. Intermittent contraction may be a sign of labour whereas a continuous contraction with uterine tenderness may suggest placental abruption. Renal tenderness should be tested on both loins. Speculum and digital vaginal examination should be performed if labour is suspected.

Investigations

Blood inflammatory markers should be interpreted with caution: baseline white cell count is raised in pregnancy ($6.0–16.0 \times 10^9$/L) and may rise even further (to around 20.0×10^9/L) following administration of corticosteroids or with the onset of labour. C-reactive protein (CRP) is a more reliable marker of inflammation.
- MSU for dipstick and culture
- 24 hour urine collection for total protein
- CRP
- FBC, U+Es, LFTs, LDH, uric acid, and coagulation screen in suspected pre-eclampsia
- Kleihauer–Betke test may be useful in suspected mild abruption with no fetal compromise
- Fetal fibronectin in vaginal secretions has a good negative predictive value for preterm labour

- Serum amylase
- Arterial blood gases for the critically ill patient.

Imaging

Ultrasound is the modality of choice. Ionizing radiation may be used when benefits outweigh the risks, especially beyond the first trimester.

- Obstetric ultrasound often does not identify the cause of pain. It is however useful as a non-invasive test of fetal wellbeing
- Abdominal ultrasound
  - adnexal pathology
  - liver, gallbladder, bile ducts
  - kidneys, ureters
  - bladder residual post micturition
- Transvaginal ultrasound for cervical length in suspected preterm labour
- Plain abdominal X-ray if there is suspicion of bowel obstruction
- MRI or CT if indicated (usually in consultation with other disciplines, i.e. general surgery, urology, radiology)

Management

Conservative management

In cases requiring hospitalization intravenous rehydration, analgesia, and antiemetics are the mainstay. H2 receptor antagonists are often useful.

Inflammatory causes

Broad-spectrum antibiotic treatment including anaerobic cover is necessary in cases of septic miscarriage and chorioamnionitis. A history of prelabour rupture of the membranes (PROM) should raise the index of suspicion, but chorioamnionitis can also occur with no history of PROM. Treatment with antibiotics should not delay the decision for delivery of the fetus regardless of gestational age, as the maternal condition can deteriorate rapidly and severely. Antibiotic treatment is also used for cholecystitis and postpartum endometritis or wound infection. Pyelonephritis usually responds to intravenous cephalosporins, with the addition of aminoglycoside in severe cases. Gastroenteritis is often viral and responds to conservative measures alone. Degenerating fibroids may require large doses of opioid analgesia.

Urological causes

Urine retention at 12–16 weeks because of a gravid retroverted uterus can be resolved with catheterization. Pyelonephritis should be treated aggressively with intravenous antibiotics as above. Ureteric obstruction and hydronephrosis may sometimes necessitate percutaneous nephrostomy or retrograde ureteric stenting.

Pre-eclampsia and HELLP syndrome

Clinical and biochemical evidence of severe pre-eclampsia with acute epigastric pain should trigger a protocol of intensive obstetric care. This should include blood pressure control with antihypertensives, seizure prophylaxis with magnesium sulphate, fluid restriction, frequent monitoring of haematological and biochemical profile, and planned delivery. Acute epigastric pain and HELLP syndrome may also present postpartum.

Fatty liver of pregnancy

Much less common than HELLP syndrome, it is associated with pre-eclampsia in only 50% of cases. Quick progression to hepatic and renal failure as well as DIC often warrants management in an intensive care setting.

Preterm labour

Corticosteroids to aid fetal lung maturation should be considered at 24–34 weeks' gestation. In the absence of fetal compromise, tocolysis may be given for up to 24 hours to allow steroids to take effect or while undertaking *in utero* transfer.

Placental abruption

Management should be dictated by maternal and fetal condition and the progress of labour. Delivery of fetus may need to be expedited if there is fetal compromise. Antepartum, postpartum haemorrhage, and DIC are potential complications that require haemodynamic monitoring of the mother and prompt resuscitation with intravenous fluids and/or blood products.

Pancreatits

More than half of the cases are gallstone related. Management and monitoring is identical as in the non pregnant state.

Postpartum pseudo-obstruction (Ogilvie syndrome)

Intravenous rehydration and nasogastric suction are necessary. Abdominal X-rays to monitor colonic diameter are indicated. Gross distension at around 9–12 cm is a sign of impending perforation. Colonic decompression with colonoscopy may be attempted. Rarely a caecostomy may be necessary.

Surgical management

Laparoscopy

This is the treatment of choice for ectopic pregnancy in the stable patient. Salpingectomy can be performed if the contralateral tube is healthy. Salpingostomy may be preferable if the contralateral tube is damaged or absent. Following laparoscopic salpingostomy β-hCG levels should be monitored as there is an 8% chance of persistent trophoblast.

Laparoscopy in the first trimester may also be necessary in cases of suspected ovarian torsion. Salpingoophorectomy has been traditionally advocated. However, several case reports and case series now support the option of detorsion and sparing of the affected ovary even in the presence of blue-black ischaemic changes.

Advanced gestation has traditionally been considered a contraindication for laparoscopy. However, recent case series suggest that this may be a safe option in experienced hands, even in the third trimester. Open laparoscopic entry (Hasson technique) or Veress needle insufflation at the midclavicular line below the left costal margin (Palmer's point) may be safer techniques in the presence of a large gravid uterus. An intra-abdominal pressure of 12–15 mmHg is usually well tolerated by the fetus. Appendicectomy and cholecystectomy may be performed using the laparoscopic route.

Laparotomy

Laparotomy is the treatment of choice for the acute surgical abdomen at any gestation when conservative treatment fails. Typical examples include open appendicectomy, cholecystectomy in cases of severe or recurrent cholecystitis, and laparotomy for bowel obstruction. It is also the most expedient treatment of ruptured ectopic gestation when the patient is haemodynamically compromised.

If laparotomy needs to be performed electively (large ovarian cyst) it is best performed in the early second trimester when the uterus is smaller and the risk of preterm delivery is reduced.

Delivery of fetus

In advanced pregnancy the decision to deliver the fetus in the course of managing severe abdominal pain emergencies may be based at any of the following considerations:
- delivery in order to optimize the resuscitation and cardiorespiratory stabilization of a critically ill mother
- in the stable mother, because of fetal compromise (abruption)
- in order to terminate the underlying pathological process (i.e. pre-eclampsia, acute fatty liver of pregnancy).

Further reading

Augustin G, Majerovic M. Non-obstetrical acute abdomen during pregnancy. Eur J Obstet Gynecol Re-prod Biol 2007;31:4–12.

Sivanesaratnam V. The acute abdomen and the obstetrician. Baillières Best Pract Res Clin Obstet Gynaecol 2000;14:89–102.

Sharp HT. The acute abdomen during pregnancy. Clin Obstet Gynecol 2002;45:405–13.

Nelson-Piercy C. *Handbook of obstetric medicine*, 3rd edn. Informa Healthcare 2006.

Internet resources

www.emedicine.com (needs free registration)

Patient resources

www.babycenter.com/0_abdominal-pain-during-pregnancy_204.bc

Amniotic fluid embolism

Definition

Amniotic fluid embolism (AFE) or 'anaphylactoid syndrome of pregnancy' is a life-threatening obstetric emergency that is characterized by acute hypotension or cardiac arrest, acute respiratory arrest (hypoxia), or coagulopathy occurring during labour, Caesarean section or evacuation of retained products of conception or within 30 minutes postpartum, in the absence of any other potential explanation for the symptoms and signs observed.

It continues to cause significant maternal and fetal morbidity and mortality and remains an unpredictable, unpreventable, and a rapidly progressive disorder.

Epidemiology

True incidence of AFE is unknown and about 10-fold variation in estimated incidence has been reported. Estimated incidence varies between 1 in 8000 and 1 in 30 000 pregnancies. Maternal mortality has been reported to be about 80%. However, recently, with advances in intensive supportive therapy, the maternal mortality has been estimated to be between 16% and 30%. Recently, the UK Obstetric Surveillance System (UKOSS) has reported a case fatality rate of 17% for AFE. Recent Confidential Enquiries into Maternal and Child health (Vlies 2007) reported a mortality rate of 25%. Approximately 50% of women who die because of AFE do so within the first hour of onset of symptoms and about 50% of those who survive this acute 'cardiorespiratory' phase, develop coagulopathy later. Although, early recognition and aggressive supportive therapy has reduced maternal mortality, many women (7%) sustain permanent neurological damage. The US and UK amniotic fluid registers have reported neonatal survival rates of 79% and 78%, respectively.

AFE exclusively occurs in women and does not have any racial predisposition. Although it was earlier suggested that 'older, multiparous' women were more susceptible, recent data from the UK amniotic fluid register does not substantiate this.

Pathophysiology

Exact aetiopathogenesis is still unknown. It has been postulated that amniotic fluid and fetal cells, lanugo, hair, etc., enter the maternal circulation and are carried to distant sites (e.g. lungs). Occlusion of pulmonary vasculature may result in symptoms similar to pulmonary venous thrombo embolism. These 'fetal materials' may also possibly trigger an anaphylactic reaction to fetal antigens. This may result in mast cell degranulation leading to the release of histamines and other mediators like tryptase as well as activation of the complement pathway. It is not always possible to identify fetal material or components of amniotic fluid in maternal circulation in patients with AFE, and conversely, material of fetal origin is often found in patients with no evidence of AFE.

Once the maternal system is exposed to a 'trigger' from the fetoplacental unit, usually there are two phases of pathophysiological response. Phase I is characterized by intense pulmonary artery vasospasm with pulmonary hypertension resulting in hypoxia and elevated right ventricular pressure. This acute hypoxic insult leads to myocardial and pulmonary capillary damage, left ventricular failure, and acute respiratory distress syndrome. Acute hypoxia may also trigger seizures. If this early Phase 1 is not managed appropriately by supportive measures, the mortality is very high.

Phase II is a 'haemorrhagic phase' that usually follows the early hypoxic phase (Phase 1) and is characterized by disseminated intravascular coagulation (DIC) leading to massive obstetric haemorrhage, bleeding from the skin and mucosal surfaces as well as into internal organs. Associated uterine atony, possibly due to the toxic effects of fibrin degradation products (FDPs) on myometrium, often worsens existing obstetric haemorrhage due to coagulopathy. FDPs can also depress the myocardium leading to 'pump failure'. The margin between Phases 1 and II may not be always well demarcated and some women may in fact present with massive coagulopathy.

Clinical approach

Symptoms and signs

AFE is unpredictable and is considered to be unpreventable and hence, should be clinically suspected when there is any sudden, unexpected collapse during late pregnancy, labour (oxytocin augmentation, precipitous labour), Caesarean section, obstetric procedures such as evacuation of retained products of conception or amniocentesis or amniofusion or within 30 minutes of these. Classical symptoms and signs include sudden onset of breathlessness with or without cyanosis, cough, altered level of consciousness with or without tonic, clonic seizures, acute hypotension, evidence of pulmonary oedema as well as fetal bradycardia. These are usually followed by evidence of consumption coagulopathy.

Investigations

Full blood count (FBC), clotting profile, liver and renal function tests to exclude other possible causes, chest X-ray (pulmonary oedema), and electrocardiograph (ECG) may show ST segment changes and evidence of right ventricular strain. Pulse oximetry and arterial blood gases (ABG) are useful to determine the degree of hypoxia. Pulmonary artery catheter to estimate the wedge pressure is useful in supportive management

Diagnosis

It has been recommended that the following four criteria should be met prior to making a clinical diagnosis of AFE:
- acute hypotension or cardiac arrest
- acute hypoxia (breathlessness, cyanosis, seizures)
- evidence of DIC or massive haemorrhage in the absence of other possible explanations
- All of these occurring during labour, Caesarean section, evacuation of retained products of conception or within 30 minutes postpartum with no other possible explanation for these findings.

Management

Once the diagnosis AFE is made, a multidisciplinary approach should be employed with input from anaesthetists, haematologists, physicians, and intensive therapists to optimize the outcome. Patients often require admission to an intensive treatment unit (ITU) for multi-organ support.

Supportive treatment

This involves maintenance of airway, breathing, and circulation. If the patient has 'collapsed', cardiopulmonary resuscitation (CPR) may be required and this should be with a left lateral tilt to reduce the compression of the inferior vena cava by the gravid uterus. Oxygen should be administered via a facemask and if necessary, the patient should be intubated to allow adequate ventilation. Acute hypotension should be aggressively treated with crystalloids and colloids. Massive haemorrhage necessitates replacement of blood and blood products.

Specific treatment

Inotropes such as digoxin may need to be administered in cases of myocardial pump failure to improve cardiac output. Dopamine infusion may help to improve renal perfusion as well as to improve myocardial contractility. Coagulopathy should be aggressively treated with blood transfusion and blood products such as platelets, cryoprecipitate and Recombinant Factor VII.

Obstetric treatment

Management of massive of postpartum haemorrhage requires oxytocics such as oxytocin bolus, infusion, prostaglandin-F2-α, and rectal misoprostol to control bleeding. Algorithms such as 'HAEMOSTASIS' have been proposed to aid logical and systematic approach to the management of atonic postpartum haemorrhage and may help clinicians to adopt a stepwise approach. Rarely, if the patient has sustained a cardiorespiratory arrest prior to bleeding and efforts to resuscitate are unsuccessful, a perimortem Caesarean section should be performed within 5 minutes of cardiac arrest. This is done to resuscitate the mother but is also likely to help in fetal salvage. This will reduce compression of the aorta and inferior vena cava by the gravid uterus and, thereby, would help improve venous return and cardiac output. Delivery of the baby is likely to reduce the oxygen consumption by the fetoplacental unit and improve the oxygenation of the mother.

AFE with cardiorespiratory arrest is an unpredictable and unpreventable obstetric emergency. Owing to the high maternal mortality, many cases are diagnosed by a post-mortem examination confirming histological evidence of components of amniotic fluid in the maternal lungs. However, a high index of suspicion is required to make a clinical diagnosis. Familiarity with adult resuscitation and 'maternal collapse drills' as well as regular skills and drills training in the management of massive obstetric haemorrhage and a multidisciplinary approach are likely to improve outcome.

Further reading

Clarke SL, Hankins GD, Dudley DA, et al. Amniotic fluid embolism: analysis of the national registry. Am J Obstet Gynecol 1995;172:1158–69.

Gilbert WM, Danielsen B. Amniotic fluid embolism: decreased mortality in a population-based study. Obstet Gynecol 1999;93:973–7.

Lim Y, Loo CC, Chia V, Fun W. Recombinant factor VIIa after amniotic fluid embolism and disseminated intravascular coagulopathy Int J Gynaecol Obstet 2004;87:178–9.

O'Shea A, Eappen S. Amniotic fluid embolism. Int Anesthesiol Clin 2007;45:17–28.

Tuffnell DJ. Amniotic fluid embolism. Curr Opin Obstet Gynaecol 2003;15:119–22.

Tuffnell DJ. United kingdom amniotic fluid embolism register. Br J Obstet Gynaecol 2005;112:1625–9.

UKOSS. Amniotic fluid embolism. In: United Kingdom Obstetric Surveillance System (UKOSS). Oxford: National Perinatal Epidemiology Unit 2008.

Vlies R. Amniotic fluid embolism. In: Saving mothers' lives: reviewing maternal deaths to make motherhood safer 2003–2005. London: CEMACH 2007: Chapter 5. www.cemach.org.uk

Antepartum haemorrhage

Definition
Antepartum haemorrhage (APH) is bleeding from the genital tract from the time of viability of pregnancy for extra uterine survival to the time of delivery of the baby.

Incidence
APH occurs in 3.5% of all pregnancies.

The incidence varies with age, parity, and social class.

In approximately half of all women presenting with APH, a diagnosis of placental abruption or placenta praevia will be made; no firm diagnosis will be made in the other half even after investigations.

Causes
- Placenta praevia
- Placental abruption
- Antepartum haemorrhage of indeterminate origin
- Vasa previa
- Show
- Bleeding from the lower genital tract:
  - vaginal infection/cervicitis
  - vulvovaginal varicosities
  - tumours
  - trauma.

Prognosis
Major APH is a significant cause of perinatal morbidity and mortality. It is also a cause of maternal morbidity and mortality.

Minor APHs cause significant maternal anxiety especially if no cause is found.

Management
Management of any patient with bleeding in late pregnancy should be in a hospital with facilities for blood transfusion, Caesarean delivery, neonatal resuscitation and intensive care.

Key points in the management of APH
- APH is largely unpredictable and a patients condition may deteriorate rapidly
- Priority is to resuscitate the mother
- Establish fetal viability and wellbeing
- Digital assessment of the cervical dilataion is contraindicated unless placenta previa has been excluded.

History
- Gestation and parity
- Amount and character of bleeding
- Association of abdominal pain and uterine contractions
- History of rupture of membranes or previous vaginal bleeds
- Presence and nature of fetal movements
- History of trauma or recent coitus
- Information from scan on placental site.

Examination
- General assessment of patient: distressed, pale, unconscious
- Maternal pulse, blood pressure, and respiratory rate
- Abdominal examination: fundal height, presence of tenderness and uterine contractions, fetal lie and presentation
- Vaginal assessment: if placenta praevia has not been excluded then vaginal examination is contraindicated. If placenta praevia has been excluded then speculum examination of the cervix is useful to exclude cervical causes.
- Fetal assessment with cardiotocography (CTG) or ultrasound.

Investigations and immediate management
This will obviously depend on the severity of the bleeding and the condition of the mother:
- i.v. access with wide bore cannula
- blood for FBC, group and save or cross-match if heavy blood or evidence of compromise
- if abruption is suspected, coagulation screen and urea and electrolytes.
- i.v. fluids
- if fetal demise with diagnosis of abruption, a significant intrauterine bleed should be anticipated and hence consider blood transfusion.

Subsequent management
This will depend on the condition of the patient and fetus, the amount of bleeding and the likely cause:

expectant management if no sign of maternal or fetal compromise
- immediate delivery if maternal or fetal compromise
- individualized management in cases of intrauterine death

Placental abruption (see Chapter 10.12).
Placenta praevia (see Chapter 10.13).

Antepartum haemorrhage of indeterminate origin
The exact cause of bleeding in late pregnancy remains unknown in about half of cases of antepartum haemorrhage. The woman typically presents with painless vaginal bleeding without ultrasound evidence of placenta praevia. Placenta praevia can be excluded by an ultrasound scan, but the diagnosis of placental abruption is based on clinical signs and symptoms, and is difficult to confirm in mild cases. Perinatal morbidity is increased in these cases.

In some cases there is separation of a normally sited placenta from its margin leading to bleeding from the marginal sinuses. The pregnancy continues as normal however there may be repeated small bleeds.

Investigations
Speculum examination will exclude local causes. Ultrasound shows a normally situated placenta and a possible retroplacental clot at its margin

Management
Management is largely conservative.

Key points
- 15–20% women presenting with APH without a firm cause labour and deliver in the next 2 weeks. Steroids should be considered if the gestation is <34 weeks.
- Once the bleeding has settled and the woman has been observed as an inpatient for 24–48 hours, outpatient management is appropriate.

- If pregnancy is beyond 37 weeks' gestation and the bleeding is recurrent or associated with fetal growth restriction, labour induction is the management of choice
- Anti-D administration is required to Rhesus-negative mothers.

- There is a higher risk of low birthweight babies and meconium staining in labour.

Further reading

Ngeh N, Bhide A. Antepartum haemorrhage. Current Obstet Gynae 2006;16:79–83.

Cancer in pregnancy

Definition
Malignancy diagnosed during pregnancy and the puerperium. Diagnosis up to 1 year postpartum is used for maternal mortality data.

Epidemiology
This is a rare clinical problem affecting approximately 1 in 1000 pregnancies. It is no more common than in the non-pregnant state. Although rare, malignant disease as a cause of indirect maternal death is over-represented in the confidential enquiry into maternal and child health (CEMACH).

Pathology
Nearly all cancer types have been reported during pregnancy. By far the commonest types encountered are
- breast cancer
- lymphoma (usually Hodgkin's)
- cervical cancer
- acute leukaemia
- melanoma.

Aetiology
Cancers occur for the same reasons they occur outside pregnancy. The pregnant state does not appear to influence the initiation or progression of cancers including hormone-responsive ones such as breast cancer, despite the large physiological changes.

Clinical approach
Cancers are a heterogeneous group of conditions and the following are the major considerations if diagnosed in pregnancy:
- the effect of pregnancy on the disease
- the risk to the mother if diagnosis and/or treatment is delayed
- the effects of chemotherapy and/or radiotherapy on the fetus, including radiological and nuclear investigations
- the effect of the disease on the outcome of the pregnancy
- the timing of delivery including the risk of prematurity, if delivered early, to start treatment
- the risks of treatment on the children and their subsequent development.

They require true MDT input to try and optimize the outcome for mother and baby including obstetricians, midwives, oncologists, specialized nursing staff, and radiologists. The options upon diagnosis are
- termination of pregnancy (TOP) and commencement of treatment: TOP will not improve the prognosis *per se*, it will only allow prompt treatment if cancer is diagnosed in early pregnancy
- delay in treatment until fetal survival is likely
- treatment with surgery, chemo/radiotherapy during pregnancy: in general the cancer should be treated as would be the case outside of pregnancy. Cervical cancer may be different as it will usually involve uterine surgery or pelvic irradiation.

The effect of pregnancy on the disease
- Cohort studies repeatedly state that for all cancers studied there appears to be an equivalent outcome in

pregnancy when matched with non-pregnant controls. This includes breast cancer, leukaemias, cervical cancer, and melanoma.
- Delays in diagnosis have been reported due to unwillingness to aggressively investigate symptoms in pregnant women, although prognosis is generally unchanged. The exception to this is acute leukaemia: delay in diagnosis and treatment will usually lead to maternal and fetal death due to the aggressive nature of the disease.
- Data are based on small cohorts, often retrospective.

The effects of chemotherapy and/or radiotherapy on the fetus
Chemotherapy
Evidence from studies consistently supports the following regarding chemotherapy in pregnancy:
- All chemotherapeutic agents have caused teratogenesis in animal models: they are contraindicated in the first trimester.
- Intrauterine growth restriction (IUGR), small for gestational age (SGA), preterm delivery, and IUD have all been reported but are unusual.
- Use of chemotherapy in the second and third trimesters appears generally safe.
- Use of 'safer' lower doses should be avoided as they put the mother at risk of undertreatment: if she needs treatment, treat her properly!
- Delivery should be avoided within 2–3 weeks of chemotherapy to allow maternal bone marrow recovery and fetal excretion of drugs.
- Information on breastfeeding is almost non-existent and therefore breastfeeding is *contraindicated* during chemotherapy.
- Data on many individual agents are largely unknown and need to be judged on a risk–benefit principle.

Radiotherapy and radiological investigations
The literature supports the following:
- teratogenesis is recognized above threshold doses of 0.1–0.2 Gy in the first trimester
- mental retardation is recognized above 0.1 Gy between 8 and 25 weeks
- supradiaphragmatic radiotherapy with shielding appears to be safe in pregnancy
- pelvi-abdominal radiotherapy is contraindicated
- X-ray, CT and MRI in the diagnostic range are safe (well below threshold doses).

The effect of the disease on the outcome of the pregnancy
- Pregnancies are generally unaffected by malignancy *per se* as long as maternal wellbeing is maintained.
- In the presence of cachexia and carcinomatosis, fetal outcome is worse including IUGR, IUD and premature delivery.
- Individual chemotherapy regimes can rarely cause problems as above: regular growth scans are required.
- Transplacental metastases have been reported but are very rare.
- Early delivery may need to be planned to initiate treatment: a decision on mode of delivery can generally be made for normal obstetric indications.

The risks of treatment on the children and their subsequent development

- There is no consistent information to suggest an excess of long-term developmental or malignant morbidities for children exposed to antineoplastic agents *in utero*.
- There is however evidence of long-term deleterious effects on intellectual development and a small increase in secondary malignancies in children exposed to radiation above threshold doses.
- The long-term reproductive ability of children exposed to chemo- or radiotherapy is largely unknown, although some offspring in the largest series studied have reproduced successfully.

Conclusion

All the above data are based on small numbers and mainly retrospective data, although it is generally reassuring concerning general prognosis and treatment. No clinician will see many of these cases and therefore each case needs to be managed on an individual basis and the development of registers for pregnant cancer patients may help to inform international experience.

Further reading

Hayes K. Cancer and its management in pregnancy. JPOG 2006:149–55.

Cardonik E, Iacobucci A. Use of chemotherapy during human pregnancy. Lancet Oncol 2004;5:283–91.

Weisz B, Meirow D, Schiff E, *et al.* Impact and treatment of cancer during pregnancy. Expert Rev Anticancer Ther 2004;4:889–902.

Lewis G, Drife J (eds). *Saving mothers lives. confidential enquiry into maternal deaths and child health 2003–5.* London: RCOG Press 2007.

Doll D, Ringenberg Q, Yarbro J. Antineoplastic agents and pregnancy. Semin Oncol 1989;16:337–45.

Patient resources

www.cancer.gov/

health.yahoo.com/breastcancer-treatment/breast-cancer-and-pregnancy-treatment-patient-information-nci-pdq/healthwise–ncicdr0000062970.html

www.cancer.org/docroot/CRI/content/CRI_2_6x_Pregnancy_and_Breast_Cancer.asp

www.siteman.wustl.edu/PDQ.aspx?id=664&xml=CDR257535.xml

www.cooperhealth.org/content/pregnancyandcancer.htm

Fibroids in pregnancy

Definition
These are uterine leiomyomata recognized during pregnancy.

Epidemiology
- Fibroids are found in up to 40% of women before the age of 40.
- Fibroids are recognized in up to 4% of all pregnancies
- They are more common in:
  - women over 40
  - women of Afro-Caribbean origin
  - pregnancy after assisted conception.

Pathology
See Chapter 13.3, Fibroids. Fibroids do respond to oestrogen and may enlarge in pregnancy, although there are no consistent data to back this up.

Aetiology
See Chapter 13.3, Fibroids.

Clinical approach
History
- May have known fibroids
- The majority are asymptomatic and incidental scan findings
- Abdominal pain is the commonest symptom in pregnancy
- Previous myomectomy will need discussion regarding mode of delivery (see below).

Examination
- Usually not obvious on clinical assessment: scan only.
- May be 'large for dates'.
- May be palpable on the uterus if large and/or multiple.
- Fetal malpresentation may rarely occur, e.g. breech, transverse, or oblique lie if lower segment or cervical fibroid.
- May be tender to palpate if in pain (usually discrete tenderness over fibroid).

Investigation
Abdominal ultrasound is usually the only investigation necessary. Transvaginal ultrasound is occasionally used to identify cervical fibroids. Magnetic resonance imaging is not usually necessary.

Clinical features
The majority of pregnancies are unaffected by fibroids. The evidence on fibroids in pregnancy is controversial, as most of the published work is based on case–control studies that have significant confounding factors.
  On balance there appears to be
- an association with subfertility (probably causal in 2–3% of cases, if submucosal, once other causes are excluded). Intramural and serosal fibroids do not appear to have a proven effect
- an association with miscarriage if submucoosal. Rates appear to be higher with fibroids versus no fibroids, but may be related to older age
- a small absolute increase in preterm delivery, malpresentation and Caesarean delivery

- a small increase in the rate of postpartum haemorrhage
  - no convincing evidence for any causal relationship with
  - increased perinatal morbidty or mortality
  - placenta praevia/abruption or IUGR
  - labour dystocia
  - retained placenta or endometritis.

Management
Subfertility and fibroids
Evidence for surgery for fibroids is of poor quality generally but overall appears to suggest
- some improvement in pregnancy rates
- best results seem to be with hysteroscopic resection for submucosal fibroids.

Miscarriage
Evidence for surgery for fibroids is of very poor quality and conflicting. Surgery to reduce the risk of further miscarriage for submucosal fibroids should only be performed on a case by case basis.

Antenatal care
Conservative
Reassurance that risks and complications are rare is usually all that is required. Routine monitoring of fibroid size or morphology is not necessary, nor is extra fetal growth monitoring. Antenatal care should be advised according to standard principles. There are no medical or surgical treatment options specifically for fibroids in pregnancy. In general 'leave them alone!'
  Special obstetric input will be required with
- significant fibroid pain
- abnormal fetal lie and where Caesarean section (CS) is required
- previous myomectomy.

Significant fibroid pain
This is the commonest clinical problem encountered with fibroids in pregnancy and is usually in the third trimester. Excessive fibroid growth, degeneration and necrosis due to 'outgrowing its blood supply' are often cited (and biologically plausible) but have no convincing evidence to support them. The pain's aetiology is poorly understood. It may be mild and self limiting but more commonly is severe and requires hospital admission. Torsion of a pedunculated fibroid is very rare and no more common than in the non-pregnant population.

Management of fibroid pain
- Exclusion of other causes of abdominal pain is vital, especially
- placental abruption
- acute appendicitis/ovarian torsion
- UTI.
- The diagnosis is one of exclusion and is clinical.
- A mild pyrexia and vomiting may be present.
- A leucocytosis is not uncommon.
- Ultrasound will identify fibroids easily if unknown. Cystic changes are commonly seen but can also be seen within fibroids outside of pregnancy.
- Symptomatic treatment is required for pain relief. Commonly used agents are paracetamol and codeine

derivatives. Buprenorphine, pethidine, and morphine may be required for severe pain.

- NSAIDs, although ideal, are generally avoided due to adverse effects on fetal renal and ductus function. They may be used off licence for a short time in refractory cases
- The majority of episodes are self-limiting (5–10 days)
- A few cases are prolonged and are very difficult to manage—pain team involvement may be helpful
- Surgery (myomectomy) for chronic unremitting pain has been described with successful results, but is not recommended due to concerns about uterine surgery during pregnancy ('a last resort').
- The pregnancy is unaffected.

Abnormal lie or presentation

- This is rare but occurs with significant lower segment/ cervical fibroids
- TA and TV ultrasound with clinical assessment will help to show the relationship of presenting part and fibroid and exclude other causes, e.g. placenta praevia!
- A decision regarding the mode of delivery can be delayed until 37 weeks
- Elective CS at 39 weeks is the only safe mode of delivery if there is persistent obstruction.

Caesarean section with fibroids

- An experienced surgeon should be present.
- The ultrasound findings are a guide only and may not truly reflect the number and size of fibroids present—expect more than you think!
- Pfannensteil incision is generally preferred, but midline may be required if fibroids are large and/or multiple.
- There is a risk of upper segment incision being required if a fibroid is occupying the whole lower segment.
- The fibroid(s) should be avoided wherever possible and uterine incision kept clear of them as excess bleeding may occur.
- Difficulty delivering the baby may occur with multiple large fibroids—be prepared and have a plan B!
- Rarely myomectomy may be necessary at the same time to facilitate delivery or in the event of bleeding.
- Increased blood loss should be anticipated—cross-match blood.
- The absolute risk of hysterectomy is still very low and probably no more than for women without fibroids.

Previous myomectomy

- Previous myomectomy *per se* is not associated with any adverse pregnancy outcomes.
- Previous myomectomy in the non-pregnant state cannot be viewed the same as previous CS.
- Operative difficulty, especially bleeding and adhesions, should be anticipated if CS is required

- Evidence of poor quality suggests that;
- uterine rupture during pregnancy is negligible
- uterine rupture in labour is very low and successful vaginal delivery can be encouraged in the majority—labour should be managed empirically as for previous CS
- Uterine rupture may possibly be more common (very little convincing data)if
  - the endometrial cavity was breached
  - multiple uterine incisions were made
  - more than one previous myomectomy.

Generally elective CS is recommended in these circumstances, although a trial of vaginal delivery is not unreasonable if a woman is fully informed

Postpartum care

Generally no specific extra care is required because of fibroids. The following can generally be advised:

- fibroid pain usually improves rapidly after delivery
- if fibroids have caused pain in one pregnancy they are more likely to do so in a future pregnancy
- obstructing fibroids will very likely do so again requiring repeat CS
- no fibroid monitoring is generally required unless they cause ongoing gynaecological symptoms
- future pregnancies are not likely to be significantly affected by fibroids.

Further reading

Okolo S. Incidence, aetiology and epidemiology of uterine fibroids. In: Arulkumaran S (ed.) *Best practice and research: clinical obstetrics and gynaecology*, vol. 22:4. Elsevier 2008: 557–88.

Khaund A, Lumsden MA. Impact of fibroids on reproductive function. In: Arulkumaran S (ed.) *Best practice and research: clinical obstetrics and gynaecology*, vol. 22:4. Elsevier 2008: 749–60.

Klatsky PC, Tran NC, Caughey AB, *et al.* Fibroids and reproductive outcomes: a systematic literature review from conception to delivery. *Am J Obstet Gynecol* 2008;357–66.

Coronado GD, Marshall LM, Schwartz SM. Complications in pregnancy, labor, and delivery with uterine leiomyomas: a population-based study. *Obstet Gynecol* 2000;95:764–9.

Qidwai GI, Caughey AB, Jacoby AF. Obstetric outcomes in women with sonographically identified uterine leiomyomata. *Obstet Gynecol* 2006;107:376–82.

Manyonda I (eds). Uterine fibroids. In: *Best practice and research: clinical obstetrics and gynaecology*, vol. 22:4. Elsevier 2008.

Patient resources

www.nhsdirect.nhs.uk/articles/article.aspx?articleId=161

www.patient.co.uk/showdoc/23068738/

www.womenshealthlondon.org.uk/leaflets/fibroids/fibroidsre-sources.html

www.femalepatient.com/pdf/patob_0506.pdf

Obstetric cholestasis

Definition

Obstetric cholestasis (OC), also called intrahepatic cholestasis of pregnancy, is a liver disease of pregnancy that affects approximately 1 in 200 pregnant women in the UK. It causes maternal pruritus in association with impaired liver function and raised serum bile acids and usually resolves within 12 weeks of delivery. Fetal complications include spontaneous preterm delivery, fetal anoxia, meconium-stained liquor, and intrauterine death.

Epidemiology

The prevalence of OC varies in different ethnic groups, ranging from 0. % of Caucasians, to 1.5% of UK Asians, and up to 5% of native Chileans. The condition is more common in multiple pregnancy and in the winter months.

Aetiology

OC has a complex aetiology with genetic, endocrine, and environmental components. Each will contribute to a different extent in individual women affected by OC. The aetiology of the fetal complications is likely to relate to the extent of the raised serum bile acids in the mother and fetus (Glantz et al. 2004).

Genetic factors

Evidence for a genetic aetiology comes from pedigree studies and mutation screens (Dixon et al. 2008). A small number of cases are caused by heterozygous mutations in biliary transport proteins (MDR3, BSEP, FIC1, MRP2) or the principal bile acid receptor (FXR). It is likely that genetic variation in the genes that encode these proteins, and others that influence bile homeostasis, also confers susceptibility to cholestasis in pregnancy.

Endocrine factors

Gestational rises in oestrogen and progesterone and their metabolites are likely to cause cholestasis in susceptible individuals (Reyes et al. 2008). A subgroup of women who had previously had OC develop symptoms of cholestasis when given oral contraceptives or in the latter half of the menstrual cycle. Also women with OC have higher levels of cholestatic oestrogen and progesterone metabolites in the serum and urine when pregnant. In vitro experiments have shown that these metabolites impair biliary excretion, thus implicating them in the aetiology of OC.

Environmental factors

OC is commoner in the winter months in Chile and Scandinavia. It occurs more frequently in women who are seropositive for hepatitis C and following ingestion of some antibiotics, e.g. co-amoxiclav or erythromycin (Geenes et al. 2009).

Aetiology of fetal complications

The largest study to date demonstrated that fetal complications (spontaneous preterm delivery, fetal anoxia and meconium-stained liquor) rarely occur if serial measurement of maternal fasting serum bile acids does not demonstrate levels >40 µmol/L. However, once the maternal bile acids rise to >40 µmol/L the risk of pregnancy complications rises with each µmol/L increment above this level. Several additional studies have demonstrated a similar association between maternal serum bile acid levels and fetal risk.

In vitro studies have shown increased myometrial contractility in the presence of bile acids, and animal studies report increased rates of preterm delivery and meconium-stained amniotic fluid following infusion of bile acids. Administration of bile acids to in vitro cultured cardiomyocytes causes abnormal rhythm of contraction, leading to the hypothesis that raised fetal serum bile acids may result in a potentially fatal fetal arrhythmia.

Fetal autopsies are characterized by changes consistent with acute anoxia, and do not show evidence of chronic uteroplacental insufficiency. OC placentas have histological abnormalities consistent with hypoxic insults, and are consistent with the changes seen in placentas from a rodent model of OC. Meconium-stained amniotic fluid is reported in almost all OC-associated intrauterine deaths. The presence of meconium may also contribute to fetal anoxia.

Prognosis

The maternal prognosis is usually good. It is important to exclude alternative underlying diagnoses. If none is present, the pruritus and hepatic impairment usually resolve 2 weeks after delivery. OC commonly recurs in subsequent pregnancies (Williamson et al. 2004). Affected women have an increased risk of gallstones, non-alcoholic cirrhosis and autoimmune hepatitis in later life (Ropponen et al. 2006).

Clinical approach

Diagnosis

The diagnostic criteria used for OC vary in different studies. Ideally liver transaminases and serum bile acids should be measured. It is of value to measure serum bile acids as they have been shown to relate to fetal outcome (Glantz et al. 2004). Pruritus may precede biochemical abnormalities by several weeks (Kenyon et al. 2001) or alternatively the serum bile acids may be raised before symptoms are present, reflecting the aetiological heterogeneity of the condition. Therefore it is advisable to perform regular blood tests to assess the serum bile acid and transaminase level.

History

It is important to ensure there is no evidence of other liver diseases, e.g. infectious hepatitis, acute fatty liver of pregnancy, or pre-eclampsia with hepatic impairment. Otherwise, the history should ascertain the following:

- duration and location of pruritus. This classically occurs in the latter weeks of pregnancy, although the condition can present in the first trimester. The pruritus is most commonly perceived on the palms, soles and 'all over' the body and is not associated with a rash (apart from excoriations). However the localization of pruritus can be variable
- changes in the colour of urine/faeces
- family history
- multiple pregnancy or assisted conception
- risk factors for hepatitis C
- symptoms of cholecystitis
- cholestatic reactions to drugs in the past.

Examination

It is important to examine the skin for jaundice and to exclude a dermatological condition.

Investigations

OC is a diagnosis of exclusion. Pruritus and abnormal liver function can occur in women with a variety of other diagnoses, including diseases within the pre-eclampsia spectrum and infectious hepatitis. It can also be the presenting feature of biliary obstruction. It may also be complicated by postpartum haemorrhage secondary to malabsorption of vitamin K. Therefore, it is important to perform investigations to exclude these diagnoses/complications, including

- ultrasound of the liver and biliary tree
- hepatitis C serology
- clotting screen
- pre-eclampsia bloods.

Management

General points

Once the diagnosis of OC has been confirmed the management strategy should include treatment of the maternal disease, fetal surveillance, and decisions about delivery. If there is a concurrent disease process, this should be treated.

Medical

- Ursodeoxycholic acid (UDCA) is the drug for which there is the most robust supporting data from clinical trials. It is a relatively hydrophilic bile acid that is found in small quantities in humans. It has been used successfully to treat cholestatic diseases outside pregnancy and is becoming increasingly popular as a treatment for OC. UDCA has several modes of action, including induction of bile acid excretion pathways, enhanced secretion of cholestatic oestrogen metabolites, and antiapoptotic effects. Most studies of the efficacy of UDCA in the treatment of OC have been small, although one included 130 cases randomized to receive UDCA, dexamethasone, or placebo (Glantz et al. 2005). UDCA has consistently been shown to improve maternal pruritus serum bile acids and transaminases (Geenes et al. 2009). However, no studies have been powered to establish whether it protects against the adverse fetal outcomes associated with OC.
- Aqueous cream with 2% menthol is a useful topical treatment that relieves pruritus. This is valuable for women who find the OC-associated itch extremely unpleasant, and it can help women get to sleep if they are suffering insomnia as a consequence of pruritus.
- Other drugs that have been used to treat OC include dexamethasone, S-adenosy methionine, cholestyramine, guar gum, and perioral activated charcoal. Although some small studies have reported maternal responses to these drugs none has consistently been shown to improve maternal symptoms and biochemical abnormalities.
- Vitamin K is often given with the aim of reducing the likelihood of postpartum haemorrhage, as this complication is thought to relate to vitamin K malabsorption secondary to steatorrhoea. There have been no clinical trials to evaluate whether this treatment is effective.

Maternal and fetal surveillance

- Once the diagnosis of OC has been established it is advisable to continue to monitor the maternal liver transaminases and serum bile acids. This will allow evaluation of the extent of the fetal risk (i.e. given the data relating fetal adverse events to maternal serum bile acid levels) and will ensure maternal wellbeing, given that pruritus and hepatic impairment may be the presenting features of other diseases, e.g. acute fatty liver of pregnancy.
- There is no evidence that regular fetal surveillance with cardiotochography facilitates the prediction of which OC pregnancies will be complicated by intrauterine death. However, this practice may reassure affected women and clinicians responsible for their care at the time it is performed.
- One study reported good fetal outcomes for OC pregnancies with a policy of routine amnioscopy at 36 weeks of gestation in addition to standard monitoring for fetal wellbeing (Roncaglia et al. 2002), but this approach may be more invasive than most obstetricians would choose.

Timing of delivery

- Some studies have reported good fetal outcomes with a policy of induction of labour at 38 weeks of gestation (Roncaglia et al. 2002). This policy has been adopted by a large proportion of clinicians in the UK as the fetal deaths appear to cluster after 37 weeks (Williamson et al. 2004). However, there have been no prospective studies to evaluate this practice.
- It is important to consider the risk of neonatal respiratory distress following delivery at 38 weeks of gestation, and to discuss the risks and benefits of this practice for the fetus/neonate with the mother. The neonatal risks of early delivery are considerably lower if the mother has undergone labour, and thus induction is likely to be associated with lower rates of respiratory distress than elective Caesarean section.

Postnatal care

Women whose LFTs remain abnormal 2 weeks after delivery should have further investigations and referral to a hepatologist.

The recurrence rate for OC is high. Women with a previous singleton pregnancy have a 70% chance of recurrent cholestasis in a subsequent pregnancy. The risk is lower following a multiple pregnancy.

Parous sisters and daughters of affected women have a 20-fold increased risk of developing OC.

Contraceptive advice

A subgroup of women who have had OC develop cholestasis following administration of ethinyl oestradiol or the combined oral contraceptive pill. Therefore, it is important to consider the risks of hormonal contraceptives. Ideally, affected women should use alternative forms of contraception, and if they use oral contraceptives they should have their liver function tests monitored.

Further reading

Dixon PH, Williamson C. The molecular genetics of intrahepatic cholestasis of pregnancy. Obstet Med 2008;1:65–71.

Geenes VL, Williamson C. Intrahepatic cholestasis of pregnancy. World J Gastroenterol 2009;15:2049–66.

Glantz A, Marschall HU, Lammert F, Mattsson LA. Intrahepatic cholestasis of pregnancy: a randomized controlled trial comparing dexamethasone and ursodeoxycholic acid. Hepatology 2005;42:1399–405.

Glantz A, Marschall HU, Mattsson LA. Intrahepatic cholestasis of pregnancy: Relationships between bile acid levels and fetal complication rates. Hepatology 2004;40:467–74.

Kenyon AP, Piercy CN, Girling J, et al. Pruritus may precede abnormal liver function tests in pregnant women with obstetric cholestasis: a longitudinal analysis. Br J Obstet Gynaecol 2001;108:119.

MacKillop L, Williamson C. Diseases of the liver, biliary system and pancreas. In: Creasy, Resnik (eds) Maternal and fetal medicine, 6 edn. Elsevier 2008.

Nelson-Piercy C, Williamson C. Hepatic and gastrointestinal disorders. In: Greer I, Nelson-Piercy C, Walters B (eds) Maternal medicine, 1st edn. Elsevier 2007.

Reid R, Ivey KJ, Rencoret RH, Storey B. Fetal complications of obstetric cholestasis. BMJ 1976;1:87.

Reyes H. Sex hormones and bile acids in intrahepatic cholestasis of pregnancy. Hepatology 2008;47:37.

Roncaglia N, Arreghini A, Locatelli A, et al. Obstetric cholestasis: outcome with active management. Eur J Obstet Gynecol Reprod Biol 2002;100:167–70.

Ropponen A et al. Intrahepatic cholestasis of pregnancy as an indicator of liver and biliary diseases: a population-based study. Hepatology 2006;43:72.

Williamson C, Sund R, Riikonen S, et al. Clinical outcome in a series of cases of obstetric cholestasis identified via a patient support group. Br J Obstet Gynaecol 2004; 111:676–81.

Internet resources

www.britishlivertrust.org.uk

Patient resources

www.ocsupport.org.uk

Ovarian cysts in pregnancy

Definition
Ovarian cysts diagnosed or known about during pregnancy.

Epidemiology
Ovarian cysts are very common findings and their incidence is related to how commonly ultrasound is used throughout pregnancy. In early pregnancy attenders, rates of 5–10% are quoted for cysts >25 mm diameter. Cysts >5 cm are seen in approximately 1–2%.

Pathology
All types of ovarian cyst have been described in pregnancy, but the most common are
- functional (presumably mainly corpus luteal) cysts (50–70%):may appear haemorrhagic
- dermoid cysts (10%)
- endometriomata (5–10%).

Malignancies are very rare and probably found in <1% of ovarian cysts in pregnancy. Much of the data arise from tertiary referral centres that quote rates up to 5%, but these are biased and highly selected high-risk groups. The majority of these tend to be borderline tumours.

Aetiology
The aetiology of most cysts is no different to the non-pregnant state. Corpus luteal cysts develop in the persistent CL necessary for successful pregnancy. The types of cyst that predominate reflect the types of cyst that are common in young women.

Clinical approach
History
- May have a known cyst.
- The vast majority are asymptomatic and incidental scan findings in early pregnancy or at booking/anomaly scans.
- Abdominal pain is the commonest presenting symptom in early pregnancy and may reflect haemorrhage, rupture or more rarely torsion.
- Severe pain, vomiting and collapse are usually indicative of an acute cyst accident.
- Symptoms of overt malignancy are rarely ever seen.

Examination
- Most will have no obvious findings (scan only)
- May be palpable abdominally or on vaginal assessment
- Significant tenderness and peritonism may be present with rupture or torsion.

Investigation
TV ultrasound is the imaging modality of choice in early pregnancy. Abdominal ultrasound is usually used beyond the first trimester. Imaging in late pregnancy may be more difficult due to cyst position behind the gravid uterus.
- High-quality ultrasound is the key to diagnosing and managing most cysts in pregnancy
- Experienced operators use pattern recognition which is highly reliable in the right hands
- Positive diagnosis of benign lesions is very reliable
- Positive diagnosis of borderline or malignant lesions is less good.

MRI is very good, and safe after the first trimester, at identifying tissue content, e.g. fat in dermoids, blood in endometiomas/haemorrhagic cysts. MRI may be useful if there is doubt as to the diagnosis of the nature of the cyst after ultrasound.

CA125, AFP, and β-hCG are all elevated in pregnancy and should be used very cautiously as they usually represent false positives.

Clinical features
The majority of pregnancies are completely unaffected by ovarian cysts and vice versa. The evidence on the effect of cysts in pregnancy is based on mainly retrospective cohort studies which may have significant confounding and bias.

On balance it appears that
- no extra specific obstetric care is required and women can be reassured
- obstructed labour is not a realistic clinical problem as most cysts are very mobile and rise up with the uterus
- malignancy is very rare
- acute cyst accidents are no more common than in the non-pregnant state and absolute risk is small (3–4%)
- the majority can be managed conservatively if high-quality imaging is available
- if Caesarean section is required for obstetric indications then removal of a cyst should be anticipated and strongly considered if the clinical situation permits—an experienced surgeon should be available as there is a very large utero-ovarian blood supply.

Management
Women can be reassured that monitoring only is adequate if
- the cyst is simple in morphology
- there is a positive diagnosis of a dermoid cyst or endometrioma or absence of malignant features
- there are no acute symptoms
- there is no upper limit to size, although the likelihood of active intervention increases with cysts >10 cm
- the woman understands the risks of acute cyst accident (3–4%).

There is no consensus on 'monitoring' but it is reasonable to rescan in the second trimester if discovered in the first, and the third if discovered in the second. The majority of simple cysts (70–80%) will have resolved on rescanning. Persistent cysts (15–20%) can be rescanned 3 months postpartum. Large cysts are generally better removed electively postpartum.

Acute abdominal pain
This should be managed in the same way as outside pregnancy in the presence of a cyst. The clinical priorities are
- exclusion of ectopic pregnancy (and other causes of pain)
- resuscitation if haemodyanmically unstable due to haemorrhagic rupture
- accurate diagnosis on clinical and ultrasound parameters—haemorrhage and rupture are usually easy to diagnose and can generally be managed conservatively
- active intervention is needed when torsion is suspected.

Suspicious cysts and diagnostic difficulty

If cyst morphology is suspicious of possible malignancy or there is diagnostic difficulty.

- MRI may help to diagnose the likely aetiology.
- Cases should be referred to the cancer multidisciplinary team (MDT) or tertiary referral unit for decision-making.
- Great care in interpretation of tumour markers is required (as above).
- Ultimately cystectomy/oopherectomy/staging laparotomy may be required if significant concern exists: laparoscopic management is generally preferred if uterine size permits its use.
- The timing of surgery will depend upon the clinical concern, gestation, and maternal wishes: in advanced pregnancy this may be deferred till after delivery or performed at the time of Caesarean section.

- Evidence regarding safety of these procedures in pregnancy is generally very reassuring: the risks of miscarriage or preterm delivery are very small.

Further reading

Valentin L. Imaging in gynaecology. In: Arulkumaran S (ed.) *Best practice and research: clinical obstetrics and gynaecology*, vol. 20:6. Oxford: Elsevier 2006:881–906.

Condous G, Khalid A, Okaro, *et al.* Should we be examining the ovaries in pregnancy? Prevalence and natural history of andexal pathology detected at first trimester sonography. Ultrasound Obstet Gynecol 2004;24:62–6.

Yazbek J, Salim R, Woelfer B, *et al.* The value of ultrasound visualization of the ovaries during the routine 11–14 weeks nuchal translucency scan. Eur J Obstet Gynecol Repro Biol 2007;132:154–8.

Zanetta G, Marlani E, Lissoni A, *et al.* A prospective study of the role of ultrasound in the management of adnexal masses in pregnancy. Br J Obstet Gynaecol 2003;110:578–83.

Postnatal depression

Approximately 1 in 10 women who deliver a baby will experience postnatal depression (Oates 2003). In a third of these women, the illness will last a year or more (Cox et al 1982), when it may have wide-reaching effects on the mother and her family if not identified and treated. Certain factors appear to increase the risk of developing postnatal depression including:

- young age of mother
- family/partner conflicts
- lack of social network
- substance misuse
- unwanted pregnancy or ambivalent to it
- pre-existing mental illness (anxiety or depression)
- frequent antenatal admissions
- family history of postnatal depression.

The management of postnatal depression includes a review of risks and benefits to mother and baby of various treatments. These will include the risks of mental illness to the mother, the baby, and other family; the potential risk benefit of treating the mother with certain medications that may affect the baby via breast milk, and fully informing and involving the woman in the decision-making process. The aim of referring to a psychiatrist is to determine whether any psychiatric symptoms are present and to discuss and advise the woman on management and coordinate between midwives, health visitors, social services, and the community mental health team to agree a suitable care plan during the postnatal period.

Detection, screening, and prevention

Many mothers under-report their symptoms, either because they misattribute them to the normal consequences of childbirth, or because they feel guilty or embarrassed that they are feeling sad and miserable following the birth of their baby. For many women this is a confusing experience, as the social and cultural pressure to experience childbirth as a happy event is considerable. The diagnosis of postnatal depression can be a relief and a first step to recovery.

All women should be screened for depression at booking, during pregnancy, and at 1 and 3–4 months postpartum using the following two questions recommended by NICE (2007).

- During the past month, have you often been bothered by feeling down, depressed or hopeless?
- During the past month, have you often been bothered by having little interest or pleasure in doing things?
- A third question can be asked if the mother answers yes to either of these questions.
- Is this something you feel you need or want help with?

This should help to identify 'at risk' mothers early on. Specific screening questionnaires can also be used, such as the Edinburgh Postnatal Depression Scale (EPDS), although they are not essential to make a referral. They help identify illness severity, and response to treatment.

Clinical features

- Low mood
- Tearfulness
- Irritability or anxiety
- Low energy or excessive tiredness

- Lack of ability to enjoy things (anhedonia)
- Biological symptoms, including poor sleep, loss of appetite, and weight loss
- Cognitive symptoms, including hopelessness, low self-esteem, guilt, suicidal ideation.

Postnatal depression can present with quite specific features centring on motherhood and the baby. These can include

- feelings of guilt and inadequacy as a mother
- lack of confidence in mothering ability
- anxieties about the baby's health, sleeping or feeding, despite reassurance that the baby is well
- concern the baby is malformed or someone else's
- excessive feelings of guilt about not feeling 'maternal' towards the baby
- reluctance to feed, hold, or cuddle the baby
- thoughts of suicide, self-harm, or harm to baby.

Some mothers experience difficulty bonding with their baby, and when this happens in the context of postnatal depression it may require attention in its own right. Long-term failures of attachment can have adverse consequences for the baby.

About half of all cases of postnatal depression are missed because family or healthcare professionals assume it is only 'baby blues' and will settle. These two conditions share the same clinical features but differences between the two are discussed below.

Differences between baby blues and postnatal depression

Baby blues

- Onset around 3 days postpartum
- Incidence of up to 8 out of 10 mothers.
- Duration of 2–5 days: self-limiting.

Clinical features

- Anxiety, low mood, tearfulness, emotional lability, irritability, and confusion.

Aetiology

- Hormonal changes in oestrogen, progesterone, and prolactin are thought to be implicated because of the close temporal link between childbirth with the onset of baby blues. These affect central neurotransmission and are also associated with mood changes at other times of physiological change in premenstrual and perimenopausal women.

Treatment

- The majority of women who deliver a baby will experience baby blues. This is self-limiting and does not require any medication. It should settle spontaneously within a few days with support and reassurance from partner, family, and midwife.
- If symptoms persist after the first week after delivery and appear to be worsening, it is important to consider postnatal depression.

Postnatal depression

- Onset within 2–6 weeks postpartum
- Incidence of 1 in 10 mothers.
- Duration of weeks to months, and longer if untreated.

Aetiology

The aetiology of postnatal depression is multifactorial with physical, psychological, and social risk factors implicated.

Physical

There are possible links with obstetric factors, e.g. traumatic delivery, poor pain relief, sleep deprivation, being hospitalized

Psychological

- Family history of mental illness
- Past psychiatric history of depression unrelated to childbirth
- Previous postnatal depression (risk of recurrence is 1 in 4 in subsequent pregnancies)
- Personality factors, e.g. anxiety traits.

Social

- Poor relationship with partner
- No partner
- Poor parental relationships
- Loss of a parent at a young age
- Lack of social network, friends, extended family
- Financial or housing worries and uncertainties.

History: key points

- Current presenting symptoms. Screen for affective symptoms (low or elated mood, tearfulness, low or increased energy, sleep disturbance, anhedonia, amotivation) and psychotic symptoms (auditory hallucinations, delusions, thought disorder).
- Screen for suicidal ideation and any thoughts of harming baby.
- Past psychiatric history: first contact with psychiatric services, any history of medications taken before or during pregnancy, any history of self-harm or suicide attempts, admissions to hospital with a mental health problem, particularly if under a section of the Mental Health Act (2007).
- Medication history. What medications is the patient currently taking? What medications have they been on prior to the pregnancy and when did these stop?
- Family history to identify any history of mental disorder
- Enquire about past or current substance misuse and alcohol use.

Examination: key points

- Ensure a thorough physical examination has been done to rule out physical causes for psychiatric symptoms.
- Perinatal psychiatry opinion to confirm diagnosis by detailed mental state examination.
- Appearance and behaviour: any evidence of poor eye contact and rapport, poor self-care?
- Speech: increased/reduced rate, rhythm, volume, content?
- Mood changes: how does the patient describe their mood?
- Thoughts: any self-harm or suicidal ideas, plans or intention? Any distressing guilty ideas or paranoid thoughts?
- Perceptions: any experiences of seeing or hearing things when alone that others cannot see, hear, or accept?
- Cognition: is concentration or memory impaired? Orientation to time, place, person?

- Insight: does the patient feel they are physically or mentally unwell? Do they wish to accept treatment and if required come into hospital?

Special investigations

- Exclude other possible causes of psychiatric symptoms such as a 'hidden' organic problem such as anaemia, gestational diabetes, thyroid disease or iatrogenic causes such as steroids.
- Consider blood tests to exclude physical conditions (FBC, WBC, U&E, LFTs, TFTs, glucose)
- Consider blood serum levels of medication to check if levels are therapeutic, e.g. lithium level.

Treatment

Treatment may include psychological or biological interventions, and admission to a specialist Mother and Baby Unit may be necessary in severe cases where there is a high risk to mother or baby.

Psychological

In mild to moderate cases psychological support with guided self-help, supportive counselling or cognitive behaviour therapy (CBT) can be helpful. CBT involves a fixed number of sessions with a psychologist and structured work on the mother's thoughts, actions, and feelings.

Biological

In more severe cases additional treatment with antidepressant medication is warranted. The specific choice of medication depends on whether the woman chooses to breastfeed and every effort should be encouraged for her to breastfeed if she wishes.

When choosing an antidepressant for a breastfeeding woman, NICE 2007 guidelines advise that

- tricyclics (TCAs) and the serotonin selective reuptake inhibitor (SSRI) sertraline are present in breast milk at relatively low levels.
- the SSRIs citalopram and fluoxetine are present in breast milk in relatively high levels
- all antidepressants carry the risk of withdrawal or toxicity in neonate. These are usually mild and self-limiting.

Although most medications can enter the breast milk in small quantities, antidepressant drugs with low excretion such as imipramine, nortriptiline, and sertraline may be preferred. Sertraline 50–200 mg po od is effective and well tolerated. The timing of this can be adjusted to avoid most of the drug entering the breast milk, e.g. the dose can be taken at night after the last evening feed and before the baby's longest sleep.

With proper treatment under specialist supervision, postnatal depression usually resolves quickly and the woman is able to make a complete recovery. Most cases can be managed in the community with regular review.

However, in severe cases where there is a high risk, admission to a Mother and Baby unit is advisable to provide specialist care and preserve the attachment between mother and baby while she recovers. A mother may be more willing to accept voluntary admission to hospital if her baby can stay with her. If there is a high suicide risk or dangerous self-neglect (mother not eating or drinking) then electroconvulsive therapy (ECT) should be considered, as this can work quickly to relieve these life-threatening symptoms. If there is a high risk of harm to the mother or baby and she is unwilling to accept voluntary admission to hospital for treatment, she may need to be admitted under a section of the Mental Health Act (2007).

Untreated postnatal depression carries high morbidity and mortality, with suicide being a leading cause of maternal death in the UK (CEMACH 2007). The long-term inability of a mother to interact emotionally with her baby due to untreated depression can lead to abnormal cognitive and emotional development in the child (Nicholls *et al* 1999). Women who have had postnatal depression previously have a 1 in 4 chance of having a relapse after future deliveries and early referral to a perinatal psychiatrist and close monitoring is advised in the postnatal period after future deliveries.

Further reading

Confidential Enquiry into Maternal and Child Health (CEMACH). Saving mothers lives: reviewing maternal deaths to make motherhood safer (2003–2007). London: CEMACH 2007.

Cox JL, Connor YM, *et al*. Prospective study of the psychiatric disorders of childbirth. Br J Psychiatry 1982;140:111–7.

Davies A, McIvor R, *et al*. Impact of childbirth on a series of schizophrenic mothers. Schizophrenia Res 1995;16:25–31.

NICE Clinical guideline 45. Antenatal and postnatal mental health National Institute of Clinical Excellence Feb 2007.

Nicholls KR, Cox JL. The provision of care for women with postnatal mental disorder in the UK: an overview. HK Med J 1999;43–7.

Oates M. Perinatal psychiatric disorders: a leading cause of maternal morbidity and mortality. Br Med Bull 2003;67:219–29.

Oates M. Perinatal Maternal Mental Health Services. Royal College of Psychiatrists Council report CR88 April 2000.

Patient resources

Support group: The Royal College of Psychiatrists website has a useful information leaflet: www.rcpsych.ac.uk/pnd

Mind: www.mind.org.uk and www.pni.org.uk.

The association for postnatal illness (APNI): www.apni.org

Meet-a-mum association (MAMA): www.mama.co.uk

Puerperal psychosis

Presentation

Puerperal psychosis presents following 1 in 500 births. Onset is rapid and usually within a few days of delivery. The majority of cases are episodes of bipolar disorder triggered by childbirth in individuals who either have a history of bipolar disorder or an underlying vulnerability to bipolar disorder. Schizophrenia and psychotic depression can present as puerperal psychosis, although less commonly. Occasionally acute physical disorders such as infection or metabolic disturbances can also present with psychotic symptoms (hallucinations and delusions) and this possibility always needs to be considered.

Early symptoms of puerperal psychosis include sleep disturbance and confusion. These can be missed or mistaken for baby blues until more florid symptoms develop.

Mood disturbance is common and can include mania (elation, agitation, overarousal, overactivity, and or irritability) or depression, or a rapidly fluctuating combination of the two, a mixed affective state. About three-quarters of cases have a predominance of affective symptoms. Disorientation and perplexity are also relatively common. About one-quarter of cases will present with a more 'schizophrenia-like' picture with a predominance of psychotic symptoms. Delusional content will typically involve the patient's baby, partner, family, or staff and may have a paranoid, grandiose, or religious flavour. Auditory hallucinations are relatively common, and when they are commanding in nature suggest high risk, especially when they involve commands to harm self or baby.

In the majority of cases, puerperal psychosis is severe and requires emergency psychiatric assessment and hospital admission. High levels of unpredictability and impulsivity in the context of a fluctuating mental state suggest high risk.

Aetiology

A number of factors have been associated with an increased risk of developing puerperal psychosis following delivery:
- first birth
- previous psychiatric history (especially of bipolar disorder or puerperal psychosis)
- previous family history (especially bipolar disorder or puerperal psychosis in first-degree relative)
- single mother
- caesarean section
- previous or current perinatal death.

The close temporal relationship to delivery suggests a triggering effect of the rapid postpartum drop in pregnancy hormones, possibly by increasing dopamine sensitivity (Cookson 1982).

Women with a family history of bipolar disorder or puerperal psychosis have a higher risk of developing puerperal psychosis themselves. Women with a personal history of bipolar disorder have up to a 1 in 2 risk of a puerperal relapse if they do not receive appropriate treatment.

All women presenting for booking should be asked if they have any past or present mental health problems, any history of contact with a psychiatrist or specialist mental health team, or any family history of severe mental disorder, especially a family history of bipolar disorder or puerperal psychosis.

A thorough history and mental state examination is required, including an assessment of risk of suicide, self-harm, and harm to the baby.

Clinical approach

History: key points
- Current presenting symptoms: screen for affective symptoms (low or elated mood, irritability or hostility, tearfulness, low or increased energy, sleep disturbance) and psychotic symptoms (auditory hallucinations, delusions, thought disorder).
- Past psychiatric history: ask about first contact with psychiatric services, any history of medications taken before or during pregnancy, any history of self harm or suicide attempts, admissions to hospital with a mental health problem, particularly if under a section of the Mental Health Act (2007).
- Medication history: what medication is the patient currently taking? What medications have they been on prior to the pregnancy, and when did these stop?
- Family history: look for evidence of psychiatric illness, particularly in first-degree relatives.
- Enquire about past or current substance misuse and alcohol use.

Examination: key points
- Ensure a thorough physical examination has been done to rule out physical causes for psychiatric symptoms.
- Refer for a perinatal psychiatry or liaison psychiatry opinion to confirm diagnosis by detailed mental state examination.
- Appearance and behaviour: any evidence of poor eye contact and rapport, poor self-care? Are they distractible, confused, or unable to respond appropriately to questions?
- Speech: increased/reduced rate, rhythm, volume, content? Are they speaking very fast (pressure of speech)?
- Mood changes: how does the patient describe their mood? Do they seem elated or irritable? Is their mood labile?
- Thoughts: any self-harm or suicidal ideas, plans, or intention? Any distressing guilty ideas or delusional ideas with a paranoid, grandiose, or religious theme? Any changes to the form or flow of thought (e.g. flight of ideas)?
- Perceptions: any experiences of seeing or hearing things when alone that others cannot see, hear, or accept? Does the woman hear voices even if they are alone? What do the voices say? Do they command the woman to do things? Do they comment on the baby? Does the woman feel in control of her actions, feelings, and thoughts?
- Cognition: is there any impairment in concentration or memory? Orientation to time, place, person?
- Insight: does the patient feel they are physically or mentally unwell? Do they wish to accept treatment and if required come into hospital?

Special investigations
- Exclude other possible causes of psychiatric symptoms such as a 'hidden' organic problem such as anaemia, gestational diabetes, thyroid disease, or iatrogenic causes such as steroids.

- Consider blood tests to exclude organic conditions (FBC, WBC, U&E, LFTs, TFTs, glucose)
- Consider blood serum levels of medication to check if levels are therapeutic, e.g. lithium level.
- Consider if CT/MRI brain scan required to rule out organic pathology, e.g. brain tumour.

Treatment

This condition should be considered a psychiatric emergency due to the potential risk to the mother and baby. The associated suicide rate is in the order of 5% (Knops, 1993) and the infanticide rate is up to 4% (Altshuler et al., 1998).

The management of puerperal psychosis involves considering the risks of mental illness to the mother, the baby, and other family; the potential risk benefit of treating the mother with certain medications that may affect the baby via breast milk and fully informing and involving the woman in the decision-making process as far as possible while she is psychotic. The aim of referring to a perinatal psychiatrist is to determine the nature and degree of any psychiatric symptoms present and to discuss and advise the woman or team on the most appropriate management and coordinate between midwives, health visitors, social services, and the community mental health team to agree a suitable care plan during the postnatal period.

In those with symptoms, there is a 35 times increased risk of hospital admission for a psychotic illness within the first month of delivering a baby, (Kendell et al., 1987). In these cases, admission to a Mother and Baby unit is advisable to provide specialist care and preserve the bonding between mother and baby while she recovers. A mother may be more willing to accept voluntary admission to hospital if her baby can stay with her. If there is a high suicide risk or dangerous self-neglect (mother not eating or drinking) then electroconvulsive therapy (ECT) should be considered as this can work quickly to relieve these life-threatening symptoms. If there is a high risk of harm to the mother or baby and she is unwilling to accept voluntary admission to hospital for treatment, she may need to be admitted under a Section of the Mental Health Act (2007).

Antipsychotic or mood stabilizing medications can be used to relieve symptoms such as hallucinations, delusions, and affective disturbance. The choice of medication will depend upon individual patient circumstances and advice should be sought from a psychiatrist with special expertise in treating perinatal mental disorders. Agitation can be relieved using a short-acting low-dose benzodiazepine such as lorazepam 1–2 mg po as required. When prescribing a drug consider (NICE 2007)

- monotherapy over combination treatment
- treatment options that can allow the women to breast-feed if she wishes and is well enough to do so.

Prognosis

With treatment the majority of mothers make a good recovery and return home within a few weeks.

However, there is around a 1 in 2 chance of having a relapse after subsequent deliveries. The 10-year recurrence rate is up to 80% (Garfield et al., 2004).

A significant proportion of women who experience puerperal psychosis will also go on to develop bipolar affective disorder later in life (1 in 4).

References

Altshuler LL, Hendrick V, Cohen LS. Course of mood and anxiety disorders during pregnancy and the postpartum period. J Clin Psych 1998;59(Supp 2):29–33.

Confidential Enquiry into Maternal and Child Health (CEMACH). Saving mothers lives: reviewing maternal deaths to make motherhood safer (2003–2007). Dec 2007.

Cookson JC. Post-partum mania, dopamine and oestrogens. Lancet 1982;ii:672.

Cox JL. Connor YM, Kendell RE. Prospective study of the psychiatric disorders of childbirth. Br J Psychiatry 1982;140:111–7.

Davies A, McIvor R, Kumor RC. Impact of childbirth on a series of schizophrenic mothers. Schizophrenia Res 1995;16:25–31.

Garfield P, Kent A, Paykel ES, et al. Outcome of postpartum disorders: a 10 year follow-up of hospital admissions. Acta Psychiatr Scand 2004;109:434–9.

Kendell RE, Chalmers JC, Platz C. Epidemiology of puerperal psychoses. Br J Psychiatry 1987;150:662–73.

Knops GG. Postpartum mood disorders. A startling contrast to the joy of birth. Postgrad Med 1993;103–4.

NICE Clinical guideline 45. Antenatal and postnatal mental health National Institute of Clinical Excellence Feb 2007.

Nicholls KR. Cox JL. The provision of care for women with postnatal mental disorder in the UK: an overview. HK Med J 1999;43–7.

Oates M. Perinatal psychiatric disorders: a leading cause of maternal morbidity and mortality. Br Med Bull 2003;67:219–29.

Oates M. Perinatal Maternal Mental Health Services. Royal College of Psychiatrists Council report CR88 April 2000.

Patient resources

The Royal College of Psychiatrists: www.rcpsych.ac.uk/pnd
Mind: www.mind.org.uk and www.pni.org.uk.

Pre-eclampsia and eclampsia

Definitions

Pre-eclampsia is a multisystem disease of pregnancy defined clinically by pregnancy-induced hypertension (blood pressure (BP) of >140/90 mmHg on two occasions 4 hours apart, or one reading of >170/110 mmHg) and proteinuria (>0.3 g/24 hours) after 20 weeks' gestation.

Severe pre-eclampsia occurs with BP ≥170/110 on two occasions along with significant proteinuria (>1 g in 24 hours). Clinical features of severe pre-eclampsia may be apparent at BP <170/110.

HELLP syndrome is considered a complication of severe pre-eclampsia and is characterized by haemolysis (microangiopathic haemolytic anaemia), elevated liver enzymes (secondary to parenchymal necrosis), and low platelets (consumption).

Eclampsia is defined as the occurrence of convulsions superimposed on pre-eclampsia. Convulsions in pregnancy should be treated as eclampsia unless proven otherwise.

Epidemiology

Pre-eclampsia affects 2–3% of pregnancies. The disease is the second most common cause of maternal death in the developing world and accounts for at least 50 000 maternal deaths per year worldwide. The incidence of the disease varies according to the population studied and rates in Latin America are much higher. In developed countries it is perinatal rather than maternal mortality that is frequently the problem, and PE is the commonest cause of iatrogenic prematurity. In addition, it frequently coexists with fetal growth restriction (FGR) and placental abruption, other important causes of adverse perinatal outcome.

HELLP affects 20% of pregnancies complicated with severe pre-eclampsia (with 15% presenting in second trimester, 50% in the third trimester, and 35% postpartum).

Eclampsia complicates ~1 in 2000 pregnancies (1–2% of pre-eclampsia cases) with one-third occurring postpartum, the highest risk being the first 24–48 hours; 3% of cases will also develop HELLP.

Pathology

The aetiology of pre-eclampsia is unknown.

In early pregnancy the extravillious trophoblast invades the uterine spiral arteries transforming them from thick-walled muscular vessels to wider diameter thin-walled vessels of low resistance. This process is complete by 20–24 weeks. In women with pre-eclampsia there is failure of normal trophoblastic invasion of the myometrial spiral arteries causing them to maintain their thick wall and high resistance.

This reduction in uteroplacental perfusion and relative placental hypoxia leads to oxidative stress and there is release of antiangiogenic and other factors into the maternal circulation. The resultant vasoconstriction causes hypertension and endothelial damage leading to loss of protein from the intravascular space. This mechanism forms the common basis of the developing maternal syndrome affecting multiple systems including renal, hepatic, haematological, and cerebrovascular.

Aetiology

There is an increased chance of developing pre-eclampsia in cases of
- primigravidity
- multigravidity with a long interpregnancy interval or new partner
- previous history of pre-eclampsia
- extremes of age
- family history (increased incidence if mother and sisters affected)
- ethnic origin (more common among Africans)
- increased body mass index
- essential hypertension
- Pre-existing renal disease, diabetes mellitus, or systemic lupus erythematosus
- antiphospholipid syndrome and inherited thrombophilia
- abnormal uterine artery Doppler flow at midgestation.

Prognosis

Pre-eclampsia is the second most common cause of maternal deaths. In the UK, 18 women died from severe pre-eclampsia and its complications in the 2003–5 Confidential Enquiry. The commonest cause of substandard care is failure of antihypertensive therapy.

With HELLP, maternal mortality is 1%. Serious complications include renal failure, abruption, DIC, and pulmonary oedema. Fetal mortality rates range from 7.7% to 60%, depending on gestation at birth.

With eclampsia, maternal mortality is 1%. Serious complications include acute renal failure, which is reversible (4%), DIC (3%), aspiration/RDS (3%), intracranial haemorrhage/transient blindness, and fetal bradycardia.

Clinical approach

Diagnosis

History

Presentation can range from asymptomatic, raised BP, and proteinuria detected on routine antenatal screening, to a combination of symptoms and signs of varying severity, including
- headache, visual disturbance, epigastric and/or right upper quadrant pain
- worsening peripheral and periorbital oedema
- nausea and vomiting,
- feeling generally unwell with flu-like symptoms
- reduced fetal movements
- abdominal pain and bleeding (due to an abruption)
- evidence of cerebrovascular accidents.

In HELLP syndrome symptoms most commonly reported are epigastric pain and right upper quadrant tenderness (65%). In addition, haematuria may be reported.

In eclampsia there is a history of seizures (in the absence of known epilepsy) and postictal confusion.

Examination

BP should be checked more than once. Oedema is not necessary for the diagnosis of pre-eclampsia, but worsening facial or sacral oedema persisting after rest is significant. Mothers with pre-eclampsia may be small for dates on routine clinical palpation.

In case of severe PET there may be epigastric and right upper quadrant tenderness. Tenderness over the liver and jaundice may be signs of HELLP. Look for evidence of disseminated intravascular coagulation. Chest examination and pulse oximetry may reveal signs of pulmonary oedema.

Clonus ≥3 beats is associated with cerebral irritation, and fundoscopy may reveal papilloedema. Although checking the deep tendon reflexes has become a part of the routine clinical examination of pre-eclamptic women, the predictive value of brisk reflexes is uncertain.

With eclampsia, grand mal generalized clonic seizures will be present. It is worth noting that 20% of women are normotensive at presentation.

Investigations
Urine tests

- Urinalysis indicating ≥ +2 protein on urine dipstick is significant and quantitative measurement should follow.
- Send an MSU to rule out infection as the cause of proteinuria.
- A 24-hour urine collection for protein is the 'gold standard' quantitative measurement for proteinuria.
- Protein–creatinine ratio can be performed on a single urine sample.

Blood tests

- FBC: raised haemoglobin and haematocrit due to haemoconcentration or a low haemoglobin due to haemolysis. Platelets may also be low.
- Urea and electrolyte analysis may reveal raised urea and creatinine.
- Liver function tests may show raised transaminases. AST levels greater than 2000 IU/L are associated with disordered mental state, jaundice, and extreme hypertension.
- Urate levels normally equate to gestation (i.e. <0.30 mmol/L at 30 weeks, <0.34 mmol/L at 34 weeks) but are raised in pre-eclampsia.
- Clotting abnormalities need to be excluded if the liver function tests (LFTs) are abnormal and/or the platelets are low in severe pre-eclampsia. DIC complicates HELLP in about 20% cases.

In suspected case of HELLP, also perform
- a peripheral blood film as haemolysis is identified by an abnormal blood film, fragmented red blood cells, and raised reticulocyte count
- lactate dehydrogenase (LDH) is raised in haemolysis (>600 IU/L).

In eclampsia, also measure serum glucose, Ca^{2+} and Mg^{2+}. A toxicology screen will help to identify a differential diagnosis if that of eclampsia is in question.

Radiology

Fetal ultrasound may reveal fetal growth restriction, reduced amniotic fluid, or abnormal fetoplacental Doppler flow.

In suspected HELLP a liver ultrasound may be necessary to exclude a subcapsular haematoma.

In eclampsia, a chest X-ray may be indicated if there is low O_2 saturation or to check for aspiration after a seizure.

CT/MRI head (+/– venous angiography) is indicated if there are focal neurological symptoms or the cause for seizures is uncertain.

Counselling

The unpredictable course of pre-eclampisa and need for close monitoring of both mother and baby should be explained. Knowledge of the potential need for early delivery (with the consequent risks of prematurity and the chosen mode) is central to counselling women. If early delivery is planned, discussion with a neonatologist about what to expect would be appropriate. Prolonged hospital stay pre- and post-delivery may be necessary, which can be distressing to the woman and her family.

Management
General points

Treatment is delivery. The timing will depend on the balance of maternal and fetal wellbeing versus the degree of prematurity. All units should have protocols for the management of women with pre-eclampsia and it is important that those looking after pregnant women know them.

In most units, if pre-eclampsia is confirmed it is managed as an inpatient unless mild and stable. Close monitoring is essential since pre-eclampsia can progress rapidly and unpredictably from mild disease to a severe life-threatening condition.

Women with new-onset pre-eclampsia, those who are symptomatic, have significant hypertension (≥140/90) with ≥2+ protein on urinalysis, haematological/biochemical disturbance or fetal effects should be admitted for further assessment. Initial monitoring should include
- 4-hourly BP measurements (including mean arterial pressure calculation)
- cardiotocography (CTG) twice a day
- 24-hour urine collection for protein
- TED stockings
- daily urinalysis
- ultrasound for fetal size, liquor volume, and umbilical artery Doppler.

The primary major failing in clinical care resulting in death is inadequate treatment of BP with subsequent intracranial haemorrhage. Second, but equally important, is iatrogenic fluid overload and pulmonary oedema.

Specific treatments
Antihypertensives

Antihypertensives control BP but do not stop the disease process of pre-eclampsia. All antihypertensives reduce the risk of severe hypertension in women with mild–moderate pre-eclampsia; however, there is insufficient evidence whether there is a reduction in serious outcomes.

Treatment of hypertension should be considered when diastolic BP measurements are persistently above 105 mmHg or systolic BP is >160 mmHg. Before 28 weeks, consider starting treatment when diastolic BP is >90 mmHg.

Bed rest may be associated with reduced risk of severe hypertension and preterm birth but there is insufficient evidence to advise this.

The main concern with antihypertensive therapy is of reduced placental perfusion and consequent FGR. Sudden drops in BP should be avoided and the aim is to keep the BP >130/80 mmHg. Women on antihypertensives should have serial growth scans to detect FGR.

Angiotensin-converting enzyme (ACE) inhibitors are contraindicated because of fetal effects (oligohydramnios, renal failure, and hypotension). Diuretics should only be used for treatment of pulmonary oedema as they deplete the intravascular volume.

There is no difference in choice of drug.
- Methyldopa: α-agonist with centrally mediated effect inhibiting vasoconstriction has a long half-life and slow onset of action. It is a safe drug supported by many years of experience. There is no evidence of long-term adverse

effects in exposed fetuses. The main adverse effects are maternal drowsiness (with the sedative effect usually resolving after a week) and depression. Administration must be avoided with deranged LFTs. Treatment is initiated with a loading dose, 500–750 mg orally, followed by a maintenance dose between 250 mg bd to 1 g tds.

- Nifedipine: calcium channel blocker that inhibits influx of calcium ions in to vascular smooth muscle causing arterial vasodilatation. There is no evidence of harm to the fetus but safety data are limited compared with methyldopa. Side-effects include headache and facial flushing. Slow-release preparations should be used as standard release is more likely to cause a sudden drop in BP. The initial dose is slow-release 10 mg bd orally, which can be increased to 40 mg bd.
- Adrenoreceptor blockers: these act on the heart, peripheral blood vessels, airway, pancreas, and liver receptors. Labetalol is a combined alpha- and beta-blocker, which in addition to its cardiac effects it lowers peripheral resistance by causing arteriolar vasodilation. Past studies have highlighted the possibility of an increased risk of FGR in those treated with beta-blockers. Side-effects are few but must be avoided in asthmatics. Treatment is commenced with labetalol 100 mg bd orally, increasing to a maximum of 2.4 g per day in three or four divided doses. In management of severe hypertension, it can be administered i.v. as either a bolus or infusion.
- Hydralazine: a vasodilator with a direct relaxing effect on smooth muscle in the blood vessels, predominantly in the arterioles. Mainly used intravenously, as a bolus or infusion, in controlling severe hypertension prior to delivery. Side-effects include maternal tachycardia and further doses should be avoided with a maternal heart rate >120 bpm. Treatment is initiated with an i.v. bolus of 5 mg, which can be repeated every 15 minutes up to a total of 20 mg.

Thromboprophylaxis

While an inpatient, TED stockings should be worn.

Women with significant proteinuria are at an increased risk of thromboembolism and prophylactic low molecular weight heparin should be given.

Fetal monitoring

Maternal perception of fetal movements is a useful crude clinical guide of wellbeing.

In women with pre-eclampsia fortnightly growth US scans should be performed, as pre-eclampsia presenting prior to 36 weeks is associated with a high risk of reduced fetal growth and neonatal morbidity and mortality. If there are concerns, umbilical artery Doppler studies are arranged in the intervening week (see Chapter 7.19, IUGR)

Steroids

If delivery before 34 weeks is anticipated then consider steroids for fetal lung maturity.

Magnesium sulphate

Used in severe pre-eclampsia or eclampsia when delivery has been decided on. It is administered for 24 hours after the last seizure or delivery, whichever is latest. The MAGPIE study demonstrated that, used prophylactically, $MgSO_4$ reduces the risk of convulsions and of abruption regardless of the severity of pre-eclampsia. Side-effects and toxicity include flushing, blurred vision, slurred speech, weakness, somnolence, loss of patellar reflexes, decreased urine output, respiratory and cardiac arrest. If any of these occur or if there are recurrent convulsions, serum levels should be checked.

Treatment of toxicity involves stopping the infusion and administering $Ca^{2}+$ gluconate i.v., 1 g over 3–10 minutes.

Delivery

The decision to deliver includes maternal and fetal aspects of wellbeing. The threshold falls with gestation.

In women who are at or near term, the decision to deliver is easier. In women who are <34 weeks the risks of expectant management (eclampsia, HELLP syndrome, hepatic rupture, abruption, and IUD) have to be weighed against the risks of prematurity. Delivery needs to be considered in women with

- signs/symptoms of severe pre-eclampsia, eclampsia, or HELLP syndrome
- worsening maternal haematological or biochemical disturbance
- more than two antihypertensives needed to control BP
- static fetal growth, reduced fetal movements, oligohydramnios
- abnormal ductus venosus Doppler flow, abnormal fetal biophysical profile or computerized CTG
- end organ damage.

Mode of delivery by labour induction should be preferable.

Mild PET

In asymptomatic women with mildly raised BP not requiring treatment, normal blood results and a normally grown fetus, expectant management is possible. This is in order for the fetus to mature and is justified as long as complications of pre-eclampsia are absent.

Women may be managed as an outpatient with regular review. Most units have a Day Assessment Unit and women can be seen regularly for BP checks, urinalysis, fetal monitoring, and blood tests. Women should be aware of the symptoms and signs of severe pre-eclampsia (headache, blurred vision, vomiting, epigastric discomfort, reduced fetal movements) and must attend when present. If there is change in any clinical parameter or the woman is non-compliant then admission is justified. Close monitoring is essential as mild pre-eclampsia can develop into life-threatening severe pre-eclampsia over a short space of time. Induction of labour at term should be considered, particularly with a favourable cervix.

Moderate/severe PET

Involvement of senior obstetric and anaesthetic staff is essential. Although diastolic BP is a useful marker of severity of pre-eclampsia, it is thought to be the pressure during systole that is more important in causing intracerebral haemorrhage.

Prompt commencement of antihypertensive treatment is essential in women with severe pre-eclampsia and should be administered when BP >160/110 and/or mean arterial pressure (MAP) >125. With MAPs >145 there is loss of cerebral autoregulation with risk of cerebral haemorrhage. BP can drop suddenly with intravenous treatments and cause fetal bradycardia. Therefore, preloading with colloid (up to 500 mL) and continuous fetal monitoring is necessary with parenteral antihypertensives. Hydralazine (i.v. bolus or infusion), labetolol (i.v. bolus or infusion), or nifedipine (orally) are used for the acute management of hypertension. The aim is to maintain a BP of 140–150/80–90 mmHg.

It should be checked every 15 minutes until it is stabilized, then every 30 minutes.

Owing to the risks of fluid overload and pulmonary oedema, input should be restricted to 85 mL/hour including all infusions (oxytocin, antihypertensives, magnesium sulphate). Output needs to be monitored and in the acute situation a catheter with hourly urometer should be used. Oliguria is often seen with severe pre-eclampsia and is defined as a urine output of less than 100 mL/4 hour. Renal failure rarely complicates pre-eclampsia and in most cases diuresis occurs postpartum.

An initial 500-mL bolus of colloid can be given if necessary. However, further fluid replacement may need to be guided by invasive monitoring (central venous pressure (CVP) line), particularly in the presence of acute blood loss.

Continuous pulse oximetry will help to detect early pulmonary oedema.

In women who are at risk of seizures, particularly with CNS symptoms (severe headache, agitation, clonus), $MgSO_4$ should be administered. O_2 saturation, respiratory rate, urine output, and deep tendon reflexes should be checked hourly to monitor for toxicity.

Once BP is controlled in women with severe pre-eclampsia, delivery needs to be considered. Individual circumstances will dictate whether delivery can be delayed for the administration of steroids in preterm gestations. Conservative management at very early gestations may improve neonatal outcome but this needs to be balanced against maternal wellbeing. The mode of delivery will depend on gestation, maternal and fetal wellbeing. If <32 weeks, vaginal delivery is less successful but still worth considering. If >34 weeks, the chance of a vaginal delivery is up to 65%.

Syntocinon should be given for the third stage. Products containing ergometrine should be avoided due to the risk of further hypertension.

HELLP syndrome

The management of HELLP syndrome follows that of severe pre-eclampsia focusing on the correction of coagulation disorders and platelet levels. Involving a haematologist early is essential. Platelet transfusion is considered when the platelet count is <20 × 10⁹/L or when platelets <50 × 10⁹/L and procedure such as Caesarean section or CVP insertion is needed.

If <34 weeks, administer steroids to improve fetal lung maturity and the severity of HELLP will dictate whether delivery can be delayed for 24 hours for optimal effect. This could potentially avoid the need for general anaesthetic for Caesarean section delivery in those with an initial platelet count <80 × 10⁹/L.

If >34 weeks vaginal delivery can be attempted. However, in severe cases, delivery by Caesarean section may be warranted independent of gestation.

Regional anaesthesia is contraindicated with abnormal clotting and platelet count <80 × 10⁹/L. IM analgesia should be avoided with platelet counts <80 × 10⁹/L

Strict fluid balance is essential and a CVP line may be required. Acute renal failure is a significant complication of HELLP syndrome secondary to acute tubular necrosis.

$MgSO_4$ should be administered since eclampsia is more often seen with HELLP than severe pre-eclampsia.

Subcapsular liver haematoma can form in association with severe parenchymal necrosis leading to stretching of the capsule, which can eventually rupture. If suspected, the surgical team should be involved to decide on conservative or surgical management.

HELLP can deteriorate within the first 48 hours of delivery; therefore, monitor closely. Red cell transfusion may be needed in cases of continued haemolysis.

Eclampsia

Involvement of consultant obstetricians and anaesthetists or ITU specialists early in the management is essential. $MgSO_4$ is the anticonvulsant of choice in eclampsia and severe pre-eclampsia. It reduces the risk of recurrent seizures, maternal mortality, pneumonia, admission to ITU, baby death, or admission to the special care baby unit. It is far more effective and safe than phenytoin or diazepam. The recurrence risk is 5–20%. In such instances, serum levels should be checked and a further bolus of 2 g of $MgSO_4$ (4 g if >70 kg) can be given. If despite the further bolus and therapeutic levels there are repeated seizures, Diazepam 10 mg i.v. or a thiopentone infusion 50 mg i.v. can be administered. In extreme situations, intubation, IPPV, and muscle relaxation may be necessary.

The choice of antihypertensive should depend on local protocols and the clinicians' experience. Labetalol orally or i.v. or nifedipine orally are first-line treatments. Hydralazine i.v. can be used but has more side-effects. Each unit should have an 'eclampsia box' with the necessary medications.

Fluid restriction (1 mL/kg/hour or 85 mL/hour) and central monitoring is essential for the careful monitoring of fluid balance to avoid the serious consequences of fluid overload.

Delivery should occur after stabilization if more than 34 weeks. If <34 weeks, steroids should be given if the condition is stable. Vaginal delivery is preferable, but feasibility depends on fetal condition, presentation, and cervical favourability.

After the acute phase, thromboprophylaxis, documentation, and close monitoring are very important.

Ergometrine must be avoided for the third stage. For the treatment of massive haemorrhage, however, ergometrine can still be used, especially if the patient is shocked and other medications are unavailable.

The case should be reported to the UKOSS (UK obstetric surveillance study).

Postpartum

All women diagnosed with PET should be reviewed before discharge. Strict fluid balance and BP control should be maintained.

BP tends to fall initially. However, it tends to rise again after 24 hours, and often additional antihypertensive treatment is needed. Avoid methyldopa postnatally because of the risk of postpartum depression. Labetolol, atenolol, nifedipine, and enalapril can be used if breastfeeding.

In women with seizures, these occur postnatally in 44%. Therefore, $MgSO_4$ should be continued for 24 hours postpartum in those at risk. Women with severe pre-eclampsia should remain in hospital because of the risk of seizures, which falls after day 4.

On discharge, arrangements for regular BP checks should be made. Antihypertensives should be reduced as needed and a follow-up arranged.

Follow-up

A postnatal review should be offered to discuss events surrounding the delivery as well as advice for future pregnancies. BP and urine should be checked at the

6-week postnatal check to ensure that hypertension and proteinuria have resolved; 10–20% of women with previous pre-eclampsia will develop it again in subsequent pregnancies. If they had HELLP syndrome, there is a recurrence risk of 3–27% for HELLP and 42% risk of any degree of pre-eclampsia or eclampsia.

Future pregnancy planning

In future pregnancies, uterine artery Dopplers at 20–24 weeks are useful to counsel at-risk women. Elevated indices or bilateral notches suggest increased resistance and increased risk of pre-eclampsia, FGR and placental abruption, while normal indices reduce this risk.

A Cochrane review has shown that antenatal aspirin provides a small to moderate benefit when used for the prevention of pre-eclampsia (15% reduction in the risk of PET, 8% reduction in the risk of delivery before 37 weeks, 14% reduction in the risk of stillbirth, neonatal/infant death). The greatest reduction of risk was observed in those taking >75 mg aspirin/day; however, the subgroups were small and the reassurance about safety of aspirin in pregnancy applies mainly to lower doses.

Further reading

Abalos E, Duley L, Steyn DW, Henderson-Smart DJ. Antihypertensive drug therapy for mild to moderate hypertension during pregnancy. Cochrane Database Syst Rev 2001;2:CD002252.

Altman D, Carroli G, Duley L, et al. Magpie Trial Collaboration Group. Do women with pre-eclampsia, and their babies, benefit from magnesium sulphate? The Magpie Trial: a randomised placebo-controlled trial. Lancet. 2002;359:1877–90.

Askie LM, Duley L, Henderson-Smart DJ, Stewart LA; PARIS Collaborative Group. Antiplatelet agents for prevention of pre-eclampsia: a meta-analysis of individual patient data. Lancet 2007;369:1791–8.

Catanzarite VA, Steinberg SM, Mosley CA, et al. Severe preeclampsia with fulminant and extreme elevation of aspartate aminotransferase and lactate dehydrogenase levels: high risk for maternal death. Am J Perinatol 1995;12:310–3.

Davison J, Baylis C. Renal disease. In: de Swiet M (ed) Medical disorders in obstetric practice, 3rd edn. Oxford: Blackwell Science 1995: 226–305.

Duley L, Henderson-Smart DJ, Knight M, King JF. Antiplatelet agents for preventing pre-eclampsia and its complications. Cochrane Database Syst Rev 2004;1:CD004659.

Girling JC, Dow E, Smith JH. Liver function tests in pre-eclampsia: importance of comparison with a reference range derived for normal pregnancy. Br J Obstet Gynaecol 1997;104:246–50.

Magee LA, Duley L. Oral beta-blockers for mild to moderate hypertension during pregnancy. Cochrane Database Syst Rev 2003;3:CD002863.

Matchaba P, Moodley J. Corticosteroids for HELLP syndrome in pregnancy. Cochrane Database Syst Rev 2004;:CD002076.

Meher S, Duley L. Rest during pregnancy for preventing pre-eclampsia and its complications in women with normal blood pressure. Cochrane Database Syst Rev 2006;2:CD005939.

PRECOG Evidence used to develop the PRECOG guidelinePRECOG Evidence used to develop the PRECOG guideline. Action on pre-eclampsia. www.apec.org.uk 2004b.

RCOG Green Top Guidelines. Antenatal Corticosteroids to Prevent Respiratory Distress Syndrome. Guideline No. 7. London, RCOG Press, 2004. www.rcog.org.uk

RCOG Green Top Guidelines. The management of severe pre-eclampsia/eclampsia. Guideline No. 10A. London, RCOG Press 2006: www.rcog.org.uk

Royal College of Gynaecologists and Obstetricians. Why mothers die 2003–2005, 7th report. London: RCOG Press www.cemach.org.uk

Rumbold AR, Crowther CA, Haslam RR, et al. ACTS Study Group. Vitamins C and E and the risks of preeclampsia and perinatal complications. N Engl J Med 2006;354:1796–806.

Sarris I, Bewley S, Agnihotry S (eds). Training in obstetrics and gynaecology. Oxford: Oxford University Press 2009.

Scottish obstetric guidelines and audit project. The management of mild non-proteinuric hypertension in pregnancy. Guideline update, March 2002.

Sibai B, Dekker G, Kupferminc M. Pre-eclampsia. Lancet 2005; 365:785–99.

Sullivan CA, Magann EF, Perry KG Jr, et al. The recurrence risk of the syndrome of hemolysis, elevated liver enzymes, and low platelets (HELLP) in subsequent gestations. Am J Obstet Gynecol 1994;171:940–3.

Wilson BJ, Watson MS, Prescott GJ, et al. Hypertensive diseases of pregnancy and risk of hypertension and stroke in later life: results from cohort study. BMJ 2003;326:845.

Yamasmit W, Chaithongwongwatthana S, Charoenvidhya D, et al. Random urinary protein-to-creatinine ratio for prediction of significant proteinuria in women with preeclampsia. J Matern Fetal Neonatal Med 2004;16:275–9.

Internet resources

www.rcog.org.uk
www.cemach.org.uk
www.apec.org.uk

Patient resources

www.patient.co.uk/showdoc/23069028/
www.rcog.org.uk/womens-health/clinical-guidance/pre-eclampsia-what-you-need-know
www.pre-eclampsia.co.uk
www.preeclampsia.org
www.pre-eclampsia-society.org.uk

Premalignant conditions of the genital tract in pregnancy

Definition
Cervical intraepithelial neoplasia (CIN) diagnosed or already known about during pregnancy.

Epidemiology
CIN is relatively common in young women and is present in 1–4% of pregnancies. It is no more common than in the non-pregnant state.

Pathology
The pathology due to HPV acquisition is no different to the non-pregnant state (see Chapter 14.3, Cervical dysplasia and human papillomavirus).

Aetiology
See Chapter 14.3, Cervical dysplasia and human papillomavirus. Pregnancy does not alter the natural history of CIN, despite large changes to the cervix

Clinical approach
History
- May have known CIN
- Asymptomatic and incidental smear finding in the vast majority
- In cases of vaginal bleeding that is *not* due to CIN as it is a preclinical disorder, look for other causes.

Examination
- CIN is not visible on routine speculum examination and requires colposcopy ± cervical biopsy as for non-pregnancy
- Cervical changes due to pregnancy need to be borne in mind when assessing the cervix at colposcopy:
- large transformation zone and ectropion
- cervical oedema
- increased and thickened cervical mucous.

Investigation
Abnormal smears should be referred for colposcopy as when not pregnant. Generally, cervical biopsy is unnecessary.

Clinical features
Pregnancies are unaffected by CIN and vice versa. Women can be reassured that there is no association with obstetric complications.

Management
Should smears be taken in pregnancy?
There is general agreement that
- cervical smears are not taken routinely as part of pregnancy care
- if the pregnancy coincides with their 3-year interval smear and the smear history is normal then preference is for a postnatal smear at 3 months
- if they are significantly over their 3-year interval, a smear should be taken in the second trimester

- if there has been an abnormal smear prior to pregnancy and the smear is due, a smear should be taken in the second trimester.

Abnormal smears
Abnormal smears should always be referred for colposcopy as when not pregnant. The aims of colposcopy in pregnancy are
- colposcopic exclusion of invasive disease
- delay of biopsy or LLETZ (large loop excision of transformation zone) till after delivery.

The rate of cervical cancer in pregnancy is very low and data from retrospective cohort studies support the safety of delay in treatment once invasion is excluded.
- If ≤CIN 1, repeat colposcopy 3 months postpartum.
- If CIN 2/3, repeat colposcopy in third trimester or 3 months postpartum if already in late pregnancy.
- Follow-up postpartum is very important as regression during pregnancy is unlikely.

When should a biopsy be taken?
If invasion is suspected then a diagnostic biopsy is necessary. Choice of biopsy (punch/loop/wedge) is arbitrary but haemorrhage should be anticipated (up to 25%) and managed accordingly.

LLETZ should be considered non-therapeutic as rates of residual disease are very high (at least 50%), i.e. diagnostic only.

Follow-up is therefore essential in all pregnant women with abnormal cytology.

Cervical glandular intraepithelial neoplasia
The management of cervical glandular intraepithelial neoplasia (CGIN) is controversial and difficult even outside of pregnancy. Again abnormal glandular cells should be referred for colposcopy with the aim of excluding invasive disease and delaying biopsy or treatment till 3 months postnatal.

Other premalignant conditions
Vaginal, vulval, and peri-anal intraepithelial neoplasia (VAIN, VIN, and PAIN) are all very rare in pregnancy and should be managed as outside of pregnancy. They are unaffected by pregnancy and vice versa. Excision or definitive treatment can invariably be left till after delivery unless invasive disease is suspected.

Further reading
Douvier S, Filipuzzi L, Sogot P. Management of cervical intra-epithelial neoplasm during pregnancy. Gynecol Obstet Fertil 2003:31:851–5.

NHSCSP publication no 20. April 2004. Colposcopy and Programme Management. Guidelines for the NHS Cervical Screening Programme.

Selleret L, Mathevet P. Precancerous lesions during pregnancy: diagnostic and treatment. J Gynaecol Obstet Biol Repro 2008: 37(Suppl1):S131–8.

Preterm labour

Definition
Preterm delivery (PTD) is the birth of a viable fetus before 37 completed weeks (or 259 days) of gestation. Spontaneous preterm labour is the precursor of one-third of all PTD. A further third of preterm births follow preterm prelabour rupture of membranes and the rest are medically indicated.

Epidemiology and importance
The worldwide incidence of PTD ranges between 5% and 13%. In the developed economies there is evidence of an increasing trend of PTD during the last decade, attributed to higher order pregnancies resulting from assisted conception techniques. A further contributor is the greater willingness of modern obstetricians to 'rescue/salvage' fetuses at earlier gestations. There is a marked racial disparity in the incidence of preterm delivery. In the USA, 8.8% of White and 18.9% of Black births occur before 37 completed weeks.

Preterm births account for more than 75% of perinatal mortality in normally formed babies. Infants who survive preterm delivery are at increased risk of subsequent neurodevelopmental deficits and lung disease. Advances in neonatal intensive care have led to an increase in the number of infants that survive PTD. For example, of the 10 241 white singleton babies born weighing less than 1000 g (22–28 weeks of gestation) in the USA during 1960, only 67 (0.65%) survived. Today, babies in this category can expect at least an 80-fold higher rate of survival. Only a reduction in the rate of PTD can be expected to translate to a significant reduction in perinatal mortality and morbidity and in the cost of neonatal care. Unfortunately, modern obstetric care continues to fail on this front because the major contributing pathological processes remain unrecognized and/or untreated, in spite of advances in diagnostics and therapeutics. Without a greater understanding of these underlying factors, there is very little chance of progress towards the prevention of PTD.

The cost of acute hospital care for preterm infants in the UK is approximately £35 000 per infant. Among neonates born ≤28 completed weeks of gestation, this is estimated to be £500 000. In the USA, the current annual cost of care of premature babies by March of Dimes is $26.2 billion. After discharge from hospital, the healthcare and social services continue to incur substantial costs for their special needs, education, and long-term disability. These cost estimates exclude the hidden costs of disruption to family life, emotional and psychological stress, childcare costs for existing children, transportation to and from the hospital, and loss of earnings on the part of the parents. For infants weighing less than 900 g, cost–benefit analyses studies indicate that the total costs per survivor are in excess of the total average lifetime earnings per survivor.

Clinical assessment
The clinical diagnosis of preterm labour is unreliable. A policy of intervention with the onset of uterine activity prior to changes in the cervix exposes many women to unnecessary and potentially harmful treatment. On the other hand, withholding treatment until clinical evidence of cervical change may result in late institution of essential treatment. At present there are no sensitive and specific tests capable of predicting preterm labour and none of the currently available interventions, including tocolysis, antibiotic therapy, bed rest, and cervical cerclage, has been shown conclusively to prevent PTD and improve perinatal outcome. These approaches are reactive and ineffective against a process that is driven by a cascade mechanism.

A detailed and comprehensive history is a useful adjunct to the assessment of the risk of PTD. Prior history of spontaneous PTD or second trimester miscarriage suggests a significantly increased risk of recurrence. The magnitude of this risk is directly related to the number of prior PTD or late miscarriage, and the outcome of the immediate preceding pregnancy (Table 9.12.1). Prior history is, however, of no value in women in their first pregnancy. Other factors include history of cervical surgery for CIN disease, late terminations of pregnancy, collagen diseases, lupus anticoagulant, current multifetal gestation, stressful lifestyle/occupation, use of recreational drugs, and history of urinary tract infections. Yet, over 50% of women with PTD display no identifiable clinical risk factors. Evidence has now accumulated that at least 70% of 'idiopathic spontaneous preterm labour' is attributable to subclinical genital tract infections, mostly atypical micro-organisms such as *Mycoplasma hominis*, *Ureaplasma urealyticum*, anaerobic species, and a host of other subpathogenic organisms associated with bacterial vaginosis. These organisms are non-pyrogenic and not easily detected on conventional microbiological techniques. Clinical assessments including bedside tests and microbiological investigations may therefore be falsely reassuring and misleading.

There may be uterine activity or irritability, sometimes only evident on the tocometer. The maternal heart should be auscultated to exclude obvious cardiac murmurs. These women are candidate recipients of combinations of corticosteroid and vasoactive tocolytic agents with a risk of cardiac failure and pulmonary oedema. The presence of pyrexia, uterine irritability, or tenderness associated with leucocytosis or fetomaternal tachycardia suggests clinical chorioamnionitis. There may be offensive vaginal discharge. Clinical chorioamnionitis is, however, present in only 12% of women with proven intra-amniotic infection. Vaginal examination is essential to exclude rupture of fetal membranes, assess the state of the cervix, obtain cervicovaginal samples for sexually transmitted pathogens and group B Streptococcus (GBS). For optimal detection of GBS colonization, samples should be obtained from the lower third of the vagina, incorporating a perineal sweep and rectal or peri-anal samples. This is then placed in a transport medium and transported rapidly to the laboratory for plating. Failure to follow these steps results in failure to detect as much as 65% of cases of GBS colonization. Bedsides urine tests for protein, leucocytes and nitrites should be performed and antibiotic therapy commenced if there is suspicion of urinary tract infection. This should take cognisance of the most likely pathogen in the local population and subsequently reviewed with sensitivity results.

About one-third of the cervix is supravaginal and inaccessible to the examining fingers. Furthermore, the process of cervical effacement and dilatation starts at the internal os and may not be observed by speculum-assisted visualization of the cervix or digital palpation. If the facilities and expertise are available, transvaginal sonographic examination of the cervix may help to refine the risk of progression to PTD. An inverse correlation exists between

Table 9.12.1 Risk of preterm delivery based on prior pregnancy outcome (Hoffman 1995)

First pregnancy	Second pregnancy	Third pregnancy	RR
Term	4.4%		1.0
Preterm	17.2%		3.0
Term	Term	2.6%	0.6
Preterm	Term	5.7%	1.3
Term	Preterm	11.1%	2.5
Preterm	Preterm	28.4%	6.5

cervical length and the risk of PTD. Between 24 and 28 weeks' gestation, cervical length less than 2.5 cm is associated with a 6–10-fold increase in the risk of PTD. Fetal presentation should be confirmed also, as the accuracy of clinical determination decreases with early gestational age. Estimation of fetal weight and amniotic fluid can be made. Application of Doppler waveform analysis may assist in distinguishing the growth-restricted preterm fetus from its appropriately grown counterpart. Occasionally, an unsuspected abruption or fetal anomaly may be diagnosed.

Principles of management

Optimal neonatal services

The availability of specialist personnel, equipped for and skilled in advanced neonatal resuscitation with round the clock capability for ventilation of the very premature infant and back up laboratory services, is essential in ensuring good neonatal outcome. Neonatal survival rates including intact survival are much higher in such centres than in relatively less well equipped and staffed units. Unfortunately, this level of care is neither available nor sustainable in all obstetric units. The current practice of transferring women at risk of PTD to regional units involves relocation of mother and baby to centres far away from home with further disruption to family life. There are knock-on implications also for the training of resident obstetricians working in the transferring hospitals.

Corticosteroids

Antenatal maternal steroid injection at ≤32 weeks gestation is associated with a 60% reduction in the risk of respiratory distress syndrome, 30–40% reduction in the risk of major intraventricular haemorrhage and necrotizing enterocolitis. These beneficial effects act synergistically to produce an overall reduction in perinatal morbidity and mortality. The corticosteroid of choice supported by published evidence is betamethasone 12 mg given intramuscularly in two doses, 24 hours apart. Weekly antenatal steroid administration to maintain these beneficial effects should be discouraged, as there are no data at present to support its use in this way. Moreover, evidence from experimental animal studies document a host of harmful effects associated with weekly steroid administration, including altered central nervous system development, impaired growth/low birthweight, necrotizing enterocolitis, placental abnormalities, adrenal suppression, and precipitation of maternal diabetes.

Tocolysis

Tocolysis as a sole intervention does not improve neonatal outcome nor significantly delay preterm birth. On the other hand, it may be associated with significant fetomaternal morbidity and mortality. It is therefore reasonable not to use tocolysis if the risks are judged to outweigh the benefits. The current accepted indications for the use of tocolysis include delaying delivery for 24–48 hours to initiate or complete corticosteroid administration, or for administered steroids to take effect, controlling uterine activity during in utero transfer to other units for gestations <32 weeks. Tocolysis is contraindicated in advanced labour, placental abruption, chorioamnionitis, and known sensitivity to the tocolytic agent. The efficacy of the available tocolytic agents is comparable. The β-sympathomimetic drugs are associated with marked cardiovascular and occasionally life-threatening side-effects. This unfavourable side-effect profile has raised the profile of the more patient-friendly, albeit more expensive, oxytocin receptor antagonist atosiban as the tocolytic of first choice. Calcium channel antagonist are marginally superior to the β-agonists in terms of efficacy, can be administered orally, and have fewer maternal side-effects, but in the UK are not licensed for this indication. Other alternatives include prostaglandin synthase inhibitors such as indomethacin and topical glycerine trinitrate (GTN). Indomethacin use is associated with premature closure of the ductus arteriosus, cerebral and renal vasospasm, and necrotizing enterocolitis. Except for mild to moderate headaches, GTN has no other significant side-effect, but the evidence base supporting its use is very slim.

Antibiotic administration

In women presenting with preterm labour with intact membranes, studies of amniotic fluid colonization by microbes suggest a mean colonization rate of approximately 8%, in contrast to 30–40% in women presenting with preterm prelabour rupture of membranes (pPROM). Since the presence of micro-organisms within the choriodecidual space may provoke the onset of preterm labour prior to the invasion of the amniotic cavity, these studies underestimate the role of infection in preterm labour and pPROM. Moreover, the observed incidence of amniotic fluid colonization is likely to be greater if more sensitive DNA amplification-based detection techniques are used. Antibiotic therapy has consistently been shown to be of no benefit in preterm labour with intact membranes and might indeed be harmful in the long term. Intrapartum antibiotic prophylaxis in the form of penicillin G is of proven benefit for the prevention of early-onset group B streptococcal disease in preterm infants.

The role of amniocentesis

The increased recognition of the role of intrauterine infection in the process of pPROM and preterm labour has led to calls for routine amniocentesis and cordocentesis for culture and demonstration of markers of infection/fetal host inflammatory response and to achieve better case selection for antibiotic therapy. At present, there is no evidence that the use of amniocentesis for this indication improves perinatal outcome. It is unknown whether fetal damage has already occurred at the time of presentation and what, if any, intervention could reverse or potentially prevent such damage.

Prediction of preterm delivery

Although PTD is a 'multifactorial' disease associated with potentially avoidable epidemiological risk factors, neither the elimination of each of these risk factors nor the treatment or prediction of the presenting symptoms such as preterm labour, cervical insufficiency, pPROM have been shown to reduce the incidence of PTD. Evidence exists to suggest that chronic pathophysiological events occur prior to the clinical diagnosis of preterm labour or pPROM. Proinflammatory cytokines have been demonstrated in the second trimester amniotic fluid of pregnancies destined for preterm delivery. Ultrasound scan may show morphological changes in the cervix such as shortening and funnelling several weeks or months before the onset of preterm labour. Other biochemical products including fetal fibronectin in the cervicovaginal fluid and raised maternal salivary oestriol may be detected for a considerable length of time prior to the onset of spontaneous labour. The challenge is to develop sensitive and specific tests that reliably detect these changes before they become irreversible and find effective interventions that are capable of arresting the process of preterm labour to enhance the effectiveness of current interventions such as maternal corticosteroid administration, short-term tocolytic therapy and transfer to a tertiary care centre.

Transvaginal ultrasound scan measurement of the cervix

Transvaginal ultrasound scan is a reliable and reproducible way of assessing the cervix. The length of the cervix is inversely related to the risk of preterm delivery. At 28 weeks of gestation, cervical length measurements of 40 mm or less, 35 mm or less, 30 mm or less, 26 mm or less, 22 mm or less, and 13 mm or less are associated with a relative risk of preterm delivery of 2.80, 3.52, 5.39, 9.57, 13.88, and 24.94 respectively. Despite this ability of cervical length measurement to predict preterm labour, its routine application is not recommended because of the lack of proven treatments that will improve outcome. The picture is different in women at high risk of PTD presenting with symptoms of preterm labour.

Bacterial vaginosis

Bacterial vaginosis is a condition of unknown aetiology characterized by abnormal ecological alteration of the vaginal flora. It is present in 10–25% of pregnant women, with the higher figures reported amongst ethnic Black populations. Over 50% of women with bacterial vaginosis are asymptomatic and may be recognized only by screening. Bacterial vaginosis is associated with significant obstetric complications, including midtrimester pregnancy loss, PTD, chorioamnionitis, postpartum endometritis, and neonatal sepsis. Trials of antibiotic treatment of bacterial vaginosis to prevent PTD in low- and high-risk women have yielded conflicting results. However, studies of antibiotic treatment of bacterial vaginosis initiated early in the second trimester of pregnancy showed a reduction in the risk of second trimester miscarriage and PTD in a general and unselected obstetric population.

Fetal fibronectin

Fetal fibronectin (fFN) is a basement membrane protein produced by the fetal membranes, which binds the placenta and membranes to the decidua. It is normally present in cervicovaginal fluid until about 20 weeks' gestation as the gestational sac attaches itself to the uterus. Beyond 20 weeks fFN in the cervicovaginal fluid is <10% and rare after 24 weeks, when it is regarded as a marker of disruption of the chorioamnion and the underlying decidua by inflammation with or without infection. In contrast to other potential predictors of PTD, the presence of fFN in the cervicovaginal fluid provides direct evidence of pathological changes at the fetomaternal interface. Furthermore,

fFN production by human chorionic cells is stimulated by bacterial products and inflammatory mediators and cytokines. The detection of fFN in the vagina has been shown to predict preterm delivery. Conversely, its absence is also associated with a reduced risk of PTD. The clinical implications of a positive test have not been evaluated fully because of the lack of effective intervention to reduce PTD. The negative predictive value of fFN to identify symptomatic women who are at low risk of PTD ranges between 69% and 92%. It improves the diagnostic accuracy in symptomatic women with uterine activity and reduces the high frequency of false-positive diagnosis of and intervention for preterm labour. Routine screening of low risk, asymptomatic women with fFN test is not recommended, because PTD in this population is so low that the test loses its usefulness.

Salivary oestriol

A surge in oestriol levels is observed 3 weeks prior to the onset of term, preterm, and post-term birth. This has rekindled interest in the measurement of salivary oestriol as a normal physiological marker for the onset of parturition. The signal for parturition appears to be given when the threshold concentration of oestriol exceeds 2.1 ng/mL. Clinical application is limited by its diurnal variation, and false-positive tests associated with gingival disease and rare placental disorders such as sulphatase and aromatase deficiencies.

Home uterine contraction monitoring

A number of small studies conducted in heterogeneous populations of women with variable risk factors for PTD reported that women with increased uterine activity had preterm labours more frequently than those with normal uterine contraction frequency. Since then, over 15 randomized controlled trials of variable design and quality have been published with conflicting results. Although the US FDA approved the home uterine contraction monitoring device for women with prior history of preterm birth, its role in the prevention of PTD is yet to be established. Furthermore, the US Preventive Services Task Force performed an independent review and concluded that the device was not effective. At present the use of this device as a tool for preventing PTD is not recommended.

Conclusions

Preterm labour is only a symptom of an underlying disorder and not a diagnosis in itself. Current therapeutic approaches assume a single pathway model. There are no proven predictive tests for spontaneous PTD. As a result, clinical management is poorly targeted with many women receiving unnecessary treatment while over 50% of women delivering their babies preterm display no recognizable risk factors. The lack of effective intervention capable of arresting the process of preterm labour also contributes to the slow progress in the development of sensitive and specific clinical tools for the detection of preterm labour.

Although the survival of preterm babies has improved dramatically in recent years, the rates of adverse sequalae have remained static and may be rising. Most spontaneous PTD <32 weeks gestation are linked to subclinical chorioamnionitis. The inflammatory mediators and cytokines are also key players in the genesis of long-term neurodevelopmental delays. The downregulation of the immune response exerted by antenatal steroids may well explain some of the benefits, although this was unintended. Perhaps in future the treatment of preterm labour will include agents that suppress the inflammatory process.

Further reading

Creasy RK. Preterm birth prevention: where are we? Am J Obstet Gynecol 1993;168:1223–30.

Walker DJ, Feldman A, Vohr BR, Oh W. Cost-benefit analysis of neonatal intensive care for infants weighing less than 1,000 grams at birth. Pediatrics 1984;74:20–5.

Carr H, Hall MH. The repetition of spontaneous preterm labour. Br J Obstet Gynaecol 1985;92:921–8.

Hoffman JD, Ward K. Genetic factors in preterm delivery. Obstet Gynecol Surv 1999;54:203–10.

Lettieri L, Vintzileos AM, Rodis JF, et al. Does idiopathic preterm labor resulting in preterm birth exist? Am J Obstet Gynecol 1993;168:1480–5.

Iams JD, Goldenberg RL, Meis PJ, et al. The length of the cervix and the risk of spontaneous premature delivery. N Engl J Med 1996;334:567–72.

Romero R, Quintero R, Oyarzun E, et al. Intraamniotic infection and the onset of labor in preterm premature rupture of the membranes. Am J Obstet Gynecol 1988;159:661–6.

Wenstrom KD, Andrews WW, Hauth JC, et al. Elevated second-trimester amniotic fluid interleukin-6 levels predict preterm delivery. Am J Obstet Gynecol 1998;178:546–50.

Iams JD, Goldenberg RL, Meis PJ, et al. The length of the cervix and the risk of spontaneous premature delivery. N Engl J Med 1996;334:567–72.

Ugwumadu A, Manyonda I, Reid F, Hay P. Effect of early oral clindamycin on late miscarriage and preterm delivery in asymptomatic women with abnormal vaginal flora and bacterial vaginosis: a randomised controlled trial. Lancet 2003;361:983–8.

Lamont RF, Duncan SL, Mandal D, Bassett P. Intravaginal clindamycin to reduce preterm birth in women with abnormal genital tract flora. Obstet Gynecol 2003;101:516–22.

Jackson GM, Edwin SS, Varner MW, et al. Regulation of fetal fibronectin production in human chorion cells. Am J Obstet Gynecol 1993;169:1431–5.

Leitich H, Egarter C, Kaider A, et al. Cervicovaginal fetal fibronectin as a marker for preterm delivery: a meta-analysis. Am J Obstet Gynecol 1999;180:1169–76.

Dame J, McGarrigle HH, Lachelin GC. Increased saliva oestriol to progesterone ratio before preterm delivery: a possible predictor for preterm labour? BMJ (Clin Res Ed) 1987;294:270–2.

Nageotte MP, Dorchester W, Porto M, et al. Quantitation of uterine activity preceding preterm, term, and postterm labor. Am J Obstet Gynecol 1988;158:1254–9.

Main DM, Katz M, Chiu G, et al. Intermittent weekly contraction monitoring to predict preterm labor in low-risk women: a blinded study. Obstet Gynecol 1988;72 :757–61.

US Preventive Services Task Force. Home uterine activity monitoring for preterm labour. Review article. JAMA 1993;270:371–6.

Paneth NS. The problem of low birth weight. Future Child 5:19–34.

Preterm prelabour rupture of membranes

Definition

Preterm prelabour rupture of membranes (pPROM) is defined as the spontaneous rupture of fetal membranes at least an hour prior to the onset of labour, and before 37 completed weeks of gestation. It occurs in 2–3% of all pregnancies and accounts for 30–40% of preterm deliveries. The role of infection in a subset of pPROM cases is well established but the role of other aetiopathogenic factors remains unclear. As a result there is considerable controversy surrounding the optimal management of pPROM.

Clinical importance

pPROM affects some 14 000 pregnancies in the UK and 140 000 in the USA. It accounts for 30–40% of preterm deliveries and is an independent risk factor for neonatal morbidity and mortality from prematurity, sepsis, and pulmonary hypoplasia. Infants born after prolonged periods of pPROM have an excess risk of long-term neurological and chronic lung disease. Subclinical intrauterine infection has been implicated as a major aetiological factor in the pathogenesis of pPROM and its associated fetomaternal morbidity. Studies of transabdominal amniocentesis following pPROM showed that the frequency of positive amniotic fluid is 25–40% with the risk of a positive culture inversely related to the gestational age at which pPROM occurred. Women with intrauterine infection have shorter latency than non-infected women, and infants born with sepsis have a fourfold increase in mortality than infants born without sepsis (Cotton et al. 1984). These findings have fuelled interest in the use of antibiotics to prevent pPROM in women at risk, to increase latency after pPROM, and as prophylaxis against neonatal morbidity such as oxygen dependency, intraventricular haemorrhage, necrotizing enterocolitis, neonatal sepsis, and mortality.

Aetiology and pathophysiology

The tensile strength of the membranes is mainly due to types III and IV collagen secreted by the epithelial cells of the amniotic membrane. In recent years, our understanding of the cellular and molecular factors that govern the structural integrity of fetal membranes and their regulation has increased and it is now clear that only a proportion of pPROM cases are infection driven. Other pathological processes such as choriodecidual fusion defects (Bryant-Greenwood and Millar 2000), fetal growth dysregulation (Cooperstock et al. 2000), activation of membrane apoptosis (Fortunato et al. 2000), upregulation of matrix metalloproteinases, and inhibition of tissue inhibitors of matrix metalloproteinases (Fortunato 1999), nutritional factors (Barrett 1994), and smoking (Barrett 1991) may be important in a significant proportion of cases of pPROM.

Diagnosis and initial assessment

The diagnosis of pPROM is made by maternal history, speculum examination and simple bedside tests. Although maternal history has an accuracy of 90% for the diagnosis of pPROM (Gaucherand 1995), it is good practice to confirm the diagnosis before applying the label of pPROM. The presence of a pool of amniotic fluid in the posterior fornix on speculum examination is confirmatory of pPROM. There may be a role for nitrazine pH-based paper testing when there is a very small amount of fluid in the posterior fornix and the observer is uncertain. However, the nitrazine test is not specific and has a false-positive rate of 17% (Gaucherand et al. 1995). The pH of vaginal fluid changes towards the alkaline range in the presence of bacterial vaginosis, other vaginitis, contamination with cervical secretion, blood, semen, or urine. In doubtful cases the patient may be asked to cough gently while visualizing the external cervical os for any trickle of amniotic fluid. An extended pad test is also useful. A panel of newer tests has been evaluated for pPROM, including fetal fibronectins and raised insulin-like growth factor binding protein-1 (IGFBP-1) in cervicovaginal secretions. These have sensitivities of 94% and 75%, respectively, and specificities of 97% (Rutanen 1993). Spontaneous rupture of membranes during the second, and early third trimesters is usually associated with a near total loss of the entire amniotic fluid pool. Therefore, ultrasound scan evidence of marked oligohydramnious or anhydramnious is highly suggestive of a diagnosis of pPROM in this context. Such an ultrasound examination should be extended to exclude fetal anomaly, evaluate the fetal growth and development, and estimate the fetal weight and presentation.

A digital vaginal examination should be avoided following a diagnosis of pPROM, unless there is a strong suspicion of labour or imminent delivery. Recent studies have shown that two or fewer digital vaginal examinations were associated with a shorter latency period but no increase in fetal or maternal infectious morbidity (Alexander et al. 2000). Thus, if one or two digital vaginal examinations were done after pPROM, this should not constitute an indication to abandon conservative management or pursue an immediate induction of labour for fear of increased risk of fetomaternal infectious morbidity.

Current management of pPROM

In many units, women with pPROM are admitted into the hospital and managed conservatively until 37 completed weeks in an attempt to increase fetal maturity. Conservative management involves 4-hourly measurements of maternal temperature, heart rate, respiratory rate, and blood pressure, daily cardiotocographs (CTGs), weekly, twice, or thrice weekly maternal white cell counts, C-reactive protein assays, and culture of vaginal swabs, all in an effort to detect intrauterine infection or chorioamnionitis. However, with histological chorioamnionitis maternal inflammatory markers are raised in only 10–15% of cases (Romero et al. 1989), suggesting that maternal markers are not sufficiently sensitive to guide clinical decisions. Furthermore, the micro-organisms usually associated with chorioamnionitis are subpathogenic, non-pyrogenic, and are often not detected on routine microbiological culture methods. For prognosis, it is fetal rather than maternal evidence of inflammation that is predictive of adverse neonatal outcome. However, the search for evidence of fetal inflammation by amniocentesis and/or cordocentesis is not routine practice and its role in reducing the risk of neonatal complications has not been adequately evaluated.

Critique of management strategies

The majority of women with infection-driven pPROM will deliver within 5 days; therefore, the value of inpatient management beyond 5 days is questionable. Outpatient care with instruction for the patient to take her own temperature and be reviewed once or twice weekly in hospital is reasonable. She should, however, be discouraged from vaginal intercourse, protected or not, and any form of intravaginal cleansing. Immersion in plain bath water is not associated with an increase in infectious morbidity. A one-off vaginal swab for pathogens, particularly group B streptococcus will suffice. There is little or no correlation between the organisms that cause amniotic fluid infection/chorioamnionitis and those isolated from the lower genital tract. Nursing women with pPROM in a head-down tilt position is unnecessary and may encourage a stagnant pool of amniotic fluid and cervicovaginal secretions with a potential for encouraging bacterial growth and multiplication. Although fetal CTG is recommended as part of the surveillance, there are no specific or reliable CTG patterns that are predictive of fetal inflammation or sepsis until very late, and neurological injuries may occur without significant CTG changes. Clinical chorioamnionitis defined as maternal fever (temperature ≥38°C) and the presence of any two or more of the following, maternal or fetal tachycardia, uterine tenderness, foul-smelling or purulent vaginal discharge, maternal leucocytosis, or raised C-reactive protein, is poorly predictive of histological chorioamnionitis, which has been shown to be more predictive of abnormal neonatal cerebral outcomes including periventricular echodensity/echolucency, ventriculomegaly, intraventricular haemorrhage, and seizures (De Felice 2001).

Timing of delivery

Expectant management until 37 weeks to improve fetal maturity is historical and based on the assumption that prolongation of pregnancy automatically translates to better fetal maturity and neonatal outcome. The risks of cord events including acute cord compression, cord prolapse, or ascending infection are not insignificant. The risks of prematurity-related morbidity including respiratory distress syndrome, necrotizing enterocolitis, grades 3–4 intraventricular haemorrhage, and mortality, diminish significantly beyond 32–34 weeks and that neonatal survival at 34 weeks in tertiary units is similar to 37–40 weeks. The increase in survival per additional week of conservative management is less than 1%.

Studies evaluating the risk–benefit analysis of induction of labour at 34 weeks found similar vaginal delivery rates, and no increase in the risk of instrumental vaginal delivery or Caesarean section (Naef et al. 1998). On the other hand, these studies documented an excess incidence of ascending infection, neonatal sepsis, cord prolapse or compression, fetal demise, and longer hospital stay in cases managed conservatively (Naef et al. 1998; Grable 2002). Therefore, the benefits of delivery at 34 weeks outweigh the risks of conservative management without increasing obstetric intervention. This balance, however, is in favour of expectant management prior to 32 weeks as delivery before 32 weeks' gestation is associated with a significant risk of gestational age-related morbidity and mortality. Therefore, unless there are concerns regarding fetal well-being, clinical or biochemical evidence of infection, women with pPROM remote from term should be managed conservatively to prolong gestation until 34 weeks to reduce the risk of gestational age related morbidity and mortality.

Antibiotic therapy to prolong latency and prevent neonatal morbidity after pPROM

Evidence from meta-analysis of randomized trials suggests that antibiotic therapy (ampicillin and/or erythromycin) delayed preterm delivery, and reduced maternal and neonatal morbidity (Mercer et al. 1994; Kenyon et al. 2004).

Routine antibiotic is therefore recommended for women with pPROM. Routine antibiotic therapy presumes an infectious aetiology, lacks guidance from microbiological cultures and sensitivity, and is based on the belief that the antibiotic somehow prevents or reverses fetal damage. Widespread use has led to an increase in erythromycin-resistant organisms even in the years leading up to the publication of the ORACLE trial (Pearlman et al. 1998; et al. 2003). This trend was attributed to increased use of erythromycin for prophylaxis against Group B streptococcus for women who were allergic to penicillin and is likely to escalate with its increased use for pPROM.

Tocolysis

Tocolysis may be applied prophylactically to prevent the onset of uterine contractions and labour in women with pPROM, or used therapeutically to abolish uterine contractions and labour after pPROM. The use of tocolysis should be individualized and restricted to those situations where there are no clinical or biochemical evidence of infection and a course of corticosteroids needed to be completed, or to allow the transfer of the woman to a tertiary centre. The choice of a tocolytic agent is a matter for local guidelines as the efficacies of the available agents are broadly similar. However, the β-adrenoceptor agonists have become less popular because of their marked cardiovascular side-effects.

Corticosteroid therapy

Initial concerns that corticosteroids may increase the risks of chorioamnionitis, postpartum endometritis, and neonatal sepsis are not supported by current evidence. Antenatal steroids reduced the risks of respiratory distress syndrome, intraventricular haemorrhage, and necrotizing enterocolitis (Harding et al. 2001). These substantial reductions in the risk of major gestational age-related morbidity translate to a significant reduction in neonatal mortality. There are few data on whether using the same dose of corticosteroid, this magnitude of benefit may also accrue for twins and other higher order pregnancies with pPROM, because of greater maternal volume of distribution. In diabetic women, the administration of corticosteroids may result in the loss of glycaemic control. The risk of this has to be carefully balanced with the potential benefit. Therefore in diabetic women with pPROM near term for example ≥32–34 weeks or in whom fetal lung maturation can be demonstrated, the value of steroid administration is questionable. Below 32 completed weeks of gestation, consideration should be given for sliding scale insulin/glucose infusion for 48–96 hours during the course of antenatal prophylactic steroid. Intramuscular betamethasone 12 mg, 24 hours apart is preferable to dexamethasone 12 mg, 12 hours apart. Betamethasone has a stronger evidence base and unlike dexamethasone, is not associated with necrotizing enterocolitis.

The role of amniocentesis

Studies of amniocentesis in pPROM women show that up to 40% (more with DNA amplification techniques) will have positive amniotic fluid cultures, and/or raised inflammatory markers at presentation, with the proportion increasing with latency. Fetal host inflammatory response rather than amniotic fluid colonization or maternal response is correlated with adverse neonatal outcome. Amniocentesis, culture of amniotic fluid and determination of the presence or absence of fetal host response may allow clinicians to select and triage cases for conservative or aggressive management. There is no evidence, however, that characterization of the amniotic fluid inflammatory status to guide management improved perinatal outcome. The timing of fetal injury is unknown and it is plausible that by the time women present with pPROM, it is already too late to reverse established inflammatory cascade. The mechanisms through which ampicillin and/or erythromycin therapy delayed preterm delivery, and reduced maternal and neonatal morbidity, remain unknown. Although the eradication of intrauterine infection, reduction/prevention of host inflammatory response, or prevention of ascending infection from the lower genital tract have all been proposed, Gomez et al. (2007) showed that antibiotic treatment very rarely eradicated microbial invasion of the amniotic cavity in patients with pPROM. An overwhelming 86% of pPROM patients with positive amniotic fluid culture and 83% with intra-amniotic inflammation maintained the same microbiological/inflammatory profile respectively, despite aggressive antibiotic therapy for 10–14 days (Gomez et al. 2007). This is consistent with data that showed poor transplacental transfer of macrolide antibiotics (Witt et al. 2003). The study also found that women with negative amniotic fluid culture or inflammation at admission developed microbial invasion of the amniotic cavity despite antibiotic therapy.

Further reading

Alexander JM, Mercer BM, Miodovnik M, et al. The impact of digital cervical examination on expectantly managed preterm rupture of membranes. Am J Obstet Gynecol 2000;183:1003–7.

Barrett B, Gunter E, Jenkins J, Wang M. Ascorbic acid concentration in amniotic fluid in late pregnancy. Biol Neonate 1991;60:333–5.

Barrett BM, Sowell A, Gunter E, Wang M. Potential role of ascorbic acid and beta-carotene in the prevention of preterm rupture of fetal membranes. Int J Vitam Nutr Res 1994;64:192–7.

Bryant-Greenwood GD, Millar LK. Human fetal membranes: their preterm delayed rupture. Biol Reprod 2000;63:1575–9.

Cooperstock MS, Tummaru R, Bakewell J, Schramm W. Twin birth weight discordance and risk of preterm birth. Am J Obstet Gynecol 2000;183:63–7.

Cotton DB, Hill LM, Strassner HT, et al. Use of amniocentesis in preterm gestation with ruptured membranes. Obstet Gynecol 1984;63:38–43.

De Felice C, Toti P, Laurini RN, et al. Early neonatal brain injury in histologic chorioamnionitis. J Pediatr 2001;138:101–4.

Fortunato SJ, Menon R, Bryant C, Lombardi SJ. Programmed cell death (apoptosis) as a possible pathway to metalloproteinase activation and fetal membrane degradation in premature rupture of membranes. Am J Obstet Gynecol 2000;182:1468–76.

Fortunato SJ, Menon R, Lombardi SJ. MMP/TIMP imbalance in amniotic fluid during PROM: an indirect support for endogenous pathway to membrane rupture. J Perinat Med 1999;27:362–8.

Gaucherand P, Guibaud S, Awada A, Rudigoz RC. Comparative study of three amniotic fluid markers in premature rupture of membranes: fetal fibronectin, alpha-fetoprotein, diamino-oxydase. Acta Obstet Gynecol Scand 1995;74:118–21.

Gomez R, Romero R, Nien JK, et al. Antibiotic administration to patients with preterm premature rupture of membranes does not eradicate intra-amniotic infection. J Matern Fetal Neonatal Med 2007;20:167–73.

Grable IA. Cost-effectiveness of induction after preterm premature rupture of the membranes. Am J Obstet Gynecol 2002;187:1153–8.

Harding JE, Pang J, Knight DB, Liggins GC. Do antenatal corticosteroids help in the setting of preterm rupture of membranes? Am J Obstet Gynecol 2001;184:131–9.

Kenyon S, Boulvain M, Neilson J. Antibiotics for preterm rupture of the membranes: a systematic review. Obstet Gynecol 2004;104:1051–7.

Manning SD, Foxman B, Pierson CL, et al. Correlates of antibiotic-resistant group B streptococcus isolated from pregnant women. Obstet Gynecol 2003; 101:74–9.

Mercer BM, Miodovnik M, Thurnau GR, et al. Antibiotic therapy for reduction of infant morbidity after preterm premature rupture of the membranes. A randomized controlled trial. JAMA 1997;278:989–95.

Naef RW, III, Allbert JR, Ross EL, et al. Premature rupture of membranes at 34 to 37 weeks' gestation: aggressive versus conservative management. Am J Obstet Gynecol 1998;178:126–30.

Pearlman MD, Pierson CL, Faix RG. Frequent resistance of clinical group B streptococci isolates to lindamycin and erythromycin. Obstet Gynecol 1998;92:258–61.

Romero R, Sirtori M, Oyarzun E, et al. Infection and labor. V. Prevalence, microbiology, and clinical significance of intraamniotic infection in women with preterm labor and intact membranes. Am J Obstet Gynecol 1989;161:817–24.

Rutanen EM, Pekonen F, Karkkainen T. Measurement of insulin-like growth factor binding protein-1 in cervical/vaginal secretions: comparison with the ROM-check Membrane Immunoassay in the diagnosis of ruptured fetal membranes. Clin Chim Acta 1993;214:73–81.

Witt A, Sommer E, Cichna M, et al. Placental passage of clarithromycin surpasses other macrolide antibiotics. Am J Obstet Gynecol 2003;188:816–9.

Prolonged pregnancy

Definition

Prolonged or post-term pregnancy has traditionally been defined as the pregnancy continuing beyond two weeks after the expected date of delivery. Prolonged pregnancy is known to be associated with risks of intrauterine growth restriction, intrauterine death, macrosomia, and an increased incidence of operative deliveries.

Confirmation of prolonged pregnancy

It is essential to ascertain the expected date of delivery, as dating error is the commonest cause of prolonged pregnancy. The estimated date of delivery, in normal pregnancies, is calculated as 280 days (40 weeks) from the date of the last menstrual period (assuming regular 28-day menstrual cycle). This is more likely to be accurate when

- there was no hormonal contraceptive use or breastfeeding for 3 months preceding the last menstrual period
- if the date of last menstrual period was certain
- when it matches with the ultrasound estimated date of delivery.
- Where the date of the last menstrual period was not available or uncertain or differs from the dating from ultrasound parameters in the absence of chromosomal or other abnormalities, the estimated date of delivery is calculated from the following ultrasound parameters:
- from crown–rump length (CRL) measured between 11 and 14 weeks
- from head circumference in the second trimester

It is difficult to ascertain the expected date of delivery by ultrasound parameters after 20–24 weeks. Hence, National Institute for Health and Clinical Excellence (NICE) guidelines recommend that all pregnant women in the UK should be offered an ultrasound scan between 11 and 14 weeks, and that the due date estimated is based on this scan regardless of the menstrual dates.

Incidence

Incidence of prolonged pregnancy reduced from 10.3% to 3.7% when the date was estimated from an ultrasound before 24 weeks. A meta-analysis found reduced rates of induction of labour for post-term pregnancy (OR 0.68, 95% CI 0.57–0.82) among women who underwent sonographic gestational age assessment in early pregnancy (before 24 weeks).

Risk factors for prolonged pregnancy

Primiparity and prior post-term pregnancy are the most common identifiable risk factors. Placental sulphatase deficiency is a rare postulated cause. Male gender has been shown to be predisposing to prolongation of pregnancy. The reduced risk of recurrence of post-term birth observed with the change in the male partner suggests that the timing of birth may be determined by paternal genes. Being parous appears to have a protective effect on fetal mortality in prolonged pregnancy.

Risks of prolonged pregnancy

With continued fetal growth, there is a higher risk of big babies. This increases the chances of fetopelvic disproportion and shoulder dystocia. The amniotic fluid volume gradually decreases, increasing the risk of intrapartum cord compression. The ageing placenta may fail to support the baby. Rate of meconeum passage is high.

Perinatal mortality

Data derived from accurately dated pregnancies show an increased perinatal mortality rate from 41 weeks. The rate increases from 2–3/1000 at 40 weeks to 4–7/1000 after 42 weeks. The rates of fetal loss per 1000 ongoing pregnancies are 0.7, 2.4 and 5.8 at 37, 40 and 43 weeks. Post-term babies who are small for gestational age are at an increased risk of perinatal death compared with those who are appropriately grown.

Perinatal morbidity

There is an increased risk of meconium aspiration syndrome, macrosomia, low Apgars, Neonatal hypoglycemia, seizures, respiratory distress, and admission to neonatal intensive care unit.

Labour abnormalities

The incidence of prolonged labour, abnormal fetal heart rate pattern, operative delivery, shoulder dystocia, perineal trauma, and postpartum haemorrhage is increased in prolonged pregnancies (Table 9.14.1).

Assessment of post-dated pregnancy

Thorough history, examination, and appropriate investigations should be undertaken to exclude complications such as small for gestational age babies, congenital anomalies, malpresentation, pre-eclampsia, etc. NICE guidelines recommend that vaginal examination and membrane sweeping should be offered to all nulliparous women after 40 weeks and parous women at 41 weeks; this has been shown to reduce the rate of post-term pregnancy. Vaginal examination will aid in assessing the favourability of the cervix using Bishop's score. Membrane sweeping is a minimally invasive method which helps in the onset of spontaneous labour.

Monitoring

The goal of monitoring is to reduce the risk of fetal death by detecting signs of hypoxic fetal compromise. At the same time, the clinician has to balance this against the risks of unnecessary intervention induced labour. There is insufficient evidence to recommend routine monitoring between 40 and 42 weeks. After 42 weeks, twice weekly fetal monitoring with cardiotocographic assessment (non-stress test) and amniotic fluid assessment are recommended as a good practice point. However, there is limited evidence to showing benefit of these tests. Doppler assessment of umbilical artery is not shown to be useful in monitoring post-dated pregnancies. In general, there is

Table 9.14.1 Risks of post-term pregnancies (data from Eden et al. 1987)

	Post-dates (born after 42 weeks) (%)	Control (born at 40 weeks) (%)
Oxytocin stimulation	14.2	2.8
Shoulder dystocia	2.8	0.8
Meconeum-stained liquor	17.6	8.3
Caesarean section	26.5	19.4

insufficient evidence to recommend any particular monitoring in post-term pregnancies to reduce the adverse outcome.

Management

The Cochrane review (Gülmezoglu et al. 2006) concluded that routine induction after 41 weeks reduces perinatal mortality without any increase in the Caesarean section rate. It would be prudent to discuss the risks and benefits of labour induction versus expectant management at 41 weeks so that the woman can make an informed choice. If the woman chooses to wait spontaneous labour onset beyond 42 weeks, twice weekly fetal monitoring is recommended.

Methods of induction of labour

This has been summarized in section 10.9 Induction of labour.

Risk of recurrence

It is estimated to be 20%, increasing with increasing gestational age at index pregnancy (30% for a gestational age of 44 weeks).

Practice points

1. Routine pregnancy dating using early ultrasonography reduces the incidence of post-term pregnancies.
2. Appropriate fetal wellbeing tests in prolonged pregnancy are largely unknown.
3. Small fetuses in prolonged pregnancies are at a higher risk of serious adverse outcome.

4. Currently, the only policy of demonstrable benefit is induction of labour after 41 weeks, but the exact timing is still uncertain.

Further reading

Agency for healthcare research and quality. Management of prolonged pregnancy. Evidence report/Technology assessment. Number 53.

Crowley P. Interventions for preventing or improving the outcome of delivery at or beyond term. Cochrane Database Syst Rev 2006;4:CD000170.

Eden R, Seifert L, Vinegar A, Spellacy W. Perinatal characteristics of uncomplicated postdate pregnancies. Obstet Gynecol 1987;69:296–9.

Gülmezoglu AM, Crowther CA, Middleton P. Induction of labour for improving birth outcomes for women at or beyond term. Cochrane Database Syst Rev 2006;4:CD004945.

Hilder L, Costeloe K, Thilaganathan B. Prolonged pregnancy: evaluating gestation-specific risks of fetal and infant mortality. Br J Obstet Gynaecol 1998;105:169–73.

Hilder L, Sairam S, Thilaganathan B. Influence of parity on fetal mortality in prolonged pregnancy. Eur J Obstet Gynecol Reprod Biol 2007;132:167–70.

NICE guidelines. Antenatal care for the healthy pregnant women. National Colloborating Centre for women's and children's health. March 2008.

NICE guidelines. Induction of labour. National Colloborating Centre for women's and children's health. July 2008.

Olsen A, Basso O, Olsen J. Risk of recurrence of prolonged pregnancy. BMJ 2003;326:476.

Puerperal sepsis

Definition
The International Classification of Diseases (ICD-10) defines puerperal fever as a rise in temperature of greater than 38.0°C sustained for more than 24 hours or recurring between the end of the first and tenth day of childbirth, miscarriage, or termination of pregnancy. It can develop into puerperal sepsis, which is a serious and life threatening septicaemia. The United Kingdom Confidential Enquiry into Maternal and Child Health reported that in 2003–5 genital tract sepsis accounted for 14% of direct causes of maternal death, making puerperal fever a significant factor in maternal death. The most common infection causing puerperal fever is genital tract sepsis. Other types of infection that can lead to sepsis after childbirth include urinary tract infection, mastitis, and respiratory tract infection.

Aetiology
It is a polymicrobial condition that affects a small minority of women, suggesting that the pathogenesis involves more than just a source of potentially pathogenic bacteria. Endometritis is most commonly caused by *Staphylococcus aureus* and group A streptococcus, specifically *Streptococcus pyogenes*, which is responsible for most cases of severe hemolytic streptococcal illness although other types B, C, D, and G may also cause infection. Group B streptococcus usually causes less severe maternal disease. Other causal organisms, in order of prevalence, include staphylococci, coliform bacteria, anaerobe bacteria, chlamydia bacteria, mycoplasma, and, very rarely, *Clostridium welchii*.

Endometritis
Endometritis is the commonest puerperal infection and usually presents within 5 days of delivery.

Risk factors
- Caesarean section (27% versus 1.2% in women who had vaginal delivery)
- Multiple vaginal examinations during labour
- Prolonged rupture of membranes
- Use and duration of internal monitoring devices
- Prolonged labour
- Group B streptococcal colonisation
- Anaemia, diabetes mellitus, obesity.

Diagnosis
Criteria for diagnosis include fever, with or without chills and rigors, uterine tenderness, with or without abdominal pains, purulent or foul-smelling lochia, leucocytosis, and exclusion of another focus of infection. There may be tachycardia. Localizing signs may be absent if the infection is due to group A or B streptococcus. Obtain cervical and vaginal samples for culture.

Treatment
If febrile and unwell, use intravenous broad-spectrum antibiotics with anaerobic cover, for example cephalosporin or clindamycin and gentamycin.

Septic pelvic thrombophlebitis
This is thought to be due to bacterial injury to the pelvic (ovarian) venous endothelium. The diagnosis should be considered in any patient with a persistent temperature despite appropriate antibiotic therapy and prior soft tissue pelvic infection.

Clinical features
- Persistent fevers may be the only presentation
- Progressively worsening abdominal pain usually right more than left
- Nausea, vomiting or abdominal distension may be present
- Bowel sounds may be normoactive or absent
- Tachycardia
- Tachypnoea and respiratory distress if pulmonary embolus has occurred
- The thrombosed ovarian vein (usually right) may be palpable as an abdominal or adnexal mass.

Investigations
- Ultrasound scan
- CT scan

Treatment
- Broad-spectrum antibiotic therapy
- Anticoagulation with heparin was a traditional adjunct to therapy but this is no longer recommended
- Surgical ligation/excision of the affected vein is reserved for patients with acute abdomen or not responding to medical therapy

Urinary tract infection
This is a common cause of postpartum pyrexia and is usually caused by *Escherichia* coli, although enterococci, group B streptococci and other gram-negative aerobic bacilli may occasionally be responsible. Symptoms include dysuria, frequency, nocturia, fever, backache, and physical examination may reveal tenderness in the renal angles. A clean catch specimen of urine for culture is helpful in diagnosis. Sterile pyuria may reflect bladder inflammation from trauma during labour and delivery.

Risk factors
- Physiological hydroureter of pregnancy
- Asymptomatic bacteriuria
- Intrapartum catheterization.

Treatment
Parenteral cephalosporin and gentamycin initially until urine cultures and antibiotic sensitivities become available

Mastitis and breast abscess
Staphylococcus aureus is the main causative agent of sporadic, epidemic, and endemic mastitis. Fever, malaise, and breast pain and tenderness are the usual presenting features. Breast abscess may develop in untreated cases.

Treatment
A penicillinase-resistant penicillin such as flucloxacillin or erythromycin should be administered. Other measures include breast support, ice packs, and analgesics. Breastfeeding should continue unless abscess develops.

Wound and episiotomy infections
Around 5–15% of Caesarean section wounds become infected depending on the definition of wound infection used. The presence of erythema, induration, pain, and fluid exudate are suggestive signs. If the wound breaks down, debridement, and secondary closure is now recommended instead of the traditional approach of debridment and

dressing, and allowing healing by secondary intention. Clinicians should maintain a high index of suspicion in order to recognize life-threatening wound complications such as necrotizing fasciitis, clostridial myonecrosis (gas gangrene), and non-clostridial bacterial synergistic gangrene (Meleney gangrene).

A simple episiotomy infection usually presents with localized erythema, oedema, and exudate, which are limited to the surrounding skin and subcutaneous tissue. If the findings are more extensive, a deeper infection may be present. The wound should be opened, explored, drained, and debrided, and appropriate antibiotics administered.

Most of these will heal by granulation but if perineal muscles or the anal sphincter is involved, the wound should be resutured once the infection settles down, in about 5–10 days. The patient should avoid sexual intercourse and have sitz baths three or four times daily.

Further reading

Gwyneth Lewis (ed.). Saving Mothers' Lives: Reviewing maternal deaths to make motherhood safer–2003–2005. The Seventh Report of the Confidential Enquiries into Maternal Deaths in the United Kingdom. www.cemach.org.uk/getattachment/8f5c1ed8-fdf3–489b-a182-e53955bec07b/Saving-Mothers–Lives-2003–2005_full.aspx:+CEMACH. page 97.

Care in labour

Analgesia and anaesthesia in obstetrics 364
Breech 368
Brow presentation 371
Cord prolapse 372
Episiotomy and obstetric perineal trauma 374
Face presentation 376
Fetal surveillance in labour 378
Home birth 384
Induction of labour 386
Labour 390
Maternal collapse 394
Meconium-stained liquor 398
Placenta praevia 402
Placental abruption 406
Postpartum haemorrhage 408
Prelabour rupture of membranes at term 412
Resuscitation of the newborn 414
Retained placenta 418
Shoulder dystocia 420
Shoulder presentation 424
Uterine inversion 426

Analgesia and anaesthesia in obstetrics

Analgesia for labour

Definition

Although labour and delivery can be extremely painful, not every woman's experience is the same. Regional analgesia, non-regional techniques, and pharmacological agents are used to provide pain relief for the parturient. Non-regional methods of labour analgesia include acupuncture, aromatherapy, hydrotherapy (birthing pool), transcutaneous electrical nerve stimulation (TENS), sterile water blocks, relaxation and breathing techniques, and massage. The most frequently used pharmacological agents are Entonox (50% nitrous oxide in oxygen) and meperidine (pethidine), but morphine and other opioids such as fentanyl, diamorphine, and remifentanil are also increasingly used. Epidural and spinal analgesia provide very effective and reliable pain relief by blocking the transmission of pain signals through spinal nerves in or near the spinal cord.

Epidemiology

Pain relief not facilitated by regional anaesthesia is still most frequently used during labour, although an increase in the uptake of epidural analgesia can be seen in many parts of the world. The type of labour analgesia used can be significantly influenced by the woman's epidemiological, cultural, or religious background.

Non-regional techniques

TENS has been put forward as a way of providing analgesia by blocking the transmission of pain signals through stimulation of $A\beta$-fibres and local release of β-endorphines. However, there is no evidence that TENS is more effective than placebo; TENS has minimal side-effects and may be appropriate for women who decline all other methods of pain relief in labour. Equally, there is no clear evidence that aromatherapy, acupuncture, hydrotherapy, and sterile water blocks are effective to relieve pain in labour; and only continuous support throughout labour and delivery has been shown to have a positive influence on analgesia requirements and the spontaneous vaginal delivery rate.

Pharmacological agents

Nitrous oxide mixed 50:50 with oxygen (Entonox), which has been used in obstetric practice for over a century, is widely available and provides analgesia within 60 seconds of inhalation. Besides its clear advantages, ease of use, a very short half-life and its safety profile, nitrous oxide can have significant side-effects such as drowsiness, disorientation, and nausea, and current evidence suggests that it provides only incomplete analgesia in most women. Nitrous oxide can be useful in places where other analgesic options are limited or unavailable. The phenylpiperidin derivate Meperidine (Pethidine), which can be given by a registered midwife without a physician's prescription, is usually administered intramuscularly (0.5–1.0 mg/kg). Despite its still widespread use many investigators have suggested that Meperidine provides merely sedation rather than analgesia, and that Pethidine is less efficacious than Entonox. Like any other opioid, Meperidine causes dose-dependent respiratory depression, pruritus, and obstipation and can delay gastric emptying; the metabolite Normeperidine has convulsant properties. Meperidine crosses the placenta and the highest fetal plasma concentration can be measured 2–3 hours after its maternal intramuscular administration.

Babies of women who have received meperidine in labour have been shown to be sleepier and less able to establish breastfeeding despite normal Apgar scores. Morphine, diamorphine, fentanyl, and remifantanil do not have convulsant effects but tend to be less frequently used for labour analgesia. Fentanyl, and especially remifentanil, have been successfully used with patient-controlled analgesia (PCA), for example in cases where regional analgesia is not available or is contraindicated. Remifentanil is an ultra-short-acting opioid that is rapidly hydrolysed by unspecific esterases; it does not accumulate even after prolonged infusions. Bolus doses of 0.25–0.5 μg/kg with a 1–3-minute lockout interval have been used successfully. However, careful instruction of all staff and the patient herself, as well as close monitoring of both parturient and neonate, is essential; supplementary oxygen may be required in some cases.

Regional techniques

Uterine pain is transmitted to the dorsal horns of T10–L1 of the spinal cord via sensory fibres, vaginal pain via the S2–S4 nerve roots; neuraxial techniques can effectively attenuate or completely block the transmission of pain signals.

Indications for regional techniques in labour
These include

- maternal request
- obstetric reason (e.g. pre-eclampsia, twin pregnancy)
- maternal cardiovascular, respiratory or neurological disease (e.g. mitral or aortic regurgitation; asthma; intracranial lesions)
- anticipated operative delivery.

Contraindications (absolute) for regional techniques in labour
These include

- maternal refusal
- severe hypovolaemia/haemorrhage
- allergy to local anaesthetics
- local infection at site of insertion
- systemic sepsis
- known clotting disorder, coagulopathy (a platelet count $>80 \times 10^9$/L and normal clotting will be adequate in most cases).

Oral or written consent should be obtained prior to performing any regional technique. Ideally, discussions about neuraxial analgesia should take place antenatally, as many women are unable to recall information which is given during labour.

Epidural analgesia

Like any other neuraxial regional technique, epidural analgesia requires secure i.v. access, a full lateral or sitting position of the parturient, a sterile technique and monitoring of the fetal heart rate. The maternal blood pressure should be measured at 3–5-minute intervals for at least 20 minutes after every bolus of local anaesthetic is administered.

The combination of spinal and epidural analgesia (CSE) will achieve a rapid onset of very effective pain relief but can be technically more challenging.

Recent studies clearly indicate that epidural analgesia does not result in an increase in the Caesarean section rate; it may, however, cause an increase in the operative vaginal delivery rate. Careful management of epidural analgesia is paramount to its success rate. Side-effects such as hypotension, motor block, unilateral or 'patchy' blocks, total spinal, fetal bradycardia, and maternal respiratory depression can be avoided by

- gentle and 'appropriate' administration of low concentration local anaesthetics (e.g. Bupivacaine 0.075–0.125%), supplemented with opioids (e.g. Fentanyl 2 µg/mL). Patient-controlled epidural analgesia (PCEA) with or without a continuous background infusion can be superior to bolus administration of local anaesthetics
- regular assessment of height and quality of the block (e.g. Bromage scale)
- insertion of soft and multiport epidural catheters into the epidural space (approximately 5 cm of catheter should be positioned within the epidural space)
- limiting intrathecal opioids to small doses if spinal analgesia or combined spinal epidural (CSE) analgesia is used.

The most frequent side-effect of epidural, spinal, or CSE analgesia is mild hypotension but a fall in systolic blood pressure of only 10–20% is usually accepted. If more severe hypotension occurs, it has to be treated without delay:

- left lateral tilt in order to prevent, treat or avoid aortocaval compression
- administration of 100% oxygen, vasoconstrictors such as phenylephrine (e.g. 100 µg bolus) and crystalloid fluid through a large bore cannula.

Severe complications of regional techniques are rare; global or partial failure of epidural analgesia is the most frequently experienced complication. If positioning towards the failing side, manipulation of the catheter itself and top-ups with more potent local anaesthetics (e.g. bupivacaine 0.25%) are unsuccessful, the epidural has often to be re-sited. It is even more important to check the quality of the block regularly if an operative vaginal delivery/Caesarean section is anticipated. The insertion of an epidural catheter can lead to a marked rise in maternal temperature; however, the reason for this and the significance for mother and fetus remain uncertain. Postdural puncture headache (PDPH) occurs in less than 1% of all paturients who have received neuraxial analgesia. Loss of cerebrospinal fluid through the punctured dura with stretching of the meninges is thought to cause this headache. If the dural puncture is recognized while the epidural puncture is performed, the 'epidural' catheter can be passed into the intrathecal space and subsequently used as a 'spinal catheter'; further top-ups should then be given only by an anaesthetist. Pain relief will be excellent and the incidence of PDPH is thought to be reduced. PDPH can be seen in 70–85% of cases of accidental dural puncture and occurs typically 24–48 hours after the event. Late management includes the prescription of oral analgesics (e.g. paracetamol and/or diclofenac); aggressive fluid administration and strict bed rest do not appear to be beneficial. Therapeutic blood patches are currently thought to be efficacious in up to 85% of cases, but definitive advice on the timing and the volume to be injected must await further evidence.

A 'total spinal', nerve damage, and back pain are discussed in the next chapter Anaesthesia in obstetrics. Local anaesthetics given in too large doses, or accidentally injected intravenously, can provoke cerebral convulsions or cause apnoea, unconsciousness and cardiac arrest. Intralipid 20% has been successfully used in patients to treat, in combination with standard cardiopulmonary resuscitation, local anaesthetic toxicity.

For women with pre-eclampsia epidural analgesia is usually the method of choice. Dramatic increases in blood pressure associated with contraction pain are avoided and the uteroplacental perfusion may be improved. It is important to obtain a platelet count (and test for normal clotting parameters in more severe cases) prior to the epidural or spinal puncture; current guidelines recommend a platelet count of at least 80×10^9/L.

Paturients who receive prophylactic (or therapeutic) low molecular weight heparin (LMWH) must wait at least 12–24 hours after their last dose of LMWH before neuraxial analgesia or anaesthesia can be performed safely.

Anaesthesia in obstetrics

Anaesthesia is mainly required for Caesarean sections and instrumental deliveries but can also be necessary postpartum (e.g. removal of retained placenta). General anaesthesia or, far more frequently, regional anaesthetic techniques are used to eliminate pain and inhibit motor activity almost completely during obstetric operations.

Anaesthetists are involved in the care of paturients in 25–75% of cases. This number obviously correlates with the local Caesarean section rate and the demand for epidural analgesia during labour. Regional anaesthesia is the method of choice for elective and most emergency Caesarean sections. Regional anaesthesia rates well above 90% or even 95% are not unusual in places where modern obstetric anaesthesia is practised.

Spinal anaesthesia and CSE are most commonly used for elective Caesarean sections.

Epidural anaesthesia

Epidural anaesthesia is typically established by using epidural catheters, already *in situ* for labour analgesia, for the injection of stronger local anaesthetics (e.g. Bupivacaine 0.5%). Rapid haemodynamic effects are less likely to occur with epidural or CSE anaesthesia and are frequently performed in women who would not tolerate sudden changes in peripheral vascular resistance (e.g. maternal cardiovascular disease).

Technique

Regardless of the regional technique planned, informed consent must be obtained prior to the procedure and maternal refusal is an absolute contraindication for regional anaesthesia.

Good intravenous access with at least one large bore cannula (14G or 16G) must be established and the parturient should also have received antacid prophylaxis. For elective surgery 150 mg ranitidine is commonly given orally 12 hours and 2–4 hours before surgery, combined with 10 mg metoclopramide orally 2–4 hours before surgery and, immediately prior to the procedure, 30 mL of 0.3 M sodium citrate orally. For emergency cases 50 mg ranitidine and 10 mg metoclopramide is injected slowly i.v., combined with 30 mL of 0.3 M sodium citrate orally.

Neuraxial anaesthesia is typically performed in the lumbar region between L2 and L3, L3 and L4, or L4 and L5 of the vertebral segments of the spine. The full lateral position can be associated with less hypotension and is probably slightly more comfortable for the patient. Many anaesthetists prefer the parturient to be in the sitting position which makes anatomical landmarks along the spine easier to identify.

Neuraxial anaesthesia can cause significant hypotension by the inhibition or an almost complete blockade of the sympathetic nerve system. Crystalloid solutions have been commonly administered for 'pre-loading' the patient's intravascular space. However, the effect of spinal or epidural anaesthesia on the incidence of hypotension reported in the literature is not consistent. The use of colloid solutions appears to be more efficacious but the potential for side-effects such as anaphylaxis and the additional costs involved must also be considered. Hypotension should be treated promptly to avoid side-effects such as dizziness, nausea, and vomiting for the mother, and potential risks such as hypoperfusion of the placenta and acidaemia for the fetus. Phenylephrine (50–100 μg i.v. bolus) is usually very effective and has recently been shown to be associated with fetal acidosis less often than is ephedrine (Table 10.1.1).

Epidurals which are only partly effective in labour will be unlikely to provide good anaesthesia for instrumental or surgical deliveries. These epidurals shouldn't be topped up prior to the procedure and spinal anaesthesia would provide better (and safer) anaesthesia in these cases.

Severe complications after epidural, spinal or (CSE) anaesthesia are rare; the incidence of temporary and permanent nerve damage is probably in the region of 1 in 10 000 and 1 in 50 000 respectively. Neurological deficits can also result from prolonged vaginal or instrumental deliveries (lithotomy position) and studies have shown that neurological symptoms after general anaesthesia are as (un-)common as they are after regional anaesthesia.

A 'total spinal' can occur if too much local anaesthetic has been injected into the intrathecal space and is characterized by a rapid onset of weakness of arms and respiratory muscles, followed by apnoea, cardiovascular depression, and unconsciousness; it is rare (1 in 5000–1 in 50 000) but must be treated immediately with intubation of the trachea and ventilation of the patient; cardiovascular support with vasoactive drugs is often also necessary.

Back pain is frequently reported to be a typical complication after neuraxial anaesthesia but several controlled trials appear to show that 'new, long-term postpartum back pain is not caused by intra-partum epidural analgesia or anaesthesia'. The annual prevalence of back pain among women of reproductive age is reported to be up to 50% and can increase to 76% during pregnancy (Table 10.1.2).

General anaesthesia

General anaesthesia is commonly reserved for patients who are unsuitable for regional techniques, where there is immediate threat to the life of mother or fetus

Table 10.1.1 Comparison epidural and spinal anaesthesia

Epidural anaesthesia	Spinal anaesthesia
Epidural space	Intrathecal space
Large doses of LA	Small doses of LA
Slow onset	Rapid onset
Fall in blood pressure ↑↑↑	Fall in BP only ↑–↑↑
Technically more difficult	Easier to perform
'Anaesthetic top-up' after labour analgesia possible	Single shoot technique (de novo)
Intraoperative top-ups	No top-ups
Poorer quality of block	Very dense block

Table 10.1.2 Complications of regional anaesthesia

Early	Late(r)
Hypotension	Urinary retention
High block	Respiratory depression
Total spinal	Postdural puncture headache
Nausea and vomiting (due to hypotension)	Nausea and vomiting (due to opioid supplement)
Failure	Infection at puncture site
Bleeding	Encephalitis, meningitis
Paraesthesia (when epidural/spinal is inserted)	Temporary or permanent nerve damage

(Category I Caesarean sections), or for other emergencies. Indications for general anaesthesia include

- maternal request
- need for immediate delivery/surgery (e.g. Category I Caesarean section)
- regional anaesthesia is contraindicated (severe haemorrhage, clotting disorder, eclampsia)
- failed or insufficient regional block (pre- or intra-operative conversion to general anaesthesia).

Technique

At term, the risk for aspiration of gastric content is significantly higher in pregnant women and antacid prophylaxis and a 'rapid sequence induction of anaesthesia' (RSI) are obligatory in order to minimize this risk. Sufficient pre-oxygenation with 100% oxygen in the left lateral tilt position, intubation and subsequent ventilation with 50% oxygen, as well as keeping the maternal blood pressure at a stable level are all measures to avoid hypoxaemia or hypoperfusion of the uteroplacental unit. Careful assessment of the woman's airway is very important but it is interesting to know that difficult and failed intubations occur in parturients with approximately the same frequency as in non-pregnant patients (grade 3 or 4 laryngoscopy in 1–6% of cases, failed intubations in 0.1–0.6% of cases). Obstetric anaesthetists have to manage difficult airways only infrequently because most procedures are nowadays performed under regional anaesthesia. It is therefore essential that equipment for difficult intubations is up to date, always available and that all anaesthetic staff are familiar with a difficult airway drill.

In contrast to general anaesthesia for Caesarean sections, regional anaesthesia techniques allow the woman to be awake during the delivery of her baby, and the partner can also be present. There are additional advantages such as a slightly reduced peri-operative blood loss, improved 1-minute Apgar scores in infants born by Caesarean section and better and more prolonged analgesia after neuraxial blockade. However, current data do not support the view that maternal mortality is higher in patients who receive general anaesthesia. The individual patient's situation and risk factors, and the experience of the anaesthetist, should determine the technique to be used. In women with pre-eclampsia for instance, regional anaesthesia is considered to be safe as long as platelet count and clotting remain within the normal range; blood pressure changes after epidural or spinal anaesthesia are typically less severe in pre-eclamptic patients, and general anaesthesia carries

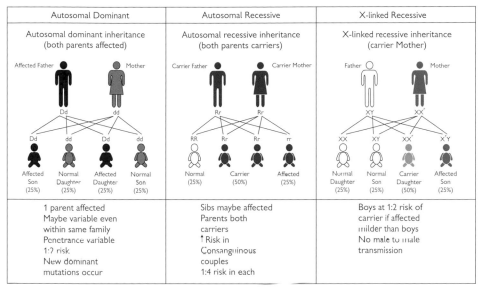

Autosomal Dominant	Autosomal Recessive	X-linked Recessive
Autosomal dominant inheritance (both parents affected)	Autosomal recessive inheritance (both parents carriers)	X-linked recessive inheritance (carrier Mother)
Affected Father / Mother Dd / dd Dd — Affected Son (25%) dd — Normal Daughter (25%) Dd — Affected Daughter (25%) dd — Normal Son (25%)	Carrier Father / Carrier Mother Rr / Rr RR — Normal (25%) Rr — Carrier (50%) rr — Affected (25%)	Father / Mother XY / XX′ XX — Normal Daughter (25%) XY — Normal Son (25%) XX′ — Carrier Daughter (50%) X′Y — Affected Son (25%)
1 parent affected Maybe variable even within same family Penetrance variable 1:2 risk New dominant mutations occur	Sibs maybe affected Parents both carriers ↑ Risk in Consanguinous couples 1:4 risk in each	Boys at 1:2 risk of carrier if affected milder than boys No male to male transmission

Fig. 7.7.1 Mendelian inheritance patterns.

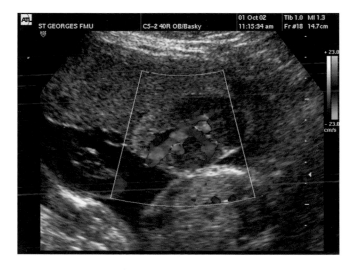

Fig. 7.22.1 Ultrasound image showing a placental chorioangioma, with colour Doppler blood flow within it.

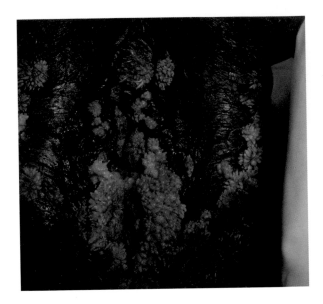

Fig. 8.20.2 Extensive genital warts in a pregnant woman presenting with a CD count of 170 cells/mm³.

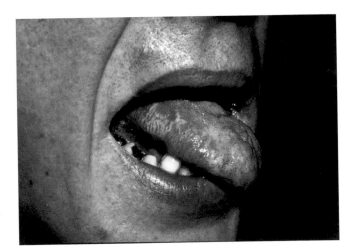

Fig. 8.20.3 Hairy oral leukoplakia is seen as white patches on the side of the tongue in HIV infection with often only moderate immunosuppression. The brown discolouration is related to smoking.

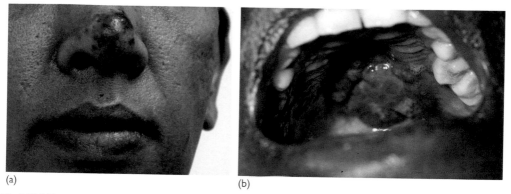

(a)   (b)

Fig. 8.20.4 Kaposi's sarcoma on the face (a) and large lesion on the palate (b). When this occurs multiple lesions are usually present in the gut and lungs as well.

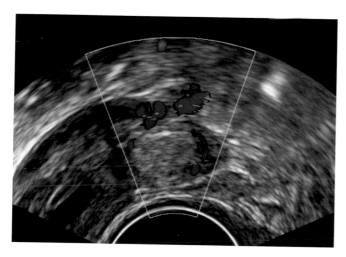

Fig. 12.9.2 A sonogram showing the right ovary (O) and a small hyperechoic solid structure adjacent to its medial pole (E). The swelling was highly vascular on Doppler examination, which helped to confirm the diagnosis of a tubal ectopic pregnancy.

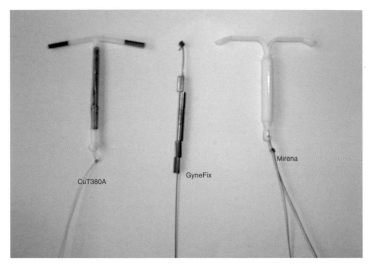

Fig. 12.18.1 Copper and progestogen-containing intrauterine devices.

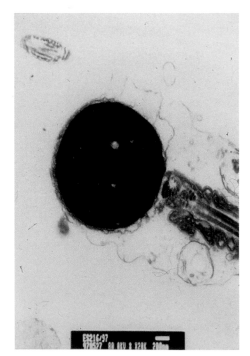

Fig. 12.22.1 Electron micrograph of a spermatozoon exhibiting the lack of an acrosomal membrane. The patient's concentration of sperm was in excess of 20 million per millilitre and greater than 60% of sperm were motile. The couple would require intracytoplasmic sperm micro-injection to achieve a pregnancy.

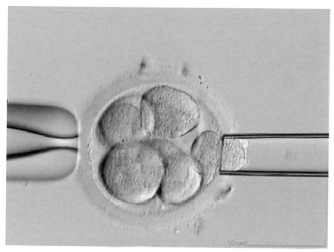

Fig. 12.32.1 Single cell being removed as a biopsy from a day 3 human preimplantation morula for genetic testing.

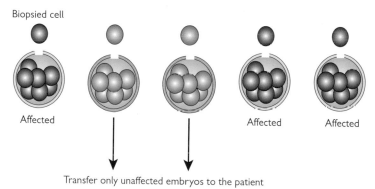

Biopsied cell

Affected

Affected

Affected

Transfer only unaffected embryos to the patient

Fig. 12.32.2 Principle of preimplantation genetic testing.

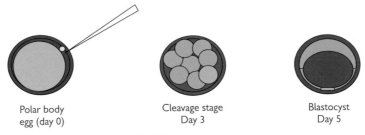

| Polar body | Cleavage stage | Blastocyst |
| egg (day 0) | Day 3 | Day 5 |

Fig. 12.32.3 Stages at which biopsy can be undertaken for PGD.

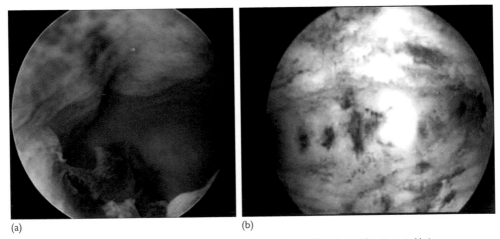

(a) (b)

Fig. 15.2.2 (a) Endometrial cavity seen at hysteroscopy prior to Novasure ablation; (b) endometrial cavity post ablation.

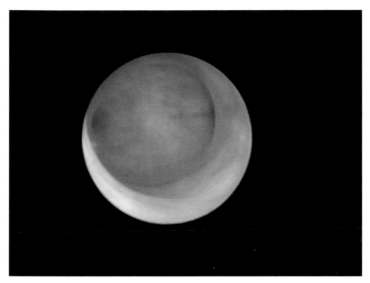

Fig. 15.3.3 Normal uterine cavity.

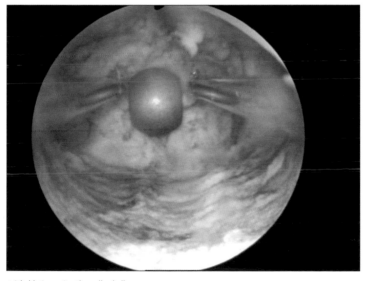

Fig. 15.3.4 Endometrial ablation using the roller ball.

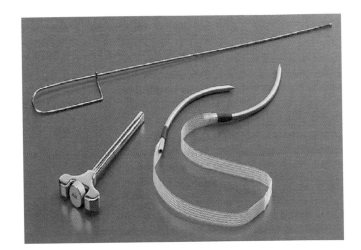

Fig. 15.5.1 Transobturator tape with needle.

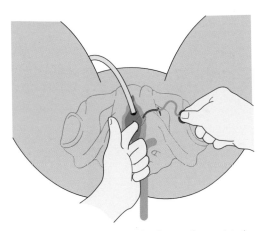

Fig. 15.5.2 Placement of tape via the obturator foramen into the vaginal incision.

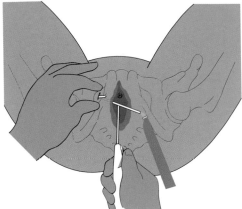

Fig. 15.5.3 Placement of tape via the vaginal funnelling into the obturator space.

the significant risk of uncontrolled pressure responses to laryngoscopy and intubation.

Anaesthesia-related maternal (and neonatal) mortality is nowadays extremely low and aspiration of gastric contents, a major cause of maternal deaths in the 1950s, is fortunately a rare occurrence. However, there is still a certain amount of controversy about whether paturients should be allowed to eat during labour. Recent studies indicate that the intake of solid food leads to an increased risk of vomiting and aspiration, especially if opioids are administered during labour. Until more evidence is available, it appears rational to restrict solid foods but allow calorie-containing clear fluids such as energy drinks) for maternal comfort.

Further reading

Comparative Obstetric Mobile Epidural Trial (COMET) Study Group UK. Effect of low-dose mobile versus traditional epidural techniques on mode of delivery: a randomised controlled trial. Lancet. 2001;358:19–23.

Halpern SH, Douglas MJ (eds). *Evidence-based obstetric anesthesia.* Oxford: Blackwell Publishing 2005.

Hodnett ED, Gates S, Hofmeyr GJ, et al. Continues support for women during childbirth. Cochrane Database Sys Rev 2003;3.

Horlocker TT, Wedel DJ, Benzon H, et al. Regional anesthesia in the anticoagulated patient: defining the risks (the second ASRA Consensus Conference on Neuraxial Anesthesia and Anticoagulation). Reg Anesth Pain Med 2003;28:172–97.

Lee A, Ngan Kee W D, Gin T. A quantitative, systematic review of randomized controlled trials of ephedrine versus phenylephrine for the management of hypotension during spinal anesthesia for cesarean delivery. Anesth Analg 2002;94:920–6.

O'Sullivan G, Liu B, Shennan AH. Oral intake during labor. Int Anesthesiol Clin 2007;45:133–47.

Rosenblatt MA, Abel M, Fischer GW, et al. Successful Use of a 20% Lipid Emulsion to Resuscitate a Patient after a Presumed Bupivacaine-related Cardiac Arrest. Anesthesiology 2006;105:217–8.

To WW, Wong MW. Factors associated with back pain symptoms in pregnancy and the persistence of pain 2 years after pregnancy. Acta Obstet Gynecol Scand. 2003;82:1086–91.

Wilson MJ, Cooper G, MacArthur C, et al.; Comparative Obstetric Mobile Epidural Trial (COMET) Study Group UK. Randomized controlled trial comparing traditional with two 'mobile' epidural techniques: anesthetic and analgesic efficacy. Anesthesiology 2002;97:1567–75.

Internet resources

The Obstetric Anaesthetists' Association (OAA): www.oaa-anaes.ac.uk

International Journal of Obstetric Anesthesia (IOJA). www.elsevier.com/wps/find/journaldescription.cws_home/623045/description#description

Breech

Definition

A malpresentation in which the fetus is in longitudinal lie and the presenting part is buttocks (or 'breech'), with the head occupying the upper pole of the uterus.

Epidemiology and predisposing factors

The incidence of breech presentation at term is between 3% and 4% and shows an inverse relationship with the gestational age. It is estimated that about 25% of fetuses would present by breech and 28 weeks and this figure falls to 5% at 34 weeks, suggesting that there is a progressive 'spontaneous version' to cephalic presentation as the pregnancy advances.

The main factors that result in spontaneous version to cephalic presentation include progressive calcification of the fetal skull bones (i.e. the head becomes heavier and therefore sinks down due to gravity, occupying the lower pole); gradual reduction of the amniotic fluid volume as the gestation advances that enables the uterus to exert its 'piriform' shape (i.e. in earlier gestations, due to the relatively large amniotic fluid volume, the uterus loses its 'piriform' shape and becomes 'globular', thereby allowing the fetus more flexibility with regard to lie and presentation); as the fetus grows, the larger (and bulkier) breech is forced to occupy the more spacious upper pole, whereas the head moves down to occupy the smaller lower pole of the 'piriform' uterus. It has been postulated that 'fetal kicking' plays an important role in facilitating spontaneous version and therefore an intact and functioning neuromuscular system appears to be essential for this process.

Predisposing factors

Prematurity is the commonest cause of breech presentation as the mechanisms described above that result in spontaneous version to cephalic presentation, gradually operate over time, with advancing gestation. Hence, it is obvious that earlier the gestation, greater the chance of breech presentation.

Factors that alter any of the variables that have been described are likely to predispose to breech presentation. These include alterations in amniotic fluid volume (oligo- or polyhydramnios), changes in uterine shape that eliminate the 'piriform effect' (congenital malformations such as septate or bicornuate uterus, fibroids in the lower segment, placenta praevia, cornual implantation of the placenta), and fetal factors that alter the normal anatomy such as congenital malformations (e.g. hydrocephalus that makes the head bulkier than breech), intrauterine growth restriction (smaller baby has more 'space' to occupy, nullifying the restrictive effects of piriform uterus), and multiple pregnancy. Abnormalities of the central nervous system or neuromuscular defects can affect fetal 'kicking movements' that may prevent spontaneous version.

True cephalopelvic disproportion (CPD) due to a contracted pelvis (rare) and congenital uterine anomalies may predispose to recurrent breech presentation. This term is used when three or more consecutive pregnancies are complicated by breech presentation (also termed 'habitual breech').

Types of breech

There are three main types of breech presentation.

Frank breech (or extended breech)

This is the commonest type of breech presentation (60–70%) that is characterized by flexion at the hip joint and extension at the knee joint. It is the commonest breech in primigravidae and possibly reflects firm (i.e. previously unstretched) uterine and abdominal wall muscles that do not allow enough intrauterine space for the fetus to flex its knees. Frank breech is ideal when vaginal breech delivery is contemplated because it is firmly applied to the cervix during labour. This enables good cervical dilatation during labour and does not allow any free space between the breech and the cervix, resulting in reduced incidence of cord prolapse. In fact, the incidence of cord prolapse with frank breech is similar to cephalic presentation (0.5%).

Complete breech (or flexed breech)

Characterized by flexion at both hip and knee joints. Common in multigravidae possibly due to lax abdominal and uterine muscles (due to stretching and loss of tone as a consequence of previous pregnancies) that allows sufficient space for the fetus to flex the knees. It is also common in cases where there is an increase in the intrauterine space–fetus ratio, such as polyhydramnios or intrauterine growth restriction. Complete breech is not very well applied to the cervix and hence it is a poor dilator of the cervix during labour and has an increased risk of cord prolapse (5%) as compared to frank breech.

Footling presentation (incomplete breech)

Characterized by extension at both hip and knee joints, the feet being the presenting part. Sufficient intrauterine space is essential for the extension to occur both at knee and hip joints and hence, footling breech presentation is common in extreme preterm fetuses. Footling breech is associated with significant perinatal morbidity and mortality due to increased incidence of cord prolapse (15%) and head entrapment. The latter is due to the possibility of the feet and trunk passing through a partially dilated cervix, up to the neck of the fetus, and the head being 'entrapped'. This is especially common in a preterm fetus that has a relatively larger head–trunk ratio than a term fetus.

- Knee presentation is very rare and is characterized by extension at the hip joint and flexion at the knee joints. Risks are similar to footling breech presentation.
- When breech presentation occurs in the absence of any obstetric (maternal and fetal) or medical complications, it is termed 'uncomplicated breech'. Conversely, when any of these risk factors (e.g. previous Caesarean section, placenta praevia, intrauterine growth restriction) coexist, it is termed 'complicated' breech presentation.

Pathophysiology

In contrast to cephalic presentation, the largest and least compressible part (i.e. the fetal head) presents last during vaginal breech delivery. This has many implications.

- It is possible for the fetal body to be passed through a partially dilated cervix, especially in case of a preterm fetus with footling presentation. This may lead to head entrapment, fetal hypoxia and fetal demise.
- The base of the skull which presents in breech presentation consists of skull bones, which are fused, as opposed to bones of the cranial vault in cephalic presentation, which are joined by membranous sutures. The latter facilitates moulding (overriding of skull bones on each other) and helps in the correction of mild degrees of cephalopelvic disproportion. Hence, in breech presentation, the fetal skull bones do not have the capacity to

undergo moulding and this may result in fetopelvic disproportion.

- Absence of moulding and relatively quicker delivery than cephalic presentation may result in sudden 'compression–decompression' injury to the fetal brain, especially, if the delivery of after-coming head is not controlled. This may result in intracranial haemorrhage and possible long-term neurological sequelae.
- Owing to rapidity of delivery as well as malconducted breech delivery, especially by inexperienced birth attendants, fetal injuries may occur. These include fracture of the femur, dislocation of the hip, soft tissue injury (rupture of liver, spleen), fracture of humerus and injury to the spinal cord (including laceration and complete transaction of the spinal cord) as well as skull fractures and intracranial haemorrhage.
- Sentinel hypoxic events during labour such as cord prolapse may cause hypoxic–ischaemic encephalopathy. Preterm fetuses with breech presentation may not have the necessary physiological reserve to cope with hypoxia and also have increased risk of birth trauma.

Clinical approach

History
History of uterine anomalies, previous breech presentation, placenta praevia, and fibroids should raise a clinical suspicion of abnormal lie and malpresentation, including breech presentation.

Clinical examination
On abdominal palpation, hard and round head will be felt in the upper pole of the uterus and is ballotable, whereas the soft, 'more bulky' breech will be felt in the lower pole. On auscultation, fetal heart sounds are audible usually at or above the umbilicus (fetal heart is located closer to the fetal head). In cases of undiagnosed (or misdiagnosed) breech presenting in labour, an irregular, broad, soft tissue mass may be felt on vaginal examination. The presence of the anal orifice in the same plane as bony prominences on either side (ischial tuberosities) may help differentiate a breech presentation from a cephalic presentation. In the latter, the mouth and two bony prominences on either side (malar eminences) are on different planes (like a triangle). It is also sometimes possible to elicit a 'sucking response' if the examiner's finger is inserted into the mouth of the fetus during a vaginal examination in face presentation as opposed to a 'gripping action' in case of breech presentation due to the constriction of the anal sphincter.

Investigations
Ultrasonography is the gold standard to confirm the diagnosis of breech presentation. This may also provide additional information such as number of fetuses, estimated fetal weight (EFW), the amniotic fluid volume, location of the placenta, presence of nuchal cord, hyper-tension of fetal head, and other information such as coexisting soft tissue masses (e.g. fibroids), which may aid in planning the mode of delivery. Earlier, some advocated radiological (X-ray) and CT pelvimetry to exclude fetopelvic disproportion prior to planning a vaginal delivery. However, there is no evidence to support this and these investigations are not recommended in current practice.

Management
There are three management options: vaginal breech delivery (spontaneous, assisted, and breech extraction);

external cephalic version (ECV) and elective Caesarean section.

Vaginal breech delivery
The Term Breech Trial by Hannah et al. (2000) concluded that vaginal breech delivery is associated with increased perinatal mortality, neonatal mortality, and serious neonatal morbidity compared with an elective Caesarean section (1.6% versus 5%; RR 0.33, 95% CI 0.19–0.56; p<0.0001). Serious maternal risks or complications were similar in both groups. In the light of this evidence and based on the guidelines and recommendations by various professional bodies (RCOG, ACOG), clinical practice has undergone a dramatic (and potentially irreversible) shift. Women should be informed of the findings of the Term Breech Trial and an elective Caesarean section should be recommended at term. However, in the following circumstances, a vaginal breech delivery may still be appropriate:

- the patient, after considering the risks and benefits, makes an informed choice to have a vaginal birth
- preterm breech deliveries (the findings of the Term Breech Trial is applicable for 'term' fetuses only)
- previously undiagnosed breech presentation in advanced labour (risks of an emergency caesarean section to both the mother and her baby may outweigh any potential benefits)
- a patient who has been planned to have an elective Caesarean section for breech presentation is admitted in advanced labour. It is estimated that up to 10% of women may go into labour prior to the date of their planned (elective) caesarean section
- twin pregnancy with second twin presenting by breech. The Term Breech Trial is applicable to singleton pregnancies at term
- in centres where facilities for an elective Caesarean section are not freely available (e.g. developing countries).

If vaginal breech delivery is contemplated, there are three approaches:

- spontaneous breech delivery (especially in multipara)—clinician does not perform any manoeuvres and allows nature to take its course
- assisted vaginal breech delivery (AVBD) is recommended. Delivery of the baby up to the level of the umbilicus is unaided (sometimes Pinard's manoeuvre in an extended breech to flex the knee). Assistance is then offered for the delivery of the shoulder, especially in cases of extended or nuchal arms (Lovset's manoeuvre) and the 'after-coming' head (Burns–Marshall technique, Mauriceau–Smellie–Viet (MSV) technique or the use of forceps). It is important not to pull in haste (may cause extension of the fetal head or nuchal arms), hold the fetus on the pelvic brim and not the abdomen (avoids injury to intraperitoneal organs), avoid hyperextension of the neck (avoids cervical spine injury), and to have a controlled delivery of the 'after-coming' head (avoids intracranial haemorrhage due to sudden compression–decompression injury)
- breech extraction refers to an accelerated process of delivering the fetus by pulling on the feet, with no or minimum effort by the mother. It is contraindicated in modern obstetric practice due to potential fetal and maternal trauma. However, when there is cord prolapse or acute fetal distress of the second twin, after the delivery of the first twin, this procedure may be attempted to expedite delivery if the cervix is fully dilated.

External cephalic version (ECV)

This refers to 'manipulation of the fetus through the mother's abdomen, with a view to turning the fetus from breech to cephalic presentation, thereby to avoid a caesarean section'.

- ECV should be offered at term (ideally 37–38 weeks, when there is sufficient amniotic fluid).
- Contraindications for normal delivery should be excluded (placenta praevia, hyperextended head, previous uterine scars, large fetus (>4 kg), clinically inadequate pelvis, and growth-restricted fetus). In addition, absolute contraindications include major uterine abnormality, multiple pregnancy, ruptured membranes, abnormal cardiotocograph (CTG), and significant antepartum haemorrhage within the preceding 7 days.
- Overall success rate of ECV is between 50–60% and this may be improved, especially in primigravidae by tocolysis (terbutaline 0.25 μg subcutaneously) 20 minutes prior to the procedure.
- Fetal heart rate should be monitored both before (to assess fetal wellbeing) and after (to detect complications) the procedure.
- Women should be informed of potential risks, including placental abruption, fetomaternal haemorrhage (may require Anti-D if Rhesus negative), cord accidents, and, rarely, uterine rupture. The chance of an emergency caesarean section is about 0.5%.
- Women should be informed that there is a spontaneous reversion rate (to breech presentation) of 5% and the possibility of intrapartum emergency Caesarean section.

Elective Caesarean section

Lower segment Caesarean section (LSCS) should be offered to all patients who have had a failed ECV or have declined ECV, as well as those who have an absolute contraindication for vaginal delivery or ECV.

- Adequate exposure is essential to facilitate a 'non-traumatic' delivery. The manoeuvres during a Caesarean section are similar to assisted vaginal breech delivery: the breech, trunk and shoulders, as well as the 'after-coming' head should be delivered in that order, using the same manoeuvres, where necessary (Pinard's to deliver the legs, Lovset's to deliver the shoulders, Burns–Marshall or obstetric forceps to deliver the 'after-coming' head). In cases of extended head ('star-gazing'), flexing the head prior to delivery is likely to make delivery easier.
- It may be prudent to use tocolysis in established labour (especially late first stage or second stage of labour) to abolish uterine contractions and to facilitate easy delivery during caesarean section.

Post 'Term Breech Trial'

- A 2-year follow up study by the Term Breech Trial Group has concluded that there is no significant difference with regard to neurodevelopmental delay between the vaginal and planned Caesarean section groups, at 2 years of age. Subsequently, Glezerman (2006) has suggested that analysis of the original and new data gives rise to serious concerns as far as study design, methods, and conclusions are concerned (with respect to the original 'Term Breech Trial'). In a substantial number of cases, there was a lack of adherence to the inclusion criteria. There was a large interinstitutional variation of standard of care; inadequate methods of antepartum and intrapartum fetal assessment were used, and a large proportion of women were recruited during active labour.

- More recently, an observational prospective study with an intent-to-treat analysis concluded that in units where planned vaginal delivery is a common practice and when strict criteria are met before and during labour, planned vaginal delivery of singleton fetuses in breech presentation at term remains a safe option that can be offered to women.
- In light of recent studies that further clarify the long-term risks of vaginal breech delivery, the American College of Obstetricians and Gynecologists (ACOG) recommends that the decision regarding mode of delivery should depend on the experience of the healthcare provider.
- Despite of its shortcomings, the Term Breech Trial was a randomized controlled trial that concluded that vaginal breech delivery is associated with an increased perinatal morbidity and mortality compared with an elective Caesarean section. Hence, before a vaginal breech delivery is planned, women should be informed that the risk of perinatal or neonatal mortality or short-term serious neonatal morbidity may be higher than if a Caesarean delivery is planned, and the patient's informed consent should be documented. Failure to do so may have medicolegal implications.

Further reading

ACOG Committee Opinion No. 340. Mode of term singleton breech delivery. Obstet Gynecol 2006;108:235–7.

Chandraharan E, Arulkumaran S. Acute tocolysis. Curr Opin Obstet Gynecol 2003;17:151–6.

Glezerman M. Five years to the term breech trial: the rise and fall of a randomized controlled trial. Am J Obstet Gynecol 2006; 194:20–5.

Goffinet F, Carayol M, Foidart JM, et al. PREMODA Study Group. Is planned vaginal delivery for breech presentation at term still an option? Results of an observational prospective survey in France and Belgium. Am J Obstet Gynecol 2006;194:1002–11.

Hannah ME, Hannah WJ, Hewson SA, et al. Planned caesarean section versus planned vaginal birth for breech presentation at term: a randomised multicentre trial. Lancet 2000;356:1375–83.

Royal College of Obstetricians and Gynaecologists. Pelvimetry: clinical indications. Green-top Guideline No. 14. London: RCOG 1998.

Royal College of Obstetricians and Gynaecologists. External cephalic version and reducing the incidence of breech presentation. Green-top Guideline No. 20a. London: RCOG 2006.

Royal College of Obstetricians and Gynaecologists. Vaginal breech delivery. Green-top Guideline No. 20b. London: RCOG; 2006.

Whyte H, Hannah M, Saigal S. Term BreechTrial Collaborative Group. Outcomes of children at 2 years of age in the Term Breech Trial. Am J Obstet Gynecol 2003;189:S57.

Internet resources

Breech presentation: www.patient.co.uk/showdoc/40000237/

Patient resources

Turning a breech in your womb (external cephalic version): Information for you: www.rcog.org.uk/resources/public/pdf/PITurningECV0208.pdf.

A breech Baby at the end of pregnancy: information for you: www.rcog.org.uk/resources/public/pdf/PIBreechBaby0208.pdf.

Brow presentation

Definition

A rare malpresentation in which the area between the orbital ridges (inferiorly) and bregma (superiorly), becomes the presenting part. This is due to deflexion (i.e. partial extension) of the fetal neck, which results in the largest diameter of the fetal skull, the mentovertical diameter (13.5 cm) to be the engaging diameter. Hence, there is no mechanism of labour in persistent brow presentation as the mentovertical diameter is larger than all the diameters of the bony pelvis. The denominator for brow presentation is the forehead (frontum).

Epidemiology

It is difficult to estimate the true incidence of brow presentation as the vast majority change into face or vertex presentations during labour. Reported incidence varies from 1 in 3000–1 in 500 (0.03–0.5%). Predisposing factors are similar to face presentation and include multiparity, cephalopelvic disproportion (CPD), uterine malformation, abnormalities in amniotic fluid volume (polyhydramnios or oligohydramnios). Conditions that cause deflexion of the fetal head such as congenital goitre or branchocoele, multiple cord round the fetal neck ('nuchal cord') and rarely musculoskeletal abnormalities that cause spasm (or shortening or contracture) of the muscles of the extensor compartment of the neck may also predispose to brow presentation.

Mechanism of labour

Brow presentation may undergo further flexion to become a vertex presentation or further extension to become a face presentation. Prerequisites for such favourable outcomes are roomy pelvis, average size fetus, and strong and effective uterine contractions. Absence of favourable factors results in a persistent brow presentation. There can be no mechanism of labour because the mentovertical diameter (13.5 cm) is larger than the dimensions of the pelvis and hence, there can be no progress of labour. Prompt diagnosis and timely Caesarean section is necessary to improve maternal and perinatal outcome. Rarely, if the fetus is preterm or macerated, vaginal birth may still be possible with persistent brow presentation.

Clinical approach

Diagnosis of a brow presentation may be difficult prior to the onset of labour. The presence of a high (non-engaged) head at term and prominent occiput should alert the clinician. As in face presentation, there is a groove between the occiput and the fetal back. However, unlike the face presentation where the entire fetal head is felt at the same side as the fetal spine due to extension, the head is felt on both sides of the fetal spine due to deflexion (partial extension). An ultrasound scan may be performed antenatally or during labour to help diagnose or exclude abnormalities of amniotic fluid (oligo- or polyhydramnios), placenta praevia, congenital abnormalities (anencephaly, branchocoele, fetal goitre). Doppler examination may be helpful when nuchal cord is suspected.

On vaginal examination during labour, the root of the nose, orbital ridges, frontal sutures, and anterior fontanelle can be palpated. Unlike the face presentation, the mouth and chin cannot be felt on vaginal examination.

Management

Brow presentation should be clinically suspected in any multipara with a non-engaged head at term or in early labour. Owing to 'ill-fitting' presenting part, membranes may herniate and rupture early leading to increased risk of cord prolapse. Hence, the patient should be counselled about this possibility and advised to attend early in labour if brow presentation is suspected or diagnosed antenatally. Sometimes, persistent decelerations on a cardiotocograph, despite of a high fetal head may arouse clinical suspicion of brow presentation. This is because repeated pressure on the eyeballs during contractions may stimulate parasympathetic nervous system, leading to decelerations of the fetal heart rate.

During early labour, in the absence of unfavourable factors that have been discussed earlier, vaginal delivery can be anticipated, especially if CPD and fetal macrosomia have been excluded. Optimum uterine contractions may change brow presentation into a face presentation (extension) or vertex presentation (flexion). However, up to 33–50% of brow presentations may present with secondary arrest or failure to progress, despite adequate contractions. Emergency Caesarean section is the safest mode of delivery in such cases. In cases of preterm infants (i.e. very small) and a roomy pelvis in the presence of good uterine contractions and anterior brow presentation, vaginal delivery may be possible. Similar to mentoposterior face presentation, there is no mechanism of labour in posterior brow presentation. During Caesarean section, care should be taken to flex the fetal head prior to delivering through the uterine incision to avoid extension of the incision at the uterine angles. As in face presentation, atonic or traumatic postpartum haemorrhage may occur following delivery and these should be anticipated and managed appropriately.

Further reading

Bashiri A, Burstein E, Bar-David J, Levy A, Mazor M. Face and brow presentation: independent risk factors. J Matern Fetal Neonatal Med 2008;21:357–60.

Chandraharan E, Arulkumaran S. Operative delivery, shoulder dystocia and episiotomy. In: Arulkumaran S, Penna LK, Bhasker Rao K (eds) The management of labour, 2nd edn. Orient Longman 2005.

Stitely ML, Gherman RB. Labor with abnormal presentation and position. Obstet Gynecol Clin N Am 2005;32:165–79.

Cord prolapse

Definition

Cord prolapse (or prolapse of the umbilical cord) occurs when a loop of umbilical cord lies below the presenting part and the membranes have ruptured. Cord presentation refers to the presence of a loop of cord below the presenting part when the membranes are intact. Occult cord prolapse is said to occur when a loop of umbilical cord lies alongside the presenting part.

Epidemiology

It has been estimated that overall, cord prolapse occurs in 1 in 3000 deliveries. However, the incidence of cord prolapse is believed to vary with the nature of the presenting part and the lie of the fetus. The incidence is estimated to be 0.5% with cephalic and frank breech presentations; 5% with complete breech; 15% with footling breech presentations; and 20% with transverse lie. It is difficult to estimate the exact incidence of occult cord prolapse. Variable decelerations on the cardiotocograph suggest cord compression and are known to occur in over 50% of established labour. These are often transitory and often disappear with changes in the maternal position. Hence, it would appear that occult cord prolapse is quite common during labour and often goes undiagnosed.

Risk factors

- Unstable lie (transverse lie) /malpresentation such as breech (especially a footling breech)
- Polyhydramnios
- Prelabour rupture of membranes, especially in preterm pregnancies
- Twins and higher order multiple pregnancy
- High presenting part in labour (e.g. true or relative cephalopelvic disproportion or CPD, placenta praevia and rarely fibroids in the lower segment of the uterus)
- Obstetric interventions: artificial rupture of membranes (ARM), fetal blood sampling (FBS), or application of a scalp electrode or pulse oximeter when the presenting part is high
- Multiparity (predisposes to abnormal lie and malpresentations)
- Long umbilical cord (rare).

Pathophysiology

Prolapse of the umbilical cord may result in two detrimental processes that may reduce the oxygen supply to the fetus. First, there may be a mechanical effect due to the compression of the umbilical cord between the presenting part (head, breech) and the maternal birth passage. Second, there may be a physiological effect of umbilical cord spasm, as the fetal blood vessels (umbilical arteries and vein) are exposed to the cold air. Both these processes would threaten to reduce the blood supply from the placenta to the fetus, resulting in acute fetal hypoxia. Degree of fetal hypoxia and the resultant neurological damage (risks of cerebral palsy, long-term neurological sequelae, and neonatal death) would depend on the degree of cord compression, placental reserve, ability of the fetus to withstand the acute hypoxic stress (preterm, post-term, and growth-restricted fetuses may not effectively cope with hypoxia), and the time interval between cord prolapse and delivery.

Diagnosis

- In frank or overt cases of cord prolapse, the umbilical cord can be seen protruding from the introitus or loops of cord can be seen or palpated within the vagina during a vaginal examination.
- Occult cord prolapse is often suspected based on abnormalities of the fetal heart rate (repeated variable decelerations) seen on a cardiotocograph (CTG). Rarely the umbilical cord may be felt beside (not below) the presenting part on vaginal examination.
- Cord presentation may be diagnosed when loops of cord are palpated through an intact membrane.
- Ultrasound examination (especially colour Doppler) may help identify a loop of cord below the presenting part and hence, may help in the diagnosis of cord presentation prior to the onset of labour. This is not routinely used in clinical practice as it has poor sensitivity and specificity. However, is selected cases such as polyhydramnios and vasa praevia (insertion of the umbilical cord on to the fetal membranes that results in cord vessels traversing fetal membranes below the presenting part), Doppler may be a useful tool.

Management

Cord prolapse is an acute obstetric emergency and is considered to be a sentinel hypoxic event during labour. Delay in delivery would increase the chances of hypoxic injury to the fetus and worsen the outcome. Principles of management involves a rapid assessment of fetal viability (Pinard's fetoscope, Dopplertone, ultrasound examination to confirm fetal heart activity) and immediate delivery by the safest and most appropriate method. If the fetus is viable, institute measures to avoid further cord compression to improve oxygenation until delivery. Neonatal resuscitation is an important aspect of management as there is a likelihood that the neonate would be born in a poor (asphyxiated) condition.

- If the fetus is dead at the time of diagnosis of cord prolapse or on admission (e.g. transfer from home or another unit with cord prolapse), then no further intervention is needed. The woman and her partner should be informed and sympathies expressed. Labour should be allowed to progress, anticipating a vaginal birth unless there is a maternal indication (transverse lie or major degree placenta praevia) that necessitates a Caesarean section.
- If the fetus is viable (i.e. fetal heart rate is present), the safest and most appropriate mode of delivery should be contemplated with a view to deliver the fetus within the shortest possible time. This would necessitate an immediate vaginal examination to assess the dilatation of the cervix and the station of the presenting part.
- In the first stage of labour (i.e. cervix is not fully dilated) or if the cervix is fully dilated, but the presenting part is high (above the ischial spines) an immediate (Category 1) Caesarean section should be performed. However, prior to the operative procedure, the clinical situation may be reassessed by performing a vaginal examination, as some labours progress rapidly (e.g. multigravida with 9 cm or fully dilated cervix with the vertex below spines). In such situations the safest and quickest option may be an assisted vaginal delivery.

- In the second stage of labour (i.e. fully dilated cervix and presenting part below the spines) an instrumental delivery (ventouse or forceps) could be attempted as this is likely to be the safest and most expedient mode of delivery. However, difficult rotational deliveries are best avoided, especially in the presence of fetal heart rate abnormalities associated with cord prolapse as birth trauma may compound the detrimental effects of hypoxia, leading to an unfavourable outcome.
- Immediate (Category 1) Caesarean section should be carried out in cases of cord prolapse occurring with an abnormal lie (e.g. transverse lie) or breech presentation. In cases of cord prolapse of the second twin (after the birth of first twin) a breech extraction may be attempted as this is likely to be the safest and most expedient method in this situation.

Measures to improve fetal outcome prior to delivery

Measures to improve oxygenation to the fetus include reducing the chances of vasospasm, relieving cord compression, and reducing the intensity and frequency of uterine contraction to allow for 'intrauterine resuscitation'.

- Reduce the chance of vasospasm by gently replacing the cord within the vagina and retaining it inside the vagina with a warm saline pack. This is likely to reduce the exposure to cold air that triggers the spasm of the cord vessels. However, excessive handling of the cord itself may trigger a spasm.
- Relieve cord compression by placing the patient in an exaggerated Simms position with the hips and buttocks elevated by a wedge or pillow. This is likely to mobilize the presenting part away from the cord due to the effect of gravity. The foot-end of the bed could be elevated to achieve the same results.
- The clinician who diagnosed cord prolapse could insert two fingers into the vagina in order to push up the presenting part during contractions. This may be useful when cord prolapse is diagnosed in a 'home birth' situation while awaiting additional help to transport the patient to the hospital.
- Urinary bladder could be catheterized with a 16G Foley catheter and approximately 500 mL of normal saline be instilled into the bladder via a standard giving set. The balloon is then inflated and the catheter clamped. A 'full bladder' displaces the presenting part upwards, thus relieving the pressure on the umbilical cord. This method eliminates the need for the examiner's fingers to displace the presenting part. However, the clamp should be removed prior to Caesarean section to avoid inadvertent bladder injury.

- Acute tocolysis (Terbutaline 0.25 mg subcutaneously) may be attempted to abolish uterine contractions. This is likely to improve uteroplacental blood flow and, hence, fetal oxygenation.

Anticipation and prevention of cord prolapse

- Cord prolapse should be anticipated in the presence of risk factors and measures should be taken to minimize its occurrence. In the presence of polyhydramnios, a controlled artificial rupture of membranes (ARM) should be attempted. A 'stabilizing induction' may allow the presenting part to fit in snugly within the pelvis at the time of rupture of membranes and thereby reduce the space available for cord prolapse.
- Early diagnosis of cord prolapse is likely to improve the outcome. Vaginal examination should be performed in the presence of repeated variable decelerations, especially after ARM, application of fetal scalp electrode or fetal blood sampling as the displacement of the presenting part during these procedures may predispose to cord prolapse.

Risk management issues

It is important to explain the events and the possible causes to the patient and her partner and this discussion should be clearly documented in the notes. Cord blood gases (arterial and venous pH, base excess, PO_2, and PCO_2) should be determined and documented. An incident report form should be completed and regular audit of Category 1 Caesarean sections should be carried out to determine whether the 'decision-to-delivery' interval standards are met.

Further reading

Chamberlein G, Steer P. ABC of labour care: unusual presentations and positions and multiple pregnancy. *BMJ* 1999;318:1192–4.

Chandraharan E, Arulkumaran S. Acute tocolysis: Review Article. Curr Opin Obstet Gynecol 2003;17:151–6.

Chandraharan E, Arulkumaran S. Prevention of birth asphyxia: responding appropriately to cardiotocograph (CTG) traces. Best Pract Res Clin Obstet Gynaecol 2007;21:609–24.

Critchlow CW, Leet TL, Benedetti TJ, Daling JR. Risk factors and infant outcomes associated with umbilical cord prolapse: A population-based case control study among births in Washington state. Am J Obstet Gynecol 1994;170:613–8.

Katz Z. Management of labour with umbilical cord prolapse: a 5 year study. Obstet Gynaecol 1998;72:278–81.

Murphy DJ, MacKenzie IZ. The mortality and morbidity associated with umbilical cord prolapse. Br J Obstet Gynaecol 1995;102:826–30.

Prabulos AM, Philipson EH. Umbilical cord Prolapse; so far so good. J Reprod Med 1998;43:129–32.

Episiotomy and obstetric perineal trauma

Definition

Perineal trauma may occur spontaneously during vaginal birth or intentionally when a surgical incision (episiotomy) is made to facilitate delivery.

Perineal trauma is classified as follows:

- first degree: laceration of the vaginal epithelium or perineal skin only
- second degree: involvement of the perineal muscles (bulbocavernosus, transverse perineal) but not the anal sphincter
- third degree: disruption of the anal sphincter muscles which should be further subdivided into 3a, <50% thickness of external sphincter torn; 3b, >50% thickness of external sphincter torn; 3c, internal sphincter also torn
- fourth degree: a third degree tear with disruption of the anal epithelium as well.

Episiotomy is a surgical incision made with scissors or a scalpel into the perineum in order to increase the diameter of the vulval outlet and facilitate delivery.

There are two main types of episiotomy incision:

- a midline episiotomy is an incision from the midpoint of the posterior fourchette directed vertically towards the anus
- a mediolateral episiotomy is an incision from the midpoint of the posterior fourchette directed 40 to 60 degrees away from the midline.

Incidence

Perineal trauma is dependent on variations in obstetric practice including rates and types of episiotomies, which not only vary between countries but also between individual practitioners within hospitals.

- In the UK approximately 85% of women sustain some form of perineal trauma during vaginal delivery and of these 69% will require stitches
- In centres where mediolateral episiotomies are practised, the rate of obstetric anal sphincter injuries (OASIS) occurs in 1.7% compared to 12% in centres practising midline episiotomy.

Indications for episiotomy

- To accelerate vaginal delivery in cases of fetal distress.
- Reduce the occurrence of multiple lacerations in the presence of a thick or rigid perineum.
- To facilitate manoeuvres during shoulder dystocia.
- To minimize severe perineal trauma during a forceps delivery.
- In situations where prolonged 'bearing down' maybe harmful for the mother (e.g. severe hypertensive or cardiac disease).

Management and repair of perineal trauma

Ensure that the wound is adequately anaesthetized prior to commencing the repair with 10–20 mL of lignocaine 1% injected evenly into the perineal wound. If the woman has an epidural it may be 'topped-up' and used to block perineal pain during suturing instead of injecting local anaesthetic. Repair of obstetric anal sphincter trauma should be undertaken in theatre, under general or regional anaesthesia.

First-degree tears and labial lacerations

Women should be advised that in the case of first-degree trauma, the wound should be sutured in order to improve healing, unless the skin edges are well opposed.

Episiotomy and second-degree tears

Perineal trauma should be repaired using the continuous non-locking technique to reapproximate all layers (vagina, perineal muscles, and skin) with absorbable polyglactin 910 material (Vicryl rapide).

The steps in Fig. 10.5.1 should be followed

- The first stitch is inserted above the apex of the vaginal laceration and the vaginal wound is closed with a loose, continuous, non-locking technique down to the hymenal remnants. Insert the needle through the skin at the fourchette to emerge in the centre of the perineal wound.
- Check the depth of the trauma and close the perineal muscle (deep and superficial) with continuous non-locking stitches.
- At the inferior end of the wound, bring the needle out just under the skin surface reversing the stitching direction. Continue to take bites of tissue from each side of the wound edges until the hymenal remnants are reached. Secure the finished repair with a loop or Aberdeen knot placed in the vagina behind the hymenal remnants.

Third- and fourth-degree tears

- Intraoperative antibiotics should be administered.
- In the presence of a fourth-degree tear, the torn anal epithelium is repaired with interrupted Vicryl 3/0 sutures with the knots tied in the anal lumen.
- The internal anal sphincter should be identified and if torn, repaired separately from the external anal sphincter. The ends of the torn muscle are grasped with Allis forceps and an end-to-end repair is performed with interrupted sutures (3-0 PDS (Polydioxanone) or 2-0 Vicryl (polyglactin-Vicryl)).
- The torn ends of the EAS therefore need to be identified and grasped with Allis tissue forceps. When the EAS is only partially torn (Grade 3a and some 3b) then an end-to-end repair should be performed using two or three mattress sutures. If there is a full thickness EAS tear (some 3b, 3c, or fourth degree), either an overlapping or end-to-end method can be used with equivalent outcome, although in experienced hands superior results have been reported with the overlap technique.
- The perineal muscles should be sutured to reconstruct the perineal body in order to provide support to the repaired anal sphincter.
- Finally, the vaginal skin should be sutured and the perineal skin approximated with a Vicryl 2-0 subcuticular suture.

Basic principles after repair of perineal tears

- Check that complete haemostasis is achieved and confirm that the finished repair is anatomically correct.
- A rectal and vaginal examination should be performed to confirm adequate repair so as to ensure that no other tears have been missed and that a suture is not inadvertently placed through the rectal mucosa. Confirm that all tampons or swabs have been removed.
- Detailed notes should be made of the findings and repair.

Postoperative care

- The use of broad-spectrum antibiotics and laxatives is recommended following third- and fourth-degree tears

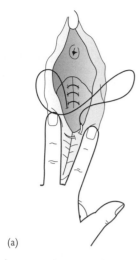
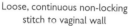
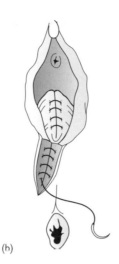
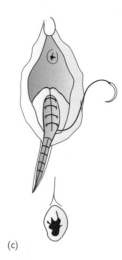

(a)

Loose, continuous non-locking
stitch to vaginal wall

(h)

Loose continuous non-locking
stitch to perineal muscles

(c)

Closure of skin using a
loose subcutaneous stitch

Fig. 10.5.1 Continuous suturing technique for mediolateral episiotomy. Sultan AH, Thakar R. Repair of episiotomy, first and second degree tears. In Sulatn AH, Thakar R, Fenner D (eds) *Perineal and anal sphincter trauma* (2009); 20–32. With kind permission of Springer Science Business and Media.

- All women who have had obstetric anal sphincter repair should be reviewed 6–12 weeks postpartum by a senior clinician.

Further reading

Carroli G, Belizan J. Episiotomy for vaginal birth. Cochrane Database Syst Rev 1999;3:CD00081.

Intrapartum Care. NICE Clinical Guideline. Guideline 55 2007 Available from: URL: www.nice.org.uk/CG055

Kettle C, Hills RK, Ismail KM. Continuous versus interrupted sutures for repair of episiotomy or second degree tears. Cochrane Database Syst Rev 2007;4:CD000947

Sultan AH, Thakar R, Fenner D (eds). *Perineal and anal sphincter trauma*. London: Springer 2007

Henderson C, Bick D (eds). *Perineal care: an international issue.* Wiltshire: Quay Books 2005

Royal College of Obstetricians and Gynaecologists. *Management of third and fourth degree perineal tears following vaginal delivery.* Guideline No 29. London, RCOG Press 2007.

Royal College of Obstetricians and Gynaecologists. *Methods and materials used in perineal repair.* Guideline No. 23. London: RCOG press 2004.

Sultan AH, Thakar R. Third and fourth degree tears. In: Sultan AH, Thakar R, Fenner D (eds) *Perineal and anal sphincter trauma.* London: Springer-Verlag 2007: 33–51.

Internet resources

www.perineum.net

www.patient.co.uk/showdoc/40000277

Face presentation

Definition

A malpresentation in which the presenting part is the face bounded superiorly by orbital ridges (glabella), laterally by the malar eminences and inferiorly by the chin (or mentum). The head is hyperextended and the chin forms the denominator with submentobregmatic diameter as the presenting diameter.

Epidemiology

Overall incidence of face presentation is approximately 1 in 500 births (0.5%). Incidence increases in the presence of fetal congenital malformations (15%) such as iniencephaly or dolichocephalic head. Anencephaly is associated with an increased incidence of face presentation (30%) because of the absence of vault of the fetal skull. Other predisposing factors include multiparity, cephalopelvic disproportion (CPD), uterine malformation, and abnormalities in amniotic fluid volume (polyhydramnios or oligohydramnios). Any condition that causes hyperextension of the fetal neck is likely to predispose to face presentation. These include congenital goitre or branchocoele, multiple cord round the fetal neck ('nuchal cord'), and rarely musculoskeletal abnormalities that cause spasm (or shortening or contracture) of the muscles of the extensor compartment of the neck. Primary and secondary face presentation refers to diagnosis of face presentation during the antenatal period and labour, respectively.

Mechanism of labour

Mentum or chin is the denominator in face presentation. And the engaging diameter is submentobregmatic, which is similar to the biparietal diameter in vertex presentation (9.5 cm). When chin is anterior (i.e. in relation to the iliopectineal eminence), it is termed left or right mentoanterior (LMA or RMA) position. Similarly, if the mentum is posterior (i.e. in relation to the sacroiliac joints) it is termed left or right mentoposterior (LMP or RMP) positions. If the chin is along the transverse diameter of the pelvis, it is termed mentolateral (ML) or mentotransverse (MT).

The largest diameter of the skull (biparietal diameter or BPD) is about 7 cm behind the advancing face presentation during labour. This means that the BPD engages only when the face is at +2 or +3 station (i.e. almost crowning the vulva). Failure to appreciate this anatomical fact may lead to increased perinatal and maternal morbidity due to earlier intervention to expedite vaginal delivery when the largest diameter is still above the pelvic brim.

The majority of face presentations occur during labour, secondary to extension of a brow presentation, in the presence of strong and effective uterine contractions in the presence of an adequate pelvis. Mentoanterior positions are delivered by flexion. Mentoposterior positions (LMP, RMP, or direct) behave similar to occipitoposterior positions (OP) and hence, need to undergo a long anterior rotation (three-eighths of a circle) during labour, prior to delivery. The chance of a successful long rotation is only about 45–65% during the second stage of labour. Failure of this long anterior rotation makes further progress of labour impossible in mentoposterior positions (except in cases of extreme prematurity or macerated fetus).

- In mentoposterior positions, delivery should occur by extension. However, the head is already maximally extended and hence, further extension is not possible.

- As the length of the sacrum is about 10–12 cm and that of neck is only 5 cm, the shoulders enter the pelvis and become impacted while the head is still in the pelvis, thus the labour is obstructed. Entry of the thorax into the pelvis makes it difficult for the sternobregmatic diameter (18 cm) to enter the pelvis.

Clinical approach

Primary face presentation is diagnosed prior to the onset of labour. On abdominal palpation, the cephalic prominence is on the same side as the fetal back, with a 'groove' separating the occiput from the spine. The occiput is above the level of the sinciput. If face presentation is suspected on clinical examination prior to the onset of labour it may be confirmed by ultrasound examination. Intervention is not necessary because, in the absence of any predisposing factors such as nuchal cord or congenital goitre, the majority of these would revert to vertex presentation during labour. It is reasonable to expect that effective uterine contractions during labour in the presence of an adequate, roomy pelvis may aid conversion of the face presentation to a more favourable vertex presentation.

Secondary face presentation is diagnosed during labour. Abdominal examination may reveal the above findings. However, vaginal examination is more reliable. Orbital ridges, malar eminences, and the mouth can be felt. Clinically, face presentation can be differentiated from breech presentation as the mouth and malar eminences on either side form three angles (or apices) of a triangle. In contrast, the anal orifice and ischial tuberosities on either side are on a straight line in breech presentation. Also, inserting the tip of the finger into the mouth enables the palpation of hard gums and may stimulate fetal sucking. In breech presentation, if the tip of examiner's finger is inadvertently introduced into the anus, a 'gripping' action of the anal sphincter may be elicited. Sometimes it may be difficult to palpate the mouth and malar eminences due to gross oedema of the face (called 'tumefaction'), which is similar to 'caput' in a vertex presentation. In this situation, the eyeballs, nose, and lips are swollen.

Role of ultrasound

In modern obstetric practice, an ultrasound scan can be performed antenatally or during labour to confirm face presentation. Ultrasonography can also help diagnose or exclude abnormalities of amniotic fluid (oligo- or polyhydramnios), placenta praevia, and congenital abnormalities (anaencephaly, branchocele, fetal goitre). Doppler examination may be helpful when nuchal cord is suspected.

Management

An elective Caesarean section should be offered if there is clinical evidence of contracted pelvis (i.e. true CPD), if the ultrasound scan identifies any predisposing factor that may preclude a vaginal delivery, or if there are any absolute contraindication for vaginal delivery (major degree placenta praevia). In all other cases, after careful counselling, a vaginal birth may be attempted with careful monitoring of the fetal heart rate as well as progress of labour. The presence of strong, effective uterine contractions is essential for progress of labour and for successful internal rotation. Hence, judicious use of oxytocin to achieve effective uterine contractions is not contraindicated.

Overall, the success rate of vaginal delivery for face presentation is about 60–70% and about 10–20% require an emergency Caesarean section during labour.

Mentoanterior face presentation

Approximately 60–70% of fetuses with face presentation have mentoanterior position and approximately 90% of these will achieve a vaginal birth. Labour may be prolonged compared with vertex presentation because the face is a poor dilator of the cervix compared with the occiput. An episiotomy may be indicated to avoid perineal tears and gain adequate access. Prolonged second stage of labour (or fetal distress in the second stage) may warrant a forceps delivery (ventouse or vacuum delivery is contraindicated in face presentation), if CPD has been excluded. The operator should understand the anatomy prior to application of the forceps blades. The mouth (face presentation) substitutes for the posterior fontanelle (vertex presentation), whereas the chin or mentum (face presentation) substitutes for the occiput (vertex presentation). The direction of traction should be downward initially to maintain extension until the chin passes under the symphysis. The direction of traction should then be gradually changed (i.e. forceps handle elevated) to allow the delivery of the fetal head by flexion. Utmost care must be taken to avoid hyperextension of the fetal head during delivery, as this can result in injury to cervical spine.

Mentolateral (ML) or mentotransverse (MT) position

Ten to 12% of fetuses with face presentation have a mentotransverse position. If rotation to the mentoanterior position does not occur during labour, an emergency Caesarean section is indicated. This is because deep transverse arrest is common and there may not be further progress of labour. Manual rotation to the mentoanterior position under a general anaesthetic and forceps delivery (Thorn's manoeuvre) and rotation with Kielland's forceps have been described. However, these are likely to have a limited role in modern obstetric practice.

Mentoposterior (MP) position

20–25% of fetuses with face presentation have a mentoposterior position during labour. With strong uterine contractions and adequate pelvis, 45–65% of these will rotate to a mentoanterior position. Persistent mentoposterior despite strong and effective uterine contractions and an adequate pelvis is an indication for an emergency Caesarean section. As mentioned earlier, the mechanism of labour is not possible due to anatomical factors. However, in early labour, a conservative approach is entirely acceptable if the fetal heart rate is normal and true CPD is excluded. In such cases, judicious use of oxytocin can be used to achieve optimum uterine contractions, sufficient to achieve internal rotation to the mentoanterior position. It is wise to perform a Caesarean section if there is lack of progress for 3–4 hours despite good contractions with oxytocin infusion. Manual rotation and Kielland's rotation have been described but these are associated with perinatal and maternal morbidity, especially in inexperienced hands. In modern obstetric practice, a Caesarean section is the preferred option for persistent mentoposterior face presentation.

Delivery during Caesarean section

A Caesarean section should be performed or supervised by an experienced obstetrician. Flexion of the head should be attempted prior to delivery through the uterine incision. Uterine angles should be carefully inspected to exclude angular extensions.

Postpartum complications

These include complications because of prolonged labour and genital tract trauma, both of which may result in postpartum haemorrhage. The neonate may have laryngeal oedema as an extension of facial oedema ('tumefaction') and may need resuscitation after birth. The neonate should also be examined to exclude injury to the cervical spine, especially if hyperextension during delivery was suspected. Parents should be reassured that the facial oedema, which is cosmetically very unappealing, will settle with time.

Further reading

Chandraharan E, Arulkumaran S. Operative delivery, shoulder dystocia and episiotomy. Chapter In: Arulkumaran S, Penna LK, Bhasker Rao K (eds) The management of labour, 2nd edn. Orient Longman 2005.

Gee H. Malpresentation and malposition. In: James DK, Mahomed K, Stone P, Wijngaarden, Hill LM (eds) Evidence-based obstetrics. Saunders 2003.

Nassar AH, Fayyumy R, Saab W, et al. Grandmultiparas in modern obstetrics. Am J Perinatol 2006;23:345–9.

Sahid S, Sepulvida W, Dezerega W. Iniencephaly: prenatal diagnosis and management. Prenat Diagn 2000;20:202–5.

Vialle R, Pietin-Vialle C, Ilharrebode B. Spinal cord injuries at birth: a multicenter review of nine cases. J Matern Fetal Neonatal Med 2007;20:435–40.

Fetal surveillance in labour

Definition
Fetal surveillance is recommended in labour with the intention of detecting fetal hypoxia prior to the development of asphyxial damage in the fetus. The ideal fetal surveillance would have a high sensitivity (detect all fetuses with developing hypoxia) and a high specificity (be reassuring about all fetuses with no hypoxia). The test should also be easy to perform, not interfere with labour progress, and have a high acceptability to women. Unfortunately the ideal monitoring technique does not currently exist.

Currently available diagnostic tests include
- fetal blood sampling (FBS) for pH and base-excess
- FBS for lactate (this is less well validated than pH and is less widely used but requires a small sample of fetal blood)
- neonatal assessment after delivery (Apgar scores, cord blood pH, neonatal outcome).

As the available diagnostic tests are expensive and invasive they are used selectively. Therefore, routine fetal surveillance in labour aims to identify a group of fetuses with a high chance of developing hypoxia so that a diagnostic test can be used.

Currently available screening tests
Universal
- Maternal history: to assess for risk factors
- Observation of amniotic fluid for meconium
- Intermittent auscultation (IA)

In women with a low-risk that their fetus will develop hypoxia, evidence shows that routine use of continuous fetal monitoring increases the rate of intervention in labour (assisted vaginal delivery and Caesarean section) with no improvement in neonatal morbidity and mortality when compared with intermittent auscultation. Any abnormality detected in any of these screening tests requires that a higher level of screening be implemented.

Selective
- Continuous electronic fetal monitoring using a cardiotocograph (CTG).
- Analysis of the ST segment of the fetal ECG (STAN) used in combination with the CTG.

Epidemiology
Abnormalities of the fetal heart rate are very common; 75% of cardiotocographs will show at least one abnormality during labour and almost 1 in 5 will show a serious abnormality. 1 in 10 CTGs show recurrent decelerations and more than 1 in 20 fetuses will have a period of prolonged deceleration during labour. A true hypoxic event occurs in only 3/1000 labours so most observed CTG abnormalities are false positives. Unfortunately, some CTGs are misdiagnosed or are false negatives (falsely reassuring) as intrapartum deaths occur (0.75/1000 births) in the UK and neonates exhibit clinical features of ischaemic brain injury (hypoxic ischaemic encephalopathy) in 2.25/1000 neonates (ischaemic injury can occur due to other causes).

Worldwide, the World Health Organization has estimated that 1 million infants die each year as a result of birth asphyxia with about the same number surviving with long-term neurological disability.

Pathology
- Hypoxaemia describes a common situation where there is a reduction in placental or cord blood flow causing a reduction in the level of oxygen in the peripheral arterial circulation of the fetus. This occurs as a normal part of labour as uterine contractions reduce blood flow to the placenta. Fetuses are able to cope with hypoxaemia for relatively long periods of time without injury occurring. Fetal growth and activity reduces but the oxygen delivery to tissues is maintained and so no metabolic acidosis develops. Hypoxaemia due to cord compression is also associated with an increase in carbon dioxide levels and the appearance of respiratory acidosis.
- Hypoxia describes the situation where the blood flow is interrupted for more prolonged periods and as a result there is a reduction in the delivery of oxygen to the peripheral tissues The fetus may show some stress response (such as a developing tachycardia) but there are mechanisms to allow this situation to occur for short periods of time (hours) without fetal damage. The fetus must switch to anaerobic metabolism to create energy from glucose and stored glycogen. The byproduct of this process is lactic acid and thus a metabolic acidosis develops. Buffering will allow a normal pH to be maintained for a period of time. Some fetuses have lower reserves of glycogen and/or a lower ability to buffer if metabolic acidosis occurs (preterm, infants of diabetic mother, growth restricted fetuses).
- Asphyxia describes the situation where the oxygen delivery fails to such an extent that there is reduction in oxygen delivery leading to metabolic acidosis in the tissues due to anaerobic metabolism in addition to hypoxia. This causes critical organ damage with fetal demise *in utero* or damage. Neonates who have been asphyxiated suffer multi-organ failure after delivery with a high risk of mortality. Asphyxial injury to the brain results in hypoxic ischaemic encephalopathy (HIE). The severity of the injury is variable but there is a significant risk of cerebral palsy in survivors of a severe asphyxial episode.
- Fetal infection reduces the reserve to cope with hypoxia and certain fetal heart rate changes may occur in the presence of significant fetal infection.
- Fetal anaemia either acute (due to fetomaternal haemorrhage) or chronic (due to parvovirus or red-cell immunization) causes the characteristic findings of a sinusoidal pattern on a cardiotocograph. A fetus with anaemia is at greater risk of hypoxia and also has a very reduced reserve to cope with hypoxia as haemoglobin acts as a buffer in metabolic acidosis.

Aetiology
- Acute hypoxia occurs as a result of sudden reduction in placental/cord blood flow and develops rapidly over minutes. Most causes are irreversible once the process begins. Management requires rapid delivery or reversal of the acute insult in cases of hyperstimulation, if the fetus is viable, to prevent death or damage:
- uterine dehiscence

- cord prolapse (with cord spasm or compression)
- critical cord compression (e.g. the cord along side the fetal head as it descends in the second stage)
- significant abruption with detachment of a large area of the placenta or due to uterine hypertonia
- hypertonic uterine contractions secondary to the administration of prostaglandins or oxytocin.
- Chronic hypoxia occurs due to a reduction in the placental blood flow over a long period. It can occur in any condition where there is placental vascular disease. The common examples are fetal growth restriction and recurrent antepartum haemorrhages. The fetus will cope with this for a significant period of time by redistributing blood to vital organs, reducing growth and activity, and by buffering against the lactic acid formed during low levels of anaerobic metabolism. However, the point can be reached where the disease process worsens or the ability to buffer is exhausted and lactic acidosis develops. Surveillance with fetal Dopplers in the antenatal period helps to detect the point where decompensation becomes likely so that delivery can be recommended in the fetus that is viable. This will allow the diagnosis of chronic hypoxia prior to the onset of labour in most cases. A fetus with chronic hypoxia will not cope with the reduction in placental blood flow that occurs during labour and fetal heart rate abnormalities are seen. A reduction in variability in the trace of any fetus at the onset of labour may be ominous if it does not improve with time, and there is a risk of poor outcome, as it suggests a significant degree of metabolic acidosis and a failure of compensatory mechanisms.
- Gradually developing hypoxia is the most common type of intrapartum hypoxia. Early recognition that the fetus may be at risk of developing hypoxia allows interventions aimed at improving the fetal condition. This type of hypoxia develops in labour as a result of recurrent cord compression. Cord compression occurs to some degree in all labours but is worsened by a number of clinical situations:
- strong contractions (e.g. in the second stage or during administration of oxytocin)
- oligohydramnios (e.g. following ruptured membranes or in post-term pregnancy)
- cord around the neck in the first or the second stage

Prognosis

Prolonged reduction in oxygenated cerebral blood flow due to any cause can result in an acute brain injury with the clinical features of hypoxic ischaemic encephalopathy (HIE). Asphyxial birth injury due to hypoxia during labour is only one cause of HIE. The severity of the injury is related to the length of time of hypoxia but certain fetuses may also be more susceptible to injury due to less fetal reserve (such as in fetal growth restriction).

The mortality from severe HIE is 50–75% with over half of the deaths occurring in the first week of life. Of infants who survive with a diagnosis of severe HIE, 80% will have severe complications, 10–20% will have mild or moderate complications, and up to10% will develop normally. In infants surviving with moderate HIE there is a 30–50% chance of serious long-term complications and 10–20% risk of minor complications, with 30–70% of infants developing normally. The infants with mild HIE invariably develop normally with no complications. The sequelae of

HIE include mental retardation, epilepsy, and cerebral palsy.

Clinical approach
Decide what surveillance should be recommended
Risk assessment
- The antenatal and intrapartum history must be assessed for all women in labour to allow appropriate monitoring to be recommended. The presence of risk factors for pathologies that may increase the risk of fetal hypoxia should be considered:
  - increased risk of cord compression: breech, oligohydramnios, strong contractions due to syntocinon or induction of labour
  - reduced retroplacental pool of blood as in cases of suspected fetal growth restriction, pre-eclampsia, diabetics, antepartum or intrapartum haemorrhage, severe maternal disease
  - reduced fetal reserve; prematurity, fetal infection, fetal anaemia, multiple pregnancy, growth restriction
  - increased risk of severe acute hypoxic event, e.g. scar rupture during vaginal birth after Caesarean section
  - at times monitoring is needed for maternal reassurance: previous stillbirth or other poor pregnancy outcome may result in a maternal desire for the fetus to be monitored as closely as possible.

Meconium
- If the membranes have ruptured then the liquor can be assessed for the presence of meconium. The presence of meconium has an independent association with poor fetal outcome and therefore if present it necessitates a review of the recommendations for fetal surveillance.

Recommend appropriate monitoring
Intermittent auscultation
- If the woman has no risk factors (low risk) and there is no meconium then intermittent auscultation should be recommended. If this is acceptable to the woman it is recommended that the operator listen for one minute soon after a contraction using a pinnard stethoscope or a hand-held Doppler machine. This should be done every 15 minutes in the first stage of labour and every 5 minutes in the second stage of labour. Continuous electronic fetal monitoring should be commenced if any of the following occur:
  - a baseline abnormality
  - any audible deceleration (variable or late)
  - new meconium staining of the liquor is observed
  - a new risk factor develops during the course of labour (such as oxytocin therapy or intrapartum haemorrhage)

Continuous electronic fetal monitoring
- If the woman has risk factors then continuous fetal monitoring should be recommended. The reasons for this should be discussed with her and the fact that it may reduce her mobility in labour. Some women may decide that they wish to decline continuous monitoring and request intermittent auscultation. As long as the woman understands the implications of this decision her wishes should be supported.
  - Cardiotocograph (CTG) will be used in the majority of situations. It can be used with an external transducer

and does not require the membranes to be ruptured. A fetal scalp electrode may be used but this is only required if a good quality trace cannot be obtained from the external transducer.

- ST analysis of the fetal ECG (STAN) can be used if resources are available for this and the cervix is sufficiently dilated for a fetal scalp electrode to be connected (with amniotomy if the membranes are intact).

Effective interpretation of CTG

FIGO and the UK (NICE/RCOG) guidelines

- FIGO published guidelines for the interpretation of fetal monitoring in 1985 and these were the most commonly used guidelines worldwide. They continue to be used in many countries. In the UK the NICE guidelines published in 2008 along with the Intrapartum Care guidelines are used. These are built on and refined from the recommendations made by FIGO. It is important that local guidelines are developed and adhered to by healthcare professionals working in that unit. The following describes the guidelines for interpretation recommended in the UK.
- Assessment of four features of the fetal heart rate tracing.

Baseline

This describes the average level of the fetal heart rate in between contractions. It should be observed over a period of 5–10 minutes to allow the true baseline to be established. In the presence of significant accelerations or recurrent decelerations it may be difficult to be certain of the true baseline within this time frame and a longer period of monitoring maybe required. If the mother reports associated fetal movements it makes recurrent decelerations less likely than recurrent accelerations. The baseline is associated with gestation and this should be considered when the level of the baseline is reviewed. A preterm fetus may have a heart rate at the upper limit of normal whereas a post-term fetus may have a baseline at the lower limit of normal. The converse may occur but should prompt more careful scrutiny of the clinical risk factors and the other features of the CTG.

A tachycardia develops slowly over a period of time (hormonally mediated) and may be a sign of developing fetal hypoxia but can also indicate fetal infection if the rise of baseline rate is associated with no recurrent decelerations. It may occur if a woman develops pyrexia or is dehydrated.

A bradycardia develops suddenly (mediated via the vagal nerve) and is a sign of acute hypoxia. If a bradycardia does not show signs of recovery over a 6–9-minute period, urgent delivery is required. A fall in the baseline that recovers should be described as a prolonged deceleration, this may indicate intermittent severe fetal hypoxia due to placental or cord issues but may also occur due to maternal hypotension such as following an epidural top-up or following a period where the woman has been overly supine such as a vaginal examination.

Variability

This describes the variation in the fetal heart occurring three to five times per minute giving a 'spiky' appearance to the CTG. This is caused by interplay of the fetal autonomic nervous system, which acts continuously to maintain the heart rate within normal limits. Variability is normally more than 4bpm and less than 25 bpm. Variability that is persistently outside these limits has a high correlation with fetal hypoxia. Persistently reduced variability suggests a hypoxic effect on the autonomic nervous system and is associated with a poor prognosis. Reduced variability that is intermittent is of no clinical significance and may occur as part of a normal fetal sleep–wake cycle and even if persistent is not abnormal in the presence of definite accelerations. A CTG with persistently increased variability >25 bpm is known as saltatory. This type of pattern is uncommon but may have an association with fetal hypoxia or fetal fitting and should be managed based on the other features of the trace and the clinical situation.

Accelerations

An acceleration is a rise of the fetal heart rate of 15 bpm or more for 15 seconds or more. They occur in response to fetal movements or other stimulation of the fetus and are almost always a sign of fetal wellbeing. Accelerations should be intermittent and if they occur without a period of normal baseline for a prolonged period (more than 90 minutes) they should be considered to be a saltatory pattern CTG (see Variability). Accelerations become less common during active labour, which may reflect the mild hypoxaemia that occurs in fetuses in normal labour

Decelerations

A deceleration is a transient fall in the fetal heart rate of 15 bpm for 15 seconds or more. If the deceleration lasts for longer than 60 seconds it is defined as a prolonged deceleration. A fall in the fetal heart rate that does not recover is a bradycardia (see Baseline).

There are four types of deceleration that may be seen:

- Early decelerations occur due to fetal head compression with consequent stimulation of the vagal nerve. They require a significant degree of head compression and are only seen in the late last 1st stage or more commonly the second stage when the contractions are expulsive and the head is deeply engaged. As they represent a physiological response of the fetus to an ongoing standard stimulus they are of the same size and shape. The deceleration must occur within the time that the contraction occurs with a return to normal baseline by the end of the contraction. Fetuses experiencing early deceleration have normal cord blood flow and placental gas transfer and thus early decelerations are benign.
- Variable decelerations occur due to cord compression. During this type of deceleration the blood flow between the fetus and the placenta is interrupted and thus a short period where the level of carbon dioxide rises and the oxygen saturation falls is inevitable. As this is a dynamic process with movement of the mother and fetus between contractions they may vary in appearance from one contraction to the next. This type of deceleration shows that the fetus has the physiological reserve to respond to intermittent period of hypoxia. The deceleration will have a transient small rise on the baseline immediately before and after the deceleration (shouldering). The deceleration must occur within the contraction with return to baseline by the end of the contraction.
- Atypical variable decelerations occur due to cord compression but have lost the features to reassure that the fetus has a good physiological reserve to cope with the intermittent period of hypoxia caused by the cord compression. Atypical features include:
- a loss of the pre and post shouldering

Table 10.7.1 Description of the features of the fetal heart rate (FHR) tracing

Feature	Baseline (bpm)	Variability (bpm)	Decelerations	Accelerations
Reassuring	110–160	>5 (or <5 for <40 minutes or for any time period if accelerations+)	None	Present
Non-reassuring	100–109	<5 (for 40 to 90 minutes)	Early or variable (should be present with >50% contractions for 90 minutes)	The absence of accelerations on an otherwise normal CTG is of uncertain significance
	161–180		Single prolonged (<3 minutes)	
	(Reassuring if all other features reassuring)			
Abnormal	<100	<5 (for >90 minutes)	Atypical variable or late (for >50% contractions over 30 minutes)	
	>180		Single prolonged (>3 minutes)	
	Sinusoidal (>10 minutes)			

- a biphasic deceleration (a second deceleration occurs before the first has fully recovered)
- the variability during the deceleration is reduced
- the deceleration is slow to recover lasting beyond the contraction subsiding
- the depth of the deceleration >60 beats and the duration >60 seconds.
- Late decelerations occur due to an abnormality in the retroplacental pool. During every contraction the blood flow into the placenta is reduced. In normal circumstances the fetus is able to maintain normal oxygen levels by gas transfer with a residual volume of oxygenated blood contained in the retroplacental area. In certain situations the retroplacental pool is reduced so that the oxygen levels of the fetus fall during the contraction. The late deceleration shows the fetus responding to the hypoxia. The retroplacental pool is reduced in conditions such as fetal growth restriction, recurrent antepartum haemorrhage with loss of placental area due to infarcts, or in conditions such as diabetes where the placental structure may be abnormal. A fetus in this situation will develop a progressive metabolic acidosis. There is no reliable way of improving the retroplacental pool. Reducing oxytocin, hydration, and positioning of the mother may help in some situations. In the others, early delivery to avoid hypoxia in labour is the only option.

Categorize CTG

The CTG should be reviewed with assessment of all four features and then categorized to decide on further management (Table 10.7.1).

Normal CTG: all four features are reassuring
Suspicious CTG: one non-reassuring feature
Pathological CTG: any two non-reassuring features or any single abnormal feature

Management of CTG following interpretation and categorization

Normal CTG

The risk factors should be reviewed as a CTG may have been commenced unnecessarily in a low risk situation and

may be discontinued with conversion to intermittent auscultation to allow the woman to mobilize more effectively.

No specific action is required if the CTG is normal. Occasional variable decelerations in early labour should prompt early action to try to alter the maternal position to relieve cord compression in the anticipation that the degree of cord compression may increase as the labour progresses.

Although the baseline may not show a frank tachycardia a rise in the baseline of 20 bpm during monitoring should prompt a review of the clinical situation with consideration of the need to screen the woman for infection or to improve her hydration.

Suspicious CTG

A full risk factor reassessment should occur. The likely reserve of the fetus to withstand hypoxia should be considered. The woman's parity, current cervical dilatation, progress in labour and the presence of heavy meconium are also important in deciding further management. A suspicious CTG in early labour in a primigravida woman with a fetus likely to have poor fetoplacental reserve (such as severe growth restriction) requires that the option of delivery should be considered as the probability of developing significant hypoxia is high.

In all other women efforts should be made to try to improve the fetal condition:

- rehydration of the mother with intravenous crystalloid
- administer antipyretic drugs such as paracetamol
- administer antibiotics after appropriate maternal screening if infection is suspected
- change maternal position to avoid the supine dorsal position with use of a lateral (left or right), an upright position or all-fours as these position will reduce caval compression but more importantly reduce cord compression (e.g. cord positioned between the maternal sacrum and the fetal head)
- review of oxytocin therapy to ensure that the contraction frequency is no more than four or five contractions every 10 minutes.
- avoidance of episodic hypotension if this is seen to be precipitating factor in an abnormal fetal heart rate as

occurs sometimes following epidural top-ups or vaginal examination in the dorsal position.

A plan should be clearly documented of when the trace will be reviewed again and it is imperative that this review occurs with earlier review if the trace deteriorates further.

Pathological CTG
The management is as for a suspicious trace with the addition of either
- assessment of the fetus for acidaemia by fetal blood sampling (FBS)
- delivery of the fetus by assisted vaginal delivery or Caesarean section. If assisted vaginal delivery is possible but is technically (especially mal-positions) difficult fetal blood sampling should be performed first. Delivery is more appropriate than fetal blood sampling if there is heavy meconium staining and delivery is unlikely to occur in a reasonable time period of a few hours (i.e. in very early labour). Likewise delivery rather than fetal blood sampling should be considered in situations with a poor fetal reserve (infection or prematurity) unless there is a realistic expectation that delivery will occur soon. The ultimate decision will depend on the whole clinical picture in complex cases such as these.

Fetal blood sampling
General comments
- FBS should be performed with the woman in left lateral as lithotomy position increases maternal postural hypotension. If a fetal blood sample cannot be achieved due to early cervical dilatation or the level of the fetal head is high, then delivery rather than fetal blood sampling is appropriate.
- FBS is an intrusive and uncomfortable assessment and the appropriate verbal consents must be obtained from the mother. If a woman declines FBS and the trace is pathological then delivery must be undertaken.
- The cervix must be at least 3 cm dilated with ruptured membranes. BS can occasionally be achieved at dilatations of less than 3cm. The membranes may be ruptured if FBS is required. Membranes were often ruptured to "see the colour of the liquor" if a trace was abnormal. If the trace is suspicious, presence of thick scanty meconium may prompt delivery but amniotomy may also worsen the condition of the fetus by increasing the frequency and severity of cord compression.
- The head should be fixed within the pelvis. A presenting part that moves out of the pelvis on pressure risks increasing cord prolapse during the procedure or immediately after if the cord was in the vicinity of the fetal head.
- FBS can be performed on a breech but should only be done following review by a senior obstetrician as the plan for vaginal delivery should be reviewed. In current practise, Caesarean section is preferred in such situations.

Contraindications to FBS include
- Lack of maternal consent
- Maternal HIV, hepatitis B (including low-infectivity) or hepatitis C infection
- Known maternal immunothrombocytopaenia (gestational thrombocytopaenia is not a contraindication) as this may cause a low fetal platelet count
- Possible fetal bleeding disorder (e.g. male fetus in a haemophilia carrier)

- Non-recovering prolonged deceleration (bradycardia) or pre-terminal CTG pattern (absent variability with recurrent decelerations)
- Independent reason for early delivery
- Grade 3 meconium with a pathological CTG is a relative contra-indication to FBS unless it is expected that either spontaneous or assisted vaginal delivery is likely to be possible within a short time period.

Management of result from first FBS
Normal>7.25
Repeat in no later than 1 hour if CTG abnormality persists

Repeat sooner if the CTG deteriorate or there is heavy meconium or other risk factor for poor fetal reserve to compensate for developing hypoxia (such as infection, growth restriction, prematurity). If the CTG returns to normal a further fetal blood sample is not required.

Borderline 7.20–7.25
Repeat in no more than 30 minutes. As FBS takes an average of 18 minutes to perform the sampling procedure should be commenced almost immediately.

If the CTG deteriorate during this time delivery should be undertaken rather than repeat fetal blood sampling. If there is heavy meconium or other risk factor for poor fetal reserve to compensate for developing hypoxia (such as infection, growth restriction, prematurity) arrangements to expedite delivery should be made with repeat fetal blood sampling only to assess fetal condition if assisted vaginal delivery is possible. If the CTG returns to normal with acceleration a further fetal blood sample is not required but normalisation with the absence of accelerations still requires fetal blood sampling.

Abnormal <7.20
Arrangements should be made for immediate delivery by the quickest possible method. A straightforward assisted vaginal delivery is not contraindicated and may be quicker than delivery by caesarean section but a mid-cavity rotational delivery should be avoided unless the woman is multigravid. Delivery should be achieved in the minimum time required to ensure safety for the woman with standard recommendations to aim for a decision to delivery interval of no more than 30 minutes. Spinal anaesthetic is not contraindicated but the time taken to do this must be considered in relation to the pH result from fetal blood sampling and likelihood of further deterioration.

Terbutaline 0.25 mg s.c. should be considered to reduce contraction frequency and strength as this may help to improve the fetal condition while preparations are made for delivery.

Failure to obtain result
If the fetus responded to the FBS procedure with an acceleration and the CTG remains stable or has improved, then an immediate repeat of the procedure can be performed.

If the fetus did not accelerate in response to the procedure or there has been further deterioration in the appearances of the CTG then immediate delivery should be undertaken.

Management of a result from a second and subsequent FBS
If the pH result remains stable then a further sample is only required if the CTG deteriorates with new abnormalities or worsening of existing abnormalities, e.g. rise in baseline

rate, increase in depth and duration of the deceleration and reduction of baseline variability.

A third fetal blood sample is rarely indicated as in most cases the whole picture of the labour may suggest delivery. A senior obstetrician should be involved in the decision to perform a third fetal blood sample.

Further reading

Gibb D, Arulkumaran S. *Fetal monitoring in practice*. Churchill Livingstone 2007.

Guidelines for the use of fetal monitoring (FIGO news). Int J Gynecol Obstet 1987;25:159–67.

NICE guideline on fetal surveillance during labour 2001.

NICE intrapartum care guideline 2007 (Chapter 13).

Internet resources

RCOG guidelines 2001 www.rcog.org.uk/index.asp?pageid=695

NICE guidelines 2007 www.nice.org.uk/cg055

FIGO guidelines: www.onlinetog.org/cgi/reprint/1/2/18.pdfRCOG

Patient resources

MIDIRS: www.choicesforbirth.org/booklets.php?id=2

NICE: www.nice.rg.uk/guidance/cg00/publicinfo/pdf/english

Home birth

Definition

Home birth refers to giving birth at one's home, away from the hospital, midwifery-led unit, or a birth centre. The concept is based on the notion that childbirth is a normal physiological process and, hence, is most likely to succeed in a non-medicalized environment (i.e. home) surrounded by family and friends. Home birth may also facilitate the involvement of fathers in planning and attending the home-birth, which may lay the foundation for their engagement in both childbearing and child rearing in the future.

Epidemiology

Prior to 1900, about 90% of births worldwide occurred at home. Recent figures suggest that home birth rate in the UK remains at about 2–3% and this figure has not changed significantly over the last 10 years. It has been suggested that if all women were given a choice, about 8–10% of women may opt to have a home birth. There is evidence to suggest that about 16% of women who have planned for home birth may need to be transferred to the hospital to manage complications (4% antenatally and 12% during labour). In primigravidae, the rate of transfer is about 40%. It has been recognized that financial constraints, culture, beliefs and attitudes of organizations, and lack of competent staff contribute to low home birth rate in the UK.

Eligibility criteria

Home birth should be recommended to 'low-risk women' without any medical, obstetric, or fetal conditions that may necessitate closer monitoring and intervention. The health-care system should be able to provide resources (trained and competent community midwives) and supporting services (facilities for transport to a hospital in emergency). Women should be fully counselled regarding their birth choices, which include a home birth, birth in a midwifery-led unit or a birth centre, and birth in hospital with obstetric input. Women with risk factors such as pre-eclampsia, diabetes mellitus, heart disease, malpresentation, previous uterine scars, and fetal complications such as intrauterine growth restriction (IUGR) and any other medical, obstetric, or fetal complications should be advised to have a hospital birth. This is because closer monitoring and therapeutic interventions may be necessary to improve maternal and/or fetal outcome in these situations. Hence, a risk assessment should be carried out both in the antenatal period as well as at the onset of and during labour, to identify any risk factors that may necessitate transfer to a hospital unit. It is important to realize that risk assessment tools do not have sufficient predictive value and risk assessment is a dynamic process throughout pregnancy and labour.

Antenatal preparation

Woman should develop confidence in the safety of the home environment. Continuity of care with her community midwife, attending antenatal classes and considering the options for pain relief (hypnotherapy, yoga, aromatherapy, acupressure bands, Transcutaneous electric nerve stimulation or TENS machine) are of paramount importance.

Apart from required cloths for the mother and baby, birthing stool, birthing pool or a birth ball may be used at home to facilitate labour.

Advantages of home birth

Home birth avoids unnecessary medicalisation of a normal physiological process and enables the woman to labour at home in the comfort of her familiar environment, with the support of family and friends. It gives greater control for her and her partner over the birthing experience. Hospital acquired infections and other inconveniences (food, environment, disturbance from parturients) are minimized. Home birth also facilitates bonding and a quicker return to normal life.

In low-risk women, there is evidence to suggest that home birth reduces the requirement for analgesia, obstetric interventions (instrumental vaginal delivery and caesareans sections) and improves maternal satisfaction. There is no significant difference in maternal or fetal complications between home births and hospital births.

Possible complications

These include failure to progress in first or second stage of labour, fetal distress, intrapartum abruption, maternal collapse, requirement for analgesia, shoulder dystocia, and postpartum complications such as postpartum haemorrhage, inversion of uterus, maternal collapse, gential tract trauma, and retained placenta. Neonatal complications include cardiorespiratory collapse or meconium aspiration. Women should be counselled about the rare possibility of fetal compromise (rarely, intrapartum fetal death), maternal compromise due to postpartum haemorrhage as well as the possibility of transfer to the hospital. They should be made aware that these life-threatening complications are rare but immediate operative interventions may not be available, as in the hospital setting, but arrangements would be made to receive the case quickly by ambulance transfer.

It is recommended that at least two midwives are present during a home birth, especially during the second stage of labour to manage these complications. It is good practice to inform the labour ward of the local hospital about women who are actively labouring at home, so that staff can anticipate a potential admission.

- Failure to progress in first stage of labour can be initially managed by amniotomy. If there is further delay (at least 2 cm of cervical dilatation in 4 hours in active stage of labour), the woman should be transferred for augmentation of labour. Similarly, failure to progress in second stage of labour (2 hours in a primigravidae and 1 hour in a multigravida without epidural anaesthesia) would require transfer to an obstetric unit.
- If the woman does not cope with pain and requires stronger analgesia, transfer may need to be considered.
- If intermittent fetal heart rate monitoring (every 15 minutes during first stage of labour and every five minutes during second stage of labour, after a contraction) reveals evidence of decelerations and if delivery is not imminent, immediate transfer to the closest maternity unit should be arranged. Intravenous fluids and changing the position (e.g. left lateral position) may help improve placental circulation during transfer. Similarly, if meconium staining of liquor is noted, the woman should be transferred for continuous electronic fetal heart rate monitoring (EFM).
- Shoulder dystocia and neonatal cardiorespiratory resuscitation are emergencies that need to be managed by

midwives in attendance. It is paramount that midwives who conduct home births regularly update themselves on skills and drills on shoulder dystocia, and neonatal resuscitation. In both these situations, transfer to a hospital is unlikely to improve perinatal outcome as delay in treatment may cause irreversible hypoxic injury.

• Postpartum haemorrhage (atonic, traumatic, or due to retained placenta or coagulopathy) needs immediate measures to resuscitate the patient. Insertion of large-bore intravenous cannulae, administration of oxytocin or ergometrine and intravenous fluids as well as uterine massage can be performed by the attending midwives prior to transfer.

Dilemma: maternal choice versus safety

Clinicians may be faced with a situation whereby a woman who is at high risk, requests a home birth, against medical advice. In the author's experience, women with previous Caesarean section, intrauterine growth restriction, breech presentation and known group B streptococcal (GBS) colonization of the vagina have all requested a home birth. If the woman has the capacity to consent or to refuse treatment, after careful counselling, maternal choice should be respected. It is good practice to refer the woman to another colleague for counselling. Clear and detailed documentation of the discussion should be made in the mother's hand-held maternity notes, with emphasis of potential complications and outcome.

Home birth: future challenges

Following the confidential survey carried out by the National Birthday Trust, it was anticipated in 1999 that the home birth rate in the UK would rise to 4–5% in the following decade. Unfortunately, the recent joint statement by the Royal College of Obstetricians and Gynaecologists (RCOG) and the Royal College of Midwives (RCM) in 2007, suggests that that the home birth rate is still round 2% and, hence, has not changed dramatically over the last decade. In contrast, about a third of all births occur at home in some Scandinavian countries. Financial constraints, shortage of competent and experienced community midwives, concerns about safety by both staff and patients, as well as inherent negative attitude towards home birth, are some of the factors that have prevented an increase in home births in the UK.

Recently, National Drivers such as National Service Framework (NSF) and the National Institute of Clinical Excellence (NICE) have emphasized the importance of home birth as a choice that should be offered to all low-risk women. There is no doubt that for a group of low-risk women, home birth would remain the safest and the best option. Every effort should be made by all clinicians to promote home birth for these women, to improve their birth experience.

Further reading

Anderson RE, Murphy PA. Outcomes of 11,788 planned home births attended by certified nurse-midwives. A retrospective descriptive study. J Nurse Midwifery 1995;40:483–92.

Christiaens W, Gouwy A. Bracke P. Does a referral from home to hospital affect satisfaction with childbirth? A cross-national comparison. BMC Health Service Res 2007;12;7:109.

Department of Health. The National Service Framework for Children and Young People. Maternity Services. Standard 11. London: Department of Health; 2004 www.dh.gov.uk/assetRoot/04/09/05/23/04090523.pdf.

Janssen PA, Lee SK, Ryan FM, et al. Outcomes of planned home births versus planned hospital births after regulation of midwifery in British Columbia. CMAJ 2002;166:315–23.

Janssen PA, Lee SK, Ryan EM. An evaluation of process and protocols for planned home birth attended by regulated midwives in British Columbia. J Midwifery Womens Health 2003;48:138–45.

Johnson KC, Daviss BA. Outcomes of planned home births with certified professional midwives: large prospective study in North America. BMJ 2005;330:1416.

Mehl-Madrona L, Madrona MM. Physician- and midwife-attended home births. Effects of breech, twin, and post-dates outcome data on mortality rates. J Nurse Midwifery 1997;42:91–8.

Olsen O. Meta-analysis of the safety of the home birth. Birth 1997;24:4–13.

RCOG/RCM. Home births. Royal College of Obstetricians and Gynaecologists/Royal College of Midwives Joint statement No.2, April 2007.

Royal College of Midwives. Home birth hand book: Vol. 1: Promoting home birth. London: RCM 2002.

Royal College of Midwives. Home birth hand book: Vol. 2: Practising home birth. London: RCM 2003.

Patient resources

www.homebirth.org.uk
www.homebirth.net

Induction of labour

Definition
Induction of labour is defined as the artificial initiation of labour at any point after viability of the fetus (24 weeks). Cervical ripening is referred to as the process of cervical effacement and softening that precedes cervical dilatation.

Frequency
Induction rates vary hugely worldwide, and have increased rapidly over the last three decades. Quoted national rates vary between 1% and 40%, although individual units quote rates as high as 55%. In a recent English survey, the rates in units varied from 13% to 44% (median 26%, HCC 2008).

Indications
Irrespective of the country studied, the commonest causes of induction are post-date pregnancy (Chapter 9.14, Prolonged pregnancy) and hypertension (Chapter 8.22, Hypertension). Other causes included ruptured membranes (Chapter 10.16, Prelabour rupture of membranes), fetal compromise, maternal disease, intrauterine fetal death, and maternal request (see below) make up the remainder.

Risks of induction
- Induction of labour is associated with an increased risk of Caesarean section (CS) (typically ×1.5; Cammu 2002). However, this effect occurs primarily as a result of the indication for induction: in randomized controlled trials (RCTs) of elective induction at term for maternal request the risk of Caesarean section appears to be reduced (NCCWCH 2007).
- Uterine hyperstimulation after low-dose prostaglandin induction occurs in about 5% of women (one-third of these will have fetal heart rate abnormalities). It can be rapidly reversed with β2-adrenergic therapy (e.g. terbutaline 250 µg subcutaneously) without maternal or fetal complications.
- In well-resourced settings, uterine rupture is a complication usually only found in women who have had a previous CS. In women undergoing VBAC (after a single delivery by CS) the rupture rate of 1 in 210 in spontaneous labours is increased to 1 in 70 in women induced with prostaglandins (Smith 2004). The rupture rate in women induced with amniotomy and oxytocin alone, or in women who have also previously delivered vaginally, was not significantly increased.

Pharmacological methods
Dinoprostone (PGE2)
- In women with an unfavourable cervix, vaginal PGE2 improves cervical status and reduces the need for oxytocin augmentation. The risk of hyperstimulation is, however, increased (×4) over placebo rates.
- Vaginal prostaglandin tablets and gel are equally effective, but intracervical prostaglandins result in a slower induction. The three have otherwise no difference in maternal or fetal outcomes. Oral prostaglandins are also effective, but have a high rate of gastrointestinal side-effects.

Oxytocin
- When combined with artificial rupture of membranes (ARM), oxytocin is as effective as vaginal dinoprostone for labour induction but with less maternal satisfaction. There are no differences in hyperstimulation rates.
- When used alone, oxytocin is less effective than vaginal prostaglandins for induction of women with either intact or ruptured membranes.
- Oxytocin is usually used for labour augmentation following induction, or with ARM following cervical priming. The only alternative for this indication is oral misoprostol (see below).

Misoprostol
- Misoprostol (an orally active PGE1 analogue) is effective for labour induction when used at low dose. Its price and heat stability make it an attractive option.
- Although 25 µg vaginal pessaries are available in some countries, most misoprostol tablets are 200 µg. To obtain small doses, the tablets need to be cut and this makes dosaging inaccurate. A more accurate regimen is to dissolve a 200 µg tablet in 200 mL water – this solution is stable at room temperature for at least 24 hours. The solution should be stirred before every use.
- Oral misoprostol solution (20 µg 2 hourly) is as effective as vaginal dinoprostone, and has a lower CS rate. Vaginal misoprostol (25 µg 4 -hourly) had equivalent outcomes to vaginal dinoprostone.
- Titrated oral misoprostol solution has also been used during induced labour for augmentation (instead of oxytocin). Women are given 5–20 µg orally every 1–2 hours to keep contractions at 3 in 10 minutes. This regimen is commonly used following induction with oral misoprostol solution, and appears to be as effective and safe as oxytocin (Hofmeyr 2001).

Mifepristone
- Mifepristone is a progesterone antagonist that sensitizes the uterus to prostaglandins.
- When used alone, it results in labour in only 50% of women after 48 hours.
- When given 24–48 hours before induction in women with intrauterine fetal deaths, it reduces the induction to delivery interval.
- There are reports of neonatal antiglucocorticoid effects, as well as fetal renal and hepatic dysfunction when used with live fetuses. Its use is therefore restricted to women with intrauterine fetal deaths.

Others
- Vaginal nitric oxide donors (e.g. isosorbide mononitrate, or glyceryl trinitrate) also induce labour, but are much slower than vaginal dinoprostone (with corresponding lower rates of hyperstimulation). There is a high rate of mild maternal side-effects (headache in 90%), but maternal satisfaction is higher than for dinoprostone. Their gentle uterine effects may make them suitable for outpatient cervical ripening (Osman 2006)
- Oral corticosteroids, intracervical hyaluronidase injection, and oestrogens have all shown some effect, but there is not enough RCT evidence to comment on their safety and efficacy.

Surgical methods
Amniotomy
- Amniotomy is rarely used alone for induction. When combined with oxytocin it is as effective as vaginal dinoprostone (see above).

- Amniotomy may be a useful adjunct to allow visualization of liquor and placement of a fetal scalp electrode.

Transcervical balloon catheter

- A Foley catheter may be inserted through the cervix (manually or using 'sponge holders') and the balloon filled to 30–50 mL. The catheter is then taped to the inner thigh under slight tension. Some also infuse saline extra-amniotically at 50 mL/hour. When the catheter falls out, an ARM is performed and oxytocin commenced.
- Balloon catheters appear to be as effective at labour induction as vaginal prostaglandins, with comparable rates of uterine hyperstimulation.

Laminaria tents

- Laminaria tents are made from sterile seaweed or synthetic hydrophilic materials, and are introduced into the cervical canal. As these devices absorb water, they increase in diameter and so stretch the cervix.
- Laminaria appear to be as effective at labour induction as vaginal prostaglandins, but with a reduced incidence of uterine hyperstimulation. This may make them safer for women who have had a previous CS.

Non-pharmacological methods

Membrane sweeping

- Membrane sweeping involves inserting a finger through the cervical os and sweeping it around between the chorion and the uterine wall to release prostaglandins.
- The clinical effects of membrane sweeps are to reduce the need for formal induction of labour (especially in multiparous women) and to increase the rate of spontaneous labour, if performed more than once from 38 weeks of gestation. In view of this it is recommended in the UK for all women at clinic visits following their due date and before formal induction (NCCWCH 2008).
- If the cervix will not admit a finger it may not be possible to do a formal membrane sweep. In such cases massaging around the cervix in the vaginal fornices may achieve a similar effect.
- A small amount of bleeding is common following the procedure.

Complimentary and natural methods

- Herbal medicines, acupuncture, enemas, castor oil, and homeopathy have all been used for labour induction. There are Cochrane reviews of all these interventions, but all find insufficient scientific research to recommend their use.
- Sexual intercourse has been subjected to two randomized trials, but neither has shown any benefit in clinical outcome.
- There is some evidence to support breast stimulation as an induction method.

Clinical approach

Prior to induction

- The indication and gestation should be rechecked.
- Fetal health should be rechecked just prior to induction, usually using electronic fetal heart rate monitoring.
- The modified Bishop score (Table 10.9.1) should be assessed to decide on the need for pre-induction cervical ripening. A Bishop score of 8 or more indicates a 'ripe' or favourable cervix.

During induction

- Induction of labour should ideally be carried out in settings with electronic fetal monitoring, facilities for accurately measuring infusion rates, and access to emergency CS.
- Outpatient induction is an option, but methods with low rates of hyperstimulation should be used (e.g. mechanical methods, nitric oxide donors or controlled release prostaglandins). RCTs suggest no difference in clinical outcome, but higher maternal satisfaction rates (Biem 2003).
- Inductions should ideally be started in the morning as they are associated with higher maternal satisfaction and lower operative vaginal delivery rates.
- Electronic fetal heart rate monitoring should be conducted before and after every drug administration, and once contractions start. Once in labour, most women have continuous monitoring. The only exception is women who have had an uncomplicated pregnancy (i.e. they have no fetal indication for induction) and who have not needed oxytocin augmentation (NCCWCH 2008).
- Induced labours are more painful than spontaneous labours. However, women (and staff) can be reassured that administering epidural analgesia prior to painful contractions or in early labour has no adverse effects on clinical outcomes and increases maternal satisfaction.

Special indications

Intrauterine fetal death (IUFD)

- Without therapy 90% of women with an IUFD will deliver within 3 weeks. In the absence of abruption, the risk of clotting disorders is low for the first 2 weeks.
- Standard dinoprostone or oxytocin regimens may be used at term, or gemeprost 1 mg 3 h
- Mifepristone 200mcg given orally 48 hours prior to induction may reduce the time to delivery.
- Vaginal misoprostol is useful in that its dose can be adjusted according to gestation. Lower doses of misoprostol are needed for labour induction following IUFD. A typical regimen (Gómez 2007) is:
- 13–17 weeks: misoprostol 200 µg 6 hourly (×4)
- 18–26 weeks: misoprostol 100 µg 6 hourly (×4)
- >26 weeks: misoprostol 25-50 µg 4 hourly (×6)
- There is an increased risk of chorioamnionitis following IUFD and so ARM should be delayed as long as possible to prevent ascending infection.

Maternal request for induction of labour (37–40 weeks)

- Despite being widely discouraged, there is no evidence that the outcomes are any worse for women induced without medical indication. Indeed the limited evidence suggests that the CS rate may actually be decreased, albeit with increased operative vaginal delivery rates. It obviously prevents stillbirths following the induction date, although these are very rare (Gulmezoglu 2006).

Suspected fetal macrosomia

- Diagnosis is an initial problem—only about 50% of babies >4 kg are detected with either ultrasound or palpation.
- From the limited RCT evidence, there is no reduction in delivery complications, and the need for CS is doubled (Sanchez-Ramos 2002). However, shoulder dystocia is rare even in suspected macrosomia (5% in the Cochrane meta-analysis) and so it would take very large studies to demonstrate an effect.

Table 10.9.1 Bishop score table. The score for each factor is added giving a score between 0 and 13

Bishop score	Factor				
	Dilatation (cm)	Cervical length (cm)	Station	Cervical consistency	Cervical position
0	<1	<4	−3	Firm	Posterior
1	1–2	2–4	−2	Average	Mid/anterior
2	2–4	1–2	−1/0	Soft	–
3	>4	>1	+1/2		–

High risk inductions

Previous Caesarean section

- The risk of uterine rupture in spontaneous labourers with a previous CS is around 1 in 210. Induction of labour with prostaglandins increases this risk to around 1 in 70 (and possibly even higher with misoprostol). The risk is not increased in those who have had a previous vaginal delivery (even if induced with prostaglandins) or in those suitable for ARM/oxytocin (Smith 2004).
- Successful vaginal delivery is achieved in approximately 70% of spontaneously labouring women undergoing VBAC. This is reduced in women undergoing induction (to 50%) and in those with an unfavourable cervix.
- The use of intrauterine pressure catheters does not prevent uterine rupture.

'High head' (controlled 'ARM')

- Induction of labour when the head is high in the pelvis increases the risk of cord prolapse and malpresentation. Medical methods (e.g. dinoprostone) should therefore always be used initially.
- When ARM is necessary, this should be performed along with fundal pressure. With polyhydramnios, it is useful to keep the examining hand in the vagina until the liquor has drained and the head descended. The woman should sit upright after the ARM to encourage head descent.
- If the head is very high, some practitioners prefer to conduct the ARM in theatre so that CS can rapidly be carried out in the event of a cord prolapse.

Induction in low resource settings

- Induction indications in low resource settings are similar to those in high resource settings, except that there are fewer inductions for fetal reasons (e.g. IUGR).
- With limited resources for fetal monitoring, induction is more hazardous for mother and baby and the threshold for induction is consequently raised. In these settings the stillbirth rate is doubled and need for neonatal resuscitation increased fourfold (Dujardin 1995). This reflects both the lack of monitoring and the fact that the women being induced have more advanced clinical disease.
- In these settings there are great benefits to the use of oral misoprostol solution for induction as it is cheap, requires no infusion apparatus, and can be continued at low dose (typically 5–20 μg/hour) through labour in place of oxytocin (Kundodyiwa 2009).

Failed induction

- In around 15% of women it is not possible to do an ARM even after cervical ripening with 2 doses of prostaglandin.
- Management options depend on the urgency and indication for the induction. If low risk and no urgency, then the induction process may be repeated after a 24–48-hour rest period. If more urgent, then alternative induction methods may be attempted or a CS performed.

Frequently asked questions

- Can cervical ripening be performed as an outpatient?
- This has been done safely, but experience is limited (see above). A CTG is done after the dinoprostone is inserted, and the woman returns once contractions start or at the time of next planned dose.
- Are induced labours more painful?
- Yes: analgesic requirements are higher in induced labours.
- Does the use of an epidural early in the induction have any adverse effects on labour outcome?
- No. Early, rather than late, administration of epidural analgesia does not prolong labour or increase the incidence of instrumental or caesarean section births. There is no benefit in waiting until labour has started to give epidural (NCCWCH 2008).

Further reading

Beukens P. *Overmedicalization of maternal care in developing countries*. Antwerp: ITGT Press; 2001.

Biem SR, Turnell RW, Olatunbosun. A randomized controlled trial of outpatient versus inpatient labour induction with vaginal controlled release prostaglandin-E2: effectiveness and satisfaction. J Obstet Gynaecol Canada 2003;25:23–31.

Cammu H, Martens G, Ruyssinck G, Amy J. Outcome after elective labor induction in nulliparous women: A matched cohort study. Am J Obstet Gynecol2002;186:240–4.

Dujardin B, Boutsen M, De Schampheleire I, et al. Oxytocics in developing countries. Int J Gynaecol Obstet 1995;50:243–51.

Gómez Ponce de León C, Wing D, Fiala C. Misoprostol for intrauterine fetal death. Int J Gynecol Obstet 2007;99(Suppl. 2):S190–3.

Gülmezoglu AM, Crowther CA, Middleton P. Induction of labour for improving birth outcomes for women at or beyond term. Cochrane Database Syst Rev 2006;4: CD004945.

Hofmeyr GJ, Alfirevic Z, Matonhodze B, et al. Titrated oral misoprostol solution for induction of labour: a multi-centre, randomised trial. Br J Obstet Gynaecol 2001;108: 952–9.

Kundodyiwa T, Alfirevic Z, Weeks A. Low dose oral misoprostol for induction of labor: a systematic review. Obstet Gynecol 2009; 13:374–83.

National Collaborating Centre for Women's and Children's Health (NCCWCH). Induction of Labour. London: RCOG Press; 2008.

Osman I, MacKenzie F, Norrie J, et al. The 'PRIM' study: A randomized comparison of prostaglandin E2 gel with the nitric oxide donor isosorbide mononitrate for cervical ripening before the induction of labor at term. Am J Obstet Gynecol 2006;194:1012–21.

Sanchez-Ramos L. Expectant management versus labor induction for suspected fetal macrosomia: a systematic review. Obstet Gynecol 2002;100:997–1002.

Smith GC. Factors predisposing to perinatal death related to uterine rupture during attempted vaginal birth after caesarean section: retrospective cohort study. BMJ 2004;329:375.

Internet resources

Health Care Commission 2008 (HCC): www.healthcarecommission.org.uk/healthcareproviders/nationalfindings/surveys/healthcareproviders/surveysofpatients/maternityservices.cfm

www.misoprostol.org

Labour

This section covers the management of normal labour and slow labour. Other sections cover the complications of labour, place of birth (Chapter 10.8, Home birth), fetal assessment (Chapter 10.7, Fetal surveillance in labour), analgesia (Chapter 10.1, Analgesia and anaesthesia in obstetrics), episiotomy (Chapter 10.5, Episiotomy and obstetric perineal trauma), Caesarean section (Chapter 11.2, Caesarean section), and operative vaginal delivery (Chapter 11.5, Ventouse delivery).

Definitions

Labour is defined as painful contractions with progressive cervical change (NCCWCH 2007). The *latent phase* of labour is a period of time during which there are painful contractions and some cervical changes (effacement or dilatation up to 4 cm dilated). The *established first stage* is when there are regular painful contractions and progressive cervical dilatation from 4 cm. The *passive second stage* is the finding of full dilatation prior to involuntary expulsive contractions. The *active second stage* occurs when there are expulsive contractions or active pushing with full dilation or the head is visible. The *third stage* of labour is from the time of birth of the baby to the expulsion of the placenta and membranes.

Schools of labour management

Labour management has varied hugely over the years in response to scientific advances, public health priorities, fashion, and opinion-formers. The major schools are listed below.

Medicalized labour (1950s)

This school arose in an attempt to reduce the very high maternal and fetal complication rates. Proponents believed that complications of labour could be largely resolved by the use of medical technology. As such, it advocated the extensive, and largely uncritical use of all available technology such as episiotomy, electronic fetal monitoring, and operative vaginal delivery.

Natural labour (1950s to date)

In response to the increased medicalization of labour, an alternative school grew up that recognized the dangers of medical intervention in normal labours. Leaders such as Kitzinger and Odent promoted the benefits of home and water birth, relaxation, and physiology.

Active management of labour (1970–90)

This regimented style of labour management was developed in the National Maternity Hospital in Dublin. It was characterized by clearly defined protocols for the diagnosis of labour (painful contractions with a fully effaced cervix, ruptured membranes, or show) and the early diagnosis of dystocia (hourly vaginal examinations for the first 3 hours), which was treated with oxytocin. The impressive outcome data from this hospital seemed to provide evidence of its benefit and 'active management' became extensively practiced worldwide.

Evidence-based labour management (1990 to date)

The arrival of the Cochrane Database of Pregnancy and Childbirth in the late 1980s injected a new rigour into the assessment of evidence, and Thornton and Lilford went on to challenge the use of active management (Thornton 1994). An RCT of 'active management' finally showed it to provide no benefit on labour outcomes (Frigoletto 1997).

Since then, the evidence-based medicine (EBM) school has been largely unchallenged.

This chapter is written using EBM methods and draws extensively on the 2007 guidelines from the UK National Institute of Clinical Excellence (NICE), produced by the National Collaborating Centre for Women's and Children's Health (NCCWCH 2007).

Assessment of labour progress

Clinical examination

- Although helpful in assessing labour progress, vaginal examinations should be minimized due to discomfort and the risks of infection. The risk of postpartum endometritis has been found to be closely related to the number of internal examinations after membrane rupture.
- The digital vaginal assessment of head descent is notoriously difficult. The use of abdominal palpation may improve accuracy, but is difficult in the obese or tense. A new device called the StationMaster has been shown to increase the accuracy of assessment in clinical models (Awan 2009).
- Likewise, the accuracy of digital cervical dilation is poor, especially between 4 and 8 cm dilatation (Awan 2009). An electronic device called Birthtrack increases accuracy but is invasive.

The partogram

- The partogram (Fig. 10.10.1) is based on the original cervicogram, developed by Friedman in the 1950s. Philpott (1972) added an 'action line' set 4 hours to the right of the alert line to aid the correct timing of intervention.
- A cluster RCT of partogram versus no partogram found that use of the partogram halved the rate of prolonged labour and use of oxytocin while increasing the rate of spontaneous birth (Anon 1994). Recent studies show that placement of the action line 2 hours to the right of the alert line (rather than 4 hours) increased intervention without improving clinical outcomes.
- With increasing lengths of the second stage in epidural labours, a second-stage partogram might help to predict and time for delivery intervention (Sizer 2000). Efforts so far have been hampered by difficulties in accurately assessing head descent.

First stage of labour

Normal progress

- In nulliparous women, the average latent phase lasts 7 hours (upper limit 15 hours) and the active first stage lasts 8 hours (upper limit 19 hours). In multiparous women, the average length of the active first stage is 5 hours (upper limit 15 hours). The NICE guideline suggests that a rate of less than 0.5 cm/hour in the active phase should be used as a cut off for intervention rather than the customary 1 cm/hour (NCCWCH 2007).

Optimizing outcomes

- Clinical intervention is not advised where labour is progressing normally.
- Birth at home and in birthing centres (Chapter 10.8) are all associated with an increased chance of normal birth.
- Routine amniotomy shortens the length of labour but has no other beneficial effects on outcome.
- Early oxytocin use has not been shown to be of benefit:

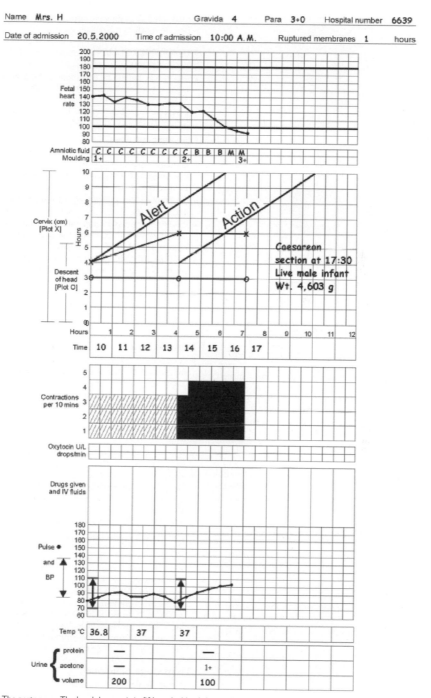

Fig. 10.10.1 The partogram. The head descent is in fifths palpable abdominally, and the shading of the contractions relates to the duration of the contractions.

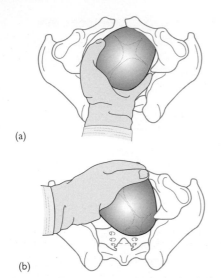

(a)

(b)

Fig. 10.10.2 Manual rotation for correcting malposition in the second stage of labour.

it increases the pain without beneficial effects on labour outcome.

- One-to-one midwifery care was originally thought to be a minor part of the active management of labour package. But when the various components were unpicked, this proved to be the only component that significantly improved clinical outcomes with reductions in analgesia use, operative delivery, and low APGAR scores (Thornton 1994). The Cochrane analysis now shows that the care is at least as effective if the continuous support is provided by a friend rather than member of staff.

Managing delay
- Prolonged latent phase (over 18 hours in a nulliparous woman) is best treated with reassurance and analgesia. Use of oxytocin in this situation increases the need for Caesarean (CS) and poor outcomes in the neonate without benefit.
- Primary dysfunctional labour (progress of under 0.5 cm/hour) should be treated with amniotomy and oxytocin with continuous fetal heart rate monitoring (NCCWCH 2007). NICE's suggested timeline for nulliparous women (in hours) is
- Time 0: diagnosis of labour
- 4 hours later: if less than 2 cm progress→amniotomy
- 2 hours later: if less than 1 cm further dilated→oxytocin
- 4 hours later: if less than 2 cm progress on oxytocin → consider the option of further augmentation or CS.
- There are multiple oxytocin regimens available and conflicting evidence as to their relative benefits. Infusion rates should be increased every 30 minutes until there are around four contractions in every 10 minutes.
- Secondary arrest of labour (cessation of progress following normal active phase dilation) is usually caused by disproportion and or malposition of the fetal head. Improving contraction strength with oxytocin may help to correct the disproportion, although the risk of a CS remains high.
- Late secondary arrest with delay between 7 and 10 cm is

associated with difficult instrumental vaginal deliveries, despite reaching full dilatation.

Second stage of labour
Normal progress
- The mean length of the second stage in primigravid women (without epidurals) is 54 minutes with an upper limit (mean +2 SD) of 2 hours 22 minutes. For mutigravid women the mean is 18 minutes, with an upper limit of 60 minutes (NCCWCH 2007).

Optimizing outcomes
- Lying in a supine position increases both pain and the need for operative vaginal delivery. Women should be encouraged to adopt any other position that they find comfortable.
- Techniques for reducing perineal trauma are discussed in Chapter X.
- *Epidurals* are associated with an increased need for operative vaginal deliveries but provide higher rates of maternal satisfaction with analgesia.
- In primiparous women with epidurals, the use of routine oxytocin in the second stage of labour can reduce the need for non-rotational forceps delivery.
- Primiparous women with epidurals have fewer rotational or mid-cavity operative interventions when pushing is delayed for 1–2 hours or until they have a strong urge to push

Managing delay
- A diagnosis of delay is made after 2 hours of pushing in a nulliparous or after 1 hour in a multiparous (NCCWCH 2007).
- Oxytocin can be used in nulliparous women if contractions are poor. Oxytocin should not be used (or with extreme caution based on contractions observed) for delay in multiparous women due to the risk of uterine rupture.
- Caesarean section (Chapter 11.2) or instrumental delivery (Chapter 11.3) are the definitive treatments for delay. The choice of instrument depends on operator experience. Operative vaginal delivery should not be attempted if the head is more than one-fifth palpable abdominally.
- Manual rotation is sometimes used to improve outcomes with malposition during the second stage, but there is little evidence to support its use. It should be undertaken with care due to the risks of fetal trauma and cord accidents. The classic technique is to slide the fingers right behind the occiput so that the head can be flexed and rotated at the same time (Fig. 10.10.2). The operator's right hand is used for LOPs and the left hand for ROPs (Donald 1979). It has been used both prophylactically at the start of the second stage (Le Ray 2007) and as an alternative to rotational operative delivery after delay.

Third stage of labour
Normal physiological progress
- The median length of third stage is 15 minutes if physiologically managed and 8 minutes if actively managed (Rogers 1998).
- For a physiologically managed third stage the third stage is prolonged if it lasts over 60 minutes. This time limit is reduced to 30 minutes when prophylactic oxytocics are used (NCCWCH 2007).

- Median measured blood loss in a physiological third stage is 496mls with 17% loosing over 1000 mL of blood (Hoj 2005).

Physiology

- Four phases of the normal third stage are described (Herman 1993). In the latent phase there is contraction of the entire uterus except for the retroplacental myometrium. The length of this phase determines the length of the third stage. This is followed by phases of retroplacental contraction, placental detachment, and expulsion.
- The retroplacental contraction compresses the radial arteries as they pass through the myometrium, thus cutting off the blood supply to the placental site and minimising haemorrhage.

Optimizing outcomes

Active management package

- Classic active management is a combination of routine oxytocic use, early cord clamping, and controlled cord traction using the Brandt–Andrews method. In view of the adverse effects of early cord clamping, FIGO has now amended this package to replace the early cord clamping with uterine massage (FIGO 2003).
- In an actively managed third stage, the median measured blood loss is reduced with only 3% loosing over 1000 mL.
- Multiple oxytocics have been studied. Oxytocin 10 IU i.m. (effective in 2 minutes, lasts 15 minutes) is now the oxytocic of choice as it combines high efficacy with few side-effects (FIGO, NCCWCH 2007). Ergometrine 500 µg i.m. (effective in 6 minutes, lasts 30 minutes) is slightly more effective than oxytocin, but causes vomiting and hypertension, and, when given i.v., retained placenta. Syntometrine 1 ampoule i.m. (contains 5 IU of oxytocin and 500 µg of ergometrine) combines the benefits and side-effects of both. Misoprostol 600 µg po (effective in 8 minutes, lasts 120 minutes) is less effective than oxytocin 10 IU i.m., but is heat stable and easy to administer.

Timing of cord clamping

- The neonate receives about 30% of its final blood volume in the first 3 minutes after delivery from the placenta.
- Early cord clamping reduces neonatal cord haemoglobin concentrations and the rate of hyperbilirubinaemia, but increases the rate of neonatal anaemia (with associated reduced iron stores for up to 6 months of age). This could have important public health implications in populations with already high rates of iron deficiency anaemia.
- In premature babies, early cord clamping increases the rate of intraventricular haemorrhages and the need for transfusion to treat anaemia and hypotension.
- There is no known benefit to the woman of early cord clamping in terms of reduced postpartum haemorrhage outside of the active management package. Indeed, small trials of cord drainage suggest that it might even have benefits by reducing the rate of retained placenta.

Controlled cord traction

- This was introduced as part of the active management package so as to reduce the rate of retained placenta. In the Brandt–Andrew's method once there are signs of placental separation (a small gush of blood and lengthening of the cord) the cord is held taut while the other hand on the abdomen presses the uterus away.
- There are dangers of cord traction: premature cord traction may cause bleeding by separating the placenta

from an uncontracted myometrium, and overenthusiastic traction may detach the cord from the placenta.
- The first major trial of controlled cord traction is currently in progress and is expected to finish in 2010.

Uterine massage

- Postnatal uterine massage has only been investigated in one small trial and this showed some reduction in blood loss.

Managing delay

Retained placenta is covered in Chapter 10.18.

Further reading

Akmal S, Kametas N, Tsoi E, et al. Comparison of transvaginal digital examination with intrapartum sonography to determine fetal head position before instrumental delivery. Ultrasound Obstet Gynecol 2003;21:437–40.

Anonymous. Managing complications in pregnancy and childbirth. A guide for midwives and doctors. Geneva: WHO 2006.

Anonymous. World Health Organization partograph in management of labour. World Health Organization Maternal Health and Safe Motherhood Programme. Lancet 1994;343(89:1399–401.

Awan N, Rhoades A, Weeks AD. The validity and reliability of the StationMaster: a device to improve the accuracy of station assessment in labour. Eur J Obstet Gynecol Reprod Biol 2009; 145:65–70.

Chalmers I, Enkin M, Kierse MJNC (eds). Effective care in pregnancy and childbirth. Oxford: Oxford University Press 1989.

Crichton D. A reliable method of establishing the level of the fetal head in obstetrics. S Afr Med J. 1974;48:784–7.

Donald I. Practical obstetric problems, 5th edn. London: Lloyd-Luke 1979.

FIGO/ICM. Prevention and treatment of post-partum haemorrhage: new advances for low resource settings. A joint statement of the International Confederation of Midwives (ICM) and International Federation of Gynaecology and Obstetrics (FIGO). Available at: www.figo.org/docs/PPH%20Joint%20Statement%202%20English.pdf

Frigoletto FD Jr, Lieberman E, Lang JM, et al. A clinical trial of active management of labor. N Engl J Med 1995;333:745–50.

Gülmezoglu AM, Villar J, Ngoc NT, et al. WHO multicentre randomised trial of misoprostol in the management of the third stage of labour. Lancet 2001;358:689–95.

Herman A, Weinraub Z, Bukovsky I, et al. Dynamic ultrasonographic imaging of the third stage of labor: new perspectives into third-stage mechanisms. Am J Obstet Gynecol 1993;168:1496–9.

Høj L, Cardoso P, Nielsen BB, et al. Effect of sublingual misoprostol on severe postpartum haemorrhage in a primary health centre in Guinea-Bissau: randomised double blind clinical trial. BMJ 2005;331:723.

Kitzinger S. The new pregnancy and childbirth, 4th edn. London: Dorling Kindersley 2003.

Le Ray C, Serres P, Schmitz T, et al. Manual rotation in occiput posterior or transverse positions: risk factors and consequences on the cesarean delivery rate. Obstet Gynecol 2007;110:873–9.

National Collaborating Centre for Women's and Children's Health (NCCWCH). Intrapartum Care. London: RCOG Press 2007.

O'Driscoll K, Meagher D, Boylan P. Active management of labour, 3rd edn. London: Mosby 1993.

Odent M. Birth and breastfeeding: rediscovering the needs of women during pregnancy and childbirth. Forest Row: Clairview Books 2003.

Philpott RH, Castle WM. Cervicographs in the management of labour in the primigravida. II. The action line and treatment of abnormal labour. J Obstet Gynaecol Br Commonw 1972; 79:599–602.

Rogers J, Wood J, McCandlish R, et al. Active versus expectant management of third stage of labour: the Hinchingbrooke randomised controlled trial. Lancet 1998;351:693–9.

Sizer AR, Evans J, Bailey SM, Wiener J. A second-stage partogram. Obstet Gynecol. 2000;96:678–83.

Thornton JG, Lilford RJ. Active management of labour: current knowledge and research issues. BMJ 1994;309:366–9.

Maternal collapse

Definition
Maternal collapse can occur for many underlying reasons. It describes a reduction in the level of consciousness related to cerebral hypoperfusion or a primary neurological insult. If not promptly diagnosed and managed then there is a significant risk of serious long-term morbidity and mortality.

Epidemiology
- The UK confidential enquiry into maternal death gives prevalence of maternal death due to specific conditions. Data regarding the incidence of maternal collapse where the woman recovers is less good as the condition is not a single entity. Likewise data regarding the incidence worldwide is very poor, as in most developing countries figures are not collected. Overall like maternal death, collapse is a very rare occurrence in developed countries and this creates issues related to training. The World Health Organization (WHO) publishes statistics on maternal mortality by country and these data are a stark reminder of the inequities in healthcare that exist around the world.
- Pregnancy is an independent risk factor for a number of conditions that can cause collapse:
  - thromboembolism (pulmonary embolus) 5× increase in risk
  - ischaemic stroke 9× increase in risk in the puerperium
  - haemorrhagic stroke 26× increase in risk
  - subarachnoid haemorrhage 20× increase in risk.
- The incidence of some of the important causes of collapse in pregnancy in developed countries are
  - cardiac arrest in pregnancy 1 in 30 000 pregnancies
  - myocardial infarction 1 in 10 000
  - amniotic fluid embolism 1 in 8000–20 000
  - septic shock 1 in 800
  - massive postpartum haemorrhage (blood loss of more than 1500 mL) 1 in 200
- Certain maternal characteristics are associated with an increased risk of collapse: increased maternal age, social deprivation, late booking, lack of antenatal care, pre-existing maternal disease (e.g. cardiac, diabetes), maternal obesity (BMI >30), asylum seekers.
- Drugs used during pregnancy may result in maternal collapse due to toxicity or anaphylaxis:
  - magnesium (eclampsia/pre-eclampsia)
  - antibiotics (group B Streptococcus prophylaxis/pyrexia treatment)
  - lignocaine/bupivicaine (epidural and local anaesthetic)
  - synthetic prostaglandins (postpartum haemorrhage possibly due to coronary artery spasm)
  - latex (gloves, catheters)
  - blood products (blood transfusion, coagulation factors).
- A past medical history of certain conditions increases the risk of collapse in pregnancy:
  - pre-existing cardiac disease increases the risk of collapse due to ischaemia, arrhythmia, or cardiac failure
  - Marfan's syndrome increase the risk of aortic dissection

- essential hypertension cardiomyopathy
- inherited thrombophilia pulmonary embolism

Prevention
Appropriate antenatal care
All women should be seen by a healthcare professional at an early stage in pregnancy to allow a full history to be taken; in the UK this visit is recommended to occur before the end of the thirteenth completed week of gestation. This will allow the identification of risk factors increasing the risk of a disease process occurring that will result in collapse. This allows the care of the pregnancy to be planned with optimization of underlying disease and the use of prophylactic treatments to reduce the chances of collapse occurring. Pre-conception counselling and support should be offered to all women of childbearing age with any serious pre-existing medical or mental health problem. This should include women with significant risk factors such as obesity.

Modified obstetric early warning systems
Early warning signs of impending maternal collapse often go unrecognized, and this has led to the recommendation that modified early obstetric warning system (MEOWS) with the routine use of early warning charts that allow changes in vital signs to be flagged up and referred are used in all units. Such charts are already used in critical care units.

Training skills and drills
Maternal collapse although very serious is a rare occurrence even in a busy maternity unit, and individuals will have only rare exposure to clinical occurrences. It is therefore essential that all units have regular 'skills' training sessions and that mock 'drills' of maternal collapse are scheduled to allow staff to practise management and reflect on this process. There are now a number of courses that aim to teach the essential skills and team working.

Aetiology
Maternal collapse may be due to a number of different causes (see individual entries).

Non-serious causes
Although these are common, more serious causes of collapse must always be considered prior to making these diagnoses:
- hyperventilation
- vasovagal attack (faint).

Potentially life-threatening causes of collapse
Haemorrhagic causes
- Massive antepartum haemorrhage (abruption or placenta praevia)
- Massive intrapartum haemorrhage (abruption or uterine rupture)
- Massive postpartum haemorrhage (uterine atony, genital tract trauma including uterine rupture, retained placenta)
- Rupture of a splenic artery aneurysm,
- Liver capsule rupture
- Ruptured aortic aneurysm.

Neurological (cerebral)
- Eclampsia

- Haemorrhagic stroke
- Ischaemic stroke
- Subarachnoid haemorrhage
- Cerebral arterial/venous thrombosis.

Cardiac/pulmonary
- Tension pneumothorax
- Amniotic fluid embolism
- Pulmonary embolism
- Severe pulmonary oedema (pre-eclampsia)
- Cardiomyopathy
- Myocardial infarction
- Dissecting aortic aneurysm
- Pre-existing cardiac disease
- Heart failure or arrhythmia.

Non-haemorrhagic
- Hypoglycaemia
- Uterine inversion
- Septic shock
- Drug toxicity
- Anaphylaxis
- Anaesthetic complications
- Suicide attempts (poisoning).

Prognosis

In developed countries maternal mortality is a rare event. In the UK, the confidential enquiry into maternal death collects statistics regarding death due to particular conditions. However, the morbidity associated with maternal collapse is less well documented. Prompt management will improve prognosis and reduce the risk of long-term disability.

Clinical approach

In cases of collapse, history taking, examination, and resuscitation must all occur simultaneously to reduce delay in diagnosis and management. This is often called the *primary survey*.

Team-working is essential and a call for help from other disciplines is essential and should be immediate:
- osenior obstetrician
- ojunior obstetrician(s) to assist and for training
- oexperienced anaesthetist
- senior midwife
- junior midwife to assist and for training
- porter to take sample to laboratory
- recorder to note times of steps in resuscitation
- the cardiac arrest team may be requested if respiratory or cardiac arrest is suspected at the time of collapse
- the appropriate specialists (e.g. neurologist, cardiologist) should be involved in management early where specific pathologies are suspected.
- the laboratory should informed if a major obstetric haemorrhage is suspected.

Diagnosis
History
- A history should be obtained from people witnessing the collapse as the behaviour leading up to the event may give indicators to the underlying cause.
- All history taking is simultaneous with assessment and resuscitation, which must be commenced without delay.

- Antenatal or intrapartum risk factors should be established from a relative or midwife. An individual not essential to resuscitation can review the notes and report to the resuscitation teams relevant findings.

Examination
Initial examination is based on the identifying life-threatening problems to allow appropriate resuscitation. However the possible causes of collapse must be identified as soon as possible to allow appropriate management.
- Is the woman responsive?
- Is she fitting?
- Pulse, BP, capillary filling time, heart auscultation?
- Respiratory rate, tracheal position, auscultation for air entry.
- Abdominal palpation for rebound/guarding, uterine tenderness, tone and size.
- Vaginal examination for bleeding &and cervical dilatation.
- Fetal heart auscultation to assess whether fetus is alive.

Monitoring
- Intravenous access must be established using wide-bore peripheral cannulae or central venous line.
- Pulse, non-invasive blood pressure, oxygen saturation, and ECG monitoring should be commenced in all cases.
- A urinary catheter should be inserted after initial resuscitation.
- Consider arterial and central venous pressure lines.
- Fetal monitoring is a secondary consideration to maternal monitoring. Fetal hypoxia will occur if the mother is hypotensive for any reason. Maternal resuscitation must always take priority over any fetal consideration, and ultimately the best way to resuscitate the fetus is to resuscitate the mother. Delivery should only be considered once the woman has been stabilized or if cardiac arrest has occurred and resuscitation is unsuccessful at 5 minutes.

Investigations
- Group and cross-match.
- A full blood count, coagulation screen, full liver and renal profile and C-reactive protein (CRP) should be sent in all women
- Selective investigations depending on differential diagnosis
- Arterial blood gases
- A bedside assessment of blood glucose (backed-up by a laboratory sample)
- A 12-lead ECG
- Chest X-ray
- Abdominal/pelvic ultrasound to assess fetal position and presence of free fluid
- Consider need for specialist investigations CT/MRI, CTPA, echocardiography

Management and immediate resuscitation
Assessment and resuscitation occur simultaneously with the aim of identifying life-threatening problems in the order that they will cause death. It is imperative that the steps are performed in order with movement onto the next step only once any identified problem has been corrected.

Tilt
A 30-degree left lateral tilt should be instituted for all women greater than 20 weeks' gestation. A tilt is recommended for

collapse in the immediate puerperium when a clot-filled uterus may still cause significant caval compression. This can be achieved by the use of a wedge or by manual displacement if a wedge is not available.

Step A **A**IRWAY

- Visually assess airway by looking in mouth.
- Suction if necessary to clear secretions or vomit.
- Consider possible airway obstruction.
- Causes of airway obstruction (rare in pregnancy):
  - severe pre-eclampsia with swelling of the tongue and larynx
  - post-fitting tongue oedema due to biting
  - smoke inhalation
  - trauma (road traffic accident).
- In an unconscious or semi-conscious woman the tongue may fall back and a head tilt/chin lift manoeuvre or a jaw thrust may improve the patency of the airway.
- An airway adjunct such as an oropharyngeal (Guedel) airway can be considered in an unconscious woman but may not be tolerated in a conscious or semi-conscious woman).
- The airway must remain patent and if breathing and circulation are confirmed the woman should be moved into the 'recovery' position.

Step B **B**reathing

- The respiratory system should be assessed, initially by looking, listening, and feeling for evidence of spontaneous respiration (no more than 10 seconds).
- If not breathing a respiratory arrest is diagnosed and a cardiac arrest call should be made.
- Commence assisted ventilation with a pocket mask or a bag and valve mask.
- Intubation should be performed as soon as an anaesthetist arrives to give assistance.
- Causes of respiratory arrest:
  - drug toxicity (lignocaine or magnesium sulphate)
  - total spinal anaesthesia
  - amniotic fluid embolism
  - anaphylaxis.
- A witnessed respiratory arrest may not progress to cardiac arrest if effective assisted ventilation is commenced promptly. However, an untreated respiratory arrest will rapidly progress to collapse (cerebral hypoxia) and cardiac arrest (myocardial hypoxia).
- If breathing spontaneously commence high-flow oxygen (facemask with a non-rebreathing bag gives 60% oxygen) at 15 L/minute should be administered.
- If breathing is occurring respiratory rate (normal 12–20) and oxygen saturation (normal >95%) should be checked and if these are abnormal repeat a full respiratory examination (with chest expansion observation, percussion and auscultation).

Step C **C**irculation

- The pulse should be checked (simultaneous to the assessment of breathing by checking the carotid pulse).
- The blood pressure, pulse (normal <100 bpm), and capillary refill time (normal <2 seconds) should be assessed. The signs of hypovolaemia are masked in pregnancy until late; thus a tachycardia and fall in systolic BP indicate that a 30% (2000 mL) loss of circulating blood volume has already occurred.

- If there is no pulse commence cardiac compressions 100/minute at a ratio of 30 compressions to one assisted ventilation breath. In a single operator resuscitation chest compressions can be performed without ventilation until more help arrives.
- Causes of cardiac arrest:
  - ongoing airway obstruction or respiratory arrest
  - hypovolaemia due to haemorrhage
  - myocardial infarction
  - magnesium toxicity.
- If cardiopulmonary resuscitation does not succeed in restoring circulation by 5 minutes after the diagnosis of cardiac arrest then perimortem Caesarean section should be performed. In gestations of 20–24 weeks a hysterotomy should be performed to aid maternal resuscitation. At gestations below 20 weeks emptying the uterus is not necessary, as it does not cause significant caval compression.
  - The choice of incision should be that which the operator feels able to perform most rapidly.
  - Cohen's abdominal/uterine entry should be used to achieve rapid delivery.
  - A paediatrician should be requested to attend delivery if the fetus is of a viable gestation but it is stressed delivery in this situation is to improve the chances of successful resuscitation in the mother and not for fetal distress.

If there is a pulse present but the clinical signs and history suggest hypovolaemia fluid resuscitation should commence with crystalloid solutions. Colloid may be required if hypotension persists and cross-matched blood is not yet available.

Step D **D**isability

- Initial assessment of consciousness using the AVPU scale
  - A **a**lert
  - V response to **v**erbal command
  - P response to **p**ain
  - U **u**nresponsive
- The Glasgow coma scale (Table 10.11.1) is a more precise tool to assess the level of consciousness and assess any deterioration with time; it should be performed in any woman scoring VPU or where a neurological problem is suspected.

Further management

Immediate considerations

- Ongoing fluid resuscitation:
  - Is there a risk of fluid overload?
  - What blood products might be required?
- Is there a need for surgical intervention?
  - Laparotomy for delivery, management of uterine atony, suspected intra-abdominal bleeding or sepsis
  - Examination under anaesthesia for retained placenta, genital tract trauma or uterine atony.
- Should antibiotics be given?
  - Treatment of sepsis
  - Prophylaxis.

Table 10.11.1 Glasgow Coma Scale

Response	Description	Score
Eye opening	Spontaneous (open with normal blinking)	4
	Eye opening to speech on request	3
	Eye opening only to pain stimulus	2
	No eye opening despite stimulation	1
Verbal	Orientated, spontaneous speech	5
	Confused conversation but answers questions	4
	Inappropriate words but recognizable	3
	Incomprehensible sounds/grunts	2
	No verbal response	1
Motor	Obeys commands/moves limbs to command	6
	Localizes (e.g. moves upper limb to stimulus)	5
	Withdraws from painful stimulus on limb	4
	Abnormal flexion or decorticate posture	3
	Extensor response, decerebrate posture	2
	No movement to any stimulus	1

- Where will the woman be best managed now?
  - High dependency unit
    Suspected major system failure (renal, liver etc.)
  - Intensive care unit
    If ventilated.

Ongoing management
- This is sometimes called the *secondary* survey and is a full assessment and review that occurs after initial resuscitation and management. It involves the formulation of a definitive management plan and may involve other medical specialists and more complex investigations.
- During this time it is essential that airway, breathing, and circulation are re-evaluated regularly and appropriate support continued. Full re-evaluation is especially important if any new deterioration occurs in the woman's condition.
- Follow-up/recurrence/future pregnancy planning
  - It is essential that the woman and her family be debriefed following any episode of collapse. This should be performed as soon as feasible after the event with repeat sessions if required
  - Professional counselling may be required to reduce post-traumatic stress. The risks of recurrence in a future pregnancy must be discussed and any preventative strategies that can be used in a future pregnancy.
  - Contraceptive advice should be offered to women who do not wish to have further children.

Further reading

Al-Shabibi N, Penna L, Postpartum collapse. Curr Obstet Gynaecol 2006;16:72–6.

Clarke J, Butt M. Maternal collapse. Curr Opin Obstet Gynecol 2005;17:157–60.

Lewis G. Saving mother's lives 2003–2005. London: CEMACH publications 2007.

Howell C, Grady K, Cox C. *Managing obstetric emergencies and trauma: The MOET course manual.* RCOG Press 2007.

Internet resources

www.alsg.org
www.also.org.uk
www.resus.org.uk
www.cemach.org.uk

Patient resources

www.jessicastrust.org.uk

Meconium-stained liquor

Definition
Meconium is the sterile material produced by the fetal digestive tract. It is composed of material ingested by the fetus from the amniotic cavity, such as epithelial cells, lanugo, blood, amniotic fluid and is pigmented by bile. The majority of fetuses will not pass meconium *in utero* with passage occurring in the first few days after birth. A minority of fetuses pass meconium *in utero*, resulting in the amniotic fluid becoming stained with meconium.

Obstetric convention grades meconium:
- Grade 1 describes a large volume of amniotic fluid lightly stained with meconium.
- Grade 2 describes a good volume of amniotic fluid heavily stained with meconium.
- Grade 3 describes absent or reduced volume of amniotic fluid so that the meconium is very thick.

The terms light, moderate and heavy are equally acceptable. Whatever classification is used visual assessment has poor accuracy with studies showing high interoperator variability in grading.

Epidemiology
Meconium stained liquor (MSL) occurs in 8–20% of all births after 34 weeks. The incidence increases with gestation with an incidence of more than 30% after 42 weeks' gestation. Conversely, the incidence is lower in gestations below 34 weeks with an incidence of less than 5%. There are no other demographic associations and the incidence is expected to be the same worldwide.

Aetiology
Meconium is passed due to active peristalsis of the fetal gut. Abnormal peristalsis of the bowel may occur due to an external stress, resulting in increased sympathetic drive in the fetus.

Normal variant
- Peristaltic activity in the bowel increases as central nervous system and gastrointestinal tract matures and thus the passage of meconium may occur without any particular stimulus as a part of normal physiology in some term fetuses. The incidence of MSL increases as gestation increases and may be normal in any fetus beyond 34 weeks' gestation. MSL is usually only lightly (grade 1) stained as a normal variant.
- Passive pressure on the fetal abdomen can cause passage of meconium. Breech presentation may be associated with the passage of meconium in the late first stage and second stage due to pressure on the fetal abdomen as it descends in the pelvis. The meconium staining may appear moderate to heavy in this situation but is obviously fresh in nature.
- Women with obstetric cholestasis may have an increased incidence of MSL before and during labour, with a number of studies suggesting an incidence of up to 25% in term pregnancies and 18% in preterm pregnancies. The reasons for this increase are unknown.

Abnormal
- Many fetuses show an adrenergic stress response to developing hypoxia; this causes a developing tachycardia and may result in an increase in gut peristalsis with the development of intrapartum MSL; the staining is usually moderate to severe (grades 2 or 3) in these situations.

Not all fetuses with subacute hypoxia will pass meconium. Fetuses who experience a sudden severe hypoxic event such as uterine rupture may not pass meconium, and the absence of MSL in the presence of an abnormal fetal heart rate patterns in not reassuring.
- The passage of meconium has an association with perinatal infection. Fetal infection may result in a stress response with the passage of meconium. In addition to this, infection reduces the ability of a fetus to compensate for developing hypoxia. In preterm gestations, MSL has an association with listeria infection. However, this association is not strong and infections with common agents such as group B streptococcus need not present with MSL.

Prognosis
The majority of labours complicated by MSL have normal outcomes, but the presence of MSL increases the risk of a number of adverse neonatal outcomes. The risk of poor outcome increases with the grade of meconium seen in the liquor (see Management).

Meconium aspiration
- MSL is a risk factor for meconium aspiration syndrome. Meconium aspiration most likely occurs as a result of fetal gasping *in utero*. A fetus will gasp in response to sudden severe hypoxia or when a gradual onset subacute hypoxia becomes severe. MSL meconium aspiration can be a life-threatening condition and is known to account for 2% of perinatal deaths. It is more likely to occur with heavy MSL than with light MSL but it can occur with both types. It may not be initially apparent at birth and therefore neonatal protocols should recommend increased surveillance of babies with MSL in labour. This will result in longer hospitalization for the majority of mothers and their babies where meconium aspiration does not occur.

Poor condition at birth and hypoxic ischaemic encephalopathy
- A fetus that is becoming hypoxic may pass meconium and thus MSL is a risk factor for poor neonatal outcome (low pH, low APGAR scores, neonatal seizures). Heavy MSL also implies a relative oligohydramnios, which has an association with placental insufficiency and more profound cord compression during labour. Fetal heart rate monitoring remains a valid tool even in the presence of meconium

Cerebral palsy
- As both meconium aspiration and severe hypoxic ischaemic encephalopathy (HIE) are associated with a long-term risk of mental retardation and cerebral palsy, this means that MSL is a risk factor for this outcome. However, the link is weak with MSL a common occurrence and cerebral palsy a rare outcome (3/10 000 births in England and Wales). However, among infants with meconium aspiration, recent research has suggested a risk of about 20% for cerebral palsy or global developmental delay.

Clinical approach
Diagnosis
History
- Elicit history suggesting ruptured membranes.

- Confirm gestational age and history of onset of labour.
- Review antenatal history for risk factors for fetal hypoxia, chorioamnionitis or obstetric cholestasis.

Examination
- Maternal observations for signs of infection (pyrexia or tachycardia)
- Meconium staining can be assessed by looking at the colour of the liquor on a (white) pad. A speculum examination is only required if the diagnosis is uncertain or a high vaginal swab is required.
- Review of fetal heart rate pattern (if on continuous monitoring).

Differential diagnosis
- Women who have had antepartum haemorrhage can have greenish liquor due to blood products contaminating the liquor or a greenish discharge from blood breakdown products.
- Bile staining of the amniotic fluid may occur in fetuses with bowel obstruction (who are less likely to pass meconium).
- Vaginal infections such as thrush can cause a creamy greenish discharge.

Initial management

Initial management decisions at diagnosis
- If there is MSL (light or heavy staining) following prelabour rupture of membranes after 34 weeks' gestation, arrangements should be made for stimulation of labour as soon as possible. Conservative management is contraindicated for heavy MSL and is controversial even in light MSL at gestations above 37 weeks. Labour can be induced with prostaglandin or an oxytocin infusion, but continuous monitoring must be carried out throughout.
- If meconium is suspected with preterm prelabour rupture of membranes there is a high risk of perinatal infection. Clinical signs of infection should be reviewed (uterine tenderness, maternal or fetal tachycardia, pyrexia, offensive vaginal discharge) and investigations to assist in diagnosing chorioamnionitis should be sent (vaginal swab, white cell count, and C-reactive protein). In the absence of signs of infection, steroids should be given and labour stimulated after the course has been completed. If there is a high risk of chorioamnionitis, then delivery should be expedited even though the course of steroids has not been completed. Induction of labour in not absolutely contraindicated but the decision regarding mode of delivery should take into consideration the current likely fetal condition and the length of time likely to allow vaginal delivery. There is no evidence that Caesarean section improves the prognosis of an infected fetus as long as fetal hypoxia does not occur; however, an infected fetus is more likely to become hypoxic and thus if a long and difficult labour is anticipated (e.g. an unfavourable cervix in a primigravida) then delivery by lower segment caesarean section (LSCS) may offer benefits for neonatal prognosis.
- There is no evidence that amnio-infusion in women with MSL reduces the risk of meconium aspiration or other poor fetal outcomes, and it is not recommended for routine clinical practice.
- If the woman is in active labour management decisions depend on the grading of the liquor.

Grade 1 meconium
Review antenatal and intrapartum history carefully. Consider whether continuous electronic fetal monitoring (EFM) should be recommended if the labour is being monitored by intermittent ausculation. If any fetal heart rate abnormality is suspected, electronic fetal monitoring should be recommended immediately. If there are clinical factors that can explain the presence of meconium (usually postterm pregnancy) then the labour can be managed in the same way as a pregnancy with non-MSL; however, if the meconium staining increases the possibility of infection or hypoxia EFM must be considered immediately and the management plan changed accordingly. If any risk factor (or borderline risk factor) exists recommend fetal monitoring. If no risk factors exist intermittent ausculation can be continued but must be performed strictly according to guidelines for the first and second stages of labour (see Chapter 10.7, Fetal surveillance in labour) and the liquor should be reassessed regularly to see if the level of meconium staining is increased.

Grades 2 and 3 meconium
Continuous fetal heart rate monitoring should be recommended and commenced without delay.

Further management
This depends of the fetal heart rate pattern.

Normal fetal heart rate
- No specific action is required but continuous monitoring should be continued. Regular vaginal examinations must be performed to ensure the labour is progressing normally. If labour progress is poor, then augmentation with syntocinon can be considered to reduce the length of labour. The risk of oxytocin is that subacute hypoxia is more likely to develop and so it is important that the fetal heart rate remains normal.

Suspicious fetal heart rate pattern
- The usual actions should be performed to try to improve the fetal heart rate pattern (see Section 10.7 Fetal surveillance). Syntocinon should be reduced or stopped if the uterus is contracting more than 4 in 10. Fetal blood sampling should be performed and repeated if normal in 30 minutes if the heart rate abnormality persists. If the repeat shows any deterioration in the pH and increase in the base excess then delivery should be expedited unless spontaneous delivery is likely in a short time (for example a multigravid woman in the late first stage). Any abnormal pH or base excess requires plans to be made for immediate delivery. If there is poor labour progress, syntocinon can only be considered if the pH of the fetus is stable.

Pathological fetal heart rate pattern
- A fetal blood sample can be considered if it is likely that vaginal delivery will be possible in a short time. However, if vaginal delivery is unlikely for a few hours and especially if there is con current poor labour progress, delivery by Caesarean section should be undertaken without fetal blood sampling. If an uncomplicated assisted vaginal delivery is possible, this should be recommended instead of fetal blood sampling. Oxytocin therapy should not be continued until the results of blood sampling are available.

Management in special situations
Prematurity
- Meconium staining is very rare in gestations below

34 weeks. If MSL is noted then the possibility of chorioamnionitis should be considered even in the absence of any other clinical signs. Antibiotics are routinely prescribed in all preterm labours and consideration should be given to broad-spectrum antibiotics. Continuous fetal heart rate monitoring should be recommended and if the fetal heart rate pattern becomes suspicious delivery by caesarean section is recommended due to the reduced fetal reserve to cope with hypoxia. In cases of preterm prelabour rupture of membranes, a change in the colour of the liquor to green requires urgent review as the passage of meconium in this situation may be the first sign of chorioamnionitis. The diagnosis can be difficult as sometimes a greenish discharge may occur in the absence of passage of meconium (possibly due to the breakdown of blood in the cervical canal).

Home birth

- If grade 2 or 3 MSL is diagnosed during a homebirth, then transfer to hospital should be arranged unless the woman declines or transfer is impractical (e.g. second stage of labour). If grade 1 meconium is diagnosed then the clinical situation should be reviewed, including consideration of the ease that transfer to hospital can be arranged. Transfer to hospital is not mandatory if the woman is low risk with clinical features supporting the likelihood of the meconium being a normal variant (post-term pregnancy) and transfer can be achieved rapidly if required, but the threshold for transfer should be reduced if the labour progress is slow or any other problem develops. If the labour continues at home, careful auscultation of the fetal heart must occur throughout labour, neonatal resuscitation equipment should be available and checked, the hospital should be aware of the situation and in case of very heavy (grade 3) meconium an ambulance should be on standby for immediate neonatal transfer to hospital.

Gastroschisis and other fetal bowel obstruction

- The amniotic fluid may appear green in cases of fetal bowel obstruction but in these cases the passage of meconium is very unlikely, as the fetus is unable to ingest significant material to produce large volumes of meconium. The green staining in this situation most likely represents staining with bile. However, aspiration of bile stained liquor can also cause a severe aspiration syndrome and therefore severe fetal hypoxia must be avoided to prevent fetal gasping so that the finding should be managed as if it were heavy MSL.

Counselling

- If a woman declines continuous electronic fetal monitoring in spite of recommendation the reasons for monitoring should be discussed and documented. The association between MSL and meconium aspiration should be discussed and the importance of prompt diagnosis of hypoxia to try to prevent fetal gasping. Intermittent ausculation should be continued, but the woman must be informed that this may not diagnose subtle indicators of fetal hypoxia and result in a delay of up to 15 minutes of detecting even serious changes in the fetal heart rate.

Neonatal resuscitation

General comments:

- The need for a paediatrician/neonatal nurse practitioner to be present at delivery should be considered in any birth with light MSL. If the electronic fetal monitoring or intermittent auscultation is normal attendance is not mandatory.
- A paediatrician/neonatal nurse practitioner should be requested to be present at delivery of all babies with heavy MSL even if the monitoring is normal. If the fetal heart rate monitoring is abnormal the chance that the baby will require advanced neonatal resuscitation is increased, and appropriately experienced personnel should be asked to be present at the birth.
- Suctioning of the nose and mouth on the perineum prior to the delivery of the shoulders is not beneficial and is not required. As part of resuscitation the upper airway should only be suctioned if thick meconium is seen in the mouth.
- Further resuscitation depends on the condition of the baby

Depressed

A baby with a low heart rate and no breathing requires a trained individual to carry out suction under direct vision during laryngoscopy. Depending on the response to resuscitation these infants may require admission to a neonatal unit for careful observation.

Good condition

No suction or additional resuscitation is required in a vigorous baby.

Postnatal neonatal observation by midwifery team

The midwifery team performs neonatal observations after delivery and any abnormality requires urgent referral to a neonatologist for review. No special maternal observations are required.

Heavy meconium

The baby should be observed closely for signs of respiratory distress with observations at 1 and 2 hours and then 2 hourly until 12 hours of age. Observations should include general wellbeing and feeding, and assessment of heart rate, respiratory rate, temperature, capillary refill, muscle tone, and chest movements.

Light meconium

The baby should be observed at 1 and 2 hours as above, but if all is normal no special review is required after this.

Recurrence/future pregnancy planning

Women can be reassured that meconium is not a recurrent problem and that the risk in future pregnancy is the same as that in the general population. Induction of labour at 41weeks reduces the incidence of meconium aspiration and women who have experienced this outcome in a pregnancy may wish to discuss this option in future pregnancies.

Further reading

Beligere N, Rao R. Neurodevelopmental outcome of infants with meconium aspiration syndrome: report of a study and literature review. J Perinatol 2008;28(Suppl 3):S93–101.

Clinical Effectiveness Support Unit, The use of electronic fetal monitoring, RCOG press 2001.

Gibb D, Arulkumaran S. *Fetal monitoring in practice*. Churchill Livingstone 2007.

National Collaborating Centre for Women's and Children's Health, Intrapartum Care: care of healthy women and their babies during childbirth-clinical guideline, RCOG press 2007.

Rao S, Pavlova Z, Incerpi MH, Ramanathan R, Meconium-stained amniotic fluid and neonatal morbidity in near-term and term deliveries with acute histologic chorioamnionitis and/or funisitis. J Perinatol 2001;21:537–40.

Xu H, Mas-Calvet M, Wei SQ, et al. Abnormal fetal heart rate tracing patterns in patients with thick meconium staining of the amniotic fluid: association with perinatal outcomes. Am J Obstet Gynecol 2009;200:283.e1–7.

Internet resources

www.nice.org.uk/nicemedia/pdf/IPCNICEGuidance.pdf

www.rcog.org.uk/files/rcog-corp/uploadedfiles/NEBEFMGuideline-Final2may2001.pdf

Patient resources

www.patient.co.uk/showdoc/40000245/

www.pregnancy.about.com/od/laborcomplications/a/meconium.htm

Placenta praevia

Definition
The implantation of a placenta in the lower uterine segment. This can cause potentially life-threatening antepartum and postpartum haemorrhage.

Incidence
Four or five per 1000 pregnancies.

Aetiology
Unknown cause.

Risk factors
- Previous uterine scars
- Smoking
- Advanced maternal age
- Grand muliparity
- Recurrent miscarriage
- Low social class
- Infertility treatment.

Associations with placenta praevia
- Placental abruption
- Congenital malformations
- Abnormal presentations
- Preterm delivery

Clinical presentation
History
- Painless vaginal bleeding, which may be catastrophic
- May be associated with labour
- Abdominal pain may occur as 10% of cases will have associated abruption, making diagnosis difficult
- In 30–50% of cases there may be no antenatal vaginal bleeding
- Usually normal fetal movements
- In most cases, a low placenta has already been identified at the 21–23-week scan.

Examination
- General condition and vital signs
- Abdominal assessment including lie of fetus to exclude malpresentation
- Fetal assessment: unlikely to show signs of compromise unless maternal compromise
- Vaginal examination is contraindicated as may exacerbate bleeding. Therefore, inspection should be carried out to quantify blood loss.

Investigations
- Full blood count
- Blood grouping and cross match
- Ultrasound to confirm placental site, presentation (Fig. 10.13.1)

Diagnosis
Placenta praevia is diagnosed with ultrasound, which is safe, accurate, and convenient. Transvaginal ultrasound is superior to the transabdominal approach and is safe (Fig. 10.13.2). Prior to routine use of ultrasound in antenatal care, the diagnosis was made on clinical examination in theatre.

Screening for placenta praevia
The 20–22-week anomaly scan provides a screening test to predict the likelihood of placenta praevia at delivery.

Traditionally it is routine practice to repeat the scan in later pregnancy if the placenta is found to be low lying at 20–22 weeks. Evidence shows that unless the placental edge reaches or overlaps the internal os, the placenta is likely to have moved by the third trimester. The placenta is known to migrate as the pregnancy progresses and explains why midpregnancy ultrasound overdiagnoses placenta praevia. This apparent migration is due to the differential growth of the lower and the upper part of the uterus. The average rate of migration is 4.1 mm/week. In cases with significant overlap (>10 mm) the rate of migration was minimal at 0.1 mm/week. The rate of migration was higher if the placental edge is thin.

All cases where the placenta is less than 2 cm from the internal os at the anomaly scan should have a scan at 36 weeks.

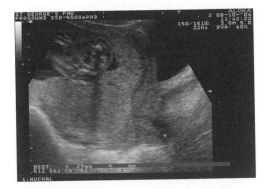

Fig. 10.13.1 Abdominal ultrasound scan carried out at 22 weeks shows the placenta implanted over the internal os.

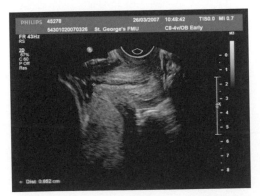

Fig. 10.13.2 Transvaginal scan showing the proximity of the placental edge to the internal os. The distance is measured by the markers.

Counselling

Women found to have a low-lying placenta at their anomaly scan should be advised

- that the majority of placentas will move by term and allow vaginal delivery
- if the placenta is anterior and there is a previous Caesarean section, it is more likely to remain low
- to seek medical advice if vaginal bleeding
- they should not have coitus in pregnancy if there is a history of vaginal bleeding
- need for rescan at 36 weeks

If a woman is confirmed to have placenta praevia at term it is essential to provide counselling on:

- the mode of delivery
- the possible need for blood products
- the potential need for additional surgical measures to control bleeding such as hysterectomy.

Management

In 30–50% of cases of placenta praevia, there will be no antepartum bleeding. The RCOG guideline in the management of placenta praevia recommends extensive counselling of these women to assess their suitability for outpatient management and to consider factors such as proximity to hospital.

In the case of women who present with antepartum haemorrhage their management will depend on:

- the degree of bleeding and maternal compromise
- gestation.

Conservative management

- This is appropriate if the fetus is not mature and the bleeding is not compromising the mother.
- Corticosteroids should be administered before 34 weeks to promote fetal lung maturity.
- Tocolysis may be considered if there is no evidence of active bleeding and no fetal compromise.
- Transfusion of blood and blood products may be required.
- Anti-D is needed for Rhesus-negative mothers.
- The RCOG recommends that women who bleed with placenta praevia after 34 weeks be hospitalized until delivery.

Mode of delivery with placenta praevia

A trial of vaginal delivery is appropriate if the placental edge is at least 2 cm away form the internal os. If the placental edge is less than 2 cm from the os Caesarean section at 38 weeks is recommended

Caesarean section for placenta praevia

- Senior consultant obstetrician should be present
- Senior anaesthetist
- Availability of HDU facilities
- Counselling and obtain consent
- Usually able to perform traditional lower uterine segment Caesarean section
- May be surgically challenging due to poorly formed lower uterine segment and dilated veins
- Knowledge of whether the placenta is anterior or posterior. If anterior, it can usually be swept off the uterine wall and not cut in order to deliver the fetus
- May require additional procedures to control bleeding such as use of haemostatic balloon, uterine artery ligation, brace sutures and hysterectomy if intractable bleeding (Section 10.15, Postpartum haemorrhage.
- Be prepared for placenta accreta
- Increased incidence of postpartum haemorrhage.

Advice for future pregnancies

The risk of recurrence is low.

Placenta accreta

Definition

An abnormally firm attachment of placental villi to the uterine wall.

Incidence

Varies from 1 in 540 to 1 in 70 000. The incidence has increased by 10-fold, probably due to the increased caesarean section rate.

Pathology

Abnormally deep attachment of chorionic villi to the uterine wall with the absence of the normal intervening decidua basalis

There are three variants:

- placenta accreta, where the placenta is attached directly to the myometrium
- placenta increta, where the placenta extends into the myometrium
- placenta percreta, where the placenta extends through the entire myometrium.

Risk factors include

- Placenta praevia
- Previous Caesarean section
- Advanced maternal age
- Grand multiparity
- Previous vigorous curettage
- Myomectomy
- Submucous myoma
- Asherman's syndrome
- A short Caesarean to conception interval

Prognosis

Placenta accreta is associated with a 7% mortality rate in addition to increased morbidity caused by massive blood transfusion, infection, and damage to adjacent organs. The recent CEMACH report highlighted the need for women who have had previous Caesarean section and placenta praevia in their subsequent pregnancy to have further investigations to try and identify placenta accrete. This is with a view to developing safe management strategies for their delivery.

Diagnosis

Imaging using ultrasound has limited ability to exclude placenta accreta. Anticipation of placenta accreta in cases with identifiable risk factors is likely to be the most useful strategy.

Presence of multiple linear irregular vascular spaces within the placenta on ultrasound has the highest positive predictive value for prospective identification of placenta accreta. In the largest series, placental lacunae with turbulent flow was associated with a 80–90% sensitivity for detection of placenta accrete. Colour Dopplers and magnetic resonance imaging have not been sufficiently studied, but may be helpful.

Management
- Adequate counselling pre-delivery regarding possible hysterectomy
- Availability of blood and blood products
- Experienced obstetrician with other specialists available
- Pre-surgery radiologically assisted cannulation of uterine arteries for embolization should there be massive bleeding
- Leaving placenta *in situ* and tying off the umbilical cord if there is no bleeding to conserve the uterus
- There is no evidence for use of methotrexate in cases of placenta percreta if placenta was left behind after delivery

Vasa praevia

Definition
Fetal blood vessels unsupported by either the placenta or umbilical cord traverse the membranes in the lower segment of the uterus.

Incidence
Approximately 1 in 6000 deliveries.

Prognosis
If these vessels precede the presenting part they can rupture and lead to fetal haemorrhage. The perinatal loss rate has been reported as high as 33–100%.

Diagnosis
Can be diagnosed by ultrasound showing echogenic parallel or circular lines near the cervix representing the umbilical cord. This finding can be confirmed using Doppler.

Higher incidence in women who have had a low-lying placenta in second trimester which later recedes.

Women may present with intrapartum bleeding, and cardiotocography (CTG) abnormalities if antenatal diagnosis has been missed.

Management
If a prospective diagnosis has been made, delivery by Caesarean section at or near term is recommended. Emergency Caesarean will be needed if the diagnosis is made intrapartum.

Antepartum identification of vasa praevia leads to significant improvement in perinatal mortality.

Further reading

Placenta previa and placenta previa accreta: Diagnosis and mamangement. Green top guideline No. 27, Royal College of Obstetricians and Gynaecologists, 2005.

Bhide A & Thilaganathan B. Recent advances in the management of placenta previa. Curr Opin Obstet Gynecol 2004;16:447–51.

Saving mothers lives. The Seventh Report of the Confidential Enquiries into Maternal Deaths in the United Kingdom, 2007: www.cemach.org.uk

Internet resources

Causes of Maternal Mortality: www.maternityworldwide.org/causes.html.

Placental abruption

Definition
Complete or partial separation of a normally implanted placenta.

Incidence
0.52–1.29% of all pregnancies.
30–35% of cases of antepartum haemorrhage with recognized causes are due to placental abruption.

Complications of placental abruption
Fetal
- Prematurity
- Hypoxia
- Death
- Hypoxic brain injury.

Maternal
- Hypovolaemia due to blood loss
- Coagulopathy
- Renal failure
- Postpartum haemorrhage.

Pathology
Placental abruption is multifactoral
- An association of reduced invasiveness of the cytotrophoblast, which leads to inadequate placentation
- Dysregulation of the maternal immune response
- Folate deficiency has been shown to have an association

It is postulated that arterial spasm followed by relaxation and subsequent venous engorgement and arteriolar rupture into the decidua basalis with the accumulation of blood clot causes the separation of the placenta.

Two of the potential mechanisms of abruption are:
- acute inflammation-related conditions
- chronic inflammation or vascular dysfunction.

Risk factors for placental abruption
Pre-pregnancy
- Previous history of abruption
- Previous Caesarean section
- Uterine malformations

During pregnancy
- Smoking
- Alcohol abuse
- Placenta praevia
- Pre-labour rupture of membranes
- Hypertension/pre-eclampsia
- Cocaine use
- Choriomanionitis
- Positive uterine artery Doppler screen in the second trimester.

Other risk factors for abruption have historically been reported but not conclusively proven in large series on abruption. These include
- assisted conception
- polyhydramnios and oligohydramnios
- maternal diabetes
- uterine trauma
- external cephalic version
- short umbilical cord and velamentous insertion of cord

- coagulation defects
- invasive intrauterine procedures like amniocentesis.

Clinical presentation
History
- Painful vaginal bleeding is the most common presentation. This occurs in 70–80% of patients and may be very heavy. In other cases, there may be no vaginal bleeding if the abruption is concealed.
- Abdominal pain.
- Reduced or absent fetal movements.

Examination
- Tender and irritable uterus is the classical clinical feature.
- The uterus may be tonically contracted making fetal palpation difficult.
- Signs of shock: pallor, tachycardia, hypotension.
- Coexisting hypertension may mask fall of blood pressure due to blood loss.
- Signs of fetal distress may be present if the fetus is alive. The fetus may be dead at presentation.

Investigations
- Full blood count
- Coagulation screen
- Blood for grouping and cross match
- Urea and electrolytes
- Assessment of fetal wellbeing.

Diagnosis
- The diagnosis is based on the clinical presentation and examination findings
- Ultrasound is not sensitive in the diagnosis of abruption but is useful to exclude placenta praevia, confirm fetal viability, and presentation

Management
The management will be depend on the grade of abruption and the gestation. Severe cases of placental abruption can make the mother very unwell.
- Delivery is usually required in cases of placental abruption. Conservative management is rarely justified other than in the very minor abruptions.
- Replace blood volume.
- In women presenting with placental abruption and intrauterine fetal death, preparations for blood transfusion should be commenced as there is likely to have been a major placental separation with significant retroplacental blood loss.
- Look for and correct clotting abnormality.
- Involve senior obstetrician.
- Multidisciplinary team involvement of anaesthetist, haematologist, and neonatologist. In cases of severe bleeding an interventional radiologist and vascular surgeon may be needed.
- Decision regarding delivery.

Vaginal delivery
May be appropriate if
- abruption occurs near term and the maternal and fetal condition is reassuring
- abruption occurs in labour and delivery can be expedited

- if there is fetal demise and Caesarean delivery is to be avoided
- there are no other contraindications to vaginal delivery such as abnormal lie or previous Caesarean section
- complications such as disseminated intravascular coagulation (DIC), which increase the risks of blood loss with surgical management

if vaginal delivery is attempted there must be close surveillance of maternal and fetal condition during labour as the clinical picture may deteriorate rapidly.

Caesarean delivery
Is appropriate for
- abruption with signs of significant fetal compromise
- abruption which has significantly compromised maternal condition such that waiting for vaginal delivery could be life-threatening
- in cases of fetal demise if there is a failed attempt at vaginal delivery. This may occur if the uterus becomes atonic as a result of blood infiltrating the myometrium (Couvelaire uterus)

Care of the baby
- In most cases, there is insufficient time for benefit with antenatal steroid administration.
- Neonatologists should be alerted to anticipate birth of a preterm (if the abruption is in preterm period) and hypoxic baby.

Counselling
Counselling is difficult due to the unpredictable nature of abruption. However, it is important to keep the mother and her partner well informed, including the need for blood products and the potential need for additional haemostatic measures such as uterine artery ligation or hysterectomy.

With all deliveries there must be provision made for
- NNU facilities for the birth of a potentially hypoxic or acidaemic fetus.
- The need for HDU/ITU facilities for the mother.

Management of complications
Delay in treating abruption increases the risk of hypovolaemic shock, coagulation failure, renal failure and post partum haemorrhage.

In cases of concealed abruption the degree of shock may be out of proportion with the blood loss seen before delivery.

Disseminated intravascular coagulation
The progressive separation of the placenta releases thromboplastin-like substances that activate the coagulation cascade. This activation consumes coagulation factors, which leads to secondary thrombocytopenia. Which in turn triggers the formation of fibrin degradation factors and D dimers.

Complications of DIC
These include
- renal failure
- pulmonary hypoperfusion
- PPH
- postpartum pituitary necrosis.

Clinical signs of DIC
Bleeding from multiple sites, e.g. wound, venepuncture, gums.

Diagnosis of DIC
- Prolonged prothrombin time (PT) and partial thromboplastin time (PTT)
- Low fibrinogen (<100 mg/dL)
- Reduced antithrombin III levels
- Presence of fibrin degradation products (FDP) (above 10 µg/mL)
- Thrombocytopenia
- Raised D dimers.

Treatment
- Aimed at removing the cause by delivering the fetus and placenta by the least traumatic route.
- Replacing clotting factors (frozen plasma and cryoprecipitate) and platelets

Vaginal delivery is preferable because of increased surgical risks due to coagulation failure.

Renal failure
Acute renal failure can occur due to
- hypovolaemia (pre-renal) due to inadequate or delayed volume replacement
- acute tubular or cortical necrosis (renal)

postpartum haemorrhage (also see Section 10.15,

Postpartum haemorrhage
Postpartum haemorrhage should be anticipated. In 2% of cases of placental abruption the uterus will become hypotonic and resistant to oxytocics. The third stage of labour should be managed actively.

Advice for subsequent pregnancies
Increased risk of recurrent abruption should be explained. Smoking cessation where appropriate. There are no known predictors apart from the risk factors. There is some evidence of the benefit of Folic acid and multivitamin supplementation in reducing the recurrence.

Further reading
Nilsen RM, Vollset SE, Rasmussen SA, et al. Folic acid and multivitamin supplement use and risk of placental abruption: a population-based registry study. Am J Epidemiol 2008;167:867–74.

Smith GC, Yu CK, Papageorghiou AT, et al. Fetal Medicine Foundation Second Trimester Screening Group. Maternal uterine artery Doppler flow velocimetry and the risk of stillbirth. Obstet Gynecol 2007;109:144–51.

Postpartum haemorrhage

Definitions

Postpartum haemorrhage (PPH) is most commonly defined as an estimated blood loss from the genital tract greater than 500 mL following a vaginal delivery or in excess of 1000 mL after a Caesarean section. Major PPH is usually defined as blood loss of 1000 mL or more after a vaginal delivery. According to the Royal College of Obstetricians and Gynaecologists Green Top guideline on Prevention and Management of Postpartum Haemorrhage, major PPH can be considered to be moderate (1000–2000 mL) or severe (>2000 mL). The Scottish Confidential Audit of Severe Maternal Morbidity defines an estimated blood loss ≥2500 mL, or transfused 5 or more units of blood, or received treatment for coagulopathy (fresh frozen plasma, cryoprecipitate, platelets) as 'major haemorrhage'. These definitions are rather arbitrary as visual assessment of blood loss is unreliable. The effect that haemorrhage has on the woman depends not only on the amount, but also on the rapidity of blood loss, on her blood volume and any underlying health factors. For this reason a definition would include any blood loss that causes a significant haemodynamic change. Primary PPH occurs within the first 24 hours after delivery, and secondary PPH occurs between 24 hours and 6–12 weeks postpartum.

Epidemiology

Postpartum haemorrhage (PPH) occurs in 5–15% of deliveries. PPH is the most common cause of maternal mortality and accounts for one-quarter of all maternal deaths worldwide. Fourteen million cases of PPH occur each year with a case fatality rate of 1%. In the UK, PPH is the third most common cause of maternal mortality and accounts for 10.6% of all direct maternal deaths according to the Confidential Enquiries into Maternal and Child Health.

Aetiology and risk factors

The major aetiological factors of PPH are uterine atony (tone), retained placental tissues (tissue), membranes or blood clots, genital tract trauma (trauma), and coagulation abnormalities (thrombin).

Overdistension of the uterus due to multiple pregnancy, polyhydramnios, or fetal macrosomia is a common risk factor for PPH by increasing the risk of uterine atony. Other risk factors for PPH include placental abruption or placenta praevia, antepartum haemorrhage, pre-eclampsia, obesity, coagulation disorders, primigravidity, chorioamnionitis, prolonged rupture of membranes, fibroid uterus, previous Caesarean delivery, induction of labour, prolonged labour, instrumental delivery, and prior PPH. However, PPH can occur even in women without identifiable risk factors.

Pathophysiology

Following delivery of the fetus, myometrial contraction results in placental separation and constriction of the blood vessels by retracting myometrial fibres ('living ligatures'). Uterine atony or retained placenta causes a failure of this mechanism and bleeding from the placental bed. Young and healthy women can compensate for moderate blood loss without demonstrating any haemodynamic changes. When up to 20% of the blood volume is lost, the perfusion of non-vital organs and tissues is decreased, with pale and cool skin as a common clinical feature. Moderate shock occurs when 20–40% of the blood volume is lost

resulting in decreased perfusion of visceral organs (liver, the gut, and kidneys) resulting in oliguria or anuria, hypotension, and tachycardia. When 40% or more of the blood volume is lost, severe shock results in decreased perfusion of the essential organs, the heart and brain, leading to restlessness, coma, and possibly cardiac arrest.

Prevention

Prevention of PPH may be feasible with identification and modification of risk factors antenatally, and appropriate management of labour and delivery. Anaemia or other health conditions should be diagnosed and treated. Women with risk factors for PPH should have their haemoglobin levels as well as general health status optimized in anticipation of PPH and should be delivered in centres with transfusion facilities and an intensive care unit (ICU). However, it is not possible to predict and prevent all cases of PPH, as only 40% of women who develop PPH have an identified risk factor.

Active management of the third stage of labour consists of administration of uterotonic agents, controlled cord traction and uterine massage after delivery of the placenta. The aim of these interventions is to facilitate the delivery of the placenta by increasing uterine contractions and to prevent uterine atony and PPH. This approach reduces the risks of PPH, postpartum anaemia, blood transfusion requirements, prolonged third stage of labour, and use of therapeutic drugs for PPH. The International Confederation of Midwives (ICM) and the International Federation of Gynecology and Obstetrics (FIGO) advocate active management of the third stage of labour for all women. It is recommended that active management should be routine for maternity hospitals and births at home or birth centres.

Oxytocin is a first-line uterotonic agent in active management as it is effective 2–3 minutes after injection and has minimal side-effects. Other uterotonics include ergometrine maleate, ergometrine with oxytocin 5 IU/mL (Syntometrine, Alliance Pharmaceuticals), misoprostol, or carbetocin. Misoprostol (Cytotec, Pfizer), a prostaglandin E1 analogue, is more stable than oxytocin and has been administered by oral, sublingual, and rectal routes; however, misuse of misoprostol can lead to significant maternal morbidity and even death. The main side-effects are nausea, vomiting and diarrhoea, shivering, and pyrexia. A Cochrane review on the use of prostaglandins for the prevention of PPH concluded that neither intramuscular prostaglandins nor misoprostol is preferable to conventional injectable uterotonics as part of the management of the third stage of labour, especially for low-risk women. Carbetocin is a long-acting oxytocin agonist, which has been used for the prevention of PPH. Intramuscular carbetocin has longer duration of action than intramuscular oxytocin, but there is insufficient evidence that intravenous carbetocin is as effective as oxytocin to prevent PPH. A Cochrane review suggests that carbetocin is associated with reduced need for additional uterotonic agents and uterine massage, and there are no significant differences in adverse effects between carbetocin and oxytocin.

Although the active management of the third stage of labour originally included early cord clamping, delayed cord clamping is associated with less anaemia, intraventricular haemorrhage, and late-onset sepsis, especially in preterm infants. As there is little evidence to suggest that the timing of cord clamping has an impact on the incidence of PPH, the collaborative ICM/FIGO group decided not to include early cord clamping in the active management protocol. The cord may be clamped at the time the baby is dried and wrapped and passed to the mother to breastfeed.

FIGO also advises that if oxytocin or misoprostol are unavailable, skilled birth attendants should use physiological (or expectant) management of the third stage. This means that cord traction should not be applied before the uterus has contracted and placental separation has begun. The placenta should be allowed to be delivered without interference. Early or prophylactic interventional radiology for the prevention of PPH should be considered for high-risk cases.

Treatment

Medical management

Early diagnosis, prompt resuscitation, and restoration of the blood volume lost are essential in the initial management of PPH. Major PPH should be managed by a multidisciplinary team approach with senior obstetricians, anaesthetists, midwives, and theatre staff. Haematologists, blood bank staff, hospital porters, and the intensive care unit should be alerted.

General resuscitation measures include assessment of the woman's haemodynamic status, level of consciousness, blood pressure, heart rate, and oxygen saturation. Two large-bore cannulae should be inserted and blood samples taken for full blood count, group, and cross-match (the number of units will depend on the severity of haemorrhage), coagulation screen, and renal and liver profiles.

Fluid resuscitation should be based on the volume and rapidity of blood loss. A total volume of up to 2l of warmed Hartmann's solution be given rapidly and followed by up to a further 1.5 L of warmed colloid until cross-matched blood is available, as most of the infused fluid shifts from the intravascular to the interstitial space.

A systematic examination to identify the cause of PPH should be undertaken simultaneously with resuscitation and treatment measures. Assessment of the uterine size and tone should be followed by vigorous uterine massage and administration of uterotonic agents if the uterus is atonic. Uterine massage, manually or bimanually, is a simple and very effective first-line measure and reduces bleeding even if the uterus remains atonic, allowing resuscitation to take effect. Manual exploration of the uterine cavity is essential to exclude or remove retained placental tissues and membranes and is best done with sufficient anaesthesia. If bleeding persists despite a well-contracted uterus, examination under anaesthesia should look for cervical or vaginal lacerations, as these may extend into the uterus or the broad ligament or they may cause pelvic haematomas. If retained tissue or trauma is excluded and bleeding continues despite a well-contracted uterus, a coagulation disorder as a possible cause should be excluded.

Uterotonic agents

As uterine atony is the most common cause, medical management consists of slow intravenous oxytocin (10 units) or ergometrine (0.5 mg), methergine 0.2 mg intramuscularly, oxytocin infusion, 15-methyl PGF2α (Carboprost or Haemabate) intramuscularly or intramyometrially, dinoprostone vaginally or rectally, or misoprostol.

Oxytocin, can be administered as slow intravenous bolus of 5 units or as an infusion (40 units in 500 mL of 0.9% normal saline, infused at a rate of 125 mL/hour) in order to maintain uterine contractions. Although there are no absolute contraindications, an antidiuretic effect may develop with high doses.

Ergometrine is an ergot alkaloid. Hypertension and cardiac disease are contraindications as ergometrine can potentially cause severe hypertension and myocardial ischaemia.

Carboprost (Haemabate; Pfizer, Pharmacia & Upjohn, Kalamazoo, MI) is a prostaglandin F2 analogue, which is administered intramuscularly or intramyometrially. It is a second-line agent for uterine atony (0.25 mg repeated every 15 minutes to a maximum dose of 2 mg). This is 80% to 90% effective in arresting PPH in cases that are refractory to oxytocin and ergometrine. It has bronchoconstrictive properties and is contraindicated in asthma. Side-effects include diarrhoea, vomiting, fever, headache, and flushing.

Dinoprostone (Prostin) is a prostaglandin E2 analogue that may be given vaginally (may get washed off with blood) or rectally. It can cause temperature elevations. It should be stored at −20°C (−4°F) and brought to room temperature before use. This is a limitation for its use in acute severe haemorrhage.

Misoprostol is a synthetic prostaglandin E1 analogue. As the time taken for peak serum concentration of oxytocin is much shorter than oral misoprostol, which reaches its serum peak concentration at 20 minutes, a combination of these two agents could provide a sustained uterotonic effect. However, a Cochrane review concluded that there is insufficient evidence that the addition of misoprostol is superior to the combination of oxytocin and ergometrine.

Recombinant activated factor VII (rFVIIa, NovoSeven; Novo Nordisk, Bagsvaerd, Denmark) has originally been used in treating haemorrhage in patients with haemophilia or other bleeding disorders. It has also been used in non-haemophilic haemorrhage, including life-threatening obstetric haemorrhage and may be considered as an alternative haemostatic agent when the standard treatment is ineffective.

Transfusion

Blood and blood product transfusion should be commenced if bleeding continues, if the estimated blood loss is over 30% of the blood volume, or if the patient is haemodynamically unstable despite aggressive resuscitation. Group-specific or O group, Rh-negative blood should be transfused until cross-matched blood becomes available. Dilutional coagulopathy occurs when approximately 80% of the original blood volume has been replaced. Four units of fresh frozen plasma (FFP) should be administered with every 6 units of blood transfused (12–15 mL/kg or total 1l). Platelet concentration should be more than $50 \times 10^9/L$ or more than $80–100 \times 10^9/L$ if surgical intervention is likely. Cryoprecipitate should be administered if there is disseminated intravascular coagulation (DIC) or if the fibrinogen level is less than 1 g/L.

Surgical management

Ongoing bleeding indicates the need to transfer and assessment in the operating theatre. Bimanual compression and direct pressure over lacerations may help control bleeding while resuscitation continues and preparations are made for surgical intervention. Obstetricians must consider all available interventions to stop haemorrhage, including balloon tamponades compression sutures, uterine artery embolization, pelvic devascularization, or radical surgery.

Uterine tamponade

Uterine balloon tamponade has been used as a prognostic test ('tamponade test') and is therapeutic, with success rates between 70% and 100%. The anterior lip of the cervix is secured with a sponge forceps and a balloon catheter (usually a Sengstaken-Blakemore catheter) is inserted into the uterine cavity. The balloon is then filled with warm sterile water or a warm saline solution until it becomes visible in the cervical canal. When the pressure exceeds that of the pressure with which blood is entering the uterine cavity, the bleeding should stop. If there is no bleeding, the 'tamponade test' result is successful and no further fluid is added. The 'tamponade test' allows the obstetrician to identify which women will require laparotomy. Advantages include easy and rapid insertion with minimal anaesthesia, rapid identification of failed cases and painless removal. No immediate complications such as bleeding or sepsis, or long-term sequelae such as menstrual problems or problems with conceiving have been reported in women who underwent uterine tamponade. If bleeding continues despite the 'tamponade test', laparotomy and compression suture should be next step.

Compression sutures

In cases of PPH at the time of Caesarean section or in cases of failed 'tamponade test', if haemostasis is achieved with bimanual compression of the uterus, compression sutures are likely to arrest haemorrhage. The ease of application is an advantage, and fertility is preserved. The obvious disadvantages are the need for laparotomy and usually hysterotomy (although some modified types to the original 'B-Lynch' suture technique have avoided this surgical step). Complications are extremely rare and include erosion through the uterine wall, pyometra, and uterine necrosis.

Pelvic devascularization

Failure of compression sutures to arrest haemorrhage warrants stepwise pelvic devascularization by ligation of the uterine, ovarian, and finally internal iliac arteries. This procedure is usually effective but it can be time-consuming. Ligation of internal iliacs can be technically challenging and carries risks of surgical injury. Prerequisites include a haemodynamically stable patient and surgical expertise. The reported success rates vary between 40% and 100%. When arterial ligation fails, hysterectomy is usually associated with higher morbidity than a hysterectomy without previous attempted arterial ligation.

Uterine artery embolization

Arterial embolization has success rates as high as 70–100% and the potential of preservation of fertility. Prophylactic embolization may have a role in a planned Caesarean section with a morbidly adherent placenta. Complications include haematoma formation, infectious complications, contrast-related side-effects, and ischaemia resulting in uterus and bladder necrosis. The requirement of equipment and an interventional radiologist are limitations of this procedure.

A systematic review of the management of PPH when medical measures fail showed that the success rates for arresting PPH are as high as 84.0% for balloon tamponade, 90.7% for arterial embolization, 91.7% for compression sutures, and 84.6% for pelvic devascularization (including uterine or internal iliac artery ligation). As none of these methods is significantly superior to any other, the choice should depend on the availability of facilities, the degree of ongoing bleeding, the estimated blood loss, and the haemodynamic status of the woman.

Hysterectomy

Subtotal or total abdominal hysterectomy is usually the last resort in the management of PPH and should not be delayed if the conservative measures have failed. Hysterectomy is associated with numerous postoperative complications, including urinary tract injury, fistula formation, bowel injury, vascular injury, pelvic haematoma, and sepsis. Subtotal hysterectomy may not be effective when the cause of the bleeding is at the lower segment, cervix, or vaginal fornices.

Further reading

CEMACH. *Saving mothers' lives: reviewing maternal deaths to make motherhood safer. 2003–2005.* The Seventh Report of the Confidential Enquiries into Maternal Deaths in the United Kingdom. CEMACH: London 2007.

Clinical Management Guidelines for Obstetrician-Gynecologists. ACOG Practice Bulletin: Number 76, October 2006: Postpartum Hemorrhage. Obstet Gynecol 2006;108:1039–47.

Condous GS, Arulkumaran S, Symonds I, et al. The 'tamponade test' in the management of massive postpartum hemorrhage. Obstet Gynecol 2007;101:767–72.

Doumouchtsis SK, Papageorghiou AT, Arulkumaran S. Systematic review of conservative management of postpartum hemorrhage: what to do when medical treatment fails. Obstet Gynecol Surv 2007;62:540–7.

Doumouchtsis SK, Papageorghiou AT, Vernier C, Arulkumaran S. Management of postpartum hemorrhage by uterine balloon tamponade: prospective evaluation of effectiveness. Acta Obstet Gynecol Scand 2008;87:849–55.

Gulmezoglu A, Forna F, Villar J, Hofmeyr G. Prostaglandins for preventing postpartum haemorrhage. Cochrane Database Syst Rev(3) 2007;CD000494.

Lalonde A, Daviss BA, Acosta A, Herschderfer K. Postpartum hemorrhage today: ICM/FIGO initiative 2004–2006. Int J Gynaecol Obstet 2006;94:243–53.

Mousa HA, Alfirevic Z. Treatment for primary postpartum haemorrhage. Cochrane Database Syst Rev 2007;1:CD003249.

Penney G, Kernaghan D, Adamson L. Scottish Confidential Audit of Severe Maternal Morbidity. 3rd Annual Report 2005, Scottish Programme for Clinical Effectiveness in Reproductive Health.

Prendiville WJ, Elbourne D, McDonald S. Active versus expectant management in the third stage of labour. Cochrane Database Syst Rev 2009;3:CD000007.

Rabe H, Reynolds G, Diaz-Rossello J. Early versus delayed umbilical cord clamping in preterm infants. Cochrane Database Syst Rev 2004;4:CD003248.

Ramanathan G, Arulkumaran S. Postpartum hemorrhage. J Obstet Gynaecol Can 2006;28:967–73.

Razvi K, Chua S, Arulkumaran S, Ratnam SS. A comparison between visual estimation and laboratory determination of blood loss during the third stage of labour. Aust NZ J Obstet Gynaecol 1996;36:152–4.

RCOG. *The role of emergency and elective interventional radiology in postpartum haemorrhage.* Good Practice Guidelines. London: RCOG 2007.

Royal College of Obstetricians and Gynaecologists (RCOG) *Prevention and management of postpartum haemorrhage.* Green Top Guideline No 52. London: RCO 2009.

Su L, Chong Y, Samuel M. Oxytocin agonists for preventing postpartum haemorrhage. Cochrane Database Syst Rev 2007;3:CD005457.

WHO. *Maternal mortality in 2000: Estimates developed by WHO, UNICEF, and UNFPA.* Geneva: Department of Reproductive Health and Research 2004.

WHO. *WHO Recommendations for the prevention of postpartum haemorrhage.* Geneva: WHO 2007.

World Health Organization (WHO) *The World Health Report 2005. Make every mother and child count.* Geneva: WHO.

Patient resources

www.patient.co.uk/showdoc/40000261/

Prelabour rupture of membranes at term

Definition

Prelabour rupture of membranes (PROM) at term is defined as spontaneous rupture of fetal membranes for an hour or more before the onset of labour at or over 37 completed weeks of gestation. The time from rupture to the onset of labour has been variably defined in clinical studies.

Epidemiology

The incidence of PROM ranges between 5% and 20% depending on the series and the method of dating of the pregnancies studied. The natural history of PROM is the spontaneous onset of contractions and labour within 24 hours in 60–80% of cases. After the first 24 hours, the rate of onset of spontaneous labour falls off to an additional 5% per day.

Aetiology

Unlike preterm PROM, term PROM is a physiological event in the vast majority of cases. Indeed a proportion of PROM near term (≥34 weeks' gestation) is believed to be of physiological origin. In a small but significant proportion of cases of term PROM, lower genital tract or intra-amniotic infection, abruption, or trauma may be the cause of the membrane rupture.

Diagnosis and initial assessment

The diagnosis of PROM is frequently made on the basis of maternal history alone, sometimes with erroneous results, particularly in nulliparous women. A speculum examination and simple bedside tests may be required in equivocal cases. Although maternal history was found to have an accuracy of 90% for the diagnosis of PROM, it is good practice to confirm the diagnosis before instituting the management steps for PROM. The presence of a pool of amniotic fluid in the posterior fornix on speculum examination is confirmatory of PROM, provided that copious but clear and viscid cervical secretion has been excluded. There may be a role for nitrazine pH-based paper testing when there is a very small amount of fluid in the posterior fornix and the observer is uncertain. However, a positive nitrazine test is not specific for PROM and has a false-positive rate of 17%. The pH of the normally acidic vaginal fluid changes to alkaline if there is vaginitis, bacterial vaginosis, contamination with cervical secretion, blood, semen, or urine. In doubtful cases the patient may be asked to cough gently while visualizing the external cervical os for any trickle of amniotic fluid. An extended pad test is also useful. A panel of newer and more sensitive/specific tests based on insulin-like growth factor binding protein-1 (IGFBP-1) in cervicovaginal secretions have been evaluated.

A digital vaginal examination should be avoided after PROM unless there is a strong suspicion of labour or imminent delivery. In our institution we obtain a low vaginal and peri-anal swab for group B streptococcal colonization in all women that present with PROM. The colour of the amniotic fluid is documented and the presentation of the fetus confirmed.

Clinical questions associated with term PROM

- Should PROM be managed expectantly in the first instance or by induction of labour on diagnosis?
- If induction of labour is indicated, what agents should be used, what route and for how long?
- If conservative management is selected, how long is it safe without increasing the risk of infection?
- Is monitoring or surveillance indicated during expectant management, and what tests are appropriate?
- How frequently should these tests be applied and what tests results should prompt an intervention?
- Who should be performing these tests?

Management of term PROM

The most frequently discussed aspect of the management of term PROM is the risk of feto-maternal infectious morbidity. However, there are other risks such as acute cord prolapse and acute cord compression. Furthermore, there are resource implications associated with aggressive and immediate induction of labour for PROM and these should be appraised by the individual maternity unit, in the context of its activity level. Provided that vaginal delivery is appropriate, immediate induction of labour should be undertaken if there is evidence of chorioamnionitis, non-reassuring fetal status, meconium staining of the amniotic fluid, abruption, or evidence of other maternal compromise.

The risk of serious neonatal infection with term PROM is 1% compared with 0.5% for babies born to women with intact membranes. However, the evidence reviewed by the NICE Guideline Development Group (GDG) suggests that maternal and fetal outcomes were similar between those that were managed with planned induction of labour and those managed expectantly. The GDG recommended that induction of labour is appropriate 24 hours after term PROM as expectant management up to 24 hours is not associated with a significant increase in neonatal infection rates, and approximately 60% of women with term PROM will go into spontaneous labour within 24 hours. Women who elect to be managed expectantly should be advised to monitor their own temperature readings every 4 hours during waking hours and to report immediately any alteration in the colour or smell of their vaginal loss. They should be advised that sexual intercourse may increase the risk of infection. The fetal heart rate and movement should be reviewed every 24 hours after term PROM, and any reduction of fetal movements brought to the attention of the clinical team. Delivery should be conducted in the hospital with access to neonatal services if labour has not started after 24 hours of term PROM. The baby should be observed for at least 12 hours for any signs of infection.

The current NICE guidelines advise against intrapartum antibiotic prophylaxis even with PROM over 24 hours unless the woman displays evidence of infection, in which case a full course of intravenous broad-spectrum antibiotic should be administered. The baby should be referred for specialist neonatal care immediately after birth. Asymptomatic term babies born to women with term PROM >24 hours should be monitored closely for the first 24 hours. Elements of these recent guidelines are at odds with the risk-based approach for the prevention of early-onset GBS disease. With the exception of infection, there are no differences in other neonatal outcomes between immediate induction of labour and expectant management for up to 96 hours following term PROM.

There are no differences in instrumental vaginal delivery rates or Caesarean section rates between immediate induction and expectant management for up to 96 hours after term PROM. There is significant increase in the risk of maternal infectious morbidity including chorioamnionitis and endometritis with expectant management over 24 hours. There is no data on fetal or maternal outcomes with expectant management beyond 96 hours as the vast majority of women would have delivered by this stage.

Further reading

Intrapartum care: care of healthy women and their babies during labour. NICE clinical guideline 55. www.nice.org.uk/CG55

Resuscitation of the newborn

Introduction

Resuscitation of the newborn infant differs from that of any other age group. The newborn is small, wet, and therefore prone to getting cold and has lungs that contain lung liquid. Therefore the approach to resuscitation needs to be adapted to their needs.

Although the majority of infants will not require resuscitation at birth, approximately 3–5% of newborn infants may need some support. Most of the time, the potential need for resuscitation can be anticipated from the maternal and obstetric history such as the presence of a congenital anomaly on the antenatal scans, preterm gestation, fetal distress (for example as indicated by an abnormal cardiotocograph trace or abnormal fetal scalp blood sample), or by the presence of meconium. In these cases trained members of the midwifery and/or neonatal team should be present prior to delivery. Very occasionally a newborn infant may be unexpectedly delivered in poor condition and while the neonatal team are being alerted, resuscitation must be commenced.

Physiology

The primary reason for need for resuscitation in the newborn infant differs from that in adults. Whereas adults requiring resuscitation will normally have had a cardiac event, the newborn infant's heart is healthy and it will usually be a hypoxic or ischaemic event initially that will have compromised the newborn. Therefore, particular attention to management of the airway and breathing is imperative.

In normal circumstances, the process of labour and delivery will aid most resorption of lung liquid, but the first breaths a newborn takes are vital in making that transition from *in utero* to *ex utero* life. If the newborn does not breath at birth, or has an inadequate respiratory effort such as gasping or apnoea, then unless additional help is given, there will be a fall in PaO$_2$, a rise in PaCO$_2$, and a rise in lactic acid; this will result in a fall in heart rate and also antagonize the ability to respond to resuscitation when it is initiated.

The process of compromise will initially start with a transition from regular breathing to 'primary apnoea'. At this stage the infant may then go into a phase of gasping. The effect of gasping may be enough for the infant to 'resuscitate itself' or if given resuscitation in the form of airway management should respond quickly. After the gasping phase 'terminal apnoea' follows. At this stage there will normally already have been a significant compromise to the infant with a low PaO$_2$, high PaCO$_2$, high levels of lactic acid, and a slow heart rate. This infant will need more resuscitative measures if airway management is not sufficient.

Equipment needed

The items mentioned are not an exhaustive list and when faced with the delivery of the newborn infant out of the hospital setting making a note of the time, drying the infant, and considering providing warmth with skin to skin contact between the infant and mother may be all that is needed. Using a piece of string to tie the umbilical cord should also be undertaken while awaiting help to arrive.

In a planned delivery at home, midwives will take with them a bag–valve–mask device with facemasks, oral airways, a laryngoscope, a small oxygen cylinder and suction with catheters at least size 12Fr. They should also have cord clamps, scissors, and disposable gloves.

In the hospital setting, all of this equipment should be more easily available including a resuscitaire to provide a flat surface, which is also able to provide warmth, radiant heat, a clock, pressure limited delivery of air/oxygen, and suction. In addition, face masks, oral airways, laryngoscopes, and endotracheal tubes should be present. Equipment for placement of an umbilical venous catheter should also be made available if required and also drugs.

Priorities

Warmth

Maintaining temperature is imperative and indeed hypothermia is associated with worsening morbidity and mortality. Therefore, when present at the delivery of any newborn, irrespective of it's need or not for resuscitation, drying the infant, disposing of the wet towels, and wrapping the infant with a dry warm towel is necessary before further steps are taken. After drying and wrapping, the infant should be immediately assessed. The assessment comprises respiratory effort, heart rate, tone, and colour. Based on this assessment, the need for resuscitation will be determined. Should resuscitation be required, call for help early. Starting the clock on the resuscitaire when the baby is born should also be undertaken in order to guide resuscitation and also for documentation.

Airway

Newborn infants have a large occiput and when placed on the resuscitaire or a hard surface the tendency is for the head to flex forward thereby obstructing the airway. To overcome this, place the head in the neutral position by extending the neck very slightly (Fig. 10.17.1). This will result in the plane between the nose and mouth being parallel to the plane of the ceiling. This is different from adults in whom you tilt the head and apply a chin lift. Sometimes this simple manoeuvre is all that is needed in order to assist the newborn's respiratory effort, although there are further airway manoeuvres one can apply (see below).

If, having placed the head in the neutral position, the baby's respiratory effort remains poor or absent, with a heart rate that is slow (<100 bpm) five inflation breaths will need to be given. The idea of these inflation breaths is to overcome the initial stiffness of the lungs, which will still have some lung liquid present. Therefore, these breaths are given with pressures set at 30 cmH$_2$O each lasting 2–3 seconds. These breaths are given using a bag and mask, or preferably a pressure-limited 'Tom Thumb' or other ventilation device. The reason for five breaths is that the initial

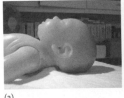 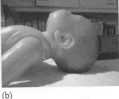

(a)   (b)

Fig. 10.17.1 Newborn infants have a large occiput and when placed on the resuscitaire or a hard surface have a tendency for the head to flex forward thereby obstructing the airway (a). Placing the infant's head in the 'neutral position' opens the airway (b). Care must be taken not to overextend the head.

two or three breaths may only help in pushing lung liquid out of the alveoli and not expand the lungs with air. In order to give these breaths effectively, the right size of mask should be used, which covers the nose and mouth but does not go over the end of the chin or on the eyes. Once these five inflation breaths are given, reassess the situation to see if this has aided the infant. While assessing tone, colour and respiratory effort the important sign of effective inflation breaths will be a rise in heart rate. If there is no rise in heart rate and the chest was not seen to move while giving five inflation breaths, other airway manoeuvres must be considered to open the airway and ensure the infant receives the inflation breaths.

Other airway manoeuvres include a single-handed jaw thrust, whereby the third or fourth finger of the hand used to keep the facemask on the infant is placed behind the angle of jaw and pushed up. This will aid opening the airway by bringing the lower jaw in line with the upper jaw and helping to bring the tongue, which may have propped backwards into the airway, out of the way. Having carried out this manoeuvre, five inflation breaths should again be given. If this does not result in a rise in heart rate or help is available, and if help is available, the two-person jaw thrust can be attempted, where by one person applies the jaw thrust behind both jaw angles and holds the facemask in place while the other gives the inflation breaths.

If this does not work or there is no help available, if competent, the larynx and vocal cords should be directly visualized using a laryngoscope placed in the left hand and suction should be performed if a blood clot, vernix, or meconium is seen. Alternatively, if there is no obstruction, an appropriately sized oral airway should be placed using the laryngoscope or a tongue depressor should be performed.

To size an oral airway the length should be equal to the distance from the midline of the lips to the angle of the jaw. The airway is inserted in the anatomical position that is desired, i.e. it is not rotated in the mouth because of the fragile palate.

Following these manoeuvres, five inflation breaths should be given. One can only feel reassured if there is a rise in heart rate or you visualize chest movement. If, using these manoeuvres, the chest wall moves with the inflation breaths but there is no rise in heart rate you then need to undertake chest compressions. You may at any of these points intubate if trained and skilled to do so.

Breathing

Having made sure that the chest wall has moved with the inflation breaths, if there is a rise in heart rate but the newborn continues not to breath or has poor respiratory effort, ventilation breaths should be given. These breaths are to 'breath for the baby' and are therefore given with shorter inspiratory times and a quicker rate of 30 breaths per minute. Having overcome the initial stiffness of the lungs, pressure given should also be reduced to a pressure sufficient to get chest wall movement (normally around 20–25 cmH$_2$O).

If after 30 seconds the infant is still not breathing effectively, you may need to consider admission of the infant to the neonatal unit for ventilation and further management.

There is growing evidence from both animal and human studies that resuscitation of infants with room air is as effective as 100% oxygen. There is a theoretical risk that 100% oxygen can cause tissue damage via free radicals. Tan et al. (2008) undertook a Cochrane review looking at air versus oxygen for resuscitation of infants at birth. They concluded that if you choose to resuscitate using air, supplementary oxygen should be available as a back-up.

Some devices are now available which allow you give a set positive end expiratory pressure (PEEP) as well as a peak inspiratory pressure, such as the Neopuff. There is a theoretical benefit to the infant for using PEEP, as this establishes and maintains functional residual capacity. Although there have been several papers showing the benefit particularly in preterm infants where there is an association between absence of functional residual capacity and subsequent respiratory distress syndrome in those requiring ventilation, a Cochrane review undertaken in 2003 and recently updated in 2008 concluded that there was insufficient evidence to determine the efficacy and safety of PEEP in ventilation breaths given during resuscitation of the newborn infant and that further randomised clinical trials were needed.

Circulation

If despite good chest movement with inflation breaths, there is no rise in heart rate, chest compressions must be given. The aim of these chest compressions is to move oxygenated blood from the lungs to the coronary arteries. The best method for administering chest compressions is to encircle the whole of the infant's chest with both hands and place the tips of your thumbs just below and imaginary inter nipple line (Fig. 10.17.2).

The compressions need to compress the chest by one-third and are given at a ratio of one ventilation breath to three chest compressions. After approximately 15 cycles or 30 seconds, the infant must be assessed with regards to colour, tone, respiration, and heart rate. If the heart rate has improved (>60/minute) then chest compressions can stop and depending on the respiratory effort ventilation breaths may or may not need to be continued.

If however despite good airway management with chest movement and chest compressions the heart rate does not increase, drugs should be considered.

Drugs

If you need to obtain vascular access and give drugs, the outcome for this newborn infant is likely to be poor. The drugs used in resuscitation are sodium bicarbonate, adrenaline, and dextrose. Occasionally volume (0.9% sodium chloride or O Rhesus-negative blood) can be given particularly if there is an obvious history of blood loss. Refer to the BNF for children for appropriated drug doses. The best method of administering drugs is via central access. In the newborn infant, this will be by way of a catheter that has been inserted into the umbilical vein of the cord. Alternatively an intra-osseous needle may be used.

If access is difficult the only drug that can be given via an endotracheal tube is adrenaline but due to variable absorption the efficacy of this route is questionable and therefore it is not recommended if alternative access is available.

Preterm infants

Infants born prematurely will have less reserve, and therefore attention to temperature control is important. For those born at 30 weeks' gestation or less, immediately placing the body of the infant (without prior drying) into a plastic bag/wrap under a radiant heater has been shown to improve maintenance of normothermia. Preterm infants are more likely to require stabilization rather than resuscitation. The approach to resuscitation is exactly the same as the approach to that of a term newborn.

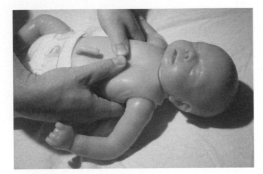

Fig. 10.17.2 Position of hands for cardiac compression in a newborn infant.

Owing to the fragility of their lungs, pressures required to inflate their lungs and move the chest wall will be less and if inflation breaths are required, starting with pressures of 20–25 cmH$_2$O should be adequate. Having given inflation breaths due to prematurity, their respiratory effort may not be sufficient and hence intubation by a trained and skilled member of the team may need to be undertaken. One may consider using a device that is able to provide PEEP when delivering ventilation breaths. If intubation is required, administration of surfactant at this time via the endotracheal tube should be considered. Having stabilized the infant, they should be transferred to the neonatal unit for ongoing assessment and management.

Meconium aspiration

Most babies that pass meconium *in utero* are either term or post-term. The presence of meconium is normally an indicator of fetal stress. The fetus must be gasping in order to aspirate meconium.

If a newborn cries at delivery, despite the presence of meconium, it will imply that the infant has an open airway and therefore no action is required. If however the infant is born with no respiratory effort (i.e. apnoeic), there may have been a period of gasping *in utero* and this infant is at risk of meconium aspiration. Therefore, it is important, having firstly paid attention to keeping the infant warm, to directly visualize the larynx and vocal cords in order to suction any large plugs of meconium that may be present. Having directly visualized the cords and either assessed that there is no obstruction or removed the obstruction to the normal approach to newborn resuscitation can proceed.

Known congenital problems

The majority of antenatal problems, such as oesophageal atresia with a tracheo-oesophageal fistula or a congenital diaphragmatic hernia, that could alter the approach to resuscitation will be picked up antenatally and these should be delivered at an appropriate tertiary centre if indicated.

However, potential congenital problems with the airway, such as Pierre-Robin sequence, can be difficult to pick up on an antenatal scan and therefore the use of adjunct airways may be required if an infant needing resuscitation fails to inflate their chest with airway positioning and jaw thrust. Insertion of an appropriately sized oral airway or a nasopharyngeal airway can aid the maintenance of a patent airway by preventing the tongue, which is large in relation to the size of the oral cavity, flopping backwards, and occluding the larynx.

Stopping resuscitation

The Resuscitation Council (UK) has suggested that if there are no is signs of life after 10 minutes of continuous and adequate resuscitation then discontinuation of resuscitation may be justified. This is supported with data published by Patel and Beeby (2004), which looked at outcome of term newborn infants who had resuscitation beyond 10 minutes. Twenty-nine babies were included in their observation study. 20/29 babies died before leaving hospital. Of the nine who were discharged alive, eight had severe disability and one had moderate disability.

Summary

Newborn resuscitation follows a systematic stepwise approach with emphasis placed on temperature control and airway. The majority of newborn infants will not need resuscitation but should they do so, the vast majority will respond when airway and breathing are managed. It is estimated that more aggressive resuscitation will be required in 1 in 2000 deliveries. In the small minority who need further resuscitative measures the outcome of resuscitation is likely to be poor, and good documentation of time of birth

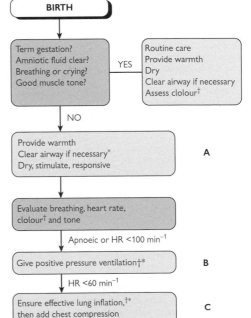

Newborn Life Support

BIRTH

Term gestation?
Amniotic fluid clear?
Breathing or crying?
Good muscle tone?

— YES →

Routine care
Provide warmth
Dry
Clear airway if necessary
Assess clolour†

↓ NO

Provide warmth
Clear airway if necessary*
Dry, stimulate, responsive   **A**

↓

Evaluate breathing, heart rate, clolour† and tone

Apnoeic or HR <100 min⁻¹

Give positive pressure ventilation†*   **B**

HR <60 min⁻¹

Ensure effective lung inflation,†*
then add chest compression   **C**

HR <60 min⁻¹

Consider adrenaline etc.   **D**

*Tracheal intubation may be considered at several steps
†Consider supplemental oxygen at any stage if cyanosis persists

Fig. 10.17.3 Newborn life support. With permission from the Resuscitation Council UK.

and intubation, cardiac compressions, and administration of drugs will help with further management and the counselling of parents. An approach to newborn resuscitation may be summarized in Fig. 10.17.3 by the algorithm provided by the Resuscitation Council.

Further reading

Barber CA, Wyckoff MH. Use and efficacy of endotracheal versus intravenous epinephrine during neonatal cardiopulmonary resuscitation in the delivery room. Paediatrics 2006;118:1028–34.

Bhatt DR, White R, Martin G, et al. Transitional hypothermia in preterm newborns. J Perinatol 2007;27:S45–S47.

Morley CJ, Davis PG. Advances in neonatal resuscitation: supporting transition. Arch Dis Child Fetal Neonat Edn 2008;93:F334–F336.

National Institute for Health and Clinical Excellence (NICE). *Intrapartum care: management and delivery of care to women in labour.* Clinical Guidelines (UK) 2007:42.

O'Donnell C, Davis P, Morley C. Positive end-expiratory pressure for resuscitation of newborn infants at birth. The Cochrane Database Syst Rev 2008;2:CD004341.

Patel H, Beeby PJ. Resuscitation beyond 10 minutes of term babies born without signs of life. J Paediatr Child Health 2004;40:136–8.

Saugstad OD. Practical aspects of resuscitating newborn infants. Eur J Pediatr 1998;157:S11–S15.

Soll RF. Heat loss prevention in neonates. J Perinatol 2008;28:S57–S59.

Tan A, Schulze A, O'Donnell CPF, Davis PG. Air versus oxygen for resuscitation of infants at birth. Cochrane Database Syst Rev 2008;2:CD002273.

Upton CJ, Milner AD. Endotracheal resuscitation of neonates using rebreathing bag. Arch Dis Child 1991;66:39–42.

Internet resources

Resuscitation Council (UK) 2008 www.resus.org.uk.

BNF for children. www.bnfc.org

Retained placenta

Definition
A retained placenta occurs when the placenta fails to deliver 30 minutes following delivery of the fetus with active management of the third stage or 60 minutes with a physiological third stage (NCCWCH 2007).

Epidemiology
The retained placenta (RP) rate is dependent on both definition and third–stage management. It also varies historically and geographically, with rates increasing with time and degree of industrialization (Weeks in press). In actively managed third stages, rates of around 1 in 200 are typical for the developing world (or the UK in the 1950s) while current rates in the USA and UK are around 1 in 50. The reason for this is unclear, but may relate to the association between retained placenta and induction, previous uterine surgery, and birth position (see Aetiology below).

Pathology
Three types of retained placenta are recognized, with the first two being readily distinguished on ultrasound. The quoted frequencies are taken from retained placentas at a mean of 3 hours postpartum in the Release Study (Weeks et al. 2008).

Placenta adherens (60%)
Caused by a failure of contraction of the retroplacental myometrium. On ultrasound, a thin layer of myometrium can be seen behind the retained placenta (the remainder of the myometrium is thickened and contracted). At manual removal of placenta (MRP), the placenta is easily separated from the myometrium.

Trapped placenta (15%)
Where the placenta is already expelled from the uterus, but trapped behind the cervix. On ultrasound, the uterus is seen to be empty with a thick, contracted myometrium throughout. The placenta is seen external to the uterine body, held in the lower segment by a closed cervix.

Placenta accreta (25%)
Caused by invasion of the placenta into (or through) the underlying myometrium. The invasion can be localized or widespread. Most commonly the placenta can still be manually removed, but there is a small area that is 'torn away' rather than separated, or it needs to be removed 'piecemeal'.

Aetiology
The strongest association of RP is with gestational age but increased rates of RP are also found with delivery in a labour bed (rather than standing or squatting), pre–eclampsia, previous termination of pregnancy, extremes of parity or age, use of oxytocin, non–Asian race, and midwifery deliveries (Coombs and Laros 1991). In addition to these, RP has also been found to be associated with induced labour, previous uterine injury, and uterine abnormalities. These studies suggest that interventions common in the most developed countries (labour induction, use of oxytocin, termination of pregnancy) may be contributing to their high RP rates.

Delivery of the placenta is much faster with active management of the third stage. However, by 60 minutes most placentas have been expelled in both groups, and there is no difference in the need for manual removal. The one exception is when intravenous ergometrine is used as prophylactic when the MRP rate is greatly increased (relative risk 19.5, 95% CI 2.6–145.4) (Hammar et al. 1990; Prendiville et al. 2000).

Lack of patience in the third stage of labour can lead to iatrogenic RP due to a snapped cord, or haemorrhage due to partial removal of an undetached placenta. It is therefore crucial that the signs of separation are awaited and undue cord traction avoided. In an audit of RPs in Liverpool, UK, 20% of all RPs had snapped cords. Once this is done it becomes very difficult to extract the placenta, even if it detaches from the uterus, and a MRP is needed.

Prognosis
The prognosis for RP is dependent on the facilities available for treatment. Although in the UK there has only been one death since 1967 from a RP following vaginal delivery, studies from the developing world have found much higher mortality rates. In the South African confidential enquiry into maternal deaths, there were 13 RP deaths in 1999, the single biggest contributor to death from PPH (NCCEMD 1999).

Clinical approach
Diagnosis
Authorities disagree about the time limit for a normal third stage. In developed countries the time taken for 95% of placentas to expel is around 15 and 50 minutes for actively managed and physiological third stages respectively (Prendiville et al. 2000). Blood loss increases after an actively managed third stage of 18 minutes, but waiting for a further 30 minutes leads to the delivery of a further 40% of placentas (Carroli and Bergel 2007). Most authorities suggest that a diagnosis of RP be made at 30 minutes, but that a vaginal examination is performed prior to transfer to theatre for MRP in case of spontaneous delivery in the meantime.

The differentiation between a placenta that is 'trapped' or adherent (placenta adherens) is not easy unless ultrasound is used. Clues to a trapped placenta will be if the fundus feels small and contracted, or if the edge of placenta is palpable through a tight cervical os. In contrast, with placenta adherens the fundus is usually soft and wide. Placenta accreta is rare in women having a vaginal delivery, and will usually be discovered only at the time of attempted MRP.

Ultrasound can be used to differentiate between a trapped and adherent placenta. With a trapped placenta the uterus is empty with a clear endometrial echo. The placenta can be seen lying outside the uterine body within a distended lower segment. In contrast, with an adherent placenta the myometrium will be thickened in all areas, except where the placenta is attached, where it will be very thin or even invisible.

General management
- Women with RPs are at high risk of postpartum haemorrhage and so should be transferred to a high-risk area with an intravenous line in situ.
- Care should be taken in making further attempts at cord traction to remove the placenta as it can lead to a snapped cord or further haemorrhage.

Medical management
- Infusions of oxytocin have been widely used for the treatment of RP, even though they make a MRP more

difficult by contacting the cervix. This treatment has never been subjected to a randomized trial, although there is some evidence that intravenous prostaglandins may be beneficial (van Beekhuizen et al. 2006). Given the lack of convincing evidence and the potential difficulties that they cause, it would seem sense to reserve their use for those women who bleed while awaiting MRP.

- The use of umbilical vein injections have been recommended widely (NCCWCH 2007, Carroli and Bergel 2001). This technique allows the oxytocic to be directed specifically at the area with the contractile failure, while sparing the remainder. However, emerging data from the Release Study (RCT of 577 women having intraumbilical injections of either oxytocin 50 IU or water) show no benefit of oxytocin. There appears therefore to be no benefit of intraumbilical oxytocin injection.

- Intraumbilical prostaglandins may cross the placenta more efficiently and there is some evidence that they may be an affective alternative. However, more research is needed before they can be recommended.

- Glyceryl trinitrate (GTN) may be effective for the management of RP. This was based on numerous observational studies, most of which used intravenous boluses of 50–200 μg. Sublingual GTN tablets (1 mg, as used for angina) have also been shown to be effective in a small randomized trial (Bullarbo et al. 2005). A large trial is needed to confirm these findings.

Surgical management

- MRP is the standard management for RP and it is recommended that this is carried out at around 30 minutes postpartum to keep blood loss to a minimum. A wait of 90 minutes will however lead to the delivery of 55% of placentas without the need for MRP and with a median extra blood loss of only 400 mL (Release Study data). There is therefore a balance to be achieved for each woman to keep intervention and blood loss to a minimum.

- If the cervix is tightly closed when it comes to the manual removal, uterine relaxation may be achieved with the aid of GTN in an intravenous bolus of 50–500 μg or 1 mg sublingually. Marked uterine relaxation occurs after 30–40 seconds and the uterus recovers its tone after 1–2 minutes.

- MRP following either vaginal delivery or CS carries with it an increased risk of endometritis and bleeding. Full aseptic procedures should therefore be followed and a prophylactic broad-spectrum antibiotic used. MRP should also be followed by the use of a long-acting oxytocic (ergometrine or oxytocin infusion).

Recurrence

Following a RP in any previous pregnancy there is an overall recurrence rate of 6.25% (Hall et al. 1985). The risk of RP in the second pregnancy rises from 2% to 4.8% if there was a RP in the first.

Further reading

Bullarbo M, Tjugum J, Ekerhovd E. Sublingual nitroglycerin for management of retained placenta. Int J Gynaecol Obstet 2005;91: 228–32. Erratum in Int J Gynaecol Obstet 2006;92: 337.

Carroli G, Bergel E. Umbilical vein injection for management of retained placenta. Cochrane Database Syst Rev 2001;4: CD001337.

Combs CA and Laros RK. Prolonged third stage of labour: morbidity and risk factors. Obstet Gynecol 1991;77:863–7.

Hall MH, Halliwell R, Carr-Hill R. Concomitant and repeated happenings of complications of the third stage of labour. Br J Obstet Gynaecol 1985;92:732–8.

Hammar M, Boström K, Borgvall B. Comparison between the influence of methylergometrine and oxytocin on the incidence of retained placenta in the third stage of labour. Gynecol Obstet Invest 1990;30:91–3.

National Collaborating Centre for Women's and Children's Health (NCCWCH). Intrapartum Care. Care of healthy women and their babies during childbirth. London: RCOG Press 2007.

National Committee for Confidential Enquiries into Maternal Deaths (NCCEMD). Second Interim Report on Confidential Enquiries into Maternal Deaths in South Africa. www.doh.gov.za/docs/reports/1999/interim-rep.pdf

Prendiville WJ, Elbourne D, McDonald S. Active versus expectant management in the third stage of labour. Cochrane Database Syst Rev 2000;3:CD000007.

van Beekhuizen HJ, de Groot AN, De Boo T, Burger D, et al. Sulprostone reduces the need for the manual removal of the placenta in patients with retained placenta: a randomized controlled trial. Am J Obstet Gynecol 2006;194:446–50.

Weeks AD. Alia G, Vernon G et al. Umbilical vein oxytocin for the treatment of retained placenta (RELEASE study); a double blind randomised controlled study. Lancet 2010;375:141–7.

Shoulder dystocia

Definition

Shoulder dystocia is defined as 'a delivery that requires additional obstetric manoeuvres to release the shoulders after gentle downward traction has failed. It occurs when either the anterior or, less commonly, the posterior fetal shoulder impacts on the maternal symphysis or sacral promontory'. Shoulder dystocia has also been defined as a prolonged head–to–body delivery time (e.g. more than 60 seconds), although many birth attendants usually await the next contraction after the delivery of the head to deliver the shoulders.

Epidemiology

The incidence of shoulder dystocia ranges between 0.2% and 3% of births. Significant variations have been observed in different populations. In North America and the UK the incidence is 0.6% and in African American women it is 2.6%.

Pathophysiology

Shoulder dystocia occurs due to a 'mismatch' between the fetal shoulder dimensions and the maternal bony pelvis. During vaginal delivery the fetal head descends through the pelvic brim in an occipito-transverse position. The shoulders rotate and are accommodated in the pelvic inlet at an oblique position as this has a larger diameter than the anteroposterior. The posterior shoulder descends first followed by the anterior one. If the fetal shoulders remain in an anteroposterior position or descend simultaneously, then the anterior shoulder becomes impacted behind the symphysis pubis and rarely the posterior shoulder behind the sacral promontory. Although at this stage the fetal head is delivered, the fetal chest remains compressed and respiratory efforts cannot be initiated. As the uterus is contracted, blood flow to the fetus is impeded. Delay in completing the delivery may result in fetal asphyxia, as the umbilical cord pH falls by 0.04 units per minute.

Complications

Fetal

Severe cases of hypoxia can result in permanent brain injury and death. The rates of perinatal mortality secondary to shoulder dystocia are 0–2.5%. The risk of fetal hypoxic injury depends on the fetal condition prior to the occurrence of shoulder dystocia and on the time required for the completion of delivery.

Brachial plexus injury is a common fetal complication with wide variations in the reported incidence from 4% to 40%. In the majority of cases the injury is transient and will resolve within a year, with less than a 10% rate of persistent injury.

Fractures are also common and are usually clavicular or humeral. Clavicular fractures complicate 3–9.5% of shoulder dystocia cases. Most of these fractures heal well without sequelae.

Maternal

Postpartum haemorrhage and vaginal and perineal injuries are common maternal complications. Shoulder dystocia is one of the most significant risk factors for anal sphincter injuries. Uterine rupture is a rare complication, which may occur following fundal pressure.

Risk factors

The large majority of cases occur in the absence of risk factors. Antenatal risk factors include a previous pregnancy complicated by fetal macrosomia, gestational diabetes or shoulder dystocia, pre-existing or gestational diabetes mellitus, maternal obesity or excessive weight gain, multiparity, and prolonged gestation. Induction of labour is also a risk factor for shoulder dystocia.

Intrapartum risk factors include a prolonged first stage of labour, secondary arrest, a prolonged second stage of labour, oxytocin augmentation, and assisted vaginal delivery. The incidence of shoulder dystocia is increased by approximately 35–45% in assisted deliveries of non-diabetic and diabetic mothers. Sequential use of instruments is associated with even higher rates.

Fetal macrosomia

The risk of shoulder dystocia increases significantly with increased birthweight. Nesbitt et al. (1998) conducted a large population-based study and reported the following rates of shoulder dystocia for unassisted births of non-diabetic mothers: 5.2% for birthweight 4000–4250 g, 9.1% for 4250–4500 g, 14.3% for 4500–4750 g, and 21.1% for 4750–5000 g.

Although fetal macrosomia is the most significant risk factor and associated with most of the other risk factors (maternal diabetes, multiparity, previous macrosomic infant, prolonged gestation, maternal obesity, or excessive weight gain), almost half of the cases of shoulder dystocia occur in infants <4000 g. Additionally, clinical fetal weight estimation is inaccurate and late pregnancy ultrasound scans for estimation of fetal weight have a low sensitivity.

Maternal diabetes

There is a positive association between maternal hyperglycaemia and the risk of shoulder dystocia. Nesbitt et al. (1998) found that the risk of shoulder dystocia for unassisted births to diabetic women was 8.4%, 12.3%, 19.9%, and 23.5% when the birthweight was 4000–4250 g, 4250–4500 g, 4500–4750 g, or >4750 g, respectively. The risk of shoulder dystocia for assisted births to diabetic mothers was even higher: 12.2% for infants 4000–4250g, 16.7% for those 4250–4500g, 27.3% for those 4500–4750g, and 34.8% for those 4750–5000g.

Prediction and prevention

Although shoulder dystocia is largely unpredictable, statistical models have been developed to predict the risk. Parameters used in these models are birthweight, maternal height and weight, gestational age, and parity. Some studies suggest that it is possible to identify combinations of factors that are associated with shoulder dystocia and neonatal injury. In general, the presence of multiple risk factors appears to be a predictor for shoulder dystocia.

Identification of risk factors and an antenatal care plan that aims to modify them may reduce the incidence of shoulder dystocia. For example, tight control of glucose levels in diabetic pregnant women may reduce the risks of fetal macrosomia and shoulder dystocia. When risk factors are present, a plan for delivery should include a senior midwife and an experienced obstetrician available at the second stage, which may facilitate a successful management.

Mode of delivery

Induction of labour has been considered as an option for managing suspected macrosomia, thus reducing the risk of shoulder dystocia and subsequent birth trauma. However, early induction of labour for non-diabetic women with suspected fetal macrosomia does not appear to improve either maternal or fetal outcome.

The RCOG guidelines do not recommend elective Caesarean section for suspected fetal macrosomia (estimated fetal weight >4500 g) in non-diabetic women. Elective Caesarean section can be considered in diabetic women when the estimated fetal weight is >4500g and in non-diabetic women when the estimated fetal weight is >5000 g. Elective Caesarean section can be discussed with the parents in cases of a previous birth affected by shoulder dystocia, brachial plexus injury, or associated asphyxial injury.

Prophylactic manoeuvres at delivery (McRoberts manoeuvre and direct suprapubic pressure) have been considered for the prevention of shoulder dystocia, but there are no clear findings to support or refute their use.

Recurrence of shoulder dystocia

The recurrence risks vary between 11.9% and 16.7%. In a large population study by Moore et al. (2008), the annual incidence of primary and recurrent shoulder dystocia was 2.3% and 13.5% respectively. This study highlighted birthweight ~3500 g, assisted vaginal delivery and severe shoulder dystocia in the previous delivery as the most significant independent risk factors for recurrence. The only identifiable risk factor may often be the prior history itself.

Management of shoulder dystocia

The aim of management should be prevention of fetal asphyxia, while avoiding fetal and maternal injury (Fig. 10.19.1). The attending midwife or obstetrician should be able to recognize a shoulder dystocia immediately and proceed through a stepwise sequence of manoeuvres to expedite delivery.

First-line manoeuvres

McRoberts manoeuvre

The woman is on supine position with the hips acutely flexed and the knees close to the chest. This position straightens the lumbosacral angle, allowing descent of the posterior shoulder. The maternal pelvis is rotated cephalad and the pelvic inlet is now perpendicular to the direction of the maternal expulsive forces. This manoeuvre has success rates as high as 90%.

Directed suprapubic pressure

Continuous or 'rocking' (cyclical compression/relaxation) pressure on the posterior aspect of the anterior shoulder may facilitate its rotation to an oblique position, adduction of the shoulders and a reduction of the bisacromial diameter (Fig. 10.19.2).

Second-line manoeuvres

Delivery of the posterior arm

The hand enters the vagina posteriorly and gentle pressure is applied at the antecubital fossa to flex the fetal forearm, which is then grasped and swept across the fetal chest. With this manoeuvre, delivery of the posterior arm may be achieved, allowing the anterior arm to rotate posteriorly or descend behind the symphysis pubis as Kung et al. (2006) showed that the shoulder dimensions are reduced by 2.5 cm with this manoeuvre, especially in larger fetuses.

Rubin's manoeuvre

If the posterior arm is not deliverable, rotation can be attempted by placing two fingers in the vagina behind the anterior shoulder. The shoulder is pushed forward and the bisacromial diameter rotates into an oblique position. If unsuccessful, this can then be combined with the Woods' screw manoeuvre.

Woods' screw

Two fingers are inserted vaginally, on the anterior aspect of the posterior shoulder and apply pressure aiming to rotate the fetus towards the same direction as the Rubin's manoeuvre.

Reverse Woods' screw

Two fingers are placed behind the posterior shoulder and an attempt is made to rotate in the opposite direction to the original Woods' screw.

All these manoeuvres aim to rotate the shoulders 180 degrees and enable delivery by bringing the anterior shoulder posteriorly. Recent studies have indicated that insertion of the whole hand in the vagina may enable better thrust on the shoulder and facilitate rotation (Crofts et al. 2008) (Fig. 10.19.3). It has also been suggested that knowledge of the concepts that underlie manoeuvres and the practical details of their execution is much more effective

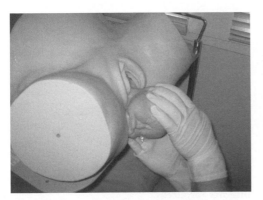

Fig. 10.19.1 Downward traction should be avoided.

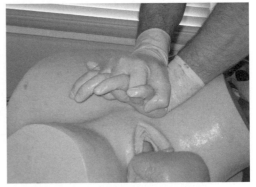

Figure 10.19.2 Directed suprapubic pressure.

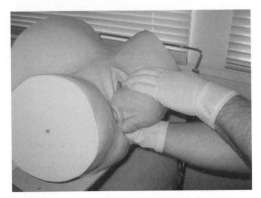

Fig. 10.19.3 Insertion of the whole hand posteriorly in the vagina.

than knowledge of the precise definitions or eponyms of each manoeuvre.

All-fours
With the woman on her hands and knees, gentle traction is applied aiming to deliver the posterior shoulder first, which may descend downwards due to gravity and to a possible increase of the anteroposterior diameter of the maternal pelvis.

Clavicular fracture
This manoeuvre will reduce the bisacromial diameter, but may be associated with brachial plexus injury or vascular and soft tissue fetal trauma.

Third-line manoeuvres
Zavanelli manoeuvre
The fetal head is flexed, restitution is reversed, the head is rotated back to the occipitoanterior position, and replaced into the uterine cavity. Tocolytics can be used along with general anaesthetic agents for uterine relaxation. The fetus is then delivered by Caesarean section. High success rates up to 92% have been reported, but this manoeuvre is associated with significant fetal and maternal morbidity, including fetal injuries and deaths, uterine and vaginal rupture. It is likely that most injuries are not necessarily due to the procedure itself but may occur following other unsuccessful manoeuvres and prolonged fetal hypoxia. Nevertheless, this manoeuvre should only be performed in cases of severe shoulder dystocia unresponsive to first- and second-line manoeuvres and the fetal condition should be

Table 10.19.1 Modified 'HELPERR' algorithm (obtained from ALSO programme manual)

H	call for **H**elp (midwives, senior obstetricians, neonatologists, anaesthetist)
E	evaluate for **E**pisiotomy
L	flex **L**egs (McRoberts' manoeuvre)
P	suprapubic **P**ressure (continuous or rocking)
E	**E**nter (internal rotational manoeuvres)
R	**R**emove the posterior arm
R	**R**oll the patient on all fours

evaluated first, taking into account the potential irreversibility of fetal asphyxia.

Symphysiotomy
This procedure requires a degree of surgical expertise and is associated with significant risks of lower urinary tract injury. It should only be used as a last resort manoeuvre. The patient is in a supine position and the thighs are abducted no more than 45° from the midline. A urethral catheter is inserted and the urethra is displaced laterally. Following local infiltration with lignocaine, a vertical stab incision is made on the symphysis with a scalpel. Cutting through the fibres by rotational movement of the blade usually allows partial separation of the symphysis and the anterior fetal shoulder to be disimpacted.

Training
As for all the obstetric emergencies and especially the rare ones with high morbidity and mortality rates, regular training sessions for the management of shoulder dystocia with fire drills and the use of mannequins should be organized by all obstetric units. Unit protocols should advise a multidisciplinary and systematic approach. Algorithms and mnemonics such as the HELPERR algorithm (Table 10.19.1) are commonly used and may facilitate a prompt and sequential use of the manoeuvres.

Further reading
American College of Obstetricians and Gynecologists. Shoulder dystocia. ACOG practice bulletin clinical management guidelines for obstetricians–gynecologists. Number 40. Obstet Gynecol 2002;100:1045–50.

Athukorala C, Middleton P, Crowther CA. Intrapartum interventions for preventing shoulder dystocia. Cochrane Database Syst Rev 2006;4:CD005543.

Belfort MA, Dildy GA, Saade GR, et al. Prediction of shoulder dystocia using multivariate analysis. Am J Perinatol 2007;24:5–10.

Cheng YW, Norwitz ER, Caughey AB. The relationship of fetal position and ethnicity with shoulder dystocia and birth injury. Am J Obstet Gynecol 2006;195:856–62.

Crofts JF, Fox R, Ellis D, et al. Observations from 450 shoulder dystocia simulations: lessons for skills training. Obstet Gynecol 2008;112:906–12.

Dyachenko A, Ciampi A, Fahey J, et al. Prediction of risk for shoulder dystocia with neonatal injury. Am J Obstet Gynecol 2006;195:1544–9.

Kung J, Swan AV, Arulkumaran S. Delivery of the posterior arm reduces shoulder dimensions in shoulder dystocia. Int J Gynaecol Obstet 2006;93:233–7.

Mehta SH, Blackwell SC, Chadha R, Sokol RJ. Shoulder dystocia and the next delivery: outcomes and management. J Matern Fetal Neonatal Med 2007;20:729–33.

Moore HM, Reed SD, Batra M, Schiff MA. Risk factors for recurrent shoulder dystocia, Washington state, 1987–2004. Am J Obstet Gynecol 2008;198:e16–24.

Nesbitt TS, Gilbert WM, Herrchen B. Shoulder dystocia and associated risk factors with macrosomic infants born in California. Am J Obstet Gynecol 1998;179:476–80.

Royal College of Obstetricians and Gynaecologists (RCOG) Shoulder dystocia. Guideline No 42. Green Top Guidelines. London: RCOG 2005

Spong CY, Beall M, Rodrigues D, Ross MG. An objective definition of shoulder dystocia: prolonged head-to-body delivery intervals and/or the use of ancillary obstetric maneuvers. Obstet Gynecol 1995;86:433–6.

Internet resources
www.erbspalsygroup.co.uk

Shoulder presentation

Definition

It is a malpresentation in which one of the fetal shoulders occupies the lower pole of the uterus and is the first to engage when labour commences. It is associated with an abnormal lie (i.e. transverse lie), in which the fetal spine is at right angles to the long axis of the uterus) with the head in one iliac fossa and the breech occupying the other iliac fossa. In this situation, one of the shoulders comes to occupy the lower pole of the uterus. Acromion process of the scapula is the denominator and depending on its relationship to the ilio-pectineal eminence (right and left) and sacro-iliac joints (right and left), the following positions are described:

- left scapulo (or dorso): anterior
- right scapulo (or dorso): anterior
- left scapulo (or dorso): posterior
- right scapulo(or dorso): posterior

However, there is *no* mechanism of labour in transverse lie as the engaging diameter (fetal back) cannot enter the pelvic brim, except in rare cases of extreme prematurity or in a macerated fetus, in which an acute angulation of the fetal spine is possible (i.e. folding of the fetal trunk).

Epidemiology

Transverse lie with shoulder presentation occurs in about 2–3% of pregnancies in early gestations. However, at term, only about 0.3% of fetuses have shoulder presentation (1 in 300 deliveries).

Predisposing factors

Any factor that hinders a longitudinal lie may predispose to transverse lie and shoulder presentation. The majority of transverse lie (over 90%) occur in multipara due to laxity of the abdominal wall muscles as well as the uterine myometrium that enables the uterus to lose its piriform shape. Similarly, alterations in amniotic fluid volume (polyhydramnios) as well as other factors that obliterate the piriform shape of the uterus (congenital malformations such as arcuate or subseptate uterus, fibroids in the lower segment, major degree placenta praevia) would prevent the fetus from assuming a longitudinal lie. True or relative cephalopelvic disproportion will also reduce the space available in the longitudinal axis of the uterus, thereby forcing the fetus to assume a transverse lie.

Fetal factors are congenital malformations, prematurity, intrauterine growth restriction (smaller baby has more 'space' to occupy, nullifying the restrictive effects of piriform uterus) and multiple pregnancy. Approximately 40% of transverse lie (i.e. shoulder presentation) is associated with multiple pregnancy and a majority of these involve the second twin. In about a third of cases, no specific cause for transverse lie could be identified.

Natural history of shoulder presentation

- Spontaneous rectification—it is estimated that approximately 80% of transverse lie diagnosed antenatally may correct itself to a longitudinal lie, by the onset of labour. Absence of predisposing factors (placenta praevia, contracted pelvis) increases the chances of spontaneous rectification. It is called spontaneous rectification when the vertex becomes the presenting part and spontaneous version when the presenting part is breech.

- Spontaneous evolution—in the presence of strong uterine contractions, head is retained above the pelvic brim, the neck elongates and the breech descends into the pelvis, followed by the trunk and 'after coming head'. This is similar to spontaneous version but occurs in the pelvis after the onset of uterine contractions.

- Spontaneous expulsion is common if the fetus is dead (is macerated) or is extremely small (<800 g) in the presence of a roomy maternal pelvis. With strong uterine contractions, the trunk of the fetus folds on itself (termed 'conduplicato corpore'). Fetus gets expelled with the head, thorax and trunk doubled on itself.

- Impacted shoulder presentation occurs in cases of neglected shoulder presentation with obstructed labour. Pathological 'obstruction ring' (Bandl's ring) is often present and marks the demarcation of the dilating and stretching lower uterine segment and the contracted upper segment. This ring can be felt (as well as often seen) through the anterior abdominal wall. Bandl's Ring rises as the obstruction worsens indicating that the lower uterine segment is thinned out and overstretched, and, hence, may rupture if prompt delivery is not undertaken. Fetal heart rate is often absent and the mother's condition worsens (dehydration, ketoacidosis, sepsis, and shock). Hand or cord prolapse may be noted.

Clinical approach

Transverse lie (shoulder presentation) should be anticipated in the presence of known predisposing factors. If this is suspected on clinical examination, an ultrasound scan should be performed to confirm the findings.

Antenatal period

- Abdomen may look 'transversely stretched' during inspection.
- Symphysio-fundal height (SFH) is less than the period of gestation.
- On palpation, there is an 'empty lower pole' (i.e. no fetal part can be palpated in the suprapubic region on Pawlik's grip)
- Fetal head can be palpated in one iliac fossa and breech in the other, with fetal back lying transversely between the head and the breech.
- Fetal heart rate is best heard on one side of the umbilicus (close to the fetal head).

During labour

- In addition to the above clinical findings, if a vaginal examination is performed in early labour (after excluding placenta praevia by an ultrasound examination), a 'bogginess' will be felt due to the absence of a presenting part (head or breech) within the pelvic cavity.
- After the rupture of membranes, it may be possible to feel the side of the thorax (rib cage may feel like 'grid-iron'), scapula, axilla as well as the clavicle. These fetal parts are felt very high because of the inability to engage during labour, due to the larger dimensions.
- During late labour, especially with 'neglected shoulder presentation', cord prolapse or prolapse of the fetal arm may be observed. There may be signs of obstructed labour, including a Bandl's Ring (an oblique groove that appears between the dilating lower segment and contracting upper segment).

- In cases of prolapse of the arm through the vagina, the dorsum of the supinated hand points towards the back and the thumb points towards the head.

Role of ultrasound scan

In modern obstetric practice, an ultrasound scan can be performed antenatally or during labour to confirm or to exclude a shoulder presentation and to diagnose or exclude abnormalities of amniotic fluid (polyhydramnios), placenta praevia, congenital abnormalities (anencephaly), uterine malformation (arcuate or subseptate uterus), and the lie of the second twin in multiple pregnancy. Ultrasonography can also help to identify the position of the fetal back (dorso-superior or dorso-inferior). Doppler may help diagnose the presence of the cord above the cervix (a cord presentation).

Management

As there is no mechanism of labour in shoulder presentation and the significant risks of cord prolapse and uterine rupture, patients should not be allowed to go into labour, if shoulder presentation (i.e. transverse lie) is diagnosed antenatally or early in labour.

- Conservative approach is recommended up to 37 weeks, anticipating spontaneous version to cephalic (or breech) presentations. Patient should be advised to present early, if she develops painful uterine contractions or rupture of membranes. This will help avoid neglected shoulder presentation and to exclude cord prolapse (or arm), respectively.
- After 37 weeks, patient should be counselled regarding the pros and cons of different management options, which include external cephalic version (ECV), stabilizing induction, and elective Caesarean section. Internal podalic version (IPV) is an accepted option for second twin, after the vaginal delivery of the first twin.
- ECV may be attempted with the view to converting transverse lie to cephalic presentation. In the light of the Term Breech Trial (Hannah et al 2008), conversion to breech is no longer recommended. Tocolysis (terbutaline 250 μg subcutaneously) may be administered to relax the myometrium, prior to ECV. Contraindications should be excluded (please refer to 'breech presentation) and the woman should be counselled to attend early in labour, even after a successful ECV as there is a 5% chance of spontaneous reversion after ECV.
- For unstable lie or persistent transverse lie, a stabilizing induction may be tried. This involves conversion to cephalic presentation by ECV and commencing oxytocin infusion to 'push the head into the pelvis). Once the fetal head enters the pelvic brim and is fixed by progressive uterine contractions, an amniotomy (artificial rupture of membranes (ARM)) should be performed. Examiners fingers should be placed in the opening after the membranes are ruptured to prevent a sudden gush of amniotic fluid. Such a 'controlled ARM' may help avoid cord prolapse and also may help recognise an occult cord prolapse early. The examining fingers can be withdrawn once the fetal head rests on the fingers.
- Elective caesarean section should be offered if ECV or stabilizing induction fails or if the patient declines these options and chooses to have an elective caesarean section, after weighing the pros and cons. Elective Caesarean section is recommended in the presence of contra-indications to ECV.

- Emergency Caesarean section should be performed if a patient with transverse lie presents in advanced labour. If the patient presents in early labour with intact membranes, tocolysis with terbutaline and stabilizing induction may be attempted.
- Caesarean section for transverse lie should be performed by or under the supervision of an experienced obstetrician. Failure of the formation of lower segment may necessitate a low vertical or a 'J shaped' incision. The membranes should not be ruptured early to prevent the uterine walls clamping on to the fetus that may make delivery through the uterine incision difficult. Fetal feet could be grasped through the membranes and the fetus may be delivered by breech.
- In the presence of additional risk factors (advanced labour, neglected shoulder presentation, major degree placenta praevia), a classical (upper segment) caesarean section should be considered. If the patient presents in advanced labour with an impacted shoulder, acute tocolysis (terbutaline 250 μg subcutaneously) could be tried to abolish uterine contractions to facilitate delivery.
- In developing countries, neglected shoulder presentation with intrauterine death may still occur due to lack of easy access to the healthcare system. In such cases, the mother may have ketosis, dehydration, chorioamnionitis, and septic shock due to prolonged and obstructed labour. In such cases, performing a Caesarean section increases the risk of maternal morbidity and mortality, especially if facilities are not available for intensive treatment therapy after surgery, to provide multi-organ support. Destructive operations such as decapitation with a Blond–Heidler saw or decapitation hook, and evisceration and decompression of the fetus may be safer options in these circumstances. However, it is important to recognize that destructive operations performed by inexperienced hands can also result in maternal morbidity and mortality due to unintended trauma (uterine perforation and injury to adjacent organs).

Further reading

Chandraharan E, Arulkumaran S. Operative delivery, shoulder dystocia and episiotomy. In: Arulkumaran S, Penna LK, Bhasker Rao K (eds) The management of labour, 2nd edn. Orient Longman 2005.

Chandraharan E, Arulkumaran S. Acute tocolysis: Review Article. Curr Opin Obstet Gynecol 2003;17:151–6.

Chhabra S, Bhagwat N, Chakravorty A. Reduction in the occurrence of uterine rupture in Central India. J Obstet Gynaecol 2002;22:39–42.

Fox AJ, Chapman MG. Longitudinal ultrasound assessment of fetal presentation: a review of 1010 consecutive cases. Aust NZ J Obstet Gynaecol 2006;46:341–4.

Hannah ME, Hannah WJ, Hewson SA, et al. Planned caesarean section vs planned vaginal birth for breech presentation at term: a randomised multicentre trial. Term Breech Collaborative Group. Lancet 2000;356:1375–83.

Nassar N, Roberts CL, Cameron CA, Olive EC. Diagnostic accuracy of clinical examination for detection of non-cephalic presentation in late pregnancy: cross sectional analytic study. BMJ 2006 16;333:578–80.

Seffah JD. Maternal and perinatal mortality and morbidity associated with transverse lie. Int J Gynaecol Obstet1999;65:115.

Sharma JB. Evaluation of Sharma's modified Leopold's maneuvers: a new method for fetal palpation in late pregnancy. Arch Gynecol Obstet 2009;279:481–7.

Uterine inversion

Definition

Uterine inversion is a complication of the third stage of labour. After delivery of the fetus, the uterus is partially or completely inverted and protrudes through the cervix, in or outside the vagina. Puerperal uterine inversion can occur after a vaginal delivery or Caesarean section. It can be acute (<24 hours postpartum), subacute (>24 hours postpartum), or chronic (>1 month postpartum). Chronic, non-puerperal uterine inversions can occur rarely and are usually associated with uterine tumours. A simple classification categorizes uterine inversion by severity in four degrees. The first degree (incomplete) involves extension of the inverted fundus to the cervical ring. In second-degree (incomplete) inversion the fundus protrudes through the cervical ring but the inverted uterus remains within the vagina. In the third degree (complete) the inverted fundus extends to the introitus. The fourth degree is a total inversion where the vagina is also inverted (Figs 10.21.1 and 10.21.2).

Epidemiology

Uterine inversion is rare with a reported incidence varying between 1 in 2000 and 1 in 6400 deliveries. An even lower incidence of 1 in 20 000–25 000 deliveries has also been reported. The introduction of active management of the third stage of labour may have led to a significant decrease in the incidence of uterine inversion.

Aetiology

The most common cause is excessive cord traction on an umbilical cord before complete placental separation. Downward traction on the fundus, usually in combination with uterine atony, results in partial or complete prolapse of the uterine wall through the dilated cervix. A short umbilical cord, fundal implantation of the placenta, morbidly adherent placenta, or uterine anomalies are contributing factors.

Clinical presentation

Uterine inversion is often associated with major life-threatening haemorrhage in 94% of cases and shock disproportionate to the estimated blood loss with bradycardia due to increased vagal tone. Other symptoms and signs include acute lower abdominal pain in the

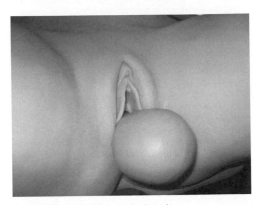

Fig. 10.21.2 Fourth-degree uterine inversion.

third stage. The placenta may or may not be *in situ*. The uterus is not palpable abdominally. In partial inversion there may be a uterine dimple palpable suprapubically. Pelvic examination may reveal a mass in or outside the vagina.

Management

Early recognition, rapid, systematic assessment, and simultaneous initiation of resuscitation and management measures are essential, as delay may result in severe morbidity or mortality. Treatment consists of aggressive fluid and blood replacement and appropriate manoeuvres to replace the uterus.

Help

Assistance, including an experienced obstetrician, an anaesthetist, and a senior midwife, is summoned immediately. The blood bank should be notified urgently, and blood and blood products requested.

Assessment and resuscitation

The level of consciousness should be ascertained and airway maintained. Continuous monitoring of blood pressure, pulse, respiratory rate, oxygen saturation, and urine output is mandatory. Oxygen administration should be commenced. Two wide-bore intravenous cannulae are inserted to enable fluid resuscitation and blood transfusion. Blood samples are sent for urgent full blood count, cross-match of 4–6 units, and clotting screen. Intravenous crystalloid infusion is commenced. If the patient is in shock with bradycardia, intravenous atropine is administered. Syntocinon infusion should be stopped until the uterus is replaced. At the same time, appropriate analgesia is administered and preparations are made for transfer to theatre.

Non-surgical management

Replacement of the uterus should be attempted without delay and concurrently to anti-shock measures, as resuscitation may not be successful until the inversion is corrected. Replacement is also more likely to be achieved if attempted before the development of a constriction ring and oedema of the uterus. Immediate non-surgical measures are successful in the vast majority of cases of uterine inversion. The uterine fundus can be replaced manually or by hydrostatic pressure.

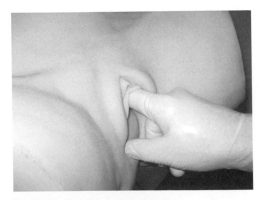

Fig. 10.21.1 Third-degree uterine inversion.

Manual replacement (the Johnson manoeuvre)

This should be attempted preferably under general anaesthesia. The uterus may require relaxation for successful manual replacement. Different regimes of tocolytic agents have been used including magnesium sulphate (4–6 g intravenously over 20 minutes), terbutaline (250 µg subcutaneously), ritodrine or a volatile agent for general anaesthesia. The inverted uterus may be replaced by applying constant pressure with the palm on the fundus and the tips of the fingers at the uterocervical junction. The tension that is applied on the uterine ligaments may widen the constriction ring and allow the repositioning of the uterus through the cervix (Fig. 10.21.3).

If the placenta is still *in situ*, it is not removed until fluid resuscitation has been commenced, and anaesthesia has been administered. Once the uterus is repositioned, the tocolytic agent is discontinued and a hand is kept in the uterine cavity until intravenous oxytocin is given and the uterus is contracted. Then, if still *in situ*, the placenta is removed and the cavity is gently explored to exclude retained placental tissues or trauma. Bimanual compression may be applied at this stage to improve uterine tone and arrest haemorrhage. After the uterus is well contracted, continuous monitoring is necessary to exclude haemorrhage or recurrence of inversion.

Hydrostatic replacement (O'Sullivan's technique)

If the attempt to replace the uterus manually immediately is unsuccessful, the woman is transferred to the operating theatre and placed in lithotomy position. Uterine rupture must be excluded and 2 L of warm normal saline are infused into the vagina via a giving set. A silastic ventouse cup may be attached to the giving set. The ventouse cup is placed just inside the introitus and the fluid ran under gravity from a height of 2 m maintaining a seal manually.

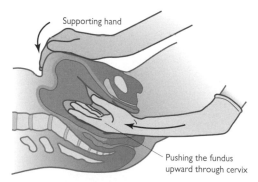

Supporting hand

Pushing the fundus upward through cervix

Fig. 10.21.3 Reduction of uterine inversion. The inverted uterus is replaced by applying firm pressure with a gloved hand. Taken from Sarris et al., *Training in obstetrics and Gynaecology* (2009), with permission from Oxford University Press.

The hydrostatic pressure that is developed will distend the vaginal walls and the constriction ring and push the uterine fundus upwards.

Surgical management

Laparotomy is the next step if manual attempts fail, usually due to a dense constriction ring around the cervix. In the Huntington's procedure, after laparotomy, tenaculum or Allis forceps are placed on the fundus of the inverted uterus and gentle traction is applied.

The fundus is pushed from the vagina upwards and simultaneously pulled abdominally. A traction suture placed in the inverted fundus may facilitate replacement. An alternative technique involves passing the suture through the whole thickness of the uterus threading it through a small plastic tube to avoid pulling through the myometrium.

If the constriction ring still prohibits replacement, a longitudinal incision posteriorly, will release the constriction and allow uterine placement (Haultain's technique). Laparoscopically assisted replacement has also been described. The uterine incision is repaired after replacement. Uterotonics should be commenced after repositioning to keep the uterus contracted.

Prevention

Uterine inversion may be prevented by avoiding mismanagement of the third stage. Traction on the umbilical cord should not be excessive and not be applied before the placenta is separated.

Further reading

Baskett TF. Acute uterine inversion: a review of 40 cases. J Obstet Gynaecol Can 2002;24:953–6.

Bhalla R, Wuntakal R, Odejinmi F, Khan RU. Acute inversion of the uterus. Obstet Gynaecol 2009;11:13–18.

Brar HS, Greenspoon JS, Platt LD, Paul RH. Acute puerperal uterine inversion. New approaches to management. J Reprod Med 1989; 34:173–7.

Calder AA. Emergencies in operative obstetrics. Baillieres Best Pract Res Clin Obstet Gynaecol 2000;14:43–55.

Livingston SL, Booker C, Kramer P, Dodson WC. Chronic uterine inversion at 14 weeks postpartum. Obstet Gynecol 2007;109:555–7.

MOET Managing Obstetric Emergencies and Trauma, The MOET Course Manual. London: RCOG Press 2003.

Paterson-Brown S. Obstetric emergencies. In: Edmonds DK (ed.) *Dewhurst's textbook of obstetrics and gynaecology*. Oxford: Blackwell Publishing 2007:145–58.

Shamsudin F, Morton K. Novel correction technique of chronic puerperal inversion of the uterus. J Obstet Gynaecol 2007;27:197–8.

Thomson AJ, Greer IA. Non-haemorrhagic obstetric shock. Baillieres Best Pract Res Clin Obstet Gynaecol 2000;14:19–41.

Vijayaraghavan R, Sujatha Y. Acute postpartum uterine inversion with haemorrhagic shock: laparoscopic reduction: a new method of management? Br J Obstet Gynaecol 2006;113:1100–2.

Internet resources

www.patient.co.uk

Common obstetric techniques, procedures, and surgery

Balloon tamponade *430*
Caesarean section *434*
Forceps delivery *446*
Uterine compression sutures *452*
Ventouse delivery *456*

Balloon tamponade

Definition
The insertion of a balloon device into the genital tract to control bleeding from the placental bed, and/or lacerations in the uterus, cervix, and vagina, by means of pressure effect when the balloon is inflated with fluid. The commonest application is in the treatment of primary postpartum haemorrhage (PPH), but various forms of balloon tamponade have been used to treat bleeding from ectopic cervical pregnancy, vaginal laceration following delivery, and lacerations of the lower uterus and cervix following gynaecological procedures.

Epidemiology
The actual incidence of the use of balloon tamponade in the management of PPH, and occasionally for the management of bleeding from a cervical pregnancy or lower genital tract laceration, remains unknown. There are only anecdotal case reports and small case series in the literature, but this most likely represents under-reporting.

Pathology
PPH is the third most common cause of maternal mortality worldwide and accounted for 10% of the direct maternal deaths in the UK. There has been a progressive increase in the risk factors for PPH, such as the increasing prevalence of mothers with advanced age, multiple pregnancy, and a scarred uterus. Excessive bleeding can occur from a failure of the placental bed blood vessels to be occluded by the contracting myometrium. This can be consequent to the following:
- inadequate uterine contraction after the complete expulsion of the placenta, as in the case of uterine atony.
- inability of the uterus to contract effectively:
  - partial separation of the placenta:
    - morbidly adherent placenta (e.g. placenta accreta, placenta increta)
    - inadequate, inappropriate, or delayed administration of oxytocic agent for the management of the third stage.
  - completely separated placenta trapped inside the uterus due to:
    - premature contraction of the cervix
    - failed controlled cord traction following breaking of the cord
    - narrowing, elongation, or distortion of the lower uterine segment after child birth from intramural (e.g. uterine fibroid) or extramural (e.g. non-pregnant horn of a bicornuate uterus) compression
    - external pressure from a pelvic mass (e.g. distended urinary bladder)
    - lacerations of the genital tract—from the uterus down to the vagina
  - coagulapothy:
    - disseminated intravascular coagulation (e.g. severe pre-eclampsia, abruptio placentae)
    - consumptive coagulopathy resulting from the delayed, inadequate, or failure, of administration of blood product replacement in the management of postpartum haemorrhage.

Balloon tamponade can be used in almost any form of PPH, either as the primary surgical treatment or in conjunction with brace compression sutures. In PPH in which inadequate uterine contraction and retraction is a significant factor, or despite satisfactory uterine contraction, bleeding still continues from the placental bed or repaired lacerations, direct compression from within the uterus by a balloon device to produce a tamponade effect can often control the bleeding. In order for balloon tamponade to be effective, the uterus has to be able to contract in response to oxytocic stimulation, without or with the additional use of brace compression sutures on the uterus to prevent it from stretching. In the case of cervical pregnancy or cervical laceration in a non-pregnant uterus, direct compression of the bleeding site by balloon tamponade is often sufficient by itself to control the bleeding.

Aetiology
PPH is usually categorized into four major groups as follows:
- uterine atony (tone)
- retained products of conception (tissue)
- genital tract lacerations (trauma)
- coagulopathy (thrombin).

Sometimes, a combination of causes can be found. Irrespective of the underlying cause(s), ineffective and/or delayed treatment can lead to consumptive coagulopathy, so that even when the primary cause is eliminated, bleeding continues unless the coagulopathy can be corrected.

Risk factors for postpartum haemorrhage
- Abruptio placentae
- Placenta praevia
- Multiple pregnancy
- Pre-elcampsia
- Nulliparity
- Previous PPH
- Obesity
- Caesarean section
- Retained placenta
- Instrumental vaginal delivery
- Prolonged labour (>12 hours)
- Big baby (>4.0 kg)
- Vaginal lacerations and episiotomy
- Uterine fibroid.

Prognosis
Apart from mortality, PPH and its direct complications, together with the short- and long-term sequelae of various forms of treatment, can lead to serious maternal morbidity including end organ damage such as renal failure, Sheehan's syndrome, and the effects of hysterectomy. Balloon tamponade is a safe treatment modality without creating any lasting effects since its use is usually restricted to 24 hours and the balloon can be deflated and removed any time without causing additional trauma or residual harm to the patient. In tying the patient over the critical period, balloon tamponade not only can save lives but also provides the opportunity for other forms of treatment and full resuscitation. No significant side-effects have been reported in association with the use of balloon tamponade.

Advantages of using balloon tamponade
- Easy administration and removal.
- Can ascertain effectiveness quickly.
- Allows continual assessment of blood loss that is drained through the catheter lumen.
- Can reduce the need for hysterectomy and other surgical procedures via laparotomy.
- The success rate of balloon tamponade is generally high in the reported cases/series, varying from 70% to 100%, with an average rate of around 80%.

Clinical approach
Devices
The use of a number of devices has been reported, including devices 'borrowed' from other uses to purposely designed devices.

Sengstaken–Blakemore tube or Sengstaken–Blakemore oesophageal catheter
This is the most frequently reported device used for this purpose. Originally designed to stop bleeding from oesophageal varices, the Sengstaken–Blakemore (SB) tube consists of two balloons: a gastric and an oesophageal balloon. If a SB tube is used, the tip of the catheter distal to the gastric balloon is first cut off close to the gastric balloon to ensure a close fit. If a Sengstaken–Blakemore oesophageal catheter (SBOC) is used, the catheter distal to the oesophageal balloon is cut off before use. Then the anterior lip of the cervix is grasped with ring forceps and the portion of the catheter with the balloon(s) is then inserted through the cervix into the uterine cavity. If the SB tube is used, either the gastric or the oesophageal balloon can be inflated with normal saline with the aim to fill up the uterine cavity completely and compress against the uterus from within. Therefore, the volume can vary from as little as 50 ml in case of placenta accreta and a well-contracted uterus, to as much as 300 mL in an atonic uterus, until the uterus is firm on abdominal palpation and the bleeding has been arrested, or until the balloon dilates the cervix and becomes visible at the internal cervix. If no or minimal bleeding is observed the 'tamponade test' is considered positive and the device can be kept *in situ* using rolled gauze packed in the vagina. If bleeding cannot be controlled then further surgical treatment is required.

Bakri tamponade balloon
This is designed for temporary management of lower segment bleeding and is less effective in the presence of uterine anatomical anomalies. For transvaginal placement, the recommendation is to insert the balloon portion beyond the internal os and under ultrasound guidance. For transabdominal placement following Caesarean delivery, the recommendation is to pass the inflation port of the balloon via the uterine incision, and then the shaft is pulled out through the uterus, cervix, and finally into the vagina until the deflated balloon base is in contact with the internal cervical os. The uterine incision is closed, taking care to avoid puncturing the balloon. The balloon is then inflated with sterile water or normal saline according to the product label for maximum inflation volume. Gentle traction is applied to the balloon shaft to ensure proper contact between the balloon and tissue surface and tension can be maintained by securing the shaft to the inner aspect of the patient's thigh or to a weight not exceeding 500 g; or the balloon can be kept in place by vaginal packing.

Rüsch urological hydrostatic balloon
This is designed as a hydrostatic (bladder distension) catheter. For application the catheter is inserted through the cervical canal into the uterine cavity and the balloon is then distended with 250–300 mL of normal saline. The distal end of the catheter shaft is pulled out of the vagina to achieve tamponade effect.

Foley catheter
The principle and method of application of the Foley catheter is similar to that of the other balloon catheters. However, for the postpartum uterus, the balloon of a Foley catheter is usually too small to be effective, and the use of multiple Foleys is cumbersome without any guarantee of effectiveness even if the catheters are enclosed in an overbag. Blood collected inside the uterus cannot be drained when using an overbag and therefore further haemorrhage is concealed. Therefore the use of the Foley catheter should be considered only in the absence of the other devices.

Condom hydrostatic tamponade
This simply involves the use of a single condom tied to a catheter introduced into the uterine cavity and then inflated with 250–300 mL of normal saline until the bleeding is controlled. The proximal end of the catheter is then folded and tied with thread to keep the saline from escaping. Rolled gauze is then packed into the vagina to keep the inflated condom in place for 24–48 hours. The disadvantage of this device is that any further bleeding inside the uterus may remain undiagnosed until much later. In addition, condoms are not readily available in the delivery suite or operation theatre. However, in a primary care setting, this may be the only available means to control bleeding for the transfer of patients to a better equipped centre for further management.

Application
- The whole placenta, or the bulk of the placenta in case of placenta accreta, should have been removed first.
- The patient is placed in the lithotomy position in the operation theatre. General or regional anaesthesia is preferred, but not necessarily so, for this procedure, which can be performed under sedation and other forms of analgesia.
- A Foley catheter is placed in the bladder for continuous urinary drainage.
- The balloon portion of the catheter is then inserted through the cervix in case of vaginal delivery. In case of Caesarean delivery, the balloon portion is placed inside the uterine cavity under direct vision with the rest of the catheter and injection portal pushed into the vagina through the cervix and then led outside the vagina by an assistant. If the uterine incision has been closed already, the device can be introduced, as in the case following vaginal delivery, by an assistant, with the rest of the catheter and the injection portal led outside the vagina while the surgeon observes the progress. Further surgical treatment can be carried out immediately if the tamponade test fails.
- The balloon is inflated with warm normal saline, with the objective to completely fill up and compress against the uterine cavity or the site of bleeding. The volume is therefore variable according to the degree of uterine volume.
- The presence of bleeding from inside the uterus can be gauged from the amount of blood drained from the

drainage port of the catheter, which can be collected in a graduated bag connected to the opening of the catheter.

- The balloon and catheter is secured in place by means of gauze rolls soaked with iodine or antibiotic packed into the vaginal canal until there is no room for the catheter to move about. The packing should be performed gently so as to avoid superficial abrasion to the already oedematous or raw surface of the vagina and cervix. Excessive packing should be avoided so as to prevent excessive stretching and iatrogenic laceration to the tissues of the lower genital tract.
- After packing and stabilization of the balloon, the position of the uterine fundus and outline of the uterus should be traced with a marking pen on the abdominal wall (after closure of the abdomen first in case of Caesarean delivery) so as to identify changes in the uterine size and shape, which could reflect blood collection inside the uterus or the development of broad ligament haematoma, hence calling for further actions.
- The balloon should be kept for at least 12 hours, but not more than 24 hours. The pack and the balloon can be removed in phases, first the pack and then the balloon. For removal, the balloon should be deflated by aspiration of the contents followed by gentle withdrawal from the uterus. There is no need for swabbing the balloon for culture afterwards.
- In case of deterioration of vital signs, or evidence of continued and unabated bleeding, or features suspicious of an enlarging pelvic collection, tamponade treatment should be considered a failure and other measures should be undertaken.
- The findings and procedure should be clearly documented in the notes and the condition explained to the patient afterwards, especially in the case of placenta praevia and accreta, where placental fragments may be left behind.

Postoperative management

- Adequate and appropriate analgesia is necessary
- Prophylaxis for deep vein thrombosis should be undertaken. Initially physiotherapy and compression stockings can be prescribed. Anticoagulant therapy should be avoided for the initial 24–48 hours for obvious reasons. The patient should be encouraged to ambulate within 24 hours and to start walking around, with help if necessary, after the first day or removal of the balloon device. Anticoagulant therapy with prophylactic dose of unfractionated heparin or low molecular weight heparin should be commenced afterwards according to the protocol for the prophylaxis against postoperative thromboembolism.
- Bladder drainage with the Foley catheter should be maintained until the balloon is removed, and preferably until the sensation of the lower abdomen and perineum has returned (in case of epidural analgesia and patient controlled analgesia).
- Prophylactic antibiotic should be given, covering both aerobic and anaerobic organisms, and commencing with intravenous injection for the first 24–48 hours then continuing with oral treatment. If fragments of placental tissue remain inside the uterus, or if the Foley catheter is still required beyond the first 24 hours, or if there is any

suspicion of endometritis, antibiotic prophylaxis should be continued for 1 week or until the culture results are available, or until symptoms and signs of infection have completely subsided. Otherwise, the antibiotic treatment can be discontinued after 72 hours.

- Attention should be paid to maintain fluid balance, and to avoid fluid overload.
- Oral intake can be resumed gradually as for other postoperative patients. Constipation frequently occurs in the first few days. To avoid straining at defecation, stool softeners and bulk agents can be prescribed from the time oral intake is allowed until discharge from hospital.
- Before discharge, the patient should be warned about the potential problems, including infection and secondary postpartum haemorrhage, if fragments of placental tissue are left in situ. Early postnatal visit should be arranged to assess the condition. Further investigations including ultrasound assessment may be required. Follow-up visits should be arranged until return of menstruation. Sheehan syndrome may need to be excluded if there is prolonged amenorrhoea in the absence of breast feeding.

Further reading

ACOG Practice Bulletin: Clinical Management Guidelines for Obstetrician-Gynecologists Number 76, October 2006: postpartum hemorrhage. Obstet Gynecol 2006;108:1039–47.

Akhter S, Begum MR, Kabir J. Condom hydrostatic tamponade for massive postpartum hemorrhage. Int J Gynecol Obstet 2005;90:134–5.

Condous GS, Arulkumaran S, Symonds I, et al. The 'tamponade test' in the management of massive postpartum hemorrhage. Obstet Gynecol 2003;101:767–72.

Dabelea V, Schultze PM, McDuffie RS Jr. Intrauterine balloon tamponade in the management of postpartum hemorrhage. Am J Perinatol 2007;24:359–64.

Danso D, Reginald P. Combined B-Lynch suture with intrauterine balloon catheter triumphs over massive postpartum haemorrhage. Br J Obstet Gynaecol 2002;109:963.

Doumouchtsis SK, Papageorghiou AT, Vernier C, Arulkuraman S. Management of postpartum hemorrhage by uterine balloon tamponade: prospective evaluation of effectiveness. Acta Obstet Gynecol Scand 2008;87:849–55.

Ferrazzani S, Guariglia L, Triunfo S, et al. Successful treatment of post-cesarean hemorrhage related to placenta praevia using an intrauterine balloon. Two case reports. Fetal Diagn Ther 2006;21;277–80.

Frenzel D, Condous GS, Papageorghiou AT, McWhinney NA. The use of the 'tamponade test' to stop massive obstetric haemorrhage in placenta accrete. Br J Obstet Gynaecol 2005;112:676–7.

Fylstra D, Coffey MD. Treatment of cervical pregnancy with cerclage, curettage and balloon tamponade: a report of three cases. J Reprod Med 2001;46:71–4.

Johanson R, Kumar M, Obhrai M, Young P. Management of massive postpartum haemorrhage: use of a hydrostatic balloon catheter to avoid laparotomy. Br J Obstet Gynaecol 2001;108:420–2.

Okeahialam MG, Tuffnell DJ, O'Donovan P, Sapherson DA. Case report. Cervical pregnancy managed by suction evacuation and balloon tamponade. Eur J Obstet Gynecol Reprod Biol 1998;79:89–90.

Ramanathan G, Arulkumaran S. Postpartum haemorrhage. Curr Obstet Gynaecol 2006;16:6–13.

Royal College of Obstetricians and Gynaecologists (RCOG) *Placenta praevia and placenta praevia accrete.* Clinical Green top Guidelines. London: RCOG 2005.

Seror J, Allouche C, Elhaik S. Use of Sengstaken-Blakemore tube in massive postpartum hemorrhage: a series of 17 cases. Acta Obstet Gynecol Scand 2005;84:660–4.

Tattersall M, Braithwaite W. Balloon tamponade for vaginal lacerations causing severe postpartum haemorrhage. Br J Obstet Gynaecol 2007;114:647–8.

Internet resources

www.cookmedical.com

Patient information and contacts

www.rcog.org.uk

Caesarean section

Definition
Caesarean section (CS) refers to a form of operative delivery in which the infant is delivered through the abdomen via skin and uterine incisions.

Epidemiology
There is a progressive increase in the prevalence of CS worldwide. The increase in primary CS rates was attributable to a number of factors, including changes in practice and perceived benefits for the mother and infant, changes in maternal anthropometric characteristics such as older age, higher pre-pregnancy body mass index (BMI) and gestational weight gain, short stature, increased fetal size, the increased incidence of a scarred uterus, and the lower threshold for Caesarean versus other forms of operative vaginal delivery, especially in the presence of obstetric complications. The changing medicolegal climate also plays direct and indirect roles. In the USA, the overall rate for primary CS in 2002 was 25.8% and 13.3% for first child versus second child or later. The rate showed a progressive increase from 17.8% in women <20 years old to 52.4% in women >40 years old for the first child, and from 11.3% to 23.8% respectively for the second child and after. The changing maternal and fetal risk profiles means that there is no such thing as an ideal CS rate, and any target rate set must be realistic and reviewed periodically for appropriate adjustments.

Pathology
Maternal morbidity associated with CS increases with increasing number of CSs. There are direct and indirect maternal and perinatal morbidities, which could lead to mortality if overlooked or mismanaged.

Direct maternal morbidity
Compared with vaginal delivery, both elective and intrapartum CS are associated with increased risk of severe maternal morbidity. However, when compared with induction of labour at term, CS without labour was associated with less early postpartum haemorrhage and composite maternal morbidity, whereas the highest morbidity was found in the CS in labour group. The occurrence of serious or multiple morbidities may necessitate admission to the intensive care unit, and the rate for the first to the sixth or later CS was 1.85%, 0.57%, 0.54%, 1.58%, 1.94%, and 5.62% respectively. The rate of major complications was 4.3%, 7.5%, and 12.5% for the second, third, and fourth or more CS respectively. Overall, women with multiple CS have increased risk of excessive blood loss, dense adhesions, placenta accreta, and hysterectomy.

Infection
- Metritis and endometritis: the rate was shown to be highest in the first (5.98%) and sixth or later (6.74%) CS, but much lower for the second to fifth CS (1.55–2.96%)
- Wound infection: this is a common complication especially for emergency CS, and the rates varied from 1.53% for the first CS to 3.37% for the sixth or later CS.
- Septicaemia
- Chest infection.

Haemorrhage
- Uterine atony
- Uterine lacerations

- Poor surgical techniques
- Underlying pathologies, e.g. uterine fibroids.

Surgical trauma and injuries to neighbouring organs
- Bladder injury/cystotomy: the rates increase from 0.13%, 0.09%, 0.28%, 1.17%, 1.94%, to 4.49% respectively from the first to the sixth or later CS.
- Ureteric injury: the rates increase from 0.03%, 0.01%, 0.02%, 0.07%, 0.39% to 1.12% respectively from the first to the sixth or later CS.
- Bowel injury: the correlation with the number of CS is more variable, from 0.11%, 0.06%, 0.13%, 0.34%, 0%, to 1.12% respectively from the first to the sixth or later CS.
- Omental injury.

Hysterectomy
The risk is correlated with the number of CS, and the rate increases from 0.65%, 0.42%, 0.90%, 2.41%, 3.49% to 8.99% respectively from the first to the sixth or later CS, and the corresponding odds ratios from the second to the sixth or later CS were 0.7, 1.4, 3.8, 5.6 and 15.2 respectively.

Wound complications
- Haematoma
- Pain
- Dehiscence: the rate is generally low <0.5% with no correlation with the number of CS
- Granulation tissue/keloid formation
- Cosmetic problems.

Chest/respiratory complications
- Ventilator care: the rate was 1.0%, 0.21%, 0.24%, 0.69%, 0.78%, and 1.12% from the first to the sixth or later CS.
- Aspiration
- Pulmonary oedema

Anaesthetic complications
This is becoming rare with the improvement of anaesthetic techniques and new medications. The complications are generally related to the mode of anaesthesia.
- General anaesthesia: complications include aspiration, hypoxia due to wrong or failed intubation, hypertensive complications associated with intubation, and prolonged paralysis due to missed underlying medical conditions like myasthenia gravis.
- Regional anaesthesia: failure due to ineffective or partial block, dural tap in epidural anaesthesia, and haematoma. Rarely is there persistent pain at the needle insertion site. Extremely rarely is nerve injury.

Indirect maternal morbidity
Fluid overload
- Fluid loading for epidural anaesthesia
- Intravenous oxytocin infusion
- Intravenous infusion of other medications

Postpartum anaemia
Postpartum drop in haemoglobin is usually greater following CS than vaginal delivery due to the inevitably higher blood loss, and can be aggravated by factors that necessitated the CS in the first place, such as antepartum haemorrhage. The need for transfusion for ≥4 units was 1.05%,

0.48%, 0.77%, 1.59%, 2.33%, 10.11%, from the first to the sixth or later CS. The associated factors include
- effect of antepartum and intraoperative haemorrhage
- overlooked antenatal anaemia
- haemodilution due to excessive intravenous fluid administration
- underlying haemoglobinopathies
- wound haematoma: this should always be looked for in case of an inexplicable drop in postpartum haemoglobin.

Postoperative venous thromboembolism
The rates of deep vein thrombosis varied from 0.14–0.27% but it was shown to be as high as 1.12% at the sixth or later CS. The rates of pulmonary embolism varied between 0.08% and 0.39%; it was similarly shown to be increased to 1.12% at the sixth or later CS.

Constipation and intestinal obstruction
- Postoperative ileus is correlated with the number of CS, and increases from 0.66%, 0.45%, 0.68%, 0.90%, 1.55% to 3.37% respectively from the first to the sixth or later CS. The predisposing factors include
- intrapartum CS for failure to progress
- previous bowel adhesions
- postoperative immobilization.

Healing of the uterine incision
Union of the uterine incision occurs almost invariably, but the strength of the scar may be influenced by certain factors. Infection/endometritis and haematoma formation are thought to influence the strength adversely. The effect of the method of closure however remains unclear. Anatomically, there is a correlation between scar thickness determined ultrasonographically and clinically at CS. Since antepartum scar thickness correlates inversely with the risk of intrapartum rupture, it is possible to predict intrapartum rupture. The healing and strength between one- versus two-layer closure remains controversial. Although outcomes in vaginal birth after CS (VBAC), as well as the thickness of the scar up to 6 weeks postpartum, were reported to be equivalent between the two methods, one-layer closure was also reported to be associated with increase in uterine 'windows' at repeat CS, and increase the odds of rupture at VBAC. However, the true impact between these two methods on the outcome of subsequent pregnancies can only be regarded as inconclusive in view of the small sample sizes in these reports and the number of confounding factors that could not be taken into account.

Maternal mortality
Maternal death is consistently shown to be increased following CS, being four- to 10-fold greater than that following vaginal delivery. There was a correlation with the number of CS, being highest (0.19%) for the first CS and decreasing to 0.05–0.07% for the third and later CS.

Direct perinatal morbidity
Fetal/neonatal injuries occur in CS (overall incidence 1.1%), especially in intrapartum CS, and the rate for second stage (2.8%) was significantly higher than that for first stage (1.2%) operation. Difficult delivery of the neonate was associated with multiple CS.

Birth trauma due to manipulation (incidence per 1000)
- Cephalhaematoma (2.4)
- Fracture of clavicle (0.3) and long bones (0.2)
- Facial nerve palsy (0.3)

- Skull fracture (0.2)
- Brachial plexus injury (0.2)
- Intracranial haemorrhage (0.1)
- Internal organ injuries (very rare)
- Bruising and ecchymosis.

Surgical injuries (incidence per 1000)
- Skin lacerations (7.3)
- Surgical incisions on limbs, face, scalp, and buttocks requiring treatment (rare).

Indirect perinatal morbidity
Iatrogenic prematurity
- Misdiagnosis of fetal growth restriction
- Elective procedure for recurrent indications but with wrong dates
- Underlying fetal anomalies.

Respiratory complications
- Hyaline membrane disease/respiratory distress syndrome—the rate was increased from 0.16% to 0.47% in the vaginal versus CS groups (OR 3.0), and to 0.2% in the elective CS group (not significant).
- Transient tachypnoea of newborn—the rate was increased from 1.1% for vaginal deliveries to 3.5% for all CS, and 3.1% for elective CS (OR 3.3 and 2.8 respectively).
- Persistent pulmonary hypertension—the rate was increased from 0.08% for vaginal delivery, to 0.4% and 0.37% for total and elective CS (OR 4.9 and 4.6 respectively).

Breastfeeding and weight loss
- CS is one of the factors in delayed onset of lactation (>72 hours), which in turn contributes to excess neonatal weight loss.

Factors affecting likelihood of adverse maternal and perinatal outcomes
- Maternal obesity: adverse perinatal outcome is increased with increasing maternal BMI, which also increases the difficulty of the operation and the risk of most peri- and postoperative complications.
- Timing of operation: elective CS before labour is associated with the lowest maternal and perinatal risks, especially in high-risk cases where adequate preparations can be undertaken to prevent complications. The incidence of fetal injury was 0.5% for elective repeat CS. For intrapartum CS, maternal and neonatal morbidity is increased in the second compared with first stage CS, including uterine atony, uterine incision extension, cystotomy, and neonatal injury.
- Indications for CS: most indications were associated with a low rate of fetal injury between 0.7% and 1.5%. The exception is failed instrumental delivery (ventouse or forceps), both for primary CS (6.9%), and for CS for failed VBAC (1.7%).
- Type of uterine incision: the incidences of fetal injury for 'T' or 'J' incision, vertical incision, and low transverse incision were 3.4%, 1.4%, and 1.1% respectively.
- Speed of the delivery: among neonates with injuries, the rate was correlated with the skin incision to delivery interval. The rate of injury decreased from 1.9% for an interval of ≤3 minutes, to around 1.0% for intervals of 6 minutes or more.

• Decision–incision interval: one study revealed that 65% of the primary emergency CS began within 30 minutes of the decision to operate. Maternal morbidity was not related to this factor, but neonatal compromise in the form of umbilical arterial pH <7.0 and intubation in the delivery room was significantly more common (4.8% versus 1.6%, and 3.1% versus 1.3% respectively) in cases where the interval was ≤30 minutes compared with >30 minutes. This may be related to the indication for CS.

Aetiology

A number of conditions are associated with increased likelihood of CS for medical reasons. There are a number of general conditions such as anthropometric parameters that are associated with, and on occasions become indications for, CS. These conditions probably act as surrogates for other underlying conditions. There are some factors which have been utilized as predictors of CS, but which by themselves are not true indications. Indications should be reserved to describe specific conditions in which the maternal and/or fetal risks are so significantly increased that vaginal birth is not an acceptable option.

Factors associated with increased risk of CS

Maternal weight, BMI, and obesity
A significant linear association between maternal BMI and risk of CS has been demonstrated, with the leanest mothers having the highest rate of vaginal delivery, while CS rates increased with increasing BMI, being highest in the morbidly obese, when confounding factors such as gestational diabetes, delivery ≥37 weeks, maternal height <150 cm, primiparity, and maternal age ≥35 years were controlled for.

Maternal age
The incidence of CS is correlated with maternal age in both nulliparous and multiparous women. This relationship disappears after adjustment for obstetric predictors and risk factors only in multiparous women. Patients' preference and obstetricians' practice could be important determinants, as the acceptable levels of risk, the threshold for intervention, and the trade-offs involved in the decision could well be influenced by maternal age, which serves as a surrogate for factors such as the type of conception, previous fertility history, and the likelihood of future pregnancies.

Maternal stature
In general, maternal stature is inversely correlated with the likelihood of CS, but there is no universal definition of short stature or consensus on a certain height measurement below which CS is absolutely warranted.

Past obstetrical and gynaecological history
There are several aspects that impact on the risk of CS in the current pregnancy.
• Presence of uterine scar—a previous myomectomy or hysterotomy scar is thought to increase significantly the risk of uterine rupture in subsequent pregnancies, especially if the scar involves the whole thickness of the uterine wall and if labour is allowed.
• Previous Caesarean delivery (see Prognosis)
• Poor obstetrical history: in the absence of any definite complication in the current pregnancy, a reduced threshold, or an excuse, for intervention rather than any genuine medically proven mechanism, is likely to be the underlying reason.

• History of infertility: the attitude towards, and the perception and acceptability of risk in the patient and /or obstetrician probably play greater roles than any genuine medical reasons.

Conception through fertility treatment
A number of factors usually interact in the individual patient, including past medical history, maternal age and anthropometrical factors. There is also increased risk of obstetrical complications associated with IVF pregnancies, so that overall, IVF pregnancies especially are associated with increased risk of CS.

Predictors of CS
These are factors that do not constitute indications for CS per se, but which are associated with higher risk of CS through certain mechanisms, such as malposition and cephalopelvic disproportion, that play a common yet variable role according to the individual patient. These apply more to induced than to spontaneous labour, especially in the situations of prelabour rupture of the membranes and prolonged latent phase.
• Nulliparity
• First stage >12 hours
• Epidural analgesia
• Clinical chorioamnionitis
• Internal fetal monitoring
• Fetal weight ≥4000 g
• Labour induction
• Labour augmentation with oxytocin
• Advanced maternal age (≥35 years)
• Latent phase ≥12 hours
• Meconium-stained liquor.

Indications for CS
Maternal (relative rather than absolute)
• Uterine anomalies
• Uterine fibroids
• Uterine scars
• Contracted/deformed pelvis
• Cardiorespiratory complications
• Severe hypertension
• Neurological conditions
• Previous pelvic trauma/anal sphincter damage
• Cervical factors.

Maternal benefits of CS
The main benefit is the prevention of deterioration in the physical condition or development of complications that are attributable to the physical stress of the labour and delivery process. The rationale behind performing CS for preserving/protecting sexual function and health through the avoidance of perineal/vaginal trauma and scarring is questionable in the absence of previous third/fourth-degree tear. Although there is some evidence that there is a protective effect in the first 3 months postpartum, there is little evidence to support any long-term difference or benefits of CS in this aspect.

Fetal/neonatal
• Cephalopelvic and fetopelvic disproportion.
• Congenital anomalies.
• Malpresentation and abnormal fetal lie: abnormal fetal lie such as transverse and oblique lie, and compound and brow presentation are absolute indications for CS.

Although CS for breech presentation has been controversial, current evidence is in favour of planned CS in breech presentation for better perinatal and neonatal outcomes.

- Impaired placental function and fetal growth restriction: a small fetus is by no means an indication for CS, since there is reduced risk of disproportion. However, for suspected fetal growth restriction with evidence of placental insufficiency, such as absent/reversed umbilical end diastolic flow, the fetus is most unlikely to be able to tolerate the stress of labour and vaginal delivery.
- Placenta praevia: even for minor praevia, if there is any obstruction to the descend/engagement of the fetal head, CS should be performed.
- Fetal distress/hypoxia/compromise
- Multifetal pregnancy.

Fetal/neonatal benefits of Caesarean section

In infants born to nulliparous women, the risk of intracranial haemorrhage is higher among those delivered by ventouse extraction (OR 2.7), forceps delivery (OR 3.4), and intrapartum Caesarean section (OR 2.5), with no significant difference among these three groups when compared with infants delivered spontaneously. However, the risk among infants delivered by CS before labour was not higher. This suggested that abnormal labour is the common risk factor for intracranial haemorrhage. Overall risk in breech presentation and risk of intrapartum fetal death in cephalic presentation are reduced by CS.

Prognosis

Maternal and infant wellbeing

Elective CS was shown to be associated with a significantly lower rate of maternal and fetal complications than vaginal birth. Birth experience, as assessed by the Salmon Test, was significantly better in elective CS than vaginal delivery, but was worse in women with emergency CS and worst in women with vacuum delivery. For the next pregnancy, 83.5%, 74.3%, 66%, and 30.1% respectively would choose the same mode of birth for vaginal, elective CS, medically indicated CS, and emergency CS.

Pelvic structures and function

Urinary incontinence

When compared with nulliparous women, women with previous CS have increased risk of stress or mixed type of urinary incontinence (adjusted OR 1.5 for any incontinence, 1.4 for moderate or severe incontinence). However, compared with CS, vaginal delivery is associated with further increase in urinary incontinence (adjusted OR 1.7 for any incontinence and 2.2 for moderate or severe incontinence).

Faecal incontinence

At 6 years after their first delivery, women who had CS, or those who had exclusive CS, showed less risk of persistent faecal incontinence than women who had spontaneous vaginal delivery.

Sexual function and health

CS is thought to protect sexual health after childbirth by avoiding perineal trauma. A study in primiparous women revealed that when compared with vaginal delivery, CS was protective against dyspareunia-related symptoms, but only for the first 3 months after delivery. At 6 months, there were no significant differences in dyspareunia-related symptoms, sexual response-related symptoms, and postcoital problems.

Future fertility

There are few data regarding the effect of one previous CS on subsequent fertility, but there is no evidence to suggest that the uterine scar impacts on the chances of subsequent conception. There is however increased risk of miscarriage and ectopic pregnancy.

Future pregnancy outcome

Pregnancy complications

- Stillbirth: it has been reported that women who had a previous CS have increased risk of a subsequent unexplained antepartum stillbirth, but this association could not be proven in a subsequent study.
- Placenta praevia: this risk is highly correlated with parity and the number of previous CS, and the rate increases from 1.33%, 1.14%, 2.27%, 2.33%, and 3.37% after the first to the sixth or later CS. In general, the risk for placenta praevia in the second pregnancy after a previous CS was 1.17 to 1.5, and 1.7 if the second pregnancy was within 1 year after the CS.
- Placental abruption: the rate of abruption after one previous CS was 0.95% versus 0.74% in women with a vaginal delivery, and the risk for abruption after one or two consecutive CS was 1.3–1.4. The risk for a second pregnancy within 1 year after a CS was 1.5.
- Placenta accreta/increta/percreta: the incidence of placenta accreta increased progressively from the second to the sixth or later CS, being 0.31%, 0.57%, 2.13%, 2.33%, and 6.74% respectively, and the odds ratio was 1.3, 2.4, 9.0, 9.8, and 29.8 respectively. The occurrence of placenta accreta was influenced by the coexistence of placenta praevia. The rates for the second to the sixth or later CS with and without placenta praevia were 11%, 40%, 61%, 67%, and 67%, versus 0.2%, 0.1%, 0.8%, 0.8% and 4.7%, respectively. The presence of placenta accreta increased comorbidities that included injury to other pelvic organs, thromboembolic complications, and intensive care unit admission.
- Scar dehiscence/uterine rupture: the overall rate of symptomatic rupture was 0.7%, and the rates of rupture were reported to be 1.5% versus 0.5% versus 0.3% in women without vaginal birth versus vaginal birth prior to CS versus prior VBAC. The rate of uterine rupture in VBAC was similar between women with multiple or single prior CS, being 0.9% and 0.7% respectively. One study found that for spontaneous labour, the rupture rate was 0.5% before and 1.0% after 40 weeks, while the corresponding figures for induced labour were 2.1% and 2.6% respectively. In contrast another study reported that the rupture rate increased significantly from 0.4% before to 2.1% after 40 weeks for spontaneous labour, without any corresponding increase in the rate of CS, or maternal and perinatal morbidity.

Labour and trial of scar (VBAC)

- Effect of previous vaginal deliveries: previous vaginal delivery and VBAC are associated with higher rates of successful VBAC in the index pregnancy. One study found that the success rates were 70.1%, 81.8% and 93.1% in women with no vaginal delivery, one vaginal delivery before the previous CS, and a prior VBAC respectively, whereas the rates of third/fourth degree tears and operative vaginal deliveries were 8.5%, 2.5% and 3.7%, and 14.7%, 5.6% and 1.9% respectively.

- Number of previous CS: although some reports suggested that VBAC can be an option in women with two previous CS, most obstetricians have reservations due to the higher rates of complications and morbidity.
- Maternal BMI: in general, the success rate of VBAC diminishes with increasing BMI, from 83.1% in the underweight to 68.2% in the obese categories, and obese women have half the likelihood (OR 0.53) compared with underweight women. As well, there is increased risks of uterine rupture/scar dehiscence, composite maternal morbidity, and neonatal injury.
- Induced labour: this increases the early postpartum haemorrhage (OR 1.66), CS (OR 1.84), and NICU admission for the neonate (OR 1.69). The limited literature also suggested that using prostaglandin analogues like misoprostol for labour induction increased significantly the risk of uterine rupture (9.7%).

Gestational age at VBAC: it was reported that the rate of CS increased significantly from 25% to 33.5% and from 33.8% to 43% before and after 40 weeks for spontaneous and induced labour respectively. Another study showed no significant difference in the CS rates for spontaneous labour before (34.1%) and after (40.4%) 40 weeks, but labour induction increased these figures significantly to 64.6% and 52% respectively. In general, the success rate for VBAC was not increased in spontaneous labour after 40 weeks compared with induced labour before 40 weeks, so that the advantage of awaiting for spontaneous labour to occur after 40 weeks is really to avoid induction, which may increase the risk of uterine rupture.

- Other outcomes: there is increased risks of endometritis (2.9% versus 1.8%) and blood transfusion (1.7% versus 1.0%), but the greater risk is one of neonatal hypoxic-ischaemic encephalopathy (0.08% versus 0%), the majority of which was related to uterine rupture, when compared with repeat elective CS. As for the type of previous uterine incision, the limited literature suggested that a prior lower segment vertical incision is similar to a transverse incision with respect to maternal perinatal safety and the likelihood of successful outcome.

Repeat CS

The difficulties in repeat CS are related to the number of previous CS, and the incidences of complications are correlated with the number of previous operations. Multiple prior CS was associated with increased rates of hysterectomy (0.6% versus 0.2%), transfusion (3.2% versus 1.6%), and overall maternal morbidity (OR 1.41)

Preterm (<37 weeks) birth in repeat CS

There was increased risk of preterm birth after the first CS, the rate from the second to the sixth or later CS was 14.6%, 12.8%, 16.7%, 19.1%, and 31.8% respectively.

Clinical approach

General approach

The general principles that apply to all surgical procedures also apply here, such as aseptic technique, minimal and gentle tissue handling, good haemostasis, avoiding excess suture material, eradication of dead space, appropriate tension and proper apposition, avoiding strangulation of tissue, and avoiding the introduction of talc powder or other foreign material into the wound.

Decision to delivery interval

For emergency CS, the decision-to-delivery interval should be clearly recorded. The generally acceptable interval is <30 minutes. In one study, the decision-to-incision times of more than 30 minutes could be found in 35% of the cases of emergency primary CS, mostly for non-reassuring fetal heart rate tracings, but this was not associated with neonatal compromise in 95% of the infants. However, the basic rule is that the interval should be as short as possible without compromising maternal safety. Obviously for critical situations such as suspected placental abruption or uterine rupture, the aim is for prompt delivery before the fetus has suffered from significant hypoxic injuries.

Anaesthesia

General anaesthesia (GA) was the norm for CS, but regional anaesthesia (RA) is becoming more popular and acceptable due to its effectiveness and greater safety for both mother and infant. The incidence of GA and RA varies in different centres, but in centres where both are available, RA is usually administered to 80–90% of the cases, with spinal anaesthesia being preferred to epidural anaesthesia due to the former's quicker onset of action and minimal side-effects. The failure rate of RA is generally low (around 3%), and is related to increased maternal size, preoperative risk, rapid decision–incision interval, and intrapartum CS. In general, women with the greatest preoperative risk were sevenfold more likely to receive GA. While anaesthetists are responsible for obtaining the patient's consent for anaesthesia, the operator should have a clear picture of the local anaesthetic practice for a better collaboration between the two services, especially for high risk-patients in whom special considerations such as intrapartum fluid restriction, use of anticoagulants, bleeding tendency, control of blood pressure, etc., have to be discussed and finalized beforehand.

Prevention of infection

Infectious morbidity is a major concern, since this factor cannot be easily controlled or prevented by the operator. The measures that have been examined or recommended are as follows.

Skin preparation

The most commonly used preparation for skin scrub is povidone-iodine scrub (7.5%) or solution (10%). Another preparation is parachlorometaxylenol. No significant difference in the effect was shown between these preparations.

Vaginal preparation

Preoperative vaginal scrub with povidone-iodine decreases the risk of postoperative endometritis (OR 0.44), but there is no effect on the overall risk of postoperative pyrexia or wound infection.

Antibiotic solution

This can be used for irrigation of the pelvis and subcutaneous tissue at the time of uterine and fascial closure, and this has been reported to reduce significantly the incidence of endometritis.

Preparations

The patient should be placed on the table at a lateral tilt of about 15° to avoid supine hypotension. The arms should be placed on boards set at almost right angles to the body to facilitate intravenous access. The bladder should be catheterized with a Foley catheter, which is then secured to the inner aspect of the left thigh and connected to a graduated urine bag, before skin preparation. It should be confirmed that urine is free flowing into the urine bag, and that the catheter should not be pulled taut or the balloon could traumatize the bladder neck and urethra. Prior shaving of the pubic hair is controversial and objected by some, but excessive hair above the mons pubis can easily get into the wound and interfere with the application of the dressing, and trimming of the hair to skin level may be preferred on an individual basis. The incision site should be cleansed with povidone-iodine or chlorhexidine gluconate, commencing from the intended line of incision and moving outwards to cover the entire lower abdomen up to the level of the umbilicus. Disposable drapes with an adhesive film and fluid collection pouch spreading is preferred if available. Otherwise, sterile towels/drapes should be applied to create two layers secured together with towel clips and exposing only the immediate site of the incision. The suction catheter and its connection, as well as the diathermy pen and its connection, should be tested to be functioning before the commencement of the operation. In case of regional anaesthesia, skin sensation in the lower abdomen must be tested before the scalpel is applied to the skin.

Skin incision

The standard incision is either a vertical or a suprapubic/lower abdomen transverse incision.

Vertical incision

This is a subumbilical midline incision the length of which should be related to the estimated size of the fetal head and the thickness of the abdominal wall. Although the incision may be extended upwards if more room is needed later, this is usually unnecessary if the aforementioned factors are taken in consideration, unless there are major complications. This incision is supposed to be easier with a faster speed of abdominal entry and causes less bleeding, but there is a greater risk of postoperative wound dehiscence and later incisional hernia. Burst abdomen may also occur, mostly in patients with repeated vertical incisions and thin abdominal wall/rectus muscle or previous incision hernia. The scar is less cosmetically acceptable especially in individuals prone to keloid formation.

Following the cutting of the skin, one can open up the linea alba or move laterally to open up the right (for a right-handed surgeon standing on the patient's right side) rectus sheath. The muscle is reflected laterally to allow access of the posterior sheath, which is then opened allowing access to the peritoneum. Any torn and bleeding perforating vessels should be cauterized. The peritoneum should be lifted up with artery forceps to ensure there is a window without any bowels adhering to the intended site of peritoneal entry. The peritoneum is then incised with scalpel and the opening enlarged with fingers, taking care to look and feel for any structures that may be adhering to the peritoneum, which should be avoided. Abdominal packing is indicated only if the bowel loops are protruding and getting into the surgical field, or to correct for dextro-rotation or to stabilize the uterus during preterm delivery or delivery of a very growth restricted fetus. In case of chorioamnionitis or meconium-stained amniotic fluid, packing may prevent spillage of the liquor into the abdominal cavity. Nevertheless, the routine placement of abdominal packs can cause problems including trauma to the bowel and the uterine appendages, especially in the presence of pelvic/abdominal adhesions. For most CS performed at term, the gravid uterus usually will be closely

apposed to the abdominal incision and fill up any space in between so that packing is not necessary or may even be difficult.

For a repeat vertical incision, it is preferable to incise along the previous scar, removing the keloid in the process. The procedure is similar to the aforementioned except that during the sharp dissection along the rectus sheath, care must be exercised to look for and avoid cutting right through to any adherent tissue below, which may be bowel loops, the gravid uterus, or omentum. Locate a window and open this up using artery forceps and scalpel, enlarging it by stretching with the index fingers, and then with scissors if necessary and only after exclusion of adherent organs. Look for the window as close to the umbilicus as possible to avoid opening into the adherent and stretched bladder instead, since it is not possible to know in advance whether the bladder is pulled upwards underneath the rectus sheath. Adhesions should be freed by sharp and blunt dissection and bleeding vessels transfixed with stitches. Diathermy should be avoided as far as possible.

Lower transverse skin incisions

The advantage of this type of incision is that it is adequate for the great majority of CS (but this is obviously dependent on the surgeon's skills and experience), is cosmetically more acceptable, and is associated with less pain especially during ambulation in the first few days after delivery. Furthermore, there is minimal chance of incisional hernia and of burst abdomen. The types of incisions are described below.

- Pfannenstiel incision: this is the classical skin incision. It is a crescent-shaped suprapubic incision at/above the pubic hairline (or at two fingers' breadths above the pubic symphysis) and curving slightly upwards at both ends towards the anterior superior iliac spines, and ideally placed along a natural fold of skin. The length should be assessed as adequate to allow easy passage of the fetal head. The dissection is carried through the subcutaneous tissue to the rectus sheath, which is incised transversely, and the incision is extended laterally with the fascial edges elevated under tension with toothed clamps to allow sharp and blunt dissection of the underlying muscles. The rectus muscles are separated in the midline with blunt dissection. Any bleeding vessels are electrocoagulated. The peritoneum is opened in the midline with sharp dissection and then extended longitudinally to expose the intraperitoneal contents.

- Joel Cohen incision: this is a straight horizontal incision placed at a higher level (3 cm above the pubic symphysis). The subcutaneous tissue and rectus sheath are opened only for about 3 cm in the midline, and the rectus sheath incision is extended laterally and separated from the muscles with blunt dissection using fingers. The rectus muscles are separated in the midline by stretching caudally and cranially with the index fingers, and then the muscles, fascia, and subcutaneous tissues are pulled gently and evenly to both sides by means of the index and middle fingers of the operator and assistant to create an appropriately sized orifice that will allow the head to be delivered. The peritoneum is similarly opened by means of stretching longitudinally with the fingers. The advantages of this approach is that it is restrictive in the use of sharp dissection and respect the anatomical structures with minimal tissue trauma and quicker postoperative recovery, less febrile reaction, less bleeding in the abdominal wall, less need for antibiotics and analgesics, fewer peritoneal adhesions and less scarring, and earlier return of bowel function. It is also quicker and suitable for emergency CS. This method is also known as the Misgav Ladach method, and is endorsed as the incision of choice by NICE.

- In practice, an approach combining the best of both methods or slight modifications can be applied depending on the circumstances. The Joel Cohen skin incision could create an unsightly guttering effect in an erect posture especially in women with certain amount of abdominal subcutaneous fat.

Uterine incision

Classical

This is seldom used but may be necessary for abnormal lie and presentation, especially in relation to a major placenta praevia or lower segment uterine fibroid(s) that displaces the fetus upwards towards the fundus, or fetal problems such as a large tumour that causes fetal malpresentation and abnormal lie. In the case of placenta praevia with suspected placenta accreta, this approach can avoid disturbing the placenta which is left in situ to be dealt with by uterine artery embolization and/or methotrexate treatment. In this way, excessive bleeding and potential hysterectomy with risk of injury to the lower urinary tract can be avoided. This is a vertical incision in the upper segment, preferably made along the midline, the length of which depends on the fetal size and indication. The incision can sometime extend spontaneously with manipulation at delivery; therefore, avoid making the initial incision up to the fundus.

Lower segment transverse

Also known as Kerr's incision, the uterovesical fold of peritoneum is opened with sharp dissection and the bladder is pushed downwards gentle to expose the lower segment of the uterus. Sharp dissection may be necessary if there are adhesions. A 2–3-cm curvilinear incision is made in the midline of the exposed lower segment about 2–3-cm below the peritoneal reflection, avoiding the rupturing of the membranes so that the amniotic fluid will not be drained before the infant is delivered. The incision is extended laterally with gentle traction using the index fingers hooked below the uterine wall and avoiding extension to the broad ligaments.

Lower segment vertical

Also known as DeLee's incision, a similar-sized incision is made at the same spot but in a longitudinal manner, and the orifice is enlarged by stretching of the two sides laterally with the index fingers, carefully avoiding the lower end extending into the cervix and vagina.

Extension of the initial incision

This may be necessary in the case of a poorly formed lower segment or for the delivery of a preterm infant especially with malpresentation. A J-extension to the lower segment incision is, usually from the end of the incision on the side opposite to that of the operator and extending towards the upper segment, or a U-extension at both ends may be necessary to enlarge the incision to create more room for the manipulation and delivery of the infant. This can be done with a pair of heavy curved scissors. Never direct an extension downwards towards the cervix and bladder. Inverted T-extension should be avoided unless there is no amniotic fluid and/or the infant is stuck with transverse lie/compound presentation.

Delivery of the fetus in singleton pregnancy

Cephalic presentation

The position and degree of flexion of the fetal head should be determined preferably before cutting the membranes, and the subsequent steps should be decided before the fingers are inserted into the uterus. Once the membranes are cut, try to insert the fingers of the right hand alongside the fetal head/face to below the vertex and rotating the head to an occipital anterior position simultaneous with upward traction and correction of any asynclitism and deflexion. For a high head, low cavity forceps with no/minimal pelvic curve should be used to deliver the head. This is followed by the rest of the trunk but avoid hasty delivery of the shoulders especially for a macrosomic infant, as extensive tearing of the angles of the Kerr's incision, especially into the broad ligament and/or downwards towards the cervix and bladder, can occur with disastrous consequence.

Breech presentation

The type of breech and position of the sacrum should be determined before attempted manipulations, and similar manoeuvres to those for vaginal delivery are used. Avoid excessive pressure applied to the body or the limbs during traction/rotation, as injury to the internal organs and fractures of the limb bones are known complications. Forceps can similarly be used for delivery of the after-coming head.

Transverse/oblique lie

It is most important to avoid cutting the membranes and draining the amniotic fluid if abnormal lie is known before the uterine incision. The author's preference is to perform external podalic version first, then ask the assistant to stabilise the fetus and apply fundal pressure to bring the fetal limbs to the level of the uterine incision, preferably into the fetal sac that is already bulging out, before cutting the membranes with a toothed clamp held by the left hand. The right hand is inserted immediately into the hole to grasp the legs/feet, and the infant is delivered as for breech extraction with the help of fundal pressure by the assistant and before most of the amniotic fluid is drained. In case external podalic version fails, then internal podalic version is performed immediately after cutting the membranes. The importance of help by the assistant in turning and stabilizing the fetus during the process cannot be overemphasized, and the operator should brief the assistant thoroughly and provide the appropriate instructions at the right time. External cephalic version often does not work here, because the actual space within the uterine cavity is usually diminished due to decreased volume of the intrauterine fetal sac from the herniation through the uterine incision, even if the membranes remain intact. The author has encountered a number of occasions when the fetus remained stuck in transverse lie or developed compound presented when the membranes are cut following external cephalic version, as the fetal head is not low enough to act as a stopper to prevent most of the amniotic fluid from gushing out under pressure as soon as the membranes are cut.

Obstruction to delivery

Occasionally there is obstruction to delivery due to an extended limb, an umbilical cord that is extremely short thus causing the malpresentation or cord encirclement of the neck or limbs, or unsuspected submucosal fibroids. In case of difficulty in the delivery, a quick exploration of the fetal parts/posture and environment should be done, and the situation amended immediately by the appropriate manoeuvre. The cord may need to be clamped and cut before the infant can be delivered.

Delivery of the fetuses in multifetal pregnancy

Twins with cephalic/cephalic presentation

This is done as for singleton pregnancy with cephalic presentation, but the first twin to be delivered should be the one closer to the uterine incision, who is not necessarily the presenting twin by vaginal examination.

Twins with cephalic/breech presentation

The cepphalic-presenting twin should be delivered first, for locked twins can still occur if the breech-presenting twin is delivered first as there is no means of manipulating the breech-presenting twin if the head is obstructed by the body or head of the remaining twin. Under no circumstance should the sac of the remaining twin be cut in an attempt to free the stuck first twin, for this will only create more difficulty with the fetal parts of both twins entangled and locked together. If the breech-presenting twin is closer to the uterine incision if it is easy it should be pushed up and out of the way by the operator, and kept in place by the assistant, before the operator proceeds to deliver the cephalic-presenting twin.

Twins with breech/breech presentation

In this situation, the procedure is similar to that in delivering twins with cephalic–cephalic presentation, with the one closer to the incision to be delivered first. The second twin can be pushed out of the way until after the first twin is delivered.

Monoamniotic twins

The situation depends on the presentation and follows the aforementioned principles. The cord of the first twin may need to be clamped and divided before the infant is out of the uterus as the cords are often intertwined. Since there is only one sac, the amniotic fluid will be drained out quickly and there should be minimal delay in the delivery of the second twin.

Higher order multifetal pregnancy

Before the uterine incision is made, the fetuses should be carefully palpated to ascertain their lies and positions. Prior ultrasound assessment may not be helpful since the order of presentation relative to the uterine incision may not be the same as that at the time of the scan. Again, deliver the fetus closest to the uterine incision first. Then examine the remaining sacs to determine which fetus should be next. The sac closest to the incision should be the next fetus to be delivered and this is again facilitated by manipulating the remaining fetus(es) out of the way. This process is repeated until all the fetuses are delivered.

Delivery of the placenta

Cord traction following spontaneous separation

This is similar to the controlled cord traction following vaginal delivery.

Manual removal

This is similar to the manual removal method after vaginal delivery. Manual removal is associated with more operative blood loss, a greater drop in postoperative haemoglobin, and shorter operative time, but there is no difference in the incidence of endometritis, wound infection or need for blood transfusion.

Exploration of the uterus

After the delivery of the placenta, the uterine cavity should always be explored digitally to ensure that no placental tissue is left behind, especially in the case of marginal or velamentous insertion of the cord, or in multifetal pregnancy. If morbidly adherent placental tissue is encountered, treatment options depend on the site and size of the adherent tissue, the degree of bleeding, and uterine contraction. Small irregular fragments or a rough placental bed can be left alone if bleeding is minimal, especially if the uterus is contracting well. Large pieces of tissue, especially in the lower segment, have to be dealt with either locally by means of figure-of-eight sutures, or compression sutures with/without the addition of balloon tamponade (see relevant sections) after attempted removal of the bulk of the adherent tissue. Overzealous digital evacuation of adherent tissue, especially at the sites of scars of previous surgery, should be avoided since it may result in accidental perforation, or attenuation of the wall leaving only the serosa.

Repair of the uterus

- Uncomplicated lower segment incision: traditionally the lower segment incision is closed in two layers with absorbable synthetic sutures after the angles of the incision are first secured. The first layer should be a continuous non-locking suture involving at least two-thirds of the thickness of the myometrium from the decidual side but including as little decidua as possible. This layer of suture should be able to stop bleeding from myometrial vessels into the uterine cavity, the diagnosis of which may be delayed until the time of the vaginal examination after the operation. The second layer should be a continuous imbricating suture that includes the rest of the myometrium up to the serosa level, with the aim of proper closure of the incision and assurance of haemostasis, especially of the vessels that develop around previous uterine incision scars. A single layer closure should be reserved for totally uncomplicated cases or in the context of trials.

- Classical incision: a three-layer closure is preferred. The first layer should be interrupted stay sutures that include the angles and are placed about 1–1.5 cm apart, involving the inner half of the myometrial layer, and which is used to hold together the cut edges of the uterus. These are left untied until after the second continuous layer is inserted, which involves most of the myometrial layer. The first layer is sutured with the help of pressure from both sides provided by the assistant. The suture of the second layer is then tightened to take up the slack as the uterus usually has contracted somewhat by this time so that the second layer suture will be lax. The second layer is tied at both ends to achieve haemostasis. The third layer is a continuous imbricating suture that closes the remaining myometrium and serosa for final haemostasis.

- Tears in the upper or lower flap: a two-layer closure with continuous sutures is recommended. The apex of the tear must be identified and secured before most of the thickness of the tear is closed with the first layer. The second layer ensures proper closure and complete haemostasis. The repair should not extend into the incision proper or it can lead to distortion and impaired healing of the incision.

- Tears at the angles: it is important to stop any bleeding with haemostatic clamps first and then inspect the tear and the neighbouring structures, especially looking out for the ureters, before repair. Sharp dissection to mobilise the ureter out of harms way may be necessary. The tear should be repaired by figure-of-eight sutures placed at the exact site, and avoid over-repair with excessive sutures or including too much neighbouring tissue, as tying of the suture may pull the neighbouring tissue together and lead to kinking of the ureter and obstruction.

- Placental bed: bleeding vessels from the placental site can be tackled by figure-of-eight sutures, especially in the case of placenta praevia. Failure to achieve haemostasis may result in uncontrollable postpartum haemorrhage necessitating hysterectomy or uterine artery embolization.

Caesarean myomectomy

The traditional teaching is against myomectomy at the time of CS. However, myomectomy may be necessary because the fibroid(s) may cause significant distortion of the uterus and/or the uterine incision so that closure becomes difficult or that the union would not be expected to be satisfactory. Fibroids may also produce a ball-valve effect causing obstruction to the discharge of lochia, or interfere with uterine contraction resulting in persistent haemorrhage. Apart from anecdotal cases, a retrospective case–control study of 47 pregnancies with Caesarean myomectomy compared with 94 pregnancies without removal of the fibroids demonstrated that there was no need for hysterectomy, and no difference in the puerperal complications, postoperative haemoglobin, need for transfusion, or prolonged hospitalization in the myomectomy group, despite the fact that the myoma diameter in this group was significantly larger (7.9 cm versus 5.9 cm), and that 22.0% and 29.5% of the removed myomas were multiple and intramural/submucosal respectively.

EXIT procedure

The *ex utero* intrapartum treatment (EXIT) procedure was designed to ensure continuous oxygen supply through the placenta to a fetus who is having airway obstruction from congenital or iatrogenic causes, for which treatment in the form of establishing a patent and adequate airway for subsequent breathing has to be initiated during the time of birth and before separation of the placenta. This involves an elective delivery by CS with the appropriate teams standing by for immediate surgical treatment of the fetus as soon as the fetal head and part of the upper trunk are delivered outside the uterus. The mother has to be put under deep inhalational anaesthesia with/without concomitant tocolytic treatment to maintain total uterine relaxation until a patent airway is established in the fetus, who is then delivered and transferred to the receiving neonatal surgical team for further management. For the mother, the CS is completed as usual. The main maternal risk is bleeding from the hysterotomy.

Inspection of pelvic organs

After closure of the uterus a systematic and careful inspection of the pelvic organs, especially the bladder, should be performed before closure of the abdomen. It is not unknown that accidental cystotomy is discovered only at this stage. High-risk situations include previous CS or pelvic surgery, and pelvic/bowel/omental adhesions from any cause found at the time of surgery. Injury to the ureters may also occur especially if there is an extension of one of the angles of the incision or following repair of a

haematoma. The tubes and ovaries must be inspected, in case an ovarian cyst/tumour is missed during pregnancy. Any ovarian tumours, especially solid tumours, found at CS should be removed for histological examination. If malignancy is suspected, frozen section should be arranged immediately and the oncologist be consulted for a proper assessment, staging, and further surgery if necessary.

Repair of the bladder/omentum/bowel

In case injuries to these organs are found, a proper assessment by an experienced surgeon is mandatory. Bleeding from omental vessels can be persistent and troublesome. Repair should be carried out only by an experienced surgeon, and a general surgeon should be consulted if necessary.

Postpartum management

Postpartum urinary retention, defined as a post-void residual bladder volume of ≥150 mL on ultrasound scan, can be as high as 24%, and the incidence of overt and covert retention were 7.45 and 16.7% respectively. The associated factors include morphine-related analgesia, multiple pregnancy and low BMI.

Further reading

Alderdice F, McKenna D, Dornan J Techniques and materials for skin closure in caesarean section. Cochrane Database Syst Rev 2003;2:CD003577.

Alexander JM, Leveno KJ, Hauth J, et al. Fetal injury associated with cesarean delivery. Obstet Gynecol 2006;108:885–90.

Alexander JM, Leveno KJ, Rouse DJ, et al. Comparison of maternal and infant outcomes from primary cesarean delivery during the second compared with first stage of labor. Obstet Gynecol 2007;109:917–21.

Allen VM, O'Connell CM, Baskett TF. Maternal morbidity associated with caesarean delivery without labor compared with induction of labor at term. Obstet Gynecol 2006;108:286–94.

Armson BA Is planned cesarean childbirth a safe alternative? CMAJ 2007;176:475–6.

Asakura H, Nakai A, Ishikawa G, et al. Prediction of uterine dehiscence by measuring lower uterine segment thickness prior to the onset of labor: evaluation by transvaginal ultrasonography. J Nippon Med Sch 2006;67:352–6.

Aslan H, Unlu E, Agar M, Ceylan Y. Uterine rupture associated with misoprostol labor induction in women with previous caesarean delivery. Eur J Obstet Gynecol Reprod Biol 2004;113:45–8.

Barau G, Robillard P-Y, Hulsey TC, et al. Linear association between maternal pre-pregnancy body mass index and risk of caesarean section in term deliveries. Br J Obstet Gynaecol 2006;113:1173–7.

Barrett G, Peacock J, Victor CR, Manyonda I Cesarean section and postnatal sexual health. Birth Issues Perinat Care 2005;32:306–11.

Bhattacharya S, Campbell DM, Liston WA, Bhattacharya S. Effect of body mass index on pregnancy outcomes in nulliparous women delivering singleton babies. BMC Public Health 2007;7:168–76.

Björklund K, Kimaro M, Urassa E, Lindmark G. Introduction of the Misgav-Ladach caesarean section at an African tertiary centre: a randomized controlled trial. Br J Obstet Gynaecol 2000;107:209–16.

Bloom SL, Leveno KJ, Spong CY, et al. Decision-to-incision times and maternal and infant outcomes. Obstet Gynecol 2006;108:6–11.

Bloom SL, Spong CY, Weiner SJ, et al. Complications of anesthesia for caesarean delivery. Obstet Gynecol 2005;106:281–7.

Bouchard S, Johnson MB, Flake AW, et al. The EXIT procedure: experience and outcome in 31 cases. J Pediatr Surg 2002;37:418–26.

Bujold E, Bujold J, Hamilton EF, et al. The impact of a single-layer or double-layer closure on uterine rupture. Am J Obstet Gynecol 2002;186:1326–30.

Chapman SJ, Owen J, Hauth JC. One- versus two-layer closure of a low transverse caesarean: the next pregnancy. Obstet Gynecol 1997;89:16–8.

Darj E, Nordström M-L. The Misgav Ladach method for caesarean section compared to the Pfannenstiel method. Acta Obstet Gynecol Scand 1999;78:37–41.

Declercq E, Menacker F, MacDorman M. Maternal risk profiles and the primary cesarean rate in the United States, 1991–2002. Am J Public health 2006;96:867–72.

Delaney T, Young DC. Spontaneous versus induced labor after a previous caesarean delivery. Obstet Gynecol 2003;102:39–44.

Dewey KG, Nommsen-Rivers LA, Heinig MJ, Cohen RJ. Risk factors for suboptimal infant breastfeeding behaviour, delayed onset of lactation, and excess neonatal weight loss. Pediatrics 2003;112:607–19.

Dunsmoor-Su R, Sammel M, Stevens E, et al. Impact of socioeconomic and hospital factors on attempts at vaginal birth after cesarean delivery. Obstet Gynecol 2003;102:1358–65.

Durnwald C, Mercer B. Uterine rupture, perioperative and perinatal morbidity after single-layer and double-layer closure at cesarean delivery. Am J Obstet Gynecol 2003;189:925–9.

Fatusic Z, Kurjak A, Jasarevic E, Hafner T. The Misgav Ladach method—a step forward on operative technique in obstetrics. J Perinat Med 2003;31:395–8.

Gareen IF, Morgenstern H, Greenland S, Gifford DS. Explaining the association of maternal age with cesarean delivery for nulliparous and parous women. J Clin Epidemiol 2003;56:1100–10.

Gates S, McKenzie-McHarg K, Hurley P. Effects of surgical techniques of caesarean section on maternal health. Fetal and Maternal Medicine Review 2001;12:105–37.

Getahun D, Oyelese Y, Salihu HM, Ananth CV. Previous cesarean delivery and risks of placenta previa and placental abruption. Obstet Gynecol 2006;107:771–8.

Grobman WA, Gilbert S, Landon MB, et al. Outcomes of induction of labor after one prior caesarean. Obstet Gynecol 2007;109:262–9.

Guise J-M, McDonagh MS, Osterweil P, et al. Systematic review of the incidence and consequences of uterine rupture in women with previous caesarean section. BMJ 2004;329:1–7.

Hassiakos D, Christopoulos P, Vitoratos N, et al. Myomectomy during caesarean section A safe procedure? Ann NY Acad Sci 2006;1092:408–13.

Henderson J, Petrou S. The economic case for planned caesarean section for breech presentation at term. CMAJ 2006;174:1118–9.

Hendler I, Bujold E. Effect of prior vaginal delivery or prior vaginal birth after caesarean delivery on obstetric outcomes in women undergoing trial of labor. Obstet Gynecol 2004;104:273–7.

Hibbard JU, Gilbert S, Landon MB, et al. Trial of labor or repeat caesarean delivery in women with morbid obesity and previous caesarean delivery. Obstet Gynecol 2006;108:125–33.

Hibbard JU, Ismail MA, Wang Y, et al. Failed vaginal birth after a cesarean section: how risky is it? I. Maternal morbidity. Am J Obstet Gynecol 2001;184:1365–73.

Holmgren G, Sjöholm L, Stark M. The Misgav Ladach method for caesarean section: method description. Acta Obstet Gynecol Scand 1999;78:615–21.

Joseph KS, Young DC, Dodds L, et al. Changes in maternal characteristics and obstetric practice and recent increases in primary caesarean delivery. Obstet Gynecol 2003;102:791–800.

Juhasz G, Gyamfi C, Gyamfi P, et al. Effect of body mass index and excessive weight gain on success of vaginal birth after caesarean delivery. Obstet Gynecol 2005;106; 741–6.

Kacmar J, Bhimani L, Boyd M, et al. Route of delivery as a risk factor for emergent peripartum hysterectomy: a case-control study. Obstet Gynecol 2003;102:141–5.

Khosla AH, Dahiya K, Sangwan K. Cesarean section in a wedged head. Indian J Med Sci 2003;57:187–91.

Kiran TSU, Chui YK, Bethel J, Bhal PS. Is gestational age an independent variable affecting uterine scar rupture rates? Eur J Obstet Gynecol Reprod Biol 2006;126:68–71.

Kulas T, Habek D, Karsa M, Bobić-Vuković M. Modified Misgav Ladach method for ceasrean section: clinical experience. Obstet Gynecol Invest 2008;65:222–6.

Landon MB, Hauth JC, Leveno KJ, et al. Maternal and perinatal outcomes associated with a trial of labor after prior caesarean delivery. N Engl J Med 2004;351: 2581–9.

Landon MB, Spong CY, Thom E, et al. Risk of uterine rupture with a trial of labor in women with multiple and single prior cesarean delivery. Obstet Gynecol 2006;108:12–20.

Levine EM, Ghai V, Barton JJ, Strom CM. Mode of delivery and risk of respiratory diseases in newborns. Obstet Gynecol 2001;97:439–42.

Liang CC, Chang SD, Chang YL, et al. Postpartum urinary retention after cesarean delivery. Int J Gynecol Obstet 2007;99:229–32.

Liston FA, Allen VM, O'Connell CM, Jangaard KA. Neonatal outcomes with caesarean delivery at term. Arch Dis Child Neonatal edn 2008;93:F176–F182.

Locatelli A, Regalia AL, Ghidini A, et al. Risks of induction of labour in women with a uterine scar from previous low transverse caesarean section. Br J Obstet Gynaecol 2004;111:1394–9.

Lydon-Rochelle M, Holt VL, Easterling TR, Martin DP Cesarean delivery and postpartum mortality among primiparas in Washington State, 1987–1996. Obstet Gynecol 2001;97:169–74.

MacArthur C, Glazener C, Lancashire R, et al. Faecal incontinence and mode of first and subsequent delivery: a six-year longitudinal study. Br J Obstet Gynaecol 2005;112:1075–82.

Magann EF, Dodson MK, Ray MA, et al. Preoperative skin preparation and intraoperative pelvic irrigation: impact on postcesarean endometritis and wound infection. Obstet Gynecol 1993; 81:922–5.

Naef RW 3rd, Ray MA, Chauhan SP, et al. Trial of labor after caesarean delivery with a lower-segment, vertical uterine incision: is it safe? Am J Obstet Gynecol 1995;172.1666–73.

Nisenblat V, Barak S, Griness B, et al. Maternal complications associated with multiple caesarean deliveries. Obstet Gynecol 2006;108:21–6.

Nygaard I. Urinary incontinence: is cesarean delivery protective? Semin Perinatol 2006;30:267–71.

Raatikainen K, Heiskanen N, Heinonen S. Transition from overweight to obesity worsens pregnancy outcome in a BMI-dependent manner. Obesity 2006;14:165–71.

Ramadani H. Cesarean section intraoperative blood loss and mode of placental separation. Int J Gynecol Obstet 2004;87:114–8.

Rortveit G, Daltveit AK, Hannestad YS, Hunskaar S, for the Norwegian EPINCONT Study Urinary incontinence after vaginal delivery or cesarean section. N Engl J Med 2003;348:900–7.

Rozenberg P, Goffinet F, Phillippe HJ, Nisand I. Ultrasonographic measurement of lower uterine segment to assess risk of defects of scarred uterus. Lancet 1996;347:281–4.

Sachs BP, Castro MA. The risks of lowering the caesarean-delivery rate. N Engl J Med 1999;340:54–7.

Schindl M, Birner P, Reingrabner M, et al. Elective cesarean section vs spontaneous delivery: a comparative study of birth experience. Acta Obstet Gynecol Scand 2003;82:834–40.

Shipp TD, Zelop CM, Repke JT, et al. Labor after previous caesarean: influence of prior indication and parity. Obstet gynecol 2000;95:913–16.

Silver RM, Landon MB, Rouse DJ, et al. Maternal morbidity associated with multiple repeat ceasrean deliveries. Obstet Gynecol 2006;107:1226–32.

Simm A, Ramoutar P. Caesarean section: techniques and complications. Cur Obstet Gynecol 2005;15:80–6.

Smith GCS, Pell JP, Dobbie R. Caesarean section and the risk of unexplained stillbirth in subsequent pregnancy. Lancet 2003; 362:1779–84.

Society of Obstetricians and Gynaecologists of Canada (SOGC). Clinical practice guidelines. Guidelines for vaginal birth after previous caesarean birth. Number 155. Int J Gynaecol Obstet 2005;89:319–31.

Srinivas SK, Stamilio DM, Stevens EJ, et al. Predicting failure of a vaginal birth attempt after caesarean delivery. Obstet Gynecol 2007;109:800–5.

Starr RV, Zurawski J, Ismail M. Preoperative vaginal preparation with povidone-iodine and the risk of postcesarean endometritis. Obstet Gynecol 2005;105:1024–9.

Tanik A, Ustun C, Cil E, Arslan A. Sonographic evaluation of the wall thickness of the lower uterine segment in patients with previous caesarean section. J Clin Ultrasound 1996;24:355–7.

Towner D, Castro MA, Eby-Wilkens E, Gilbert WM. Effect of mode of delivery in nulliparous women on neonatal intracranial injury. N Engl J Med 1999;341:1709–14.

Varga P, Bódis J. Comparative evaluation of the Misgav Ladach caesarean section with two traditional techniques. The first four years' experience. Acta Obstet Gynecol Scand 2001;80:90–2.

Villar J, Carroli G, Zavaleta N, et al. Maternal and neonatal individual risks and benefits associated with caesarean delivery: multicentre prospective study. BMJ 2007;335:1025–36.

Villar J, Valladares E, Wojdyla D, et al. Caesarean delivery rates and pregnancy outcomes: the 2005 WHO global survey on maternal and perinatal health in Latin America. Lancet 2006;367:1819–29.

Witter FR, Caulfield LE, Stoltzfus RJ. Influence of maternal anthropometric status and birth weight on the risk of cesarean delivery. Obstet Gynecol 1995;85:947–51.

Wood SL, Chen S, Ross S, Sauve R. The risk of unexplained antepartum stillbirth in second pregnancies following caesarean section in the first pregnancy. Br J Obstet Gynaecol 2008;115:726–31.

Xavier P, Ayres-De-Campos D, Reynolds A, et al. The modified Misgav-Ladach versus the Pfannenstiel-Kerr technique for cesarean section: a randomized trial. Acta Obstet Gynecol Scand 2005; 84:878–82.

Yang Q, Wen SW, Oppenheimer L, et al. Association of caesarean delivery for first birth with placenta praevia and placental abruption in second pregnancy. Br J Obstet Gynaecol 2007;114: 609–13.

Zelop CM, Shipp TD, Cohen A, et al. Trial of labor after 40 weeks' gestation in women with prior cesarean. Obstet Gynecol 2001;97:391–3.

Internet resources

www.babycenter.com
www.childbirth.org
www.netdoctor.co.uk

Patient information and contacts

www.americanpregnancy.org
www.babycenter.com
www.questia.com
www.pregnancy-info.net

Forceps delivery

Definition

This refers to a form of operative vaginal delivery by means of an instrument called the obstetric forceps. The forceps are made with metal and consist of two halves (left and right). Upon assembly they produce a cradle for the fetal head, and upon traction along the handle that is connected by a shank to the cradle, will result in the controlled delivery of the fetal head, to be followed by the rest of the infant.

Epidemiology

There has been a declining rate of forceps delivery in many centres due to a combination of factors that include the perceived higher maternal and fetal risks with forceps delivery, an increasing popularity with ventouse delivery, and the progressive loss of skills in forceps delivery. The rate of forceps delivery can be as low as <1% in some centres and up to 5–6% in others.

Pathology

The obstetric forceps have certain characteristics that serve to fulfil its designed purpose. It can create complications if improperly handled. The four essential parts of a pair of obstetric forceps are the blades, which are usually fenestrated; the shank that connects the blades to the handles; the handles that are grasped by the operator's hand to exert the traction force; and a lock located at the junction between the shanks and handles by means of which the two halves of the forceps can be assembled and kept in position. Some forms of forceps include an axis traction handle that is attached to the shank and through which an effective traction force along the axis of the birth canal can be exerted by only one hand. The two halves are usually numbered so that upon assembly, the two halves can be checked to ensure that these belong to the same pair and will fit perfectly upon assembly.

The risk–benefit balance is related to the level of skills of the operator. The following factors in the design and use of forceps contributes to the potential risks to infant and mother.

- It will take up space inside the birth canal after application.
- It has a rigid structure and the length varies in different models. Therefore its insertion into the birth canal which is mostly filled up with the fetal head requires manipulation and manoeuvring which can be difficult.
- Each blade consists of a cephalic curve, and a pelvic curve. Both curves are of standard shape and dimensions for each particular model of forceps. But neither the size and shape of the baby's head, nor the size, shape, and angulation of the birth canal, are standard in all cases. Therefore, even in skilful hands, the application of forceps can traumatise the baby's head and the birth canal.
- Traction on the fetal head is responsible for the delivery process. The force exerted by the forceps on the skull can be considerable and underestimated by the operator, since there is no means of gauging the force in practice. Therefore in difficult cases, excessive force exerted will increase the risk of traumatic injuries.
- Proper and adequate training is required in order to acquire the necessary skills involved in the use of the different models of forceps. This is sometimes overlooked.
- Fetal intracranial injury and maternal perineal tear can both be attributable to the forces of labour and the fetus being propelled through a rigid or inadequate passage. If forceps delivery is undertaken, the blame is often laid on the use of forceps.

In view of these factors, it is hardly surprising that forceps delivery has been credited with a high risk of traumatic injuries to both infant and mother. However, in skilful hands, injuries on the baby's scalp and face are largely cosmetic and will heal without sequelae, while maternal genital tract tears can be repaired with good results. Anal sphincter damage and incontinence with faeces and flatus however are increased with forceps delivery. Nevertheless, it cannot be proven beyond doubt that the true culprit is forceps delivery, rather than the conditions for which forceps delivery is indicated.

Aetiology

Forceps delivery is now considered only when there is a high probability of successful vaginal delivery, and as an alternative to ventouse delivery. Since the safety of Caesarean section has improved greatly, high-forceps is totally abandoned. Mid-forceps is seldom performed when there is no major concern about cephalopelvic disproportion and the operator is very experienced. Almost all forceps delivery now belonged to low-forceps or outlet forceps, and the choice between forceps and ventouse in instrumental delivery depends as much on the indications as on the preference of the operator. The only difference is that forceps delivery can be applied for the aftercoming head in the occasional vaginal breech delivery. The types of forceps remaining in use include the following:

- outlet to low forceps
  - Wrigley's forceps
  - Simpson's forceps
  - Neville-Barnes forceps
  - Piper's forceps
- mid-cavity rotational forceps
  - Kielland's forceps.

Indications for forceps delivery

- To hasten or control delivery in case of cephalic presentation in the following situations:
  - prolonged second stage of labour
  - suspected fetal distress
  - poor maternal efforts or unconscious mother
  - to eliminate or minimize the need for maternal efforts, e.g. mothers with severe myopia, severe hypertension, intracranial pathologies, etc.
  - delivery of the cephalic-presenting second twin when the head is engaged and the cervix is fully dilated and there is failure to progress or concerns about the fetal condition.
- To control the delivery of the aftercoming head in breech delivery.

Contraindications for forceps delivery

- Incompletely dilated cervix
- Unknown fetal position
- Station above the ischial spines
- Operator is inexperienced in forceps delivery
- Clinical cephalopelvic disproportion.

Prognosis

Maternal

Forceps delivery is associated with increased risk of vaginal lacerations and third- and fourth-degree perineal tears (see Chapter 10.5, Episiotomy and obstetric perineal trauma), primary postpartum haemorrhage and vaginal/perineal haematomas, and other postpartum problems secondary to these problems such as pain leading to urinary retention and deep vein thrombosis due to decreased ambulation. However, one study in the USA reported that postpartum haemorrhage was more likely with ventouse than forceps delivery. Long-term morbidity is related to the pelvic floor and perineal injury.

At 6 years after the first delivery, those women delivered by forceps had a twofold higher risk of persistent faecal incontinence than women who had spontaneous vaginal delivery.

Infant

Neonatal complications and injuries that can be attributed directly to forceps delivery are trauma to the fetal head, including skull fractures, intracranial and intracerebral haemorrhage, and subdural haematoma. Indirect complications include shoulder dystocia due to haste in the delivery of the trunk, and the associated brachial plexus injury and clavicular fracture. One study in the USA showed that neonatal mortality, intracranial and retinal haemorrhage, and feeding difficulty, were comparable between forceps and ventouse delivery, but forceps delivery is more likely to be associated with birth injuries, neonatal seizures, and need for assisted ventilation, but less likely to have shoulder dystocia.

Clinical approach

Prerequisites for forceps delivery

In deciding for forceps delivery, the first consideration should be the skill and experience of the operator. Forceps delivery should be considered a surgical procedure and as such, it should be organized similarly with an operator, an assistant, a circulating nurse, a trained person for neonatal resuscitation, appropriate analgesia, the patient should have an intravenous drip or at least an intravenous access, and an aseptically prepared delivery trolley with a specially designated prepacked set of instruments. If the operator is inexperienced, the assistant should be the well experienced supervisor. The circulating nurse should be able to provide any additional equipment, administer medications, and to summon help where necessary. The person for neonatal resuscitation should be adequately trained to handle an infant born in a poor condition. For a patient receiving epidural analgesia, top up will be required if the effect is wearing off, or regional analgesia should be given if forceps delivery is planned beforehand. In case of emergency situation, adequate local anaesthetic should be infiltrated into the perineum in anticipation of an episiotomy. Nowadays, bilateral pudendal block is rarely given and if this is deemed necessary, regional analgesia may be preferable. Under normal circumstances, consent for the possible use of forceps delivery should have been obtained at an early stage, together with the consent for an episiotomy. In case this is not yet done, or the patient raises concerns, written consent may be preferable unless the decision is made urgently to avoid major compromise to the fetus.

The prerequisites for forceps delivery
- The fetal head must be engaged
- The cervix must be fully dilated
- The position of the head must be ascertained
- The shape of the pelvis should be assessed, and the adequacy of the outlet determined, making sure that the pelvis is not convergent
- The bladder should be empty
- The analgesia is effective
- The delivery team is ready and standing by.

Examination prior to the application of forceps

Abdominal palpation

Irrespective of the entries in the notes or partogram, the operator must perform a complete examination, starting with the abdominal examination. The operator should determine
- the amount of fetal head palpable above the pelvic brim in fifths (none or 0/5 should be palpable)
- the position of the anterior shoulder (this helps the subsequent manual rotation if necessary and reduces the risk of shoulder dystocia due to misdiagnosis of restitution and external rotation of the fetal head)
- whether the bladder is distended
- that the fetal size is not too large.

Only when these points are satisfied should forceps delivery proceed. In case of doubt, a trial of forceps can be organized in the operating theatre. In case more than one of these points are not satisfied, one should consider abandoning the procedure, since there are much greater risks of fetal hypoxia and injury, and maternal trauma, if forceps delivery fails and a caesarean section was required.

Vaginal examination

An aseptic approach should be adopted. If the bladder is still palpable, or it is uncertain if the bladder is empty enough, the bladder should be drained with a disposable catheter which is removed afterwards. Do not use a self retaining Foley catheter as the balloon can be dragged along by the descending fetal head leading to forceful dilation and damage to the bladder neck and urethra, resulting in complete urine incontinence. Then perform the vaginal examination to determine
- full dilatation of cervix
- station
- position
- flexion
- asynclitism
- caput and moulding of the fetal head
- the shape and size of the bony pelvis and whether the pelvis is convergent.

Forceps delivery should not be performed if station is above the ischial spines in the absence of moulding, three-plus moulding despite a station of 1–2 cm below the ischial spines, a grossly deflexed or asynclitic head, and a convergent pelvis with an outlet that cannot admit the clenched fist of the operator. In case of doubt, the procedure should be organized in the operating theatre as a trial of forceps.

The choice of forceps

This should be dependent on the type of application and the findings on vaginal examination, and the experience that the operator possesses for different types of forceps. For outlet or lift-out forceps delivery, either Wrigley's or Simpson's forceps can be used. However, with the marked pelvic curve in Wrigley's forceps, its application should be restricted to direct, or almost direct occipital anterior position, with or without manual rotation. Simpson's forceps have minimal pelvic curve, and so it can be applied for both occipital anterior and posterior positions. For low cavity forceps, Neville-Barnes forceps is preferred, because the very short shank in Wrigley's and Simpson's forceps means that after application, the entire shank and even part of the handle may have gone inside the vagina, thus rendering traction difficult. Piper's forceps are reserved for delivery of the aftercoming head of the breech. The long curved shanks ensure that after application of the blades, the handle is still beyond the level of the buttocks so that the trunk of the baby will not interfere with the operator as long as it is supported by the assistant. As well, the wide gap between the shanks ensures that the umbilical cord, dangling below the baby's abdomen, will not be crushed by the shanks upon locking.

Kielland's forceps belong to a category by itself. There is a slight backward pelvic curve, long overlapping shanks with a sliding lock, and on each anterior surface of the finger guard at the front of the handle of each side is a knob that denotes the anterior surface and serves as reference point for the occiput. The sliding lock allows the correction of asynclitism.

Always check the number imprinted on the handle of the forceps to ensure the two blades belong to the same pair, and then assemble the forceps to ensure that the pelvic and cephalic curves are symmetrical and the shanks can come together to lock, before application. In case of doubt, exchange for another pair of forceps. There should never be more than one pair of the same type of forceps on the delivery trolley in case of a mix-up of the blades. When ready the blades are liberally lubricated with KY jelly or Hibitane cream, then assembled again and placed on the trolley ready for use.

The application of forceps for traction in cephalic presentation

When ready for application, the pair of forceps is held with the right hand and the handles and shanks are disassembled with the left hand, which is then used to grasp the handle of the left blade. The forceps blades should be applied with the head in the occipital anterior (OA) position. Heads not in the OA position can be rotated manually. Manual rotation usually involves an initial upward motion to disimpact the head before rotation to as direct OA as possible, meanwhile avoiding deflexion and asynclitism. The head is then held in place with the same hand involved in rotation while the other hand is used to apply the first (left) blade. In this manoeuvre, ensure that the umbilical cord does not slip down or past the fetal head to be compressed by the fetal head later.

The first blade to be applied is the left blade. For forceps with a pelvic curve, the handle should be held with the end pointing skyward and lying in the palm of the left hand, the shank positioned above the maternal right groin and parallel to the right inguinal ligament, and the tip of the blade resting on the palm of the right hand the fingers of which are inside the vagina steadying the fetal head (especially after rotation). The first blade should be inserted after a uterine contraction, and never at the onset or height of a uterine contraction. With a gentle sweeping motion, the left hand describes an arc through the air, pushing the tip of the blade along the inside of the right hand which is used to retract away the vaginal wall and to assist the blade to negotiate the cephalic and pelvic curve. If a left mediolateral episiotomy has been made beforehand for whatever reason, the dorsum of the right hand forms a shield before

the opened vaginal wall prevent the blade to cause further extension of or splitting up the wound further.

When the tip of the blade reaches the level of the proximal interphalangeal joints of the fingers, the fingers should bend with the finger tips pushing the fetal head medially thus creating room for the blade to advance. When the tip of the blade reaches the tip of the fingers, the fingertip of the index finger should slip into the fenestrum of the blade to maintain the pressure on the fetal head, while the tip of the blade should remain pressed against the tip of the middle finger. Then the fingers of the right hand are used to properly position the blade alongside the fetal head, advancing with the middle and ring fingers as the leading point and guiding the tip of the blade until the blade is in place. The index finger is used not only to create room but also to feel for the facial structures and the ear to ensure the correct positioning of the blade.

This approach will ensure the correct application of the blade and minimize both maternal and fetal trauma. If the fetal head rotates, descends or ascends, the movements will be detected by the index fingers, and the hand can make fine adjustments to allow the blade to be properly applied against the face without excessive force or pressure which can cause injuries. The feeling for the ear can also confirm the position and proper application of the first blade. Only when the blade is in place should the right hand withdraw slowly, with the left hand maintaining the position of the handle in the correct position. In case the baby is small or the pelvis very roomy, the mother can be asked too bear down slightly so that the downward pressure will keep the blade in place as the right hand withdraws as if it is squeezed out by the maternal effort, while the application of the fetal head against the cephalic curve of the blade will help to maintain its position.

With the left blade now in place and kept in position with the left hand with/without some maternal bearing down effort, the right blade is then applied using the same method, only with the sides reversed. The operator's left hand is inserted into the vagina and the right blade is inserted in between contractions, i.e. the process is a repetition of the other side.

Once the right blade is in place, the shanks and handles should be almost alongside, and slight adjustment of one or the other side should allow the handle to lock. If the handles are not in alignment, the side that is at an angle should be brought into alignment gently by shifting the entire side anteriorly or posteriorly alongside the fetal head, and pushing upwards and then the handles are likely to lock. The operator must not forcibly move the maligned handle into apposition with the other handle as this will not work and could cause trauma at the point of the base of the blade which becomes the fulcrum of such movements. Exerting pressure on the underlying fetal skull could result in a depressed fracture. If the shanks and handles are parallel but at different levels, the handle at the lower level should be gently pushed upwards, moving slightly anteroposteriorly as necessary, to bring the handles together and lock. Correct application is confirmed when the sagittal suture is perpendicular to the shanks and the posterior fontanelle is 3 cm above the plane of the shanks and only one finger can be admitted between the blade and the head on either side. When these conditions are satisfied traction can commence.

In case the handles cannot be locked together, the right blade should be retrieved for reapplication. Sometimes even the left blade may need to be reapplied, and in this instance, the fetal head usually would have changed its position so that the complete process of assessment and application has to be repeated again. If the forceps fail to lock a second time, the operator should suspect the following conditions: incorrect diagnosis of position, asynclitism, or failure to diagnose cephalopelvic disproportion. If difficulties are encountered with correct application, the procedure should be abandoned and a Caesarean section should be performed.

Traction for cephalic presentation

Traction should be gentle and along the axis of the birth canal, using both hands. The hand that is holding onto the handle exerts horizontal traction force, while the other hand is placed on the shanks before the first hand and exerts vertical downward force. Traction should be synchronized with uterine contractions and maternal bearing down efforts. Traction can be applied with the operator standing or sitting. Although the sitting position is preferred by many, one study demonstrated that more traction force is generated in the sitting position, so that this should be borne in mind during the procedure.

An episiotomy can be made, if it is felt to be necessary, at the time when the head is about to crown. As the head crowns, the other hand can be removed from the shanks. Traction should be maintained at a reduced level and the direction of pull should be guided by the degree of movement of the crowning head to become progressively upwards. In this way, the direction of traction is dictated by the direction of the path of least resistance, and inappropriately excessive horizontal traction, which may pull the occiput against the inferior pubic rami, or inappropriately excessive downward force, which may result in overstretching and tearing of the perineum, can both be avoided.

The head is delivered, controlling the rate so that it does not pop out. Once the jaws can be reached, the blades are first loosened by relaxing the grip on the handles, and then removed in the opposite order to application. Pushing the perineum below the emerging head will help a smooth controlled delivery of the head. Do not pull on the head excessively or too rapidly, as this will pull the shoulders, especially the anterior shoulder, to become impacted against the pubic bones thus creating iatrogenic shoulder dystocia. Once the head is delivered, allow time for restitution of the head so that the true position of the shoulders can be gauged. Then allow time for external rotation of the head which signifies engagement of the shoulders, before delivery of the anterior shoulder is attempted. Undue haste in delivery of the shoulders is the main reason for shoulder dystocia and brachial plexus injury in an otherwise normal sized baby through an adequate pelvis.

During delivery of the head and the shoulders, an assistant should guard the perineum to prevent sudden and excessive stretching along the episiotomy which could result in a third or fourth degree tear.

The application of forceps for rotation and traction in cephalic presentation

Kielland's forceps are rarely used nowadays, as the indications are very limited and there has been much publicity about the associated maternal and fetal risks. If midcavity traction or rotation is required, ventouse delivery is usually preferred due to its higher safety margin and technical ease in its performance. The method of application of Kielland's forceps is not covered in this chapter.

The application of forceps for the aftercoming head in breech delivery

Piper's forceps is designed for the delivery of the aftercoming head in breech delivery. Following the delivery of the shoulders and arms, the fetal back is rotated to face upwards with the chin posterior, which can be confirmed by digital examination. An assistant supports the trunk and the limbs of the baby with a towel sling held by the assistant. The trunk should not be pulled upwards out of the way in order to avoid injury to the neck. The left blade is applied first with the operator in a sitting or kneeling position so that his/her vision is in line with the perineum and not obscured by the baby's trunk. This is facilitated by the assistant carrying the baby's trunk to the mother's right horizontally. The left blade is applied, as described before, to the right side of the baby's face, its position adjusted if necessary to allow for the slight variation of the position of the baby's occiput. If resistance is encountered, the tip of the blade is introduced more posteriorly and then wandered around to the side of the head. The right blade is then applied in a similar manner. After locking the shanks the baby is allowed to straddle the forceps, with the handles held in the upturned palm of the right hand and the middle finger inserted in the space between the shanks.

Downward traction is made with the operator in the same position until the chin appears at the outlet. The handles are then elevated with traction, following the pelvic curve to bring the suboccipital region under the pubic arch. This is facilitated by using the index and middle fingers of the left hand to press on the suboccipital region, which also serves to protect the neck with the splinting effect. If resistance is encountered, the handles are depressed and then elevated again during gentle traction. Extraction of the head is achieved by maintaining the handles close to the horizontal and the blades in place. During delivery of the head, the occiput serves as the fulcrum for flexion. As the head is delivered, the assistant can hold the baby while the operator removes the blades from the baby's head. The cord is clamped and divided and the baby is transferred to the resuscitaire.

Trial of forceps

In case of suspected cephalopelvic disproportion, or unfavourable pelvis, the forceps delivery should be organized as a trial of forceps. The anaesthetist should be alerted and the operating theatre prepared as for an emergency Caesarean section with the scrub and circulating nurses standing by. Blood should be sent for group and save. An intravenous drip should be set up and adequate regional analgesia be ensured. The woman should be prepared as for emergency general anaesthesia with ranitidine and sodium citrate given orally beforehand. The procedure is performed on the operating table with the woman in lithotomy position

Following application of the forceps, the three-pull rule (= over three contractions) should be strictly followed. The trial must be abandoned if delivery has not occurred, or is not imminent, and there is unsatisfactory descent by the third pull. The delivery should be converted to an emergency Caesarean section.

Procedures after successful delivery

Following each delivery, the following should be checked in addition to the routine examination:
- any extension of the episiotomy, vaginal and perineal tears, and third and fourth degree perineal tears

- cervical lacerations
- bleeding from above the cervix (this could be due to uterine lower segment tears or uterine rupture).

Vaginal and perineal tears, and episiotomy should be dealt with as described in the relevant chapters.

The baby should be resuscitated if necessary by a paediatrician. In case the forceps delivery is performed for fetal reasons, paired umbilical cord artery and venous blood should be taken for measurement of pH and blood gases. The placenta and membranes should be checked. In case of vulval perineal oedema or haematoma, an indwelling Foley catheter should be inserted for continuous drainage. The woman should be re-examined 1 hour later for evidence of vulvovaginal haematoma before she is transferred to the postnatal ward.

The indications, type of procedure, time and duration, and outcome of the delivery should be clearly documented in the notes. Any maternal and neonatal injuries must be recorded and where necessary diagrams can be drawn to indicate the site and extent of the injuries. The mother should have a clear picture of what has happened, since misunderstanding or misinformation, especially if injuries are present, can become the basis of future litigation.

Abandoning delivery ('failed forceps')
Forceps delivery should be considered unsuccessful under the following circumstances:
- if the blades could not be applied or locked
- if there was no progress after three pulls.

Further reading
Demissie K, Rhoads GG, Smulian JC, et al. Operative vaginal delivery and neonatal and infant adverse outcomes: population based retrospective analysis. BMJ 2004;329:1-6.

Dennen PC. Dennen's forceps deliveries, 3rd edn. Philadelphia: F.A. Davis 1989.

Johanson RB, Menon V. Vacuum extraction versus forceps for assisted vaginal delivery. Cochrane Database Syst Rev 1998;4:CD000224.

Leslie KK, Dipasquale-Lehnerz P, Smith M. Obstetric forceps training using visual feedback and the isometric strength testing unit. Obstet Gynecol 2005;105:377–82.

MacArthur C, Glazener C, Lancashire R, et al. Faecal incontinence and mode of first and subsequent delivery: a six-year longitudinal study. Br J Obstet Gynaecol 2005;112:1075–82.

Patel RR, Murphy DJ. Forceps delivery in modern obstetric practice. BMJ 2004;328:1302–5.

Royal College of Obstetricians and Gynaecologists (RCOG) Operative vaginal delivery. Guideline No. 26. London: RCOG 2005.

Useful websites
www.emedicine.com

Patient resources
www.rcog.org.hk

Uterine compression sutures

Uterine compression sutures are sutures applied externally to the body of the uterus in various patterns and involving either the upper or lower segments or both, so as to act as a brace to facilitate uterine contraction and retraction. The tightening of the sutures also produces a compression effect. Together these two actions will help to control postpartum haemorrhage from the uterus, and possibly avoiding the need for hysterectomy as a life-saving procedure.

Epidemiology

The actual incidence of the use of this treatment in the management of postpartum haemorrhage remains unknown. There are only anecdotal case reports and small case series in the literature and most likely represent under-reporting. In the experience of one centre, compression sutures were performed in 1 per 1126 deliveries over a 7-year period. All were carried out at Caesarean delivery, with an incidence of 1 in 221 Caesarean deliveries in labour and 1 in 637 elective Caesarean deliveries.

Pathology

In cases of normal placentation, uncontrolled haemorrhage from the placental bed can occur due to a failure of occlusion of the placental bed blood vessels by the contracting myometrium if uterine atony develops. In cases of abnormal placentation, such as placenta accreta/increta, retained adherent placental tissue interferes with haemostasis in the placental bed, and the additional effect of uterine atony, whether as a primary or secondary event, would aggravate the situation. Therefore, correcting uterine atony and promoting uterine contraction play key roles in controlling postpartum haemorrhage. The myometrial response to uterotonic agents is quite variable, but it can be enhanced by external compression of the uterus. Hence, manual compression and massaging the uterus is effective in some cases. When this approach fails, the application of compression sutures may be considered, as this can reduce the uterine size and provide sustained compression force.

Compression sutures can be used in almost any form of postpartum haemorrhage, either as the primary surgical treatment or in conjunction with balloon tamponade. In postpartum haemorrhage in which inadequate uterine contraction and retraction is a significant factor, compression sutures result in direct occlusion of intramyometrial vessels, in addition to providing a scaffolding to facilitate the uterus to contract under the stimulation of uterotonics. For bleeding from placental bed vessels in the case of placenta praevia, and from the ragged placental bed in the case of placenta accreta, compression sutures applied externally over the bleeding site can also control the bleeding by similar mechanisms. Any residual bleeding can then be controlled by means of balloon tamponade.

Aetiology

After delivery of the fetus and placenta, immediate haemostasis is achieved by occlusion of the arcuate and spiral arteries of the placental bed by means of contraction of the myometrial fibres in the uterine body. Hence, bleeding from the placental bed in the case of placenta praevia and abruption is less easily or well controlled. Direct application of haemostatic figure-of-eight or other forms of sutures is often successful, but on occasions, more extensive application of sutures to compress the vascular supply of the bleeding site is necessary. The variety of compression sutures reported in the literature can be applied to deal with bleeding from an atonic uterus to bleeding from localized sites in an otherwise well-contracted uterus.

The indications for compression sutures include
- uterine atony
- placenta praevia
- abnormal placentation, such as placenta accreta, increta and percreta.

Prognosis

As absorbable suture material is used there is no risk of the threads causing long-term problems. However, there are several potential complications.

The first is avascular necrosis, usually involving partial thickness, of the uterine wall. The second is the problem of using non-absorbable sutures that become loose in the abdomen after the uterus has involuted. The third is the slipping of the sutures after application, causing problems such as bowel obstruction and strangulation of pelvic organs by cutting off the blood supply to the tissue/organs trapped within the loose loops. For absorbable sutures, there is no long-term problem to the uterus or pelvic organs as these would disappear eventually. Successful pregnancy has been reported following the application of compression sutures to control postpartum haemorrhage.

For the B-Lynch suture, more than 1300 cases have been performed with very few reported failures, which have been attributed to delayed application, defibrination syndrome, and technical problems. Among the handful of reported cases with postoperative imaging studies or follow-up assessment, no defects were found inside the uterine cavity, and suture erosion through the uterus was reported once. Successful pregnancies resulting in term deliveries have been reported in a number of reports.

For the square suture first described by Cho et al. (2000), uterine drainage and involution may be affected, and blood-filled pockets may result, although ultrasound imaging in one case reported patency of the uterine canal 2 weeks after surgery. Delayed complications include pyometra and uterine synechiae with partial obstruction of menstrual flow. Four subsequent pregnancies occurred in the original series of 23 cases. Partial thickness necrosis of the uterine wall has been reported in a case following combined B-Lynch and Cho-square sutures.

Information on the long-term morbidity and outcome, including menstrual and fertility issues, of the other techniques is scanty.

Clinical approach

The use of uterine compression sutures should be considered when there is major postpartum haemorrhage, defined as estimated blood loss in excess of 1000 mL or more. Rather than as a last resort, this procedure should be considered whenever the uterus has to be conserved and conservative/medical methods are unsuccessful, especially following Caesarean delivery for placenta praevia, when the abdomen is already opened. In case of vaginal delivery, balloon tamponade can be tried first, followed by compression sutures if the former has failed. Compression suture can be combined with balloon tamponade, producing the uterine 'sandwich'. A number of compression sutures have been reported in the literature. These are described below.

B-Lynch suture

First described by C. Balogun-Lynch, the B-Lynch suture is the most frequently reported, and probably the most widely applied, compression suture technique worldwide. The technique is described below.

Testing for efficacy

With the patient in the semi-lithotomy position, an assistant, standing between the patient's legs, swabs the vagina to determine the extent of the bleeding. The operator then exteriorizes the uterus and applies bimanual compression of the whole uterus down to the level of the cervix. If the bleeding is stopped, then the suture has a good chance of successfully arresting the haemorrhage.

Suture application following Caesarean delivery

With an second assistant maintaining the bimanual compression, the operator displaces the bladder inferiorly and the first stitch is inserted 3 cm below the lower margin of the lower segment uterine incision on the patient's left side, then threaded through the uterine cavity to emerge 3 cm above the upper uterine incision margin and approximately 4 cm from the lateral border of the uterus. The suture is then brought over the fundus vertically to the posterior side, maintaining the same 4 cm distance from the lateral border, and the needle is reinserted at the level of insertion of the uterosacral ligament into the uterine cavity. The needle is then brought horizontally across the cavity to the other side of the posterior uterine wall, exiting the cavity through the wall, thus bringing the suture outside the posterior wall. The suture is again brought over the fundus onto the anterior right side of the uterus. The needle then enters and exits the anterior wall at the corresponding points on the right side. During this process, the assistant maintains the compression as the suture is applied to ensure progressive and uniform tension to be applied as the suture compresses the uterus, and to avoid slippage. The ends of the suture are placed under tension and tied with a double throw after the lower segment incision is closed to ensure that the corners of the incision are secured and included in the repair of the incision without leaving any bleeding points. The first assistant then confirms that vaginal bleeding is controlled and then abdomen is closed.

Suture application following vaginal delivery

A hysterotomy is recommended to ensure that the uterine cavity is empty, exclude abnormal placentation, and remove large blood clots. The uterine incision also provides the anatomical landmark for the correct application of the suture and to ensure maximum and even distribution of the compression, without the risk of accidentally obliterating the lumen. In case of placenta accrete, increta, or percreta, an additional figure-of-eight or transverse compression suture can be applied to the bleeding site before the application of the longitudinal suture.

Suture material

A monocryl suture is recommended because it is user and tissue friendly with uniform tension distribution and is easy to handle.

Square suture

First described by Cho et al. (2000), this involves the placement of multiple full thickness square sutures applied with a straight number 7 or number 8 needle to approximate the anterior and posterior uterine walls, especially in areas with heavy bleeding, and achieving haemostasis by compressing the haemorrhagic site. The original report involved the use of chromic '1' catgut. It was successful in all the 23 cases that were delivered by Caesarean section.

Vertical suture

There are some variations to this method of suturing.

- In Hayman's technique, the primary vertical compression sutures are applied in a similar fashion to the B-Lynch technique except that the left and right side are placed separately without the need to open up the uterine cavity, and the knots are tied over the fundus. Horizontal cervical isthmic sutures can be applied if necessary. Although quicker to perform, this method does not allow the uterine cavity to be explored.

- In the technique described by Nelson and Birch (2006), performed after a Caesarean section, a number '2' vicryl suture threaded through a large needle was inserted 2 cm below the uterine incision in a similar manner to the B-Lynch technique, and then brought up vertically and exits the anterior wall 2 cm above the uterine incision. Then the suture was passed through the fundus 3–4 cm medial to the cornual region and 2–3 cm below the superior aspect of the fundus. The needle and suture are then brought back through the posterior aspect of the lower segment and joined anteriorly after exiting below the uterine incision. The process is repeated on the other side. The suture is tied while bimanual compression of the uterus is done by an assistant. The uterine incision is then closed after bleeding has been seen to be controlled.

- Another form of short vertical sutures described by Tjalma and Jacquemyn (2004) involves the placing of sutures 2 cm apart in rows of four, with the needle passing from the anterior through the posterior wall and then back to the anterior wall, exiting anterior wall about 1 cm medial to the point of initial entry; the thread is then tied.

- A variation of this approach used in a case of relaparatomy after Caesarean section for placenta praevia is reported by Muppala et al. (2006), in which four parallel vertical sutures were applied to the lower segment without reopening the uterine incision, using number '1' vicryl suture mounted on a curved round bodied needle. The sutures were placed anteroposteriorly just above the attachment of the uterosacral ligaments, each being 1.5–2 cm apart, and the exit point is 2 cm cranial to the entry point in the anterior wall.

- A similar but modified procedure has been described by Hwu et al. (2006) in the management of bleeding from placenta praevia or accreta during Caesarean section. This involves two parallel vertical sutures that are placed 3 cm medial to the right and left borders of the lower segment respectively. The 40-mm curved round needle is inserted 2–3 cm above the upper margin of the cervix into the uterine cavity, then into the middle layer of the posterior wall of the lower segment 2–3 cm above the upper cervical margin. The needle then travels for 3–4 cm vertically upwards within the middle layer of the posterior wall and exits the uterine cavity and anterior wall at a point 2–3 cm below the uterine incision. Each suture is tied individually as tightly as possible, and the uterine incision is closed in the usual manner.

U-suture

This was described by Hackethal et al. (2008), using a Vicryl '0' suture and an XLH needle with the curve straightened manually. For an interrupted single U-suture, the needle is inserted at the anterior wall through to exit at the posterior wall, then passed back through the anterior wall forming a horizontal U that includes 2–4 cm of tissue, and the thread is joined by a flat double knot tied while the uterus is compressed bimanually by an assistant. The number of suture required depends on the size of the uterus and persistence of bleeding, and usually 6–16 U-sutures in horizontal rows starting from the fundus and ending at the cervix are required.

One variation of the U-suture is the isthmic-cervical apposition described by Das et al. (2005), which is applied only in the lower segment and essentially involves the two horizontal isthmic-cervical sutures of the Hayman technique.

Transverse suture

This was described by Ouahba et al. (2007) and involves four sutures. First an absorbable suture on a big round needle is inserted from the serosa of the anterior wall to the serosa of the posterior wall through the cavity of the uterus on one side in the lower segment. The needle is then brought to a point 8 cm across from the exit of the suture and inserted again from the posterior to the anterior wall on the other side. The ends of the suture are brought to the midpoint of the anterior wall and a flat double knot is tied as tightly as possible, thus forming a loop to compress the uterus. To facilitate the procedure, the uterine walls should be compressed to reduce the thickness and distance between the anterior and posterior walls. A second suture is placed likewise across the middle of the uterine body. The third and fourth sutures are placed 2–3 cm medially in the left and right horns. If bleeding continues, hysterectomy should be performed. This method was used to treat 20 women with postpartum haemorrhage due to uterine atony not responding to medical management, including 17 who had a Caesarean delivery. Hysterectomy was only required in one woman who had developed disseminated intravascular coagulopathy.

Postoperative management

This is along the lines of the management of postpartum haemorrhage using balloon tamponade. If balloon tamponade is used in conjunction, the balloon catheter is removed following the same protocol. If compression sutures alone are used, uterotonic agents should be maintained until bleeding is controlled for several hours, the duration of uterotonic infusion is dependent on the underlying cause(s) and the patient's condition. The sequence of events and the procedure should be clearly documented in the clinical record, which should include a diagram describing the positions/sites of the applied sutures. This will facilitate explanation to the patient afterwards and the preparation of any medical report in the future.

Since absorbable sutures are used, there is no need to remove them at a later date. However, maternal vital signs and symptoms should be monitored for the rare complications such as pyometra. Postnatal follow-up should be more frequent, the first visit preferably at 2 weeks postpartum. There is no recommendation for routine ultrasound examination of the uterus and the uterine cavity in the postnatal period, but this should be arranged if there is any suggestion of complications or if the uterus fails to involute at the normal rate.

Further reading

Akoury H, Sherman C. Uterine wall partial thickness necrosis following combined B-Lynch and Cho square sutures for the treatment of primary postpartum hemorrhage. J Obstet Gynaecol Can 2008;30:421–24.

Allam MS, B-Lynch C. The B-Lynch and other uterine compression suture techniques. Int J Gynecol Obstet 2005;89:236–41.

Balogun-Lynch C, Whitelaw N. The surgical management of post partum haemorrhage. Fetal Matern Med Rev 2006;17:105–23.

Baskett TF. Uterine compression sutures for postpartum hemorrhage. Efficacy, morbidity, and subsequent pregnancy. Obstet Gynecol 2007;110:68–71.

Chen C-P, Chang T-Y, Yeh L-F, et al. Sonographic appearance of the uterus after simple square suturing for rapid control of postpartum hemorrhage and preservation of fertility. J Clin Ultrasound 2002;30:189–91.

Cho JH, Jun HS, Lee CN. Hemostatic suturing technique for uterine bleeding during cesarean delivery. Obstet Gynecol 2000;96:129–31.

Das C, Mukherjee P, Choudhury N, et al. Isthmic-cervical apposition suture: an effective method to control postpartum hemorrhage during cesarean section for placenta previa. J Obstet Gynecol India 2005;25:143–9.

El-Hamamy E, B-Lynch C. A worldwide review of the use of the uterine compression suture techniques as alternative to hysterectomy in the management of severe postpartum haemorrhage. J Obstet Gynaecol 2005;25:143–9.

Habek D, Kulas T, Bobić-Vuković M, et al. Successful of the B-Lynch compression suture in the management of massive postpartum hemorrhage: case reports and review. Arch Gynecol Obstet 2006;273:307–9.

Hackethal A, Brueggmann D, Oehmke F, et al. Uterine compression U-sutures in primary postpartum hemorrhage after cesarean section: fertility preservation with a simple and effective technique. Hum Reprod 2008;23:74–9.

Hayman R, Arulkumaran S, Steer PJ, et al. Uterine compression sutures: Surgical management of postpartum haemorrhage. Obstet Gynecol. 2002;99:502–6

Hwu Y-M, Chen C-P, Su H-S, Su T-H. Parallel vertical compression sutures: a technique to control bleeding from placenta previa or accrete during cesarean section. Obstet Gynecol Surv 2006;61:82–3.

Muppala H, Basama FMS, Hamer F. Re-laparotomy and parallel vertical-compression sutures and prostaglandins for massive intraperitoneal haemorrhage following caesarean section for placenta praevia. Internet J Gynecol Obstet 2006;5(2).

Nelson GS, Birch C. Compression sutures for uterine atony and hemorrhage following cesarean delivery. Int J Gynecol Obstet 2006;92:248–50.

Nelson WL, O'Brien JM. The uterine sandwich for persistent uterine atony: combining the B-Lynch compression suture and an intrauterine Bakri balloon. Am J Obstet Gynecol 2007;196:9–10.

Ochoa M, Allaire AD, Stitely ML. Pyometra after hemostatic square suture technique. Obstet Gynecol 2002;99:506–9.

Ouahba J, Piketty M, Huel C, et al. Uterine compression sutures for postpartum bleeding with uterine atony. Br J Obstet Gynaecol 2007;114:619–22.

Tjalma WAA, Jacquemyn Y. A uterus-saving procedure for postpartum hemorrhage. Int J Gynecol Obstet 2004;86:396–7.

Wu H-H, Yeh G-P. Uterine cavity synechiae after hemostatic square suturing technique. Obstet Gynecol 2005;105;1176–8.

Internet resources

www.obgmanagement.com

Patient information and contacts

www.rcog.org.hk

Ventouse delivery

Definition
Ventouse delivery refers to a form of operative vaginal delivery in which a cup-type device is applied to the fetal head and kept in place through the creation of a vacuum between the cup and scalp. Traction on the cup is then applied to bring about descent and rotation of the fetal head with the aim to assist the delivery of the fetal head, working in conjunction with uterine contractions and maternal bearing down effort.

Epidemiology
Among most centres, the overall operative vaginal delivery rate is around 12–20%. There is a trend of increasing ventouse delivery and decreasing forceps delivery, with a ratio that varied from 2:1 to 5:1 or more between ventouse to forceps delivery, and the reported rate of ventouse delivery varied from 7% to 15%.

Introduction
The ventouse device consists of a cup, made with either metal or plastic, and connected to a suction system through which vacuum suction can be generated by means of an electric or hand pump. The negative pressure generated within the cup sucks in the fetal scalp which will completely fill up the space within the cup by forming an artificial caput or chignon. It was originally thought that 10 minutes are required for an effective chignon to form, but it is now known that only 2 minutes are required. Traction may commence after 1 minute without compromising efficiency and safety. The recommended vacuum pressure is 80 kPa (600 mmHg). Traction on the cup can be exerted by means of a handle or a metallic chain connected to a handle, and this in turn pulls the fetal head along, eventually achieving delivery through the combined effects of uterine contractions and maternal expulsion efforts.

For the expulsive phase of vaginal birth, the forces acting on the fetal head has been estimated to be between 8 kg and 15 kg. Traction force of 10 kg or less has been shown to be sufficient for ventouse delivery without dislodgement of the cup.

For the infant, scalp laceration may occur along the rim of the cup or on the chignon within the cup if the cup is manipulated or rotated artificially, or if excessive traction force is exerted at an angle from the vertical axis of the cup, or if the cup becomes dislodged due to inappropriately exerted force or leakage in the system. Leakage can occur around the rim of the cup due to incorrect direction of traction, inappropriate manipulation, or accidental trapping of maternal tissue, and will result in failed traction or cup dislodgement. If the cup is incorrectly positioned over one of the fontanelles, the negative pressure may cause intracranial injuries and haemorrhage, especially if the cup becomes dislodged. There is no evidence that reducing the vacuum pressure between contractions or keeping the vacuum pressure to <80 kPa will reduce the risk of scalp injuries.

Following delivery of the head, if time is not allowed for restitution and external rotation, the shoulders will not yet have engaged. Attempts to deliver the anterior shoulder can lead to shoulder dystocia. In addition, shoulder dystocia can occur in undiagnosed disproportion. Shoulder dystocia, and incorrect manipulation of the head in the delivery of the shoulders even in the absence of shoulder dystocia, can result in brachial plexus injury and fracture of the clavicle.

Maternal injuries can occur due to several mechanisms. Trapping of vaginal or cervical tissue within the cup during application may occur. If this is not realized and the negative pressure is built up, the trapped maternal tissue will tear when traction is performed. The tear may be longitudinal, circumferential, or spiral, depending on the direction of the traction relative to the trapped tissue and whether rotation occurs. The vaginal tear may extend from the episiotomy, sometimes in a radial manner, especially if the episiotomy is made prematurely or the direction is inappropriate. Third or fourth degree tear may also occur, especially if there is undiagnosed disproportion, prolonged downward traction, or failure of guarding of the perineum. Rarely, a cervix tear may occur if the traction was applied before full cervical dilatation or if a rim of cervical tissue is inadvertently trapped inside the cup.

The likelihood of neonatal and maternal trauma is therefore related to the degree of skill of the operator and the difficulty of the procedure. Both factors also influence the likelihood of achieving successful vaginal delivery, which in turn can account for some of the occurrence of maternal and neonatal injuries. Difficulty can be anticipated by the risky nature of the procedure and it can be categorized accordingly.

Low-risk procedure
Procedure performed for suspected non-reassuring fetal status, delay in the second stage, or need to shorten the second stage, epidural analgesia with poor maternal effort, and with the station being low or at the outlet with visible caput

Moderate-risk procedure
Procedure performed for indications such as evidence of fetal compromise, delay in second stage due to suspected cephalopelvic disproportion or malposition (occipital posterior or transverse, or occipital anterior >45°), severe moulding, and maternal distress or exhaustion, weak infrequent contractions, and with the station being low or mid with the caput not visible. Other associated risk factors of neonatal injury include nulliparity, delivery requiring more than three pulls, and dislodgment of the cup.

Indications
Ventouse delivery is performed for indications similar to those of forceps delivery except that midcavity rotation (autorotation) is largely performed with ventouse rather than forceps nowadays. Also, ventouse delivery can be attempted in very skilful hands for situations that are absolutely contraindicated for forceps delivery.

Indications for ventouse delivery
- Suspected fetal distress
- Suspected maternal distress/fatigue
- Lack of progress in the second stage of labour
  - with epidural analgesia: ≥3 hours in nulliparas and ≥2 hours in multiparas
  - without epidural analgesia: ≥2 hours in nulliparas and ≥1 hour in multiparas;
- Malposition in the absence of or minimal moulding and station below spines
- Delivery of the cephalic-presenting second twin (in this

instance the procedure can be attempted even when the cervix may appear to have shrank, as long as the cup can be applied correctly without trapping any cervical tissue. A smaller sized metal cup, e.g. No. 4 may be preferred here).

Contraindications for ventouse delivery
- Cephalopelvic disproportion
- Brow, face or breech presentation
- Station at/above ischial spines and/or caput not visible at introitus (twin two is exception to this rule), and/or with 2-plus moulding, or station at 0 to 2 cm below spines but with 3-plus moulding
- Fetal position undetermined or uncertain
- Suspected or confirmed bleeding tendency or coagulation defect in the fetus
- Absence of or deficient maternal efforts/expulsive powers/cooperation
- Incomplete cervical dilatation (twin two is exception to this rule, see above).

Prognosis
In general ventouse delivery is associated with fewer maternal and neonatal traumatic injuries, but some studies nevertheless have reported more birth trauma associated with ventouse delivery. Compared with forceps delivery, ventouse delivery was associated with less general and regional anaesthesia, Caesarean delivery, and more vaginal deliveries. Neonatal cephalhaematoma and retinal haemorrhage are associated more with ventouse delivery. The failure rates of rigid and soft cups are 9% and 16% respectively, and the rates for dislodgement are 10% and 22% respectively. Soft cups are associated with less scalp injury, but there is no reduction in the risk of cephalhaematomas.

Possible injuries can be direct and indirect and can occur in both the mother and neonate in the same case.

Maternal injury
- Lacerations to the genital tract, including cervical, vaginal and perineal first and second degree tears. Even with an episiotomy, ventouse delivery may still be associated with radial tears in the vagina/perineum.
- Anal sphincter injury in the form of third- and fourth-degree tears.
- Cervical laceration.

Neonatal injury
- Injuries to the scalp and skull, including scalp blisters and lacerations, cephalhaematoma (as high as 10.8–11.5%), subaponeurotic haemorrhage, and skull fracture (5.0%).
- Intracranial injuries, including retinal haemorrhage, subdural haematoma, subarachnoid haemorrhage, and tentorial tear; intracranial haemorrhage can occur in up to 0.87%.
- Brachial plexus injury, can be associated with shoulder dystocia following ventouse delivery. The risk was increased with the time required for ventouse extraction.

In singleton, neonatal deaths were associated with cranial trauma. Cranial traumatic injury was almost always associated with physical difficulty at delivery and the use of multiple instruments. The use of ventouse as the primary or only instrument did not prevent this outcome. Subaponeurotic (subgaleal) haematoma has been strongly related to delivery or attempted delivery by ventouse extraction. It has been shown that ventouse extraction was associated with increased risk of subarachnoid haemorrhage and cephalhaematoma compared with forceps delivery. However, it was also shown that while infants delivered by ventouse extraction had higher rate of subdural or cerebral haemorrhage compared with infants delivered spontaneously, there was no significant difference from that associated with forceps use. The common risk factor for haemorrhage was actually abnormal labour.

Clinical approach
When operative delivery is indicated, the choice between ventouse and forceps delivery is related not only to the medical indications and contraindications, but to the status, experience, and perception of the operator as well. It has been shown that even among the same group of specialists with similar expertise, ventouse delivery tended to be used in less difficult cases in women with higher parity and shorter labour compared with forceps delivery. There are also different preferences in the choice of the ventouse cups.

Ventouse delivery is thought to be an easier and safer procedure with less risk of maternal and fetal injuries, in many centres. This method is used by family physicians as well, while forceps delivery is restricted to obstetricians. Appropriate level of skill is required to achieve the best outcome, and ventouse delivery should not be taken light-heartedly. In obtaining consent it is best to provide explanation for performing forceps and ventouse delivery, since forceps delivery may have to be used in case of failed ventouse delivery.

Type of ventouse devices available
Soft anterior cups
- Silc cup
- Standard Mityvac cup
- Soft-touch cup
- Kiwi ProCup.

Rigid anterior cups
- Malmstrom cup
- Bird Anterior original (chain) cup
- Bird Anterior New Generation (string) cup
- O'Neil Anterior cup
- M-Style Mityvac cup
- Flex cup
- Kiwi OmniCup.

Posterior cups
- Bird Posterior original (chain) cup
- Bird Posterior New Generation (string) cup
- O'Neil Posterior cup
- Kiwi OmniCup
- M-select Mityvac cup.

Usually, only a few types of devices are available in any given hospital, and most obstetricians are familiar with only a few of these devices. It is recommended to focus on learning the use of and become proficient in one type each of the anterior and posterior cup before embarking on trying other cups. Some cups have an indicator (a knob in metallic cups) to show the position of the occiput. This allows tracking of the rotation of the occiput if the cup is correctly placed with the indicator in the direction of the occiput.

The prerequisites for ventouse delivery

Essentially this is a checklist to ensure that contraindications have been excluded.

- The fetus is in cephalic presentation and the fetal head is engaged.
- The fetus is at or near term and the estimated birthweight is ≥2500 g.
- The exact position of the head should be ascertained.
- There are no fetal contraindications to the use of negative suction pressure on the fetal scalp, such as suspected bleeding tendency and thrombocytopenia.
- Uterine contractions are present, and if the contractions are weak and infrequent, then the uterus is responding to augmentation with oxytocin infusion.
- The mother is conscious and able to bear down spontaneously or following instructions if she is under the effect of epidural analgesia, and that there are no maternal contraindications to bearing down.
- The analgesia is effective.
- The cervix should be fully dilated, but in skilful hands, ventouse delivery can be performed with cervical dilation of 8–9 cm in multiparas.
- There is no obstruction or narrowing in the birth canal that could result in difficulties or failure of the procedure. The shape of the pelvis should be assessed, and the adequacy of the outlet determined, making sure that the pelvis is not convergent.
- The bladder should be empty.
- The delivery team is all ready and standing by, including a staff member (nurse/midwife, obstetrician, or neonatologist) assigned to resuscitate the neonate.

Examination prior to cup application

- Abdominal palpation: this should be performed as in the case of forceps delivery to determine the amount of fetal head palpable above the pelvic brim and the side of the fetal back. Similarly, in case of doubt, a trial of ventouse can be organised in the operating theatre. In case the findings on abdominal examination are non-reassuring, the operator should consider abandoning the procedure, since there are much greater risks of fetal hypoxia and injury, and maternal trauma, if ventouse delivery fails and forceps or caesarean delivery is required instead.
- Vaginal examination: again the same approaches to forceps delivery should be applied here. At times, the large caput or significant moulding may make the diagnosis of the position, or the degree of deflexion and asynclitism, difficult to ascertain. In this instance, a trial of ventouse delivery can still be performed.

The choice of the ventouse cup and instrument check

This should be dependent on the type of application and the findings on vaginal examination. For low-risk procedure, a soft or rigid cup can be chosen. For high-risk procedure, a rigid cup is preferable. For mid-cavity, or occipital posterior and transverse position, the posterior cup should be chosen. For metal cups, different sizes may be available, and for a normal size or large fetus, the No. 5 cup (5 cm diameter) should be chosen. Whatever the choice, always check the instruments, the connection, and the working of the pump before application.

The application of the ventouse cup

Location of the 'flexion point'

In applying the ventouse cup, it is important to ascertain the flexion point, which is about 3 cm anterior to the posterior fontanelle on the sagittal suture. This point represents the leading end of the completely flexed and normally moulded head as it descends the birth canal. If the ventouse cup is properly placed over the flexion point and traction is applied, the fetal head diameters would be optimal for delivery with no need for any manoeuvring or manipulation of the fetal head through the point of traction.

Placement of the cup

The following process can be used to facilitate placement of the cup over the flexion point. During the vaginal examination, first locate the posterior fontanelle with the middle finger and then place the index finger about 3 cm from the middle finger along the sagittal suture. Then the middle finger is moved to join the index finger, the tip of the former now resting on the flexion point. The hand is supinated with the palm facing upwards. The index finger is then moved towards the palmar surface along the middle finger until the tip reaches the level of the posterior fourchette. The length of the middle finger as marked by the tip of the index finger represents the distance inside the vagina that the ventouse cup must be inserted to achieve a correct application. If in order to keep the finger tip on the flexion point the middle finger remains buried in the vagina up to the carpometacarpal joint, then the fetal head is too high for an attempted instrumental vagina delivery which should therefore be abandoned.

Building up the vacuum pressure

Once the cup is properly placed, the negative pressure can be built up to the recommended 80 kPa in one step, although the traditional teaching is to build this up stepwise over 3–6 minutes.

The traction for cephalic presentation

Number and duration of tractions

The traction force and number of pulls are influenced by all the factors that determine the success or otherwise of vaginal delivery. Therefore restricting the number of pulls to 'three' in the completion of the delivery process may not be practicable, especially in the presence of epidural analgesia and a restrictive approach to episiotomy. One study showed that only 27% of the deliveries were completed within three pulls. It is recommended to divide the process into a descent and an outlet phase. A higher traction force and greater number of pulls may be required for the outlet phase than is the case for the descent phase, and 84% of the deliveries were completed by three pulls each of the descent and outlet phase (six pulls in total) without increase in significant adverse outcomes. In terms of the time duration, most deliveries were completed in 15 minutes and almost all in 20 minutes. However, if progress is not observed in the first three pulls, the procedure should be abandoned even if the time duration is much less than 15 minutes.

Method of traction for occipital anterior position

Traction should be synchronized with uterine contraction and maternal bearing down efforts. The fingertips of the dominant hand should be used to hold onto the crossbar of the traction device, and the traction force, being limited by the fingertips, should be generated from the elbow and shoulder rather than from the whole body. The traction force exerted should be smooth and steady along the axis of the birth canal and not jerky or wagging sideways or up and down. By ensuring that the handle remains perpendicular to the outside of the cup, the direction of traction will be along the axis of the birth canal. The axis will change from downwards to horizontal. Only when the head crowns should the traction be directed upwards.

During traction the other hand should provide counter-traction with the thumb on the cup and the index finger is placed on the scalp to reflect the descent of the head. Counter-traction should be given until the head is delivered. Traction should stop once the uterine contraction is over and/or the mother stops bearing down. No difference in the time required for delivery, incidence of method failure, or maternal and neonatal complications, could be demonstrated between continuous traction to maintain fetal station with the same negative suction pressure versus intermittent traction with reduction in negative suction pressure between contractions.

As the head crowns, avoid pulling too hard or rapidly, because the resistance due to the resistance of the perineum can lead to dislodgement of the cup, and time should be allowed for the completion of autorotation. Episiotomy, if indicated, should be made at this point.

Traction for occipital posterior and transverse positions
The procedure is similar to traction for occipital anterior position, but the most important point is the correct placement of the posterior cup at the flexion point (flexing median application). Flexion of the head and anterior autorotation of the head occurs in >90% of the cases as long as there is flexing median application, whereas autorotation occurs in only 30% if the application is deflexing. There is no need to manipulate the cup or the handle in attempts to rotate the head, which could actually cause more failures (cup dislodgement).

Failed ventouse delivery
Failure can be in form of failure to descend with tractions or dislodgement of the cup. The commonest cause of failure is incorrect technique as 80% of the cases of failed ventouse delivery would have delivery completed with forceps. Other causes include persistent occipital posterior or transverse position, midcavity procedure, deflexing and paramedian application of the cup, use of inappropriate cup, traction before full cervical dilatation, and undiagnosed cephalopelvic disproportion. In the latter instance there is increased risk of fetal intracranial injury and laceration to the maternal genital tract.

Following failure of ventouse delivery, there should be a reappraisal of the likelihood of vaginal delivery. If the fetal head is visible at the introitus, forceps delivery may be attempted.

Trial of ventouse delivery
In case of suspected cephalopelvic disproportion, or unfavourable pelvis, the ventouse delivery should be organized as a trial of ventouse. The same preparations for a trial of forceps apply here. The same three-pull rule for initial progress is similarly followed, but progress is assessed not only in terms of descent but also of flexion and rotation of the head as reflected by the indicator on the cup. The trial must be abandoned if delivery has not occurred, or is not imminent, or there is no suggestion of flexion or rotation that should have occurred, by the third pull. The cup must be detached before the emergency Caesarean section is performed. If an episiotomy has been made already, this can be packed and repaired later after the baby has been delivered.

Procedures after successful delivery
Following ventouse delivery, the genital tract and perineum should be checked, and tears and episiotomy repaired, in the same way as following forceps delivery.

The baby should be resuscitated in the same way and documentation of neonatal acid–base status performed. A thorough examination of the neonate should be conducted to look for any injuries which, if present, should be clearly documented. The placenta and membranes should be checked to make sure it is complete. In case of vulval or perineal oedema or haematoma, an indwelling Foley catheter should be inserted for continuous drainage for the first 24 hours. The patient should be re-examined one hour later for evidence of vulvovaginal haematoma before being transferred back to the postnatal ward.

Training in ventouse delivery
Ventous delivery is often considered as an easy procedure. Emphasis on the proper and adequate training in its use is wanting. Ventouse delivery was shown to be associated with a relatively high failure rate, which was related in part to suboptimal application and inappropriate positioning of the cup. Apart from possible difficulty in the accurate application of the cup due to caput or malposition, poor assessment of the orientation and position of the fetal skull might also have played an important role, thus underscoring the need for improvement in training methods.

Further reading

Bofill JA, Rust OA, Schorr SJ, et al. Morrison JC. A randomized trial of two vacuum extraction techniques. Obstet gynecol 1997;89:758–62.

Cargill YM, MacKinnon CJ. Guidelines for operative vaginal birth. SOGC Clinical Practice Guidelines. J Obstet Gynaecol Can 2004;26:747–53.

Chadwick LM, Pemberton PJ, Kurinczuk JJ. Neonatal subgaleal haematoma: associated risk factors, complications and outcome. J Paediatr Child Health 1996;32:228–32.

Chan CCT, Malathi I, Yeo GSH. Is the vacuum extractor really the instrument of first choice? Aust NZ J Obstet Gynaecol 1999;39:305–9.

Gilbert WM, Nesbitt TS, Danielsen B. Associated factors in 1611 cases of brachial plexus injury. Obstet gynecol 1999;93:536–40.

Johanson RB, Menon V. Vacuum extraction versus forceps for assisted vaginal delivery. Cochrane Database Syst Rev 2007;4:CD000224.

Mollberg M, Hagberg H, Bager B, et al. Risk factors for obstetric brachial plexus palsy among neonates delivered by vacuum extraction. Obstet Gynecol 2005;106:913–18.

O'Mahony F, Settatree R, Platt C, Johanson R. Review of singleton fetal and neonatal deaths associated with cranial and cephalic delivery during a national intrapartum-related confidential enquiry. Br J Obstet Gynaecol 2005;112:619–26.

Simonson C, Barlow P, Dehennin, et al. Neonatal complications of vacuum-assisted delivery. Obstet Gynecol 2007;109:626–33.

Towner D, Castro MA, Eby-Wilkens E, Gilbert WM. Effect of mode of delivery in nulliparous women on neonatal intracranial injury. N Engl J Med 1999;341:1709–14.

Vacca A. Reducing the risks of a vacuum delivery. Fetal and Maternal medicine Review 2006:17:301–15.

Vacca A. Vacuum-assisted delivery. Baillieres Best Pract Res Clin Obstet 2002;16:17–30.

Wen SW, Liu S, Kramer MS, et al. Comparison of maternal and infant outcomes between vacuum extraction and forceps deliveries. Am J Epidemiol 2001;153:103–7.

Internet resources

www.emedicine.com
www.aafp.org

Patient resources

www.rcog.org.hk

Part 3

Gynaecology

Reproduction *463*
Benign and urogynaecology *599*
Benign, premalignant, and malignant tumours in
  gynaecology *639*
Common gynaecological procedures and surgery *687*

Reproduction

Ambiguous genitalia *464*
Anatomy of female pelvis *468*
Chronic pelvic pain *476*
Contraception *478*
Disorders of sex development *482*
Donor insemination *484*
Heavy menstrual bleeding *486*
Dysmenorrhoea *488*
Ectopic pregnancy *490*
Embryo freezing *494*
Emergency contraception *498*
Endometriosis *500*
Female infertility *502*
Fertility in survivors of childhood malignancy *508*
Imaging in reproductive medicine *512*
Induction of ovulation *514*
Intracytoplasmic sperm injection *518*
Intrauterine devices *520*
In vitro fertilization *524*
In vitro oocyte maturation *528*
Malformations of the genital tract *532*
Male subfertility *536*
Menopause and hormone replacement therapy *542*
Menorrhagia *550*
Menstrual cycle: physiology *554*
Miscarriage: early *556*
Oocyte donation *560*
Oligomenorrhoea and amenorrhoea *562*
Ovarian hyperstimulation syndrome *566*
Paediatric and adolescent problems *570*
Polycystic ovary syndrome *574*
Preimplantation genetic diagnosis *578*
Premature ovarian failure *580*
Premenstrual syndrome *582*
Psychosexual problems *584*
Recurrent miscarriage *590*
Termination of pregnancy *594*

Ambiguous genitalia

Definition
The genitalia are considered ambiguous when they are atypical in appearance and it is not possible to assign gender merely by inspection of the genitalia.

Incidence
About 1 in 4000 births.

Aetiology
Normal sexual differentiation
Genetic sex is determined at the time of conception when the ovum is fertilized by a spermatozoa containing either X or Y chromosome. The developing gonad is indifferent until about 7 weeks of gestation and both sexes develop Müllerian and Wolffian ducts.

In a male fetus, the SRY (sex determining region of the Y chromosome) and testes-determining factors (TDFs) promote the differentiation of the gonad into testes. Ovarian development was considered to be a default position in the absence of the SRY gene, although recently ovarian-determining genes have been found.

Hormonal production by the developing testes determines phenotypic sex. The Sertoli cells produce anti-Müllerian hormone (AMH), which cause regression of the Müllerian duct. Around 8 weeks, the Leydig cells produce testosterone, which promotes the development of the Wolffian duct into the epididymis, seminal vesicles, and the vas deferens. Testosterone is converted by the enzyme 5-α-reductase to dihydrotestosterone (DHT), which causes the growth of the phallus, fusion of the urethral folds to create an opening at the tip of the penis, and fusion of labioscrotal folds to form the scrotum. Masculinization of the external genitalia is complete by 14 weeks and the penis, similar in size to the clitoris at 14 weeks, starts to grow from 20 weeks until birth.

In the female fetus, the absence of AMH causes the development of the Müllerian ducts into the Fallopian tubes, uterus, and upper portion of the vagina. In the absence of androgens, the urogenital sinus develops into the clitoris, labia, and the lower part of the vagina.

Pathophysiology of ambiguous genitalia
The older terminology for ambiguous genitalia included true hermaphroditism, pseudo-hermaphroditism, and intersex. These terminologies are generally unhelpful as a descriptor of the phenotypic abnormality and are considered pejorative by patient groups. Following international consensus, the terminology used for these conditions is disorders of sex differentiation (DSD).

The pathophysiology of the conditions that lead to ambiguous genitalia are essentially caused by overviriliza-tion of an XX fetus (XX, DSD) or undervirilization of an XY fetus (XY, DSD).

As the development of the female external genitalia is essentially an autonomic process, genital ambiguity in a female fetus with normal ovaries can only happen when it is exposed to an environment where there is an excess of androgens. This can occur because of abnormalities in the fetal adrenal gland or placenta, or because of effects of exogenous androgens in the maternal circulation, which crosses the placenta.

The development of the male external genitalia is an active process and undervirilization of the external genitalia can cause genital ambiguity. This can be due to abnormalities in testicular development, failure to convert testosterone into dihyrotestosterone, which is the androgen responsible for virilization of the external genitalia (5-α-reductase deficiency), or abnormalities in the androgen receptor (androgen insensitivity syndrome (AIS)).

In some cases, testicular and ovarian tissue may be present in the same individual. This condition previously called true hermaphroditism is now termed ovo-testicular DSD.

The causes of ambiguous genitalia are listed in Table 12.1.1.

Congenital adrenal hyperplasia
Congenital adrenal hyperplasia (CAH) is the most common cause of virilization of a female fetus. It is most commonly due to 21 hydroxylase deficiency, an autosomal recessive disorder that leads to glucocorticoid and miner-alocorticoid deficiency. This leads to excessive production of adrenocorticotropic hormone (ACTH), adrenal hyper-plasia, accumulation of precursors prior to the enzymatic defect, and excess production of androgens due to diversion of the precursors along the androgen pathway.

This commonly presents as ambiguous genitalia in a female fetus, salt-losing crisis in male fetuses, or a general failure to thrive. In female fetuses, the clitoris is enlarged, the labia partially fused and rugose, and a common uro-genital sinus is present instead of separate urethral and vaginal orifices. The internal genitalia are those of a normal female.

Androgen insensitivity syndrome
This syndrome is due to an abnormality of the androgen receptor. Despite the presence of normal levels of androgens, the phenotype is either female or ambiguous.

Complete AIS (CAIS) was previously known as testicular feminization syndrome. This terminology is considered offensive by patient groups and is no longer recommended. The typical presentation of CAIS is of primary amenorrhoea at puberty with normal breast development and pubertal growth spurt. There is absence or scanty pubic and axillary hair, the vagina is often underdeveloped and the uterus and Fallopian tubes are absent.

Table 12.1.1 Causes of ambiguous genitalia

Normal female XX karyotype	Congenital adrenal hyperplasia (CAH)
	Maternal exogenous androgens (progestogens)
	Maternal endogenous androgens (ovarian/adrenal tumours)
	Placental aromatase deficiency
Normal male XY karyotype	Mixed gonadal dysgenesis
	Partial androgen insensitivity syndrome (PAIS)
	5-α-reductase deficiency
	Defects in testosterone biosynthesis: 17 β-ketosteroid hydroxylase deficiency
	Leydig cell hypoplasia
Congenital anomalies	Cloacal extrophy
	Microphalia
	Severe hypospadias

CAIS can also present as bilateral inguinal hernias in female infants, which is otherwise a rare condition and should prompt investigation to exclude CAIS.

It should be noted that CAIS does not present as ambiguous genitalia, as the phenotype is of a normal female infant.

Partial androgen insensitivity syndrome (PAIS) encompasses a spectrum of conditions where there is partial response to androgens during development. It often presents as ambiguous genitalia with penoscrotal hypospadias, micropenis, and a bifid scrotum. In the most severe cases, it may present as isolated clitoromegaly only marginally varying from CAIS. In the mildest form, it may present as isolated hypospadias which may be severe.

5-α-reductase deficiency

This often presents with either ambiguous genitalia or phenotypically female infants who go on to develop significant virilization at puberty and in some cases to change of gender. The underlying cause is a defect in the enzyme 5-α-reductase, which coverts testosterone to the more potent DHT, which is required for virilization of the external genitalia. At puberty, virilization occurs under the influence of testosterone. The condition is inherited as an autosomal recessive trait and it is more common in some geographical areas such as the Dominican Republic.

The phallus is small and the urethral opening is situated in the perineum. The vagina is absent or inconspicuous and the testes are usually present in the inguinal region.

Clinical approach

Diagnosis

History

- Maternal drug intake: progestogens cause virilization in a female fetus and cyproterone causes undervirilization in a male fetus.
- Maternal history of virilization during pregnancy: in placental aromatase deficiency, the fetal androgens which are not metabolized by the placenta cross into the maternal circulation and cause virilization.
- Family history: AIS is X linked, CAH-autosomal recessive. 5-α-reductase deficiency and 17 β-hydroxysteroid dehydrogenase deficiency is more common in consanguineous couples. Family history of neonatal deaths, problems at puberty and unexplained infertility may point to underlying syndromes.

Examination

- General examination of the infant should be carried out to exclude other morphological abnormalities that may point to a syndrome complex.
- Rarely, the mother may show signs of virilization suggesting either a functional tumour (adrenal/ovarian) or placental aromatase deficiency.
- Abnormal skin hyperpigmentation is suggestive of CAH as the increased production of ACTH stimulates melanocyte production.
- Assessment of the phallus requires care, as chordee is usually present resulting in the phallus appearing smaller than it actually is.
- The position of the urethral orifice should be ascertained, although this may be difficult to determine until the infant voids. This may be present either on the phallus or on the perineum, the position determines the degree of hypospadias.

- The colour and rugosity of the labioscrotal folds should be assessed: hyperpigmentation is suggestive of CAH and rugosity is suggestive of exposure to androgens.

The presence or absence of a vagina

- Palpation of the gonad requires practise and patience. With the thighs abducted, gentle palpation of the inguinal region starting above the inguinal ring towards the external genitalia is performed. The presence of a palpable gonad in this region indicates a male infant, as in cases of ambiguous genitalia in female infants, the ovaries are in their normal intra-abdominal position.

Investigations

The investigations to be undertaken in cases of ambiguous genitalia are listed in Table 12.1.2. As CAH is the most common cause of ambiguous genitalia, initial investigations should focus on excluding this condition. Simultaneous determination of sex chromosome status should be carried out using fluorescent *in situ* hybridization (FISH).

Counselling

- Ambiguous genitalia constitutes one of the most distressing situations for parents because of the uncertainty regarding the most basic identity of their newborn child.
- It is advisable to avoid speculation regarding the gender. Instead, parents should be told that there is a problem identifying the gender and further investigations are required.
- Counselling of the parents should be performed by an experienced member of the team who will care for the child.
- Once the diagnosis has been established, a further discussion should occur with the parents regarding the long-term prognosis, including the need for hormonal treatment and impact on future fertility.
- The impact of prenatal exposure of androgens on the developing female brain may impact on future behaviour and gender identity.
- As many causes of ambiguous genitalia have an inherited basis, the parents should be informed regarding the inheritance pattern and counselled regarding the implication for other siblings and future pregnancies.

Management

Management of CAH

- In the salt-losing form of CAH, presentation may be in the form of circulatory collapse or failure to thrive.
- Hyperkalaemia is one of the first signs, and serum electrolytes should be measured regularly.
- Replacement glucocorticoids and mineralocorticoids should be given.
- Hormonal therapy is required lifelong with additional higher doses required for surgical interventions.
- In fetuses at risk of developing CAH, CVS or amniocentesis may be considered with a view to commencing steroid therapy for affected females. Dexamethasone given prenatally suppresses the fetal hypothalamo-adrenal axis and prevents virilization in about 85% of cases. This treatment is controversial as the long-term effects of antenatal dexamethasone is unknown and should only be carried out in a specialist centre.

Assignment of gender of rearing

- Management of these children should be carried out by a multidisciplinary team that includes neonatologists,

Table 12.1.2 Investigations in cases of ambiguous genitalia

Investigation	Rationale and results
Serum 17 hydroxyprogesterone levels	Elevated in CAH (>242 nmol/L in CAH, normal <3 nmol/L)
Urea and electrolyte levels	Abnormal in salt-losing CAH
Corticotropin stimulation test (measurement of 17-OHP 60 minutes after injection of corticotropin)	Elevated in non-classic CAH (levels >45 nmol/L in CAH)
Basal and hCG-stimulated androgen levels	Elevated in AIS Elevated levels of precursors compared to testosterone in errors of testosterone production
Serum AMH levels	Absent in anorchia Reduced in dysgenetic gonads Elevated in AIS
FISH (fluorescent in situ hybridization)	To detect Y chromosome sequence: results are usually available in 6–8 hours
Karyotype	To determine genetic sex
Ultrasound	To identify the presence of uterus and identify the nature of the gonad (either intra-abdominal or inguinal)
Genitography	CAH to identify the level at which the vagina opens on to the urogenital sinus In all other cases to assess the presence of a vagina, cervix, uterus, and Fallopian tubes
CT and MRI scan	Good definition of the pelvic floor structures can be obtained with MRI. However, the need for sedation or anaesthesia to prevent movement artefact and the high quality images usually available with ultrasound limit their use
Genital fibroblast culture	To identify the extent and affinity of androgen receptors

paediatric surgeons/urologists, endocrinologists and psychologists.

- Factors influencing gender assignment include diagnosis, appearance of the genitalia, surgical options, need for hormonal therapy, fertility, parental wishes, and possibly cultural factors.
- More than 90% of 46,XX CAH and all cases of 46,XY CAIS reared as female identify with female gender. This supports the concept of raising even severely virilized female infants as female gender.
- The allocation of gender in 5-α-reductase deficiency and PAIS is more problematic. Around 60% of children with 5-α-reductase deficiency raised as girls will virilize at puberty and will have gender reassignment. About 25% of individuals with PAIS are dissatisfied with the gender of rearing whether male or female.
- Male infants with micropenis should be raised in the male gender. The severity of hypospadias is not necessarily a determining factor in gender assignment as it is often surgically correctable.

Surgery for ambiguous genitalia
- It has long been considered that children have a gender neutral identity until the age of 3 and that it is therefore necessary to assign gender by this age. Recently, this concept has been challenged as it is recognized that this is a gradual process.
- In cases of severe virilization of a female fetus, feminizing genital surgery was often carried out soon after birth. The aim was to restore the genitalia to a more 'normal' appearance allaying parental anxiety and confirming gender identity.

- Feminizing genitoplasty involves surgery to reduce the size of the clitoris, create or enlarge a vaginal orifice and reduce the size of the labia.
- Such surgery has come under the spotlight in recent years, particularly with adult patients claiming a feeling of 'being mutilated' following such surgery.
- There is growing evidence of the adverse impact of such surgery particularly on the clitoris and problems with sexual function in adulthood.
- Vaginoplasty procedures performed in children often require a revision procedure during adolescence because of stenosis.
- Clitoral surgery includes clitoredectomy (no longer recommended), clitoral recession (where the corpora are hitched under the symphysis; this can cause painful erections), and clitoral reduction (conserving the neurovascular bundle).
- The timing of such surgery is controversial and hotly debated in view of the potential adverse long-term outcomes.
- In cases of mild clitoromegaly, it is appropriate to avoid surgery.
- There are calls to defer such surgery until adolescence to enable the individual to play a major role in giving informed consent. This must be balanced against the potential psychological distress to both the individual and the parents from the uncorrected ambiguous genitalia.
- This type of surgery should only be performed in specialist centres with long-term follow up of outcomes.
- A historical difficulty in assessing the impact of such surgery has been that there has often been non-disclosure

of the condition to the affected individual. It is currently recommended that full disclosure should be made so that individuals are able to access appropriate support and information.

Gonadectomy

Gonadectomy is often required when a 46,XY infant is assigned to a female gender of rearing. This is often required to prevent virilization at puberty. Dysgenetic gonads have a significant risk of malignancy and should be removed.

The timing of gonadectomy is discussed further in Section 12.5, Disorders of sex development.

Further reading

Aaronson IA. The investigation and management of the infant with ambiguous genitalia: a surgeon's perspective. Curr Probl Paediatr 2001;31:168–94.

Berra M, Liao LM, Creighton SM, Conway GS. Long-term health issues with women of XY karyotype. Maturitas 2010;65:172–78.

Hindmarsh PC. Management of a child with Congenital Adrenal Hyperplasia. Best Pract Res Clin Endocrin Res 2009;23:193–208.

Hughes IA, Deeb A. Androgen resistance. Best Pract Res Clin Endocrin Res 2006; 20:577–98.

Lee PA, Houk CP, Ahmed SF, Hughes IA. Consensus Statement on the Management of Intersex Disorders. Paediatrics 2006;118:e488–e500.

Merke DP, Bornstein SR. Congenital Adrenal Hyperplasia. Lancet 2005;365:2125–36.

Michala L, Creighton SM. The XY female. Best Pract Res Clin Obstet Gynaecol 2009;1–10.

Rangecroft L 2003. Surgical management of ambiguous genitalia. Arch Dis Child; 88:799–801.

Zucker KJ. Intersexuality and gender identity differentiation. J Paediatr Adolesc Gynecol 2002;15:3–13.

Patient resources

Androgen Insensitivity Syndrome Support Group www.aissg.org

Intersex Society of North America www.isna.org

Anatomy of female pelvis

Introduction

A clear understanding of the anatomy of the female pelvis is essential for practising obstetricians and gynaecologists. Knowledge of specific anatomical relationships between the bony pelvis and its associated muscles and ligaments, blood vessels, lymphatics and pelvic viscera helps in the diagnosis as well as management of disorders affecting the female genital tract. Meticulous knowledge of normal anatomy as well as recognition of 'distorted anatomy' may help to avoid unintended damage to adjacent structures during pelvic surgery, such as ureteric damage, while ligating uterine arteries during a hysterectomy. Similarly, precise anatomical knowledge of pelvic vasculature may be life saving, as in ligation of internal iliac arteries during massive obstetric or gynaecological haemorrhage.

The bony pelvis

The pelvis is formed of four bones: two hip bones laterally and in front and the sacrum and coccyx behind. The hip bones are fused iliac, ischial, and pubic bones. The ischium and pubis also meet below, in the centre of the inferior ramus, to form the obturator foramen. The arcuate line that extends from the sacral promontory to the pectineal line of the pubis divides the pelvis into bowl-shaped false and a circular true pelvis. The urogenital organs lie in the true pelvis.

A low midline incision allows a direct approach into the true pelvis. The bony landmarks for the pelvic surgeon are the anterior and posterior iliac spines, the iliac crests, the pubic tubercles, and the ischial tuberosities. Fig. 12.2.1 illustrates the parts of an articulated bony pelvis.

Cooper's (pectineal) ligament overlies the pectineal line and offers a sure hold for sutures in prolapse repairs and urethral suspension procedures. The ischial spine is palpable transvaginally and provides attachment to the pelvic diaphragm and the sacrospinous ligament.

The sacroiliac joints are strong synovial joints and least prone to fractures. The pubic bones are the thinnest of the pelvic bones, are more prone to fractures, and their fragments may injure the adjacent bladder, urethra, and vagina. Diameters of the pelvic inlet, midcavity, and outlet influence the mechanism of human labour and these are given in Table 12.2.1.

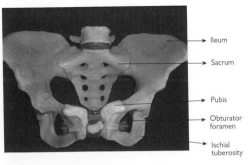

Fig. 12.2.1 The bony pelvis.

Table 12.2.1 Diameters of the pelvic planes

Plane	Anteroposterior	Oblique	Transverse
Pelvic inlet	11.5	12	13
Midcavity	12	12	12
Pelvic outlet	12	–	10.5

Soft tissues of the pelvis

Muscles of the pelvis

The pelvic floor

The pelvic floor is composed of a funnel-shaped wide and thin fibromuscular tissue forming the inferior border of the abdominopelvic cavity. It separates the structures in the pelvis from the perineum and ischeorectal fossae and extends from midway of the symphysis pubis to the coccyx and from one lateral pelvic sidewall to the other. The primary muscles of the pelvic diaphragm are the levator ani and the coccygeus.

The levator ani muscles forms the bulk of the pelvic diaphragm and has three parts named after their origin and insertion: pubococcygeus, iliococcygeus, and ischiococcygeus. It arises from the tendinous arch extending from the posterior aspect of the body of pubis, arcuate line (or the 'white line') on the obturator fascia, to ischial spine. The coccygeus is a triangular muscle that occupies the area between the ischial spine and the coccyx.

The paired levator ani muscles act as a single muscle. It is pierced in the midline by urethra, vagina, and anal canal, and, hence plays an important role in the control of urination, in parturition, and in maintaining faecal continence. Fig. 12.2.2 illustrates the muscular attachments of the pelvic floor.

Urogenital diaphragm

The urogenital diaphragm is a strong muscular membrane that lies external and inferior to the pelvic diaphragm. It occupies the area between the pubis symphysis and ischial tuberosities anteriorly and has two layers that enclose the deep transverse perineal and sphincter urethrae muscles. These muscles surrounds both the vagina and the urethra. The urogenital diaphragm reinforces the pelvic diaphragm and provides support to the urethra and maintains the urethrovesical junction.

Perineal body or the central perineal tendon

The perineal body is a pyramidal shaped fibromuscular tissue located in the midline between the anus and the vagina, forming a 'hub' for supporting the pelvic viscera. The superior border of the perineal body represents the point of insertion of rectovaginal (Denonvilliers') fascia, which extends to the underside of the peritoneum covering the Pouch of Douglas, separating the ano-rectum from the urogenital compartment. The perineal body represents the point of fusion between the free posterior edge of the urogenital diaphragm and the posterior apex of the urogenital hiatus. Virtually every muscle of the perineum (superficial and deep transverse perinei, bulbocavernosus,

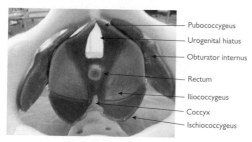

Fig 12.2.2 The muscles of the pelvic floor ('pelvic diaphragm').

- Pubococcygeus
- Urogenital hiatus
- Obturator internus
- Rectum
- Iliococcygeus
- Coccyx
- Ischiococcygeus

levator ani, external anal sphincter, striated urethral sphincter) and fascia (perineal membrane, Denonvilliers', Colles', and endopelvic) are attached to the perineal body. At its core are abundant elastin smooth muscle fibres which are richly innervated, which suggests that it may have a dynamic role in supporting the genital tract. Fig 12.2.3 illustrates the perineal body.

The perineal body is also an important part of the pelvic floor as it supports the lower vagina, and its weakness predisposes to defects such as rectocele and enterocele.

The endopelvic fascia and ligaments form a system of connective tissue interlaced with elastin, smooth muscle cells, fibroblasts, and vascular structures. It lies immediately beneath the peritoneum and is a single continuous unit with various thickenings or condensations in specific areas. Over the viscera, it merges with the visceral fascia and is very thin. This allows for displacements and changes in volume of the uterus, bladder, and rectum. Anteriorly, laterally, and posteriorly the endopelvic fascia gets condensed and thickened to form strong ligaments that support the pelvic visera. The urinary bladder and urethra are attached to the pelvic walls by pubovesical and pubourethral ligaments and the uterus by the pubocervical ligaments, lateral sacral (Cardinal), and uterosacral ligaments, respectively, to the bony pelvis.

Blood supply in the pelvis

Ovarian artery

The ovarian arteries arise from the anteriolateral aspect of the aorta just below the renal vessels and run downwards in the retroperitoneal space. The right ovarian artery crosses the anterior surface on vena cava, the lower part of the 'abdominal' ureter on the right side and then runs lateral to the ureter. It then enters the pelvis via the infundibulopelvic ligament. The left artery crosses the ureter almost immediately after its origin at just below the left renal artery and then runs in the retroperineal space,

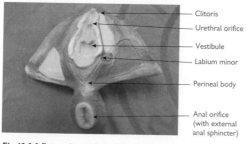

- Clitoris
- Urethral orifice
- Vestibule
- Labium minor
- Perineal body
- Anal orifice (with external anal sphincter)

Fig 12.2.3 External genitalia and the perineal body.

crossing the bifurcation of the common iliac artery at the pelvic brim to enter the infundibulopelvic ligament.

The blood supply to the ovary and lateral aspects of the fallopian tubes is derived from the numerous small branches of the ovarian artery as it passes through the mesovarium. The ovarian artery ends by anastomosing with the tubal branch of the uterine artery in the mesovarium.

Common iliac artery

The aorta bifurcates at the level of the fourth lumbar vertebra into two common iliac arteries, each being approximately 5 cm long until dividing into the external and internal iliac arteries.

The internal iliacs, or hypogastric arteries, are approximately 3–4 cm in length and are responsible for supplying structures of the pelvis. Throughout their course they are in close proximity to the ureters and divide into a larger anterior and a small posterior branches. The posterior division has three branches: the iliolumbar, lateral sacral, and superior gluteal arteries and provides blood supply to the lumbosacral and gluteal region.

The larger anterior division has parietal and visceral branches. The three parietal branches are the obturator and the terminal branches, internal pudendal, and inferior gluteal arteries. The six visceral branches include the umbilical, middle vesical, inferior vesical, middle rectal, uterine, and vaginal arteries. The superior vesical artery usually arises from the umbilical artery.

Uterine artery

The uterine artery is a branch of the anterior division of the internal iliac artery and runs medially towards the isthmus of the uterus. Approximately 2 cm lateral to the endocervix, it crosses above the ureter and reaches the lateral wall of the uterus. The ascending branch of the uterine artery courses in the broad ligament, with a tortuous route and ends by anastomosing with the ovarian artery in the mesovarium.

Throughout its tortuous course in the parametrium, the uterine artery gives off numerous branches that unite with arcuate arteries from the opposite side. Arcuate arteries develop radial branches that supply the myometrium, which give rise to basilar arteries that supply the basalis layer of the endometrium. The basilar arteries give rise to the spiral arteries that supply the functional layer of the endometrium. The descending branch of the uterine artery branches to both the cervix and the vagina. In each case, the vessels enter the organ laterally and anastomose freely with vessels from the opposite side.

Surgical management of postpartum haemorrhage includes ligation of the anterior division of internal iliac artery. Owing to extensive collateral circulation, this occlusion does not cause hypoxia of the pelvic viscera but reduces haemorrhage by decreasing the arterial pulse pressure. Fig. 12.2.4 illustrates the blood supply to the pelvis.

Vaginal artery

The vaginal artery may arise either from the anterior trunk of the internal iliac or from the uterine artery. It supplies blood to the vagina, bladder, and rectum. There are extensive anastomoses with the vaginal branches of the uterine artery to form the 'azygos plexus' of arteries of the cervix and vagina.

Internal pudendal artery

This artery is the terminal branch of the internal iliac artery and supplies branches to the rectum, labia, clitoris, and perineum.

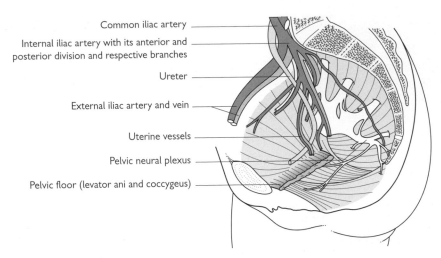

Common iliac artery

Internal iliac artery with its anterior and posterior division and respective branches

Ureter

External iliac artery and vein

Uterine vessels

Pelvic neural plexus

Pelvic floor (levator ani and coccygeus)

Fig. 12.2.4 Blood vessels of the pelvis.

Veins

The veins of the female pelvis and perineum are thin walled with few valves. The venous drainage of the pelvis begins in small sinusoids that drain to numerous venous plexuses within or immediately adjoining the pelvic organs and follow the course of the arterial supply.

The venous drainage of the ovaries is an exception. The left ovarian vein empties into the left renal vein, whereas the right ovarian vein directly drains into the inferior vena cava.

Nerve supply

The pelvis is richly innervated by both autonomic and somatic nervous systems.

Autonomic nerves

The sympathetic supply is derived from the lower part of lumber sympathetic chain and the aortic plexus which continues downwards over the bifurcation of the aorta to form the hypogastric plexus. This divides into right and left pelvic plexuses, which lie lateral to the rectum and are subdivided into anterior innervations for the bladder and urethra and posterior innervations for the uterus, cervix, vagina, sigmoid colon, and rectum.

Parasympathetic nerves

The parasympathetic nerves enter the pelvis through second, third and fourth sacral nerves. The pre-ganglionic fibres are distributed through the pelvis plexus and the parasympathetic ganglia are situated close or in the walls of the viscera. All the internal pelvic organs are supplied by the pelvic plexus. However, the ovaries and fallopian tubes are supplied directly by nerves from the pre aortic plexus travelling along the ovarian vessels.

Somatic nerves

The lumbosacral plexus and its branches provides motor and sensory innervations to the lower abdominal wall, the pelvic and the urogenital diaphragms, the perineum, hip, and lower extremity

Lymphatic drainage

Lymph nodes are arranged along the blood vessels. The structures supplied by the aorta, i.e. ovary, fallopian tubes, upper ureter, and uterine fundus drain directly to lateral aortic group of nodes.

The lymph drainage of most other structures within the pelvis is via more distant groups of lymph nodes associated with iliac vessels (i.e. internal iliac and common iliac nodes).

Anatomy of the female reproductive tract

External genitalia

External genital organs in females include the mons pubis, clitoris, urinary meatus, labia majora, labia minora, vestibule, Bartholin's glands, and periurethral glands. These are often collectively referred as the 'female perineum'.

The internal genital organs are located in the true pelvis and include the vagina, cervix, uterus, fallopian tubes, ovaries, and surrounding supporting structures.

The perineum is a diamond shape area bounded anteriorly by lower margin of symphysis pubis, posteriorly by the tip of coccyx, and laterally by the ischial tuberosities and sacrotuberous ligaments. An imaginary line joining the ischial tuberosities divides this area into an anterior urogenital triangle and a posterior anal triangle.

The urogenital triangle contains the vulva and the urethral opening, and the anal triangle includes lower end on anal canal. The external anal sphincter surrounds the anal canal and the ischeorectal fossae are on either side of the anal canal. Posteriorly, the anococcygeal body lies between the anus and the tip of the coccyx and consists of thick fibromuscular tissue supporting the rectum and lower part of the anal canal.

The vulva refers to an area that extends anteriorly from the mons pubis to the rectum, posteriorly is bounded by genitocrural folds laterally. The entire vulval area is covered by keratinized, stratified squamous epithelium.

Mons pubis: this is a triangular eminence directly anterior and superior to the symphysis pubis. It becomes hairy after puberty.

Labia majora: these are a pair of longitudinal cutaneous folds of fibroadipose tissue measuring 7–8 cm in length and 2–3 cm in width. They extend from the mons pubis anteriorly and fuse in the midline between the vagina and the anus at the posterior fourchette. The skin of the outer convex surface of the labia majora is pigmented and covered with hair follicles. The inner surface is devoid of hair follicles but is rich in sebaceous glands. Histologically, the labia majora have both sweat and sebaceous glands.

Labia minora: these are a pair of small red cutaneous folds situated between the labia majora and the vaginal orifice. Anteriorly, they separate at the clitoris to form superiorly the prepuce and inferiorly the frenulum of the clitoris. Posteriorly, they merge at the posterior fourchette. Histologically, they are composed of dense connective, elastic, and erectile tissues. The skin is rich in sebaceous glands, but it has no hair follicles or sweat glands.

Clitoris: it is a short, cylindrical, erectile organ at the superior portion of the vestibule measuring approximately 1.5–2 cm in length and 1 cm in width. The base of the clitoris consists of two crura, attached to the periosteum of the symphysis pubis. The body has two cylindrical corpora cavernosa composed of thin-walled, vascular channels that function as erectile tissue. The distal one-third of the clitoris is the glans, richly supplied by nerve endings

Hymen: this is a thin usually perforated fibrous tissue covered by stratified squamous epithelial membrane present at the entrance to the vagina.

The vestibule is the cleft between the labia minora extending from the clitoris to the posterior fourchette. The urethral meatus, vaginal orifice, and ducts of the Bartholin's glands open into the vestibule.

Urethra: This is immediately anterior to the vaginal orifice and about 2 cm beneath the clitoris. The female urethra measures 3.5–5 cm in length. The proximal two-thirds of the urethra is composed of stratified transitional epithelium, whereas the distal one-third is stratified squamous epithelium.

Internal genitalia

Vagina

The vagina is a thin-walled, distensible, fibromuscular tube that extends posterosuperiorly from the vestibule to the uterus. The vagina is attached at a higher point posteriorly than anteriorly; therefore, the posterior wall is 9 cm and the anterior is 7 cm long. The potential space of the vagina is larger in the middle and upper thirds. The walls of the vagina are normally in apposition except superiorly at the vault, where they are separated by the cervix. The vault of the vagina is divided into four fornices: posterior (deepest), anterior, and two lateral.

The axis of the upper vagina lies fairly close to the horizontal plane when a woman is standing, with the upper portion of the vagina curving toward the hollow of the sacrum. In most women an angle of at least 90° is formed between the axis of the vagina and the axis of the uterus.

Vagina supports: the vagina is held in position by the surrounding endopelvic fascia and ligaments. The lower third of the vagina is in close relationship with the urogenital and pelvic diaphragms. The middle third of the vagina is supported by the levator ani muscles and the lower portion of the cardinal ligaments. The upper third is supported by the upper portions of the cardinal ligaments and the parametrium.

Histologically the vagina is composed of four distinct layers.

- The vagina is lined by stratified, non-keratinized squamous epithelium that is firmly attached to the underlying muscle. The epithelium is thick and rich in glycogen, which increases in the post-ovulatory phase of the menstrual cycle. There are no glands in the vagina and it is lubricated from the mucus secretion from the cervix. Vaginal lubrication also occurs from a transudate produced by engorgement of the vascular plexuses that encircle the vagina.

- The second layer is of collagen and elastic tissue- lamina propria. It is composed of fibrous connective tissue. This is rich in vascular and lymphatic channels.
- The muscular layer has many interlacing fibres. There is an inner circular layer and an outer longitudinal.
- The fourth layer consists of cellular areolar connective tissue containing a large plexus of blood vessels.

Blood supply: the vagina derives its blood supply from the vaginal artery and branches from the uterine, middle rectal, and internal pudendal arteries

The nerve supply of the vagina comes from the autonomic nervous system's vaginal plexus, and sensory fibres come from the pudendal nerve. Pain fibres enter the spinal cord in sacral segments S2, S3, and S4.

The primary lymphatic drainage of the upper third of the vagina is to the external iliac nodes, the middle third of the vagina drains to the common and internal iliac nodes, and the lower third has a complex and variable distribution, including the common iliac, superficial inguinal, and pararectal nodes.

Uterus

The uterus is a thick-walled hollow fibromuscular organ located centrally in the female pelvis with the urinary bladder anteriorly and the rectum posteriorly. The fallopian tubes enter the uterine cavity at the cornua in the superolateral aspects. The uterus is often described as an inverted pear-shaped structure and is divided into the upper uterine body and lower cervix. The uterine body has a dome-shaped fundus superiorly and an isthmus inferiorly. The latter is a short area of constriction in the lower uterine segment. The lower edge of the fundus is limited by an imaginary line drawn between the attachments of each Fallopian tube. A typical nulliparous uterus measures 8 cm long, 5 cm wide, and 2.5 cm thick and weighs 40–50 g.

The uterus has three layers: the thin, external serosal layer; the middle muscular layer, the myometrium; and the inner mucous layer, the endometrium. The serosal layer is the visceral peritoneum. The peritoneum is firmly attached to the uterus in all areas except anteriorly at the level of the internal os of the cervix.

The muscular layer is 1.5–2.5 cm thick and has three indistinct layers of smooth muscle. The outer longitudinal layer is continuous with the muscle layers of the fallopian tubes and vagina. The middle layer has interlacing oblique, spiral bundles of smooth muscle, and large venous plexuses. The inner muscular layer is also longitudinal.

The endometrium is a reddish mucous membrane that varies from 1 to 6 mm in thickness, depending on hormonal stimulation. The uterine glands are tubular and composed of tall columnar epithelium. The endometrium may be divided into an inner stratum basale and an outer stratum functionale. The stratum functionale may be further subdivided into an inner compact stratum and a more superficial spongy stratum. Only the stratum functionale responds to fluctuating hormonal levels.

Blood supply: the blood supply to the uterus is the uterine artery which anastomoses with the ovarian and vaginal arteries.

The lymphatic drainage of the uterus is complex. The majority of lymphatics from the fundus and the body of the uterus go to the aortic, lumbar, and pelvic nodes surrounding the iliac vessels, especially the internal iliac nodes. However, it is possible for metastatic disease from the uterus to be found in the superior inguinal nodes transported via lymphatics in the round ligament. This is because the round ligament is attached to the fibrofatty tissue of the labia majora. Nerve supply to the uterus is via the uter-ovaginal plexus of nerves.

Cervix : the lower narrow portion of the uterus is the cylindrical shaped cervix. It is predominantly composed of fibrous tissue.

Its attachment to the vagina divides it into an upper supravaginal portion and a lower part in the vagina called the ectocervix or portio vaginalis The ureter runs about 1 cm laterally to the supravaginal cervix. The length of the endocervical canal is 2.5–3 cm and it opens proximally into the endometrial cavity at the internal os and distally into the vagina at the external os.

The ectocervix is lined by stratified squamous epithelium and the endocervix is lined by mucus-secreting columnar epithelium. The junction of these two epithelia, the 'squamo-columnar junction', is hormonal sensitive. This very active 'transformation zone is believed to be the site of origin of cervical cancers.

The arterial supply of the cervix is from the descending branch of the uterine artery. There are numerous anastomoses between these vessels and the vaginal and middle rectal arteries. The major arterial supply to the cervix is located on the lateral cervical walls at the 3 and 9 o'clock positions, respectively. Therefore a deep figure-of-eight suture through the vaginal mucosa and cervical stroma at 3 and 9 o'clock helps to reduce blood loss during procedures such as cone biopsy.

The venous drainage accompanies these arteries. The lymphatic drainage of the cervix involves multiple chains of nodes. The principal regional lymph nodes are the obturator, common iliac, internal iliac, external iliac, and visceral nodes of the parametrium. Other possible lymphatic drainage includes the following chains of nodes: superior and inferior gluteal, sacral, rectal, lumbar, aortic, and visceral nodes over the posterior surface of the urinary bladder. The stroma of the endocervix is rich in free nerve endings. Pain fibres accompany the parasympathetic fibres to the second, third, and fourth sacral segments.

Fallopian tubes

The fallopian tubes are 10 cm long, paired hollow structures representing the 'unfused' Mullerian ducts. The fallopian tubes connect the cornua of the uterine cavity and the peritoneal cavity. They arise from the superolateral portion of the uterus and travel along the upper margin of the broad ligament and end in the peritoneal cavity close to the ovary.

Each tube is divided into four anatomic sections.

1. Intramural or interstitial: 1–2 cm in length and is surrounded by myometrium. It lies within the uterine wall and forms the tubal ostia at the endometrial cavity.

2. Isthmus: the isthmus is narrow and straight and begins as the fallopian tube exits the uterus. It is approximately 4 cm in length and has the most highly developed musculature.

3. Ampulla: this is 4–6 cm in length and approximately 6 mm in diameter. It is wider and more tortuous in its course than other segments. Fertilization normally occurs in the ampullary portion of the tube.

4. Infundibulum: this is the distal trumpet-shaped portion of the tube that is in close proximity to the ovary.

The abdominal ostia of the tube have numerous irregular finger-like projections called fimbriae. One of the largest fimbriae is attached to the ovary and this is called the fimbria ovarica.

The tubal mucosa is ciliated columnar epithelium and is most prominent near the ovarian end of the tube. The mucosa of the oviduct has three different cell types: Columnar ciliated epithelial cells that account for about 25% of the mucosal secretory cells; non-ciliated 'columnar' cells that account for about 60% of the epithelial lining and are more prominent in the isthmic segment. The narrow 'peg cells' are found between secretory and ciliated cells and are believed to be a morphological variant of secretory cells.

The smooth muscle of the tube is arranged into inner circular and outer longitudinal layers. The tubes are covered by peritoneum. The vascular supply to the fallopian tubes is from the uterine and ovarian arteries, which anastomose in the mesosalpinx. The uterine arteries supply the medial two-thirds of each tube. Lymphatic drainage includes the internal iliac nodes and the aortic nodes surrounding the aorta and the inferior vena cava at the level of the renal vessels. The innervations of the tubes are from the uterovaginal and the ovarian plexus.

Ovaries

The ovaries are paired gonadal structures that lie suspended between the pelvic wall and the uterus by the infundibulopelvic ligaments laterally and the utero-ovarian ligament medially. The infundibulopelvic ligament contains the ovarian artery, ovarian veins, and accompanying nerves. It attaches the upper pole of the ovary to the lateral pelvic wall.

Inferiorly the hilar surface of each ovary is attached to the broad ligament by mesentery (mesovarium).

The ovary is the only intra-abdominal structure not to be covered by the peritoneum. During reproductive years, ovaries weigh 3–6 g and measure approximately 1.5 × 2.5 × 4 cm.

Each ovary consists of an outer cortex and an inner medulla. The ovarian surface is covered by a single layer of cuboidal epithelium, termed the germinal epithelium. This term is a misnomer because the cells are similar to those of the coelomic mesothelium, which forms the peritoneum. The germinal epithelium is not in any way related to the histogenesis of the Graafian follicles.

If the ovary is transected, numerous transparent, fluid-filled cysts are noted throughout the cortex. Microscopically these are Graafian follicles in various stages of development, active or regressing corpus luteum, and atretic follicles. The stroma of the cortex is composed primarily of closely packed cells around the follicles. These are specialized connective tissue cells that form the theca. The medulla contains the ovarian vascular supply and loose stroma.

Each of the ovarian arteries arises directly from the aorta just below the renal arteries. They descend in the retroperitoneal space, cross anterior to the psoas muscles and internal iliac vessels, and enter the infundibulopelvic ligaments, reaching the mesovarium in the broad ligament. The ovarian blood supply enters through the hilum of the ovary. The venous drainage of the ovary collects in the pampiniform plexus and consolidates into several large veins as it leaves the hilum of the ovary. The ovarian veins accompany the ovarian arteries, with the left ovarian vein draining into the left renal vein, whereas the right ovarian vein connects directly with the inferior vena cava.

The lymphatic drainage of the ovaries is primarily to the aortic nodes adjacent to the great vessels at the level of the renal veins. Nerve supply is from the ovarian plexus and uterovaginal plexus.

Ureters: the ureters are whitish, muscular tubes, 28–34 cm in length, extending from the renal pelvis to the urinary bladder. The ureter is divided into abdominal and pelvic segments.

The abdominal portion of the right ureter is lateral to the inferior vena cava. Throughout its course it is retroperitoneal and runs downwards and medially along the anteromedial surface of the psoas major muscle. It is crossed by four arteries and accompanying veins . They are the right colic artery, the ovarian vessels, the ileocolic artery, and the superior mesenteric artery.

The ureter enters the pelvis anterior to the sacroiliac joint and crosses the bifurcation of common iliac artery. There is a slight variation between the two sides of the female pelvis. The right ureter tends to cross at the bifurcation of the common iliac artery whereas usually the left ureter crosses 1–2 cm above the bifurcation. It then passes along the posterolateral aspect of the pelvis running in front and below the internal iliac artery and its anterior division medial to the obturator nerve and vessels.

Approximately at the level of the ischial spines, the ureter changes its course and runs forward and medially from the uterosacral ligaments to the base of the broad ligament, thereby entering the cardinal ligaments. In the pelvis, the ureter runs forwards and medially through the base of the broad ligament and lateral to the cervix. It is crossed superiorly from the lateral to medial side by the uterine artery. It continues forwards about 1.5 cm lateral to the cervix anterolateral to the upper part of the vagina. The ureter then runs upwards and medially in the vesical uterine ligaments to obliquely pierce the bladder wall. Just before entering the base of the bladder, the ureter is in close contact with the anterior vaginal wall and passing slightly medially enters the bladder at the trigone.

The ureteric mucosa is composed of transitional epithelium. The muscle layer has outer circular and inner longitudinal fibres and it has rich blood supply from renal, ovarian, common iliac, internal iliac uterine, and vesical arteries. These form a longitudinal plexus in the adventitia of the ureter. Nerve supply is through the ovarian and vesical plexus.

Urinary bladder

The urinary bladder is a hollow muscular organ designed for the storage of urine and lies between the symphysis pubis and the uterus. The size and shape of the bladder may vary with the volume of urine it contains. The bladder is divided into two areas which are of physiological significance.

- The base of the bladder lies directly adjacent to the endopelvic fascia over the anterior vaginal wall. It consists of urinary trigone posteriorly and a thickened area of detrusor muscle anteriorly. The three corners of the trigone are formed by the two ureteric orifices and the urethral opening into the bladder. The distance between the uretral orifices is approximately 2.5 cm when empty and 5 cm when the bladder is distended. It is innervated by α-adrenergic sympathetic fibres that maintain continence

- The dome of bladder is the remaining bladder area above the bladder base. This has parasympathetic innervations and is responsible for micturition.

The prevesical or retropubic space of Retzius is the area lying between the bladder and symphysis pubis and is bounded laterally by the obliterated hypogastric arteries. This space extends from the fascia covering the pelvic diaphragm to the umbilicus between the peritoneum and transversalis fascia. The bladder is anterior to the cervix, upper vagina, and part of the cardinal ligament. Laterally it is bounded by the pelvic diaphragm and the obturator internus muscle.

The bladder is lined by transitional cell epithelium. The muscle layer is intermeshing fibres called Detrusor muscle.

The arterial supply of the bladder originates from branches of the hypogastric (internal iliac) artery: the superior vesical, inferior vesical, and middle rectal arteries. The nerve supply to the bladder includes sympathetic and parasympathetic fibres, with the external sphincter supplied by the pudendal nerve.

Urethra

The female urethra measures 3.5–5 cm in length and extends from the bladder to the vestibule. It runs anteroinferiorly behind the symphysis pubis immediately related to the anterior vaginal wall. It crosses the perineal membrane and ends at the external urethral orifice at the vestibule about 2.5 cm behind the clitoris. The Skene's tubules, draining the paraurethral glands, open into the lower urethra. There is no true anatomical sphincter to the urethra.

The urethra contains an inner longitudinal layer and outer circular layer of smooth muscle. The perineal membrane begins at the junction of the middle and distal third of the urethra. Proximal to the middle and distal third of the urethra, voluntary muscle fibres derived from the urogenital diaphragm intermix with the outer layer of smooth muscle. This increases urethral resistance and contributing to continence. At the level of the urogenital diaphragm the urethra is encircled by voluntary muscle fibres arising from the inferior pubic ramus to form the so called external sphincter.

The mucosa of the proximal two-thirds of the urethra is composed of stratified transitional epithelium, whereas the distal one-third is stratified squamous epithelium. The distal orifice is 4–6 mm in diameter, and the mucosal edges grossly appear everted.

The vascular supply for the urethra is from the vesical and vaginal arteries and the branches from the internal pudendal artery. The nerve supply is from the vesical plexus and the pudendal nerve.

The rectum is the terminal 12–14 cm portion of the large intestine. It begins at the level of third sacral vertebrae where the sigmoid colon loses its mesentery and follows the curve of the lower sacrum and coccyx, becoming entirely retroperitoneal at the level of the recto-uterine pouch. The rectum continues along the pelvic curve just posterior to the vagina until the level of the anal hiatus of the pelvic diaphragm. At this point, it takes a sharp 90° turn posteriorly, becoming the anal canal, and is separated by the vagina by the perineal body. The rectum, unlike other areas of the large intestine, does not have taeniae coli or appendices epiploicae.

The rectal mucosa is lined by a columnar epithelium and characterized by three transverse folds that contain mucosa, submucosa, and the inner circular layer of smooth muscle. The rectum receives a rich arterial supply originating from five arteries: the superior rectal artery, which is a continuation of the inferior mesenteric; the two middle rectal arteries; and the two inferior rectal arteries.

Anal canal

The anal canal is 3 cm long and passes downwards and backwards from the rectum. At the anorectal junction the mucosa changes to stratified squamous epithelium, which continues until the anal verge, where there is transition to perianal skin. The circular muscle of the rectum continues down to form the internal anal sphincter. The lower part of the anal canal is surrounded by striated muscle fibres, the external anal sphincter.

The anal canal is slit-like when empty but distends greatly during defaecation. Anteriorly it is related to perineal body and lower vagina, whereas posteriorly it is related to the anococcygeal body. Faecal continence is primarily provided by the puborectalis muscle and the internal and external anal sphincters. The blood supply is from the superior, middle, and inferior rectal arteries and the nerve supply is from the middle rectal plexus, inferior plexus and the pudendal nerve.

Conclusion

Understanding the normal anatomy of the pelvis is vital for practising obstetricians and gynaecologists. This will help in diagnosis and management of gynaecological disorders as well as planning and performing pelvic surgery. Distortion of pelvic anatomy may result in inadvertent unintended damage to pelvic organs during surgery. Knowledge of anatomy may also help in the prevention and management of genital tract prolapse, and urinary and fecal incontinence that may result from childbirth.

Further reading

Norton PA. Pelvic floor disorders: the role of fascia and ligaments. Clin Obstet Gynecol 1993;36:926–38.

Mukhopadhyay S, Arulkumaran S. Anatomy of the female pelvis. Chapter In: *Essentials of obstetrics*. Jaypee Brothers 2004.

Chandraharan E, Arulkumaran S. Female pelvis and details of operative delivery; shoulder dystocia and episiotomy. In: Arulkumaran S, Penna LK, Rao B (eds) *Management of labour*. Orient Longman 2005.

Healy JC. Female reproductive system. In: Standring S (ed) *Grays anatomy*. Churchill Livingstone 2008.

Chronic pelvic pain

Definition

Chronic pelvic pain (CPP) is usually defined as 'constant or intermittent pain in the lower abdomen or pelvis of at least 6 months' duration'. Women with dysmenorrhoea and/or dyspareunia only are therefore excluded, as are those with pain related to pregnancy or malignancy. The definition solely considers the location and duration of the symptoms; no assumptions are made about the cause.

An alternative definition is 'non-cyclical pain of at least 6 months' duration that appears in locations such as the pelvis, anterior abdominal wall, lower back, or buttocks, and that is serious enough to cause disability or lead to medical care'.

Epidemiology

The lack of an unambiguous definition makes studying the epidemiology difficult. Until recently, studies focused on the frequency of finding pelvic pathology at laparoscopy as an explanation for CPP, and on attempts to explain the symptoms when no such pathology was found.

The best estimate of the annual prevalence in primary care, in women aged 18–50, is 37/1000: a figure similar to that for asthma and back pain. The prevalence varies with age: from 18/1000 in 15–20-year-olds to 28/1000 in women older than 60.

In a community survey, 24% of women reported having CPP in the last three months; excluding ovulation-related pain reduced the estimate to 17%.

Contributory factors to the genesis of CPP

CPP is difficult to diagnose and treat, due to the wide range of possible causes with overlapping symptoms:

- endometriosis
- pelvic inflammatory disease (PID)
- adhesions
- irritable bowel syndrome (IBS)
- interstitial cystitis (IC)
- urethral syndrome
- muscle and mechanical pelvic pain
- pelvic pain posture
- nerve entrapment
- neuropathic and referred pain
- pelvic congestion syndrome
- psychosocial factors
- psychogenic pain
- physical and sexual abuse.

Risk factors

In a recent systematic review, drug or alcohol abuse, miscarriage, heavy menstrual flow, previous Caesarean section, PID, pelvic pathology, abuse, and psychological comorbidity were associated with an increased risk of non-cyclical pelvic pain.

Initial consultation

As pain is perceived in the mind, the experience of CPP will inevitably be affected by factors in the sufferer's physical and psychological environment, e.g. coexisting illness, stress levels or beliefs about the pain.

Thus, in assessing patients with CPP, it is imperative to see the individual as a whole, and not to dichotomize pain as either organic or psychological. In addition, adequate time should be given at the initial assessment, ideally in a multidisciplinary setting. Women with CPP need to feel they have been able to tell their story and that they have been listened to and believed.

As there is frequently more than one component to CPP, assessment should aim to identify all contributory factors, rather than assign causality to a single pathology.

Many women want an explanation for the pain, especially if they already have their own theories or concerns about its origin. These should be discussed, as consultations that elicit the woman's own ideas result in a better doctor-patient relationship and improved concordance with investigation and treatment.

Initial history

This should include questions about the pain pattern and its association with other problems, e.g. psychological, bladder and bowel symptoms, as well as the effects of movement and posture on the pain.

'Red flag' symptoms (those suggestive of serious disease) should be excluded and managed as appropriate:

- rectal bleeding
- NEW bowel symptoms (>50 years old)
- irregular vaginal bleeding (>40 years old)
- post-coital bleeding
- pelvic mass
- new pain after the menopause
- suicidal ideation
- excessive weight loss.
- Completing a daily pain diary for two to three menstrual cycles may help the clinician and patient identify provoking factors or temporal associations. The information may be useful in understanding the cause of the pain.

Women should also be screened for IBS with a symptom-based tool, e.g. the Rome II criteria:

- At least 12 weeks continuous or recurrent abdominal pain/discomfort associated with ≥2 of the following:
- pain relieved by defaecation
- a change in frequency of stool
- abnormal appearance or form of stool.

Examination

The examination is most usefully undertaken when there is sufficient time to explore the woman's fears and anxieties, at which point new information may be revealed.

- Features to note include:
- signs of pelvic pathology, e.g. rectovaginal nodule of deeply infiltrating endometriosis
- patient attitude, as detachment may indicate disgust with this part of her body
- evidence of altered sensation (allodynia or hypersensitivity) before abdominal palpation is performed
- effects of movement on pain if a musculoskeletal cause is suspected
- altered sensation on vulva or perineum
- pelvic floor muscle tone
- Vaginismus, in which case more than a gentle one FINGER examination may be inappropriate.

Investigations

- The following should be considered:
- transvaginal ultrasound for an ovarian mass

- transvaginal ultrasound or MRI for adenomyosis
- if there is any suspicion of PID, appropriate samples should be taken although, ideally, *all* sexually active women less than 25 should be offered opportunistic screening for chlamydia.

Laparoscopy

Laparoscopy has been the 'gold standard' diagnostic test in CPP as it is the only way to diagnose adhesions and peritoneal endometriosis. Therefore, gynaecologists have seen it as an essential tool to assess women with CPP. However, there are problems associated with its use as a first line investigation.

- Risks of anaesthesia, bleeding and organ injury: 3.3/100 000 mortality and 4.6/1000 morbidity during diagnostic and therapeutic laparoscopy in a study of 30,000 patients. Complications needing laparotomy (approx. 25% of which were missed at the initial laparoscopy) occurred in 3.2/1000 patients.
- Laparoscopy cannot diagnose many potential causes of CPP, e.g. adenomyosis, IC and IBS.
- The presence of visible 'pathology' e.g. peritoneal endometriosis, may be coincidental and not the cause of the woman's symptoms.
- 30–50% of diagnostic laparoscopies are negative, which disappoints many women as they assume their doctor now thinks 'the problem is all in my head'.

Consequently, laparoscopy should only be performed where (a) the index of suspicion of endometriosis and/or adhesions requiring surgical intervention is high and (b) other causes have been excluded.

Microlaparoscopy or 'conscious pain mapping' may be an alternative to laparoscopy as it avoids general anaesthetic. Although it may seem to confirm particular lesions as the source of the pain, it has not been widely adopted and questions remain as to its acceptability, reproducibility and validity.

Empirical treatment

It has been suggested that women with cyclical pain should undergo a therapeutic trial using the combined oral contraceptive or a GnRH agonist for 3–6 months before being offered a diagnostic laparoscopy.

The rationale is that ovarian suppression is an effective treatment for pain associated with endometriosis (and some other causes such as pelvic congestion syndrome).

Women should also be offered appropriate analgesia to control their pain; this includes

- regular NSAIDs with or without paracetamol
- compound analgesics including opioids
- tricyclic antidepressants e.g. amitriptyline
- anticonvulsants e.g. gabapentin
- non-pharmacological modalities such as TENS may help some patients.

Condition-specific treatment

Some conditions require specific treatments, e.g. women with IBS should be offered a trial with antispasmodics as a systematic review has concluded that smooth muscle relaxants such as mebverine are beneficial in treating IBS where abdominal pain is a prominent feature. They should also try to amend their diet.

Treatment options for CPP

The options are summarized extremely well in a recent systematic review of the literature (Cheong and Stones 2006), which identified 13 relevant RCTs. These included interventions with medroxyprogesterone acetate (MPA) alone or in combination with psychotherapy, goserelin, sertraline, lofexidine hydrochloride, ultrasound scanning to aid counselling and reassurance, i.v. dihydroergotamine for acute exacerbations and the use of a Polaroid print to assist in postoperative patient consultation.

Other interventions identified were writing therapy to improve symptoms, static magnetic fields to improve pain, adhesiolysis via laparoscopy or laparotomy, and a multidisciplinary approach to investigation, including physiotherapy, psychology, and attention to dietary and environmental factors.

The best available evidence provides some support for the use of ultrasound scanning as an aid to counselling and reassurance; MPA or goserelin for pelvic congestion, and a multidisciplinary approach to assessment and treatment. Adhesiolysis provides no benefit other than in women with severe adhesions. Short-term results for presacral neurectomy (PSN) and laparoscopic uterosacral nerve ablation (LUNA) are similar, although PSN has better results in the long term. SSRI antidepressants have not been shown to be of benefit.

References

American College of Obstetricians and Gynecologists (ACOG) Practice Bulletin No. 51. Chronic pelvic pain. Obstet Gynecol 2004;103:589–605.

Chapron C, Querleu D, Bruhat M, *et al*. Surgical complications of diagnostic and operative gynaecological laparoscopy. Hum Reprod 1998;13:867–72.

Cheong Y, Stones W. Chronic pelvic pain: aetiology and therapy. Best Pract Res Clin Obstet Gynaecol 2006;20:695–711.

Latthe P, Mignini L, Gray R, *et al*. Factors predisposing women to chronic pelvic pain: systematic review. BMJ 2006;332:749–55.

Moore J, Kennedy S. Causes of chronic pelvic pain. Baillieres Clin Obstet Gynaecol 2000;14:389–402.

Royal College of Obstetricians and Gynaecologists (RCOG) *The initial management of chronic pelvic pain*. Greentop Guideline. London: RCOG 2005.

Vincent K. Chronic pelvic pain in women. Postgrad Med J 2009;85:24–9.

Williams RE, Hartmann KE, Steege JF. Documenting the current definitions of chronic pelvic pain: implications for research. Obstet Gynecol 2004;103:686–91.

Zondervan KT, Yudkin PL, Vessey MP, *et al*. Chronic pelvic pain in the community: symptomatology, investigations and diagnoses. Am J Obstet Gynecol 2001; 184:1149–55.

Internet resources

The International Pelvic Pain Society aims to educate health care professionals on how to diagnosis and manage CPP: www.pelvicpain.org/

The American Chronic Pain Society aims to facilitate peer support and education for individuals with chronic pain and their families so that they may live more fully in spite of their pain: www.theacpa.org/

European Association of Urology guideline on management of CPP: www.uroweb.org/

Summary written for Patient UK: www.patient.co.uk/showdoc/40000111/

Contraception

Definition

When conception or impregnation has been intentionally prevented by a sexually active individual through the use of various devices, agents, drugs, sexual practices and or surgical procedures it is referred to as contraception.

Epidemiology

Contraception has been practiced from time immemorial. The main objective of contraceptive provision is to permit sexually active individuals to enjoy positive aspects of their sexuality without it affecting their mental or physical health adversely.

It is estimated that about 4 million people utilize the National Health Service contraceptive services in the United Kingdom each year. Three-quarters see a general practitioner and the rest attend specialist community contraceptive ser-vices.

Pathology

Contraceptive methods may be either temporary or permanent.

Temporary methods

User dependent
- Barrier
- Oral contraceptives (combined as well as progestogen-only preparations)
- Patches (containing oestrogen and progestogen)
- Spermicides either used alone or in combination with barrier method
- Fertility awareness methods.

User independent (long-acting reversible contraception) methods
- Intrauterine devices
- Implants (progestogen only)
- Vaginal rings (oestrogen and progestogen containing)
- Progestogen only injectables.

Permanent methods
- Female sterilization methods
- Male sterilization methods.

Factors influencing choice of method
- Peer opinion
- Lifestyle
- Duration of action
- Medical complications
- Return to fertility
- Side-effects
- Safety
- Efficacy.

Barriers preventing choice of contraception
- Myths
- 'I can't be at risk' attitude
- Religious and cultural misconceptions.

Safety

Contraceptive benefits to health

Contraception helps women have a planned pregnancy and thus avoid the emotional stress involved with an unplanned one.

Worldwide, 200 million unintended pregnancies occur each year to women not using an effective method of contraception. More than half of these end in abortion, half of which may be performed in an unsafe or unhygienic way. A strong correlation has been noted between unmet need for contraception, unintended pregnancy, and unsafe abortion. Increasing access to contraception would lower the incidence of unintended pregnancy, which then leads to decreased risk to the woman of lifelong injury or death.

The risk of ectopic pregnancy is also decreased with the use of contraception. Use of a contraceptive is known to decrease ectopics by an estimated 30–280 per 100 000 annually in monogamous relationships and by 680–920 per 100 000 non-monogamous relationships.

Non-contraceptive benefits of contraception

Hormonal methods

Combined oral contraceptives
- Lighter, regular, and less painful periods
- Decreased risk of benign breast disease
- Decreased ovarian cysts
- Decrease in both ovarian and endometrial cancer
- Decrease in acne.

Hormone releasing intrauterine devices(intrauterine systems)
- Decrease in menstrual blood flow
- Induce endometrial atrophy
- Some evidence that the pain of endometriosis is decreased.

Non-hormonal

Barrier contraception
- Prevents sexually transmitted infections.

Risks

Barrier methods
- High failure rate
- Latex allergy
- High incidence of urinary tract infections with use of diaphragm

Oral contraceptives
- Bleeding irregularities in 20–30% of users.
- Mood changes, headaches, nausea, breast tenderness, or changes in libido.
- Risks of myocardial infarction in smokers increased with combined oral pill usage. Risk of death through cardiac causes increased fourfold if a smoker over 35 and using combined oral contraceptives.
- Venous thrombosis risk is raised. Risk in combined pill takers of non-fatal pulmonary embolism is 10–30/100 000 compared with 5/100 000 for non-pill users. However, in pregnancy the risk is 60/100 000.

Aetiology

Mechanism of action
- Most hormonal contraceptives such as combined oral pills, patch, vaginal ring, implant, and injectables work by inhibiting ovulation.
- Progestogen-only preparations such as the mini pill, implants, injectables, and intrauterine systems thicken the cervical mucus, preventing entry of sperm through the cervical mucus plug barrier in addition to any other mechanism attributed to them.

- Intrauterine devices (IUDs) including hormone-releasing ones render implantation in uterine endometrium impossible by creating an inflammatory reaction locally. The copper in a copper IUD is spermicidal and toxic to the ovum.
- Barrier contraceptives prevent ascent of sperm into the uterine cavity.
- Fertility awareness methods are where the woman predicts the fertile time in her cycle by interpreting symptoms and signs in her body and avoids sexual intercourse during that period.

Efficacy

The efficacy of contraceptive methods is usually quantitated by the pearl index, which is defined as the number of unintended pregnancies per 100 women per year.

The most effective methods are those that are not user dependent such as the permanent methods and the long-acting reversible contraceptives (LARCs). Their perfect use (theoretical efficacy) figures closely match typical use (actual efficacy), unlike user-dependent methods, where there is a wide discrepancy (Table 12.4.1).

Prevalence by method

In the UK according to the Office of National statistics (ONS) the pill, including the mini pill, continue to be the most popular method with 27% of 16–49 year olds choosing it. The male condom was the next popular at 22%. LARCs were used by just 8% and sterilization, including male and female methods, by 20%.

In the USA, 62% use some form of contraception. The figures for 2002 showed the most frequently used were the oral contraceptives (30.6%), male condoms (18%), female sterilization (27%), male sterilization (9.2%), and injectables (5.3%) accounting in total for 90% of use.

The National Institute for Clinical Guidelines (2005) have calculated that all LARCs are more cost-effective at 12 months of use than oral contraception, as pregnancy rates are lower with much fewer visits to the clinician.

Contraindications for contraception

Oestrogen-containing methods
- Past or current history of thrombosis
- Focal migraine
- Active disease of the liver
- Undiagnosed vaginal bleeding

Table 12.4.1 Percentage of unintended pregnancies per 100 women per year in the first year of use of contraceptive

Contraceptive	Perfect use (%)	Typical use (%)
Spermicide	18	29
Diaphragm + spermicide	6	16
Male condom	2	15
Pill	0.3	8
Injectables	0.3	3
Implant	0.05	0.05
Intrauterine system	0.2	0.2
Copper coil	0.6	0.8

- Oestrogen-dependent tumours
- Smokers over the age of 35
- Body mass index of ≥35.

Progestogen-only methods
- Bleeding abnormalities
- Hepatic adenoma or chronic liver condition such as porphyria
- Current cardiovascular disease
- Current breast cancer.

Intrauterine devices
- Undiagnosed vaginal bleeding
- Active pelvic infection
- Uterine abnormalities.

Fertility regulation procedures
- Menstrual abnormalities
- Chronic or active pelvic infection
- Immediately following childbirth, terminations, miscarriages or gynaecological surgery
- Those on medications
- Those with medical conditions such as hypothyroidism.

Sterilization procedure

Couples need to be absolutely certain of their decision: 10% are known to regret their decision and 1% seek reversal. Reasons for regret are
- marital/relationship problems
- young age
- when done as postpartum or postabortal procedures
- psychiatric illness in either partner.

Return to fertility

This is an important advantage of reversible methods. Except for injectables, where the return takes an average of 9 months, for all other methods 70–90% attempting to conceive do so within 12 months.

Research

Contraceptive vaccines are under investigation and none are clinically available. They aim to target gamete production, gamete function, or gamete outcome.

Male hormonal contraception is not currently available. It is however undergoing clinical trial. It involves injecting a hormone every 2 months to turn off sperm production. However, as this could lower testosterone production this requires a testosterone implant injection every 4 months.

Summary

Unintended pregnancy could carry significant health risks and the use of contraception helps avert it. Responsible societies aim towards ensuring all pregnancies are planned. Contraceptive measures should therefore be encouraged as an effective public measure.

Further reading

Faculty of Sexual and Reproductive Healthcare Clinical Effectiveness Unit. *Intrauterine methods of contraception.* London: FSRH CEU 2007.

Faculty of Sexual and Reproductive Healthcare Clinical Effectiveness Unit. *UK Medical eligibility criteria for contraceptive use.* London: FSRH CEU 2009.

Harlap S, Kost K, Forrest JD. *Preventing pregnancy, protecting health: a new look at birth control choices in the United States.* New York: Alan Guttmacher Institute 1991.

Mesca D, Sines E. *Unsafe abortion: facts and figures, 2006.* Washington DC: Population Reference Bureau 2006.

Mosher WD, Martinez GM, Chandra A, *et al.* Use of contraception and use of family planning services in the United States: 1982–2002. Adv Data. 2004;350:1–36.

National Institute for Health and Clinical Excellence (NICE). *Long-acting reversible contraception: the effective and appropriate use of long-acting reversible contraception.* London: NICE 2005.

The National Health Service information centre KT31 return.

Internet resources

http://www.emedicine.com

Patient resources

www.fsrh.org
www.fpa.org.uk

Disorders of sex development

Definition

Disorders of sex development (DSD) occur when the development of chromosomal, gonadal, or anatomical sex is atypical. Previous terminology used to describe this group of conditions included intersex, pseudohermaphroditism, and testicular feminization. These terms are inaccurate and misleading for clinicians and are perceived by patients as pejorative. The recent consensus statement on the management of intersex disorders recommended the adoption of the term DSD (Hughes et al. 2006). This terminology described by the consensus group encompasses a wide range of conditions and has been quickly adopted by the majority of units around the world managing this group of patients. The incidence of DSD is estimated to be in the region of 1 in 4500 births.

Congenital adrenal hyperplasia

Congenital adrenal hyperplasia (CAH) is an autosomal recessive condition occurring in approximately 1 in 13 000 births. It results from a deficiency of an enzyme for the production of cortisol. Over 90% of cases are caused by 21-hydroxylase deficiency, leading to an excess of testosterone precursors. Affected individuals will have an androgen excess, which leads to virilization in the 46,XX female fetus. This results in clitoromegaly, labial fusion, and rugosity, with a urogenital sinus and most commonly presents with ambiguous genitalia at birth. The upper vagina, uterus, fallopian tubes, and ovaries are normally formed. Management includes steroid replacement therapy and surgical treatment to the genital area. The nature and timing of genital surgery is controversial. Virilization may persist or recur in those who are inadequately treated, and individuals require lifelong steroid replacement therapy. Both under- and overtreatment may result in short stature, and girls may have oligomenorrhoea or amenorrhoea, leading to fertility difficulties.

Androgen insensitivity syndrome

Androgen insensitivity syndrome (AIS) occurs as a result of a defect in the gene coding for the androgen receptor, leading to insensitivity to circulating androgens. The condition is X-linked in two-thirds of cases, with an incidence of 1 in 40 000 births. Those with complete androgen insensitivity syndrome (CAIS) will have a 46,XY karyotype, with phenotypical female external genitalia. The vagina is blind ending and of variable length. The internal gonads are normal testes. Complete regression of the Müllerian ducts occurs and therefore no uterus is present. Partial AIS results in a variable degree of virilization, with appearances ranging from ambiguous genitalia to simple hypospadias. Management includes the creation of a vagina to facilitate penetrative intercourse and the option of elective gonadectomy with subsequent hormone replacement therapy.

Disorders of testosterone biosynthesis

Rarer DSDs include those resulting from a deficiency in any enzyme required in the biosynthesis or metabolism of testosterone.

5-α-reductase converts testosterone to the more active metabolite dihydrotestosterone (DHT). Deficiency leads to the development of an undervirilized male (46,XY). The condition is autosomal recessive and individuals have normal testes. The external genitalia may be ambiguous or phenotypically female. The majority of individuals are reared as female, although subsequent virilization may occur at puberty if the gonads have not been removed. Fertility has been reported in those reared male, but is significantly reduced.

17 β-hydroxysteroid dehydrogenase deficiency occurs when there is an absence or reduction of the enzyme converting androstenedione to testosterone. This condition is autosomal recessive, and results in a 46,XY individual with ambiguous or phenotypically female genitalia. Virilization may occur at puberty.

Turner syndrome

Turner syndrome results in gonadal dysgenesis due to the absence or anomaly of one of the X chromosomes. This includes those with 45,X, those with duplication of the long arm of the X chromosome, and those with mosaicism with one or more additional cell lineages. The incidence is approximately 1 in 3000 female births. Individuals have normal internal Müllerian structures with streak gonads and normal external female genitalia. Possible phenotypes include short stature, webbed neck, broad shield-shaped chest and drooping eyelids, although none of these features may be present. Additionally, heart defects, hypertension, obesity, diabetes, renal anomalies, Hashimoto's thyroiditis, cataracts, arthritis, and scoliosis have been associated with the condition. Primordial follicles are initially present in the streak gonads, but these appear to undergo premature apoptosis and are usually absent by adult life. The vast majority of women with Turner syndrome will require induction of puberty and long-term hormone replacement therapy. Spontaneous fertility has been reported, but is rare. Owing to the presence of a normal uterus, fertility may be possible with assisted conception techniques.

Swyer's syndrome

Swyer's syndrome, also known as pure gonadal dysgenesis, occurs as a result of bilateral dysgenetic testes. Individuals have normal 46,XY chromosomes. As the testes do not function, no testosterone is produced and hence no virilization occurs. In addition, normal internal Mullerian structures develop due to the lack of Mullerian inhibiting substance (MIS). Women are often taller than may have been expected, and this has been attributed to the presence of a Y chromosome. There is a failure of spontaneous puberty, with hormone replacement therapy being required. Fertility is possible with egg donation and assisted conception techniques.

Ovotesticular DSD

This condition was previously known as true hermaphroditism and refers to the presence of both ovarian and testicular tissue in the same individual. The karyotype is 46,XX in over 70% of cases and the gonads may be a separate ovary and/or testes and/or an ovotestis. The external genital appearance may be ambiguous, with Müllerian and Wolffian structures present internally. Asymmetry of gonads and subsequent reproductive tracts and external genitalia may occur. Fertility may be possible depending upon karyotype and phenotype.

Rokitansky syndrome

Also known as Mayer–Rokitansky–Kuster–Hauser (MRKH), this condition occurs in approximately 1 in 5000 births, and consists of the congenital absence of the uterus and upper vagina. Isolated fallopian tubes may persist with normal ovaries. The karyotype is 46,XX, with normal female external genital appearance. The vagina is blind ending and may be of variable length. As the ovaries are unaffected, puberty proceeds normally, with the development of normal secondary sexual characteristics. Individuals usually present with primary amenorrhoea, and may have no other signs or symptoms. There is an association with renal, skeletal, auditory, and cardiac anomalies. There appears to be a genetic component to the condition, but the aetiology remains elusive. Fertility is possible via *in vitro* fertilization (IVF) and a surrogate mother. Management consists of psychological support and the option of creating a vagina to enable penetrative intercourse.

Presentation of DSDs

Conditions which include ambiguous genitalia will be apparent from birth. However, those with normal external genitalia may not present until later childhood or puberty with a herniated inguinal gonad, primary amenorrhoea or progressive virilization.

Features in a neonate that would warrant further assessment include bilateral undescended testes in an apparently full-term male child, hypospadias associated with separation of the scrotal sac, or an undescended testis, ambiguous genitalia, clitoral hypertrophy, single opening urogenital sinus, or an inguinal hernia containing a gonad.

Diagnosis

CAH is the most common cause of neonatal ambiguous genitalia. Chromosomal analysis, with specific fluorescent *in situ* hybridization for a Y fragment should be performed. Serum biochemical tests can identify a block in testosterone biosynthesis. A human chorionic gonadotrophin stimulation test may be necessary to assess response. Anti-Müllerian hormone and inhibin B are also playing an increasing role in determining the presence of testicular tissue. Ultrasound scans may be of value, but the neonatal Müllerian structures can be difficult to image clearly. A laparoscopy may be performed to inspect and biopsy the gonads.

Medical management

DSDs are complex and rare conditions. It is essential that such conditions are managed within a multidisciplinary setting comprising paediatric endocrinology, urology, gynaecology, and psychology teams. Previously a policy of non-disclosure of diagnosis to patients was widespread. Patients were denied information about their condition and so the opportunity to access support groups and the option for genetic testing for unaffected relatives. This further reinforced the secrecy and shame felt by many patients. This policy is no longer practised and clinicians should disclose all information to patients as it becomes age appropriate, with concomitant psychological input. Many conditions now have peer-led support groups.

Sex of rearing

When an infant presents with ambiguous genitalia a decision as to appropriate sex of rearing is made, based upon a number of considerations: the potential for fertility, along with the likelihood of successful sexual functioning in adulthood, the outcomes of proposed surgery and the wishes of the parents.

Surgical management

For those born without a vagina and being reared female, the option of creating a vagina is considered. This is necessary for those with a uterus to allow menstrual flow, and should be achieved before puberty. However, in the absence of a uterus, these procedures can be deferred until adolescence or later, depending on the wishes of the individual. Dilation therapy should always be considered as first-line treatment. A series of plastic cones are pressed against the vaginal dimple, to stretch the skin. Over 3–6 months, a vagina suitable for penetrative intercourse can be created. Dilation has success rates of 85% and avoids the risk of surgery. For those where dilation does not work, the laparoscopic Vecchietti procedure may be performed, where an acrylic olive is positioned in the vaginal dimple and winched up over 7 days, creating a vagina through the pressure effect. Other vaginoplasty techniques include the use of skin or bowel grafts to create a tissue tube, which is then fixed to the introitus. Both carry a risk of contracture and long-term carcinoma development. Bowel vaginoplasties are associated with the excessive production of mucus, and risk the development of diversion colitis.

Clitoral surgery is offered for cosmetic reasons and is often performed at the time of vaginal surgery. However, this damages function and increasingly is avoided for those with mild to moderate clitoromegaly. Surgery is irreversible and infants are unable to give consent. Deferring a decision for surgery until the child can be involved may be appropriate, with the option of surgery at a later date.

Gonadectomy

Dysgenetic gonads carry a 30% risk of malignant change, and gonadectomy is recommended at the time of diagnosis. This includes conditions where a Y fragment is present. For conditions with normal but intra-abdominal testes, such as CAIS, the malignancy risk is much lower in the order of 2–3%. Puberty is more successful with endogenous hormones and current practice is therefore elective gonadectomy after completion of puberty. Individuals may choose to retain their gonads longer than this but screening for potential malignancies is inaccurate.

Further reading

Balen AH, Creighton SM, Davies, *et al. Paediatric and adolescent gynaecology*, 1st edn. Cambridge: Cambridge University Press 2004.

Hughes IA, Houk C Ahmed SF, Lee PA. Consensus statement on management of intersex disorders. *Arch Dis Child* 2006;91:554–63.

Internet resources

Androgen Insensitivity Syndrome: www.aissg.org

Climb CAH Support Group: www.livingwithcah.org

Donor insemination

Male factor infertility is diagnosed in a third of couples presenting to fertility clinics. Donor insemination (DI) was the only treatment available to couples where there were severe abnormalities in semen until the introduction of intracytoplasmic sperm injection (ICSI) in the mid-1990s. As long as a few viable sperm can be retrieved for ICSI, the couple are able to have a genetically related child, with IVF pregnancy rates well above donor insemination cycles. As a result, there has been a marked decline in donor insemination treatment. The number of cycles undertaken in the UK fell from 15 000 in 1996 to 4153 in 2006. Availability and regulation of treatment varies between countries; for example, donor anonymity is protected in Spain, gamete donation is prohibited in Italy, and donor payment is the norm in the USA. In 2005 the UK lifted anonymity from donors, enabling potential offspring to identify their biological father. This resulted in a significant fall in the number of volunteers willing to donate sperm; the supply of UK-sourced donor sperm is scarce and the number of donor cycles has fallen further.

Indications

- In current practice, DI is usually reserved for severe male factor infertility where sperm cannot be obtained by masturbation or surgically. Absence of spermatogenesis may be congenital (e.g. Klinefelter's syndrome) or acquired (e.g. cancer treatment). Some couples may choose DI as being less invasive and expensive than ICSI.
- Gamete donation may be used by couples who are carriers of serious inherited disease.
- Women without a male partner may be treated with DI: about a third of treatment cycles in the UK are for single women and lesbian couples.

Recruitment of donors

Guidelines for recruitment of donors and the use of donated gametes are available; in the UK there are national regulations issued by the Human Fertilisation and Embryology Authority.

Donors should be aged 18–45, in good health, and carefully screened. They must be offered independent counselling to explore the implications of donation. The great majority of donors are anonymous to the recipient (although they may be identified to their offspring). A small minority of couples have known donors. Donations are altruistic with financial compensation only for time and travel. Only 10 pregnancies are permitted per donor. As a result of these restrictions many fertility clinics in the UK have found it difficult to recruit and are importing donated sperm from overseas. Recruitment is supported by the National Gamete Donation Trust.

Screening of donors

Semen is a natural vector for a range of infectious diseases and also a potential source of inherited disorders. To minimize risk to the woman receiving the donor sperm and to potential offspring, every effort is made to screen donors for these conditions. All men donating sperm should be in good health and the initial evaluation should include a full history and clinical examination, paying attention to the presence of any genital lesions (genital warts, urethral discharge, or ulcers) which would indicate sexually transmissible infection.

Donors are screened for HIV 1 and 2, hepatitis B and C, cytomegalovirus, syphilis, gonorrhoea, and chlamydia.

Genetic screening comprises a family history, karyotype, and testing for carriage of cystic fibrosis in European donors and haemoglobinopathies in other ethnic groups. Blood group and Rhesus group are usually recorded.

To allow for the incubation period of transmissible viral infections, donated semen samples are frozen and quarantined for at least 6 months and the donor is retested before samples are released for use.

Storage of semen

Semen is cryopreserved for storage and this reduces the sperm count and motility. The main hazard to survival of sperm is intracellular ice crystal formation during freezing; the sperm are dehydrated by exposure to serially increasing concentrations of cryoprotectants to minimize osmotic shock. The resultant frozen vial or straw containing sperm and cryoprotectant is sealed and stored in nitrogen vapour in order to minimize cross-contamination with other samples in the storage tank, which is regularly topped up with liquid nitrogen. Ideally, ejaculates should contain at least 40 million sperm per millilitre to ensure adequate sperm counts after thawing. However, many clinics will now accept donors who are unable to provide such quality samples. Intrauterine insemination of prepared sperm can compensate for this.

Couples may request that samples be saved for subsequent treatment to enable them to have more than one child with the same donor. Under UK regulations, samples can be stored for 10 years.

Clinical aspects of donor insemination

Assessment of the female partner

- Full history and examination to identify any potential medical or gynaecological problems.
- Confirmation of ovulatory cycles (menstrual history, mid-luteal progesterone) and assessment of ovarian reserve (early follicular phase hormone profile, antral follicle count).
- Pelvic ultrasound scan to establish normal pelvic anatomy, preferably in the early follicular phase to determine the number of antral follicles.
- Tubal patency testing is usually performed by hysterosalpingogram.
- Screening for HIV 1 and 2, hepatitis B and C, and cytomegalovirus, and swabs to exclude genital infection including chlamydia.
- Pre-pregnancy assessment: discuss any relevant medical history, review medication, confirm rubella immunity, and ensure recent negative cervical cytology.
- Folic acid supplementation is recommended. Smoking, alcohol, diet, and exercise are discussed. Weight reduction is strongly advised for women with a BMI above 30 because of the implications for success rates and pregnancy outcome.

Counselling

Couples should see an independent counsellor to explore the implications of treatment, discuss any concerns about raising a child genetically unrelated to the male partner, and consider disclosure to the child of his or her origin.

Matching the donor

Donors are matched to the male partner so that any potential child will share as many characteristics as possible with the father. Matching will include:

- ethnicity
- hair and eye colour
- height and build
- blood group.

However, with the limited supply of donor sperm, these matching criteria may be relaxed to an extent.

The CMV status of the female partner is taken into account: CMV negative, i.e. non-immune, patients should be treated with CMV-negative donor sperm because of the small risk of congenital CMV infection.

Management of treatment cycles

Intrauterine insemination is the preferred method of delivery of donor semen as this gives better pregnancy rates than intracervical insemination of frozen-thawed semen

In women who have normal investigations, the initial cycles should be unstimulated as these women are fertile and have a significant risk of multiple pregnancy with ovarian stimulation.

However, if there is no pregnancy after three unstimulated cycles or there are any mild female factors, such as mild endometriosis, then mild ovarian stimulation with either Clomiphene or gonadotrophins may be undertaken with the aim of producing not more than three follicles in each cycle. In anovulatory women, ovulation induction is used in a similar way but the aim here is to produce a single follicle in each cycle.

If there are significant problems identified, such as tubal blockage, then IVF can be performed with donor sperm.

The law and regulation in the UK

In the UK, fertility treatment is regulated by the Human Fertilisation and Embryology Authority (HFEA), set up by an act of parliament, which issues a 'Code of Practice' and inspects and licenses clinics. The HFEA maintains a register of all gamete donors and records all donor treatment cycles carried out in UK clinics.

Welfare of the child

All couples considering fertility treatment are required to complete a 'Welfare of the Child' assessment in order to identify any potential risks to the unborn child or existing children in the family. It is very unusual for a clinic to withhold treatment.

Confidentiality

Gamete donation is a personal decision and treatment is kept private by many couples. In UK clinics the patient's consent is required for disclosure even to other medical practitioners. The donor is also protected by confidentiality and only non-identifying information can be revealed to the recipient.

Rights of the parents, donor, and child

The couple receiving treatment are the child's legal parents and their names are on the child's birth certificate.

Married couples automatically have legal rights and duties towards the child called 'parental responsibility'. Unmarried couples are advised to take legal advice to ensure that the male partner has parental responsibility. A child born to a single woman following donor insemination will have no legal father.

The donor has no legal rights or responsibilities towards the child. Conversely, the child has no claim on the donor. However, if donation has not taken place through a licensed clinic the legal position is less clear.

Children born from donor insemination have the right to obtain details of the identity of the donor from the UK national register once they reach adulthood (18 years). They may also apply to the register if they are planning to marry, to check that their partner is not genetically related (though this risk is very small because of the restricted number of donor pregnancies). Voluntary registers exist to help children born before this provision came into force.

Success rates

Live birth rates for donor insemination average 11% per cycle. This is lower than IVF but insemination is a simple treatment which can be repeated, and up to 50% of couples will conceive in 6 months. Data from the HFEA show a clear trend of reducing success rates with advancing maternal age, with a live birth rate of 13.5% for women under 30 falling to 5.3% at age 40–42.

Further reading

Byrd W, Bradshaw K. Carr B, et al. A prospective randomised study of pregnancy rates following intrauterine and intracervical insemination using frozen donor sperm. Fertil Steril 1990;53:521–7.

Hamilton MP. Working Party on Sperm Donation Services in the UK. *Human Fertility* 2008;11:147–58.

Human Fertilisation and Embryology Authority. *Code of Practice*. 2007.

Human Fertilisation and Embryology Authority. Disclosure of Donor Information Regulations (2004) Statutory Instrument 2004 No 1511. HMSO.

National Collaborating Centre for Women's and Children's Health on behalf of the National Institute of Clinical Excellence. (2004) *Fertility: assessment and treatment for people with fertility problems*. London: RCOG Press 104–6.

Practice Committee of the American Society for Reproductive Medicine and the Practice Committee of the Society for Assisted Reproductive Technology. Guidelines for Gamete and Embryo Donation. *Fertility Sterility* 2006;86:S38–50.

Tomlinson M, Barratt C. Donor insemination. In: Serhal and Overton (eds) *Good clinical practice in assisted reproduction*. Cambridge 2004:86–99.

Internet resources

www.hfea.gov.uk
www.ngdt.co.uk/
www.bica.net/

Patient resources

HFEA Guide to Infertility. Human Fertilisation and Embryology Authority, London 2008 (also available online)
www.infertilitynetworkuk.com/
www.dcnetwork.org/
www.ukdonorlink.org.uk/

Heavy menstrual bleeding

Definition

Heavy menstrual bleeding (HMB) is excessive menstrual bleeding that diminishes the woman's physical, emotional, social, and material quality of life and which can occur alone or in combination with other symptoms (NCCWCH 2007). It is frequently termed dysfunctional uterine bleeding, which is abnormal bleeding from the uterus in the absence of any identifiable pathology or pregnancy. It can also be termed menorrhagia, but these terms should be avoided where possible since they mean different things to different people.

Epidemiology

Between 4% and 51% of women experience HMB depending on the country and clinical setting of origin. In the UK, 5% of all women present with this problem. The incidence increases with both age and parity (Rybo 1966).

Pathology

HMB may be associated with the presence of fibroids, adenomyosis, endometriosis, and possibly endometrial polyps, although in many instances, no pathological features are present. HMB may be the result of either ovulatory or anovulatory cycles.

Aetiology

Disorders of endometrial function have been reported particularly related to the vasculature (Jabour et al. 2006). In particular, disordered production and metabolism of the prostaglandins has been well documented, as well as of a number of growth factors. Frequently ovarian function is normal in these women. HMB may occur in women with thyroid dysfunction and bleeding disorders, although this is unusual.

Prognosis

Heavy bleeding increases with age and is greatest during the 30s. In addition, the number of anovulatory cycles reported increases as the menopause approaches making irregular bleeding commoner. Dysfunctional uterine bleeding is cured by the menopause.

Clinical approach

Diagnosis

History

A full menstrual history should be taken, including length of bleeding, length of the cycle, the number of days of heavy bleeding, and the impact on the woman, such as flooding or the inability to get out of the house as well as the presence of other menstrual symptoms.

The presence of 'red light' symptoms must be excluded as these may indicate the presence of significant pathology. These symptoms are
- intermenstrual bleeding
- post-coital bleeding
- pelvic pain not related to the menses
- pressure symptoms.

Examination

The principal reason to carry out an abdominal examination in this context is to identify a pelvic mass.

Pelvic examination is required before a
- levonorgestrel-secreting interuterine system (LNG-IUS) fitting

- investigation for structural abnormality
- investigation for histological abnormality.

Pharmaceutical treatment can be started without examination in those where pathology is unlikely, i.e. regular heavy periods with no 'red light' symptoms

Investigations

These aim to detect whether pathology is causing the symptoms and, if present, whether the pathology is correctable (Critchley et al. 2001).

Ultrasound is the first-line diagnostic tool for identifying structural abnormalities.

It should be carried out in the following circumstances:
- the uterus is palpable abdominally
- vaginal examination reveals a pelvic mass
- pharmaceutical treatment fails.

However, hysteroscopy may be required if ultrasound is unsatisfactory or if an abnormality impacting on the cavity of the uterus is considered likely.

Endometrial biopsy

The incidence of endometrial cancer in women under 45 is extremely low. Biopsy is indicated
- when there is intermenstrual bleeding
- if the woman is aged over 45
- if there has been treatment failure
- if the woman is at high risk for endometrial cancer.

Treatment

Medical treatment

These are useful where there is no significant structural abnormality or where small fibroids only are present (Fraser et al. 1991; Lethaby et al. 2004, 2005). The main issues for consideration are
- whether contraception is required
- whether dysmenorrhoea is present
- woman's preference.

Where contraception is required, the following treatments are appropriate:
- LNG-IUS
- tranexamic acid
- non-steroidal anti-inflammatory agents or combined oral contraceptive pill
- Norethisterone 15 mg per day for days 5–26 of the cycle, or injected progestagens

Side-effects are unusual although women should be counselled about the prolonged nature of irregular bleeding when using the LNG-IUS.

Surgical treatment

Endometrial ablation

Endometrial ablation may be achieved by resecting the endometrium using a hysteroscope under direct vision or destroying the endometrium using a number of modalities (microwave, heat, radiofrequency). These latter methods (second generation techniques) do not require visualisation of the cavity and therefore less skill is required.

Ablation techniques (Cooper et al. 2005; Lethaby et al. 2005):
- are useful in women with a normal uterine cavity or very small fibroids.
- can be offered as an initial treatment for HMB if appropriate

- are NOT contraceptive and women must be advised to avoid subsequent pregnancy and to use contraception. Pregnancy, when it occurs, usually has a poor outcome.

Hysterectomy

The numbers performed for benign conditions have dropped significantly over the last ten years but it is still an appropriate option for some women, provided they are aware of all new possible alternatives (Garry et al. 2004; Maresh et al. 2002).

It should be used when:

- Other treatment options have failed, are contra-indicated or are declined.
- There is a wish for amenorrhoea
- The fully informed woman requests it and no longer wishes to retain her uterus and fertility.

The route by which hysterectomy will be performed will depend on a number of factors including the size of the uterus, its mobility and the preference of both the patient and the surgeon. Vaginal hysterectomy is to be preferred over abdominal where possible. Subtotal and total hysterectomy are both possibilities and whether the ovaries will be removed or retained also needs to be discussed.

Women who have uterine fibroids need to be counselled about the increased risk of complications over those with no fibroids.

Healthy ovaries should not be removed unless a woman specifically requests this. HRT administration should then be discussed.

Pain may start before the bleeding but usually gets better as the period progresses. It may be associated with other symptoms such as back ache, gastrointestinal symptoms or other menstrual symptoms.

Further reading

Cooper KG, Bain C, Lawrie L, et al. A randomised comparison of microwave endometrial ablation with transcervical resection of the endometrium; follow up at a minimum of five years. Br J Obstet Gynaecol 2005;112:470–5.

Critchley HO, Warner P, Lee AJ, et al. Evaluation of abnormal uterine bleeding: comparison of three outpatient procedures within cohorts defined by age and menopausal status. Health Technol Assess 2001;8:iii–iv,1–139.

Fraser IS, McCarron G. Randomized trial of 2 hormonal and 2 prostaglandin-inhibiting agents in women with a complaint of menorrhagia. Aust NZ J Obstet Gynaecol 1991;31:66–70.

Garry R, Fountain J, Mason S, et al. The eVALuate study: two parallel randomised trials, one comparing laparoscopic with abdominal hysterectomy, the other comparing laparoscopic with vaginal hysterectomy. BMJ 2004;328:129–33. [erratum appears in BMJ 2004;328:494.

Hurskainen R, Teperi J, Rissanen P, et al. Clinical outcomes and costs with the levonorgestrel-releasing intrauterine system or hysterectomy for treatment of menorrhagia: randomized trial 5-year follow-up. JAMA 2004;291:1456–63.

Jabour HN, Kelly RW, Fraser HM, Critchly HOD. 2006. Endocrine regulation of menstruation. Endocrine Rev 27:17–46.

Lethaby A, Augood C, Duckitt K. Nonsteroidal anti-inflammatory drugs for heavy menstrual bleeding. Cochrane Database Syst Rev 2004;3:CD000400.

Lethaby A, Farquhar C, Cooke I. Antifibrinolytics for heavy menstrual bleeding. Cochrane Database Syst Rev 2004;4 CD000249.

Lethaby A, Hickey M. Endometrial destruction techniques for heavy menstrual bleeding. Cochrane Database Syst Rev 2005;CD001501.

Lethaby A, Irvine G, Cameron I. Cyclical progestogens for heavy menstrual bleeding. Cochrane Database Syst Rev 2004;4:CD001016.

Lethaby A, Shepperd S, Cooke I, Farquhar C. Endometrial resection and ablation versus hysterectomy for heavy menstrual bleeding. Cochrane Database Syst Rev 2004;2:CD003855.

Lethaby AE, Cooke I, Rees M. Progesterone/progestogen releasing intrauterine systems for heavy menstrual bleeding. Cochrane Database Syst Rev 2005;4.

Maresh MJ, Metcalfe MA, McPherson K, et al. The VALUE national hysterectomy study: description of the patients and their surgery. Br J Obstet Gynaecol 2002;109:302–12.

Marjoribanks J, Lethaby A, Farquhar C. Surgery versus medical therapy for heavy menstrual bleeding. (Cochrane Review). In: Cochrane Database of Systematic Reviews, Issue 2, 2006. Oxford: Update Software.

National Collaborating centre for Women's and Children's Health (NCCWCH). Heavy menstrual bleeding. Clinical Guideline. 2007: 20–30.

Rybo G. Menstrual blood loss in relation to parity and menstrual pattern. Acta Obstet Gynecol Scand 1966;45(Suppl 7):25–45.

Internet resources

National Institute for Clinical Excellence. Fluid-filled thermal balloon and microwave endometrial ablation techniques for heavy menstrual bleeding. Technology Appraisal 78. London: NICE 2004 1–25: www.nice.org.uk

National Institute for Clinical Excellence. Impedance-controlled bipolar radiofrequency ablation for menorrhagia. London: NICE 2004: www.nice.org.uk

National Institute for Health and Clinical Excellence. Endometrial cryotherapy for menorrhagia. London: NICE 2006: www.nice.org.uk

Full Heavy menstrual Bleeding Guideline: http://nice.org.uk/CG044fullguideline

Dysmenorrhoea

Definition
Dysmenorrhoea is painful menstruation.

Epidemiology
Primary dysmenorrhoea is found particularly in teenage girls and usually starts 1 or 2 years after the menarche. It is frequently relieved following pregnancy and labour. Secondary dysmenorrhoea occurs in older women in association with pathology as described below. It may also occur in women taking hormone replacement therapy (Andersch and Milsom 1982).

Pathology
Dysmenorrhoea is often associated with endometriosis and may be the principal symptom associated with chronic pelvic pain. Other common causes are uterine fibroids or adenomyosis. In young women with dysmenorrhoea, pathology is unlikely although endometriosis does occur.

Aetiology
Primary dysmenorrhoea is related to the presence of prostaglandins. The concentration within the endometrium and myometrium is increased, particularly of those that lead to vascoconstriction and increased uterine contractility. Uterine prostaglandin production may also be increased in adenomyosis and where fibroids are present (Lumsden et al. 1984).

The posterior pituitary peptides, vasopressin and oxytocin, have also been implicated in the aetiology (Akerlund et al. 1979; Strömberg et al. 1984). It is unclear if there is an interaction between the two pathways.

Prognosis
The prognosis for primary dysmenorrhoea is good. It is very responsive to treatment and improves with age. The prognosis for secondary dysmenorrhoea depends on the cause.

History
- Identify relationship with menstrual bleeding:
  - the pain may precede the bleeding but is usually worse during the first 2 days of the menses.
- Quality of pain:
  - it is a cramping pain.
- Age of onset:
  - with onset of ovulatory cycles, 1–2 years following the menarche.
- Associated menstrual symptoms;
  - heavy menstrual bleeding is more likely in those with pathology such as fibroids
  - symptoms such as headache and gastrointestinal symptoms are common but improve as menses progress.

Examination
- Abdominal and pelvic examination will usually be normal.
- In secondary dysmenorrhoea, pelvic examination may reveal an
  - enlarged uterus (fibroids)
  - enlarged ovaries (endometrioma)
  - palpable fallopian tube (hydrosalpinx due to infection)
  - tenderness (endometriosis, pelvic inflammatory disease)
  - nodules (endometriosis).

Investigation
No investigation is required unless there
- is treatment failure
- is an abnormality detected on examination
- are other associated symptoms present suggestive of pathology.

Investigation includes either ultrasonography or laparoscopy.

Ultrasonography
This can be used to identify structural abnormality such as fibroids or uterine abnormality.

Laparoscopy
This is the best method for the diagnosis of endometriosis or pelvic inflammatory disease.

Treatment
Primary dysmenorrhoea
Non-steroidal anti-inflammatory agents (NSAIDs)
These should be taken regularly during the menses commencing with the onset of the pain or bleeding (whichever comes first and continued until the pain completely disappears. Ibuprofen, mefenamic acid, and naproxen are all effective (Dingfelder 1981; Elstrom et al. 1989; Courtland Robinson et al. 1992).

Combined oral contraceptive pill
This is useful in women desiring contraception.

These treatments decrease prostaglandin production and hence decrease uterine contractility and increase blood flow to the uterus. Of women with primary dysmenorrhoea, 80% will be treated successfully with these drugs alone or in combination.

The levonorgestrel-secreting intrauterine system (LNG-IUS) is also very valuable, even in those who do not achieve amenorrhoea (see above). However, it may be difficult to insert through a nulliparous cervix.

Vasopressin receptor antagonists have also been trialled and shown to be successful, although no oral preparations are yet available for use (Bossmar et al. 1997).

Preparations that lead to amenorrhoea will also relieve the problem. These include the gonadotrophins-releasing hormone agonists. However, long-term use is limited due to osteopenic side-effects, unless hormonal add-back therapy is coadministered. Continuous administration of progestagens may be effective and Danazol is a further option, although the use of these two therapies is often limited by side-effects.

Surgical treatment
Laparoscopic uterine nerve ablation has been advocated but the evidence of efficacy is poor and it is no longer recommended. Hysterectomy will be an appropriate option for some women and is discussed in Section 12.24, Menorrhagia.

The treatment of secondary dysmenorrhoea depends on the underlying pathology. It is usually less responsive to medical treatment unless this leads to amenorrhoea and may require surgical intervention.

Alternative treatments
Patients often enquire about the many alternative treatments such as herbal preparations, Chinese medicine, spinal manipulation, acupuncture, and many others. However, convincing evidence that they are effective is absent.

Further reading

Akerlund M, Strömberg P, Forsling ML. Primary dysmenorrhoea and vasopressin. Br J Obstet Gynaecol 1979;86:484–7.

Andersch B, Milsom I. An epidemiologic study of young women with dysmenorrhea. Am J Obstet Gynecol 1982;144:655–60.

Bossmar T, Brouard R, Doberl A, Akerlund M. Effects of SR 49059, an orally active V1a vasopressin receptor antagonist, on vasopressin-induced uterine contractions. Br J Obstet Gynaecol 1997;104:471–7.

Courtland Robinson J, Plichta S, Weisman CS, et al. Dysmenorrhoea and use of oral contraceptives in adolescent women attending a family planning clinic. Am J Obstet Gynecol 1992;166:578–83.

Dawood MY. Dysmenorrhoea. Clin Obstet Gynecol 1990;33:168–78.

Dawood MY. Primary dysmenorrhea: advances in pathogenesis and management. Obstet Gynecol 2006;108:428–41.

Dingfelder JR. Primary dysmenorrhoea treatment with prostaglandin inhibitors. Am J Obstet Gynecol 1981;140:874–9.

Elstrom P, Junicka E, Laudanski T, et al. Effect of an oral contraceptive in primary dysmenorrhoea: changes in uterine activity and reactivity to agonists. Contraception 1989;40:39–47.

Hauksson A, Akerlund M, Melin P. Uterine blood flow and myometrial activity at menstruation, and the action of vasopressin and a synthetic antagonist. Br J Obstet Gynaecol 1988;95:898–904.

Lumsden MA, Kelly RW, Baird DT. Primary dysmenorrhoea: the importance of both prostaglandins E2 and F2α. Br J Obstet Gynaecol 1983;90:1135–40.

Marjoribanks J, Proctor ML, Farquhar C. Nonsteroidal anti-inflammatory drugs for primary dysmenorrhoea. Cochrane Menstrual Disorders and Subfertility Group. Cochrane Database Syst Rev 2008;4:CD001751.

Proctor ML, Latthe PM, Farquhar CM, et al. Surgical interruption of pelvic nerve pathways for primary and secondary dysmenorrhoea. Cochrane Menstrual Disorders and Subfertility Group. Cochrane Database Syst Rev 2008;4:CD001896.

Proctor ML, Roberts H, Farquhar CM. Combined oral contraceptive pill (OCP) as treatment for primary dysmenorrhoea. Cochrane Menstrual Disorders and Subfertility Group. Cochrane Database Syst Rev 2008;4: CD002120.

Strömberg P, Akerlund M, Forsling MI, et al. Vasopressin and prostaglandin in premenstrual pain and primary dysmenorrhoea. Acta Obstet Gyncecol Scand 1984;63:533–8.

Wenzloff NJ, Shimp L. Therapeutic management of primary dysmenorrhea. Drug Intell Clin Pharm 1984; 18:22–6.

Yap C, Furness S, Farquhar C. Pre and post operative medical therapy for endometriosis surgery. Cochrane Menstrual Disorders and Subfertility Group. Cochrane Database Syst Rev 2008; 4:CD003678.

Ectopic pregnancy

Definition

The word ectopic is derived from the Greek word *ektopos*, which means out of place; an ectopic pregnancy is defined as implantation of a fertilized ovum outside the uterine cavity. It is an important cause of morbidity and mortality in women of reproductive age and is responsible for 75% of pregnancy related deaths in the first trimester (CEMACH 2007).

An ectopic pregnancy should be suspected in any woman of reproductive age, with a positive pregnancy test, presenting with abdominal pain and/or vaginal bleeding.

Epidemiology

Over 10 000 ectopic pregnancies are diagnosed annually in the UK, with an overall incidence of 11 in 1000 pregnancies (CEMACH 2007). However, it is likely that the number of ectopic pregnancies in the population is much higher, as many of them follow a benign course and tend to resolve spontaneously without causing significant clinical symptoms. Despite an increase in the incidence, the mortality due to ectopic pregnancies remains stable at 3.4% of all maternal mortalities in the UK (CEMACH 2007).

Aetiology

The main cause of ectopic pregnancy is damage to the tubal epithelium, which leads to implantation into the Fallopian tube. In cases with no evidence of anatomical tubal damage, the cause of ectopic pregnancy may be a dysfunction in the tubal smooth muscle activity secondary to an altered oestrogen–progesterone ratio (Pulkkinen and Talo 1987). This may adversely affect the transport of the fertilized egg into the uterus.

A number of risk factors have been identified which increase the risk of an ectopic gestation (Ankum *et al.* 1996). These include

- history of previous ectopic pregnancy
- pelvic inflammatory disease/chlamydia infection
- early age of intercourse and multiple partners
- history of infertility
- previous pelvic surgery
- IUCD *in situ* or sterilization failure
- use of emergency contraception
- assisted conception
- increased maternal age.

The most common site of an ectopic pregnancy is the Fallopian tube, accounting for nearly 95% of the cases. Other possible sites include the interstitial segment of the tube, cervix, deficient Caesarean section scar, ovary, and abdominal cavity.

Clinical approach

History: key points

The most common symptom of ectopic pregnancy is irregular vaginal bleeding, which typically starts at the time of expected menstruation. Abdominal pain is a late clinical feature, which usually indicates the presence of intra-abdominal bleeding. The location of pregnancy in the tube usually determines the clinical presentation. The majority of the tubal ectopics are ampullary, and they present relatively early with vaginal bleeding and pain. In ectopics that are located more proximal to the uterus, such as isthmic and interstitial pregnancies, early warning signs are often absent and they may present with sudden rupture and severe haematoperitoneum.

A careful history should include the duration and severity of symptoms and the presence or absence of risk factors. A urine pregnancy test is usually positive, but negative results do not rule out the possibility of ectopic pregnancy in women with typical clinical presentation. Some women with ruptured ectopics may predominantly complain of gastrointestinal symptoms. This may delay the diagnosis and treatment, as has been previously described in cases with fatal outcomes.

Examination: key points

Abdominal and vaginal examination can be unremarkable, or may demonstrate signs of acute abdomen with rebound tenderness. Cervical excitation and/or adnexal tenderness may be found on bimanual pelvic examination. Where transvaginal ultrasound is available, bimanual pelvic examination adds little to the diagnosis and does not need to be routinely carried out. Women with a positive pregnancy test and clinical signs of intra-abdominal bleeding and cardiovascular instability should be operated on without delay, regardless of the imaging results.

Investigations

Transvaginal ultrasound

This is the front-line investigation in assessing haemodynamically stable patients with a suspected ectopic pregnancy. The majority of clinically significant ectopic pregnancies can be diagnosed on ultrasound scan prior to surgery (Condous *et al.* 2005).

In the past an ectopic pregnancy was suspected in women with a positive pregnancy test and an 'empty uterus' on ultrasound scan. In modern practice an ectopic pregnancy should be directly visualized on ultrasound examination. The diagnosis of ectopic pregnancy is based on the detection of an adnexal swelling separate from the uterus and the ovaries. The morphology of ectopic pregnancy varies, but in most cases, an extrauterine gestational sac with or without a yolksac or embryo can be seen (Fig. 12.9.1). With high resolution ultrasound equipment an ectopic pregnancy is often seen as nonhomogeneous solid swelling that moves separate from the ovary on palpation (sliding organ sign) (Timor-Tritsch and Rottem 1987) (Fig. 12.9.2).

The presence of an intrauterine pregnancy cannot be used to rule out the possibility of a concomitant ectopic pregnancy in women with clinical symptoms suggestive of an ectopic pregnancy. In some cases bleeding into the empty uterine cavity may create features on ultrasound scan suggestive of an early intrauterine pregnancy, which can cause diagnostic errors and delay in the diagnosis of ectopic.

Biochemical markers

The measurement of serum β-human chorionic gonadotropin (β-hCG) and progesterone may aid the diagnosis in women with a high index of suspicion for ectopic pregnancy, in whom a pregnancy is not visualized on the ultrasound scan.

Serum β-hCG

In a normal intrauterine pregnancy, serum hCG doubles every 1.4 days before 5 weeks' gestation and 2.4 days between 5 and 7 weeks. A slow rise in β-hCG indicates an abnormal pregnancy; however, it does not discriminate between early intrauterine miscarriages and ectopic pregnancies. Also, β-hCG levels show a normal rate of increase in some ectopic pregnancies.

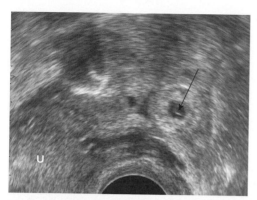

Fig. 12.9.1 An ultrasound scan showing an empty uterus (U) and a small gestational sac with a yolk sac in the left adnexa (arrow). These findings were conclusive of a left tubal ectopic pregnancy.

Serum progesterone

The production of progesterone from the corpus luteum responds rapidly to changes in hCG production from the trophoblast. Measurements of serum progesterone can therefore be used to assess viability of pregnancy. Serum progesterone of >60 nmol indicates a normal rise in hCG levels, usually associated with normal intrauterine pregnancies. Low progesterone level <20 nmol/L is a highly sensitive and specific test to identify spontaneously resolving failed pregnancies and can be used to reduce the need for further follow up for women in whom pregnancies cannot be located on ultrasound scan (Banerjee et al. 2001).

Many diagnostic algorithms have been described to aid in the management of pregnant women in whom ultrasound scan fails to identify the location of pregnancy. None of them has been compared in prospective randomized trials and individual units should choose between them on the basis of local expertise and experience.

Laparoscopy

Until recently, laparoscopy was considered to be the test of choice for the diagnosis of ectopic pregnancy. However, with the improvement of ultrasound diagnosis the role of laparoscopy has evolved from primary diagnostic to a primary treatment modality for ectopic pregnancies.

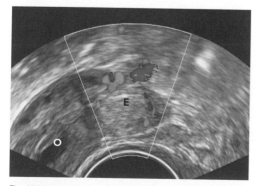

Fig. 12.9.2 A sonogram showing the right ovary (O) and a small hyperechoic solid structure adjacent to its medial pole (E). The swelling was highly vascular on Doppler examination, which helped to confirm the diagnosis of a tubal ectopic pregnancy. See also colour plate section.

Management

Surgery

Laparoscopy has become the mainstay of surgical management of tubal ectopic pregnancy in haemodynamically stable patients. The rates of subsequent intrauterine pregnancy appear to be similar after laparoscopy or laparotomy. However, a minimally invasive approach offers obvious advantages over laparotomy, including shorter hospital stay, less postoperative pain, and faster recovery (Lundorff et al. 1991; Murphy 1992).

Salpingectomy is the excision of a Fallopian tube containing the ectopic pregnancy and is preferred when the contralateral tube is healthy. It should also be considered in the presence of a large ectopic pregnancy, ipsilateral tubal pathology or haemorrhage after attempts at tubal conservation.

Salpingotomy is a procedure in which the Fallopian tube is conserved by removing the ectopic pregnancy through a linear incision. It is attempted if there is evidence of contralateral tubal damage and the woman desires further pregnancies. There is a high risk of intraoperative and postoperative bleeding and a 10–15% risk of persistent trophoblast, which may require further surgical/medical treatment (Hajenius et al. 2007).

It is unclear whether future reproductive outcomes are better after salpingotomy; however, the data from observational studies show slightly higher rates of intrauterine pregnancies after tubal conservation (Bangsgaard et al. 2003). A prospective randomized trial that aims to address this issue is currently under way (Mol et al. 2008). Until then the choice between the two approaches should be decided on an individual case basis.

Medical management

Methotrexate is the most commonly used drug for the medical management of ectopic pregnancy. It is a folic acid antagonist that inhibits DNA synthesis and cell division in the trophoblast. It can be given either systemically or locally within the ectopic gestational sac. When given as a single dose there is a small risk of side-effects such as gastritis, alopecia, nausea, vomiting, hepatic or renal impairment, leucopenia, and thrombocytopenia.

There are strict selection criteria for patients suitable for methotrexate administration:

- minimal clinical symptoms
- certain ultrasound diagnosis of ectopic
- no evidence of embryonic cardiac activity
- size <5 cm
- no evidence of haematoperitoneum on ultrasound
- low serum β-hCG <3000 IU/L.

According to recent studies, one-third of all tubal ectopic pregnancies fulfil this criteria and 65–82% of them have successful treatment with methotrexate (Hajenius et al. 1997; Sowter et al. 2001). Hence medical treatment can be used to successfully manage 25–30% of women diagnosed with tubal ectopic pregnancy.

Expectant management

The use of expectant management of ectopic pregnancy is based on the observation that many ectopic pregnancies have a tendency to resolve spontaneously without causing any clinical symptoms. Expectant management is a suitable option for motivated patients with minimal clinical symptoms who are willing to attend for repeated follow-up visits. According to current literature, the success of expectant management is largely predicted by initial serum β-hCG levels. In women in whom an ectopic pregnancy is visible on the scan and who present with serum β-hCG levels <1500 IU/L, spontaneous resolution rates of 60–70% have been reported (Elson et al. 2004).

Future pregnancies and recurrence

Studies have demonstrated tubal patency rates of 92% after expectant management, resulting in subsequent intra-uterine pregnancy rates of 89% (Fernandez et al. 1991). This is similar to the intrauterine pregnancy rates with salp-ingotomy and is significantly higher than those following salpingectomy (66%) (Bangsgaard et al. 2003)

Ectopic pregnancy recurs in 6–16% cases with previous history, and therefore these women may be offered an early scan at 5–6 weeks' gestation in future pregnancies (Dubuisson et al. 1990).

Further reading

Ankum WM, Mol BW, Van der Veen F, et al. Risk factors for ectopic pregnancy: a meta-analysis. Fertil Steril 1996;65:1093–9.

Banerjee S, Aslam N, Zosmer N, et al. Expectant management of early pregnancies of unknown location: a prospective evaluation of methods to predict spontaneous resolution of pregnancy. Br J Obstet Gynaecol 2001;108:158–63.

Bangsgaard N, Lund CO, Ottesen B, et al. Improved fertility following conservative surgical treatment of ectopic pregnancy. Br J Obstet Gynaecol 2003;110:765–70.

CEMACH. Saving Mother's Lives: The Seventh Report on the Confidential Enquiries into Maternal and Child Health in the United Kingdom. 2007:92–3.

Condous G, Okaro E, Khalid A, et al. The accuracy of transvaginal ultrasonography for the diagnosis of ectopic pregnancy prior to surgery. Hum Reprod 2005;20:1404–9.

Dubuisson JB, Aubriot FX, Foulot H, et al. Reproductive outcome after laparoscopic salpingectomy for tubal ectopic pregnancy. Fertil Steril 1990;53:1004–7.

Elson J, Tailor A, Banerjee S, et al. Expectant management of tubal ectopic pregnancy: prediction of successful outcome using deci-sion tree analysis. Ultrasound Obstet Gynaecol 2004;23:552–6.

Fernandez H, Lelaidier C, Baton C, et al. Return of reproductive performance after expectant management and local treatment for ectopic pregnancy. Hum Reprod 1991;6:1474–7.

First trimester pregnancy complications. Clin Obstet Gynecol 2007;50:1–154.

Hajenius PJ, Engelsbel S, Mol BW, et al. Randomized trial of sys-temic methotrexate versus laparoscopic salpingostomy in tubal pregnancy. Lancet 1997;350:774–9.

Hajenius PJ, Mol F, Mol BW, et al. Interventions for tubal ectopic pregnancy. Cochrane Database Syst Rev 2007;1:CD000324.

Lundorff P, Thorburn J, Lindblom B, et al. Fertility outcome after conservative surgical treatment of ectopic pregnancy evaluated in a randomized trial. Fertil Steril 1992;57:998–1002.

Mol F, Strandel A, Jurkovic D, et al. The ESEP study: salpingostomy versus salpingectomy for tubal ectopic pregnancy; the impact on future fertility: a randomised controlled trial. BMC Women's Health 2008;8:11.

Murphy AA, Nager CW, Wujek JJ, et al. Operative laparoscopy versus laparotomy for the management of ectopic pregnancy. Fertil Steril 1992;57:1180–5.

Problems in early pregnancy: advances in diagnosis and management. London: RCOG Press 1997.

Pulkkinen MO, Talo A. Tubal physiologic consideration in ectopic pregnancy. Clin Ostet Gynecol 1987;30:164–72.

Sowter MC, Farquhar CM, Gudex G, et al. An economic evaluation of single dose methotrexate and laparoscopic surgery for the treat-ment of unruptured ectopic pregnancy. Br J Obstet Gynaecol 2001;108:204–12.

Timor-Tritsch IE, Rottem S. Transvaginal ultrasonographic study of the Fallopian tube. Obstet Gynaecol 1987;70:424–8.

Internet resources

www.earlypregnancy.org.uk

www.rcog.org.uk (Guideline 21:Management of Tubal Ectopic Pregnancy)

Patient resources

www.ectopic.org.uk

www.miscarriageassociation.org.uk

www.patient.co.uk/showdoc/23069044

Embryo freezing

Definition

Embryo freezing is the cryopreservation of embryos created using in vitro fertilization (IVF) and stored at very low temperatures (−196°C) for future use. Cellular metabolism and embryonic development stops when cells are cooled and can resume on thawing, provided embryos survive the freezing and thawing processes with the majority of their cells intact.

Epidemiology

The first pregnancy following freezing and thawing of a human embryo was reported in 1983. In 2006 there were 737 679 births in the UK of which 8280 (1.12%) were born following fresh IVF cycles and 1375 (0.2%) were born following frozen embryo replacement cycles. A total of 7911 frozen embryo replacement cycles were performed in the UK in 2006, with a live birth rate of 17.4% per cycle (all ages).

Advantages of embryo freezing

- The use of superovulation regimes in IVF cycles stimulates the development of multiple follicles and the collection on average of 8–12 eggs, resulting in 5–9 embryos per cycle after fertilization by IVF or intracytoplasmic sperm injection (ICSI). The best one or two embryos (<40 years) or one to three embryos (≥40 years) are normally transferred in a fresh treatment cycle. Good quality surplus embryos can be stored for future use. The ability to freeze embryos increases the cumulative live birth rate per egg collection following transfer of frozen thawed embryos, without the need for further superovulation and egg collection.
- If the fresh cycle is successful and results in a live birth, frozen thawed embryos can result in the delivery of a sibling without the need for another fresh cycle.
- When patients have over-responded to stimulation, elective cryopreservation of all embryos and replacement at a later date can be used as a strategy to minimize the risk of a patient developing severe ovarian hyperstimulation (OHSS), as pregnancy in a fresh treatment cycle is a risk factor.
- Embryo cryopreservation can be used as a method of fertility preservation by women about to undergo cancer treatment that is likely to impair their ovarian function and reserve of eggs.
- The costs of simple frozen embryo replacement cycles are considerably less than the cost of a further fresh cycle.
- Effective freezing programmes are essential to the proposed move towards single embryo transfer to minimize the risk of multiple pregnancy following IVF treatment.

Legal aspects and regulation in the UK

- Freezing and storage of human embryos and gametes can only take place in units that have been licensed by the Human Fertilisation and Embryology Authority (HFEA).
- Valid consent to store embryos must be obtained from both partners, and if one partner withdraws consent embryos can no longer be kept in storage.
- If the embryo(s) have been created using donor eggs or sperm, the embryos may only be stored if the donor has also consented to the storage of embryos created using their donated gametes.

- The duration of storage is specified on the consent form and is usually 5 years in the first instance. It can normally be extended to 10 years if necessary, and for patients who have undergone cancer treatment likely to permanently impair their fertility gametes and embryos can be stored to the age of 55 years.
- It is illegal for embryos to be stored without valid consent so it is very important for patients to keep in contact with units if they move or their circumstances change. If the first 5-year storage period has expired without patients using the embryos and it is not possible to contact the couple, the embryos must be allowed to perish.

How and when are embryos frozen?

Challenges of freezing embryos

- Human embryos contain cells that are relatively large and the main constituent of the cytoplasm is water. On cooling below freezing, temperature ice crystals start to form damaging intracellular structure and cellular membranes.
- The concentration of solutes within cells also increases, which can be toxic.
- The microtubules of metaphase spindles are also temperature sensitive and depolymerize on cooling.
- The highest risk time for cellular damage is during the freezing or thawing processes. An embryo must have at least 50% of its cells intact following thawing to retain the potential for further development.
- Once embryos are frozen, if conditions are kept stable, they can remain in storage for many years without further deterioration.
- Embryos are stored in liquid nitrogen tanks or dewars, which require careful maintenance to ensure they remain topped up. Many IVF units use alarm systems to alert the embryology team in the event of failure of a tank and a drop in liquid nitrogen levels that could jeopardize the stored embryos.
- Many patients' embryos are stored in one dewar, and careful labelling of straws and ampoules is essential, together with regular audits of stored material.

Use of cryoprotectants

Cryoprotectants are used during the freezing of embryos to increase cell survival. The use of glycerol as a cryoprotectant for human sperm was first described in 1949. Since that time other cryoprotectants have also been used including propanediol (PROH), dimethylsulphoxide (DMSO), and ethylene glycol. Cryoprotectants decrease the freezing point of solutions and reduce the amount of salts and other solutes present in the remaining liquid phase, reducing the incidence of lipoprotein denaturation. Some protocols also use high concentrations of sucrose together with cryoprotectants to assist the dehydration of cells and reduce the risk of ice crystals forming.

Stage of embryo development for freezing

Embryos may be stored soon after fertilization at the pronuclear (1 cell) stage, after early cleavage, or at the blastocyst stage

a. Pronuclear stage zygotes are relatively stable with high survival rates after freezing and PROH is often used as the cryoprotectant with sucrose. This is often the stage chosen to freeze embryos when all embryos are going to be stored without a fresh transfer (e.g. fertility preservation or reducing OHSS risk). When pronucleate embryos are thawed they are allowed to continue their development for a further 1–5 days before transfer to the uterus. Survival rates of around 70% are expected following pronucleate stage freezing with pregnancy rates of 17–31%.

b. Most embryos have been frozen at the cleavage (2–8 cell) stage following the transfer of fresh embryos 2 or 3 days after egg collection. DMSO or PROH are used as cryoprotectants at this stage. Cryopreservation of day 2 embryos has been shown to be associated with a 30% reduction in implantation potential.

c. Extended culture of embryos to the blastocyst stage of development is becoming more common in IVF units. Blastocyst culture allows identification of the embryo or embryos that have the best potential for continued development and implantation. This helps selection of a single embryo for replacement into the uterus to reduce the risk of multiple pregnancy. Other surplus blastocyst embryos can be cryopreserved by slow freezing or vitrification (see below). If this approach is adopted there are usually fewer embryos available for transfer and freezing as many human embryos exhibit developmental arrest before the blastocyst stage. Pregnancy rates as high as 60% per transfer have been reported following transfer of thawed vitrified blastocysts.

Slow cooling or vitrification

Embryos are stored in ampoules or vials in the freezing solutions and traditionally have been slow cooled to –30 to –40°C before being plunged into liquid nitrogen. To try and reduce the risk of ice crystal formation during cooling, an alternative approach of vitrification has been used. Vitrification uses high concentrations of cryoprotectants and sucrose and rapid cooling to –196°C resulting in a solid glass like state without ice crystal formation. Survival rates of 70–90% are reported following vitrification, with better embryonic survival, development, and pregnancy rates.

Frozen embryo replacement cycles

Frozen thawed embryos can be replaced in natural cycles or artificially controlled cycles using hormone replacement therapy (HRT).

- In natural cycle replacement ultrasound is used to identify the dominant follicle and endometrial development. Ovulation is either detected by monitoring for the luteinizing hormone (LH) surge or initiated using an injection of LH or human chorionic gonadotrophin (hCG) once the follicle reaches 17–22 mm diameter. Embryos are thawed and transferred the appropriate number of days after ovulation depending on the stage at which they were frozen. The appropriate endometrial changes for implantation are produced by the normal ovarian secretion of oestradiol followed by oestradiol and progesterone in the luteal phase.
- For women that do not have regular ovulatory cycles it is possible to replicate the pattern of endometrial development artificially using oestradiol orally or transdermally followed by the addition of progesterone supplementation to create a secretory endometrium. Ultrasound is used to measure endometrial thickness, which ideally needs to be 8 mm or more. Some units routinely use HRT cycles for frozen embryo replacement as it may help in planning workload. In women

Table 12.10.1 IVF and ICSI success rates 2006 UK (with permission from HFEA www.hfea.gov.uk)

Age range (years)	Live birth/cycle (fresh) (%)	Live birth/cycle (frozen) (%)
<35	31.0	20.1
35–37	26.4	18.5
38–39	18.6	16.4
40–42	11.1	9.5
43–44	4.6	9.5
>44	4.0	10.2

who are ovulatory it may be important to suppress the natural cycle using gonadotropin-releasing hormone analogues before stimulating endometrial development.

Outcome of frozen embryo replacement cycles

Success rates

The implantation potential of frozen thawed embryos is not as good as fresh (Table 12.10.1), resulting in lower pregnancy and live birth rates per cycle. There is an age-related decline in pregnancy rates as seen in fresh cycles, although the drop is less marked in women 40 years and over. This is likely to reflect the following factors:

- Patients who have sufficient embryos to freeze tend to be better prognosis patients with a higher chance of pregnancy in the fresh cycle.
- Patients who have had a live birth following a fresh cycle are more likely to have a successful outcome from a subsequent frozen cycle.
- The age at which embryos are replaced for frozen cycles may be very different from the age at which embryos were originally created. Maternal age at the time of the fresh cycle influences the proportion of embryos that are aneuploid and live birth rates.

Congenital abnormalities

Studies examining the outcome of children born following frozen embryo replacement have been reassuring, with no increase in levels of congenital abnormalities to those born following fresh IVF cycles.

Frequently asked questions

Are there any more abnormalities in babies born using frozen thawed embryos?

All pregnancies carry a small risk of babies being born with abnormalities, and studies have shown that this risk is no higher for babies born after frozen embryo replacement than after transfer of fresh embryos.

Do embryos deteriorate the longer they are kept in storage?

Some embryos do not survive the freezing and thawing process but this is due to the changes that occur to the embryo on cooling and warming. Once an embryo is frozen, studies have shown that the survival rates and pregnancy rates following frozen embryo replacement are not influenced by the length of time the embryo was stored.

Further reading

Albuquerque LE, Saconato H, Maciel, MC. Depot versus daily administration of gonadotrophin-releasing hormone agonist protocols for pituitary desensitization in assisted reproduction cycles. Cochrane Database Syst Rev 2005;1:CD002808.

Avery S, Marcus S, Spillane S, *et al.* Does the length of storage time affect the outcome of frozen embryo replacement? J Assist Reprod Genet 1995;12:675.

Balanban B, Urman B, Ata B, *et al.* A randomized controlled study of human day 3 embryo cryopreservation by slow freezing or vitrification: vitrification is associated with higher survival, metabolism and blastocyst formation. Hum Reprod 2008;23:1976–82.

Braude P. One Child at a time. Reducing multiple births after IVF. Human Fertilisation and Embryology Authority (HFEA) at www.hfea.gov.uk/docs/MOSET_report_Final_Dee_06.pdf.

Edgar DH, Bourne H, Jericho H, McBain JC. A quantitative analysis of the impact of cryopreservation on the implantation potential of human early cleavage stage embryos. Hum Reprod 2000;15:175–9.

El-Toukhy T, Khalaf Y, Al-Darazi K, *et al.* Cryo-thawed embryos obtained from conception cycles have double the implantation and pregnancy potential of those from unsuccessful cycles. Hum Reprod 2003;18:1313–18.

El-Toukhy T, Taylor A, Khalaf Y, *et al.* Pituitary suppression in ultrasound-monitored frozen replacement cycles. A randomized study. Hum Reprod 2004;19:874–9.

Granne I, Child T, Hartshorne G. Embryo cryopreservation: Evidence for practice. Hum Fertil 2008;11:159–72.

Loutradi KE, Kolibianakis EM, Venetis CA, *et al.* Cryopreservation of human embryos by vitrification or slow freezing: a systematic review and meta-analysis. Fertil Steril 2008;90:186–93.

Polge C, Smith AU, Parkes AS. Revival of spermatozoa after vitrification and dehydration at low temperature. Nature 1949;154:666.

Rama Raju GA, Jaya Prakash G, Murali Krishna K, Madan K. Neonatal outcome after vitrified day 3 embryo transfers: a preliminary study. Fertil Steril 2009;92:143–8.

Riggs R, Mayer J, Dowling-Lacey D, *et al.* Does storage time influence postthaw survival and pregnancy outcome? An analysis of 11,768 cryopreseved human embryos. Fertil Steril 2010;93:109–15.

Son WY, Yoon SH, Yoon HJ, *et al.* Pregnancy outcome following transfer of human blastocysts vitrified on electron microscopy grids after induced collapse of the blastocoele. Hum Reprod 2003;18:137–9.

Stachecki J, Garrisi J, Sabino S, *et al.* A new safe, simple, and successful vitrification method for bovine and human blastocysts. Reprod Biomed Online 2008;17:360–7.

Takahashi K, Mukaida T, Goto T, Oka C. Perinatal outcome of blastocyst transfer with vitrification using cryoloop: a 4-year follow-up study. Fertil Steril 2005;84:88–92.

Trounson A, Mohr L. Human pregnancy following cryopreservation, thawing and transfer of an eight-cell embryo. Nature 1983;305:707–9.

Vanderzwalmen P, Bertin G, Debauche Ch, *et al.* Births after vitrification at morula and blastocyst stages: effect of artificial reduction of the blastocoelic cavity before vitrification. Human Reprod 2002;17:744–51.

Emergency contraception

Ninety per cent of unplanned pregnancies are user related and 50% of women who present for a termination of pregnancy are current or recent users of a contraceptive. The need for a preventative post-coital method was recognized in ancient times and has been cited in medical folklore. Modern emergency contraceptives are either oral pills that are taken within a designated time after exposure or the use of a copper bearing intrauterine device.

In countries where no licensed products exist, woman resort to DIY emergency contraception using available combined or progestogen only pills to make up the recommended effective dosage.

Types of emergency contraception

- Combined emergency hormonal contraception comprises two doses each of 100 µg of ethinyloestradiol and 500 µg of levonorgestral. The first dose is taken within 72 hours of unprotected intercourse followed by a second dose 12 hours later.
- Progestogen-only emergency hormonal contraception (PEHC) comprises a single dose of 1500 µg of levonorgestral taken within 72 hours of unprotected intercourse. This is now the predominant emergency oral contraceptive available worldwide and the only product that is available in the UK. The prescription-only product is called Levonelle 1500; the pharmacy over-the-counter product is called Levonelle One Step.
- A new emergency oral contraceptive to be introduced in 2009 is a single dose of a selective oestrogen receptor modulator that has sustained efficacy for up to 120 hours and has the advantage of being non-steroidal.
- Antiprogesterones in the form of Mifepristone have been successfully used for emergency contraception in a single dose of 10 mg used within 72 hours of unprotected intercourse. China has a licensed preparation.
- A copper-bearing intrauterine device is the most effective emergency contraceptive and can be used up to 5 days from unprotected intercourse. It has a number of other versatile features (see box).
- Ulipristal acetate 30 mg single dose is now licensed in the UK and USA for emergency contraception up to 120 hours after unprotected intercourse. Ulipristal is a selective progesterone receptor modulator and works after the LH surge to block follicular rupture, an action that the traditional levonorgestrel emergency contraception lacks.

Mechanism of action

Emergency contraceptives are not abortifacients. Hormonal emergency contraception prevents or delays ovulation when taken before ovulation and is likely to interfere with endometrial, ovarian, and tubal mechanisms in a way that prevents or disrupts fertilization. The emergency IUD works in a similar way at endometrial and tubal levels disrupting fertilization. Prevention of implantation is the exception not the rule.

Efficacy of emergency contraception

The efficacy of the PEHC was confirmed by two World Health Organization randomized controlled trials published in 1998 and 2002. At mid-cycle the risk of conception from a single unprotected intercourse can be up to 30%, with the average risk of conception for a single random act of intercourse being 4%. No cycle days can be deemed 100% safe. Efficacy is best expressed as the percentage of expected pregnancies prevented by emergency contraception. EHC prevents 8/10 pregnancies and an IUD 9/10 pregnancies. Women who take EHC within 24 hours of unprotected intercourse avoid 95% of expected pregnancies whereas those who take the pill beyond

> Special advantages of an emergency IUD.
> 1. Failure rate extremely low
> 2. Effective up to 120 hours after intercourse
> 3. Effective up to 120 hours after earliest calculated date of ovulation
> 4. Can cover multiple exposures
> 5. An alternative to hormonal methods
> 6. Provide contraception for the rest of the cycle
> 7. Can be kept as an ongoing contraceptive
> 8. Conversely can be removed with the next menses
> 9. The traditional contraindications that apply to IUDs do not apply to the IUDs intended for emergency contraception, the exception being the risk of infection which needs to be excluded, tested for, or treated prophylactically

48 hours would expect a protection rate of about 60%. Limited research suggests that this 60% protection is maintained up to 120 hours, but levonelle is not licensed for use beyond 72 hours.

The copper IUD prevents up to 99% of expected pregnancies.

Indications

The two main indications are unprotected intercourse, and condom breakage and slippage.

Special indications include missing pills.

Impact

In the UK, emergency contraception has been promoted since the early 1980s. Over 1.5 million units of emergency hormonal contraception are dispensed every year, with the majority being provided by pharmacists. Every year 5% of women aged 16–49 use emergency contraception once, with 1% using it two or more times. The expectation that emergency contraception would reduce unplanned pregnancies and abortion rates cannot be ethically tested, but there is consensus that the method has not had the predicted impact on these variables. The main reason is that access to correct information and to free provision remains patchy and couples tend to underestimate the risk of unplanned pregnancy and therefore are unlikely to resort to the method in risky situations which they wrongly perceive as being safe.

Strategies to improve access include advance provision, increasing information about the emergency IUD and promoting immediate (so-called quick start) of an ongoing method of contraception following EHC.

Safety

The emergency IUD is an extremely safe contraceptive as long as the woman is assessed for the risk of infection, preferably screened for sexually transmitted infections, and where there is a high sexually transmitted infection risk given prophylactic antibiotics. Depending on the result of the test, partner notification is also required.

The hormonal methods are also safe with the only contraindications being allergy to the component hormone, pregnancy where the method is unlikely to work, and porphyria. Inadvertent use of emergency contraception in early pregnancy is unlikely to lead to congenital abnormalities but counselling should stress the fact that a normal pregnancy outcome can never be guaranteed.

The side-effects of EHC are all minor and infrequent; they include nausea (14%), vomiting (1%), and breast pain (8%). Cycle disruption is the exception rather than the rule, with 90% of users having their next menses on time or within 7 days of the expected time of menstruation.

Counselling points

- Estimate the pregnancy risk, describe the mechanism of action, and inform the woman about the failure risk.
- Prescribe the single dose Levonorgestral EHC.
- Emphasize that the IUD is the most effective form of emergency contraception.
- Emergency contraception is not effective if the woman is already pregnant and has no abortifacient action.
- Encourage the administration of emergency hormonal contraception as early as possible within the 72-hour window.
- The use of EHC up to 120 hours is permitted but unlicensed.
- Domperidone 10 mg is the antiemetic of choice.
- Broad-spectrum antibiotics do not interact with EHC but where liver enzyme inducers are used, a double dose of Levonorgestral should be taken stat.
- The protection of emergency hormonal contraception is not prospective and the woman should abstain or use condoms until her next period.
- Any ongoing contraceptive can be started immediately, provided the woman is fully counselled.
- Multiple doses of EHC can be administered in the same cycle but tend to be much less effective than a regular ongoing method of contraception.
- There is no need to perform tests or examinations prior to prescribing EHC.
- Follow-up is desirable, usually 3 weeks post treatment. Users should be encouraged to return if subsequent menstruation is delayed or abnormal in any way.
- EHC is unlikely to increase the risk of ectopic pregnancy but the risk of an ectopic should always be high in the awareness of the practitioner.

Further reading

Anon. Faculty of Family Planning and Reproductive Health Care. Royal College of Obstetricians and Gynaecologists, Guidance April 2000. Emergency contraception: recommendations for clinical practice. Br J Fam Plann 2000;26:93–6.

Black K, Kubba A. Is there a link between ectopic pregnancy and progestogen-only emergency contraception? Trends Urol Gynaecol Sexual health 2003;8:5–6.

Croxatto HB. Emergency contraception pills: how do they work? IPPE Medical Bulletin 2002;336:1–2.

Glasier A, Baird D. The effects of self-administering emergency contraception. N Engl J Med 1998;339:1–4.

Glasier AF, Cameron ST Fine PM, et al. Ulipristal acetate versus levonorgestrel for emergency contraception a randomised non-inferiority trial and meta-analysis. Lancet 2010;375:555–62.

IPPF International Medical Advisory Panel. Statement on emergency contraception. IPPF Medical Bulletin 2004;38:1–3.

Piaggio G, von Hertzen H, Grimes DA, et al. On behalf of the Task Force on Postovulatory Methods of Fertility Regulation. Timing of emergency contraception with levonorgestrel or the Yuzpe regimen. Lancet 1999;335:731.

Raman-Wilms L, Tseng Al Wighard TS, et al. Fetal genital effects of first-trimester sex hormone exposure; a meta-analysis. Obstet Gynecol 1995;85:141–9.

Task Force on Postovulatory Methods of Fertility Regualation. Randomised, controlled trial of levonorgestrel versus the Yuzpe regimen of combined oral contraceptive for emergency contraception. Lancet 1998;352:428–33.

UNDP/UNFPA/WHO/World Bank Special Programme of Research Development and Research Training in Human Reproduction. Task Force on Post-Ovulatory Methods of Fertility Regulation. Efficacy and side effects of immediate poscoital levonorgestrel used repeatedly for contraception. 2000;61:303–8.

Von Hertzen H, Piaggia G, Ding J, et al. Low dose mifepristone and two regimens of levonorgestrel for emergency contraception: a WHO multicentre randomised trial. Lancet 2002;306:1803–10.

Webb A, Shochet T, Bigrigg A, et al. Effect of hormal emergency contraception on bleeding patterns. Contraception 2004;69:133–5.

Wilcox AJ, Dunson DB, Weinberg CR, et al. Likelihood of conception with a single act of intercourse, providing benchmark rates for assessment of pos-coital contraceptives. Contraception 2002;63:211–15.

Yuzpe AA, Percival Smith R, Rademaker AW. A multi-center investigation employing ethinylestradiol combined with DL-norgestrel as a post-coital contraceptive agent. Fertil Steril 1982;37:508–13.

Yuzpe AA. Lance WJ. Ethinylestradiol and DL-norgestrel as a post-coital contraceptive. Feril Steril 1977;28:932–6.

Internet resources

WHO emergency contraception database: www.who.int/reproductive-health/family_planning/methods.htm

Patient resources

Princeton University's emergency contraception website: http://ec.princeton.edu/

Endometriosis

Definition
Endometriosis is defined by the presence of endometrial-like tissue in sites outside the uterus, e.g. the peritoneum, ovaries, and rectovaginal septum. It produces peritoneal inflammation and fibrosis, and can lead to the formation of endometriomas (ovarian cysts) and pelvic adhesions.

Aetiology
The cause is still unknown but retrograde menstruation is probably a permissive factor. There is increasing evidence that the disease is inherited as a complex genetic trait.

Risk factors relate to oestrogen levels (smoking history and peripheral body fat) and increased menstruation (shorter cycle length and longer duration of flow).

Associated symptoms
Some or all of the following symptoms may be present:
- severe dysmenorrhoea (painful periods)
- deep dyspareunia (pain on intercourse)
- chronic, non-menstrual pain
- pain at ovulation
- dyschezia (pain on defaecation)
- infertility
- cyclical or perimenstrual symptoms (often bowel or bladder related) ± abnormal bleeding
- chronic fatigue.

However, the predictive value of these symptoms for the diagnosis is poor, as each can have other causes and many affected women are asymptomatic.

Impact on quality of life
Endometriosis has a major impact on quality of life and work productivity. Women may need multiple admissions for surgery and/or prolonged treatment with costly drugs, which often have problematic side-effects.

Associated cancers
Large cohort studies suggest that endometriosis is a risk factor for ovarian cancer and non-Hodgkin's lymphoma.

Examination: key points
- Pelvic tenderness
- Fixed retroverted uterus
- Tender uterosacral ligaments ± deeply infiltrating nodules (especially if performed during menses)
- Enlarged ovaries
- Visible lesions in the vagina or on the cervix.
- Although these findings are suggestive of the diagnosis, the examination may be normal.

Diagnosis
- Visual inspection of the pelvis at laparoscopy is the gold standard investigation to establish the diagnosis, unless disease is visible in the vagina or elsewhere.
- Histology should be obtained if endometriomas (>4 cm) or deeply infiltrating disease are present to confirm the diagnosis and exclude rare instances of malignancy. It is uncertain if histology is required for peritoneal disease.
- Disease severity is classified by a four-point scale (stage I–IV or minimal–severe) based on peritoneal lesion size and location, and the presence of endometriomas/adhesions.

Investigations
- Transvaginal ultrasound is useful to both diagnose and exclude an ovarian endometrioma; it has no role in diagnosing peritoneal disease.
- Serum CA125 may be elevated, especially in severe disease, but it is not useful as a diagnostic test.
- MRI ± ultrasound ± barium/IVP studies may allow disease severity to be assessed when other organs are involved, e.g. bowel, ureter, or bladder.

Empirical treatment
Empirical treatment for pain symptoms presumed to be endometriosis without a definitive diagnosis includes counselling, analgesia, progestagens, the combined oral contraceptive (COC), and nutritional therapy. COC use may be conventional, continuous, or in a tricycle regimen.

Treatment: endometriosis-associated pain
Hormonal treatment
Ovarian suppression with COCs, danazol, gestrinone, medroxyprogesterone acetate, or gonadotropin-releasing hormone (GnRH) agonists reduces pain. The drugs are equally effective but their side-effects and cost profiles differ.

Treatment is usually given for 6 months. Longer use is problematic for GnRH agonists because of side-effects. Symptom recurrence after treatment is common.

The levonorgestrel intrauterine system is also effective.

GnRH agonist treatment plus 'add-back' therapy
Side-effects of GnRH agonists include:
- menopausal symptoms e.g. hot flushes, headaches, loss of libido, vaginal dryness
- loss of bone mineral density that is usually reversible.

These can be prevented by using hormone replacement therapy (HRT), e.g. tibolone, as 'add-back', which allows treatment to be prolonged beyond the 6-month licence. The efficacy of the GnRH agonist is unaffected.

Surgical treatment
Ideal practice is to diagnose and treat disease surgically at the same operation, provided that informed consent has been obtained.

Ablating peritoneal lesions plus laparoscopic uterine nerve ablation (LUNA) in stage I–III disease reduces pain at 6 months compared with laparoscopy alone; the smallest effect is seen in stage I disease. However, LUNA is probably not a necessary component of the treatment.

Pain can be reduced in severe and deeply infiltrating disease by removing the entire lesions. If a hysterectomy is performed, all visible endometriotic tissue should be removed at the same time.

Bilateral salpingo-oophorectomy (BSO) at hysterectomy usually provides pain relief and leads to a reduced need for future surgery.

There is no benefit using pre- or postoperative hormonal treatment for additional pain relief.

Hormone replacement therapy
HRT is recommended after BSO in young women; the risk of recurrent disease taking oestrogen alone is small.

Adding a progestagen to HRT after hysterectomy is not necessary, unless there is residual disease present as there is a small risk of malignant transformation.

Endometriosis-associated infertility

Numerous mechanisms have been proposed to explain the association between endometriosis and infertility, e.g. anatomical distortion due to ovarian endometriomas and dense adhesions. Whether other factors are causal is still uncertain, especially in peritoneal disease. They include

- abnormal folliculogenesis
- increased sperm phagocytosis
- peritoneal fluid toxicity
- elevated serum auto-antibody levels
- altered endometrial receptivity.

Treatment

Hormonal treatment
Ovarian suppression to improve pregnancy rates in stage I–II disease is not effective and should not be offered for this indication alone. Its role in more severe disease has not been assessed.

Surgical treatment
The results of a meta-analysis indicate that ablation of lesions ± adhesiolysis in stage I–II endometriosis improves pregnancy rates compared with laparoscopy alone, but the data have been challenged because of methodological problems with the studies. There is no role for postoperative hormonal treatment.

If an ovarian endometrioma >4 cm is present, performing a laparoscopic cystectomy is preferable to drainage and coagulation, as the latter procedures are associated with a higher risk of cyst recurrence and lower pregnancy rates.

Assisted reproduction

Intrauterine insemination
Stimulated intrauterine insemination is effective in stage I–II disease.

In vitro fertilization
In vitro fertilization (IVF) is appropriate treatment for endometriosis, especially if there are other problems such as male factor infertility, or if other treatments have failed. Problems include

- decreased oocyte numbers
- difficulties with ovarian scanning and access to the follicles due to endometriomas
- increased infection rates (related to the presence of an endometrioma).

It has also been suggested that oocyte quality is affected, which might explain the lower pregnancy rates than tubal infertility reported in a meta-analysis of published studies.

However, pregnancy rates in large national databases are not lower in patients with endometriosis, which makes it difficult to decide whether the disease has an adverse effect on IVF outcome or not.

Pre-IVF ovarian cystectomy
If an ovarian endometrioma ≥4 cm is present, performing a laparoscopic cystectomy before IVF is sensible to

- improve access to follicles
- obtain a histological diagnosis
- possibly improve ovarian response
- reduce the risk of infection
- The principal risks are reduced ovarian function after surgery and the loss of the ovary.

Coping with disease

Complementary therapies
Although there is evidence that vitamin B1, acupuncture, TENS and magnesium may help primary dysmenorrhoea, the role of complementary therapies in endometriosis is unclear.

Many sufferers report that nutritional therapy, as well as homeopathy, reflexology, traditional Chinese medicine, or herbal treatments, improve symptoms of pain.

Patient support groups

Patient self-help groups provide invaluable counselling, support, and advice.

The website www.endometriosis.org/support.html gives a comprehensive list of all self-help groups in the world. Many deliver self-management programmes that may be beneficial in providing women with tools to enable them to live with a chronic disease.

Further reading

Barlow DH, Kennedy S. Endometriosis: new genetic approaches and therapy. Annu Rev Med 2005;56:345–56.

Barnhart K, Dunsmoor-Su R, Coutifaris C. Effect of endometriosis on in vitro fertilization. Fertil Steril 2002;77:6–55.

D'Hooghe T, Hummelshoj L. Multi-disciplinary centres/networks of excellence for endometriosis management and research: a proposal. Hum Reprod 2006 11;21:2743–8.

Gambone JC, Mittman BS, Munro MG, et al, the Chronic Pelvic Pain/Endometriosis Working Group Consensus statement for the management of chronic pelvic pain and endometriosis: proceedings of an expert-panel consensus. Fertil Steril 2002;78:961–72.

Kennedy S, Bergqvist A, Chapron C, et al. ESHRE guideline for the diagnosis and treatment of endometriosis. Hum Reprod 2005;20:2698–704.

Practice Committee of ASRM. Endometriosis and infertility. Fertil Steril 2006;86(5 Suppl):S156–60.

Practice Committee of ASRM. Treatment of pelvic pain associated with endometriosis. Fertil Steril 2006;86 (5 Suppl):S18–27.

Royal College of Obstetricians and Gynaecologists (RCOG) *The investigation and management of endometriosis.* Greentop Guideline. London: RCOG 2006 www.rcog.org.uk/resources

Simoens S, Hummelshoj L, D'Hooghe T. Endometriosis: cost estimates & methodological perspective. Hum Reprod Update. 2007;13:395–404.

Patient resources

Support group: Endometriosis UK, Tel. 020 7222 2781:www.endometriosis-uk.org/

Female infertility

Definition
Infertility may be defined as the inability of a couple to conceive after 2 years of unprotected intercourse, in the absence of known reproductive pathology. Approximately 84% of young couples attempting to conceive will do so within a year, and referral for further investigation is normally appropriate after this time. Around half of the remaining 'infertile' couples will conceive within the second year without treatment. No cause for infertility is found in approximately one-quarter of infertile couples, whereas 15% have multiple causes.

Diagnosis
The diagnosis of infertility can be extremely emotionally distressing and should be handled with sensitivity. The initial investigation of the infertile woman will typically include a detailed history. Consider early investigation in women aged 35 and above, or with a history of
- amenorrhoea or oligomenorrhea
- previous infertility
- treatment for cancer
- fibroids, endometriosis or pelvic inflammatory disease (PID)
- cervical dysplasia
- pelvic or abdominal surgery.

Circulating hormone levels along with ultrasound scan may distinguish between ovulatory/hormonal and obstructive/developmental disorders. Blood tests include:
- Progesterone in the mid-luteal phase of the menstrual cycle. This is day 21 of a 28-day cycle; however, in the case of irregular or long menstrual cycles the test may be conducted later and/or repeated weekly until the commencement of the next cycle. Normal values are 3–20 ng/mL (9.54–63.6 nmol/L).
- Follicle-stimulating hormone (FSH): basal day 3 (range, days 2–5). Normal values are 3.0–20.0 U/L.
- Luteinizing hormone (LH) basal day 3 (range, days 2–5). Normal values are 2.0–15.0 U/L.
- Oestradiol basal day 3 (range, days 2–5) of the cycle. Normal values are 50–145 pg/mL (184-532 pmol/L).
- Prolactin. Normal premenopausal values are 2-20 ng/mL.
- Total serum testosterone. Normal values are 6–86 ng/dL (0.21–2.98 nmol/L).
- Dehydroepiandrosterone sulphate (DHEAS). Normal pre-menopausal values are 12–535 µg/dL.
- 17-hydroxyprogesterone basal day 3 (range, days 2–5) of the cycle. Normal values are 20–100 ng/dL (0.6–3.0 nmol/L).
- Anti-Müllerian hormone (AMH). Normal values are 15–28 pmol/L (2–4 ng/mL).

Ultrasound investigation
Ultrasound scan of the pelvis can be performed transabdominally or transvaginally. Transabdominal ultrasound provides a global assessment and normally precedes transvaginal scan. Hysterosalpingo-contrast sonography (HyCoSy) using a high contrast dye medium may also be conducted to assess tubal patency.

Saline infusion sonography (SIS) is a more recent development where saline is introduced into the uterine cavity by a small catheter prior to vaginal probe ultrasound. The liquid helps create an interface with the lining of the uterus and abnormal structures can be seen on imaging.

This technique may be combined with Doppler sonography, which estimates blood flow. Ultrasound may provide information regarding
- congenital abnormalities, including enlarged uterus, absence of uterus, uterus didelphys, bicornis bicollis, bicornis unicollis, uterus subseptae, uterus arcuatus, and uterus unicornis. A septate or double vagina may occur
- uterine cavity, endometrial thickness, and myometrium evaluation
- ovarian morphology and volume, including antral follicle count, cysts solid tumours, and endometriomas
- abnormalities of the fallopian tube commonly present as adnexal masses and generally result from salpingitis, endometriosis, or peritubal adhesions. Patency of fallopian tubes may be assessed by HyCoSy
- uterine and follicular blood flow.

Sexually transmitted infections
Further investigations in women include tests for infection, especially *Chlamydia trachomatis*, which can lead to pelvic inflammatory disease or tubal occlusion. Screening should be offered prior to uterine investigations, as with other sexually transmitted diseases.

Ovulatory disorders
Premature ovarian failure
Aetiology
Premature ovarian failure (POF) is idiopathic in the majority of cases; however, known genetic causes include, Turner's syndrome, ovarian agenesis, 46XY gonadal dysgenesis, familial POF, fragile X syndrome, gonadotrophin receptor gene mutations, and galactosaemia. Possible environmental causes are chemotherapy, pelvic radiation, autoimmunity, ovarian malignancy, viruses, toxins, or surgery.

Diagnosis
It is characterized by hypergonadotrophic ovulatory failure, leading to secondary hypergonadotrophism. Diagnosis is usually by the finding of amenorrhoea and low oestrogen or progesterone in the presence of normal or high gonadotrophins (FSH and LH). Low oestrogen concentrations may result in menopause-type symptoms, but these are common to other causes of amenorrhoea and in isolation do not necessarily indicate POF. In a minority of cases ovarian failure is temporary, and so hormone measurements taken some weeks apart may be advised. Genetic diagnosis is required to confirm specific genetic causes.

Treatment
Hormone replacement therapy (HRT) using conjugated oestrogens or oestradiol valerate, which may be delivered orally or by transdermal patch. Progesterone is advised for patients with an intact uterus in order to avoid oestrogen-induced endometrial hyperplasia. Testosterone administration is rarely required when the adrenal gland continues to supply androgens. Treatments have a neutral effect on fertility but return of reproductive function, sometimes spontaneously, has been reported. Embryo or egg donation, remain an option however.

Hypothalamic/pituitary dysfunction
Aetiology
Pulsatile hypothalamic secretions of gonadotrophin-releasing hormone (GnRH) are transported along the capillary plexus in the pituitary stalk and stimulate the anterior

pituitary to secrete gonadotrophins, LH and FSH. Disorders in this axis are characterized by hypogonadotrophic hypogonadism, leading to ovulatory failure and amenorrhoea. Hypothalamic disorders account for approximately 35% of patients presenting with amenorrhoea.

Structural lesions to the hypothalamus or pituitary may lead to absence of GnRH secretion or failure of GnRH delivery to the pituitary. Constriction by tumours such as glioma and craniopharyngiomas may be the cause. Granulomas (resulting from tuberculosis or sarcoidosis) are also sometimes implicated. Other physical causes include trauma, cranial irradiation, or postpartum pituitary necrosis (Sheehan's syndrome).

Disruption of neurotransmitters that control GnRH secretion may be precipitated by stress, or sudden weight loss and malnutrition (including anorexia nervosa). In addition, strenuous exercise may inhibit GnRH secretion by the hypothalamus via the action of endogenous opioids. Similarly, drug abuse can result in suboptimal functioning of the hypothalamus.

Rarely, congenital GnRH deficiency may manifest as Kallman's syndrome, which can result from an inherited X-linked condition, an autosomal dominant condition, or as an autosomal recessive condition and can be accompanied by anosmia.

Diagnosis

Diagnosis is usually by the finding of amenorrhoea, anovulation and low oestrogen or progesterone along with low gonadotrophins (FSH and LH). If these are present consider the following causes:

- cerebral or pituitary tumours
- vascular malformations
- stress
- sudden weight loss (including anorexia nervosa)
- strenuous exercise
- drug abuse
- genetic disorders.

Treatment

Clomiphene citrate: the first line of treatment may be the anti-oestrogen, which induces ovulation by countering oestrogenic inhibition of the hypothalamus and causing the pituitary to release gonadotrophins. If alone is unsuccessful, gonadotrophins are given in order to apply stimulation directly to the ovary.

Gonadotrophin replacement: an alternative treatment involves initial pituitary downregulation using GnRH agonist/antagonist followed by gonadotrophin replacement using urinary derived menopausal human gonadotrophin (containing FSH and LH). Recombinant FSH preparations are also available. Complications include ovarian hyperstimulation syndrome (OHSS) and multiple births.

GnRH replacement: pulsatile delivery of synthetic GnRH via mini-infusion pump has been employed and has several theoretical advantages over exogenous gonadotrophins in that it enables the patients own gonadotrophins to be used for stimulation and instigates appropriate natural pituitary feedback mechanisms limiting endogenous FSH.

Hyperprolactinaemia

Aetiology

Prolactin suppresses GnRH and FSH secretion. Pituitary secretion of prolactin itself is normally suppressed by dopamine. The use of prescription drugs that block dopamine at the pituitary or deplete brain dopamine levels is a common cause of hyperprolactinaemia. These drugs include some tranquilizers, antiemetics, and antipsychotic medicines.

Alternatively, a prolactinoma directly secreting prolactin into the circulation, or other structural lesions inducing pressure on the pituitary stalk, thereby blocking the flow of dopamine to the prolactin secreting tissues, may be responsible. Stress and other mediators of neurotransmitters may also affect control mechanisms for prolactin secretion. Finally, hypothyroidism is an important cause of prolactinaemia via elevated levels of thyrotropin-releasing hormone.

Diagnosis

Symptoms of hyperprolactinaemia include
- oligomenorrhea
- amenorrhoea
- galactorrhea
- infertility.

High prolactin levels should be confirmed by repeat testing at least once before further diagnostic evaluation and treatment. It is also important to check for hypothyroidism by repeat thyroid function tests. Pituitary imaging by computerized tomography (CT) or nuclear magnetic imaging (MRI) scans may be included as part of a definitive diagnosis or ongoing surveillance of prolactinoma.

Treatment

Dopamine agonist: consider dopamine agonist treatment (e.g. bromocriptine) to restore the menstrual cycle. A more recent and long-acting dopamine agonist, cabergoline, has fewer side-effects. Surgical resection or irradiation of the prolactinoma is generally restricted to the minority of patients with low tolerance or resistance to dopamine agonists. Withdrawal of antidopaminergic drugs should be attempted followed by repeat testing where this cause is suspected.

Polycystic ovary syndrome

Aetiology

Polycystic ovary syndrome (PCOS) affects 5–10% of all women. It is a collection of symptoms rather than a tightly defined single disease, but is characterized by a lack of follicular maturation, lack of ovulation, and formation of follicular cysts within the ovaries. PCOS may also be associated with higher than normal levels of androgens along with excessive mild symptoms of hyperandrogenism, such as acne, hyperseborrhea, or hirsutism. Insulin resistance, diabetes, and obesity are all strongly correlated with PCOS.

Polycystic ovaries develop when the ovaries are stimulated to produce excessive amounts of androgens, through the release of excessive LH or through hyperinsulinaemia, in women whose ovaries are sensitive to this stimulus.

Diagnosis

Diagnosis remains somewhat controversial, but generally given the exclusion of other endocrine disorders, two of the following three criteria should be met:
- oligoamenorrhoea and amenorrhoea
- excess androgen activity
- the presence of polycystic ovaries determined by ultrasound (12 or more follicles between 2 and 8 mm in size)

In many cases the LH/FSH ratio as measured between days 2–5 of the menstrual cycle is increased, but this appears to be a specific subgroup of patients with hyperinsulinaemia and increased adrenal androgenic activity.

Patients with regular menstrual cycles should be reassured that they are likely to be ovulating. Mid-luteal progesterone levels should be obtained to determine whether ovulation has occurred in patients with regular menstrual cycles but over 1 year of infertility.

Treatment
- Lifestyle modifications: the therapeutic approach may vary according to the individual endocrinopathy, but lifestyle modifications are an appropriate starting point for many women. Lifestyle modifications should include:
  - moderate exercise (in general this should average 30 minutes sweat-inducing exercise daily)
  - a healthy diet especially in women with a BMI greater than 30 kg/m^2. Weight loss reduces testosterone and increases ovulation in many obese women
  - advice to stop smoking.
- Ovulation induction: Clomiphene is generally used as the first-line agent to induce ovulation in departments that can provide transvaginal ultrasound monitoring to minimize the chances of multiple pregnancy. Many patients, however, are Clomiphene resistant. Metformin may improve pregnancy and ovulation rates; however, evidence demonstrating it improves live birth rates when used alone, or in combination with Clomiphene is lacking. Second-line treatments available for Clomiphene resistant patients may include low-dose step-up FSH ovulation induction.
- Laparoscopic ovarian drilling (LOD): this involves destroying part of the ovary by diathermy or laser at the time of laparoscopy. This is normally reserved for anovulatory patients with normal BMI who are undergoing laparoscopy for other reasons. LOD has been shown to be no more effective than gonadotrophin treatment, but carries a far lower risk of multiple pregnancy. The long-term effects of LOD on ovarian function are not fully understood and the patient should be informed of this minor risk.
- Assisted reproduction: patients with PCOS who do not ovulate in response to Clomiphene or FSH can be offered *in vitro* fertilization (IVF). This is especially the case where another contributory factor for infertility, such as poor semen quality or tubal disease have been identified. Generally pregnancy and live birth rates of PCOS patients undergoing IVF are similar to those reported with non-PCOS patients.

Obstructive and developmental disorders

Tubal occlusion

Aetiology

Intraluminal tubal occlusions may result from salpingitis, endometriosis, or peritubal adhesions. The fallopian tubes constitute a complex organ carrying out functions supporting sperm capacitation, fertilization and maintenance of the zygote rather than being merely a conduit between ovary and uterus. Pelvic inflammatory disease, genital tuberculosis, sexually transmitted disease such as chlamydia trachomatis, gonorrhoea, intrauterine contraceptive devices, adhesions or post-surgical complications may contribute to tubal occlusion. Congenital absence or incomplete development of the fallopian tubes is also rarely encountered.

Diagnosis

Patency of fallopian tubes is most commonly assessed by HyCoSy. A catheter is passed transcervically into the uterus and held in place by a balloon before the introduction of echo contrast media, injected transcervically into the uterus, enabling the visualization of tubal patency and anatomical abnormality by ultrasound.

Another approach to the assessment of tubal patency is hysterosalpingogram (HSG). This is essentially similar to HyCoSy except a radio-contrast dye is used and visualized by X-ray. Contraindications for both techniques include, possibility of pregnancy, PID, endometriosis, urogenital infection, or recent curettage.

Laparoscopy of the pelvic cavity under general anaesthetic may be indicated in women with a history of endometriosis, PID, adhesions, or ectopic pregnancy. A methylene blue dye may also be injected transcervically during the procedure to determine tubal patency. In general, flushing the fallopian tubes with dye, ultrasound or X-ray contrast media may also have a therapeutic benefit by removing tubal occlusions.

Hysteroscopy, involving transcervical visualization of the uterine cavity by endoscopy is sometimes employed to detect intrauterine lesions such as polyps and fibroids.

Treatment
- Selective salpingography: selective salpingography in which a catheter containing a fine guidewire is passed transcervically into the fallopian tube under X-ray guidance may be considered. The procedure is similar to HSG but the fallopian tube is flushed using contrast medium that has been diluted to allow visualization of the catheter and guidewire in the uterine cavity. If a proximal fallopian tube obstruction is encountered recanalization and intratubal injection of contrast media may be attempted. This latter technique may distinguish between a tubal spasm and debris or mucal mucous plug.
- Hysteroscopic tubal cannulation: this provides a further option. It entails passing a fine guidewire through a hysteroscope introduced transcervically directly into the fallopian tube, removing any minor obstruction.
- Assisted reproductive techniques: if attempts to unblock the fallopian tubes are unsuccessful, assisted reproductive techniques such as IVF are preferred. It is likely that the presence of inflammation or hydrosalpinx is detrimental to implantation. Performing a surgical intervention such as salpingectomy, tubal occlusion, aspiration of the hydrosalpinx fluid, or salpingostomy prior to the IVF procedure in women with hydrosalpinges is thought to improve the likelihood of successful outcome.

Adhesions

Aetiology

Adhesion development occurs when damage to peritoneal surfaces induces a series of cellular and molecular tissue repair cascades, involving the fibrinolytic, immunological, and proliferative systems resulting in adhesion development. Sources of damage include, operative trauma, infection, endometriosis, PID, and allergic reaction. Adhesions may constrict or occlude fallopian tubes or the uterine cavity and are a relatively common cause of infertility.

Diagnosis

Diagnosis by pelvic ultrasound, hysteroscopy, or laparoscopy. Where adhesions occlude fallopian tubes HSG or HyCoSy may be used for diagnosis. Biopsies may be obtained for histological staging and grading.

Treatment

Hysteroscopic or laparoscopic adhesiolysis: adhesiolysis is the removal of intrauterine adhesions surgically under hysteroscopic guidance or laparoscopically depending upon extent and location.

Endometriosis

Aetiology

Ectopic endometrial tissue may form deposits attached to organs in the abdominal cavity, including the ovaries or fallopian tubes. These lesions could be sites of inflammation or obstruction, thereby impeding transport of the ovum or implantation of the zygote.

Diagnosis

Endometriosis is often asymptomatic, even in some cases where fertility is impaired. Where symptoms occur they are most commonly pelvic pain just before or during menstruation. The intensity and duration of pain can vary widely and may depend on the precise anatomic location and stage or grade of the lesions. The only certain way to establish a diagnosis for endometriosis is laparoscopic examination.

Treatment

- Laparoscopic surgical resection, ablation, and adhesiolysis: medical management of endometriosis does not enhance fertility. Mild disease may sometimes be ablated during laparoscopic diagnosis. Laparoscopic surgical ablation and resection of endometriosis is carried out. Patients with ovarian endometriomas may be offered laparoscopic cystectomy.
- Assisted reproduction techniques: this is indicated for those cases where treatment fails to restore fertility.

Uterine leiomyomas (fibroids)

Aetiology

Uterine leiomyomas are benign masses arising from the myometrium and associated connective tissues. Fibroids are clinically apparent in more than one-quarter of women, although malignant disease in the form of leiomyosarcoma is rare. Fibroids may be intramural, subserous, submucous, or cervical and possess oestrogen receptors, making them responsive to oestrogen. Fibroids can impinge on fertility by distortion and obstruction of the pelvic reproductive organs, or by interfering with implantation. Obstetric problems such as early pregnancy loss, premature labour or bleeding are uncommon.

Diagnosis

Generally symptoms relate to the size and location of the masses, small fibroids are often asymptomatic. Where symptoms are present they include heavy or painful periods, abdominal discomfort or bloating, back ache, urinary frequency/retention. Large masses may be detected by manual examination, although the standard diagnostic technique is by ultrasonography.

Treatment

- Laparoscopic/hysteroscopic/open pelvic myomectomy: fibroids are generally treated by laparoscopic surgical resection. In the case of submucous leiomyomas, ablation is via hysterocopic myomectomy, in which high frequency electrical energy is used to resect the fibroid. In cases of very large fibroids, laparotomy may be the only option.
- Non-surgical treatments: uterine artery embolization (UAE) is occlusion of the uterine artery via a catheter inserted in the femoral artery under imaging guidance. Also, radiofrequency ablation is occasionally used, which is a minimally invasive treatment involving the insertion of

a needle-like device into the fibroid through the abdomen and heating it with low frequency electrical currents.

An even more recent non-invasive method is magnetic resonance focused ultrasound, in which high intensity ultrasound is focused on the lesion causing a localized temperature rise ($>65°C$) which destroys the tissue. The focused ultrasound is guided and monitored by MRI and has the advantage over radio-techniques in that passage of ultrasound through intervening tissues has a greatly reduced negative cumulative effect.

Medical treatments with GnRH analogues or oestrogen antagonists are not indicated for the infertile patient, nor is hysterectomy, which is the definitive treatment for women not wishing to bear children.

Endometrial polyp

Aetiology

Polyps are sessile or pedunculated masses arising from the endometrium; they may be a few millimetres to several centimetres in size. Their aetiology is probably the result of oestrogen stimulation in susceptible individuals. The contribution of polyps to infertility is unclear, but large polyps may obstruct sperm or interfere with implantation or fetal growth.

Diagnosis

Hysteroscopy is the gold standard for the diagnosis of polyp. SIS is preferred to transvaginal ultrasound and HSG as minimally invasive procedures.

Treatment

- Hysteroscopic polypectomy: this is often recommended as therapy for infertility, although supporting evidence for this is unclear. Polypectomy may also be achieved by curettage.
- Assisted reproductive technology (ART): patients should be advised and educated during assisted reproductive treatment so that they have the opportunity to make informed choices regarding their treatment based on evidence as an integral part of the decision-making process. Partners should be seen together as any decisions affect both of them. Clear information regarding possible side-effects of treatment such as nausea and vomiting, headache, ectopic pregnancy, and OHSS. In addition, the possibility of multiple pregnancy carries its own risks including miscarriage, premature birth and pre-eclampsia. Current evidence suggests no increased risk of ovarian cancer in nulligravid women with a family history of ovarian cancer receiving ovulation induction.
- Intrauterine insemination (IUI): this may be considered for couples with mild male factor infertility, unexplained infertility, and mild endometriosis. The procedure is sometimes combined with ovulation induction in cases of ovarian failure.
- Semen is collected by masturbation, normally after 3 days' sexual abstinence. Sperm are usually washed by centrifugation and the most motile fraction resuspended in a small quantity of media. Prepared sperm are transferred directly into the uterus via transcervical catheter. A variation of the technique is fallopian sperm perfusion (FSP), where the sperm preparation is injected directly into the fallopian tube.
- In natural cycles, the time of ovulation may be determined by testing for the LH surge or ultrasound monitoring. Where follicular development is stimulated by Clomifene or exogenous gonadotrophins a human chorionic gonadotrophin (hCG) trigger injection of

10 000 IU is administered subcutaneously or intramuscularly. The timing of the hCG trigger is determined by ovarian ultrasound examination and is usually given when the leading follicle reaches 16–20 mm, depending upon stimulation protocol; ovulation occurs around 36 hours later.

- Success rates depend upon the underlying pathology, but may be up to 15% per cycle. A maximum of six natural or Clomifene stimulated cycles (three gonadotrophin stimulated cycles) should be offered. If no pregnancy results IVF may be considered.

In vitro fertilization

Summary
Standard protocols entail hypothalamic/pituitary down-regulation using GnRH analogues. This is followed by gonadotrophin stimulation, leading to the development of multiple oocytes, a process monitored by ultrasound and hormone testing. The final stages of follicular maturation are triggered using human chorionic gonadotrophin and mature oocytes collected. Fertilization takes place in vitro, and embryos are cultured between 3 and 5 days before transfer of a single embryo (or two embryos) to the uterine cavity under ultrasound guidance. Luteal phase support in the form of progesterone may be offered followed by pregnancy testing.

Down-regulation
Down-regulation using GnRH agonist is administered by daily nasal inhalation or injection, beginning during the luteal phase and continuing for approximately 1 week. Baseline ultrasound scan is then performed to confirm the absence of developing ovarian follicles and thin endometrium.

Ovarian stimulation
The administration of gonadotrophins (primarily FSH) then begins, coincident with a reduction in GnRH agonist. Human menopausal or recombinant gonadotrophins are available, but existing evidence does not favour one or another preparation overall. In general, higher doses of gonadotrophins are given than for IUI cycles in order to induce superovulation. The stimulation process lasts from 10–14 days and is monitored using ultrasound to allow adjustments in daily gonadotrophin dose.

hCG trigger
The final steps of ovarian maturation are triggered using hCG by injection when the leading follicles reach approximately 16 mm in diameter as determined by ultrasound.

Oocyte retrieval
Oocyte retrieval is performed approximately 36 hours after the hCG trigger. A needle is inserted transvaginally under ultrasound guidance and each mature follicle is aspirated by suction pump, between 6 and 12 oocytes are typically collected. Fresh semen from the partner is obtained and processed as for IUI on the same day as oocyte retrieval. Alternatively, a previously cryopreserved semen sample may be used, as is the case with donated sperm.

Fertilisation and embryo culture
Oocytes and prepared motile sperm are co-incubated in fertilization media overnight under tightly controlled temperature and pH. Fertilization checks are made after approximately 18 hours, the presence of two pro-nuclei confirming fertilization. Embryos are then cultured for 2–3 days before assessment and grading. At this time, the best embryos will have reached the eight-cell stage and may be selected for transfer. The remaining embryos of suitable quality can be cryopreserved.

Blastocyst culture
Embryos can be cultured for 5–6 days until they reach the blastocyst stage before transfer. There will sometimes be some embryos that fail to develop beyond day 3, so fewer embryos are likely be available for transfer; on the other hand, any embryo that develops to blastocyst in vitro is more likely to implant and survive. The decision to proceed to blastocyst depends on various factors such as the number and quality of embryos available and the pathology and history associated with the patient. If embryo biopsy for genetic testing or aneuploidy screening is intended, then blastocyst culture is essential.

Embryo transfer
Embryo transfer is performed transcervically by catheter, normally with ultrasound guidance. A maximum of two embryos may be transferred for women under 40 years old. Those patients over 40 may elect to have three embryos transferred. Transfer of a single embryo is highly desirable due to the risk of adverse health effects of multiple births on mother and child. Cryopreserved embryos from a previous stimulation cycle may be transferred after being thawed and re-established in vitro. Luteal phase support using progesterone may be provided after transfer, followed by pregnancy testing.

Intracytoplasmic sperm injection
This is indicated for male factor infertility, such as oligospermia, asthenospermia, congenital absence of vas deferens, previous vasectomy, and surgically recovered sperm. Sperm are directly injected into the oocytes microscopically via a fine glass capillary tube in vitro. Fertilization checks and subsequent steps are then carried out as normal.

Success rates
Maternal age is the primary factor predicting success rates in ART (Table 12.13.1).

Table 12.13.1 Percentage of live births per cycle started (own oocytes): summary of UK 2006 national statistics for IVF cycles

Maternal age	Fresh cycles	Frozen cycles
Under 35	31.0	20.1
35–37	26.4	18.5
38–39	18.6	16.4
40–42	11.1	9.5
43–44	4.6	9.5
Over 44	4.0	10.2

Further reading

Agdi M, Tulandi T. Endoscopic management of uterine fibroids. Best Pract Res Clin Obstet Gynaecol 2008;22:707–16.

American College of Obstetricians and Gynecologists (ACOG). Management of infertility caused by ovulatory dysfunction. ACOG Practice Bulletin, no. 34. Washington, DC: ACOG 2002.

American College of Obstetricians and Gynecologists (ACOG). Management of infertility caused by ovulatory dysfunction. Washington, DC: ACOG 2002.

Consensus on infertility treatment related to polycystic ovarian syndrome. Human Reproduction 2008;3:462–77.

Conway GS. Premature ovarian failure. Br Med Bull 2000;56:643–9.

Farquhar C, Lilford RJ, Marjoribanks J. et al. Laparoscopic 'drilling' by diathermy or laser for ovulation induction in anovulatory polycystic ovary syndrome. Cochrane Database Syst Rev 2007:CD001122.

Fischbach FT. A manual of laboratory and diagnostic tests. Philadelphia: Lippincott.

Human Fertilisation and Embryology Authority (HFEA) *HFEA facts and figures 2006: fertility problems and treatment.* London: HFEA 2008.

Human Fertilisation and Embryology Authority (HFEA). Code of practice, 6th edn. London: HFEA 2003.

National Collaborating Centre for Women's and Children's Health. Fertility: assessment and treatment for people with fertility problems. Clinical guideline 11. London: NICE 2004.

Polena V, Mergui JL, Perrot N, *et al.* Long-term results of hysteroscopic myomectomy in 235 patients. Eur J Obstet Gynecol Reproductive Biol 2007;130:232–7.

Royal College of Obstetricians and Gynaecologists (RCOG). *Long-term consequences of polycystic ovary syndrome.* Guideline No.33. London: RCOG 2007.

Silberstein T, Saphier O, van Hooris BJ, Plosker SM. Endometrial polyps in reproductive age and infertile women. IMAJ 2006;8:192–5.

Steinkeler JA, Woodfield CA, Lazarus E, Hillstrom MM. Female infertility: a systematic approach to radiologic imaging and diagnosis. Radiographics. 2009;29:1353–70.

Fertility in survivors of childhood malignancy

Introduction

As the diagnosis and treatment of childhood cancer becomes increasingly successful, there are growing numbers of survivors with a variety of treatment effects. One of the major issues for patients is the impact of their disease on reproductive function and the implication for the health of their offspring.

Cancer and its treatment may cause a spectrum of damage to the reproductive axis and the potential effects upon fertility are diverse and complex depending upon the interaction between many patient and treatment factors. Some patients are unaffected, whereas others face infertility immediately after treatment. For many patients, there appears to be a 'fertile window' and it is the difficulty in assessing an individual's risk of subfertility that leaves many patients, their families, and clinicians uncertain about a patient's reproductive potential.

It is the clinician's role to identify possible strategies to prevent subfertility, diagnose it, if and when it occurs, and explore any necessary fertility treatments.

The preservation of fertility and the treatment of subfertility in survivors of childhood cancer is a growing field of research and although many techniques of fertility preservation are in their infancy, there is a lot of promising initial data. (See the box for quick reference material).

Definition

As survival rates for children treated for cancer continue to improve, a growing population of women emerges for whom issues of fertility are paramount. Cancer therapy may disrupt the neuroendocrine axis, damage the ovaries, and impair uterine function, resulting in pubertal delay or arrest, premature ovarian failure (POF), subfertility, or ovarian insufficiency.

Epidemiology

Childhood cancer is rare, with approximately 1400 new cases per year in the UK (SIGN 2004). With long-term survival rates approaching 73%, it is estimated that 1 in 715 of the adult population will be a survivor of childhood cancer in 2010 (SIGN 2004).

One of the major issues for patients is the impact of their disease on reproductive function and the implication for the health of their offspring.

Cancer therapy may cause a spectrum of damage to the reproductive axis, and only a minority of females will develop POF failure immediately after completion of their treatment. However, fertility may be impaired even in women who are menstruating after cancer therapy. Survivors are at high risk of permanent POF with an 8% risk before the age of 40 years, compared with <1% in the general population (Sklar et al. 2006). The prevalence of POF is dependent upon the treatment given and, in the case of radiotherapy or chemotherapy, the agent used and the dose and age of patient when treatment is administered.

Ovarian failure has been reported in 90% of women after total body irradiation (TBI), and 97% of women treated with total abdominal irradiation (Wallace 2005a). Ovarian dysfunction has been reported in 19–63% of patients treated with chemotherapies for Hodgkin's lymphoma, but appears to be preserved following treatment for childhood acute lymphoblastic leukaemia (ALL) in most cases.

Pathology and aetiology

Radiotherapy and chemotherapy may affect uterine growth, damage the ovary, and hasten oocyte depletion, resulting in loss of hormone production, uterine dysfunction, and a premature menopause. Comorbidities, and their effects upon the menstrual cycle, psychological issues and social factors may also play a role.

Radiotherapy

Total body, craniospinal axis, abdominal, or pelvic irradiation potentially exposes the ovaries to irradiation. The extent of the damage is related to the radiation dose, fractionation schedule, volume treated and age at the time of treatment (Thomson et al. 2002; Wallace et al. 2003). The number of follicles present at the time of treatment determines the 'fertile window' and influences the age of POF. The human oocyte has a LD_{50} (lethal dose to destroy 50% of follicles) of less than 2 Gy (Wallace et al. 2005a). The Faddy–Gosden model for oocyte decline can be used to predict the age of ovarian failure or the estimated sterilizing dose of any radiotherapy (Fig. 12.14.1). The sterilizing dose decreases with increasing age as the remaining population of primordial oocytes falls (Wallace et al. 2005a).

Uterine function may be impaired following radiation doses of 14–30 Gy as a consequence of disruption of the uterine vasculature and direct effects on uterine musculature. This results in reduced elasticity and uterine volume (Critchley and Wallace 2005). These effects are also dose and age dependent, with the prepubertal uterus being more vulnerable (Wallace et al. 2005a).

High-dose cranial irradiation (more than 24 Gy) may manifest as delayed puberty or absent menses and can be treated with hormone replacement therapy (HRT) (SIGN 2004). Interestingly, low-dose cranial irradiation may cause precocious puberty or a gradual decline in hypothalamic-pituitary-ovarian function. Decreased luteinizing hormone

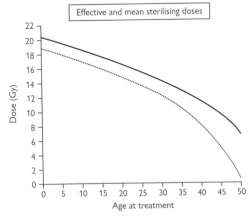

Fig. 12.14.1 The Faddy–Gosden model. The effective (red, upper) and mean (blue, lower) sterilizing dose of radiation above which premature ovarian failure occurs immediately, with no reproductive window, for a known age at treatment. Reprinted from International Journal of Radiation Oncology, Biology, Physics 62(3), Wallace et al., Predicting age of ovarian failure after radiation to a field that includes the ovaries, p. 7, copyright (2005), with permission from Elsevier.

(LH) secretion, an attenuated LH surge, and shorter luteal phases have been reported and may herald incipient ovarian failure or be associated with early pregnancy loss.

Chemotherapy

Ovarian damage is drug and dose dependent and is related to age at time of treatment, with progressively smaller doses required to produce POF with increasing age. Although the mechanism of chemotherapy-induced ovarian damage is uncertain, exhaustion of the oocyte pool is likely. Uterine function is not adversely affected by chemotherapy.

Prognosis

Pregnancy

A successful pregnancy not only depends upon a functioning hypothalamic-pituitary-ovarian axis but also on an adequate ovarian follicle reserve and a uterine cavity that is receptive to implantation and with the capacity to accommodate normal growth of the fetus to term.

If a population of oocytes survives in these women, then spontaneous ovulation and conception may occur. There are few data about the prevalence of spontaneous conception in this group of women. However, it is well documented that the offspring of such patients have no excess of congenital anomalies or other diseases (Li et al. 1979).

Advances in assisted reproduction have made pregnancy a possibility in women without ovarian function, providing there is normal uterine function. There are few data to provide an accurate prevalence of successful pregnancy with assisted reproduction. Most studies are however reassuring about reproductive outcome after chemotherapy alone. Successful pregnancy, with no excess risk of miscarriage, and healthy offspring are reported following multi-agent chemotherapy (Lee et al. 2006).

Pregnancy in all cancer survivors should be considered high risk, as pregnancy in this group is associated with an increased risk of adverse outcomes, particularly in patients with uterine dysfunction secondary to radiotherapy. Although study numbers are small, there appears to be an increased incidence of miscarriage, preterm delivery, and low birthweight neonates in women who have received radiotherapy (Lee et al. 2006). Increasing risk of preterm birth is associated with increasing radiotherapy doses (Lee et al. 2006). Low birthweight and prematurity are likely to be related to reduced elasticity of the uterine musculature with subsequent restriction of the uterine expansion required in pregnancy. Increased risk of abnormal placentation in the irradiated uterus has also been documented.

Clinical approach

Considerations prior to treatment

The potential effects of cancer therapies on fertility should first be considered at the time of diagnosis. Pubertal status should be assessed and the risk of infertility estimated. Baseline tests should be completed after consideration of the potential short- and long-term effects of the cancer's clinical course, its treatment and potential complications. If infertility is estimated to be a risk, then referral to a specialist assisted reproductive unit should be considered.

- Modern radiotherapy planning methods can be used to calculate the planned dose of radiotherapy to the ovaries. Depending on the clinical scenario the treatment can be planned to selectively avoid one ovary or modified to minimize the dose of radiation received by each ovary (Wallace et al. 2005a).

Following treatment

Girls treated for cancer should have their pubertal status and growth patterns assessed three times a year following treatment (SIGN 2004). If these parameters are below that expected for age, referral should be made. Ovarian function should be assessed using biochemical analysis of gonadotrophins and sex steroids, a menstrual history, and ultrasound examination of the uterus and ovaries. Recently anti-Müllerian hormone and inhibin B have been shown to be potential markers of ovarian reserve. Biochemical assessment before puberty is unreliable. Raised concentrations of follicle-stimulating hormone (FSH) in the early follicular phase are often seen in women who have impaired fertility, despite healthy ovulatory cycles. Results must be interpreted with care.

Primary or secondary amenorrhoea, infertility, or oestrogen-deficient symptoms should prompt investigation for POF. An elevated FSH and LH with low oestradiol, on two separate occasions is diagnostic of POF. Prolactin, thyroid function tests and an autoantibody screen should be completed to exclude other causes. Pelvic imaging is not required for diagnosis but uterine and ovarian dimensions should be measured and the endometrial thickness noted. Ultrasonic assessment of ovarian volume may be a potential predictor of reproductive potential, with volume correlating with the number of remaining follicles. In the event of a diagnosis of POF, a bone mineral density scan should be requested.

Management

All women with POF should be offered sex steroid replacement therapy to protect cardiovascular and skeletal health. This is currently offered in the convenient form of the combined OCP or HRT formulations designed for postmenopausal women. Further research is required to demonstrate the optimum formulation and dose of sex steroids that should be recommended for these younger women.

Fertility preservation

There is great awareness of the adverse effects of cancer therapy on fertility but fertility preservation techniques for children and young women remain investigational. At present, there are only two established practices of fertility preservation in female patients which are oophoropexy and cryopreservation of embryos after in vitro fertilization (Wallace et al. 2005b). Oophoropexy (surgically displacing the ovaries out of the radiation field) may preserve ovarian function but radiation-induced uterine damage may still affect the chances of successful pregnancy. Cryopreservation of embryos is only suitable for sexually mature women with a partner. Mature oocyte preservation is a potential solution for women without a partner but pregnancy rates are significantly lower as these cells sustain more damage during the freeze–thaw process than embryos (Oktay et al. 2006) Significant delays in cancer treatments may be sustained, as these techniques require ovarian stimulation with oocyte retrieval. These procedures are not without risk and the number of embryos or oocytes is also limited.

For prepubertal girls, or women without a partner, cortical ovarian tissue may be removed laparoscopically without delaying treatment, and reimplanted following successful cancer treatment (Donnez et al. 2006). There is concern, however, that this tissue may contain malignant cells capable of inducing relapse on reimplantation. Reports of embryo development following heterotopic transplantation of cryopreserved tissue and of six live births after orthotopic transplantation of cryopreserved tissue provide potential therapies for the future (Donnez et al. 2006).

Another approach to preserve fertility is the administration of a gonadotrophin-releasing hormone (GnRH) agonist. Provisional studies have demonstrated a lower rate of POF in patients treated with GnRH agonists prior to cancer treatment (<7%) in comparison to controls (>53%). They may prolong the 'fertility window' but the beneficial effects are age related.

Informed consent is required for these experimental and invasive techniques and this is challenging in young people. In the UK if the patient is less than 16 years old they must be Gillick competent if they are to make their own informed decisions. The child must demonstrate to have sufficient intelligence to understand what has been proposed.

Many women who had already undergone cancer treatment and now face infertility did not have such technologies available to them. For these women, donor oocytes are the only available option at present. Uterine function is still important and success rates may be reduced in women with radiation-induced uterine damage.

Counselling

Counselling for the patient and their family should be offered to all patients and detailed discussion with a specialist regarding the potential effects on fertility and fertility preservation techniques should be available.

Treatment of childhood cancer can have an impact on neurological, educational, and social function (SIGN 2004). Survivors are at increased risk of cognitive impairment as well as a range of psychological symptoms, including low mood and anxiety. Such problems should be reviewed at routine follow-up.

Comorbidity

In the context of management of childhood cancer survivors it is important to recognize comorbidities may exist.

Growth problems

A number of factors are responsible for impaired growth following childhood cancer. These include the disease process itself, complications of treatment (infection), direct effects during treatment (anorexia), and late effects attributable to therapy (SIGN 2004). Localized tumour treatment may affect growth of individual bones and sex steroid deficiencies may have secondary effects on growth and pubertal development (SIGN 2004).

All children should have their height, weight, BMI, and bone age measured regularly until they reach final adult height.

Dental problems

Children undergoing cancer treatment should be advised about the possible effects on orofacial and dental development. Disturbances in mineralization, the development of crowns and roots of teeth are commonly seen (SIGN 2004). Facial asymmetry has also been observed after local radiotherapy.

Cardiac problems

Anthracyclines, as well as radiotherapy to the chest, are risk factors for cardiovascular disease and monitoring using echocardiography, is therefore necessary (SIGN 2004). Mediastinal irradiation increases the incidence of coronary artery disease and myocardial infarction. The risk increases with increasing doses.

Cardiac function should be monitored during pregnancy as the hyperdynamic circulation of pregnancy may precipitate cardiac failure.

Secondary cancers

The leading cause of death among 5-year survivors is recurrence of the original cancer with a significant excess mortality rate seen due to subsequent malignancies. Breast cancer risk increases with increasing radiation dose of supradiaphragmatic radiotherapy. The risk is greater for those women treated at a younger age.

Thyroid dysfunction

Thyroid dysfunction may be due to primary damage to the gland or secondary to damage to the hypothalamic-pituitary axis. Chemotherapy is an independent risk factor for thyroid dysfunction and thyroid function tests should be checked, following treatment and annually thereafter.

Quick reference material

Cancer therapy may result in a range of disturbances to the neuroendocrine axis and may damage the ovaries and impair uterine function, resulting in diverse effects upon reproductive function

The prevalence of POF is dependent upon the treatment given, the agent used, the dose and age of patient when treatment is administered

Spontaneous ovulation and conception may occur

Offspring of cancer patients have no excess of congenital anomalies or other diseases

Reproductive outcome after chemotherapy alone is good

There is an increased incidence of miscarriage, preterm delivery, and low birthweight neonates in women treated with radiotherapy

Pregnancy in all cancer survivors should be considered high risk

Fertility preservation should be considered prior to cancer treatment

Following treatment pubertal status and growth patterns should be assessed three times a year

All women with POF should be offered sex steroid replacement therapy

Fertility preservation techniques for children and young women remain investigational

Oophoropexy (surgically displacing the ovaries out of the radiation field) may preserve ovarian function

Cryopreservation of embryos after in vitro fertilization is an established practice for fertility preservation but is limited by the age of the patient and the need for a partner

Mature oocyte preservation, cortical ovarian tissue cryopreservation, and the administration of GnRH agonists are potential solutions for fertility preservation in younger women or those without partners at the time of treatment

The only established option for preservation of male fertility is cryopreservation of spermatozoa

The possibility of germ cell transplantation offers hope to restoring fertility in the prepubertal male

There are a wide variety of potentially serious and disabling comorbidities that are recognized in the survivors of childhood cancers and careful follow-up and monitoring should therefore be arranged

Follow-up

All survivors of childhood cancer should ideally be followed up for life by a multidisciplinary team. A designated key worker should coordinate care. It is essential that all professionals involved are aware of the diagnosis and treatment received to allow vigilant observation for late effects.

Male patients

The testes are also susceptible to cytotoxic cancer treatments with the extent of damage being dependent upon the agent used and its dose. Not all damage is permanent and a proportion of men achieve parenthood spontaneously.

Radiotherapy

The degree and duration of radiotherapy-induced testicular damage depends on the field of treatment, total dose and fractionation schedule (Howell and Shalet 1998). Radiation doses as low as 0.1–1.2 Gy can impair spermatogenesis, with doses of more than 4 Gy causing permanent damage (Howell and Shalet 1998).

Chemotherapy

The effects on fertility of chemotherapies are dependent upon the drug, the dose and the age of the patient.

Fertility preservation

The only established option for preservation of male fertility is cryopreservation of spermatozoa. This is dependent on the ability of the patient to produce a specimen. Alternative invasive sperm retrieval methods may be used in boys with testes >10 mL volume who are unable to produce a sample.

Although there may be impaired spermatogenesis following cancer treatment spontaneously conceived offspring have no excess of congenital anomalies or other disease (Li et al. 1979). Modern assisted conception techniques such as intracytoplasmic sperm injection (ICSI) have allowed many men with poor semen quality to achieve parenthood.

Hormone suppression has not been shown to help reduce chemotherapy-induced testicular damage. The possibility of germ cell transplantation offers hope to restoring fertility in the prepubertal male, although techniques remain investigational.

Further reading

Critchley HO, Wallace WH. Impact of cancer treatment on uterine function. J Natl Cancer Inst Monogr 2005;34:64–8.

Donnez J, Martinez-Madrid B, Jadoul P, et al. ovarian tissue cryopreservation and transplantation: a review. Hum Reprod Update. 2006; 12:519–35.

Howell S, Shalet SM. Gonadal damage from chemotherapy and radiotherapy. Endocrinol Metabol Clin N Am 1998 27:927–43.

Lee SJ, Schover LR, Partridge AH, et al. American Society of Clinical Oncology. American Society of Clinical Oncology recommendations on fertility preservation in cancer patients. J Clin Oncol 2006;24:2917–31.

Li PP, Fine W, Jaffe N, et al. Offspring of patients treated for cancer in childhood. J Natl Cancer Inst 1979;62:1193–7.

Mertens AC, Yasui Y, Neglia JP, et al. Late mortality experience in five-year survivors of childhood and adolescent cancer: The Childhood Cancer Survivor Study. J Clin Oncol 2002;19:3163–72.

Multidisciplinary Working Group convened by the British Fertility Society. A strategy for fertility services of childhood cancer. Hum Fertil Camb 2003;6:A1–A40.

Oktay K, Cil P, Bang H. Efficiency of oocyte cryopreservation: a meta-analysis. Fertil Steril 2006;86:70–80.

Scottish Intercollegiate Guidelines Network (SIGN). Longer follow-up of survivors of childhood cancer: a national clinical guideline. SIGN 2004;76.

Sklar CA, Mertens AC, Mitby P, et al. Premature menopause in survivors of childhood cancer: a report from the Childhood Cancer Survivors Study. J Natl Cancer Survivor Study 2006;98:890–6.

Thomson AB, Critchley HO, Kelnar CJ, et al. Late reproductive sequelae following treatment of childhood cancer and options for fertility preservation. Best Pract Res Clin Endocrinol Metab 2002;16:311–34.

Wallace WH, Thomson AB, Kelsey TW. The radiosensitivity of the human oocyte. Hum Reprod 2003;18:117–21.

Wallace WH, Thomson AB, Saran F, et al. Predicting age of ovarian failure after radiation to a field that includes the ovaries. Int J Radiat Oncol Biol Phys 2005a;62:738–44.

Wallace WHB, Anderson RA, Irvine DS. Fertility preservation for young patients with cancer: who is at risk and what can be offered? Lancet Oncol 2005b;6:209–18.

Patient resources

Teenage Cancer Trust: www.teencancer.org

The United Kingdom Children's Cancer Study Group: www.ukccsg.org

Macmillan Cancerline: www.macmillan.org.uk

Imaging in reproductive medicine

Ultrasound

Ultrasound (US), transvaginal ± transabdominal, is the primary imaging modality in reproductive medicine. Diagnostic pelvic ultrasound is part of the initial assessment of patients presenting with subfertility or recurrent miscarriage and aims to

- assess ovarian morphology
- exclude significant congenital uterine anomalies
- exclude potentially associated gynaecological disease such as endometriosis and fibroids.

Further indications for US in patients undergoing treatment for subfertility include

- monitoring ovarian response and follicular growth during ovulation induction
- assessment of endometrial response during ovulation induction
- assisting with egg collection and subsequent embryo transfer
- guiding percutaneous/transvaginal aspiration of cysts which might interfere with follicle monitoring and/or egg collection
- prevention/monitoring of ovarian hyperstimulation syndrome (OHSS). OHSS is accompanied by large ovaries (up to 10 cm) containing multiple follicles and associated with ascites and pleural effusions.

Ovarian morphology

Transvaginal ± transabdominal US should be able to identify at least one ovary in over 95% of premenopausal women. Ovaries are typically oval hypoechoic masses related to the iliac vessels and contain a variable number of small cysts/follicles. Follicular growth, ovulation, and development of the corpus luteum can be monitored.

Three main types of anovulatory ovaries can be distinguished on US:

- Polycystic ovaries (PCOs): the definition of a PCO has been under debate for some time. According to a recent consensus statement a PCO is defined as an ovary with a volume of >10 mL and/or >12 cyst/follicles measuring 2–9 mm (Balen et al. 2003).
- Hypothalamic hypogonadotrophism: in contrast, hypothalamic hypogonadotrophic ovaries, typically associated with amenorrhoea due to weight loss, in athletes, or stress are small/normal in size and contain a small number of follicles, similar to adolescent, prepubertal ovaries.
- Premature ovarian failure: the ovaries are small and quiescent with no evidence of follicular activity. However, this diagnosis requires biochemical confirmation.

Congenital uterine anomalies

The ability to differentiate endometrium from myometrium allows an experienced operator to diagnose many congenital uterine abnormalities using conventional 2D ultrasound. However, it is not always possible to obtain good coronal views of the uterus, and hence differentiating arcuate from mildly subseptate uteri and subseptate from bicornuate uteri (by indentifying a fundal notch) can be difficult. 3D ultrasound overcomes this problem and has been shown to be an accurate and reproducible technique for classifiying congenital uterine anomalies (Jurcovic 1995).

Associated gynaecological disease

Endometriosis/adenomyosis

US has poor sensitivity for deep pelvic endometriosis but is able to see significant endometriomas. Typically endometriomas are cysts containing diffuse internal echoes. However, they vary in appearance from apparently simple cysts to complex multilocculated masses containing varying amounts of internal echoes with thick internal septations and irregular walls, features which can be difficult to differentiate from malignant ovarian masses. Endometriosis involving the bowel is indicated by areas of low echogenicity and irregularly thickened bowel wall.

US has an approx 80% sensitivity for the diagnosis of adenomyosis (Dijkman et al. 2000). Features include areas of heterogeneity in the myometrium, subendometrial echogenic linear striations, small myometrial cysts, and displacement of the cavity.

Pelvic inflammatory disease

US also has a low sensitivity for pelvic inflammatory disease and cannot be used to exclude tubal occlusion. Hydrosalpinges may be visualized as elongated, frequently tortuous, cystic masses, with or without incomplete septations due to residual mucosal folds but are not always detectable. The ovary maybe visible abutting the cyst or may be involved in a complex tubo ovarian mass.

Fibroids

Fibroids are perhaps the most common abnormality seen on pelvic ultrasound but their significance in patients with subfertility or recurrent miscarriage is difficult to determine. US is able to determine the approximate number, size, and location of fibroids but more importantly it can describe the relationship of the fibroids to the cavity.

Hystero contrast salpingography (HyCoSy)

HyCoSy involves cannulating the cervix and injecting an US contrast agent (e.g. Echovist or Sonovue) into the uterus while performing a transvaginal US. It is an alternative investigation to hysterosalpingography and has a similar sensitivity for the diagnosis of tubal patency (Dijkman et al. 2000). Some operators have also used saline rather than contrast. It has proved helpful when assessing the cavity for polyps and fibroids but is less accurate when assessing tubal patency.

Hystero salpingography (HSG)

Hystero salpingography (HSG) is the transcervical injection of radiographic contrast under fluoroscopic guidance and has been used for many years for the assessment of tubal patency and the shape of the uterine cavity. It is performed in the first half of the menstrual cycle, after bleeding has ceased. Complications of the procedure include

- pain (particularly if the tubes are shown to be occluded)
- infection (nowadays most units recommend routine antibiotic prophylaxis)
- vasovagal reaction due to manipulation of the cervix
- contrast allergy (very rare)

In comparison with the 'gold standard' of laparoscopy and dye insufflation, HSG has been shown to be accurate in the detection of tubal patency but is less accurate in the detection of tubal occlusion and peritubal disease. However, the fact that it does not require any anaesthetic and is well tolerated by most women means it should be the initial investigation for patients with no suspicion of tubal disease (RCOG 2004). Congenital anomalies, filling defects in the cavity due to fibroids, polyps, or adhesions are well demonstrated and the site of tubal occlusion can be seen. The absence of mucosal folds in the distended ampulla of a hydrosalpinx suggests a poor prognosis following salpingostomy. Multiple tiny contrast-filled diverticula along the isthmic portions of the tubes indicate salpingitis isthmica nodosa, which is usually caused by endometriosis or pelvic inflammatory disease and associated with an increased incidence of subfertility and ectopic pregnancy.

Selective salpingography and tubal recanalization/fallopian tube catheterization

Catheterization of the tubes has a diagnostic and therapeutic role. Simple catheterization of the cornua immediately following a conventional HSG can be used to confirm or refute tubal occlusion particularly where doubt is caused by reflux of contrast through the cervix or preferential filling of the contralateral tube. Indeed, one study showed selective tubal catheterization to be superior to laparoscopy and dye insufflation in the diagnosis of proximal tubal occlusion.

Approximately 50% of apparent cornual occlusions are due to spasm or debris and minor adhesions, and these can be cleared by either injecting contrast directly into the tube or by probing with a guidewire. Under fluoroscopic guidance, following a standard HSG, preformed catheters are used to cannulate the cornua and contrast injected. If the tube is not demonstrated a guidewire is advanced into the tube and any obstruction cleared using gentle probing movements. Subsequent injection of contrast is then used to confirm patency. Studies have shown that approximately 70% of occluded tubes can be opened in this way with a resulting pregnancy rate of 10–20%. Complications of the procedure include tubal perforation (1–10%) and tubal pregnancy (0.4–8%) but it should be noted that patients requiring the procedure are likely to have an increased risk of ectopic pregnancy even in the absence of tubal catheterization by virtue of their pre-existing tubal disease. The procedure has been approved by the National Institute for Clinical Excellence (NICE) and is recommended by the Royal College of Obstetricians and Gynaecologists for use in patients with proximal tubal occlusion (NICE 2004; RCOG 2004).

Magnetic resonance imaging

Congenital anomalies

Congenital Mullerian duct abnormalities are frequently suggested by US or HSG but accurate classification can prove difficult. Magnetic resonance imaging (MRI) has been shown to be more accurate than both these techniques and should be considered before laparoscopy/hysteroscopy if there is any doubt about the precise nature of an abnormality (Troiano and McCarthy 2004).

Associated gynaecological disease

MRI is the most accurate imaging technique for diagnosing adenomyosis. Features include widening of the so-called junctional zone (superficial layer of myometrium), high-intensity spots, asymmetrical thickening of the myometrium, and poorly defined low signal myometrial masses. Adenomyomas can be differentiated from fibroids, which is of considerable importance therapeutically.

Endometriomas are easily seen with MRI scans, which is also the most reliable technique for assessing deep pelvic endometriosis. Adhesions between the cervix, uterus and bowel are demonstrated as low signal bands causing distortion; thickening of the uterosacral ligaments is visible and rectovaginal nodules can be seen.

There are no specific features of pelvic inflammatory disease on MRI scans but the multiplanar imaging facility means that hydro- or haematosalpinges can be distinguished from other complex adnexal masses.

MRI is also of value in the management of fibroids. It can delineate the number, location, and size of fibroids and assess their vascularity and relation to overlying bowel and abdominal wall scars, important factors when considering MR-guided ablation with focused US or fibroid embolization. Focused US is only appropriate if there are less than six fibroids with diameters of <10 cm, no interposed bowel, and no anterior abdominal wall scars. These limitations do not apply to embolization.

Recurrent miscarriage

Many of the conditions described above are also of relevance to patients suffering from recurrent miscarriage. Specifically imaging is indicated to look for

• polycystic ovaries
• congenital anomalies: 2D/3D but may need confirmation with HSG or MRI scan
• intrauterine adhesions (Asherman's syndrome): suggested by highly reflective echoes in the endometrium and/or loss of the normal endometrial echo. Conventional US has poor sensitivity; HyCoSy and HSGs are more accurate and able to demonstrate the adhesions as irregular filling defects within the cavity or wall irregularity

There is currently no reliable imaging technique for diagnosing cervical incompetence in the non-pregnant patient.

Further reading

Balen AH, Laven J, Tan SL, et al. Ultrasound assessment of the polycystic ovary: international consensus definitions. Hum Reprod Update 2003;9:505–14.

Dijkman AB, Mol BWJ, van der Veen F, et al. Can hysterosalpingo-contrast-sonography replace hysterosalpingography in the assessment of tubal subfertility? Eur J Radiol 2000;35:44–8.

Jurcovic D, Geipel A, Groeberk K, et al. Three dimensional ultrasound for the assessment of uterine anatomy and detection of congenital anomalies: a comparison with hysterosalpingography and two dimensional ultrasound. Ultrasound Obstet Gynaecol 1995;5:233–7.

NICE. Fallopian tube recanalisation by guidewire. IPG 071. London: NICE July 2004.

Royal College of Obstetricians and Gynaecologists (RCOG) Fertility: assessment and treatment for people with fertility problems. London: RCOG 2004.

Troiano RM, McCarthy SM. Mullerian duct anomalies: imaging and clinical issues. Radiology 2004;233:19–34.

Induction of ovulation

The aim of induction of ovulation is to restore physiological (single follicle) ovulation in anovulatory women. Disorders of ovulation account for about 25% of causes of infertility. Most are due to an abnormal endocrine environment and are therefore treatable.

Clinical presentation of anovulation
- Amenorrhoea (>6 months)
- Oligomenorrhoea (cycle >42 days)
- Irregular menses (e.g. cycles varying between 2 and 6 weeks in duration).

Causes
The commonest cause of anovulation is polycystic ovary syndrome (PCOS) (80%). Other endocrine disorders that commonly cause anovulation are hyperprolactinaemia, isolated gonadotropin-releasing hormone (GnRH) deficiency or GnRH dysfunction secondary to weight loss or exercise.

Many other endocrine disorders are rare causes of anovulation but commonly present with menstrual abnormalities.

Endocrine disorders associated with ovulatory dysfunction
Polycystic ovary syndrome
Hypothalamic-pituitary disease
GnRH deficiency isolated or identified cause
prolactinoma
acromegaly
Cushing's
non-functioning tumours
Sheehan's syndrome
Adrenal disease
CAH
virilizing tumours
Addison's disease
Thyroid disease
hypothyroidism
hyperthyroidism

Investigation of anovulation
A small number of investigations are necessary (see box)
- FSH, LH (normal range 3–11 u/L)
- Prolactin (50–500 mu/L)
- TSH (0.5–5.0 mu/L)
- Pelvic ultrasonography to assess ovarian morphology
- Testosterone (0.5–3.0 nmol/L)
- Assessment of oestrogen status (if amenorrhoeic, patients with oligomenorrhoea have adequate endogenous E2 production)
- Serum oestradiol <75 pmol/L, endometrial thickness on ultrasound scan of <5 mm, negative progesterone

Investigation of anovulation
High FSH, low E2 = primary ovarian failure
Normal/Low FSH, low E2 = hypothalamic/pituitary disorder
Measure prolactin
Ultrasound scan with normal FSH, normal E2 (± high LH) = PCOS

withdrawal test with no menstrual bleeding after medroxyprogesterone 5 mg/day for 5 days, implies patient is oestrogen deficient.

Treatment of oestrogen-replete patients
Most patients with adequate oestrogen production will have PCOS.

Clomiphene
Mechanism of action: anti-oestrogen with negative feedback effects at the hypothalamus and pituitary causes a >50% rise above basal FSH levels with an equal rise in LH secretion.

Initial starting dose of 50mg/day on day 2 of the cycle for 5 days

Ultrasound monitoring mandatory for first cycle to establish correct dose (RCOG guidelines); 60% of patients will respond to clomiphene 50 mg, but the daily dose required can vary from 25 to 100 mg. Approximately 10% of patients are resistant (no response by day 21 of the cycle to clomiphene 50 mg followed by 100 mg.

Cumulative conception rate after nine cycles of clomiphene is 59% with a miscarriage rate of 23%, multiple (all twins) pregnancy rate of 12% (Fig. 12.16.1).

Once ovulation is confirmed by ultrasound scan and progesterone measurement, patients can be reviewed after three cycles to confirm they are still having predictable regular cycles, implying continued ovulation and additional investigations of sperm and tubal function are satisfactory.

High body mass index (BMI) is the only identified factor predicting poor response to clomiphene. BMI should be less than 30. In patients with BMI >30 a 5–10 kg weight loss is associated with a significant improvement in androgen and insulin levels and improved chance of response to clomiphene.

Alternative treatment options
Alternatives should be considered for patients resistant to clomiphene or who have not conceived after nine cycles of clomiphene.

Human menopausal gonadotrophin
Gonadotrophins LH and FSH extracted from urine, purified and reconstituted for daily injection. There are various degrees of purity with human menopausal gonadotrophin (hMG). The standard ampoule contains 75 IU FSH but the LH dose varies from 75 IU to <1 IU. With high purity

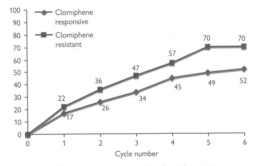

Fig. 12.16.1 Cumulative conception with clomiphene citrate.

formulations additional steps to remove urinary proteins are undertaken during manufacture. Gonadotrophins are also available as recombinant LH and FSH that have no urinary contaminants.

Ovulation induction trials have shown no difference in clinical outcome comparing urinary or recombinant preparations.

Initial hMG protocols were associated with high (20%) rates of multiple pregnancy and OHSS.

Low-dose protocol for gonadotrophin therapy
Daily dose of gonadotrophin with step-up protocol aiming to find the threshold dose that is maintained to develop a single dominant follicle. Once the dominant follicle has reached the appropriate size, ovulation is triggered with 5000 IU of hCG; no luteal phase support is given and a mid-luteal phase progesterone is taken to confirm ovulation. With this protocol, 86% of completed ovulatory cycles are unifollicular. However, 15% of cycles are abandoned due to multiple follicular development. After six cycles of treatment there is cumulative conception >50%, a miscarriage rate of 20%, and a multiple pregnancy rate (all twins) <5% (Fig. 12.16.2).

Unlike clomiphene the hMG required per cycle can vary, so each cycle must be monitored with serial ultrasound scans.

Factors affecting treatment outcome
• Endocrine profile: pretreatment LH ≥11 IU/L or testosterone ≥3 nmol/L is associated with a higher 'threshold' dose of FSH (p<0.05 (t-test)) but has no effect on the ovulation or pregnancy rates.
• BMI: a BMI ≥25 is associated with a higher 'threshold' dose of FSH (p<0.05 (t-test)) and reduced ovulation and pregnancy rates (p≤0.05 (logistic regression)).
• Clinical guidelines: hMG should be offered to patients who are resistant to clomiphene or who have ovulated but not conceived after nine cycles of clomiphene and the patient's BMI <27.

Laparoscopic ovarian diathermy
Multiple (four to eight) diathermy points to each ovary (one report of unilateral ovarian diathermy also successful). The trauma to the cortex of the ovary makes the ovaries more responsive to endogenous gonadotrophin secretion, lasts an average of 6–12 months. The reported ovulation rate is 61–100% (median 84.2%), and pregnancy rate 20–88% (median 52%).

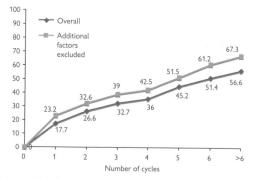

Fig. 12.16.2 Cumulative conception with hMG.

The advantages are natural ovulation with no increased risk of multiple pregnancy, and no risk of OHSS. The disadvantages are risk of adhesion formation: there are widely varying reports in the medical literature, but are probably in order of 10%. There is a theoretical risk of ovarian atrophy. A significant number of patients (up to 35%) require medical ovulation induction (with associated risks) to ovulate satisfactorily.

Risks of medical ovulation induction
There is a risk of multiple follicular development, with the risk of multiple pregnancy and ovarian hyperstimulation syndrome. With the widespread use of clomiphene more triplet and higher order births are reported following clomiphene than after hMG or IVF.

Treatment of oestrogen-deficient patients
Identifying and treating underlying cause
• Weight gain: restoring BMI to acceptable range(>19)
• Exercise: modifying or stopping exercise
• Patients with isolated (unidentified) cause for GnRH deficiency or patients who do not have resumption of a menstrual cycle despite weight gain require ovulation induction with hMG or the GnRH pump.

GnRH pump
This is the pulsatile release of GnRH using a battery operated pump giving a pulse of 5 or 10 µg of GnRH every 90 minutes. Usually given subcutaneously but can also be given intravenously. The pump is worn continuously until development of a dominant follicle. Once ovulation is triggered, the pump can be removed and luteal phase support given with hCG.

Human menopausal gonadotrophin
Compared with patients with PCOS, those with isolated GnRH deficiency have a higher hMG threshold requiring increased doses of hMG per cycle with a longer period of stimulation, a lower rate of unifollicular cycles, a higher rate of cycle cancellation because of multiple follicular development, and a lower incidence of ovarian hyperstimulation.

Both methods of ovulation induction are successful. The GnRH pump is more 'physiological'; however, both methods of stimulation have the potential for multiple follicular development and the risks of multiple pregnancy and ovarian hyperstimulation syndrome.

Hyperprolactinaemia
Patients with hyperprolactinaemia confirmed by a second measurement require MRI of the pituitary, as 50% of patients will have pituitary adenomas (usually microadenomas). Hyperprolactinaemia causes abnormalities in GnRH secretion.

Treatment is with dopamine agonists, usually bromocriptine once or twice daily. Cabergoline once weekly is an alternative for patients intolerant of bromocriptine.

Further reading
Barber TM, McCarthy MI, Wass JA, et al. Obesity and polycystic ovary syndrome. Clin Endocrinol 2006;65:137–45.

Bayram N, van Wely M, van Der Veen F. Recombinant FSH versus urinary gonadotrophins or recombinant FSH for ovulation induction in subfertility associated with polycystic ovary syndrome. Cochrane Database Syst Rev 2001;2:CD002121.

Kousta E, White DM, Franks S. Modern use of clomiphene citrate in induction of ovulation. Human Reproduction Update 3, 1997;359–65.

Legro RS, Barnhart HX, Schlaff WD, *et al.* Clomiphene, metformin or both for infertility in polycystic ovary syndrome. N Engl J Med 2007;356:551–66.

Martin KA, Hall JE, Adams JM, *et al.* Comparison of exogenous gonadotopins and pulsatile gonadotropin-releasing hormone for induction of ovulation in hypogonadotropic amenorrhea. J Clin Endocrinol Metab 1993;77:125–9.

White DM, Polson DW, Kiddy D, *et al.* Induction of ovulation with low-dose gonadotropins in polycycstic ovary syndrome: an analysis of 109 pregnancies in 225 women. J Clin Endocrinol Metab 1996;81:3821–4.

Patient resources

Infertility Network UK, Tel 08701 188088: www.infertilitynetworkuk.com

Verity: www.verity-pcos.org.uk

Intracytoplasmic sperm injection

Definition
Intracytoplasmic sperm injection (ICSI) is the micromanipulation of a sperm into the ooplasm of the oocyte by injection.

Epidemiology
ICSI was first reported in 1992 (Palermo et al. 1992). Since then it has become a mainline therapy (HFEA 2007). ICSI was performed in 47% of all UK in vitro fertilization (IVF) treatments: a total of 44 275 cycles in 34 855 women. In the same dataset, it was reported that 23.1% of all IVF/ICSI treatments resulted in a live birth. The ESHRE Capri Workshop Group (2007) reported that of all assisted reproduction treatment (ART) cycles that ICSI contributed to between 26% (Russia) to 76% (Spain) of cycles undertaken.

Success rates
Success rates with ICSI are similar to IVF and vary significantly with the woman's age (31% under 35 to 4% over 44 years) (HFEA 2008).

Clinical approach
Indications
Broadly speaking there are two important clinical situations where ICSI is indicated:
- male factor infertility (oligoasthenoteratozoospermia (OAT) to azoospermia
- failed fertilization with IVF.

The decision about what degree of OAT indicates ICSI is an arbitrary one. However, when the sperm count is normal there is no advantage to be obtained from the use of ICSI over straight IVF (Bhattacharya et al. 2001). Despite this evidence, many centres, particularly outside the UK, routinely recommend ICSI over conventional IVF (ESHRE 2007).

Bhattacharya et al. (2001) reported a failed fertilization rate of 5% with IVF and 2% with ICSI in their randomized study. Between 50% and 70% of cases of failed fertilization in IVF will have normal fertilization rates in a subsequent cycle of IVF (Kinzer et al. 2005). It is common practice, however, to recommend ICSI in this situation to maximize future fertilization chances.

Where there are no sperm present in the ejaculate (azoospermia) due to obstruction in the genital tract, sperm can be surgically retrieved from the testis or epididymis. It has also been reported that sperm can be obtained when the primary problem is with the germinal epithelium: Sertoli cell only, maturation arrest, Kleinfelter's syndrome, etc. (Palermo et al. 1998; Ramasamy et al. 2005). The numbers of sperm retrieved are, however, low and such sperm have virtually no endogenous motility and, therefore, no hope of spontaneously fertilizing an oocyte. ICSI bypasses the natural barriers to penetration and allows the nuclear DNA of that sperm access to that of the oocyte, thus permitting fertilization to occur.

ICSI is also indicated in less common procedures such as pre-implantation genetic diagnosis (PGDs) in order to decrease the chances of DNA contamination from other sperm in the molecular PCR-based laboratory techniques employed.

Counselling
As ICSI is an adjunct to IVF treatment, counselling should initially include all of the risks of IVF, such as hyperstimulation syndrome and multiple pregnancy. In addition, however, it is necessary to discuss the risks of fertility problems in any subsequent offspring and the increased rate of fetal abnormality (albeit small), in particular of the genital tract. Where OAT is profound ($<1 \times 10^6$) a karyotype should be performed and determination of any deletions in the azoospermia factor genes offered to the couple. Although these are not contraindications to ICSI they help with counselling the couple about the risks for the fertility of male offspring. Couples may wish to opt for PGD and have only female embryos transferred, although this is uncommon in the UK.

Management
To obtain sufficient oocytes, women will typically undergo an ovarian hyperstimulation cycle with follicle-stimulating hormone (FSH) injections, usually with a gonadotropin-releasing hormone (GnRH) analogue in a downregulation or 'short/boost/flare' protocol. The oocytes are usually collected under transvaginal ultrasound guidance and passed to the laboratory, where they are allowed to mature in vitro for at least 90 minutes. They are then stripped of their attached cumulus cells. This allows for closer assessment of oocyte maturity. Sperm injection should be within the next 4 hours.

The semen sample is produced by masturbation or sperm are extracted from the testis or epididymis by needle aspiration or biopsy, open or closed. The semen sample is prepared to isolate the sperm from the seminal fluids and they are then assessed for their motility and normality of appearance. Sperm taken directly from the testis and epididymis show very little movement but the presence of any movement remains the only effective way to confirm that a sperm is alive without killing it. A proportion of the sperm is placed into a medium with increased viscosity to slow their trajectories and the individual sperm for injection identified and targeted. Initially it is immobilized by crushing the tail just distal to the midpiece with the injection needle. The sperm is then aspirated into the injection needle. Simultaneously the oocyte will have been fixed with a holding pipette with the polar body either at 12 or 6 o'clock. This positioning ensures that the injection of the sperm should miss the mitotic spindle. A drop of oolema is aspirated and the sperm is then injected into the ooplasm and the needle removed.

Injected oocytes are incubated overnight and checked for normal fertilization (the presence of two polar bodies), usually the following morning. Thereafter, the procedure is as for conventional IVF.

Follow-up
It is remarkable that such fundamental manipulations of human gametes could have become a standard and widespread clinical practice without more rigorous scientific evaluation. In addition to the worries regarding IVF pregnancy complications (prematurity, low birthweight, etc.) there are concerns about fetal abnormality with ICSI: by the age of 8 years, 15 major congenital malformations had been diagnosed in 150 ICSI children compared with five in 147 matched controls (Belva et al. 2007). Bonduelle et al. (2005) reported an increase, particularly in male urogenital abnormalities. It has also been recorded that there is an increased incidence in disorders of imprinting, with the incidence of Angelman and Beckwith–Wiedemann

syndromes being greater in ICSI children than the general population (Belva *et al.* 2007). It is a sad reflection that within the UK it was only in 2005 that the first register of ART children was established and that the data collected by the HFEA are first not as well audited as could be and second not accessible to researchers under the 1990 HFE Act. Worldwide, no data have been published from any register beyond 8 years of age, despite ICSI having been in common clinical practice since the early 1990s.

Further reading

Alukal JP, Lamb DJ. Intracytoplasmic sperm injection (ICSI): what are the risks? Urol Clin North Am 2008;35:277–88.

Belva F, Henriet S, Liebaers I, *et al.* Medical outcome of 8-year-old singleton ICSI children (born >or = 32 weeks' gestation) and a spontaneously conceived comparison group. Hum Reprod 2007;22:506–15.

Bhasin S. Approach to the infertile man. J Clin Endocrinol Metab 2007;92:1995–2004.

Bhattacharya S, Hamilton MP, Shaaban M, *et al.* Conventional in-vitro fertilisation versus intracytoplasmic sperm injection for the treatment of non-male-factor infertility: a randomised controlled trial. Lancet 2001;357:2075–9.

Bonduelle M, Wennerholm UB, Loft A, *et al.* A multi-centre cohort study of the physical health of 5-year-old children conceived after intracytoplasmic sperm injection, in vitro fertilization and natural conception. Hum Reprod 2005;20:413–319.

ESHRE Capri Workshop Group. Intracytoplasmic sperm injection (ICSI) in 2006: evidence and evolution. Hum Reprod Update 2007;13:515–26.

Human Fertilisation and Embryology Authority (HFEA). *A long term analysis of the HFEA Register data 1991-2006.* London: HFEA 2007.

Human Fertilisation and Embryology Authority (HFEA). *Facts and figures 2006 fertility problems and treatment.* London: HFEA 2008.

Kinzer DR, Barrett CB, Powers RD. Prognosis for clinical pregnancy and delivery after total fertilization failure during conventional in vitro fertilization or intracytoplasmic sperm injection. Fertil Steril 2005;90:284–8.

Myers ER, McCrory DC, Mills AA, *et al.* Effectiveness of assisted reproductive technology (ART). Evid Rep Technol Assess (Full Rep) 2008;167:1–195.

Neri QV, Takeuchi T, Palermo GD. An update of assisted reproductive technologies results in the United States. Ann N Y Acad Sci 2008;1127:41–8.

Palermo G, Joris H, Devroey P, VanSteirteghem AC. Pregnancies after intracytoplasmic injection of single spermatozoon into and oocyte. Lancet 1992;340:17–18.

Palermo GD, Schlegel PN, Sills ES, *et al.* Births after intracytoplasmic injection of sperm obtained by testicular extraction from men with nonmosaic Klinefelter's syndrome. N Engl J Med 1998;338:588–90.

Practice Committee of the American Society for Reproductive Medicine. Report on management of obstructive azoospermia. Fertil Steril 2006;86:259–63.

Ramasamy R, Yagan N, Schlegel PN. Structural and functional changes to the testis after conventional versus microdissection testicular sperm extraction. Urology 2005;65:1190–4.

Sarkar NN. Intracytoplasmic sperm injection: an assisted reproductive technique and its outcome to overcome infertility. Obstet Gynaecol 2007;27:347–53.

Internet resources

www.hfea.gov.uk/

www.asrm.org/Patients/topics/icsi.html

www.britishfertilitysociety.org.uk/public/factsheets/docs/BFS-risks%20and%20complications%20of%20assisted%20conception%20.pdf

Patient resources

www.fertilityconnect.com/index.htm

http://en.wikipedia.org/wiki/Intracytoplasmic_sperm_injection

www.ivf.net/ivf/icsi_intracytoplasmic_sperm_injection-o2109.html

www.infertilitynetworkuk.com/

www.britishfertilitysociety.org.uk/public/index.html

Intrauterine devices

Definition
The intrauterine device (IUD) is a flexible rod or filament inserted into the uterus to prevent conception. Modern IUDs are medicated to enhance their contraceptive efficacy. Copper-releasing ones are referred to as IUDs or intrauterine contraceptives (IUCs) and the progestin-releasing ones are called intrauterine systems (IUS). For the purpose of this chapter all such devices will be referred to as IUD.

Epidemiology
It is estimated that about 160 million people worldwide use the IUD for contraception. In China 50% of married women who practice contraception use the IUD compared with 4% in Britain and 2% in America. Despite the variations in its usage worldwide, it remains one of the most cost-effective and reversible methods of contraception and is underused in the developed world.

The first IUD was invented and marketed by Ernst Grafenberg, a Jewish German opthalmologist turned gynaecologist in 1928. Since then the IUD has been redesigned many a time to the ones that are presently available.

Pathology
The IUD has certain characteristics that serve to fulfil its designed purpose. However, these can lead to complications if improperly chosen or handled.

In view of these factors, it is hardly surprising that IUDs have been credited with a number of ill effects and therefore are underutilized.

Mode of action
All IUDs work by preventing fertilization. A sterile inflammatory reaction occurs within the uterus, and this in turn leads to inhibition of sperm motility, reduced sperm capacitation and survival, and sperm phagocytosis.

In addition, the copper within the copper IUDs enhance a cytotoxic inflammatory reaction.

The progestins in progestin-releasing IUDs thicken the cervical mucus, which prevents sperm penetration into the uterine cavity. In addition, the decidualization and glandular atrophy caused in the endometrium prevents implantation of the blastocyst.

Shape
The framed devices are in the shape of a T, which helps conform to the shape of the uterus. This then retains the device *in utero*. There is a thread/threads attached to the end that projects through the cervix when the device is *in utero*. The presence of the thread rules out expulsion and also aids removal of the device.

The frameless device has six copper sleeves threaded on a prolene filament with a knot at one end. It is this end that is pushed into the myometrium with an introducer and helps secure it to the tissues there. The advantage of a frameless device is that it can be inserted into cavities that are distorted and unable to retain a framed device. Similarly, they are also useful in an enlarged, puerperal uterus or in a small one.

Medicated devices
Medicated devices enhance efficacy, such as copper in the copper IUDs and progestin in the progestin-releasing IUDs. The currently available copper coils have sleeves of copper on the horizontal arm, thereby increasing the available surface area of copper. This results in a much more efficient device that not only provides contraception for longer but also has a greatly reduced failure rate.

Aetiology
The modern IUD is a very effective, long-acting, safe, and easily reversible method of contraception. It has few side-

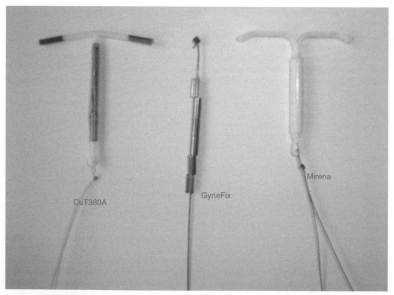

Fig. 12.18.1 Copper and progestin-releasing intrauterine devices. See also colour plate section.

effects, rarely interferes with the spontaneity of sex and offers women the privacy they seek. The types of IUD in use include the following (see also Fig. 12.18.1):

- copper IUDs
- framed devices
- copper sleeves
  - TCu380S
  - TT380 Slimline
  - TCu380A Quickload
  - MiniTT 380 Slimline
  - Flexi-T 380
- copper in stem only
  - Multioad 375
  - UT 380
  - UT 380 Short
  - NovaT380
  - Flexi-T380
- frameless devices
  - GyneFix
- progestin-releasing IUDs (also known as IUS)
  - framed device
  - Mirena
- Unmedicated (inert) IUDs
  - Lippes loop
  - Stainless steel flexible ring

Efficacy
Copper IUDs with 380 mm^2 of copper or more have a failure rate of less than 1 per 100 woman years, which is no different to the progestin-releasing IUDs.

Duration of use
The second-generation copper IUDs are known to provide efficacy for up to 10 years following insertion. If inserted after the age of 40 they can be left in place until the menopause. Frameless copper IUDs and the shorter versions of copper IUDs, such as the mini TT380A, are efficient for up to 5 years

The progestin-releasing IUDs provide contraception as well as relief from menorrhagia for 5 years. However, when used to limit endometrial proliferation as in hormone replacement therapy combinations the efficacy does not last beyond 4 years. If used for contraceptive purpose and inserted beyond the age of 45 they may be retained until the menopause.

Indications for intrauterine devices
- Most women regardless of age and parity.
- Those at low risk of acquiring sexually transmitted infections that may necessitate removal.
- Those seeking an easily reversible and effective agent.
- The copper IUD is a very effective emergency contraceptive agent. The progestin-releasing IUD cannot be used for this purpose.

Contraindications for intrauterine devices
- Uterine distortion such as bicornuate uterus
- Active pelvic infection
- Suspected pregnancy
- Wilson's disease or allergy to copper
- Unexplained uterine bleeding
- Current breast cancer: avoid progestin-releasing devices
- Active liver disease: avoid progestin-releasing devices.

Prognosis
Perforation
The rate of perforation associated with intrauterine device usage is low (0–2.3 per 1000 insertions). No major difference was noted in the incidence of perforation between the various types available.

Expulsion
About 5% of women expel IUDs and this occurs usually after within the first 3 months of insertion and more commonly during a period. The chance of expulsion is not affected to a great extent by the type of IUD inserted; however, recent studies have suggested that the risk may be increased with frameless IUDs.

Risk of ectopic pregnancy
IUDs are so effective that the absolute risk of pregnancy (intrauterine or ectopic) is very low. A previous ectopic pregnancy is no longer a contraindication to the use of these devices and the overall risk is reduced compared to women using no contraception. In fact, IUD has been shown to lower the incidence of ectopic pregnancies when compared to no contraception.

Return to fertility
IUDs have not been shown to delay a return to fertility. The mean time taken to fall pregnant following removal of either a copper or a progestin-releasing device was 3 months.

Pelvic inflammatory disease
Development of pelvic inflammatory disease (PID) is most strongly related to the background risk of sexually transmitted infections (STIs) and the insertion procedure rather than the IUD itself. Low rates of PID have been noted in IUD users of 1.6/1000 woman years. The incidence of PID was noted to be highest in the first 20 days following insertion. Thereafter the risk drops to match non-users of IUD.

Bleeding patterns and pain
Menstrual abnormalities and pain are the most common reasons for discontinuation of IUD. Copper IUDs have been noted to cause spotting, light bleeding, heavy or prolonged periods in the first 3–6 months following insertion. These symptoms are known to improve with time. Although they do not affect ovulation, a short luteal phase has been documented with these devices.

Irregular bleeding or spotting is common in the first 6 months of insertion of the progestin-releasing IUD but by 1 year amenorrhoea or light bleeding is the rule. Ovulation remains unaffected in almost 75% of women fitted with the progestin-releasing IUD.

Hormonal side-effects
Some systemic absorption does occur, and side-effects as a result are most pronounced in the first 3 months after insertion. However, from the limited evidence available there are no clinically significant differences in hormonal side-effects (acne, headache) between a copper IUD and a progestin-releasing one.

Ovarian cysts
One randomized trial has found increased incidence of ovarian cysts in progestin-releasing IUD users compared with the copper IUDs. Most resolve spontaneously and rarely become symptomatic.

Non-contraceptive benefits

The progestin-releasing IUD has found an important place in the treatment of menorrhagia, with menstrual blood loss decreasing by more than 80% in its presence. In addition, it also provides endometrial protection from the stimulatory effects of oestrogen and thus works well as the progesterone arm of hormone replacement therapy. There is also some evidence that it is useful in decreasing the pain associated with endometriosis.

The copper IUDs have in one review of case–control studies found to be associated with a reduced risk of endometrial cancer; however, the mechanism of this remains unknown.

Clinical approach

Prerequisites for IUD insertion

When deciding to have an IUD inserted, the first consideration should be the skill and experience of the operator. The Faculty of Sexual and Reproductive Health in the UK recommend that operators hold a letter of competence before undertaking these procedures. In order to maintain skills one should fit at least one device per month in an unanaesthetized woman.

IUD insertion should be considered a surgical procedure and as such should be performed under aseptic conditions. Equipment for resuscitation should be at hand and an assistant present throughout the procedure to aid the operator.

The operative technique should be explained to the patient as well as the side-effects. Verbal or written consent should be obtained prior to commencement.

A pelvic examination is important before insertion. This is the time to rule out any condition that may make insertion unsuitable. Obvious ulcers on vulva, vagina, or cervix, cervical excitation, adnexal tenderness, purulent cervical discharge, and a cervix that bleeds easily to touch all point towards a possible sexually transmitted infection or PID. Insertion should only proceed once these conditions have been ruled out. Similarly, suspicion of an excessively enlarged or distorted uterine cavity should discourage one from proceeding. If at examination, determining the size and position of uterus proves difficult, IUD insertion is best deferred. It will be impossible in such cases to ensure high placement of the coil resulting in an increased risk of perforation.

The choice of IUD

Following counselling a woman with no contraindications may opt for either a copper or progestin-containing device. However, the effects of different IUDs on menstrual bleeding may be a determining factor when making the choice. If the copper IUD is chosen then the device with the lowest failure rate and longest duration of action should be first line, namely the TCu380S in the UK. In the event of the uterine cavity length being less than 6.5 cm then a device with a shorter stem or a frameless device is chosen.

Timing of insertion

IUDs can be inserted at any time in the menstrual cycle, provided a pregnancy can be reliably excluded. Copper IUDs are effective as soon as inserted but the progestin only IUDs are not. If inserted beyond day 7 of the cycle the patient should use additional protection for 7 days.

Insertion of IUD in a conscious patient

- A 'no touch technique' should be employed throughout the whole procedure so that only clean gloves need be worn. A no touch technique implies that any instrument/object that is to be inserted into the uterine cavity should not be allowed to come into contact with unsterile surfaces and should only be held by its handle. If any manipulation is needed of the sterile IUD in its holder then sterile gloves are to be used.
- The patient is made to lie in a modified lithotomy position and a bimanual examination is performed to assess the size and lie of the uterus.
- The cervix is exposed, cleansed with aseptic solution, and grasped with a 12-inch atraumatic forceps such as Alice Tissue forceps. While stabilizing the cervix this also helps to straighten the uterocervical canal, allowing a controlled IUD insertion and correct fundal placement.
- A malleable uterine sound passed gently into the cavity helps to determine its depth and direction as well as the patency and direction of the cervical canal.
- The device is loaded into the introducer in a manner that allows that upon release it will lie flat in the transverse plane of the uterine cavity.
- The device should not be left in the introducer for a prolonged period of time as it may lose its shape.
- Once the introducer is inserted into the cavity the IUD should be released according o the manufacturer's direction
- High fundal placement is important to avoid the risk of expulsion and pregnancy. Further sounding of the canal following insertion therefore helps exclude a low-lying IUD.
- Threads are trimmed to 2.5–3 cm from the external os.

Problems at insertion

Vasovagal syncope

Severe pain leading to 'cervical shock' or vasovagal syncope is rare. It is caused by distension of the internal cervical os. In mild cases one can proceed after waiting a short while for the patient to recover; 1% local analgesic gel or a local anaesthetic injection may be applied to the cervix before resuming. In severe cases, insertion should be halted, the patient placed head down and the airway maintained. If vasovagal syncope occurs as the insertion is being completed, the IUD can be left in place while allowing the patient to recover.

Epileptic attacks

In those prone to epilepsy, fits are sometimes precipitated by the insertion. These are not a direct result of pain and usually present a few minutes after the cervical stimulus.

Perforation

Although rare, once detected or suspected immediate gynaecological reviews is necessary. Laparoscopy and or laparotomy may be necessary to retrieve the IUD.

Resuscitation measures

- IUD insertions are best carried out with a calm reassuring and unhurried approach. Patient anxieties need to be acknowledged and addressed as far as possible.
- In the event of a vasovagal attack, insertion should be deferred. The patient should remain supine but the head

end of the touch examination should be lowered and legs elevated to restore blood flow.

- A clear airway must be maintained.
- Oxygen if available should be delivered through an Ambu bag.
- In the event of persistent bradycardia, atropine should be given intravenously in at dose of 0.6 mg.
- In the rare event of a patient failing to regain her consciousness she must be transferred to the nearest accident and emergency department or intensive care unit.

Post insertion instructions

- The patient should be taught to check for the presence of threads in herself. It is best checked on a monthly basis soon after a period. The presence of threads alone implies the device has not been expelled or lost. If the threads are found to be missing it is important she seek medical help at the earliest and refrain from intercourse without alternative protection until seen.
- She should be warned to expect some degree of crampy abdominal pain, bleeding, and discharge over the next 48 hours. These can be managed symptomatically.
- There is no longer any necessity for the patient to return for a routine follow up. Provided she is capable of looking out for any untoward symptom and reporting it, the patient need return only when a removal is required.

Pelvic actinomyces and IUD

In the asymptomatic patient there is no indication for removing the IUD in case actinomyces-like organisms (ALO) are detected on swab. Again there is no need for rescreening at a later stage.

Actinomyces israeli is a normal commensal of the vagina and consideration for removal is necessary only when there are signs of infection.

STI and IUD

In the event of an STI developing with the IUD *in situ* there is no need for removal. It is unlikely for the STI to develop into PID due to presence of an IUD. Treatment can continue for the STI without the need to remove the IUD. Should PID develop, the IUD can remain in place while treatment continues. However, if the infection fails to resolve despite treatment with antibiotics, removal should be considered.

Further reading

Belhadj H, Sivin I, Diaz S, *et al.* Recovery of fertility after use of the levonorgestrel 20 mcg/d or Copper T 380 Ag intrauterine device. Contraception 1986;34:261–7.

Faculty of Sexual and Reproductive Healthcare Clinical Effectiveness Unit. *Intrauterine methods of contraception.* London: FSRH CEU 2007.

Haugan T, Skjeldestad FE, Halvorsen LE, Kahn H. A randomised trial on the clinical performance of Nova T380 and Gynae T380 Slimline copper IUDs. Contraception 2007: 75:175–6.

National Institute for Health and Clinical Excellence (NICE). *Long-acting reversible contraception: the effective and appropriate use of long acting reversible contraception.* London: NICE 2005.

Wu Shangchun, IUD: the key contraceptive method in China. Abstract, ESC. Congress, Istanbul, 2005.

Xiong X, Buekens P, Wollast E. IUD use and the risk of ectopic pregnancy: a meta-analysis of case control studies. Contraception 1995; 52:23–34.

Contraception and Sexual Health, 2004/5 ONS 2005.

Internet resources

www.emedicine.com

Patient resources

www.fsrh.org
www.fpa.org.uk

In vitro fertilization

Definition

Literally fertilization 'in glass', the term is widely used to describe the process of superovulation followed by oocyte collection, fertilization of the oocyte with sperm in a laboratory, with subsequent transfer of one or more embryos. The generic 'ART' (assisted reproductive technology) refers to all types of laboratory-based assisted conception treatments including *in vitro* fertilization (IVF), intracytoplasmic sperm injection (ICSI), intrauterine insemination (IUI), and donor insemination (DI)

Epidemiology

Infertility affects about one couple in seven in the UK. The condition is becoming more common as women defer attempts to conceive until later in life. Obesity interferes with ovulation and sexually transmitted pelvic infections affect Fallopian tube and epididymal function (Hughes *et al.* 2007; ACOG 2008). The UK Human Fertilization and Embryology Authority (HFEA) recorded over 41 000 IVF cycles in 2006 which resulted in 9,600 births and nearly 12 000 babies (Table 12.19.1).

Table 12.19.1 shows the influence of the woman's age on her chances of a live birth following IVF. The national average of 31% chance of live birth after fresh embryo transfer for women under 35 is the highest seen and reflects improvements in laboratory and clinical practice. Embryos remaining after fresh transfer can be frozen to be thawed and replaced later, usually in a natural menstrual cycle, albeit with lower chances of live birth per transfer.

In the UK, IVF contributes about 1.4% of all births. This is a modest figure compared with many Western European countries: in Denmark 6% of births are a result of IVF treatment. The proportion is rising steadily and projections suggest that some European countries will see greater than 10% of all births resulting from IVF conception by 2020.

Currently, the proportion of UK twin pregnancies resulting from IVF is above 20%. The number of triplet births arising from IVF has fallen sharply since the introduction of a 'two embryo transfer' policy for women under 40. However, twin pregnancy also carries significant excess morbidity and mortality compared with singleton birth (see www.oneatatime.org.uk). Several Scandinavian countries, Belgium, and Denmark have reduced this proportion by promoting single embryo transfer (SET) (Sunde 2007), and HFEA has now initiated a semi-voluntary code for clinics in an effort to reduce the proportion of IVF twin births in the UK.

Pathology

The pathologies that cause infertility requiring IVF treatment are multiple. IVF was first developed as a treatment for tubal disease. Damage or blockage of the Fallopian tubes can be corrected surgically but restoration of tubal patency does not necessarily result in live birth. Damage to the microstructure of the tube (epithelial cilia and surrounding smooth muscle) may be permanent and frequently leads to failure of tubal transport with persistent infertility or ectopic pregnancy. IVF bypasses the tube, with collection of oocytes from the ovary and replacement of embryos into the uterine cavity. Since the first IVF birth 30 years ago, the technique has been widely applied to all causes of infertility. Introduction of intracytoplasmic sperm injection (ICSI) in the mid-1990s revolutionized treatment of male infertility. Couples with a male factor problem now have similar chances of a live birth compared to routine IVF. Anovulatory infertility resulting from polycystic ovary syndrome is best treated with simple ovulation induction with oral agents (Clomiphene citrate, aromatase inhibitors), laparoscopic ovarian drilling, or injectable gonadotropins. Polycystic ovary syndrome carries an increased risk of ovarian hyperstimulation syndrome (OHSS) after superovulation, which should be used only for resistant cases or where other factors are also involved. Unexplained infertility is also treated with IVF following a period of 'watchful waiting', usually of at least 3 years duration if the woman is under 35 years of age (Bhattacharya 2008).

Prognosis

The most important prognostic factor in IVF treatment is the age of the woman at the time of treatment. Those under 35 years have over 30% chance of live birth per cycle, rising to 50% if 'spare' embryos can be transferred later after freeze–thaw. At age 40, IVF carries a 10% chance of live birth and births after 45 are rare (HFEA 2008). The fall in the chances of a live birth with advancing female age results from poor ovarian response to superovulation, with fewer eggs being obtained and a decline in oocyte 'quality' (increasing rates of aneuploidy and probably also increasing cytoplasmic dysfunction). Older women frequently resort to treatment with oocytes donated by younger women, which carry the potential for pregnancy and aneuploidy risk of the donor's age rather than the recipient. However, older recipients of oocyte donation are at increased risk of pregnancy complications including pre-eclampsia, premature birth, and problems in labour.

Table 12.19.1 HFEA national data for IVF, 2006 (published October 2008) (with permission from HFEA www.hfea.gov.uk)

	Success rate %	Number of patients	Number of cycles	Number of births	Number of babies
All cycles	23.1%	33051	41827	9655	11884
Under 35	*29.0%*	*14103*	*17562*	*5089*	*6440*
Fresh cycles	24.4%	29304	33916	8280	10248
Under 35	*31.0%*	*12651*	*14337*	*4447*	*5660*
Frozen cycles	17.4%	6894	7911	175	1636
Under 35	*20.1%*	*2795*	*3189*	*642*	*780*

Ageing of the male partner seems to have less impact on IVF outcome, particularly since ICSI can be used to correct for sperm dysfunction. The presence of uterine abnormalities including fibroids and congenital abnormalities can adversely affect implantation, and ovarian endometriosis is also associated with a poorer outcome in age-matched studies. Hydrosalpynx, with resultant passage of tubal fluid into the endometrial cavity, reduces pregnancy chances and pre-IVF salpingectomy or tubal occlusion is widely performed in such cases (Johnson 2004).

Clinical approach

The principle of IVF is simple. Eggs and sperm are mixed in the laboratory and the resultant embryos returned to the uterine cavity at the correct stage of the cycle. However, the complexity of practice has increased dramatically over the last two decades and ART is one of the most striking examples of successful collaboration between science and medicine.

The chances of obtaining good-quality embryos are increased if the laboratory has a number of oocytes to work with. Hence, from the 1980s onwards IVF treatment has started with superovulation, the use of injectable gonadotropins (recombinant FSH or urinary derived FSH or FSH/LH combinations) to induce multiple follicle development in the ovaries. Follicle growth is monitored by transvaginal ultrasound to count and measure the follicles. A 'mature' follicle secretes significant amounts of oestradiol into the circulation, providing a second marker of follicle growth and development. Left unchecked, rising concentrations of oestradiol would initiate an LH surge with ovulation and loss of the cohort of oocytes. Hence the practice of superovulation is combined with use of a gonadotropin-releasing hormone (GnRH) agonist or antagonist, also given by injection or, in the case of the GnRH agonist, intranasally. GnRH agonists cause an initial 'flare' in concentration of LH and FSH in serum, followed by pituitary receptor blockade and 'downregulation' of LH and FSH, thereby preventing an endogenous LH surge. The widely used 'long protocol' involves initiation of GnRH agonist in the mid-luteal phase of the cycle preceding the start of FSH superovulation. The woman will experience 2 weeks of menopausal symptoms in this period, which is followed by an ultrasound and hormonal check of downregulation (quiescent ovaries and thin endometrium on scan, suppressed concentrations of oestradiol, LH, and FSH in serum).

Over the last decade, GnRH antagonists have been introduced as an alternative to the long protocol. They act with immediate inhibition and can therefore be used in parallel with FSH superovulation without the preliminary period of downregulation. This makes the treatment cycle shorter and less unpleasant, reduces the risk of ovarian hyperstimulation, and is more cost effective than the long protocol, a process sometimes termed 'mild' IVF (Heijnen 2007).

Once ultrasound and endocrine criteria for follicle maturation have been met (usually at least two follicles of greater than 16 mm diameter), a single injection of human chorionic gonadotropin (hCG) is given. This is a cheap and simple surrogate for LH, and initiates final oocyte and follicular maturation with resumption of oocyte meiosis, expulsion of the first polar body, and progesterone synthesis by the granulosa cells. Ovulation will occur approximately 40 hours later, so oocyte collection is timed 34–36 hours after hCG administration.

In the early days of IVF, oocytes were collected laparoscopically, with the risks and organizational drawbacks of general anaesthesia and surgery. Transvaginal ultrasound-guided needle aspiration of follicles is a simpler and safer procedure, often performed with sedation and analgesia. Many units will encourage the husband/ partner to be present for egg collection. Each follicle is aspirated in turn, with the follicular fluid being passed to the embryologist, who identifies the oocyte and transfers it into culture medium using a binocular microscope. Oocyte collection takes between 15 and 45 minutes depending on the number of follicles harvested. The patient can usually return home a few hours after the procedure.

Following oocyte collection, the male partner with normal sperm parameters will produce a semen sample by masturbation. Men who do not ejaculate sperm because of previous vasectomy or other blockage to the vas or epididymis, or due to such poor spermatogenesis that sperm can only be obtained by biopsy, will need to undergo percutaneous epididymal and/or testicular biopsies. Immediate microscopy will confirm the presence of sperm in the samples. Next the IVF is performed. The oocyte is stripped of its investment of cumulus cells and exposed *in vitro* to approximately 50 000 washed sperm, allowing normal fertilization. For couples with suboptimal sperm parameters, or who have only epididymal or testicular sperm available, the ICSI procedure is performed in which a single sperm is injected into each oocyte.

Idiopathic oligospermia or azoospermia requires investigation before sperm can be used for ICSI. Male carriers of genes for cystic fibrosis may have congenital absence of the vas deferens, leading to azoospermia, and those with karyotypic abnormalities that may produce problems in their offspring may have severe oligospermia. Both conditions should be routinely screened for before IVF/ICSI is offered. Oligo or azoospermic men may also have microdeletions on the Y chromosome. Some clinics offer screening for these deletions, although they do not appear to have implications for the health of the man or his male child, apart from the risk of inheritance of the defect in spermatogenesis. Once this is explained, few patients opt for the costly testing involved in confirming or excluding this diagnosis.

One of the major areas of improvement in quality of ART over the last decade has been in the laboratory handling of gametes and embryos. Stringent incubation conditions coupled with culture media carefully designed to meet the changing metabolic needs of the early embryo as its genome is activated, have played a large part in the improvement in success rates of IVF. Embryos are generally cultured for between 2 and 5 days following oocyte collection. Culture to the blastocyst stage provides considerably more information on the morphology of the embryo, allowing improved selection of those most likely to implant after transfer to the endometrial cavity. However, such prolonged culture adds to the cost of the procedure and some women who would have had embryos for transfer on day 2 or 3 are disappointed when none survive to day 5. The optimal strategy remains a topic for debate, although the move to SET makes correct embryo selection critically important and more clinics in the UK are moving to blastocyst culture for the younger patient as a prelude to SET.

Embryo transfer is usually a straightforward procedure involving passage of a Cusco's speculum, gentle cleansing of the cervix with saline or culture medium, and transfer of the embryo(s) into the uterine cavity with a flexible catheter. This is often done under ultrasound guidance, with the optimum placement of the catheter tip approximately 1 cm from the fundus. Difficult embryo transfers are less likely to result in pregnancy: a fall in the temperature of embryos seems particularly detrimental, so it is critical to undertake a smooth and timely embryo transfer.

Once embryos have been transferred the couple have to wait for 2 weeks to know whether implantation has occurred. The luteal phase of the cycle is supported with progestagens, given vaginally or by injection. Randomized controlled trials have shown the superiority of progestagens over placebo but the optimum route and dose is not determined. Pregnancy testing is carried out by measuring hCG in a serum sample. A positive test will be repeated 7 days later, followed by early pregnancy transvaginal scan after a further week in order to detect miscarriage (blighted ovum) or ectopic pregnancy as soon as possible. Approximately 20% of IVF pregnancies will miscarry, more frequently if the woman is older, with ectopic pregnancy rates of up to 5% depending on the cause of the infertility. Both require medical intervention, which should be organized by the IVF clinic.

Complications

IVF pregnancies have lost some of their high-risk status as the numbers of women pregnant after IVF has risen. The majority of the problems in pregnancy result from the consequences of multiple pregnancy rather than from IVF treatment per se (El-Toukhy 2006). However, even IVF singleton pregnancies end slightly earlier and produce babies that are slightly lighter than matched spontaneously conceived children. Children born after ICSI appear to have a slightly higher risk of congenital malformations, particularly of the urogenital system, than do IVF or spontaneously conceived children, and some studies have raised anxiety about the frequency of disorders of imprinting after ICSI. These statistics do not mean that the technologies should be abandoned, rather that ART should only be used when necessary and not as a lifestyle choice or substitute for other simpler and more natural approaches to infertility.

The processes of superovulation, oocyte collection, and embryo transfer are generally accepted as low risk when carried out in a reputable clinic. However, some patients, particularly younger women with polycystic ovaries, are at risk of developing OHSS. This iatrogenic condition is seen in its severe form in 1–2% of IVF treatment cycles. Serious morbidities including cerebrovascular thrombosis, and renal and pulmonary failure, and some deaths have been reported. The condition results from excessively high secretion of oestrogens and of vasoactive molecules, including vascular endothelial growth factor, leading to separation of the capillary endothelial cells. Leakage of plasma water and small molecules occurs, leading first to ascites and later to pleural and pericardial effusions. At the same time the intravascular compartment is fluid depleted, with haemoconcentration and risk of thrombotic phenomena occurring. Increased intra-abdominal pressure together with intravascular dehydration results in prerenal failure and multi-organ involvement with adult respiratory distress syndrome and cardiac failure can occur (RCOG).

The best form of 'cure' is prevention. Cancellation of the treatment cycle by withholding hCG injection if an excessive number of follicles are seen on ultrasound will avoid the syndrome developing, but at the cost of an abandoned cycle. The condition worsens with further hCG stimulation so elective cryopreservation of all embryos rather than fresh embryo transfer is often used to avoid pregnancy with rising hCG and worsening of the condition. Many specific treatments have been tried without much success, and randomized trials are difficult to perform given the relative rarity of the disorder. Excessive rehydration with crystalloids should be avoided, as should diuretics. OHSS is best managed by the Reproductive Medicine team, who should maintain overall charge of clinical decisions even if the patient requires intensive care. A conservative approach with anticoagulation, careful monitoring and abdominal paracentesis, if excessive ascites develops is usually effective. Surgery should be avoided if possible as the ovaries may be hyperaemic and uncontrollable bleeding can occur.

Adjuncts to IVF

IVF allows access to embryonic DNA. Microbiopsy of one or two cells from an eight-cell embryo seems harmless. Each embryonic cell is toti-potent at this early stage and there does not seem to be any developmental detriment after biopsy. The cells can be probed with PCR or FISH (fluorescence in situ hybridization) or CGH (comparative genomic hybridization) to detect carriage of chromosomal or genetic disorders. This technique of pre-implantation genetic diagnosis has allowed families with a child affected by a serious genetic disorder such as Duchenne's muscular dystrophy or thalassaemia major to select unaffected embryos for their subsequent child. This is clearly preferable to prenatal diagnosis followed by termination of pregnancy, although the relatively low chances of pregnancy after IVF can result in a requirement for several treatment cycles before a healthy pregnancy is established. More and more non-infertile couples are likely to use IVF to access embryonic DNA in the future. New uses of IVF technology include the conception of a 'saviour sibling': an HLA matched healthy child who can act as a donor of umbilical cord stem cells for transplantation to an older affected brother or sister (Sermon 2004).

Techniques for cryopreservation of embryos and gametes have also improved dramatically over the past decade. Embryo freezing gives a second chance at pregnancy after a fresh embryo transfer cycle and can also be used to preserve fertility for young women before gonadotoxic chemotherapy or radiotherapy. Embryos can be replaced some years later after successful but sterilizing treatment is completed. However, embryo freezing requires a stable relationship with the future father of the child, and many women are not yet at this stage of life when cancer occurs. Oocyte vitrification, ultrarapid freezing with cryopreservation by glassification, has improved success rates of oocyte freezing. The frozen eggs can be thawed and fertilized by ICSI years later once treatment is complete and a stable relationship established. This is a new technique and data on effectiveness and safety are lacking. Some clinics are also offering oocyte vitrification to healthy women who wish to delay motherhood. A recent statement by the Royal College of Obstetricians and Gynaecologists has warned of the hazards of this approach: there is no guarantee that the method will work and the safety to offspring remains to be proven.

Regulation

HFEA was established following the 1984 Warnock Report. The Committee recommended a regulatory framework for this area of scientific and medical practice. It recognized the moral and the personal dimensions of advances in IVF technology and Parliament passed the Human Fertilization and Embryology Act in 1990.

The HFEA acts as regulator to provide key assurances, publishing a Code of Practice which sets out the standards for all clinics to ensure they are following both HFEA policy and the law (see below).

Functions of the HFEA

- To license and monitor fertility clinics that carry out IVF and donor insemination
- To license and monitor clinics undertaking human embryo research
- To license and monitor the storage of gametes and embryos
- To produce a Code of Practice which gives guidelines to clinics about the proper conduct of HFEA licensed activities
- To maintain a formal register of information about donors, fertility treatments and children born as a result of those treatments
- To provide relevant advice and information to patients, donors and clinics
- To review information about human embryos, the provision of treatment services and activities governed by the HFE Act.
- To monitor any subsequent developments in this area and where appropriate, advise the Secretary of State for Health on developments in these fields

Further reading

American College of Obstetricians and Gynecologists (ACOG) (The Committee on Gynecologic Practice) and the American Society for Reproductive Medicine (Practice Committee). Age-related fertility decline: a committee opinion. Fertil Steril 2008;90:486–7.

Bhattacharya S, Harrild K, Mollison J, et al. Clomifene citrate or unstimulated intrauterine insemination compared with expectant management for unexplained infertility: pragmatic randomised controlled trial. BMJ 2008;337:a716.

El-Toukhy T, Khalaf Y, Braude P. IVF results: optimize not maximize. Am J Obstet Gynecol 2006;194:322–31.

Heijnen EM, Eijkemans MJ, De Klerk C, et al. A mild treatment strategy for in-vitro fertilisation: a randomised non-inferiority trial. Lancet 2007;369:743–9.

HFEA. A long term analysis of the HFEA register data 1991–2006. London: HFEA 2008.

Hughes G, Simms I, Leong G. Data from UK genitourinary medicine clinics, 2006: a mixed picture. Sex Transm Infect 2007;83:433–5.

Johnson NP, Mak W, Sowter MC. Surgical treatment for tubal disease in women due to undergo in vitro fertilisation. Cochrane Database Syst Rev 2004;(3):CD002125. Review.

Royal College of Obstetricians and Gynaecologists (RCOG). The management of ovarian hyperstimulation syndrome Green Top Guideline number 6. London: RCOG.

Sermon K, Van Steirteghem A, Liebaers I. Preimplantation genetic diagnosis. Lancet 2004 15;363:1633–41.

Sunde A. Significant reduction of twins with single embryo transfer in IVF. Reprod Biomed Online 2007;15(Suppl 3):28–34.

Internet resources

www.hfea.gov.uk
www.oneatatime.org.uk
www.nice.org.uk
www.basw.co.uk/progar
www.progress.org.uk
www.cancerbackup.org.uk

Patient resources

www.hfea.gov.uk
www.oneatatime.org.uk
www.acebabes.co.uk
www.bica.net (British Infertility Counselling Association)
www.surrogacy.org.uk (Childlessness Overcome through Surrogacy)
www.daisynetwork.org.uk (Premature menopause support group)
www.dcnetwork.org (donor conception support group)
www.infertilitynetworkuk.com
www.miscarriageassociation.org.uk
www.multiplebirths.org.uk
www.endo.org.uk (endometriosis support group)
www.ngdt.co.uk (National Gamete Donation Trust)
www.ukdonorlink.org.uk
www.verity-pcos.org.uk

In vitro oocyte maturation

Definition

In vitro maturation (IVM) refers to a form of assisted reproductive technology. The technique is similar to *in vitro* fertilization (IVF) in many aspects. The major difference is the absence of ovarian stimulation, with exogenous gonadotropins and oocytes being collected before they attain full maturity. The immature oocytes are cultured in the embryology laboratory until they complete the maturation process, i.e. '*in vitro* maturation', and become amenable to fertilization or to cryopreservation. Upon fertilization of either fresh or frozen–thawed oocytes, the resultant embryos are transferred.

Epidemiology

IVM can, in theory, be used to treat any woman who is a candidate for IVF. Women with polycystic ovaries (PCO) or polycystic ovarian syndrome (PCOS) represent the group who achieve the highest pregnancy rates using this method, because IVM pregnancy rates correlate with the number of antral follicles and eggs collected. IVM has therefore become an established treatment for this group of patients. More recently, the indications have been extended to poor responders to ovarian stimulation for IVF or oocyte donors. IVM is also considered as an innovative fertility preservation method for patients with various diseases that preclude treatment with conventional IVF. However, compared with widespread application of IVF, IVM is still practised by relatively few clinics worldwide.

Technique

The IVM technique aims to make use of the multiple immature oocytes that already exist in the ovaries of a reproductive age woman. Early in the follicular phase, these immature oocytes are harboured in small antral follicles, and are arrested at the prophase stage of the first meiotic division. These oocytes are shown to resume meiosis upon removal from the follicle, have the capacity to complete meiotic division, and can be fertilized *in vitro*. More than 80% of oocytes were reported to resume meiosis independent of the day of the menstrual cycle and gonadotropin support in IVM culture medium.

In fact, the first pregnancy and live birth from *in vitro* matured oocytes in humans was reported in the context of a stimulated IVF cycle. However, recovery of mature oocytes following ovarian stimulation with gonadotropins and gonadotropin-releasing hormone analogues had already become the method of choice, and IVM did not attract much attention until 1991, when Cha and colleagues reported collecting immature oocytes from women undergoing gynecological surgery, fertilizing these donated oocytes following IVM and transferring the resulting embryos to a recipient woman with premature ovarian failure. The recipient delivered healthy triplet girls. Three years later, the collection of immature oocytes from women with PCOS was reported. The immature oocytes collected were matured *in vitro* with gonadotropin-enriched medium, then fertilized, and a healthy live birth following transfer of resultant embryos was reported. Currently pregnancy rates are above 30% per cycle in appropriately selected patient groups.

Indications

IVM has become an established treatment option for women with PCO or PCOS who need antiretroviral therapy (ART). Young women with PCO seem to be the best candidates for IVM treatment. Pregnancy rates seem to be significantly higher when an *in vivo* matured oocyte has been collected. However, the clinical application of IVM technology is not limited to these women alone, and can be extended to benefit other patient populations.

Over-responders to gonadotropin stimulation

IVM combined with IVF can be a valid option for patients who demonstrate an over-response to COS and are considered to be at risk of varian hyperstimulation Syndrome (OHSS) during an already started IVF cycle. Although several strategies are available for the prevention of OHSS, the only method to prevent it completely is to avoid the injection of human chorionic gonadotropin (hCG) for final oocyte maturation. However, this strategy requires cancellation of the treatment cycle, leading to frustration for both the patient and the physician. Giving the hCG injection when the leading follicle size is 12–14 mm, before the conventional hCG criteria for IVF is met, followed by oocyte collection 36–38 hours later may prove to be an effective strategy. It is possible to collect some mature oocytes together with immature oocytes at this stage of follicle development. Satisfactory high pregnancy and low OHSS rates in such women has been achieved with this strategy.

Poor responders to gonadotropin stimulation

The benefit of ovarian stimulation is the availability of a higher number of mature oocytes that can be fertilized *in vitro*, and the success of conventional IVF depends on, among other factors, the response to ovarian stimulation with exogenous gonadotropins. Unfortunately, not all women respond similarly to gonadotropin stimulation, and some fail to develop a reasonable number of mature follicles in stimulated IVF cycles. The most common cause of poor response seems to be the age-related decline in ovarian reserve, but it also occurs in some younger women. Numerous stimulation protocols have been designed to increase ovarian responsiveness. However, none has proven to provide a significant improvement over others. Given the fact that gonadotropin stimulation fails to provide the desired number of *in vivo* matured oocytes in such women, IVM in an unstimulated cycle or combined with natural-cycle IVF may provide a reasonable option.

Oocyte donation

Oocyte donation has become a recognized treatment option for women with severely decreased ovarian reserve, women of advanced reproductive age, women affected by/carriers of certain genetic disorders, women who repeatedly have poor oocyte and/or embryo quality, or multiple unexplained failed treatment cycles.

Oocyte donors are usually young women with high ovarian reserve. This places them at higher risk of early OHSS in stimulated IVF cycles. Besides the risk of OHSS, the inconvenience of the numerous injections required and the concern over the theoretical risk of cancer associated with repeated use of ovulation induction drugs are factors that may cause reluctance on the part of some potential oocyte donors. IVM can become the method of choice for oocyte donation cycles as young women with high antral follicle counts comprise the best candidates for IVM and yield good pregnancy rates. Avoiding ovarian stimulation may decrease the risks and inconvenience for oocyte donors. Such an approach may also serve to increase the availability of altruistic oocyte donors in countries where donation for a fee is not allowed.

Fertility preservation

Improvements in both diagnosis and treatment of cancer have led to an increase in numbers of cancer survivors. However, certain therapeutic agents bear the potential to permanently damage these prepubertal or reproductive age women's gonads. Chemotherapy for non-oncological conditions such as systemic lupus erythematosus, or other autoimmune disorders, surgery for endometriosis and non-malignant ovarian neoplasms, and genetic disorders such as Turner's syndrome and fragile X premutation are among other factors that can cause irreversible gonadal damage and seriously decrease future fertility potential.

The American Society of Clinical Oncology and American Society of Reproductive Medicine have endorsed IVF and embryo cryopreservation (EC) as the only methods of female fertility preservation. However, conventional IVF and embryo cryopreservation requires 2–5 weeks to complete, produces relatively high oestradiol levels, which may be deleterious in certain hormone-sensitive malignancies, and requires a male partner.

IVM expands the fertility preservation options for women who are not candidates for IVF-EC for various medical and social reasons. Women with hormone-sensitive tumours may undergo immature oocyte collection and cryopreserve resultant embryos.

IVM not only eliminates the risks and cost associated with gonadotropins but it also enables oocyte retrieval at any phase of the menstrual cycle and completion of the fertility preservation procedure in 2–10 days, preventing a delay in treatment of the primary disease.

For patients without a male partner, oocyte cryopreservation represents a less invasive option than ovarian tissue cryopreservation. Recent advances in vitrification techniques have markedly improved the efficacy of oocyte cryopreservation. Immature oocytes can also be harvested from ovarian biopsy specimens and can be vitrified following IVM. A novel fertility preservation strategy involves immature oocyte retrieval in an unstimulated menstrual cycle or from ovarian tissue biopsies, followed by IVM and oocyte vitrification or EC.

In conclusion, IVM combined with embryo or oocyte vitrification provides previously unavailable options for some patients and improves the services provided by a fertility preservation programme. Primary-care physicians and oncologists need to be made aware of the fertility preservation options in order to provide early discussion with their patients, followed by referral, if desired, to an ART centre that offers the full range of fertility preservation options.

Prognosis

Pregnancy rates

The most important determinants of pregnancy following an IVM cycle are the female age and the number of oocytes collected. Young women with PCO seem to be the best candidates for IVM treatment. In 2007, we achieved an embryo implantation rate of 15% and a clinical pregnancy rate per embryo transfer (CPR) of 36.7% in women younger than 35 years of age. However, for women aged between 35 and 40 years, implantation and CPR were 10.1% and 29.3%, respectively, in the same period. Pregnancy rates seem to be significantly higher when an *in vivo* matured oocyte has been collected. In 2009, we achieved a >50% clinical pregnancy rate in such cycles in young women with PCO. The two major changes in our protocols were delaying hCG administration until the leading follicle was 10–12 mm in size and endometrial thickness was ≥6 mm, and performing oocyte collection 38 hours after hCG injection.

Pregnancy losses

In a retrospective analysis of 1581 women who had a positive pregnancy test following ART with IVM, IVF, or ICSI in our unit during a 5-year period, biochemical pregnancy loss rates were similar among these patients (17.5% for IVM pregnancies, 17% for IVF, and 18% for ICSI pregnancies, p = 0.08). However, the clinical miscarriage rate was significantly higher in IVM pregnancies (25.3%) than in IVF (15.7%) and ICSI (12.6%) pregnancies (p <0.01). It is known that women with PCOS have higher miscarriage rates, regardless of the method of conception. Miscarriage rates reaching 25% after ovulation induction, and ranging from 25% to 37% following IVF, have been reported in such women. Therefore, the explanation of the observed higher miscarriage rate in the IVM group can be the higher incidence of PCOS in these patients. Indeed, although only 8% and <1% of women in the IVF and ICSI groups had PCOS, respectively, the incidence of PCOS in the IVM group was 80%. Critically, miscarriage rates were not different between IVM and IVF pregnancies among women with PCOS, 24.5% versus 22.8%, respectively.

Obstetric outcome

In a study comparing obstetric outcomes of pregnancies following ART and with those of spontaneous conceptions the incidence of multiple or high-order multiple pregnancies were similar among IVM (21% and 5%), IVF (20% and 3%), and ICSI (17% and 3%) pregnancies. Caesarean delivery rates of ART pregnancies were higher than spontaneous conceptions, even after exclusion of multiple pregnancies. However, the incidence of Caesarean delivery was similar among singleton pregnancies conceived with different treatments (IVM 39%, IVF 36%, and ICSI 36%). Likewise, the mean birthweights of all infants conceived with ART were similar among all ART groups, but lower than those of spontaneous conceptions. The proportion of low birthweight and very low birthweight infants was similar across ART children. Apgar scores at 1 and 5 minutes, the proportion of infants with an Apgar score ≤6 at 1 and 5 minutes, and the incidence of acidosis were all similar among IVM, IVF, ICSI, or spontaneous conception deliveries.

Congenital abnormalities, physical, and neuromotor development

Since the early days of IVF treatment, concerns have been expressed regarding the effects of *in vitro* gamete and embryo culture on the wellbeing of resultant children. Currently available data suggest an increase in the prevalence of major congenital malformations, chromosomal anomalies, and imprinting disorders in children born following AR. However, whether infertility *per se* or treatment of it is the reason for higher incidence is controversial. In a series of 55 IVM newborns, there were only two major congenital abnormalities, one case of ventriculoseptal defect, and one of omphalocele. Compared with spontaneous conceptions, the observed odds ratios (ORs) for any congenital abnormality were 1.42 (95% CI 0.52–3.91) for IVM, 1.21 (95% CI 0.63–2.32) for IVF, and 1.69 (95% CI 0.88–3.26) for ICSI. None of these were statistically significant. Interestingly, the OR was lower for IVM than for ICSI, even though ICSI was used for all IVM cases. This provides indirect evidence that the reported higher congenital abnormality rate with ICSI is due to poor sperm per se, because ICSI with normal sperm did not increase the odds of congenital abnormality to the same extent.

In a study that analysed the chromosomal constitution and mental development of 21 children born after IVM and compared these with 21 spontaneously conceived children, all of the IVM children were found to have normal karyotype and mean developmental index score, similar to controls. Another study of 46 IVM babies born to 40 women reported similar findings. The physical growth of IVM children also seems to be similar to that of spontaneously conceived children.

In summary, currently available data seem reassuring and do not suggest an increased risk of congenital malformations, physical or neurological developmental delay in IVM children.

Clinical approach

Monitoring and management of an IVM cycle

Monitoring starts with a baseline scan performed in the early follicular phase of the menstrual cycle, preferably between days 2 and 5 of a natural menstrual cycle, or a withdrawal bleed, induced with progesterone administration in amenorrheic women. The number and size of the antral follicles and endometrial texture and thickness are recorded. The uterus and ovaries are examined for any abnormalities. The antral follicle count seems to be the single most important predictor of the number of retrievable oocytes. A second scan is performed about a week later and monitoring is continued until the largest follicle has reached 10–12 mm in diameter and the endometrial thickness is at least 6 mm. At this stage, oocytes can be collected, preferably 38 hours after a single dose of hCG injection.

The decision regarding timing of oocyte retrieval requires that both the follicle size and the endometrial thickness be taken into consideration. Usually 10–14 mm is considered the optimal size for the leading follicle on the day of oocyte collection (7–12 mm on the day of hCG administration in hCG-primed cycles). However, if the endometrial thickness is <6 mm on the day of the second scan, hCG administration/oocyte collection can be delayed. Meanwhile, either oestrogen or gonadotropins can be administered to stimulate endometrial growth, depending on the size of the leading follicle. When the leading follicle is also small a short course of gonadotropins is preferred over oestrogen as the former stimulates the growth of both follicles and the endometrium. On the other hand, when the leading follicle is close to meeting the collection criteria, oestrogen is preferred as it slows down follicular growth while stimulating endometrial proliferation.

Oocyte collection procedure

The principles of transvaginal ultrasound-guided oocyte retrieval for IVM are the same as those for IVF oocyte collection with a few modifications in both the technique and the equipment. Most patients easily tolerate the procedure under conscious sedation with intravenous midazolam and

fentanyl. Paracervical block is achieved with 1% bupivacain injection after cleaning the vagina with sterile saline. As the follicles are smaller than mature follicles aspirated in IVF cycles, a smaller gauge needle (19–20G) with a shorter bevel is used. The aspiration pressure is set at 75–80 mmHg, approximately half the conventional IVF aspiration pressure, in order to minimize the risk of oocyte denudation during aspiration. This precaution is carried out because immature oocytes need the presence of surrounding granulosa cells during the nuclear maturation process. The fine-bore needle may be blocked frequently with blood-stained aspirate and ovarian stroma. Therefore, multiple punctures are often needed and flushing the needle lumen with heparinized saline between punctures is required. Sometimes external abdominal pressure may be required to fix the mobile ovaries during collection. Patients with difficult-to-reach ovaries or poor pain control may do better under limited general anaesthesia with propofol.

Embryology laboratory procedures

Similar to IVF, the follicular aspirate is first examined under a stereomicroscope to identify cumulus–oocyte complexes (COCs). Since the identification of small immature oocytes is more difficult, they can be overlooked with the conventional technique. Therefore, the follicular aspirate is filtered through a nylon mesh strainer with 70 μm pores after removal of initially identified COCs. The filtered aspirate can be re-examined after washing with HEPES buffered human serum albumin-containing medium. The maturation status of the oocytes is assessed immediately after collection; a mature oocyte at the meiosis II stage can be identified by the presence of the first polar body in the perivitelline space. The cytoplasm of immature oocytes is examined for the presence of a germinal vesicle (GV). An oocyte is defined as being at the germinal-vesicle breakdown stage if no GV can be identified in the absence of a polar body.

Oocytes reaching the MII stage on the day of collection are denuded and fertilized together with any in vivo matured oocytes, while immature oocytes are cultured in IVM medium and periodically assessed for maturation status. They are denuded and fertilized upon completion of nuclear maturation.

Although similar implantation and pregnancy rates have been reported following fertilization of in vitro matured oocytes with ICSI or IVF, ICSI has been commonly practised in IVM cycles because of a theoretical risk of zonal hardening during the in vitro culture period. Another reason for preferring ICSI over IVF in IVM cycles is some immature oocytes being denuded for assessment of polar-body extrusion. Oocytes devoid of cumulus cells can have decreased chemotactic potential for sperm in the medium. The preferred time for ICSI is 2–4 hours after polar-body extrusion.

Culture conditions for fertilized oocytes and cleavage stage embryos derived from in vitro matured oocytes are the same as those in IVF cycles. Embryo development and quality are similarly assessed, based on the number of blastomeres and the amount of anuclear fragments.

Embryo transfer

The timing of embryo transfer and the number of embryos to be transferred are dictated by the number and quality of available embryos. Embryo transfer is commonly performed on the third day after oocyte collection. Growth and quality of available embryos are evaluated with regard to fertilization time of each embryo. A group of best embryos for days is transferred using essentially the same technique as that employed in IVF cycles. In general, embryo implantation rates in IVM cycles are lower than in IVF cycles. Therefore, on average, one or two more embryos are transferred in order to maintain similar pregnancy rates. However, as expected, this fact does not seem to increase multiple pregnancy rates after IVM.

High implantation and pregnancy rates have been achieved by performing blastocyst transfers in selected IVM patients. Assisted hatching is commonly employed before embryo transfer because of the above-mentioned concerns about zonal hardening.

Luteal-phase support

The luteal-phase support protocol employed in our IVM programme includes 50 mg/day i,m. progesterone injections and oestradiol valerate 6 mg/day po in three divided doses. Luteal-phase support is continued until completion of the first trimester for pregnant patients.

Further reading

Ao A, Jin S, Rao D, Son WY, Chian RC, Tan SL. First successful pregnancy outcome after preimplantation genetic diagnosis for aneuploidy screening in embryos generated from natural-cycle in vitro fertilization combined with an in vitro maturation procedure. Fertil Steril 2006;85:1510 e9–11.

Buckett WM, Chian RC, Dean NL, et al. Pregnancy loss in pregnancies conceived after in vitro oocyte maturation, conventional in vitro fertilization, and intracytoplasmic sperm injection. Fertil Steril 2008;90:546–50.

Buckett WM, Chian RC, Holzer H, et al. Obstetric outcomes and congenital abnormalities after in vitro maturation, in vitro fertilization, and intracytoplasmic sperm injection. Obstet Gynecol 2007;110:885–91.

Cha KY, Koo JJ, Ko JJ, et al. Pregnancy after in vitro fertilization of human follicular oocytes collected from nonstimulated cycles, their culture in vitro and their transfer in a donor oocyte program, Fertil Steril 1991; 55: 109–13.

Chian RC, Buckett WM, Abdul Jalil AK, et al. Natural-cycle in vitro fertilization combined with in vitro maturation of immature oocytes is a potential approach in infertility treatment. Fertil Steril 2004;82:1675–8.

Chian RC, Buckett WM, Tulandi T, Tan SL. Prospective randomized study of human chorionic gonadotrophin priming before immature oocyte retrieval from unstimulated women with polycystic ovarian syndrome. Hum Reprod 2000;15:165–70.

Chian RC, Gulekli B, Buckett WM, Tan SL. Priming with human chorionic gonadotropin before retrieval of immature oocytes in women with infertility due to the polycystic ovary syndrome. N Engl J Med 1999;341: 1624–1626.

Chian RC, Huang JY, Gilbert L, et al. Obstetric outcomes following vitrification of in vitro and in vivo matured oocytes. Fertil Steril 2009;91:2391–8.

Child TJ, Gulekli B, Chian RC, Abdul-Jalil AK, Tan SL. In-Vitro Maturation (IVM) of Oocytes from Unstimulated Normal Ovaries of Women with a Previous Poor Response to IVF. Fertility and sterility 2000;74:S45-S.

Demirtas E, Elizur SE, Holzer H, et al. Immature oocyte retrieval in the luteal phase to preserve fertility in cancer patients. Reprod Biomed Online 2008;17:520–3.

Elizur SE, Son WY, Yap R, et al. Comparison of low-dose human menopausal gonadotropin and micronized 17beta-estradiol supplementation in in vitro maturation cycles with thin endometrial lining. Fertil Steril 2009;92:907–12.

Holzer H, Scharf E, Chian RC, Demirtas E, Buckett W, Tan SL. In vitro maturation of oocytes collected from unstimulated ovaries for oocyte donation. Fertil Steril 2007;88:62–7.

Huang JY, Buckett WM, Gilbert L, Tan SL, Chian RC. Retrieval of immature oocytes followed by in vitro maturation and vitrification: a case report on a new strategy of fertility preservation in women with borderline ovarian malignancy. Gynecol Oncol 2007;105:542–4.

Huang JY, Tulandi T, Holzer H, et al. Cryopreservation of ovarian tissue and in vitro matured oocytes in a female with mosaic Turner syndrome: Case Report. Hum Reprod 2008;23:336–9.

Huang JY, Tulandi T, Holzer H, et al. Combining ovarian tissue cryobanking with retrieval of immature oocytes followed by in vitro maturation and vitrification: an additional strategy of fertility preservation. Fertil Steril 2008;89:567–72.

Shu-Chi M, Jiann-Loung H, Yu-Hung L, et al. Growth and development of children conceived by in-vitro maturation of human oocytes. Early Hum Dev 2006;82:677–82.

Soderstrom-Anttila V, Makinen S, Tuuri T, Suikkari AM. Favourable pregnancy results with insemination of in vitro matured oocytes from unstimulated patients. Hum Reprod 2005;20:1534–40.

Soderstrom-Anttila V, Salokorpi T, Pihlaja M, et al. Obstetric and perinatal outcome and preliminary results of development of children born after in vitro maturation of oocytes. Hum Reprod 2006;21:1508–13.

Son WY, Chung JT, Demirtas E, et al. Comparison of in-vitro maturation cycles with and without in-vivo matured oocytes retrieved. Reprod Biomed Online 2008;17:59–67.

Son WY, Chung JT, Herrero B, et al. Selection of the optimal day for oocyte retrieval based on the diameter of the dominant follicle in hCG-primed in vitro maturation cycles. Hum Reprod 2008;23:2680–5.

Tan SL, Child TJ, Gulekli B. In vitro maturation and fertilization of oocytes from unstimulated ovaries; predicting the number of immature oocytes retrieved by early follicular phase ultrasonography. Am J Obst Gynecol 2002;186:684–9.

Tan SL, Chian RC, Buckett WM (eds). *In vitro maturation of human oocytes: basic science to clinical applications.* Informa Healthcare Books 2006.

Internet resources

www.mcgillivf.com
www.ivf-worldwide.com

Malformations of the genital tract

Background

The internal female genital tract develops from the two paramesonephric (Müllerian) ducts, whose caudal ends grow medially and fuse in the midline by the eighth week of embryonic life to form the uterovaginal primordium. The septum uniting the two ducts gradually regresses, leading to the formation of the uterine body and cervix and the upper part of the vagina. As the uterovaginal primordium reaches the urogenital sinus, it triggers the formation of two sino-vaginal bulbs. Their fusion forms a solid vaginal plate, which canalizes to form the vaginal lumen (Acien 1992).

Anomalies of the genital tract can occur as a result of any of the following events:

- incomplete development of a Müllerian duct: uterine agenesis, unicornuate uterus
- incomplete fusion of the paramesonephric ducts: uterus didelphys, bicornuate uterus
- failure of regression of the midline septum: septate uterus
- incomplete canalization of the vaginal plate: transverse vaginal septum, vaginal agenesis (Grimbizis et al. 2001).

Clinical approach

History: key points

- Normal development of secondary sexual characteristics.
- Primary amenorrhoea, dysmenorrhoea or cyclical pelvic pain.

Examination: key points

- Abdominal palpation may reveal a pelvic mass.
- Perineal examination to assess the presence of the vagina and its length.

Special investigations

- Magnetic resonance imaging (MRI)
- Three-dimensional ultrasound
- Intravenous urogram (IVU) to identify any associated renal anomalies
- Diagnostic laparoscopy/hysteroscopy.

Vaginal anomalies

Imperforate hymen

The hymen is the embryological remnant of a septum that forms between the sinovaginal bulbs and the urogenital sinus. The septum normally perforates late in fetal life to allow the passage of mucous and blood during menstruation. It is estimated that in 1 in 1000 females, the septum remains imperforate. This is typically an isolated anomaly, which is not associated with any other Müllerian malformations.

Presentation is usually around the time of menarche, when menstrual flow accumulates above the obstruction and leads to the formation of haematocolpos and haematometra. Cyclical pain around the time of menstruation is followed by constant pain or urinary retention as the vagina becomes more distended with menstrual blood.

A pelvic mass may be palpated abdominally, or demonstrated on ultrasound scan or MRI. This usually represents the distended vagina, which pushes the uterus upwards. On inspection of the perineum a bulging vaginal membrane of bluish hue may be visible.

Treatment consists of a cruciate incision of the membrane and excision of hymenal tissue to allow the menstrual blood to drain.

In rarer cases, an imperforate hymen may become apparent at birth, as discharge and secretions accumulate above the obstruction, leading to the formation of a mucocolpos.

Vaginal agenesis

Isolated vaginal atresia (transverse vaginal septum)

A transverse vaginal septum occurs either because of failure of canalization of the vaginal plate, or because of an incomplete union between the uterovaginal primordium and the urogenital sinus during embryogenesis. In the majority of cases, the septum lies in the upper or middle third of the vagina and usually, the higher the location of the septum the thicker it is (Rock et al. 1982). The condition presents with primary amenorrhoea and cyclical pelvic pain. The pain (as in the case of an imperforate hymen) is due to the build up of blood above the obstruction.

Surgical treatment is required in order to resect the septum and anastomose the proximal and distal edge of the vagina. Preoperatively the patient's menstruation is usually suppressed with gonadotropin-releasing hormone (GnRH) analogues in order to alleviate pain. An MRI of the pelvis will help to assess the thickness and level of the septum, as this will determine the surgical route to entertain. In cases of a thin lower septum, then a perineal approach is appropriate, whereas in cases of thicker and higher septa, it is advisable to proceed to an abdominoperineal approach, and if necessary use a graft of bowel to bridge the gap between the two portions of the vagina.

Postoperatively, the patient should perform regular dilatation, in order to prevent vaginal stenosis.

Mayer Rokitansky Küster Hauser syndrome (MRKH—combined uterine and vaginal agenesis)

This condition occurs in 1 in 5000 female births. The vagina is absent or consists of a short vaginal dimple and the uterus is absent. Often two rudimentary uterine buds can be identified on either side of the pelvis. As the patients have normal ovarian function, secondary sexual characteristics develop normally and presentation is usually in the late teenage years with primary amenorrhoea.

Clinical examination will reveal a short blind-ending vagina and the diagnosis is usually confirmed by performing pelvic imaging, usually MRI. Up to 30% of patients have associated renal anomalies and approximately 10% will have skeletal anomalies.

The condition has devastating implications for sexuality and fertility, and thus adequate specialized psychological support is required. Although women with MRKH will not be able to carry a pregnancy, they are capable of having their own genetic children via IVF and a surrogate uterus.

Treatment also involves creating a vagina to enable penetrative intercourse. In the majority of patients this can be achieved conservatively by using vaginal dilators. The patient is asked to insert vaginal moulds of gradually increasing size into the vaginal dimple and apply pressure. This method of lengthening of the vagina has been shown to be successful in 80% of patients, especially where there is adequate motivation and support (Ismail-Pratt et al. 2007).

In the minority of patients where dilation is unsuccessful, a surgical procedure is required. Various methods exist to create a neovagina and these can be divided into three categories:

- Williams vaginoplasty where a pouch is created on the perineum by suturing the labia majora. This procedure is no longer in favour, as the neovagina is external and the angle of sexual penetration is non physiological.

- Methods where the existing short vagina is lengthened by applying pressure on the vaginal dimple. The Vecchietti procedure was first described in 1965 and has since been modified to be performed laparoscopically. It consists of inserting an acrylic olive within the vaginal dimple, which is then attached to threads that pass through the rectovesical space and on to the abdominal wall. The threads are connected to a traction device that allows their gradual pulling by a centimetre a day. The patient is usually discharged after 1 week, at which time the traction device and bead are removed (Fedele et al. 2000)

- Procedures where a neovagina is created within the rectovesical space and then lined with autologous tissue graft, such as peritoneum (Davydov procedure), skin (McIndoe–Reed), or bowel (ileo- or colovaginoplasty). Both the Davydov procedure and the colovaginopastly have been modified to be performed laparoscopically (Giannesi et al. 2005).

Timing of the vaginoplasty should be carefully considered. In the absence of functioning endometrium and menstrual obstruction there is no urgency to perform an operation early. Creation of a neovagina is only required for sexual intercourse, and therefore could be delayed until the patient reaches adequate maturity to contemplate sexual activity and has the necessary understanding and motivation to perform postoperative dilation.

Longitudinal vaginal septum

A longitudinal septum can vary in length and thickness. In its extreme form, the septum extends from the cervix to the introitus and creates a true double vagina. This is usually associated with a duplication of the cervix and uterus. Rarely, one hemivagina is obstructed, leading to the formation of a unilateral haematocolpos, while menstruation flows normally from the unaffected side. In its more benign forms, the septum remains asymptomatic until the patient attempts to use tampons or becomes sexually active. Rarely, it may only become apparent on having a gynaecological examination, or during labour.

The excision of the septum is a simple vaginal procedure. However, care has to be taken to ensure that it has been fully removed, as scar tissue and stenosis may occur.

Uterine anomalies

Müllerian anomalies are commonly classified under the American Fertility Society System in seven categories, which reflect the degree of developmental failure and allow for the classification of abnormalities with similar clinical manifestations, treatment and prognosis (AFS 1988):

- Type I: hypoplasia/agenesis (vaginal, cervical, fundal, tubal, or combined)
- Type II: unicornuate uterus (with the presence of an ipsilateral rudimentary horn, or not)
- Type III: uterus didelphus
- Type IV: bicornuate uterus
- Type V: septate uterus
- Type VI: arcuate uterus
- Type VII: related to diethylstilboestrol use.

Uterine anomalies are estimated to be present in 4.3% of the fertile population (Grimbizis et al.). In their milder form, they may be entirely asymptomatic. More complex anomalies however can lead to dysmenorrhoea and obstetric complications, such as preterm labour, abnormal fetal lie

and an increased risk of Caesarean section. Because of the close embryological origin of the renal and genital tracts, uterine malformations are commonly associated with renal anomalies, such as renal agenesis, ectopy, and duplication of the collecting system (Buttram and Gibbons 1979).

Cervical agenesis

This is a rare condition occurring in approximately 1 in 80 000 females. As with other obstructive anomalies, it is associated with primary amenorrhoea and cyclical pelvic pain. Treatment has evolved over the years and now focuses on preserving fertility and anastomosing the uterine body to the vagina. A number of successful pregnancies have been reported following conservative treatment (Defarges et al. 2001) and the uterovaginal anastomosis can now be performed laparoscopically (Creighton et al. 2006).

Unicornuate uterus

A unicornuate uterus results from failure of one of the paramesonephric ducts to develop. In approximately two-thirds of cases, a rudimentary non communicating horn exists and a proportion of those contain functioning endometrial tissue (Shulman 2008). Severe dysmenorrhoea ensues as a result of obstructed menstruation and endometriosis. Although pain presents at the time of menarche, diagnosis is often delayed, as the condition is relatively rare and the patient menstruates from the unobstructed unicornuate uterus.

Treatment consists of resecting the obstructed uterine horn and this can be done laparoscopically (Strawbridge et al. 2007). Preoperative assessment, in the form of MRI and IVU is required to determine the exact level of the anomaly and the number and anatomical position of the ureters.

In management both cervical agenesis and an obstructed uterine horn, menstrual suppression with GnRH analogues is commonplace to alleviate symptoms and reduce the level of endometriosis thereby facilitating the surgical procedure.

Bicornuate uterus

This accounts for 10% of uterine anomalies. Treatment is usually not required. Traditional metroplasty techniques such as the Strassman operation may be used to unify the two cavities and restore the contour of the external uterus. However, it breaches the musculature of the uterus, potentially rendering it more feeble for carrying a pregnancy.

Septate uterus

This is the most common uterine anomaly, accounting for 50% of all. It is estimated that it affects 2–3% of the population and has a marked effect on fertility. The septum can be resected hysteroscopically but no randomized controlled trials have been performed to establish that the procedure improves reproductive outcome.

Further reading

Acien P. Embryological observations on the female genital tract. Hum Reprod 1992;7:437–45.

American Fertility Society: The American Fertility Society classification of adnexal adhesions, distal tubal occlusion, tubal occlusion secondary to tubal ligation, tubal pregnancies, Müllerian anomalies and intrauterine adhesions. Fertil Steril 1988;49:944–55.

Buttram VC Jr, Gibbons WE. Müllerian anomalies: a proposed classification (an analysis of 144 cases). Fertil Steril 1979;32:40–6.

Creighton SM, Davies MC. Cutner as laparoscopic management of cervical agenesis. Fertil Steril 2006;85:1510–15.

Deffarges JV, Haddad B, Musset R, Paniel BJ. Utero-vaginal anastomosis in women with uterine cervix atresia: long-term follow-up and reproductive performance. A study of 18 cases. Hum Reprod 2001;16:1722–25.

Fedele L, Bianchi S, Zanconato G, Raffaelli R. Laparoscopic creation of a neovagina in patients with Rokitansky syndrome: analysis of 52 cases. Fertil Steril 2000;74:384–9.

Giannesi A, Marchiole P, Benchaib M, et al. Sexuality after laparoscopic Davydov in patients affected by congenital complete vaginal agenesis associated with uterine agenesis or hypoplasia. Hum Reprod 2005;20:2954–7.

Grimbizis GF, Camus M, Tarlatzis BC, et al. Clinical implications of uterine malformations and hysteroscopic treatment results. Hum Reprod Update 2001;7:161–74.

Ismail-Pratt IS, Bikoo M, Liao LM, et al. Normalization of the vagina by dilator treatment alone in complete androgen insensitivity syndrome and Mayer-Rokitansky-Kuster-Hauser syndrome. Hum Reprod 2007;22:2020–4.

Rock JA, Zakur HA, Dlugi AM, et al. Pregnancy success following surgical correction of imperforate hymen and complete transverse vaginal septum. Obstet Gynecol 1982;59:448–51.

Shulman LP. Müllerian anomalies. Clinical Obst Gynecol 2008;51:214–22.

Strawbridge LC, Crouch NS, Cutner AS, Creighton SM. Obstructive müllerian anomalies and modern laparoscopic management. J Pediatr Adolesc Gynecol 2007;20:195–200.

Patient resources

MRKH Organization .inc, American support group for women with Rokitansky syndrome, www.mrkh.org

Male subfertility

Definition
Male subfertility can be defined where a seminal, endo-crine, genetic, or psychosexual deficiency inhibits a couple achieving a pregnancy within 12 months of attempting where no significant pathology has been identified in the female partner. Additionally, the immune system and structure of reproductive organs can also impact on male subfertility. It is also important to consider the definition of a couple's subfertility: a couple is considered as infertile if they are not able to conceive after 2 years of contracep-tive-free intercourse. Infertility is thought to affect approx-imately 14% of couples of reproductive age.

Defining male subfertility is not clear and straightfor-ward. The only true means to measure whether the male partner is fertile is to assess his ability of either achieving a pregnancy, which can be dependent on the reproductive health of the female partner, or by assessment of the defin-ing characteristics of a semen sample. It has been clearly demonstrated that the reproducibility of the basic semen analysis is not reliable, and natural pregnancy can be achieved where the male partner demonstrates a low level of sperm concentration. Confounding the problem are men who present with satisfactory sperm concentrations and possess abundant progressive motile cells but suffer from a subtle defect in the functional sperm population, inhibiting their ability to capacitate, recognize, or combine with ova or undergo the later reactions essential for fertili-zation. Unexplained or idiopathic infertility may have these subtle features; unfortunately they cannot be determined by routine semen analysis.

Epidemiology
A World Health Organization (WHO) survey demonstrat-ed from a study of 25 countries that approximately 5% of men of reproductive age suffer from male subfertility. The literature suggests that 8–15% of couples suffer from sub-fertility. Figures suggest that 30–50% of couples have a sig-nificant male factor contribution to this problem. These are conservative estimates, which increase when the pro-portion of couples who are defined as suffering from idio-pathic infertility but in fact have a male factor contribution to their inability to achieve pregnancy are included.

Aetiology
Although difficult to elucidate, there is a probable genetic basis for the aetiology of the majority of mechanical, physi-ological, and functional reasons for male factor subfertility. The genetic effect manifests itself by influencing physiolog-ical processes such as hormonal homeostasis, sperma-togenesis, and sperm quality. Applications to define subfertile phenotypes are in the developmental stages; therefore, our efforts lie with identifying markers that are apparent in response to defective gene(s) and the transfer of epigenetic information.

The clear indicators of subfertility are
- hormonal deficiencies
  - hypothalamic/pituitary or thyroid disorders
  - hypogonadotrophic hypogonadism
- testicular disorders
  - maturation arrest
  - germ cell aplasia
  - Sertoli cell-only syndrome
- defective spermatogenesis
  - azoospermia
  - low sperm concentration and motility
  - sperm dysfunction
- chromosomal abnormalities
  - Klinefelters
- varicocele (Grade 3 or greater severity)
  - systemic disease
  - liver disease
  - renal failure
  - sickle cell disease
- neurological disease
- UTI, mycoplasma and STD.

Clinical approach
Diagnosis
The WHO recommends that at least two semen analyses are performed with a time period of at least 3 months between each assessment. A detailed clinical history should be taken to determine potential pathology and to deter-mine an individualized investigation, assessment, and treat-ment programme.

History
Medical history
- Fevers (within the last 3 months)
- Recurrent chest infection, sinusitis, or bronchiectasis
- History of cystic fibrosis (agenesis of the vas deferens)
- Previous genitourinary infections in the form of orchitis (mumps, syphilis, leprosy, tuberculosis), epididymitis, (gonorrhoea, chlamydia, tuberculosis, schistosomiasis, and chronic infection of the prostate and seminal vesicle (painful ejaculation and haematospermia)
- Sport-related testicular torsion
- Chronic disorders (renal failure, liver disease, maligna-nancy, or diabetes)
- Anosmia (lack of smell), galactorrhoea, visual field defects, and sudden loss of field defects suggest signs of pituitary tumour.

Childhood disorders
- Herniorraphy or testicular torsion
- Mumps
- Precocious puberty before 9 years suggestive of endo-crine disorder
- Delayed onset of puberty (gonadotrophin deficiency)
- Cryptorchadism
- Hypospadias
- Midline defects
- End-organ androgen insensitivity.

Previous surgery
- Epididymal obstruction (Yong's syndrome)
- Testicular trauma or torsion
- Pelvic, bladder, or retroperitoneal surgery.

Fertility history
- Establish frequency and timing of vaginal intercourse.
- Duration of infertility
- History of pregnancies in present and past relationships

- Erection dysfunction
- Psychosexual dysfunction.

Social history
- Use of recreational drugs.
- Excessive alcohol or tobacco use
- Anabolic steroids
- Excessive heat from saunas, hot tubs, and work environment affects sperm production.

History of occupational hazards
- Excessive mental stress
- Exposure to testicular toxins
- Excessive exposure to heat
- Paints and solvents
- Herbicides or pesticides (ethylene dibromide, dibromochloropropane)
- Prolonged exposure to heavy metals (lead, cadmium; suppresses hypothalamopituitary axis, etc.).
- Nitrous oxide
- X-ray
- Non-ionizing and ionizing radiation.

Medications
- Antineoplastics
- Antibiotics
- Cytotoxic agents
- Suphasalazine
- Psychotropic drugs
- Antihypertensive drugs
- Cimetidine
- Nitrofurntoin
- Anticonvulsants.

Investigations
The clinical approach to assessing or considering the male contribution to the couples subfertility has traditionally fallen short compared with the time and dedication given to determining a female diagnosis. Unfortunately, examples exist where an exhaustive testing regime using expensive assays and invasive operative procedures have been performed on the female partner, which have taken years to complete, before the semen characteristics have been analysed and shown to highlight an obvious pathology.

The WHO have reassessed the values given to indicate the normal range (Table 12.22.1).

Initiate the investigation procedure by requesting at least two thorough semen analyses. They must be performed by trained staff in a recognized laboratory that employs rigorous quality control. The laboratory must have access to pathology services to enable further investigations, including collaboration with a histology service with an experienced electron microscopy team (Fig. 12.22.1). In many cases the results of a semen analysis cannot definitively assure fertility, or rule out the possibility of a man being able to sire his own children, regardless of the concentration and percentage of progressively motile sperm. Apart from some cases of azoospermia (2% of the male population are found to be azoospermic), a cautious approach should be taken when considering labelling a patient as fertile, subfertile, or sterile on the basis of the results. The semen analysis can be considered as an inexpensive starting point in determining a treatment or management strategy for a couple.

Table 12.22.1 WHO comparisons of the normal range

	Current WHO normal ranges (95% percentile confidence limit)	1999 WHO normal ranges
Volume	1.5 mL (1.4–1.7)	>2 mL
Sperm concentration	15×10^{-6}(12–16)	20×10^{-6}
Total sperm concentration	39 million per ejaculate (33–46)	$40 \times 10\ 6^{-1}$
Total motility (%)	40	50
Progressive motility (%)	32 (31–34)	25
Morphology (%)*	4 (3.0–4.0)	30
Vitality (%)	58 (55–63)	50

*Strict morphology criteria

Where medical management leads to an undefined aetiology or there is a time pressure due to the partner's age the approach from Guzick *et al.* (2001) may help direct the clinician to advising a couple whether to continue to attempt natural conception or to move directly to an appropriate type of assisted conception by considering the results in terms of ranges, not a clear-cut categorization into fertile and subfertile. Sperm concentrations of above 48.0 million per millilitre will give a good probability of pregnancy, 13.5–48.0 a moderate chance and below 13.5 significantly reduces the possibility to the point where

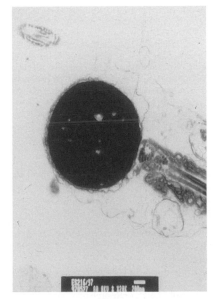

Fig. 12.22.1 Electron micrograph of a spermatozoon exhibiting the lack of an acrosomal membrane. The patient's concentration of sperm was in excess of 20 million per millilitre and greater than 60% of sperm were motile. The couple would require intracytoplasmic sperm micro-injection to achieve a pregnancy. See also colour plate section.

assisted conception should be considered immediately or counselled that pregnancy with their own sperm is unlikely. Although sometimes difficult, a man may have to consider the use of donor gametes or adoption in order to become a father.

Hormone analysis

Indications from the clinical history with a combination of semen analysis results will indicate whether evaluations of the male reproductive hormone levels are necessary. An endocrine assessment is not necessary for a man with normal semen parameters.

Evaluating the hormone profile of men with moderate to low semen samples has not been shown to improve chances of pregnancy. There seems to be no benefit prescribing supplementation with androgens or gonadotrophins. Measurements of serum testosterone and follicle-stimulating hormone (FSH) should be performed initially. A low testosterone level directs the need for a repeat assay. Assessing the level of total and free testosterone, with additional measurements of luteinizing hormone and prolactin levels, will identify whether there is a treatable endocrine pathology. An elevated FSH is a clear indication of an abnormality in spermatogenesis. Caution should be exhibited with endocrine patterns. Although abnormal hormone levels have been identified in 10% of patients who have been tested, the result is only clinically significant in less than 2% of men.

Genetic causes of male subfertility

The contribution of a genetic factor to male subfertility is not fully understood. It is considered that 15–30% of men diagnosed as subfertile have a chromosomal or single gene defect that leads to deficient spermatogenesis. The implementation of techniques such as ICSI, especially when combined with testicular surgical sperm retrieval, has provided treatment for men who would otherwise be unable to father a child. These treatment options have increased the need for an appreciation of the negative consequences and impact of inheritable mutations on the next generation. Despite the absence of evidence of an increase in imprinting disorders with the use of these technologies, there is a concern that bypassing natural selection mechanisms will have an impact on an epigenetic level.

Chromosomal analysis

An incorrect chromosomal number accounts for the majority of genetic causes for male factor infertility. Aneuploidy can lead to non-obstructive azoospermia, cryptozoospermia, and severe oligozoospermia. A karyotype is essential for men with extremely low sperm concentrations (less than 1 million sperm per millilitre) because the incidence of anueploidy is increased in this group. Klinefelter's syndrome is the most common chromosomal abnormality caused by aneuploidy, yet only a third of suffers will be diagnosed (Table 12.22.2). Spermatogenesis is normally arrested at the germ cell stage, but in some cases sperm development can be seen.

Y chromosome gene defects

Despite the presence of gene defects in many autosomal chromosomes, there is an obvious focus on the Y chromosome. The male sex chromosome contains the majority of genes that are involved in the development of the testis and that are crucial for spermatogenesis. Regions of the Y chromosome have been found to be missing or mutated in subfertile men and a clear link between subfertility and

Table 12.22.2 Genetic causes of male factor infertility. Reprinted from Fertility and Sterility, Vol. 93, Iss. 1, Flynn, K, Varghese and Agarwal, The genetic causes of male factor infertility: A review (2010), with permission from Elsevier

Genetic abnormality	Phenotype	Prevalence (%)
Chromosomal abnormalities	Azoospermia to normozoospermia	5 (total infertile population);15 (azoospermic)
Klinefelter syndrome	Azoospermia to severe oligozoospermia	5 (severe oligozoospermia); 10 (azoospermic)
Robertsonian translocation	Azoospermia to normozoospermia	0.8 (total infertile population); 1.6 (oligozoospermia); 0.09 (azoospermic)
Y chromosome microdelections	Azoospermia to oligozoospermia	10–15 (azoospermic); 5–10 (oligozoospermic)

infertility has been demonstrated. Yet care should be employed when referring men for Y chromosome microdeletion assessment, it is essential to highlight the potential of the transmission of aberrant genetic information to male offspring and perpetuating male factor subfertility but the significance of partial microdeletions is still under study and oligo- and cryptozoospermia may have other genetic origins. The NICE guidelines state that it is unnecessary to assess all patients for assessment.

DNA fragmentation

The recent sperm function literature has also placed a focus on the effects of damage to sperm DNA and a reduction in the potential to generate a healthy pregnancy. DNA damage may be caused at any point during spermatogenesis, spermiogenesis, and while cells are stored in the epididymis. There are suggestions that subfertile men have a higher proportion of sperm that have suffered DNA damage, either as a result of being marked for apoptosis during production or exposure to deleterious agents. Numerous agents can cause a negative effect on the sperm DNA despite naturally occurring protective mechanisms in the testes and seminal fluid. Sperm that have suffered damage may achieve normal levels of fertilization in IVF situations, yet there is a suggestion that embryo progression is negatively affected and spontaneous pregnancy loss may be increased. The Association of Sexual and Reproductive Medicine has stated that DNA damage is potentially detrimental to the chances of pregnancy but the testing methods and data in the literature require further analysis before this application is adopted into routine practice.

Examination

A general physical examination should be performed, initially concentrating on height, weight, and secondary sexual characteristics. This should include examination of testes, penis, and vas deferens. The Testes should be manipulated between the thumb, index, and middle finger to determine the size and consistency. In androgen-deficient men look for gynacomastia, cryptorchidism, hypospadias, and anosmia. Measurement of testicular volume is necessary. An irregular contour, induration, or abnormal consistency may suggest a previous orchitis, surgery, or malignancy. Obstructive azoospermia can be identified by assessment of the caput epididymis; if engorged, further examination by ultrasound or digital rectal examination may be necessary. The presence of a varicocele can be identified by manipulation or by observing the man while in a standing position.

Counselling

Psychological support should be provided for couples seeking fertility treatment and investigation. Support from an independent counsellor is generally recommended. The added esteem issues surrounding the label of male factor subfertility increases the potential chance of psychological stress and relationship disharmony. It is essential that the difference between virility and infertility is clearly understood by the man.

Abnormalities on the Y chromosome are thought to be associated with deficient spermatogenesis; therefore, couples undergoing assisted reproductive treatment for significantly poor sperm characteristics should have access to general genetic counselling. Further specific genetic counselling and testing should be available in cases where there is a specific genetic defect associated with failure to achieve a pregnancy.

Before a couple undergo ICSI the potential genetic risks to the resulting child should be explained in terms of the

- inherent risks of the procedure.
- potential for inheritable specific genetic defects as the cause of subfertility.

Management

Management of the potentially subfertile male should follow the clear guidance given by NICE for fertility assessments. Gonadotrophins can be utilized for men with hypogonadotrophic hypogonadism. These are effective in improving the chance of fertility without the need to resorting to assisted reproductive technology (ART):

- conservative/non-medical
- medical
- lifestyle changes
- antibiotics where infection is indicated
- diet with the addition vitamin C and E, zinc, fish oil, and selenium
- low-level fertility treatment
- intrauterine insemination
- ART.

Surgical

NICE guideline recommendations

Obstructive azoospermia can be effectively managed with surgical correction without the need to refer to assisted reproduction. Epididymal blockage can be reversed by surgery and the duct can be cleared. The chances of pregnancy are not improved by recommending that men with varicoceles are offered surgery. Potential problems associated with testicular surgery are likely to cause the production of antisperm antibodies (ASABs) in response to the breach to the blood–testes barrier.

Retrograde ejaculation

Retrograde ejaculation occurs when seminal fluid flows along the line of least resistance, after orgasm, into the bladder instead of the urethra. Failure of the bladder sphincter to close after ejaculation allows a retrograde flow of semen.

Complications after genitourinary surgery for prostate or urethral conditions can cause bladder neck muscle weakness. A common cause for retrograde ejaculation is caused by medication to treat unrelated conditions. Prescription drugs that treat high blood pressure, neurological disorders, and diabetes can affect the muscles that surround the bladder neck. General muscle relaxants can also initiate this trait. Males suffering from diabetes have been identified to have a neuropathy of the bladder sphincter.

Absence or a small ejaculate volume combined with cloudy urine after sexual intercourse can be indicative symptoms. Semen in the bladder does not cause any harm to the man and will leave the body during urination. Employing simple modifications to medication or intercourse with a full bladder can allow a couple to achieve pregnancy with resorting to ART. If necessary, successful pregnancy can be achieved with ART by preparing a sperm suspension for insemination from alkalized urine.

Complications/side-effects/sequelae

Men with idiopathic semen abnormalities and mild oligasthenoteratozoospermia should not be given antioestrogens, gonadotrophins, androgens, or kinin-enhancing drugs, since the significance in improving semen characteristics is unclear. Unnecessary use of potential carcinogens is not recommended.

Sections of the literature describe a reduced chance of pregnancy when significant levels of ASABs are identified in semen. This autoimmune response or antibody cross-reactivity can inhibit normal sperm–oocyte interaction and sperm function. NICE guidelines state that the evidence for a significant contribution to male factor subfertility is unfounded. ASAB relevance is debated and any treatment for the male is unnecessary. Corticosteroid treatment has been suggested in the past to have side-effects which outweigh any benefit in achieving pregnancy.

Despite a low rate of complication noted after corrective varicocele surgery (5%) it is recommended that the incidence of localized testicular dysfunction outweighs the benefit of redirecting venous blood flow.

Prognosis

Timely investigation and diagnosis will hopefully enable a man to contribute to a pregnancy if there is no significant pathology in the female (Table 12.22.3). The probability of pregnancy, the time involved for investigation, potential for a genetic component, and cost should be considered with the incidence of severe male factor subfertility.

Treatment options

- Time of sexual intercourse (TSI)
- Ovulation induction (OI)
- Intrauterine insemination (IUI)
- In vitro fertilization IVF
- Intracytoplasmic sperm microinjection (ICSI).

Table 12.22.3 Suggested management options in male infertility and prognosis

	Advice	Treatment	ART	Chance of live birth
Slight male factor	Try >1 year	None	Hopefully unnecessary	Good dependant on female age and aetiology
			TSI for 6 cycles	See www.hfea.gov.uk
			OI for 6 cycles	
			IUI for 6 cycles	
Significant Male Factor	Try >1 year	As necessary	IVF or ICSI depending on the sperm dysfunction	Good dependant on female age and aetiology.
	Investigate appropriately			See www.hfea.gov.uk
Obstructive Azoospermia	Immediate investigation	Surgical	Unnecessary if successful	Surgical sperm retrieval with ICSI
				Reduced chance of pregnancy in comparison to national average
				Donor gamete use may be necessary
Non Obstructive Azoospermia	Immediate investigation	As necessary		Surgical sperm retrieval with ICSI
				Reduced chance of pregnancy in comparison to national average
				Donor gamete use may be necessary
Hormone or pituitary disorders	Immediate investigation	Hormone therapy	Unnecessary if successful	Surgical sperm retrieval with ICSI
			IVF	Reduced chance of pregnancy in comparison to national average
			ICSI	
Retrograde ejaculation	Immediate investigation	Surgery	Unnecessary if successful	Good dependant on female age and aetiology
		Cessation of medication	IUI for 6 cycles	See www.hfea.gov.uk
		Medical management	IVF	
			ICSI	

Further reading

Hull M, Glazner C, Kelly NJ. et al. Population study of causes, treatment and outcome of infertility Br Med J (Clin Res Ed) 1985; 291:1693–7.

Cooper T, Noonan E, Sigrid von Eckardstein, et al. World Health Organization reference values for human semen characteristics. Human Reprod Update 2010;16:231–45.

O'Flynn O'Brien K, Varghese A, Agarwal A. The genetic causes of male factor infertility: A review. Fert Steril 2010;93:1–12.

NICE. Fertility assessment and treatment for people with fertility problems. NICE Clinical Guidelines February 2004.

Guzick DS, Overstreet JW, Factor-Litvak P, et al. Sperm morphology, motility and concentration in fertile and infertile men. N Engl J Med 2001;345:1388–93

Internet resources

www.asrm.org/uploadedFiles/ASRM_Content/News_and_Publications/Practice_Guidelines/Committee_Opiions/optimal_evaluation_of_the_infertile_male(1).pdf

www.nice.org.uk/nicemedia/pdf/CG011fullguideline.pdf
www.rcog.org.uk/files/rcog-corp/uploaded-files/NEBFertilityAlgorithm.pdf
www.rcog.org.uk/files/rcog-corp/uploaded-files/NEBFertilitySummary.pdf
www.rcog.org.uk/files/rcog-corp/uploaded-files/NEBFertilityTables.pdf
www.rcog.org.uk/womens-health/clinical-guidance/fertility-assessment-and-treatment-people-fertility-problems

Patient resources

www.hfea.gov.uk

Menopause and hormone replacement therapy

Definitions

The word menopause is derived from the Greek *menos* (month) and *pausis* (Cessation). It is defined as the last menstrual period. As such, the diagnosis can only be made retrospectively after a minimum of 1 year's amenorrhoea. Although the menopause occurs at an average age of 51, the physiological changes which result in the final menstrual period can start up to 10 years prior to this. Hormonal changes can continue long after the final menstrual period. This episode of rapid neuroendocrine change is characterized by 'the climacteric', from the Greek *klimax*, ladder, i.e. the climb to the menopause during which symptoms occur in most women.

Epidemiology

We live at a time when the population is ageing. One hundred years ago only 30% of women lived through a menopause; now, more than 90% will. Thus, the menopause transition and postmenopause is very much a condition of the twentieth and twenty-first centuries. Life expectancy is now 82 years of age for a woman living in the UK. The majority of women can therefore expect to live over a third of their lives in a menopausal state. It is estimated that 15% of women will have an early menopause below the age of 45 and 1% will have premature ovarian failure below the age of 40.

Pathophysiology

A newborn female infant has over a million follicles; the follicle cohort shrinks throughout life such that there are only a few thousand follicles left as a woman enters her 40s and few or none in the postmenopause. It is the depletion of follicles which leads to the cessation of menstruation, the cardinal sign of the menopause. Initially, ovarian failure is compensated by gonadotrophin levels starting to rise, in some women from the age of 30 years. During this time there is evidence for a reduced number of gonadotrophin receptors in perimenopausal ovaries, and inhibin production from granulosa cells falls. Decompensated failure then occurs due to the critical decline in the follicle pool leading to further rises in follicle-stimulating hormone (FSH) (10–20-fold); luteinizing hormone (LH) rises only threefold because of its shorter half-life. Oestrogen levels drop due to a reduction in follicle number and qualitative effect on granulosa cell ageing. There is permanent cessation of progesterone production. These changes have been tracked by annual sampling in large populations of women.

Premature ovarian failure/dysfunction

Premature ovarian failure is said to have occurred when menstruation ceases before the age of 40 years and early menopause before the age of 45 years. The author prefers the term premature ovarian dysfunction to signify that the transition into menopause can be lengthy and occasionally may even reverse itself. Although there are many causes of early ovarian failure, the main cause is spontaneous or idiopathic. The main identified genetic causes are Turner's syndrome and Fragile X. Recently, forkhead genes (FOX03A defect) have been discovered which lead to early follicular activation and thus premature depletion of the follicle pool. Other causes include FSH receptor polymorphisms, first characterized in Finnish populations where follicles are present but unable to respond due to the loss of the FSH receptor. The proportion of women with iatrogenic premature ovarian failure is growing as increasing numbers of women survive leukaemias, lymphomas, and gynaecological cancers due to improved surgical techniques, radiotherapy, and chemotherapeutic regimens.

Other hormonal changes

Adrenal and ovarian androgen levels start to decline from 20 years of age through to the perimenopause, stabilizing by the time of the final menstrual period. Some testosterone production continues from the ovarian theca cells. The drop in androgen levels is particularly profound in premature ovarian failure, spontaneous or iatrogenic. The main postmenopausal oestrogen is oestrone, which is produced in peripheral adipose tissue and the postmenopausal ovary by aromatization of adrenal androstenedione. The somatotrophic axis becomes less active with ageing, leading to insulin resistance and a rise in central adiposity. This in turn leads to the change in body shape from the female gynaecoid shape to the male android shape, an independent risk factor for coronary heart disease. There are a number of factors involved in perimenopausal weight gain, including genetic predisposition, socioeconomic influences, reduction in caloric need and expenditure, reduced lean body mass, and a reduction in the resting basal metabolic rate.

The menstrual cycle

Anovulatory cycles become progressively common heading towards the menopause transition. There can be continued oestrogen production in the absence of progesterone leading to endometrial proliferation, hyperplasia, and at its extreme carcinoma. As a result, menstruation can become heavy, prolonged, and unpredictable with intermenstrual bleeding.

Consequences of the menopause

Immediate

Seventy per cent of Caucasian and Afro-Caribbean women suffer from vasomotor symptoms (hot flushes and sweats), the commonest menopausal symptoms. This compares with 10–20% of Japanese and Chinese women, and may reflect cultural differences or may be diet related (isoflavone consumption). Hot flushes are thought to arise due to loss of oestrogen-induced opioid activity in the hypothalamus leading to thermodysregulation. Noradrenaline and serotonin mediate this activity, hence the rationale for using the α-agonist clonidine and the selective serotonin and noradrenaline reuptake inhibitors as alternatives to HRT. Obese women are relatively protected from these symptoms because of their production of oestrone and low sex hormone binding globulin levels, which leaves more of the free active hormone. Other typical immediate menopausal symptoms include insomnia, anxiety, irritability, memory loss, tiredness, and poor concentration. Mood disturbances can occur due to fluctuation in hormone levels, leading to perimenopausal depression. Falling oestrogen levels are thought to lead to similar falls in neurotransmitter levels such as serotonin, which trigger these symptoms. Women who have suffered from postnatal depression and premenstrual syndrome appear to be particularly predisposed to depression in the perimenopause. The menopause transition can also be associated with a significant reduction in sexuality and libido. This is not only because of decreased vaginal lubrication leading to dyspareunia, but also due to the reduction in androgen levels discussed earlier.

Intermediate

Oestrogen deficiency leads to the rapid loss of collagen, which contributes to the generalized atrophy that occurs after the menopause. In the genital tract this is manifested by dyspareunia and vaginal bleeding from fragile atrophic skin. In the lower urinary tract, atrophy of the urethral epithelium occurs with decreased sensitivity of urethral smooth muscle and a decreased amount of collagen in periurethral collagen. All this results in dysuria, urgency and frequency, commonly termed the urethral syndrome. More generalized changes are seen in the older woman as increased bruising and thin translucent skin, which is vulnerable to trauma and infection. A similar loss of collagen from ligaments and joints may cause generalized aches and pains.

Long term

Osteoporosis, cardiovascular disease, and dementia are three long-term health problems that have been linked to the menopause.

- Osteoporosis: osteoporosis is a disorder of the bone matrix resulting in a reduction of bone strength to the extent that there is a significant increased risk of fracture. These fractures cause considerable morbidity in older people, requiring prolonged hospital care and difficulties in remobilization. Osteoporosis is predominantly a disease of women, who achieve a lower peak bone mass than men and are then subjected to an accelerated loss of bone density following the menopause. The hypo-oestrogenic state leads to activation of the bone remodelling units with an excess of bone resorption relative to formation. Women lose 50% of their skeleton by the age of 70 years, but men only lose 25% by the age of 90 years. Loss of height can occur not only due to vertebral fractures but also loss of the intervertebral disc space.

- Cardiovascular: Women are protected against cardiovascular disease before the menopause, after which the incidence rapidly increases reaching a similar frequency to men by the age of 70 years. The protective effect of oestrogen in premenopausal women is thought to be mediated by an increase in high-density lipoprotein (HDL) and a decrease in low-density lipoprotein (LDL), nitric oxide-mediated vasodilatation leading to increased myocardial blood flow, an antioxidant effect on endothelial cells and a direct effect on the aorta decreasing atheroma. Cross-sectional and prospective observational studies have shown that women going through the menopause transition have elevation of cholesterol, triglyceride, and LDL levels and a reduction in HDL2 levels. A key study showed that oestrogen status was an independent predictor of atherosclerotic plaque area after controlling for age, hypertension, diabetes, etc.

- Central nervous system: oestrogen appears to have a direct effect on the vasculature of the central nervous system and promotes neuronal growth and neurotransmission. Studies have demonstrated that oestrogen may improve cerebral perfusion and cognition in women. In the long term this may prevent diseases with a vascular aetiology such as vascular dementia and Alzheimer's as the vasculature is clearly involved in this. In addition to the effect on vasculature in Alzheimer's disease, oestrogen may also intervene at the level of amyloid precursor protein. The failure to show benefit for dementia in older populations, and possibly an increased risk with HRT in some studies (Shumaker *et al.* 2003), may reflect the predominance of the prothrombotic effect of oestrogen in this age group.

Diagnosis of menopause

Prediction of ovarian reserve

Until recently, early follicular phase follicle-stimulating hormone (FSH) levels were used to predict ovarian reserve with a level of >10 IU/L indicating reduced reserve and >30 IU/L regarded as being diagnostic of the menopause. However, this test can be misleading; levels vary according to the timing of the sample and often change in subsequent cycles depending on ovarian activity. The most accurate predictors of ovarian reserve currently available appear to be measurement of anti-Müllerian hormone (AMH) production by the primordial follicles and estimation of the antral follicle count on ultrasonographic estimation. AMH is independent of the day of cycle and its predictive value is claimed to last for up to 2 years from when the sample was taken.

Diagnosis of natural menopause

The diagnosis of natural menopause can usually be ascertained from a characteristic history of the vasomotor symptoms of hot flushes and night sweats and prolonged episodes of amenorrhoea. Measurement of plasma hormone levels (oestradiol, FSH, LH) in women in their late 40s onwards with classical symptoms, are not essential as they do not change clinical management. However, in the young patient or in a woman after hysterectomy, where the diagnosis is more difficult and the metabolic implications are serious, measurement of FSH levels may be helpful, in which case repeated measurements of 15 IU/L or above may be regarded as climacteric. Women diagnosed with spontaneous premature ovarian dysfunction should, in addition to hormonal investigations, also have an autoantibody screen and karyotype performed, although the aetiology is usually idiopathic.

In patients still menstruating, persistent hot flushes and night sweats are suggestive of the climacteric, but in those patients with psychological symptoms the diagnosis may be more difficult. In such cases it may be justified to give a trial of oestrogen therapy and monitor the response before discounting a hormonal aetiology. In those women complaining of lack of energy and/or libido a free androgen index and thyroid function tests should be performed as female androgen deficiency and/or hypothyroidism may be contributing to the symptoms.

Ongoing monitoring

After the diagnosis has been established, investigations should be no more than the annual screening which is normally applicable to middle-aged women. This should include assessment of weight, blood pressure and routine cervical cytology. A recent consensus between menopause experts and cardiologists has highlighted the important role that gynaecologists can play in cardiovascular screening (see Further reading). Fasting lipid profile and insulin resistance estimation are recommended in women with risk factors, e.g. increased waist circumference or personal/family history of diabetes/cardiovascular disease.

Routine breast palpation and pelvic examination is unnecessary; these need only be performed if clinically indicated. Mammography should be performed as part of the national screening programme every 3 years unless more frequent examinations are clinically indicated. However, if a woman chooses to use HRT beyond the current age of breast screening cessation (70 years), mammographic screening should also continue. In women over 45 years of age it is best to arrange screening before starting oestrogen therapy to identify patients with sub-clinical disease. Ultrasound examination of the pelvis and/or endometrial biopsy are not a necessary prerequisite to treatment with HRT unless there is undiagnosed bleeding. In the few cases where an underlying pathology is present, bleeding will be irregular after starting treatment, indicating the need for immediate further investigation.

The best currently available measurement of osteoporosis risk is dual energy X-ray absorptiometry (DEXA) measurement of the lumbar spine and hip. Other assessment techniques such as peripheral X-ray screening, e.g. proximal phalynx and calcaneal, and ultrasound screening are improving in terms of their sensitivity and correlation with DEXA, but DEXA still remains the gold standard. Markers of bone formation and breakdown can be useful in that changes occur more rapidly than with bone density but their use is largely confined to research. The Royal College of Physicians (RCP) has issued guidelines as to which high-risk patients should be targeted for DEXA screening (see website). The RCP advises that DEXAs are performed no more than every 2 years because changes in bone mineral density are so small that they often do not exceed the margin of error of the equipment and assessor. The WHO have advised that the decision to treat osteoporosis is made by taking into account not only the bone mineral density, but also age and body mass index (see FRAX website).

Service delivery

The future delivery of menopause services should be both horizontally and vertically integrated. Vertically, in that care of the menopause patient should be in close liaison between primary, secondary, and tertiary care. Horizontally, in that care within specialist units should be multidisciplinary where patients can be cared for not only by menopause specialists but also by other affiliated specialists such as breast cancer surgeons, cardiovascular physicians, psychologists, dieticians, and nurse specialists. This is particularly important in units that look after women with premature ovarian failure and complex medical problems. Guidelines for care of menopause patients should be drawn up in collaboration with local Primary Care Trusts and key primary care specialists, in order to provide a universally high standard of management for all menopausal patients. Currently, services are threatened by lack of inclusion of menopause/HRT/osteoporosis in the new GP contract and limitation of new to follow-up ratios. Interventions

Lifestyle measures

Every woman should be encouraged to take plenty of regular exercise in addition to having a well-balanced diet and to avoid smoking. Data suggest that women who are more active tend to suffer less from the symptoms of the menopause. Not all types of activity lead to an improvement in symptoms. High impact infrequent exercise can actually make symptoms worse; the best activity is aerobic sustained regular exercise. Women who take regular weight-bearing exercise have higher bone mineral densities than sedentary controls. Exercise appears to reduce bone loss rather than reverse osteoporosis. It also improves muscle tone thus reducing falls. There is also evidence for reduction in bone loss by the daily use of calcium (approximately 1500 mg elemental calcium) and vitamin D (400–600 IU) supplements. Avoidance or reduction of intake of alcohol and caffeine can reduce the severity and frequency of vasomotor symptoms. In view of the rise in insulin resistance during the menopause transition, it is advisable that a low glycaemic index/load diet is instituted if weight gain is a problem.

Hormone therapy regimens
Dosage of oestrogen

There is general agreement now that we should be starting with the minimum effective dose of oestradiol and increasing the dose if needed to alleviate symptoms. Although there is no direct evidence that higher doses of exogenous oestrogen are associated with increased risk of breast cancer or heart disease, there is a link with venous thromboembolic risk. Importantly, lower doses of oestrogen are less likely to produce breast tenderness and bleeding problems (less endometrial stimulation), which will reduce continuance of therapy.

The dosages of currently available systemic oestrogen are as follows:

- 0.3–0.625 mg of oral conjugated equine oestrogens
- 1 mg of oral micronized oestradiol or oestradiol valerate
- 25–50 μg transdermal oestradiol
- 25–50 mg of implanted oestradiol.

Recent data suggest that the benefits of a 1-mg dose of oestradiol for symptoms and bone protection can be achieved with a 0.5 mg dose. Exceptions to this 'low dose rule' are women who suffer premature ovarian failure, who need higher doses of oestrogen to reproduce the physiological hormone levels which would have been present if the ovaries had not failed early. Sadly, very little work has been carried out to determine what the optimum route of administration or dosage is in this group of young women. The author of this section aims to set up a working group with the Royal College of Obstetricians and Gynaecologists to study this neglected area.

Route of administration

If we adhere to the principle that we should try to reproduce the most physiological state possible with a 2:1 oestradiol–oestrone ratio, then we should avoid the oral route altogether. Oral oestradiol preparations are partially metabolized to oestrone by hepatic first-pass metabolism and therefore do not fully restore this ratio. There are twice weekly or once weekly transdermal systems containing both oestrogen and progestogen that can be used either sequentially or as continuous combined HRT. The hormone is adsorbed onto the adhesive matrix, which avoids the skin reactions caused by the old alcohol reservoir patches. Oestradiol is also available as a low volume daily transdermal gel and work is ongoing to produce an oral tab/wafer that maintains the ease of oral administration while absorption avoids first-pass metabolism.

Local (vaginal) oestrogen

Recently developed vaginal HRT regimens have managed to avoid the problem of endometrial stimulation. Creams using oestriol do not produce endometrial hyperplasia and the 17β oestradiol vaginal tablet and silicone vaginal ring also provide effective relief of local symptoms without any significant endometrial effects. These preparations can be used without progestogenic opposition but are only licensed for 3 months use in the UK and 1 year in Europe. Options for local vaginal oestrogen are as follows:

- 0.01% oestriol cream and pessaries
- 0.1% oestriol cream
- 25 μg/24 hour oestradiol vaginal tablets

- 7.5 µg/24 hour oestradiol-releasing silicone ring
- Premarin cream (this preparation can potentially cause endometrial hyperplasia and should not be used without progestogenic opposition for more than 3 months).

Progestogens

Regimens

Oestrogen was originally used unopposed in non-hysterectomized women. It was noted that this led to endometrial hyperplasia in up to 30% of cases. Progestogen has therefore been added to oestrogen therapy for the last 30 years in order to avoid hyperplasia and carcinoma. It is generally accepted that women commencing HRT should start on a sequential regimen, i.e. continuous oestrogen with progestogen for 12–14 days per month. The typical dosages of the more commonly used progestogens are shown in Table 12.23.1.

Bleeding problems

If bleeding is heavy or erratic the dose of progestogen can be doubled or duration increased to 21 days. Persistent bleeding problems beyond 6 months warrant investigation with ultrasound scan and/or endometrial biopsy. After 1 year of therapy women can switch to a continuous combined regimen, which aims to give a bleed free HRT regimen and will also minimize the risk of endometrial hyperplasia. Alternatively, women can be switched to the tissue selective agent tibolone. With both these regimens there may be some erratic bleeding to begin with, but 90% of those that persist with this regimen will eventually be completely bleed free. If starting HRT *de novo* a bleed-free regimen can be used from the outset if the last menstrual period was over a year ago.

Table 12.23.1 Minimum doses of progestogen given orally in HRT as endometrial protection

Progestogen type	Sequential combined daily dosage	Continuous combined daily dosage
C19: testosterone-derived progestogens		
Norethisterone	5 mg	0.1 mg
Levonorgestrel	75 µg	n/a
Levonorgestrel (IUS)	n/a	20 µg (14 µg in development)
Norgestrel	150 µg	50 µg
C21: progesterone-derived progestogens		
Dydrogesterone*	10 mg	5 mg
Cyproterone	2 mg	1 mg
Medroxyprogesterone acetate	5 mg	2.5 mg
Micronized progesterone	200 mg	100 mg
Cyclogest pessaries	400 mg	200 mg
Crinone gel (4% or 8%)	Alternate day/ 12 days of cycle	Twice weekly

IUS, intrauterine system.
*Not currently available in UK.

Side-effects

It is vital that we maximize compliance if patients are to receive the full benefits from HRT. One of the main factors for reduced compliance is that of progestogen intolerance. Progestogens have a variety of effects apart from the one for which their use was intended, that of secretory transformation of the endometrium. Symptoms of fluid retention are produced by the sodium-retaining effect of the renin–aldosterone system, which is triggered by stimulation of the mineralocorticoid receptor. Androgenic side-effects such as acne and hirsuitism are a problem of the testosterone-derived progestogen due to stimulation of the androgen receptors. Mood swings and PMS-like side-effects result from stimulation of the central nervous system progesterone receptors.

Minimizing progestogen intolerance: the dose can be halved and duration of progestogen can be reduced to 7–10 days. However, this may result in bleeding problems and hyperplasia in a few cases (5–10%) so there should be a low threshold for performing ultrasound scans and endometrial sampling in these women. Natural progesterone has fewer side-effects due to progesterone receptor specificity and is now available in an oral micronized form, vaginal pessaries, and gel (Table 12.23.1). The levonorgestrel intrauterine system, recently granted a 4-year licence in the UK for progestogenic opposition, also minimizes systemic progestogenic side-effects by releasing the progestogen directly into the endometrium with low systemic levels. Drospirenone, a spironolactone analogue, has recently been incorporated with low-dose oestrogen in a continuous combined formulation. It is not only progesterone receptor specific but also has antiandrogenic and antimineralocorticoid properties, the former making it useful for hirsuitism and the latter for fluid retention. Also, it may have blood pressure-lowering effects. It is imperative that we continue to seek improved ways of administering the progestogens, which are important in protecting the endometrium in order to avoid progestogenic side-effects, and minimize effects on breast tissue, e.g. vaginal and intrauterine progestogens and natural progesterone. However, we still lack data about the risk of breast cancer in women using oestrogen with a levonorgestrel intrauterine system.

Risks of HRT

The Women's Health Inititiative (WHI) and Million Women Study (MWS) studies have demonstrated an excess risk of cardiovascular disease, stroke, and breast cancer in women using combined oestrogen and progestogen HRT. However, these studies were heavily criticized because their design, particularly the WHI study, where the average age of recruitment was 63 years and with an excess of obesity, hypertension, and pre-existing cardiovascular disease leading to prothrombotic problems. In contrast, a recent subanalysis of the WHI has shown that the cardiovascular risks were confined to the oldest age group. The absolute excess risk of coronary heart disease per 10 000 person years was −2 for women aged 50–59 years at randomization, −1 for those who were 60–69 years, and it increased to +19 for those in the 70–79-year age group. This shows that women in the youngest cohort (typically seen in our clinics with menopausal symptoms) had a trend towards improvement of cardiovascular risk and significant reduction in all causes of mortality. Guidance issued by the International Menopause Society has emphasized that in the WHI study the risks of breast cancer did not become significant until 7 years of usage (approximately one extra case per 1000 women per annum); they stated that for women in the normal menopause transition, the benefits of HRT far outweigh the risks and may even confer cardiovascular benefits.

Testosterone preparations/regimens

For women with distressing low sexual desire and tiredness only 100-mg implanted testosterone pellets were licensed until recently. The realization that there was an unfilled niche in the market for female androgen replacement led to the development of the 300 µg per day testosterone transdermal system to treat 'hypo sexual desire disorder'. The current licence for this product is in surgically menopausal women on concomitant oestrogen, but it is expected that licences will be granted for naturally menopausal women and women using testosterone without oestrogen. Unlicensed options include testosterone gel, which comes in 50 mg, 5-mL sachets, or tubes at a dose of 0.5–1.0 mL/day. In the author's experience if the free androgen index is kept within the physiological range there are rarely any side-effects such as hirsutism. Levels can be checked at baseline and repeated at 4–6 weeks. Alternatives to this include scaled down dosages of testosterone injections and oral preparations, although many avoid the latter route because of hepatic concerns. Concerns regarding cardiovascular and breast cancer risks have not been realized in clinical studies.

Contraindications to HRT

HRT is contraindicated in women with a history of cardiovascular disease and stroke. Although contraindicated in venous thromboembolic disease, there is some evidence that transdermal preparations are safer by avoiding first-pass metabolism.

Natural oestrogens when given to normotensive or hypertensive women do not cause an elevation in blood pressure, and when given in combination with oral progesterone may actually lower blood pressure; therefore, there is no justification for withholding HRT from hypertensive women.

Fibroids are responsive to oestrogens, and involute after the menopause. HRT may continue to stimulate these benign tumours causing some to increase in size. This can produce an increase in menstrual blood loss, but in practice does not usually represent a problem as treatment can easily be discontinued. However, in patients with a good indication who wish to continue therapy, fibroid resection or a hysterectomy is a possible compromise.

Endometriosis which is stimulated by cyclical ovarian activity can cause considerable pain and many patients with severe disease may require hysterectomy, often with bilateral oophorectomy. Unfortunately, because of a fear of using oestrogens, the ovaries are often conserved at operation and continue to stimulate the endometriosis causing continued pain in these women. Approximately 50% of women will continue to have pain until all ovarian tissue is removed, after which continuous oestrogen may be administered with a reduced risk of recurrence of endometriosis. In cases where the endometriosis has been severe and complete clearance may not have been achieved, it may be sensible to give low-dose continuous combined HRT or tibolone to reduce the risk of recurrence.

Treatment of patients with a past history of endometrial cancer is controversial, but there are reports of oestrogen use without any detrimental effects in stage I–III disease. Squamous cervical cancer is not oestrogen sensitive. There are no adverse data in ovarian cancer survivors, although there may be a very small increased risk of ovarian cancer with long-term unopposed oestrogen use in healthy women. There are no data for adenocarcinoma of the cervix, vaginal, or vulval cancer.

Breast cancer must be regarded as the principal contraindication to oestrogen treatment, but high-risk women with a strong family history of breast malignancy or those with benign breast disease should not necessarily be denied treatment. It is unclear what the precise risk of breast cancer recurrence is with HRT use. A study in breast cancer survivors using HRT was terminated because of an apparent excess risk. Unfortunately, this led to the premature termination of two other studies running concomitantly in which no excess risk had been detected. A large randomized placebo-controlled study (LIBERATE) in breast cancer survivors using tibolone recently demonstrated a marginal increase in recurrence rates (RR 1.4).

Duration of therapy

It is recognized that symptoms often return when HRT is ceased, even after many years of use. If the underpinning principle of HRT is that it should be used to improve and maintain a good quality of life, in women in whom this principle is maintained it is difficult to argue that they should have arbitrary deadlines imposed on them. Although breast cancer risks appear to be duration dependent, evidence suggests that overall mortality is actually reduced in women commencing HRT before the age of 60. Thus, duration of therapy requires careful judgement of benefits and risks on an individual basis. If therapy is to be discontinued, the dose should be reduced in a stepwise fashion over a minimum of 6 months to reduce the risk of immediate severe symptom resurgence.

Official prescribing advice

How are health professionals supposed to react to these data and advise their patients? Guidance from the Medicine's & Healthcare Products Regulatory Agency (see website) has advised that HRT should not be recommended for primary or secondary prevention of heart disease. This advice is mirrored by the European Medicine's Agency (see website) and by the North American Menopause Society (NAMS position paper). It is recommended that HRT be used merely for symptom relief in the short term at the lowest effective dose and alternatives should be considered in the long term for prevention of osteoporosis. Annual reappraisal of HRT use should be carried out with weighing up of the pros and cons on an individual basis. However, the British Menopause Society (see website) consensus statement advises that prescribing habits need not be changed by the recent studies because HRT use in the UK was primarily for symptom relief anyway rather than primary or secondary prevention. Similar statements were made by the European and International Menopause Societies (see websites).

Complementary therapies/alternatives to HRT

The concern from the recent studies regarding the risks of HRT has led to an increasing demand for alternatives to HRT for the management of menopausal symptoms. There is little scientific evidence that complementary and alternative therapies can help menopausal symptoms or provide the same benefits as conventional therapies. Yet many women use them, believing them to be safer and 'more natural', especially following the current controversies regarding HRT. The choice of treatments is confusing and, unlike conventional medicines, not much is known about their active ingredients, safety or side-effects, or how they may interact with other therapies. They can interfere with warfarin, antidepressants, and anti-epileptics with potentially fatal consequences. Some herbal preparations may contain oestrogenic compounds and this is of concern for women with hormone-dependent disease such as breast cancer. There is also concern about contaminants such as mercury, arsenic, lead, and pesticides. Legislation is soon to be introduced which will make it mandatory for herbal preparations to at least be registered with the MHRA. This will at least allow some control over what is being sold over the counter, which currently may be completely ineffective or dangerous. It is essential that alternatives to licensed preparations should be judged by similar standards.

An integrated approach to the management of vasomotor symptoms should be considered in women wanting to consider alternatives to (or contraindicated to) HRT. An algorithm drawn up by a consensus group of international experts integrating lifestyle, complementary, and pharmacological interventions is shown below (Fig. 12.23.1). Lifestyle changes and supplements such as red clover and soy isoflavones and other alternatives can be incorporated into the routine management of women with vasomotor

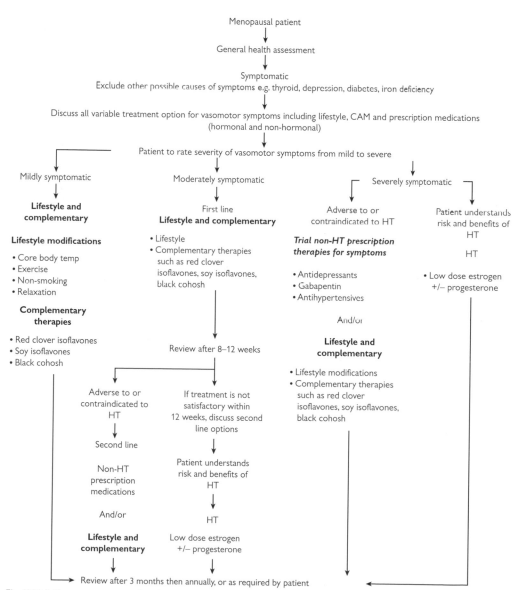

Fig. 12.23.1 Vasomotor treatment algorithm: a conservative, clinical approach.

symptoms. In conjunction with the algorithm a five-step approach is suggested:

- initial patient consultation and general health assessment
- establishment of menopause as basis of symptoms, i.e. exclusion of other conditions
- discussion of all symptom management options from very outset
- patient asked to self-rate her symptom severity
- management choice individualized based on symptom severity.

The algorithm is not intended for women with premature menopause or for those with other risk factors such as osteoporosis. It should also be remembered that certain groups of women may have contraindications to the use of complementary therapies. For instance, some women may have intolerance to soy or lignans. High-dose isoflavones should probably be avoided in breast cancer sufferers; also, those with low libido could have a deterioration due to reduction in free testosterone via SHBG. Finally, if complementary therapies have been ineffective and traditional HRT has been started there is little reason to continue the original product as this is unlikely to have an additive effect and may even interfere with the efficacy of exogenously administered hormones.

Non-pharmacological alternatives (Rees and Panay 2006)

Gels for vaginal symptoms

Replens: this vaginal bioadhesive moisturizer is a more physiological way of replacing vaginal secretions than with lubricant vaginal gels such as KY jelly. It actually rehydrates the tissues and provides a reasonable alternative to systemic or vaginal HRT.

Pharmacological alternatives

α-2 agonists

Clonidine, a centrally active α-2 agonist, has been one of the most popular alternative preparations for the treatment of vasomotor symptoms. A recent meta-analysis of the few randomized controlled trials has shown a marginal benefit of clonidine over placebo.

Selective serotonin reuptake inhibitors SSRIs/noradrenaline reuptake inhibitors SNRIs

A significant amount of evidence exists for the efficacy of SSRIs and SNRIs in the treatment of vasomotor symptoms. Although there are some data for SSRIs such as fluoxetine and paroxetine, the most convincing data are for the SNRI (venlafaxine) at a dose of 37.5 mg bd. The key effect with these preparations appears to be stimulation of the noradrenergic as opposed to the serotonergic pathways, hence the preferential effect of SNRIs. The trials demonstrate a 50–60% reduction in hot flush frequency and severity. The main drawback with these preparations (especially the SNRIs) is the high incidence of nausea, which often leads to withdrawal from therapy before maximum efficacy has been achieved.

Gabapentin

Recent work with the antiepileptic drug gabapentin has shown efficacy for hot flush reduction compared with placebo. In a recent study using gabapentin at a dose of 900 mg per day, a 45% reduction of hot flush frequency and a 54% reduction of symptom severity was demonstrated. Further work is being conducted to confirm the efficacy and safety of this preparation but for the moment its use is restricted to specialist centres. Once again, its use is limited by the frequency of often severe side-effects.

Complementary therapies: phytoestrogens

Phytoestrogens are plant substances that have effects similar to those of oestrogens. Since the first discovery of the oestrogenic activity of plant compounds, over 300 plants have been found to have phytoestrogenic activity. Preparations vary from enriched foods such as bread or drinks (soy milk) to more concentrated tablets. The most important groups are called isoflavones and lignans. The major isoflavones are genistein and daidzein. The major lignans are enterolactone and enterodiol. Isoflavones are found in soybeans, chick peas, red clover, and probably other legumes (beans and peas). Oilseeds such as flaxseed are rich in lignans, and they are also found in cereal bran, whole cereals, vegetables, legumes, and fruit. The role of phytoestrogens has stimulated considerable interest since populations, such as the Japanese, consuming a diet high in isoflavones appear to have lower rates of menopausal vasomotor symptoms, cardiovascular disease, osteoporosis, and breast, colon, endometrial, and ovarian cancers. The normal Japanese diet contains 200 mg of phytoestrogens per day compared with the average Western diet, which contains less than 1 mg. However, epidemiological studies need to be supported by data, with analyses of the isoflavone content of foods and measures of their bioavailability. The evidence from randomized placebo-controlled trials in Western populations is conflicting for both soy and derivatives from red clover, with marginal benefits demonstrated in meta-analyses of randomized trials. Similarly, there are also debates about the effects on breast cancer, lipoproteins, endothelial function, and blood pressure. Currently other studies are under way, including a European Union study (Phytos—see website), which should help quantify the relative importance and optimal doses for symptom relief, bone preserving effects, and safety.

Conclusion

Effective management of the menopause is taking on everincreasing importance in view of our ageing population. The overzealous reporting of recent clinical trials has made it imperative that physicians involved in this area can access well-balanced evidence-based information. In the author's opinion, current best practice should involve the following:

- discussion of lifestyle measures, HRT, and alternatives should take place from the outset.
- management should be individualized taking into account risks and benefits.
- the main indication for use of HRT should be for symptom relief rather than for prevention of long-term problems
- low-dose HRT should usually be commenced and increased if necessary to achieve effective symptom relief, except in premature ovarian failure where higher doses are physiological.
- androgen therapy should be considered in women with persistent low libido and energy levels
- rigid cut offs in the duration of therapy should be avoided, with regular reappraisal (at least annual) of the benefits and risks for each individual
- delivery of services should be from a multidisciplinary team if possible with close liaison with allied specialties and experts.

It is unlikely that the ultimate menopause therapy which truly has all the benefits without any side-effects and risks will ever be developed. Clinicians should therefore aim to provide the best evidence-based advice possible in order to allow women to make an informed choice about how to manage their menopause transition and beyond.

Further reading

Bjarnason NH. Postmenopausal bone remodelling and hormone replacement. Climacteric 1998;1:72–9.

Christian RC, Harrington S., Edwards WD, et al. Estrogen status correlates with the calcium content of coronary atherosclerotic plaques in women. J Clin Endocrinol Metab 2002;87:1062–7.

Davis SR, Moreau M, Kroll R, et al. Testosterone for low libido in postmenopausal women not taking estrogen. N Engl J Med 2008;359:2005–17.

Davison SL, Bell R, Donath S, et al. Androgen Levels in Adult Females: changes with Age, Menopause and Oophorectomy. J Clin Endocrinol Metab 2005;90:3847–53.

Kalu E, Panay N. Spontaneous premature ovarian failure: management challenges. Gynecol Endocrinol 2008;24:273–9.

Kenemans P, Bundred NJ, Foidart JM, et al. Safety and efficacy of tibolone in breast-cancer patients with vasomotor symptoms: a double-blind, randomised, non-inferiority trial. Lancet Oncol 2009;10:135–46.

Landgren BM, Collins A, Csemiczky G, et al. Menopause transition: annual changes in serum hormonal patterns over the menstrual cycle in women during a 9 year period prior to menopause. J Clin Endocrinol Metab 2004;89:2763–9.

Lindh-Astrand L, Nedstrand E, Wyon Y, Hammar M. Vasomotor symptoms and quality of life in previously sedentary postmenopausal women randomised to physical activity or estrogen therapy. Maturitas 2004;48:97–105.

Loprinzi CL, Kugler JW, Sloan JA, et al. Venlafaxine in the management of hot flashes in survivors of breast cancer: a randomised controlled trial Lancet 2000;356:2059–63.

Million Women Study Collaborators. Breast cancer and HRT in the Million Women Study. Lancet 2003;362:419–27.

Muscat Baron Y, Brincat MP, Galea R, Calleja N. Low intervertebral disc height in postmenopausal women with osteoporotic vertebral fractures compared to hormone-treated and untreated postmenopausal women and premenopausal women without fractures. Climacteric 2007;10:314–9.

Nardo LG, Christodoulou D, Gould D, et al. Anti-Müllerian hormone levels and antral follicle count in women enrolled in in vitro fertilization cycles: relationship to lifestyle factors, chronological age and reproductive history. Gynecol Endocrinol 2007;24:1–8.

Nelson HD, Vesco KK, Haney, et al. Non-hormonal therapies for menopausal hot flashes: systematic review and meta – analysis. JAMA 2006;295:2057–71.

Panay N Fenton A. The role of testosterone in women. Climacteric 2009;12:185–7

Panay N, Fenton A. Premature ovarian failure: a growing concern. Climacteric 2008;11:1–3.

Panay N, Studd JWW. Progestogen intolerance and compliance with hormone replacement therapy in menopausal women. Hum Reprod Update 1997;3:159–71.

Panay N, Studd JWW. The psychotherapeutic effects of estrogens Gynaecol Endocrinol 1998;12:353–65.

Panay N, Ylikorkala O, Archer DF, et al. Ultra low-dose estradiol and norethisterone acetate: effective menopausal symptom relief. Climacteric 2007;10:120–31.

Panay N. Integrating phytoestrogens with prescription medicines – A conservative clinical approach to vasomotor symptom management. Maturitas 2007;57:90–4.

Pines A, Sturdee DW, Birkhauser MH, et al. IMS Updated Recommendations on postmenopausal HRT. Climacteric 2007;10:181–94.

Powles TJ, Howell A, Evans DG, et al. Red Clover Isoflavones are safe and well tolerated in women with a family history of breast cancer. Menopause Int 2008;14:6–12.

Rees M, Mander A (eds) Managing the menopause without oestrogen. London: RSM Press 2004.

Rees M, Purdie D (eds). Management of the menopause: the handbook, 4th edn. London: RSM Press 2006.

Rees M., Panay N. The use of alternatives to HRT for the Management of menopause symptoms RCOG Scientific Advisory Committee 2006;Opinion Paper 6.

Rossouw JE, Prentice RL, Manson JE, et al. Postmenopausal hormone therapy and risk of cardiovascular disease by age and years since menopause. JAMA 2007;297:1465–77.

Salpeter SR, Walsh JM, Greyber E., et al. Mortality associated with hormone replacement therapy in younger and older women: a meta-analysis. J Gen Intern Med 2004;19:791–804.

Scarabin PY, Olger E, Plu-Bureau G. Differential association of oral and transdermal oestrogen replacement therapy with venous thromboembolism risk. Lancet 2003;362:428–32.

Shumaker SA, Legault C, Rapp SR, et al. Estrogen plus progestin and the incidence of dementia and mild cognitive impairment in postmenopausal women: the Women's Health Initiative Memory Study: a randomized controlled study. JAMA 2003;289:2651–62.

Singer D, Hunter M (eds). Premature menopause: a multidisciplinary approach. London: WileyBlackwell.

Thompson Coon J, Pittler MH, Ernst E. The role of red clover (Trifolium pratense) isoflavones in women's reproductive health: a systematic review and meta-analysis of randomised clinical trials. Focus Altern Complement Ther 2003;8:544.

Tunstall-Pedoe H. Myth and paradox of coronary risk and the menopause. Lancet 1998;351:1425–7.

Writing Group for the Women's Health Initiative Investigators. Risks and benefits of estrogen plus progestin in healthy postmenopausal women: principal results From Women's Health Initiative randomized controlled trial. JAMA 2002;288:321–33.

Internet resources

British Menopause Society site—see consensus statements: www.the-bms.org

International Menopause Society—see consensus statements: www.imsociety.org

European Menopause Society: http://emas.obgyn.net/

The medical and Healthcare Products Regulatory Agency: www.mhra.gov.uk

WHO osteoporosis fracture risk calculator: www.shef.ac.uk/FRAX/

National Osteoporosis Society—professionals and patients: www.nos.org.uk

North American Menopause Society: www.menopause.org

European Medicines Agency: www.emea.eu.int/

National Centre for Complementary and Alternative Medicine. Alternative therapies for managing menopausal symptoms: http://nccam.nih.gov/health/alerts/menopause/

The PHYTOHEALTH Network aims to establish a pan-European network of institutions dealing with safety and health effect of phytoestrogens, identification of optimal sources and processing technologies: www.phytohealth.org

The NIH Office of Dietary Supplements: http://dietary-supplements.info.nih.gov

Women's Health Initiative Website: www.whi.org

Royal College of Physicians Guidelines on Osteoporosis: www.rcplondon.ac.uk/pubs/wp_osteo_update.htm

Patient resources

Informative menopause website: www.menopausematters.co.uk

Premenstrual Syndrome website: www.pms.org.uk

National Osteoporosis Society—professionals and patients: www.nos.org.uk

Women's Health Group—including 'ask the experts': www.womens-health-concern.org/

Menorrhagia

Definition
Menorrhagia may be defined as heavy menstrual bleeding over several cycles. The traditional, objective, definition of menorrhagia is of menstrual blood loss of 80 mL or more per cycle. Measured blood loss has been shown to have little correlation with women's own perceptions of bleeding heaviness and so the clinical definition typically used is that of excessively heavy bleeding for an individual.

In practice, any blood loss that is perceived by a woman to be excessive or as having a negative impact on her quality of life warrants counselling and possibly treatment.

Epidemiology
Prevalence rates for menorrhagia of between 4% and 51% in women of reproductive years have been reported from around the world. This reflects the variety of definitions in use for the condition, the subjective nature of its reporting, and cultural differences in how bleeding is perceived. Evidence also suggests that increasing age is a risk factor for menorrhagia.

In fact, the majority of women will experience menstrual bleeding which they consider excessive at some time in their life, although this may be short-lived and self-limiting. In the UK, menorrhagia accounts for 12% of all gynaecology referrals.

Pathology
In approximately half of women presenting with menorrhagia no pathological cause will be found and their loss is therefore 'unexplained'.

Common causes include those listed below.
- Fibroids: uterine leiomyomas (fibroids) are common benign tumours of the myometrium, occurring in approximately 20% of women of reproductive age. They are associated with increased menstrual blood loss in approximately one-third of cases, with submucous fibroids distorting the uterine cavity particularly implicated. Despite this association, the presence of fibroids in a woman presenting with menorrhagia should not be assumed to be causative. In particular small intramural or subserosal fibroids may be a purely incidental finding.
- Endometrial polyps: focal overgrowth of endometrial glands and stroma to form polyps are a cause of menorrhagia, particularly in older women.
- Endometrial hyperplasia and carcinoma: malignant and premalignant conditions may present with menorrhagia, although the presence of other symptoms such as inter-menstrual bleeding may increase suspicion. The major risk factor is age, with others being related to increased oestrogenic stimulation of the endometrium, e.g. obesity, polycystic ovary syndrome, and tamoxifen therapy. Simple and complex hyperplasia carries a 1–3% risk of potential malignant change and with atypical hyperplasia the risk is approximately 20% (Table 12.24.1).
- Coagulation disorders and iatrogenic anticoagulation: conditions such as von Willebrand disease and platelet disorders as well as treatment, especially at therapeutic doses with heparin or warfarin are associated with menorrhagia.
- Medical conditions: it is thought that most chronic illness can lead to menstrual disturbance. Specific associations with menorrhagia include hypothyroidism, systemic lupus erythematosus and liver disease (Table 12.24.2).

Table 12.24.1 Risk factors for endometrial carcinoma

Raised body mass index	Late menopause
Inactive lifestyle	Unopposed estrogens
Diabetes mellitus	Prolonged irregular bleeding
Poor diet (high fat/low complex carbohydrate)	Personal/family history of breast/bowel/endometrial cancer
Early menarche	Nulliparity
Tamoxifen use	Age >40 years

- Dysfunctional uterine bleeding: this is excessive uterine bleeding that is not due to demonstrable pelvic pathology, complications of pregnancy, or systemic disease. It includes heavy bleeding due to the non-ovulatory cycles, which occur at the extremes of reproductive life, around menarche and in the perimenopause, the latter being the commonest time for women to present with menorrhagia. Dysfunctional uterine bleeding is a diagnosis of exclusion. The causes of abnormal uterine bleeding can be classified as pelvic, systemic or functional (see Table 12.24.3).

Prognosis
Prognosis is good and women can expect a significant improvement in their quality of life with appropriate management. However, it may prove more challenging to find effective treatments for those currently wishing to conceive or to preserve their fertility, as well as for those with underlying medical conditions (Table 12.24.2).

Clinical approach
Diagnosis
History, examination, and investigations should be directed towards identifying the cause and severity of menorrhagia in order to plan appropriate treatment.

History
Points to note are listed below.
- The pattern and nature of the bleeding. The use of a menstrual calendar and questions focused on the type

Table 12.24.2 Medical disorders associated with menorrhagia

Endocrine disease	Thyroid dysfunction
	Pituitary/adrenal gland abnormalities
Haematological disease	Coagulation disorders
	Platelet abnormalities
	Sickle cell disease
Autoimmune disease	Systemic lupus erythematosus
Hepatic, renal and cardiac disease	Liver disease
	Renal disease
	Cardiac disease
Metabolic disease	Gaucher's disease

Table 12.24.3 Causes of abnormal uterine bleeding

Pelvic	Uterine fibroids
	Adenomyosis
	Endometrial polyps
	Pelvic infection
	Endometrial hyperplasia
	Endometrial adenocarcinoma
	Presence of copper-containing intrauterine contraceptive device
	Uterine vascular malformations
	Myometrial hypertrophy
Systemic	Coagulation disorders, i.e. thrombocytopenia, von Willebrand disease
	Hypothyroidism
	Systemic lupus erythematosus
	Chronic liver failure
Functional	Dysfunctional uterine bleeding

and frequency of changing of sanitary products, and a measure of how day-to-day activities are disturbed may be helpful.

- The presence of associated symptoms such as intermenstrual or post-coital bleeding and abdominal or pelvic pain and pressure impact on quality of life.
- Last menstrual period and exclusion of pregnancy.
- Risk factors for endometrial carcinoma.
- Background gynaecological history, e.g. smear tests, contraception.
- Obstetric history and whether family is complete.
- General medical, surgical and drug history.

The taking of a good history should involve an exploration of the patients concerns and their aims and expectations, having sought medical help.

Examination

- General examination for signs of anaemia or thyroid disease.
- Abdominal examination to exclude a palpable fibroid uterus.
- Inspection of the genital tract including the cervix should be performed. Bimanual pelvic examination allows assessment of uterine size, mobility, tenderness, or adnexal masses.

Quantification of menstrual blood loss

Objective methods for the quantification of menstrual bleeding have been described such as the alkaline haematin method, involving the chemical extraction of haemoglobin from sanitary pads. These are no longer seen to have clinical relevance, with the emphasis now being on improving quality of life for any woman who feels her periods are problematic.

There remains a role for aids to women's own assessments of blood loss such as pictorial blood loss assessment charts and menstrual calendars.

Investigations

The majority of patients do not require the full range of investigations for menorrhagia, as described below.

Relevant tests should be carefully selected based on the history and examination findings in order to avoid unnecessary intervention and anxiety and to prevent delays in treatment.

Blood tests

A full blood count should be performed in all women with menorrhagia requiring investigation.

Serum ferritin should not be performed routinely but only where there is uncertainty as to the nature of any anaemia.

Thyroid function tests should only be performed where there are specific signs or symptoms of thyroid disease.

Testing for von Willebrand disease or other coagulation disorders should only be performed in cases where there is a history of menorrhagia from menarche or relevant family history.

A hormone profile has not been shown to be of benefit.

Assessment of the uterus and endometrium

This is required when the history and examination suggest significant structural or histological abnormalities. For example, where there is a palpable uterus or a pelvic mass, there are features suggestive of endometrial carcinoma or significant risk factors such as age over 45 years. In addition, endometrial assessment may be indicated in cases of persistent menorrhagia and failure of initial treatment.

Assessment may be by

- ultrasound
- endometrial biopsy
- hysteroscopy.

Each may be used alone or in conjunction with the other modalities. Particular methods are better at identifying particular pathologies and the choice of which tools to use will depend upon the individual presentation.

- Ultrasound: this is the first line modality for the investigation of structural abnormalities and is particularly useful for the identification and localization of fibroids. Transvaginal scanning has advantages over transabdominal scanning for the normally sized uterus. Ultrasound measurement of endometrial thickness to exclude endometrial carcinoma is of less benefit in the premenopausal woman.
- Endometrial biopsy: this must be performed where there is suspicion of histological abnormality, as described above. The pipelle endometrial sampler has become the generally accepted device for outpatient sampling. Although there is some evidence to suggest that it has comparable sensitivity for the diagnosis of endometrial carcinoma as hysteroscopically directed biopsy, concerns remain over the risk of missing serious pathology with such 'blind' sampling techniques. It also is ineffective in the removal of polyps.
- Hysteroscopy: Traditionally the 'gold standard' investigation for abnormal bleeding and suspected endometrial carcinoma, its role has been replaced in many circumstances by transvaginal ultrasound and pipelle biopsy. However, hysteroscopy remains superior to ultrasound for the detection of endometrial polyps and allows directed biopsy of suspicious lesions, although it is associated with greater patient discomfort. Furthermore, modern techniques and miniaturized scopes have led to outpatient hysteroscopy clinics, with no need for general anaesthetic and greater patient acceptability. Hysteroscopy may also be therapeutic,

with treatment to polyps, submucous fibroids or endometrial ablation possible.

Management

There are a wide variety of treatments available for menorrhagia. The woman should be an active participant in deciding management and ample time should be provided for her to make appropriate choices. High standards of communication and counselling, supported by evidence-based information are essential to allow women to make informed decisions.

Counselling

For some women simple reassurance regarding the nature of their bleeding is sufficient and no other intervention may be necessary. Specific advice that no malignancy or other serious pathology is present is often welcome

Conservative/non-medical

If the patient is coping with her menstrual loss and declines any therapeutic intervention, she can be safely discharged. Advice about ensuring adequate iron intake and the offer of review, if required, is typically all that is needed.

Medical

Recent guidelines from the National Institute for Health and Clinical Excellence have suggested that pharmaceutical therapies are considered in the order below.

First line

- Levonorgestrel-releasing intrauterine system: the slow release of progestogen prevents proliferation of the endometrium, thereby reducing menstrual blood loss. The device is also contraceptive. Following its removal fertility returns to baseline levels quickly. Side-effects may include persistent irregular bleeding together with headaches, breast tenderness, and acne, which are generally mild and transient.

Second line

- Tranexamic acid: these oral antifibrinolytic tablets help to reduce menstrual flow. They can be commenced while appropriate investigations are performed. Improvement in symptoms would be expected within three cycles. Tranexamic acid has no impact on fertility. Minor side-effects include indigestion, diarrhoea, and headache.

- Non-steroidal anti-inflammatory drugs: this group of oral medications reduce prostaglandin production. They can be used in conjunction with tranexamic acid and can also be commenced while investigations are being undertaken. Improvement in symptoms should be seen within three cycles. They are especially useful when menorrhagia and dysmenorrhoea coexist. Non-steroidal anti-inflammatory drugs are not contraceptive. Women may experience side-effects of indigestion and diarrhoea. Asthma may be exacerbated in sensitive women and gastritis may progress to peptic ulcer disease with its associated risks of gastrointestinal bleeding, perforation, and peritonitis.

- Combined oral contraceptives: as well as providing contraception, combined oral contraceptives also reduce menstrual loss by preventing proliferation of the endometrium. Fertility levels will return to baseline within a short time after discontinuation. Women on the combined oral contraceptive have an increased risk of venous thromboembolism, cerebrovascular accident and myocardial infarction.

Third line

- Oral progestogen: oral progestogens prevent proliferation of the endometrium. The recommended regime of norethisterone 15 mg daily from days 5 to 26 is not contraceptive but may adversely affect the woman's ability to conceive. Common side-effects of oral progestogens include weight gain, bloating, breast tenderness, headaches, and acne.

- Injected progestogen: injected progestogens also prevent proliferation of the endometrium. They are contraceptive and there may be a delay in return of fertility once injections cease. Injections are usually administered every 12 weeks. The side-effects are similar to oral progestogens. Long-term use can be associated with bone mineral density loss.

Fourth line

- Gonadotrophin-releasing hormone analogue: the production of oestrogen and progesterone is stopped by gonadotrophin-releasing hormone analogues, thereby inducing a temporary menopause and associated amenorrhoea. Common side-effects are those of the climacteric: hot flushes, increased sweating, and vaginal dryness. If used for greater than 6 months, add-back hormone replacement therapy is recommended to reduce the risk of osteoporosis.

Surgical and radiological

- Endometrial ablation: various techniques are now available to destroy the endometrium and thereby reduce or cease menstrual blood loss. They include the first-generation techniques of transcervical resection of the endometrium. Second-generation techniques include microwave, balloon thermal, and impedance-controlled bipolar radiofrequency ablation. Appropriate patient selection is vital: women should have no fertility desires, a uterus no greater than 10-week pregnant size, no fibroids or fibroids less than 3 cm, and no histological abnormalities of the endometrium. The procedure itself is not contraceptive but pregnancy following endometrial ablation is likely to have a poor outcome, hence effective ongoing contraception is vital. The potential intraoperative complication of uterine perforation is rare and the risk is reduced further with the second generation techniques. Women may experience vaginal discharge post endometrial ablation and increased symptoms of dysmenorrhoea, even when rendered amenorrhoeic.

- Uterine artery embolization: this interventional radiology technique is suitable for women with fibroids greater than 3 cm. Small particles are injected into the uterine arteries, which shrink the fibroids by reducing their blood supply. It is particularly useful for women who are experiencing pain and pressure symptoms associated with fibroids. This technique is likely to preserve fertility, although long-term data are limited. Persistent vaginal discharge is not uncommon post-uterine artery embolization. Women may experience pain, nausea, vomiting, and fever: the post-embolization syndrome. Rarely there may be non-target embolization resulting in tissue necrosis, haemorrhage, and infection leading to septicaemia or ovarian failure.

- MRI-guided focused ultrasound: in research trials this technique is reported to be successful in reducing unacceptable menstrual flow, especially in combination with pretreatment downregulation with gonadotrophin-releasing hormone analogue therapy.

- Hysteroscopic myomectomy: submucous fibroids can be resected hysteroscopically. The procedure preserves fertility, although intrauterine adhesions can occur post-operatively, which may impair fertility. The size of the fibroids to be resected can be reduced with preoperative use of gonadotropin-releasing hormone (GnRH) analogues. If ongoing fertility is not desired, the remaining areas of endometrium can also be resected at the same procedure. Intraoperative uterine perforation, fluid overload, and postoperative infection or fibroid recurrence (especially those fibroids with a significant intramural element) are recognized unwanted outcomes.
- Myomectomy: fibroids can be removed abdominally by either open or laparoscopic procedures. Fibroid size can be reduced preoperatively with GnRH analogues. Once again fertility is theoretically preserved but the development of postoperative pelvic adhesions adversely affects tubal functions and compromises future fertility. A myomectomy in which the uterine cavity is breached perioperatively would normally lead to the recommendation that any future successful pregnancies should be delivered by elective Caesarean section.
- Hysterectomy: previously the most common procedure performed for menorrhagia, hysterectomy is becoming increasingly uncommon due to advances in medical and alternative surgical treatments. Vaginal hysterectomy is recommended as the first-line procedure, although the route of hysterectomy must be personalized for each woman. Healthy ovaries from premenopausal women should not be removed. The surgical complications of hysterectomy include infection, haemorrhage, urinary tract or bowel injury, postoperative urinary dysfunction, and venous thromboembolism.

Complications/side-effects/sequelae

Prior to embarking on treatment for menorrhagia, it is important to explore a woman's expectations of treatment: amenorrhoea may be the perfect result for one woman but psychologically distressing for others. Relevant complications and side-effects for each treatment modality are outlined above.

Follow up/recurrence/future pregnancy planning

Some women will progress through the various treatments for menorrhagia before finally requiring a hysterectomy. However, for the majority of women, long-term relief from their menorrhagia will be provided by a levonorgestrel-releasing intrauterine system. This device needs to be changed every 5 years. It can also be used for endometrial protection for women taking oestrogen hormone replacement therapy. Hence, a device fitted for management of perimenopausal menorrhagia may have uses beyond its initial indication.

Women with menorrhagia who are currently trying to conceive have limited treatment options. In addition, those women whose symptoms do not resolve with pharmacological methods may have to consider treatments which may adversely affect their future fertility. Therefore, the importance of exploring a woman's reproductive plans prior to commencing treatment is vital.

Further reading

National Collaborating Centre for Women's and Children's Health. *Heavy menstrual bleeding.* Clinical Guideline. London: NICE 2007.

Internet resources

www.nice.org.uk
www.bnf.org
www.novasure.com/
www.microsulis.co.uk/

Patient resources

Fibroid Network, info@fibroid.co.uk, www.fibroidnetwork online.com

The Hysterectomy Association, 0871 7811141, www.hysterectomy-association.org.uk

Women's Health Concern, 0845 123 2319, www.womens-health-concern.org

Menstrual cycle: physiology

Introduction
The normal menstrual cycle can vary considerably between women and may range in length from 25 to 35 days. A woman's menstrual cycle pattern relies on a complex interaction of hormones exerted via her hypothalamic-pituitary-ovarian axis.

The menstrual cycle
Classically the 28-day menstrual cycle is used because it splits neatly into two halves, defined by the follicular and endometrial changes that occur before and after ovulation. Ovulation may still occur in cycles that are 25–35 days in length.

The first half of the cycle is marked by the start of bleeding on day 1 of the cycle. The 'proliferative phase' follows this as endometrial thickness increases under the influence of oestrogen secretion. This stage is also termed the 'follicular phase' because ovarian follicles begin to develop and mature in preparation for ovulation.

The second half of the cycle commences once ovulation has taken place. The 'secretory phase' describes the endometrial changes that take place in preparation for implantation of a fertilized egg. This stage is also termed the 'luteal phase', as the corpus luteum, left behind after ovulation, provides hormonal support to an early pregnancy.

Endocrinology
Several key hormones regulate the ovarian and endometrial changes during each cycle:
- gonadotrophin releasing hormone (GnRH)
- follicle-stimulating hormone (FSH)
- luteinizing hormone (LH)
- oestrogen
- progesterone.

The hypothalamus secretes GnRH in a pulsatile manner, and this stimulates the anterior pituitary to release the gonadotrophins FSH and LH, which in turn trigger the release of oestrogen and progesterone from the ovary. Each hormone plays an important role in the course of a normal menstrual cycle.

Follicular development
Follicular development within the ovary begins in early fetal life. 'Primordial germ cells' multiply by mitosis and differentiate to produce 7 000 000 'primordial follicles' by 32 weeks' gestation. Each primordial follicle contains a primary oocyte arrested in prophase of the first meiotic division. The primordial follicle remains in this state until menarche.

At birth the number of primordial follicles has fallen to 3 000 000 and by puberty only 40 0000 remain. At the onset of puberty 15–20 primordial follicles will differentiate into primary follicles with each menstrual cycle.

A primary follicle contains a primary oocyte surrounded by the zona pellucida and a single layer of granulosa cells. FSH induces proliferation of granulosa cells and up regulates FSH receptors to maximize this effect. LH drives the outer follicular thecal cells to differentiate into the 'theca interna' and 'theca externa'.

The normal menstrual cycle
Menarche is followed by 5–7 years period during which the menstrual cycles tend to become shorter and more regular as an abitary pattern develops. The highest incidence of anovulatory cycles is below the age of 20 years and over the age of 40 years.

At age 25, over 40% of cycles are between 25 and 28 days in length. From 25–35, over 60% are between 25 and 28 days.

Approximately 5 years before the menopause, the menstrual cycle tends to lengthen again.

A normal menstrual period may last from 2 to 7 days and results in the loss of 30–40 mL of blood. Menstrual bleeding in excess of 80 mL per cycle is associated with iron deficiency anaemia.

Endometrial cycle
Endometrium consists of two anatomical layers. The 'lamina functionalis' proliferates and is then shed each month in response to the rise and fall of oestrogen and progesterone levels. The 'lamina basalis' is unchanged but regenerates to provide the functionalis each month.

Menstrual cycle phases
Assuming a 28-day cycle the endocrine and physiological changes that occur during the menstrual cycle can be understood conveniently in five phases.

These five phases apply in all normal cycles (25–35 days). Despite a changeable cycle length the 'luteal phase' remains fairly constant (13 ± 1 day) and it is the 'follicular phase' that shortens and lengthens.

Early follicular phase (days 1–6)
- Menstruation signifies the start of the early follicular phase of the cycle as the 'lamina functionalis' is shed.
- Oestrogen and progesterone levels are low.
- Baseline FSH and LH levels rise with the influence of GnRH on the anterior pituitary.
- FSH triggers 15–20 primordial follicles to continue to grow and mature into multilaminar follicles.

Late follicular phase (days 7–14)
- Primordial follicles continue to develop into multilaminar follicles under the influence of FSH.
- FSH up regulates LH receptors on the granulosa cells.
- Granulosa cells proliferate under the influence of FSH to release oestradiol.
- Negative feedback at the pituitary level eventually causes FSH levels to fall.
- The rising oestrogen levels cause the lamina functionalis to proliferate from stem cells in the basalis layer and the endometrium thickens.
- The endometrium becomes more glandular.

Pre-ovulation and ovulation phase (days 13–14)
- The lamina functionalis and non-secretory glandular endometrium is at maximal thickness just prior to ovulation.
- High levels of oestrogen result in positive feedback at the pituitary causing a brief surge in LH and FSH levels.
- The dominant follicle, known as the graafian follicle, develops and completes the first meiotic division (Fig. 12.25.1).
- High LH levels are believed to be involved in ovulation
- At ovulation the secondary oocyte is expelled
- LH and FSH levels then return rapidly to baseline.

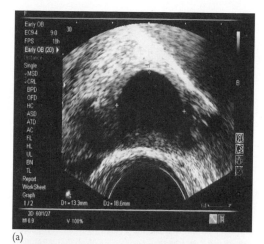

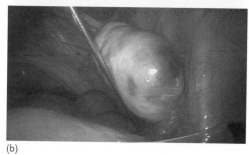

Fig. 12.25.1 A follicle on ultrasound scan (a) and at laparoscopy (b)

Early luteal phase (days 15–21)
- The granulosa and thecal cells of the dominant follicle left behind after ovulation form the corpus luteum (Fig. 12.25.2).
- Progesterone and to a lesser extent oestrogen are produced by the corpus luteum.
- Negative feedback by progesterone and oestrogen maintain FSH and LH at low levels
- The secretory endometrium forms as progesterone stimulates the secretion of glycogen, mucus and other substances.

Late luteal phase (days 22–28)
- The corpus luteum degenerates in the absence of fertilization.
- Falling oestrogen and progesterone levels remove the negative feedback effect on the pituitary gland and FSH and LH levels begin to rise
- The endometrium undergoes involution

- On days 25–26 the spiral arteries vasoconstrict
- This ischaemia causes apoptosis of the lamina functionalis and menstruation begins on or around day 28.

Clinical approach: top tips
- Most ovulatory cycles are between 25 and 35 days.
- Menstrual cycles tend to have a relatively constant 'luteal phase' of 13–14 days. It is the 'follicular phase' that usually shortens or lengthens to produce the variability in cycle length.
- Progesterone causes a rise in body temperature of half a degree Celsius. Temperature will remain elevated if pregnancy occurs and will return to normal if not.
- Luteal phase progesterone peaks 7 days before menstruation. An elevated reading (at least 21 nmol/L and preferably 32 nmol/L or more) confirms ovulation in that cycle. Hence, to test for mid-luteal progesterone subtract 7 days from the cycle length. Example: in a 40-day cycle progesterone should be taken on day 33 (40–7 = 33)
- LH dipsticks can be used to detect ovulation based on the menstrual cycle changes and LH surge.
- Note that in women with polycystic ovarian syndrome endogenously high levels of LH may give a false-positive dipstick result.
- Endometrium that has not been oestrogen primed will not be capable of a withdrawal bleed following progestagen challenge. Hence, women with amenorrhoea secondary to polycystic ovarian syndrome will have normal oestrogen levels and a withdrawal bleed after a progestagen challenge.
- Women with amenorrhoea secondary to hyperprolactinaemia or the menopause will have low oestrogen levels and no withdrawal bleed after a progestagen challenge.
- There are two rare situations when oestrogen is adequate, but there is no withdrawal bleed. In both, the endometrium is decidualized, either due to high androgen levels or high progesterone levels due to a specific adrenal enzyme deficiency.

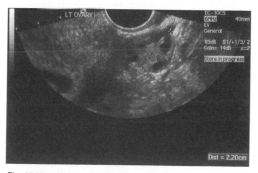

Fig. 12.25.2 A corpus luteum on ultrasound scan.

Miscarriage: early

Definition

Sporadic first trimester or early miscarriage is the commonest complication of pregnancy and is defined as a spontaneous loss of pregnancy up to 12 weeks' gestation. The European Society for Human Reproduction Special Interest Group for Early Pregnancy has published a revised nomenclature to define early pregnancy loss to improve clarity and consistency the in definitions (Table 12.26.1).

Epidemiology

Miscarriage occurs in 10–20% of clinical pregnancies (viable pregnancy defined by ultrasound examination) and is responsible for 50 000 inpatient admissions in the UK per annum (RCOG 2006). The chance of a subsequent successful pregnancy following one early miscarriage is over 95% and in women with three consecutive miscarriages is over 70%. Factors influencing the probability of a chromosomal aberration carrier status in women with sporadic miscarriages are maternal age at second miscarriage, a history of three or more miscarriages (recurrent miscarriage), and a history of over two miscarriages in the sibling or parents of either partner. The probability of carrier status in couples referred for chromosome analysis after two or more miscarriages varies between 0.5% and 10.2% and the chances of having a healthy child are as high as a non-carrier couple despite a higher risk of miscarriage (Franssen et al., 2006).

Risk factors

Assessment of women with a possible early pregnancy loss

The clinical and economic benefits of a dedicated outpatient early pregnancy assessment service are well established. Early pregnancy assessment units (EPAU) offer the advantages of efficient and high-quality service for women with threatened, inevitable early pregnancy loss. A streamlined approach to management can avoid a hospital admission altogether in 40% of cases and reduce the length of hospital stay in a further 20% (Bigrigg et al., 1991).

The National Service Framework recommends that EPAU should be universally available and easily accessible. The service should be comprehensive and appropriately staffed, with an efficient appointments system, ideally sited in a dedicated area with ultrasound equipment and easy access to laboratory facilities. The service should be available on a daily basis, with direct access for GPs and selected patient groups. Standardized information leaflets, referral and discharge letters should be available and regularly reviewed. Miscarriage is associated with significant psychological morbidity. Therefore, appropriate support and counselling offered to women after miscarriage is shown to have significant beneficial effects (Nielsen et al., 1996).

Diagnosis

Special investigations

Pelvic ultrasound examination

Transvaginal pelvic ultrasound examination is the mainstay in the diagnosis of early miscarriage. Diagnosis is based on a combination of the clinical presentation correlated with ultrasound scan findings.

- Threatened miscarriage: viable pregnancy on ultrasound examination in a patient presenting with vaginal bleeding. On vaginal examination the cervix is closed.
- Complete miscarriage: the patient presents with vaginal bleeding, the passage of tissue vaginally (products of conception) and cramping abdominal pain. On ultrasound examination the uterine cavity is empty, has a thin endometrium, and vaginal examination confirms the cervix to be closed.
- Incomplete miscarriage: the patient presents with vaginal bleeding, passing products of conception, and abdominal cramping pain. On ultrasound examination the uterus has evidence of retained products of conception (RPOC) within the uterine cavity, which measures ≥15 mm diameter.
- Early pregnancy failure: the patient presents with or without vaginal bleeding and possibly receding symptoms of pregnancy. An ultrasound examination confirms an intrauterine pregnancy; however, the following observations are made:
  - fetal pole (crown–rump length (CRL)) = 6 mm, no fetal heart activity noted
  - fetal pole CRL <6 mm, no fetal heart activity noted and no change on repeat ultrasound examination performed a week later.
  - mean sac diameter (MSD) ≥20 mm, but no fetal pole evident.
  - MSD <20 mm, no fetal pole evident or no change in scan findings after a week.

Serum progesterone concentrations

Serum progesterone can be a useful adjunct to diagnosis when an ultrasound examination suggests pregnancy of unknown location. A low serum progesterone level can be used to predict those pregnancies that are most likely to resolve spontaneously.

Human chorionic gonadotrophin

Human chorionic gonadotrophin (hCG) is a glycoprotein produced by trophoblasts and is detectable in maternal serum within days of implantation. Circulating hCG concentrations are highly variable during pregnancy and can fluctuate widely as early as 6 weeks' gestation. However, as pregnancy progresses up to 8 weeks' gestation there is a consistent doubling time over 1.94 days. Between 8 and 10

Table 12.26.1 Nomenclature of early pregnancy loss (adapted from Farquaharson et al. 2005)

Term	Definition
Biochemical pregnancy loss	Pregnancy not located on scan
Empty sac	Sac with absent or minimal structures
Fetal loss	Previous CRL measurement with subsequent loss of fetal heart activity
Early pregnancy loss	Empty sac or sac with fetus but no FHA <12 weeks
Delayed miscarriage	Early pregnancy loss
Late pregnancy loss	Loss of FHA >12 weeks
Pregnancy of unknown location	No identifiable pregnancy on scan with positive hCG

weeks gestational age (Konrad 2007), this doubling time averages 4.75 days after which it plateaus to an average of 100 000 IU/L before declining further and stabilizing at approximately 20 000 IU/L at 10–14 weeks' gestation. Serum hCG levels at these gestational ages do not help to predict outcome in women with vaginal bleeding. However, a slower rise or declining hCG concentrations during the first 10 weeks of pregnancy may indicate an ectopic or a non-viable intrauterine pregnancy.

Management

Management of all early pregnancies should be performed in a dedicated early pregnancy assessment unit (EPAU) or emergency gynaecological unit (EGU) with suitably trained personnel who can manage early pregnancy complications and are adequately trained in providing psychological support and counselling to couples suffering early miscarriages. Initial management of the patient should be focused on the patient's haemodynamic stabilization, adequate analgesia, and wellbeing. Further management would be based on the presenting symptoms, pelvic ultrasound observations, and hCG measurements.

Management of complete miscarriage
- Sympathetically inform of the diagnosis
- Offer counselling and support
- Provide information leaflets and supporting website information
- Offer open access to EGU in next pregnancy
- If repeated miscarriage, refer to the recurrent miscarriage clinic for further investigations.

Management of incomplete miscarriage
- Sympathetically inform of the diagnosis
- Offer counselling and support
- Offer the options of
  - expectant
  - medical
  - surgical management
- Counsel about all three options
- Provide written information and leaflets

Medical and expectant management should only be offered in units where women can access to 24-hour telephone advice and emergency admission if required. In terms of therapeutic intervention, patient choice should be encouraged, as it is associated with positive quality-of-life outcomes.

Expectant
If RPOC <15 mm and the patient is haemodynamically stable with minimal vaginal bleeding, she may be discharged from EPAU after reassurance but offered open access to the unit.

If RPOC ≥15 mm and the patient is haemodynamically stable with minimal vaginal bleeding, she may be reassured that there is very a high likelihood (79–96% success rate) that the miscarriage will complete within the next 3–4 weeks (Nielson et al., 1995, 1999, Sairam et al., 2001, Shelly et al., 2005).

The patient may then be allowed home with open access to EGU and reviewed in 2 weeks.

If no symptoms of infection and vaginal bleeding has subsided or discontinued she may then be discharged from care.

The advantages of expectant management are that it involves no interventional procedures and the minimal risks of infection (2%) and haemorrhage requiring blood

transfusion (0.1%) are similar to these encountered with medical and surgical management. Further, there are no morbidities that are normally associated with surgical management options.

Medical
The success rates for medical management of incomplete miscarriage average 97% (range 80–100%) (Neilson et al., 2005). However, medical management is 2.8-fold more likely to induce complete miscarriage than expectant management. Misoprostol is the drug of choice. The advantages of medical management are that morbidities normally associated with surgical management and the risks of infection (2%) and of haemorrhage requiring blood transfusion (0.1%) are minimal.

Women undergoing expectant or medical management should be informed that the completion of miscarriage may take up to 4 weeks. The provision of this information increases the acceptability of these management modes and the success rates. They should also be informed that the success rate is higher when their follow up is based on clinical findings rather than based on ultrasound examination.

Surgical
If the patient opts for surgical management, an informed consent should be obtained and information leaflets on surgical evacuation should be provided. She should be informed of the success rate of surgical evacuation as 97–100%, and the risks of anaesthesia, infection (2%), haemorrhage requiring blood transfusion (0.1%), cervical trauma (1%), and uterine perforation (0.1–0.2%) (NICE 2004; Trinder et al., 2006).

Management of early pregnancy demise or missed miscarriage
- Sympathetically inform of the diagnosis
- Offer counselling and support
- Offer the options of
  - expectant management
  - medical management
  - surgical management
- Counsel about all three options
- Provide written information and leaflets.

Expectant
The success rate varies between 25% and 85% (Bagratee et al., 2004); therefore, the patient should be advised of the higher failure rate. Expectant management for early pregnancy demise is associated with a higher risk of incomplete miscarriage and the need for emergency surgical uterine evacuation in the event of bleeding. However, there is a lower risk of infection than with surgical management. Both modes of management are equally effective and the woman's preference should be taken into consideration (Nanda et al., 2006).

It is essential that there is open access to EPAU to these women and they should be followed up within 4 weeks.

Medical
Medical evacuation of early miscarriage is an effective alternative to surgical evacuation and achieved with the use of prostaglandin analogues (gemeprost or misoprostol) with or without antiprogesterone priming (mifepristone). Efficacy rates vary widely from 13% to 96% and are influenced by factors such as type of miscarriage, gestational sac size, total dose, duration, route of administration of prostaglandin, and whether the patient's

follow-up is based on clinical or ultrasound findings. Higher success rates (70–96%) are associated with incomplete miscarriage, high dose of misoprostol (1200–1400 μg), prostaglandins administered vaginally, and clinical follow-up without routine ultrasound (Oi-Shan et al., 2006, NICE 2004, Trinder et al., 2005). The prior use of mifepristone does not significantly affect the success rates, which range from 82% to 95% (Oi San Tang et al., 2003). Vaginal misoprostol is more effective and has fewer side-effects than the oral route. The rate of expulsion of RPOC ranges between 80% and 90% in women up to 13 weeks' gestation.

If the patient opts for medical management, it is important that informed consent is obtained and relevant investigations are performed. Women ≤10 weeks' gestation on ultrasound examination can be managed as an outpatient. Women ≥10 weeks' gestation on ultrasound examination should be informed of a lower success rate and a higher risk of excessive bleeding. The usual protocol is as follows: day 1, 800 μg of misoprostol administered vaginally; day 2, the patient takes two further doses of misoprostol 400 μg 3 hours apart. The side effects of the medication are nausea, vomiting, diarrhoea, and mild pyrexia. The medication is used with caution in conditions where hypotension may precipitate severe complications (cerebrovascular disease and cardiovascular disease). The complications are those of infection (2%) and haemorrhage requiring blood transfusion (0.1%) (NICE 2004).

Women undergoing expectant or medical management should be informed that the completion of miscarriage may take up to 4 weeks. The provision of this information increases the acceptability of these management modes and the success rates (Creinin et al., 1996). They should also be informed that the success rate is higher when their follow up is based on clinical findings rather than based on ultrasound examination (Wagaarachchi et al., 2002).

All women should be provided with analgesia and offered open access to EPAU and supportive contact numbers. Follow-up examination should be arranged in 4 weeks at which a pelvic scan be performed.

- If the miscarriage is complete, the patient may be discharged with access to EPAU during her next pregnancy
- If the miscarriage is incomplete a repeat scan should be arranged in 2 weeks.
- Advise her that she may choose other management options such as surgical evacuation of uterus.
- If 6 weeks later the miscarriage is incomplete, she should be advised of alternative management options.

Following discharge the couple should be offered an appointment for counselling for psychological support (RCOG 2006).

Surgical

Women undergoing surgical evacuation should be screened for infection including *Chlamydia trachomatis* and bacterial vaginosis.

They should also have their full blood count (FBC) checked to ensure that they are not anaemic and a blood group and Rh antibody test should be performed to evaluate the need for anti-D immunoglobulin. If the patient is Rh negative she should receive 250 IU of anti-D immunoglobulin intramuscularly.

Tissue obtained at the time of miscarriage should be examined histologically to confirm pregnancy and to exclude ectopic pregnancy or unsuspected gestational trophoblastic disease.

An objective assessment of the psychological morbidity associated with expectant and surgical management of miscarriage revealed no differences related to the procedure itself. However, women with miscarriage who chose their own treatment option had the best health-related quality-of-life (HRQL) assessments compared with women who were randomized to one or other treatment modality (Nielsen et al., 1996, Wieringa-De Waard et al., 2002). It is therefore important to encourage patient choice in the management of early miscarriage.

Information on the sensitive disposal of fetal remains can be obtained from the RCOG Good Practice Guideline No. 5, *Disposal following pregnancy loss before 24 weeks of gestation*, the Stillbirth and Neonatal Death Society's (SANDS) *Pregnancy loss and the death of a baby: guide-lines for professionals* (1995) and the Institute of Burial and Cremation Administration (IBCA) *Policy document: disposal of fetal remains* (2001). The Royal College of Nursing, *Sensitive disposal of all fetal remains, guidance for nurses and midwives* is also available at www.rcn.org.uk/members/ downloads/ disposal _fetal _remains.pdf.

Expert adviser

The Recurrent Miscarriage Clinic, St Mary's Hospital, London.

Further reading

Bagratee J, Khullar V. A randomised controlled trial comparing medical and expectant management of first trimester miscarriage. Hum Reprod 2004;19:266–71.

Bigrigg MA, Read MD. Management of women referred to early pregnancy assessment unit: care and effectiveness. Br Med J 1991;302:577–9.

Creinin MD, Burke AE. Methotrexate and misoprostol for early abortion: A multicentre trial. Acceptability. Contraception 1996;54:19–20.

Farquharson RG, Jauniaux E, Exalto N. ESHRE Special Interest Group for Early Pregnancy (SIGEP). Updated and revised nomenclature for description of early pregnancy events. Hum Reprod 2005;20:3008–11.

Franssen M, Korevaar J, Fulco van der Veen, et al. Reproductive outcome after chromosome analysis in couples with two or more miscarriages: case-control study. BMJ 2006;332: 759–763.

Konrad G, First-trimester bleeding with falling HCG. Don't assume miscarriage. PMCID 2007; 53(5).

Nanda K, Peloggia A. Expectant care versus surgical treatment for miscarriage. Cochrane Database Syst Rev. 2006 Apr 19;(2):CD003518. Review.

Neilson JP, Hickey M. Medical treatment for early fetal death (less than 24 weeks). Cochrane Database Syst Rev. 2006 Jul 19; 3:CD002253.

NICE. The care of women requesting induced abortion. September 2004.

Nielsen S, Hahlin M, Möller A, Granberg S. Bereavement, grieving and psychological morbidity after first trimester spontaneous abortion: comparing expectant management with surgical evacuation. Hum Reprod 1996;11:1767–70.

Nielson S, Hamlin M. Expectant management of first-trimester spontaneous abortion. Lancet 1995;345:84–6.

Nielson S, Platz J. Randomised trial comparing expectant with medical management for first trimester miscarriage. Br J Obstet Gynaecol 1999;106:804–7.

Oi San Tang, Winnie Nga Ting Lau. A prospective randomised study to compare the use of repeated doses of vaginal with sublingual misoprostol in the management of first trimester silent miscarriages. Hum Reprod 2003;18:176–81.

Oi Shan T, Charas YT. A randomised trial to compare the use of sublingual misoprostol with or without an additional 1 week course for the management of first trimester silent miscarriage. Hum Reprod 2006;21:189–92.

Royal College of Obstetricians and Gynaecologists (RCOG) *The management of early pregnancy loss*. Green Top Guideline no 25. London: RCOG 2006.

Sairam S, Khare. The role of ultrasound in the expectant management of early pregnancy loss. Ultrasound Obstet Gynecol 2001; 17:506–9.

Shelly J, David H. A randomised trial of surgical, medical and expectant management of first trimester spontaneous miscarriage. Aust N Z J Obstet Gynaecol 2005;45:122–7.

Trinder J, Rocklehurst P. Management of miscarriage: expectant, medical, or surgical? Results of randomised controlled trial (miscarriage treatment (MIST) trial). BMJ 2006;332:1235–40.

Wagaarachchi P, Ashok P. Medical management of early fetal demise using sublingual misoprostol. Br J Obstet Gynaecol 2002;109:462–5.

Wieringa-De Waard M, Hartman E, Ankum W, *et al*. Expectant management versus surgical evacuation in first trimester miscarriage: health-related quality of life in randomised and nonrandomized patients. Hum Reprod 2002;17:1638–42.

Patient resources

Association of Early Pregnancy Units: www.earlypregnancy.org.uk

Miscarriage Association (Registered Charity No. 1076829) c/o Clayton Hospital, Northgate, Wakefield, West Yorkshire WF1 3JS. Telephone: 01924 200799: www.miscarriageassociation.org.uk.

Oocyte donation

Oocyte donation offers the prospect of pregnancy to women who are unable to use their own oocytes. The fertility potential with this treatment is high, with a low miscarriage rate being reflective of the donor's fertility status rather than the recipient. However, the process is not without risk to both parties, as the donor has to undergo an *in vitro* fertilization (IVF) cycle up to oocyte collection and the recipient then has to embark on a pregnancy that poses its own specific challenges.

Indications
Women who require oocyte donation fall into two groups.

Women with primary or secondary ovarian failure
- gonadal dysgenesis (Turner's syndrome, XY karyotype)
- premature ovarian failure (natural or iatrogenic)
- menopause.

Women with menstrual cycles
- repeated IVF failure (poor response to stimulation, persistent oocyte abnormality)
- carrier of severe genetic disease.

Recruitment of donors
There are three potential sources of donated oocytes:
- anonymous donors: altruistic individuals who volunteer, either by themselves or in response to advertisements in the media, to be oocyte donors
- known donors: women who are known to the recipient, usually sisters or friends
- 'egg sharing': women undergoing IVF treatment who donate a proportion of their oocytes, either altruistically or, more commonly, to reduce the cost of their own treatment.

Egg sharing is allowed in the UK, but direct payment to donors is limited by the HFEA Code of Practice to 'reasonable expenses'. Payment is accepted in several other countries: the American Society for Reproductive Medicine states that 'financial compensation… is justified on ethical grounds'.

There is a severe shortage of oocyte donors in the UK, with waiting lists of 1–2 years being common even in the private sector, and the demand for treatment is rising. Thus, many couples seek treatment overseas (so-called 'reproductive tourism').

Assessment of donors
- Age: the HFEA recommends that unless there are exceptional circumstances, eggs should not be taken for the treatment of others from donors aged 36 or over.
- Donors should be free of any significant medical or psychiatric history and should not have a history of familial genetic disorders.
- Donors should be provided with psychological counselling as well as a full medical examination.
- Screening: blood should be taken for hepatitis B and C, HIV, cytomegalovirus, venereal disease research laboratory (VDRL) tests, karyotype, and blood group; donors from ethnic groups susceptible to cystic fibrosis, haemoglobinopathies and Tay–Sachs disease should be appropriately screened.

Managing the donor
In general, oocyte donors (except oocyte sharers) are young, fertile women. Therefore, these women are sensitive to ovarian stimulation and the consequences of this. Careful management of the stimulation cycle is essential to minimize the risk of ovarian hyperstimulation syndrome (OHSS). The initial consultation should include information on the risk of OHSS, which in its severe form is relatively rare but can be fatal. No long-term risks of ovarian stimulation have been demonstrated. Donors must be advised on contraception to avoid unplanned pregnancy.

Managing the recipient
Women with ovarian failure
- In these women, there is no endogenous sex steroid production from the ovaries and therefore there is no oestrogen-driven development of the endometrium and subsequent decidualization by progesterone.
- Oestrogen is replaced using the oral, transdermal, or intravaginal route with ultrasound monitoring to assess the adequacy of the endometrial response, with a higher pregnancy rate associated with the 'triple layered' appearance and thickness of at least 8 mm. Oestrogen supplementation is usually required for at least 2 weeks, but individual response varies. For this reason, many fertility clinics will perform a 'dummy' endometrial preparation cycle.
- Progesterone is supplemented 1 day before oocyte collection (i.e. after hCG injection to the donor) and can be given intramuscularly or vaginally. Hormone replacement is continued until the pregnancy test.

Women with menstrual cycles
- The recipient in this situation has her own endogenous pituitary: ovarian activity and her menstrual cycle must be in synchrony with the donor in order to achieve implantation.
- Several approaches have been used, including cryopreservation of donor oocyte embryos and subsequent thawing for replacement on the appropriate day of the recipient's natural cycle.
- In contemporary practice, the preferred method is to suppress the recipient's menstrual cycle using short-acting GnRH analogues to downregulate her endogenous pituitary activity. Hormone replacement is then given as for the menopausal woman (see above). Both donor and recipient may be given the combined oral contraceptive pill to synchronize their withdrawal bleeds.

Laboratory aspects
Donated oocytes are fertilized *in vitro* with sperm from the recipient's male partner (or donor sperm) and the resulting embryos are cultured using standard laboratory protocols until transferred to the recipient's uterus.

In contrast to donor insemination, where sperm samples are quarantined before use, donor oocytes are utilized for fresh embryo transfer. Thus there is a theoretical risk of viral transmission. Recent advances in freezing technology allow vitrification of oocytes with good survival rates, and pregnancy rates approaching fresh oocytes; this raises the possibility of donor 'egg banking'. This would give a great advantage over current practice in avoiding the need to synchronize donor and recipient cycles, and also allow a quarantine period while the donor is retested for transmissible infections. Cross-border treatment might be reduced as vitrified oocytes could be imported.

Embryo transfer and maintenance of pregnancy

- Timing of embryo transfer should be based on embryonic development in the laboratory. As most oocyte donors are young and fertile, the developmental potential of their embryos is above average and a higher proportion of these embryos will be suitable for blastocyst stage transfer. These embryos have the highest implantation potential and therefore special consideration should be given to the risk of multiple pregnancy.
- Maintenance of the steroid environment is essential to support the early conceptus. Although the early placenta secretes sufficient progesterone and oestrogen to support the pregnancy independently of the corpus luteum by 6–8 weeks' gestation, oocyte recipients usually receive exogenous hormone support until at least 10 weeks' gestation.

Success rates and the outcome of pregnancy

- Oocyte donation leads to pregnancy rates above those of standard IVF. The latest published UK figures show a live birth rate of 31.5% per fresh cycle carried out in 2006, and a quarter of these were multiple births. More recent results from individual clinics show pregnancy rates around 50% per cycle.
- The age of the donor is unimportant, and pregnancy rates are maintained in older women receiving hormone replacement for uterine preparation. Women with premature ovarian failure due to pelvic irradiation have reduced pregnancy rates and poorer outcome of pregnancy consequent upon uterine irradiation.
- Donor oocyte pregnancies are obstetrically high risk. Multiple pregnancies carry their own inherent risks to both mother and babies, and these are well recognized; however, specific to oocyte donor pregnancies is the significant risk of pre-eclampsia, which can often be severe in these cases. Additionally, increasing numbers of recipients are undergoing oocyte donation because their own biological age has limited their reproductive potential. Older women are at greater risk of obstetric complications and should be considered as high risk cases. The cumulative risk of maternal age, oocyte donor pregnancy and multiple pregnancy warrant obstetrician-led care throughout pregnancy.

The law and regulation of oocyte donation

Gamete donation is strictly regulated in the UK (see Chapter 12.6, Donor insemination). Recipients of donated oocytes may be more likely to disclose their child's origins than infertile couples receiving donor insemination. Donor anonymity is protected in some countries, and this is seen as an advantage of overseas treatment by some infertile couples.

Further reading

ASRM Ethics Committee. Financial compensation of oocyte donors. Fertil Steril 2007;88:305–9.

Critchley HO, Bath LE, Wallace WH. Radiation damage to the uterus: review of the effects of treatment of childhood cancer. Hum Fertil 2002;5:61–6.

Csapo AI, Pulkkinen, MO, Ruttner B, et al. The significance of the human corpus luteum in pregnancy maintenance. I. Preliminary studies. Am J Obstet Gynecol 1972;112:1061–7.

Gosden RG. Maternal age: a major factor affecting the prospects and outcome of pregnancy. Ann NY Acad Sci 1985;442:45–7.

Human Fertilisation and Embryology Authority. A long-term analysis of the HFEA Register data (1991–2006) 2008

Human Fertilisation and Embryology Authority. Guidance on egg sharing arrangements CH(00)09 2000; www.hfea.gov.uk/en/657.html

Serhal P, Craft I. Oocyte donation in 61 patients. Lancet 1989;i:1185–7.

Serhal P, Craft I. Ovum donation: a simplified approach. Fertil Steril 1987;48:265–9.

Serhal P. Oocyte donation. In: Serhal P, Overton (eds). Good clinical practice in assisted reproduction. Cambridge 2004: 86–99.

Wiggins DA, Main E. Outcomes of pregnancies achieved by donor egg in vitro fertilization: a comparison with standard in vitro fertilization pregnancies. Am J Obstet Gynecol 2005;192:2002–6

Zaidi J, Campbell S, et al. Endometrial thickness, morphology, vascular penetration and velocimetry in predicting implantation in an in vitro fertilization program. Ultrasound Obstet Gynaecol 1995;6:191–8.

Internet resources

www.hfea.gov.uk
www.ngdt.co.uk/
www.bica.net/

Patient resources

HFEA Guide to Infertility. Human Fertilisation and Embryology Authority, London 2008 (also available online)
www.infertilitynetworkuk.com/
www.dcnetwork.org/
The Daisy Network (patient support group for premature menopause): www.daisynetwork.org.uk/

Oligomenorrhoea and amenorrhoea

Definition

Oligomenorrhoea refers to a reduction in the frequency of periods where menstrual intervals may vary between 6 weeks and 6 months.

Amenorrhoea is the complete cessation of periods for more than 6 months. Primary amenorrhoea is defined as the absence of spontaneous onset of menstrual periods by age 16 years. Secondary amenorrhoea is the absence of periods for 6 months or more when a patient has previously had regular periods and 12 months or more when the patient has had irregular cycles since her menarche.

Epidemiology

The prevalence of amenorrhea not due to pregnancy, lactation or menopause is approximately 3–4% and depends on the age group studied: 7.6%, 3.0%, and 3.7% in women aged 15–24, 25–34, and 35–44 years respectively (Münster et al., 1992).

Aetiology

The occurrence of regular monthly periods in women of reproductive age reflects cyclic ovarian activity, which is finely controlled by a sequence of hypothalamic–pituitary–ovarian interactions. Oligomenorrhoea and amenorrhoea may result from similar causes, which are more commonly due to endocrine dysfunction of the hypothalamic-pituitary-ovarian axis. In addition, amenorrhoea may be due to anatomical anomalies of the genital tract.

Women are amenorrhoeic before puberty, during pregnancy and lactation, and in the postmenopausal period. The four most common causes of amenorrhoea are: polycystic ovary syndrome (PCOS), hypothalamic amenorrhoea, ovarian failure, and hyperprolactinaemia.

Anatomical anomalies of the genital tract

These account for about 1% of cases of amenorrhoea.

Congenital
- Absence of uterus (with or without absent vagina)
- Testicular feminization syndrome
- Outflow tract obstruction (imperforate hymen or transverse vaginal septum).

Acquired
- Endometrial damage: traumatic (Asherman's syndrome), chronic endometritis (pelvic tuberculosis), endometrial resection or ablation
- Cervical stenosis (extremely rare): surgical trauma, infective
- Vaginal stenosis (extremely rare): chemical inflammation.

Endocrine dysfunction

Hypothalamic-pituitary-ovarian axis
- Ovarian
  - ovarian failure: genetic, autoimmune, post surgery/chemotherapy/radiotherapy, galactosaemia, and idiopathic
  - polycystic ovary syndrome
  - hormone-secreting tumours (rare).
- Pituitary
  - pituitary failure: adenoma, infarction (Sheehan's syndrome), infection (encephalitis), irradiation
  - hyperprolactinaemia: prolactinoma, primary hypothyroidism, chronic renal failure, and drug induced.
- Hypothalamic
  - congenital (Kallmann's syndrome)
  - functional causes: obesity, weight loss, anorexia nervosa, excessive exercise, psychological stress, debilitating illness.

Others
- Thyroid disease
- Adrenal disease.

Clinical approach

History
- Detailed menstrual history, e.g. onset of menarche, cycle length, and duration
- Sexual and contraceptive history
- Developmental age of secondary sexual characteristics, e.g. breast and pubic hair development
- Cyclical abdominal pain
- Body weight fluctuations (loss and gain)
- Hyperandrogenism, e.g. acne, excessive hair, baldness
- Presence of galactorrhoea
- Vasomotor symptoms, e.g. hot flushes, night sweats
- Symptoms of intracranial space occupying lesion, e.g. headache, vomiting, visual disturbance
- Psychological stress or excessive exercise
- Drugs history and current exposure
- History of previous surgery, e.g. surgical termination of pregnancy, endometrial ablation
- Family history of early menopause, polycystic ovary syndrome

Physical examination
- Height, weight, and body mass index (BMI)
- Secondary sexual characteristics, e.g. breast and pubic hair development
- Galactorrhoea
- Hyperandrogenism, e.g. acne, excessive hair, baldness
- Gynaecological examination: imperforate hymen, presence of uterus/vagina
- Detailed neurological (including smell and ophthalmic) examinations.

Investigations
- Urinary pregnancy test should be performed prior to any further investigation to exclude pregnancy in case of doubt.
- Pelvic ultrasound to identify the presence of a uterus and to establish ovarian morphology. Polycystic ovaries (PCO) are characterized by 12 or more follicles measuring 2–9 mm in diameter, or increased ovarian volume (>10 cm^3) (Balen et al., 2003).
- Hormonal tests including serum FSH, LH, prolactin and TSH are required to establish the endocrine causes of oligomenorrhoea/amenorrhoea. A raised prolactin level should be confirmed by repeat testing.
- Measurement of serum androgens is indicated when there is clinical evidence of hyperandrogenism such as hirsutism. Serum testosterone levels are usually elevated in patients with PCOS. When testosterone levels exceed

5 mol/L further investigations to exclude adrenal pathology are indicated. They include 17α-hydroxyprogesterone, dehydroepiandrosterone sulphate, low-dose and high-dose dexamethasone suppression, and cortisol secretion tests, along with ultrasound (US), computer tomography (CT), or magnetic resonance imaging (MRI) of the adrenal gland.

- Pituitary imaging with CT or MRI is required to detect a prolactin-producing adenoma or an empty sella. It is also indicated in patients with low gonadotrophin levels to exclude space-occupying lesions. A full assessment of pituitary hormone secretion is essential to evaluate the impairment of pituitary function. CT of the skull should be performed to exclude any space-occupying lesion around the hypothalamic and pituitary regions, which can disturb gonadotrophin secretion.

- Patients with premature ovarian failure should undergo karyotyping and autoantibody screening.

Management

The appropriate management is dependent upon accurate diagnosis and careful assessment of the individual needs of the patient. This may include treatments to promote or control fertility, improve hyperandrogenism, prevent osteoporosis, or protect the endometrium from unopposed oestrogen action.

The causes of amenorrhoea can be divided into five distinct categories (Fig. 12.28.1). Ovulation induction can be offered to anovulatory women who wish to become pregnant (Ng and Ho, 2002).

Anatomical causes

- Patients with congenital absence of the uterus do not require hormonal replacement therapy (HRT) since they have functioning ovaries. Pregnancy may be possible following in vitro fertilization (IVF) and embryo transfer to a surrogate mother.

- Those with hypoplastic or absent vagina may benefit from vaginal dilators or vaginoplasty. In girls with imperforate hymen incision and drainage should be performed.

- Hysteroscopic lysis of intrauterine adhesions and placement of an intrauterine contraceptive device followed by oestrogen therapy in the postoperative period to restore the menstrual cyclicity in patients with Asherman's syndrome (Yu et al., 2008).

- Patients with testicular feminization should undergo gonadectomy after puberty to prevent malignant transformation (dysgerminoma), which occurs in about 5% of cases. Oestrogen replacement therapy is required but not progestogens in the absence of a uterus. Careful psychological counseling is essential to achieve patient understanding of the need to remove the gonads and future hormone therapy.

- All gonads in phenotypic females containing a Y chromosome are at an increased risk of developing malignancy, and women with 46XY gonadal dysgenesis (Swyer's syndrome) should undergo gonadectomy as soon as the diagnosis is made (see Chapter 12.5 Disorders of sex development).

Hyperprolactinaemia

- The treatment of choice is dopamine agonists such as bromocriptine or carbergoline, which lower prolactin concentrations and cause shrinkage of a prolactinoma, if present. Restoration of ovulatory menstrual cycles may occur within a few months of commencing dopamine agonists and contraception will be required for women who are not planning to get pregnant.

- Surgery in the form of trans-sphenoidal pituitary adenomectomy is seldom indicated in the presence of a prolactinoma because of the high recurrence rate and possibility of pan-hypopituitarism.

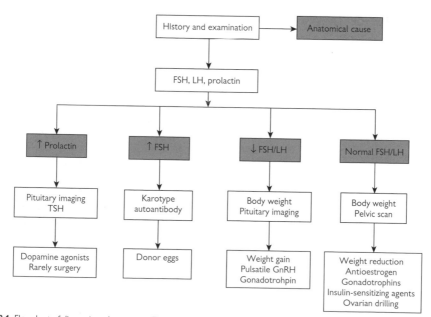

Fig. 12.28.1 Flowchart of diagnosis and treatment. This figure was published in *Gynaecology*, RW Shaw, WP Soutter and SL Stanton, Copyright Elsevier (2002) pp. 245–258.

Hypergonadotrophic hypogonadism
- These women should be offered HRT to protect their bones from the deleterious effects of endogenous hypo-oestrogenism. In women with primary amenorrhoea, HRT may help to develop the secondary sexual characteristics. In women with premature ovarian failure, HRT can help to alleviate climacteric symptoms and prevent vaginal atrophic changes which may lead to dyspareunia.
- There have been case reports of spontaneous pregnancies and successful ovulation induction therapy for women with ovarian failure. However, the only realistic treatment for these patients is the use of donor eggs in an *in vitro* fertilization treatment setting.

Hypogonadotrophic hypogonadism
- Surgery is clearly indicated in patients with central nervous system tumours.
- Patients with anorexia nervosa may benefit from psychotherapy and weight gain after extensive counselling.
- Pulsatile GnRH or gonadotrophin therapy may be offered to patients with other hypogonadotrophic causes or with persisting anovulation despite weight gain, if the patient wishes to conceive.
- HRT can be considered for those with no desire to get pregnant.

Normogonadotrophic hypogonadism
- The majority of these patients will have PCOS. The diagnosis of PCOS requires the presence of two from the following three diagnostic criteria: (i) oligo- and/or anovulation; (ii) clinical and/or biochemical features of hyperandrogenism; and (iii) the presence of polycystic ovary (PCO) morphology (The Rotterdam ESHRE/ASRM-sponsored PCOS consensus workshop group, 2004).
- Obese PCOS women will benefit from weight loss, as this will not only improve their response to ovulation induction therapies but may also result in spontaneous ovulation.
- Women with PCO usually respond well to clomiphene citrate or, failing that, to gonadotrophins for induction of ovulation. Insulin-sensitizing agents or laparoscopic ovarian drilling may be considered in those not responding to clomiphene citrate (Thessaloniki ESHRE/ASRM-Sponsored PCOS Consensus Workshop Group, 2008).
- Other causes include congenital adrenal hyperplasia, adrenal tumours and androgen-producing ovarian tumours. The patient may have clinical symptoms or signs of hyperandrogenism such as hirsutism, prompting more detailed investigations (see earlier). Congenital adrenal hyperplasia responds to corticosteroid replacement therapy. Surgical removal is required for any adrenal or ovarian tumours.

Further reading

Balen AH, Laven JSE, Tan SL, Dewailly D. Ultrasound assessment of the polycystic ovary: international consensus definitions. Hum Reprod Update 2003;9:505–14.

Münster K, Helm P, Schmidt L. Secondary amenorrhoea: prevalence and medical contact–a cross-sectional study from a Danish county. Br J Obstet Gynaecol 1992;99:430–3.

Ng EHY, Ho PC. Ovulation induction. In: Shaw RW, Soutter WP, Stanton SL (eds) *Gynaecology*, 3rd edn. Churchill Livingstone, 2003:245–58.

Practice Committee of the American Society for Reproductive Medicine. Current evaluation of amenorrhea. Fertil Steril 2008;90(Suppl 3):S219–225.

The Rotterdam ESHRE/ASRM-sponsored PCOS consensus workshop group. Revised 2003 consensus on diagnostic criteria and long-term health risks related to polycystic ovary syndrome. Hum Reprod 2004;19:41–7.

Thessaloniki ESHRE/ASRM-Sponsored PCOS Consensus Workshop Group. Consensus on infertility treatment related to polycystic ovary syndrome. Hum Reprod 2008;23:462–77.

Warren MP. Clinical review 77: evaluation of secondary amenorrhea. J Clin Endocrinol Metab. 1996;81:437–442.

Yu D, Wong YM, Cheong Y, Xia E, Li TC. Asherman syndrome—one century later. Fertil Steril 2008;89:759–79.

Internet resources

www.patient.co.uk/showdoc/40000034/

Ovarian hyperstimulation syndrome

Introduction

Ovarian hyperstimulation syndrome (OHSS) is a serious iatrogenic complication of ovarian stimulation treatment such as in vitro fertilization (IVF) and ovulation induction (OI) using gonadotrophins (follicle-stimulating hormone (FSH), luteinizing hormone (LH), human menopausal gonadotrophin (hMG), human chorionic gonadotropin (hCG)) and/or antioestrogens (clomiphene). All methods of ovulation induction can cause OHSS. It may even result from the use of oral antioestrogen, which is often unwisely used outside specialized fertility settings. On rare occasions, however, it is known to occur spontaneously in natural cycles. OHSS is a risk management issue in gynaecology as it can be potentially lethal. Moreover, there has been a stupendous rise in the number of women undergoing IVF treatment since Steptoe and Edwards pioneered its use 30 years ago. Over a million IVF cycles are being performed worldwide every year, and the incident of IVF cycles from is at least five or six times the number.

Prevalence

The prevalence of OHSS during IVF treatment varies from mild in 20–33%, moderate in 3–8% and that of severe forms in 0.5–5% of all cycles. However, there has been an alarming and disproportionate rise in the number of women developing severe OHSS (20-fold rise) compared with the total number of women having IVF treatment (sixfold increase) as more women have turned towards assisted conception treatment globally (Rizk 2006). It is generally accepted that due to inconsistencies in OHSS reporting policies compounded by the fact that OHSS may present with multisystem complications, often to medical specialties who are not familiar with this complication and lack the expertise to deal with the myriad of complications of OHSS, figures of true incidence and fatalities due to OHSS are likely to be underestimated.

Classification

OHSS is classified to aid its appropriate management and for epidemiological surveys. Based on the severity of signs, symptoms, and biochemical parameters, this syndrome has traditionally been graded into three categories as mild, moderate, and severe OHSS. Since severe OHSS causes significant morbidity and requires intensive management, it is further classified into three grades (A, B, C) the severest form of which is critical OHSS. OHSS may also occur early (3–7 days after hCG stimulus) or as late OHSS (12–17 days after hCG stimulus). However, clinical experience shows that such classifications may often be misleading since OHSS has a broad spectrum of clinical signs, symptoms, and biochemical alterations that often overlap and which may change rapidly over time.

Pathophysiology

The basic pathology is enormous cystic ovarian enlargement, pathological extravascular fluid shift, and intravascular fluid volume depletion. This exudative fluid accumulates primarily in the peritoneal cavity causing protein-rich ascites, and in pleural and pericardial cavities causing effusions. Loss of fluid into the third space causes a profound fall in the intravascular volume.

Mechanisms

Vascular endothelial growth factor

The vascular endothelial growth factor (VEGF) system, composed of ligands and receptors, plays a pivotal role in the pathophysiology of OHSS. VEGF is the prototypical member of the family of angiogenic factors which include angiopoetin, PlGF, bFGF and VEGF A, B, C, D, E which regulate physiological and pathological angiogenesis. Exposure of ovaries to hCG/LH causes a VEGF-mediated increase in vascular permeability (VP), which is cardinal to OHSS. VEGF is expressed in granulosa lutein cells of the ovary and its soluble forms are found in serum, follicular, ascitic, and pleural fluid of women with OHSS. The undisputed role of VEGF as a mediator of OHSS is exemplified by the fact that blocking VEGF action in vivo prevents development of OHSS in the murine model.

Role of oestradiol

High circulating oestradiol (E_2) concentrations are an immediate precursor of the syndrome; however, E_2 does not cause the increase VP associated with OHSS.

Ovarian renin angiotensin system

Excessive levels of ovarian derived renin, angiotensinII and aldosterone in women developing OHSS establishes a positive correlation between renin angiotensin system (RAS) and OHSS.

Cytokines

Proinflammatory cytokines (TNF-α, IL-1, 2, 6, 8, 10, 18, PG) play a role in ovarian paracrine interactions and VP. They may therefore contribute to pathogenesis of OHSS.

Kallikrein–kinin system

Tissue kallikreins are expressed in ovarian granulosa cells and are essential to inflammatory process. They may therefore contribute to the VP associated with OHSS.

Selectins and ICAM

Selectins and intracellular adhesion molecules are mediators of inflammatory reaction (sICAM) and of angiogenesis (VE-cadherin). They may cause the altered VP of OHSS.

Prediction and risk factors

Although there is now a better understanding of the pathophysiology, the treatment remains non-specific; OHSS is therefore better prevented. Predicting OHSS with known risk factors is the key to its prevention.

Prior to starting IVF

• Presence of polycystic ovaries (PCO) on pelvic ultrasound examination and/or pre treatment diagnosis of polycystic ovary syndrome (PCOS): women with PCO/PCOS respond by a profound multifollicular response (threefold higher) compared with women with normal ovaries. A higher expression of VEGF in serum and in the hyperthecotic stroma of PCO and consequently higher stromal blood flow in PCO link OHSS to PCO. Moreover, PCO is more frequently seen in women undergoing fertility treatment (40% versus 22%) than in the general population. Other predictive factors described in literature such as the necklace sign of ovaries, ovarian volume, high antral follicle count, and low intravascular ovarian resistance are largely features of a PCO. Isolated features of PCOS such as raised LH–FSH ratio, hyperandrogenism, oligomenorrhoea, and hyperinsulism have been described as risk factors for developing OHSS.

- Age, BMI and previous OHSS: younger women are more likely to develop OHSS, consistent with greater ovarian reserve/responsiveness than older women. Obese women are more likely to have a higher threshold of gonadotrophin requirement for ovarian stimulation and may therefore underrespond with standard doses of gonadotrophins. They are therefore less likely to develop OHSS. Women are more likely to develop OHSS if they have previously done so.
- Baseline serum FSH, inhibin B and AMH (anti-Müllerian hormone): these have all been investigated as markers of OHSS. Low baseline FSH and high inhibin B and AMH are markers of a greater ovarian reserve and, therefore, indirect predictors of the risk of developing OHSS.
- Genetic predisposition: FSH receptor single nucleotide polymorphism(SNP) genotype may help predict ovarian response.

During ovarian stimulation treatment
- Higher dose and longer duration of gonadotrophin treatment irrespective of the type of gonadotrophins (FSH or hMG).
- Use of GnRH analogues for pituitary down regulation increases the risk of OHSS sixfold, by abolishing endogenous LH surge thereby promoting uninhibited follicular growth when stimulated with gonadotrophins.
- Development of large number of follicles, in response to gonadotrophin stimulation. There is no agreed cut off (varies between 10 and 35) for the number of follicles that would predict OHSS. Developing >25 follicles predict OHSS with 25% positive predictive value.
- Exposure of ovaries to LH/hCG mediates VP. OHSS therefore occurs after hCG/LH administration and during pregnancy. Pregnant women develop late onset OHSS that is often severe and of longer duration.
- Greater number of oocytes retrieved which is reflective of greater ovarian responsiveness to ovarian stimulation. There is no agreed cut-off, which varies between 14 and 30; retrieving >15 oocytes has a 35% PPV.
- High E2 concentrations predict a quarter of cases of OHSS: there is no agreed cut-off for E2 concentrations that would predict OHSS. It varies widely between 2642 and 6000 ng/mL (10 000–22 020 pmol/L).
- Circulating VEGF and its receptor sflt-1 concentrations provide a non-steroidal index of ovarian response. The use of VEGF and sflt-1 measurements, however, still need to be validated prospectively and easily reproduced for its utility in clinical practice.
- High circulating concentrations of renin angiotensin, cytokines(IL-6, 8) and von Willebrand factor are observed in women developing OHSS; these however are not validated for use in clinical practice.

Prediction of OHSS by multiple markers
A combination of some or all of the above markers predicts the development of OHSS with greater accuracy.

Prevention
Identifying women at risk, judicious ovarian stimulation, and using multiple preventative factors remains the mainstay of preventing OHSS.

Prior to starting IVF
Treatment of anovulation by methods other than OI with gonadotrophins and antioestrogen:
- Lifestyle modification and weight reduction
- insulin-sensitizing agents, e.g. metformin, which increases ovarian responsiveness in hyperandrogenic, hyperinsulinaemic and often obese women with PCOS. Current evidence supports the view that co-treatment of metformin with gonadotrophins during IVF treatment in women with PCOS reduces the risk of developing OHSS.
- Laparoscopic ovarian diathermy(LOD) is a safer alternative to OI agents in women with anovulatory PCOS however current evidence does not support the view that LOD prior to IVF reduces risk of OHSS.
- Aromatase inhibitors are being used for OI at present time with no reports of OHSS. The use of ketoconazole, octreotide and pentoxyfylline has no proven benefit in reducing OHSS during OI.
- Pulsatile GnRH pump rather than hMG for OI in women with hypogonadotrophic hypogonadism causes a more physiological ovarian response.

Finally, if gonadotrophin remains the only option for OI, its judicious use and unifollicular ovulation avoids OHSS.

During IVF: prior to oocyte retrieval
- Careful regulation of dose and duration of gonadotrophins by ultrasound monitoring thereby avoiding exuberant response of ovaries.
- Current evidence suggests that the GnRH antagonist protocol of IVF results in significantly lower incidence of severe OHSS; however, the pregnancy rate is lower than the long protocol of the GnRH analogue treatment cycle.
- Cancellation of treatment cycles by withholding hCG in women with prolific ovarian response reduces the likelihood of developing OHSS. Thereafter, follicular aspiration along with continued suppression of pituitary by GnRH analogues further reduces OHSS risk.
- The use of GnRH analogues (but not rLH), to trigger ovulation instead of hCG reduces the likelihood of developing OHSS but also results in a lower clinical pregnancy rate (Griesinger et al., 2006).
- Coasting assumes the principle of withdrawing ovarian stimulation when follicular response and/or E2 concentrations reach a threshold above which the risk of developing OHSS is significant, until the E2 concentrations drops. Although coasting may reduce the risk of developing OHSS it also reduces the likelihood of pregnancy, particularly if coasting exceeds 3 days.
- Reducing the hCG dose (irrespective of human or recombinant types) reduces the severity of early-onset OHSS but not risk of developing OHSS. Current evidence does not support the view that substituting hCG with LH reduces the likelihood of developing OHSS.
- Pre-hCG unilateral follicular aspiration does not reduce the risk of developing OHSS.

During IVF: after oocyte retrieval
- Cryopreservation of embryos resulting from IVF treatment reduces the risk of developing late OHSS by eliminating endogenous hCG exposure due to a resulting pregnancy; however, it does not reduce the risk of early OHSS, which is related to ovulatory dose of hCG.

A recent Cochrane review confirms no benefit of elective cryopreservation versus fresh embryo transfer.

- Single embryo transfer in women at risk of OHSS avoids multiple pregnancies. This reduces the severity of late onset OHSS as the intensity of OHSS is related to amount of circulating endogenous hCG.
- Progesterone instead of hCG for luteal support is associated with a lower risk of developing OHSS.
- Although it is largely accepted that use of i.v. albumin does not reduce the risk of OHSS, a recent Cochrane review supports the use of i.v. albumin for preventing OHSS. The mechanism of action is twofold; first, it increases plasma oncotic pressure and secondly its binding properties may result in inactivation of vasoactive peptides which cause OHSS.
- There is insufficient evidence at the present time on the beneficial effects of hydroxylethylstarch (synthetic plasma expander), which is a safer and cost-effective alternative to albumin for preventing OHSS.
- Intravenous hydrocortisone has proven to be ineffective in preventing OHSS.
- Dopamine receptor 2 agonist, cabergoline, inactivates VEGFR and may prevent the VP of OHSS.
- *In vitro* maturation (IVM) of oocytes in women at risk of OHSS (e.g. those with PCO/PCOS) may provide a safer alternative to traditional IVF. IVM minimizes the dose and duration of ovarian stimulation and avoids hCG injection, thereby eliminating the two important risk factors of OHSS development.

Complications

OHSS may present itself with multisystem complications. Intravascular fluid depletion results in hypovolaemia (55% of all OHSS) and haemoconcentration (50% of all and 70–95% of severe OHSS), which poses a risk of thromboembolism (TE) and renal failure. Complications associated with TE occur in 0.06–10% of all severe cases of OHSS and contribute to a largest morbidity and mortality associated with OHSS. Other complications are liver dysfunction (30% of all OHSS), hepatorenal failure, pleural effusions (10–30% of severe OHSS), adult respiratory distress syndrome, and pericardial effusions resulting in cardiac tamponade. Morbidity may also be related to ovarian torsion, infection, cyst rupture, and haemorrhage prior to and during pregnancy. Complications during pregnancy in women who develop OHSS are largely related to multiple gestations and prematurity.

Diagnosis

A history of ovarian stimulation treatment in almost all women with OHSS. Early-onset OHSS occurs within 3–7 days and late-onset OHSS 12–17 days after hCG administration and is often associated with pregnancy.

Symptoms

Abdominal discomfort, pain, distension, nausea, vomiting, diarrhoea, shortness of breath, oligura, and those related to complications of severe OHSS such as TE, hepatorenal failure, and hydrothorax.

Signs

Cystic ovarian enlargement and free fluid in the abdomen diagnosed on ultrasound examination. Ovarian size does not correlate to the severity of OHSS but with larger ovaries, OHSS severity is likely to be worse. Signs related to infection and hypovolemia included hypotension, tachycardia and tachypnoea. Signs related to specific complications of severe OHSS such as TE, hepatorenal failure, ascites, and hydrothorax.

Biochemical parameters

Although biochemical alterations have traditionally been categorized in severe OHSS, in clinical practice, marginal hypoalbuminaemia, altered liver enzymes and electrolyte imbalances may be observed in women with sign/symptoms of mild and moderate OHSS. A haematocrit of >45 l/L is categorised in moderate and >55% in severe OHSS. WBC count of >15 m/l is categorised in moderate and >25 m/ml in severe OHSS. Creatinine concentration of >100 μmol/L is categorized as severe OHSS.

Management

- Centres providing IVF/OI should provide *verbal/written information* to women prior to and after undergoing treatment on the risk of OHSS, signs/symptoms expected, and advice to seek prompt expert medical advice should symptoms develop.
- *Mild and moderate OHSS* may be managed supportively in outpatient settings. It requires monitoring by ultrasound examination, blood tests (include βhCG, full blood count, electrolytes, kidney, liver function tests, and clotting profile) and relief of symptoms with analgesics and antiemetics. Optimum fluid intake is encouraged. Follow-up is mandatory until complete resolution. Strenuous exercise is to be avoided as it may cause cyst rupture or ovarian torsion.
- *Worsening signs/symptoms* requires close monitoring as *severe OHSS* requires hospitalization and multidisciplinary medical management. Critical OHSS requires ITU management.
- Monitoring by weight, abdominal girth, vital signs, fluid balance charts, blood tests as mentioned, and ultrasound examination of pelvis/abdomen/chest. Radiographic investigations may be required in complications such as TE and hydrothorax. However, it should be avoided if possible in women who are likely to be pregnant.
- Treatment modalities are aimed at maintaining fluid balance and circulation with use of intravenous crystalloids/colloids. If oligo/anuria or respiratory compromise occurs, ultrasound-guided culdocenteses/paracenteses of ascitic fluid and pleurocentesis relieve respiratory distress and maintain renal function. Use of diuretics is not advisable as it worsens the existing hypovolaemia. Heparinization is required to reduce the risk of TE. Surgical treatment of OHSS is not recommended except in complications such as ovarian torsion and haemorrhage. VEGF antagonists may in future develop as a new form of treatment for OHSS.
- Supportive counselling and reassurance should be provided to woman and family.

Conclusions

OHSS is a complication of ovarian stimulation that has risen over recent years with advances in technology and the global rise in consumerism for fertility treatment. Understanding its pathophysiology, strategies of prevention, and multidisciplinary approach to treatment are important for its appropriate management.

Surveillance

Central, judicious reporting policy of OHSS for risk management and epidemiological survey are mandatory.

Further reading

Aboulghar M, Evers J, Al-Inany H. IV albumin for preventing severe OHSS. Review Cochrane Collaboration 2008;2:1–12.

Adamson D, deMouzon J, Lancaster P, et al. International Committee for Monitoring Assisted Reproductive Technology (ICMART), World collaborative report, Fertil Steril 2006;85:1586–622.

Agrawal R, Sladkevicius P, Engmann L, et al. Serum VEGF and ovarian blood flow are increased in women with polycystic ovaries. Hum Reprod 1998;13:651–5.

Al-Inany H, Abou-Setta A, Aboulghar M. GnRH antagonist for ART. Cochrane review. Repro Med Online 2007;14:640–9.

Delvigne A, Rozenberg. Review of clinical course and treatment of OHSS. Hum Reprod Update 2003;9:77–96.

Fauser B, Diedrich K, Devroey P. (EVAR workshop). Predictors of ovarian response: progress towards individualised treatment in OI & ovarian stimulation. Hum Reprod Update 2008;14:1–14.

Griesinger G, Diedrich K, Devroey P, Kolibiankis E. GnRHa for final maturation in GnRH antagonist protocol: systematic review & meta analysis. Hum Reprod Update 2006;12:327–8.

Mathur R, Kailasam C, Jenkins J. Review of evidence base strategies to prevent OHSS. Hum Fertil 2007;10:75–85.

Rizk B. Epidemiology, pathophysiology, prevention and management of OHSS. In: Ovarian hyperstimulation syndrome. Cambridge University Press 2006:3–210.

Soares S, Gomez R, Simon C, et al. Targeting VEGF system to prevent OHSS. Hum Reprod Update 2008;14:321–33.

Paediatric and adolescent problems

Definitions

Adolescence is a variable period between childhood and adulthood characterized by rapid development in psychological, social, and biological domains (RCPCH 2003). The WHO defines adolescence as between 10 and 20 years. Children and adolescents may present with gynaecological problems that include menstrual disorders (oligo and amenorrhoea, irregular menorrhagia. and dysmenorrhoea), delayed puberty, hyperandrogenism, vulvovaginitis, labial adhesions, and sexually transmitted diseases as well as, more rarely, ovarian failure after treatment of childhood malignancy and disorders of sexual differentiation (DSD).

Thelarche (breast development) and pubarche (development of pubic and axillary hair) usually occur 1 year before menarche and before 13 years. Menarche occurs at a mean of 13 years and less than 4 years after thelarche. Most cycles initially vary between 20 and 40 days with a median cycle length of 31 days and mean length of bleeding of 5 days (WHO 1986).

Epidemiology

Nearly 25% of the UK population are children or adolescents. Up to 50% of adolescent cycles are anovular in the first year and it can take up to 7 years to establish a regular cycle.

Clinical approach

Consultation

The consultation with an adolescent can be challenging; adolescents find it difficult to volunteer information and discuss sexually related issues, whereas doctors find that mothers often dominate, daughter and mother have different agendas, and adolescents use different language and have different values and perceptions. They also mature at different rates. The gynaecologist needs to make the adolescent central to the consultation. Sensitive involvement of the parents is important, but it is also essential to respect confidentiality: ask about sexual activity away from the parent. Summarize and agree management plans with the adolescent present; avoid separate conversations with the parents.

Diagnosis

History

In addition to the normal gynaecological history, questions should include birth history, growth and pubertal milestones, relevant symptoms (galactorrohea, headaches, hyperandrogenism, weight change) a detailed family history, dieting, stress, and exercise patterns. In certain presentations (for example vulvovaginitis, prepubertal bleeding, pelvic pain) it is important to explore sensitively the possibility of sexual abuse. Gynaecologists should try to assess psychological factors that may be impacting on physical symptoms and assess the parent–child or adolescent relationship.

Examination

This should include measurement of height and weight and compared with child centile charts and BMI and waist circumference in adolescents. Record Tanner staging, and Ferriman–Gallwey scores for hirsutism. The external genitalia can be inspected, with consent, for normality and virilization. Speculum and bimanual examination should only be performed in the sexually active. Rectal examination as an alternative to vaginal examination is not indicated.

Investigations

These depend on the presentation.

In oligo/amenorrhea, investigations include a pregnancy test, measurement of LH/FSH/E2/PRL/TFTs and androgens if hirsute (testosterone and 17-hydroxyprogesterone) and an USS pelvis. An MRI of the pelvis is helpful if a Müllerian duct anomaly (MDA) is suspected. If a MDA is confirmed then the renal tracts should be visualized. Check the karyotype if there is primary amenorrhea or ovarian failure. A dexamethasone suppression test will exclude Cushing's syndrome.

In menorrhagia, measurement of haemoglobin guides management. Coagulation abnormalities (including platelet dysfunction, von Willebrand's factor deficiency) may occur in up to 47% of adolescents, so coagulation (PT, PTT, BT, PFA 100, and VWF) should be checked in those with acute menorrhagia, menorrhagia since menarche, positive bleeding history, and/or iron deficiency. In adolescents with an irregular cycle a menstrual calendar helps to clarify these; it is also a useful educational tool.

It is important to recognize rare conditions and manage or refer as appropriate.

Counselling

Management of most conditions involves patient (and parent) education, support and counselling for both the condition itself and its long-term effects on general health and fertility.

Management of individual conditions

Common conditions

Vulvovaginitis

This is a common condition in prepubertal girls and is usually secondary to poor perineal hygiene. It is important to exclude a dermatological condition (e.g. lichen sclerosus), foreign body, or sexual abuse. An EUA with vaginoscopy (use a paediatric cystoscope) is indicated if the history is suggestive of a foreign body or if there is constant offensive vaginal discharge or vaginal bleeding. Vaginal bleeding is rare in young children. The differential diagnosis includes precocious puberty, tumours, foreign bodies, or trauma.

Labial adhesions

These are common and may present as 'no vagina'. The diagnosis is made from the history and examination. No other investigations are indicated. Oestrogen cream applied at night will dissolve labial adhesions over 1–2 weeks. However, provided there is no interference with micturition, treatment is unnecessary apart from education to improve perineal hygiene. Surgical division should be avoided as this causes recurrence and scarring.

Amenorrhoea

Investigate when thelarche and pubarche are absent at 13 years or menarche delayed to more than 4 yrs after thelarche or if there is primary amenorrhoea at 15 years. Secondary amenorrhoea can be defined as no bleeds for over 6 months.

History, examination, and investigations should focus on establishing the cause. Treatment depends on the aetiology. Causes can be classified in terms of the hypothalamic pituitary ovarian pathway, for example weight-related, pituitary lesions, hyperprolactinaemia, polycystic ovarian syndrome (PCOS), ovarian failure, and DSD.

Oligomenorrhoea

Defined as cycles longer than 35 days, oligomenorrhoea is common in the first 2 years after menarche. If it fails to resolve, or bleeds are less frequent than every 3 months, further investigation is indicated. The most common cause is PCOS. Other causes include those listed above for amenorrhoea.

Hyperandrogenism

Causes include PCOS, congenital adrenal hyperplasia (CAH), Cushing's syndrome, and adrenal secreting tumours of the ovary or adrenal gland.

Polycystic ovarian syndrome

PCOS often presents during adolescence and is diagnosed when patients have two out of the following three criteria: oligo or anovulation, hyperandrogenism (clinical or biochemical) and PCO morphology on ultrasound scan following the exclusion of other aetiologies including CAH, Cushing's syndrome, or androgen secreting tumours (Fauser et al. 2004).

PCOS is managed by identifying and prioritizing the patients' concerns and being aware of their long-term risks (type 2 diabetes, insulin resistance, dyslipidaemia, and endometrial hyperplasia). In adolescents, the main concerns relate to irregular menorraghia, hirsutism, and obesity. It is generally the adolescent's mother who is concerned about her fertility. Weight loss and exercise should be encouraged in all adolescents with PCOS who have a BMI above the normal range, and those with a normal BMI should be encouraged to maintain this. If bleeds are less frequent than every 3 months then 3-monthly courses of progestogens or the combined oral contraceptive pill (COCP) should prevent the development of endometrial hyperplasia. If hirsute, then management may involve treatment with Dianette with or without additional antiandrogens (cyproterone acetate or finasteride) or spironolactone or metformin. Long-term screening of blood glucose and lipids should be considered. Evidence is lacking for the prophylactic use of metformin in adolescents with PCOS. However, there is a role for metformin in the subgroup of obese adolescents with PCOS who have signs of hyperinsulinanaemia (acanthosis nigricans) and in those with Impaired glucose tolerance.

Menstrual dysfunction

Treatment, particularly if the adolescent is anaemic, may include the OCP, tranexamic acid (TEXA), cyclical progestogens, or rarely a Mirena IUS.

The acute bleed requires immediate circulatory management, volume replacement, haemostatic agents, and/or high doses of hormones (e.g. progestogens or more rarely IV premarin) with subsequent cyclical progestogens or the COCP.

Adolescents with learning difficulties and menstrual problems can be managed with continuous COCP, Depoprovera, or a Mirena IUS.

Dysmenorrhoea/pelvic pain

Good history taking is key to the diagnosis and management of pelvic pain in the adolescent. Pregnancy and infection need to be excluded and the possibility of previous or current sexual abuse considered. Other causes of pelvic pain include endometriosis or Müllerian anomalies (for example a functioning non-communicating uterine horn), and laparoscopy to diagnose endometriosis and a magnetic resonance imaging (MRI) scan to clarify uterine anatomy may be indicated. Treatment includes

non-steroidal anti-inflammatory drugs (NSAIDs), the COCP (which can be tricycled, especially if dysmenorrhea is present), Cerazette, or a Mirena IUS.

Ovarian cysts/masses

Even large cysts may resolve in adolescents. Provided tumour markers are negative (CA125, CEA, hCG, AFP, LDH) and the patient is asymptomatic; management should initially be conservative with scan follow-up. If surgery is indicated this should be performed laparoscopically with conservation of as much ovarian tissue as possible. If tumour markers are positive, gynaecological oncologists should be involved in further management.

Premature ovarian failure

Premature ovarian failure (POF) is common after treatment of childhood malignancy and also occurs in Turner's syndrome and in some DSDs. The diagnosis is made when FSH and LH are elevated and oestradiol low on at least two occasions more than 1 month apart. Thyroid function tests, full blood count, and autoimmune screen (to include ovarian, thyroid, coeliac, adrenal antibodies, and intrinsic factor) should be checked annually. Induction of puberty using low-dose, sequentially increased oestrogen may be necessary. Consideration should be given to cryopreservation of oocytes or ovarian tissue prior to treatment for malignancy (Lobo 2005). This group of patients often requires counselling and psychological support.

Rare conditions

Precocious puberty

Menarche before 8 years is described as being 'precocious'. Investigation and management is best organized in liaison with paediatric endocrinologists so that unusual and important diagnoses can be excluded.

Delayed puberty

Normal development with amenorrhoea may be caused by outlet obstruction (imperforate hymen, transverse vaginal septum), the Mayer–Rokitansky–Kuster–Hauser (MRKH) syndrome or resistant ovaries, or premature ovarian failure. Poor or absent development may be caused by anorexia, pituitary or hypothalamic lesions, or gonadal dysgenesis (e.g. Turner's). Heterosexual development can occur in XY females, CAH, adrenal and ovarian tumours, and Cushing's syndrome.

'No vagina'

Children or adolescents who present with an 'absent vagina' may be a XY female, or have MRKH syndrome, CAH, a transverse vaginal septum, an intact hymen, or labial adhesions.

Disorders of sexual differentiation (previously referred to as intersex disorders)

Historically classification of these disorders has been confusing. A recent consensus group (Hughes et al. 2006) has attempted to clarify this. DSDs may be due to:

- abnormal genetic development
- germ cell failure
- failure to develop normal internal genitalia (Müllerian duct anomalies)
- failure to develop external genitalia (masculinization of female genitaliia or underdevelopment of male genitalia)
- deficiencies in hormonal biosynthesis.

These patients often have complex needs and are best managed in tertiary centres where there is an established multidisciplinary, multiprofessional DSD/intersex service with access to paediatric and adult endocrinologists, paediatric gynaecologists, paediatric and plastic surgeons, geneticists, and psychologists.

Management of the commoner conditions is described below. Most need genetic advice and psychological support. Disclosure of diagnoses must be handled sensitively. Currently, there is controversy over surgery, both its timing and need (Creighton and Minto 2001). A minimalist approach that aims to restore function (rather than anatomy) is increasingly favoured. HRT should be individualized and bone density monitored every two years in most conditions.

- Sex chromosome DSD, Turner's syndrome (45,X, DSD, and variants): commonly presents with poor growth as a child, or later with delayed puberty, primary, or premature ovarian failure. Management includes optimization of growth, induction of puberty, hormone replacement, and screening for other health problems (e.g. cardiac, renal, thyroid and auditory problems) (Saenger et al. 2001). A few cases need gonadectomy (which should be performed laparoscopically) if Y chromosome mosaic material is present (45,X/46,XY). Girls with Turner's should be provided with information about support groups and oocyte donation.

- 46,XY, DSD: this can be divided into disorders of gonadal (testicular) development (e.g. Swyer's syndrome) or disorders in androgen synthesis or action (complete androgen insensitivity syndrome, 5-α-reductase deficiency, Leydig cell hypoplasia).

- Swyer's syndrome (XY complete gonadal dysgenesis): presents with primary amenorrhoea or with a pelvic mass. Dysgenetic gonads require early removal as there is a high risk of malignancy. Subsequent HRT should include progestogens as these patients have a uterus. They can therefore carry a pregnancy conceived with donated oocytes and need appropriate counselling. Disclosure, genetics referral and psychological support are important.

- Complete androgen insensitivity syndrome (CAIS): this may present with inguinal herniae in a female child or with primary amenorrhoea. Disclosure is important but often difficult and psychological support helpful. Management involves laparoscopic gonadectomy, which can be deferred until after puberty, subsequent hormone replacement, with monitoring of bone density, creation of a functional vagina (generally with dilators, more rarely with surgery), genetic advice, and provision of information about support societies and surrogacy.

- 46,XX DSD: this includes disorders of ovarian development (gonadal dysgenesis) and of androgen excess (e.g. congenital adrenal hyperplasia). Other DSDs include MRKH syndrome, cloacal extrophy, and vaginal atresia.

- Congenital adrenal hyperplasia (CAH): CAH (salt losing or non-salt losing) commonly presents in the newborn with ambiguous genitalia. They are brought up as girls as they have normal internal genitalia and are potentially fertile. The main issues in the adolescent relate to menstruation, sexuality, fertility, and the need for further surgery or the use of dilators (Ogilvie et al. 2006). The effectiveness of treatment (steroids ± fludrocortisone) can be assessed by the control of the menstrual cycle and hyperandrogenism. There is currently debate about operations to restore the anatomy in babies with CAH and their timing. Many girls with CAH will require further surgery as adolescents/adults. Sexual dysfunction is common in these patients and it is important to plan surgery carefully.

- Müllerian agenesis (MRKH syndrome): this involves congenital aplasia of the uterus and upper part of vagina. Usually presents as primary amenorrhoea with normal secondary sexual characteristics. Ovaries and hormone levels are normal. A small amount of uterine tissue may sometimes be identified on MRI. Other anomalies (spinal/renal) should be excluded. Management may involve the creation of a vagina with dilators or surgery. Genetic advice is important. Surrogacy using their own oocytes can be discussed, although this has implications for resulting children. They often require psychological support.

- Müllerian duct anomalies: these include vaginal septae (longitudinal and transverse), uterus didelphys, and unicornuate uteri with rudimentary horns. MRI scans are useful in clarifying anatomy and EUAs with vaginoscopy may help in diagnosis. Remember associated renal anomalies. It is important to distinguish between an intact hymen (blue, bulging membrane) and transverse vaginal septum (pink flat vaginal skin), as excision of the latter requires a different surgical technique and patients should be referred to tertiary centres. If the septum is incompletely excised there is a high risk of vaginal stenosis and recurrence. Longitudinal septae can be excised if symptomatic. A functioning non-communicating uterine horn can cause dysmenorrhoea from haematometra and/or endometriosis and should be excised preferably laparoscopically. Management of other uterine anomalies rarely involves surgery.

Conclusions

The healthcare encounter with the child or adolescent does provide an opportunity for healthcare education; adolescents in particular need to learn how to take responsibility for their own healthcare and to use healthcare systems appropriately. Gynaecologists need to be able to manage common conditions presenting in this age group as well as recognizing rarer and more complex problems that need onward referral and multidisciplinary care.

Further reading

Creighton S, Minto C. Managing intersex. Editorial. BMJ 2001;323:1264–5.

Fauser B, Tarlatzis B, et al. The Rotterdam ESHRE/ASRM sponsored PCOS consensus workshop group. Revised 2003 consensus on diagnostic criteria and long term health risks related to polycystic ovary syndrome. Hum Reprod 2004;19:41–7 or Fertil Steril 2004;81:19–25.

General Medical Council (GMC). 0–18 years: guidance for all doctors. London: GMC 2007.

Hughes IA, Houk C, et al. Consensus statement on management of intersex disorders. J Pediatric Urology 2006;2:148–62.

Lobo, RA. Potential options for preservation of fertility in women. N Engl J Med 2005;353:64–73.

Ogilvie CM, et al. Congenital adrenal hyperplasia in adults: a review of medical, surgical & psychological issues. Clin Endo 2006;64:2–11.

RCPCH. Bridging the gaps. Intercollegiate Working party. 2003.

Saenger, P, Albertsson Wikland, K et al. Recommendations for diagnosis and management of Turner syndrome. J Clin Endo Metabol 2001;86:3061–9.

World Health Organization Task Force on Adolescent Reproductive Health. World Health Organisation multicenter study on menstrual and ovulatory patterns in adolescent girls. II. J Adolesc Health Care 1986;7:236–44.

Balen, A, Creighton SC, Davies MC, *et al.* (eds) *Paediatric and adolescent gynaecology: a multidisciplinary approach.* Cambridge: Cambridge University Press 2004.

Sanflippo JS, Muram D, Dewhurst J, Lee PA (eds). *Pediatric and adolescent gynaecology.* Philadelphia: WB Saunders 2001.

Garden AS, Topping J. *Paediatric and adolescent gynaecology for the MRCOG and beyond.* RCOG Press 2001.

Internet resources

British Society of Paediatric and Adolescent Gynaecology: www.britspag.org.uk

British Association of Paediatric Surgeons: www.baps.org.uk

British Society for Paediatric Endocrinology & Diabetes: www.bsped.org.uk

The North American Society for Paediatric & Adolescent Gynaecology: www.naspag.org/index.html

Patient resources

Turner Syndrome Society: www.tsss.org.uk

Congenital adrenal hyperplasia support group: www.ahn.org.uk

Androgen insensitivity syndrome support group: www.aissg.org

The Daisy network. A support group for Premature Ovarian Failure: www.daisynetwork.org.uk

Polycystic ovary syndrome

Definition

Polycystic ovary syndrome (PCOS) is a syndrome of ovarian dysfunction with the cardinal features hyperandrogenism and polycystic ovarian morphology (PCO) morphology. It is a clinical definition based on the presence of at least two of the following features after the exclusion of other aetiologies:

- PCO
- oligo/anovulation or oligo/amenorrhoea
- clinical or biochemical hyperandrogenism (PCOS Workgroup 2004).

This definition therefore includes women who have PCO and androgenic symptoms but regular menstrual cycles, as well as those who have the 'classical' symptoms of menstrual disturbance and hyperandrogenism. It excludes asymptomatic women who have an incidental finding of PCO.

The commonest symptoms of PCOS are irregular menses and hirsutism, with up to 75% of affected women having either or both. Acne features in up to a third. Thinning of the scalp hair in a male pattern may also be present. Obesity is not a symptom of PCOS but it is a common association.

Epidemiology

PCOS is the commonest endocrine disorder in women of reproductive age and has an estimated prevalence of 5–10% in this age group. By contrast, 23% of asymptomatic women (who therefore do not have PCOS) will have the ultrasound finding of polycystic ovarian morphology (Polson et al. 1988).

Pathology

The PCO has an increased number of antral follicles which have arrested their development at a size of less than 10 mm in diameter. This is due, at least in part, to high serum luteinizing hormone (LH) levels, high insulin levels (insulin is a weak gonadotrophin), or a combination of both. These two hormones also drive the production of androgens from the theca cells of these follicles, which is increased in those from PCO (Gilling-Smith et al. 1994).

Women with PCO are generally more insulin resistant (due to a post-receptor abnormality) and have higher insulin levels (due to hypersecretion from pancreatic beta-cells) than weight-matched controls with normal ovarian morphology, although the difference is most marked in those with irregular cycles (Robinson et al. 1993). This abnormality of insulin metabolism is thought to be one of the predisposing factors to obesity in PCOS. Obesity, which also raises serum insulin levels in response to insulin insensitivity (via a reduction in the number of insulin receptors), potentiates the abnormality. Thus the menstrual cycles of a woman with PCOS usually become more prolonged (reflecting anovulation) as her weight increases above the norm. These metabolic factors do not fully explain the appearance of the PCO. Abnormalities of follicle number and development are also present during the early, gonadotrophin-independent pre-antral stages of follicle growth (Webber et al. 2003).

Aetiology

PCOS is an inherited disorder (Franks et al. 2009), with a presentation similar to that of an autosomal dominant condition. In fact, it is likely to be polygenetic, although the genes responsible are yet to be identified.

Long-term consequences

- Diabetes: obese women with PCOS are at increased risk of gestational diabetes, impaired glucose tolerance, and diabetes. For women with a BMI ≥30 kg/m^2 the risk of developing impaired glucose tolerance is 30% per year.
- Cardiovascular disease: hypertension, an unfavourable lipid profile, and reduced endothelial elasticity are all more common in obese women with PCOS. However, a large epidemiological study did not show an increase in cardiovascular mortality in women with documented PCOS. Possible explanations for this finding include a protective effect on the cardiovascular system of PCOS, an improvement of cardiovascular risk factors by wedge resection (a procedure that had been performed on the majority of women included in the study) or that the average age of follow-up (56 years old) was too young to demonstrate any attributable mortality.
- Endometrial carcinoma: amenorrhoeic women with PCOS have an increased risk of endometrial carcinoma, especially if obese. It is not clear from the published literature whether this is due to an unopposed oestrogen effect alone or simply that this group of PCOS patients share the general risk factors for endometrial carcinoma (obesity, nulliparity, diabetes).
- Psychological: psychological morbidity is secondary to the symptoms of PCOS (particularly acne, facial hirsutism and infertility). Whether there are direct psychological consequences of elevated serum androgens associated with PCOS is unclear.

Clinical approach

Diagnosis

The diagnosis of PCOS is clinical. Investigations are aimed at excluding other causes for the symptoms.

History

- Menstrual cycle: age of menarche, cycle length, variability, duration and heaviness of bleeding. Anovulatory cycles can present with irregular vaginal spotting or episodes of prolonged or heavy bleeding.
- Weight variations and associated changes in menstrual cycle.
- Acne or hirsutism and duration of symptoms: rapidly developing hirsutism suggests an androgen secreting tumour.
- Past obstetric history: gestational diabetes, birthweight.
- Contraception and/or plans to conceive.
- Past medical history: diabetes, hypertension, thromboembolism.
- Family history: diabetes in first degree relatives.

Examination

- Weight, height, calculate BMI, ±waist circumference.
- Presence or absence of hirsutism: male pattern terminal hair growth. Enquire about any areas that have been treated by hair removal.
- Presence or absence of acne and greasy skin.
- Acanthosis nigricans (slightly raised, velvety, pigmented areas at back of neck or in axillae): a reliable indicator of insulin resistance.

- Pattern of scalp hair thinning.
- Signs of virilisation (deepening of voice, clitoromegaly) suggest other causes of hyperandrogenaemia.
- Cushingoid appearance suggests Cushing's syndrome and not PCOS.

Investigations
Blood tests
- Follicle stimulating hormone (FSH), LH, and oestradiol in early follicular phase if cycling or random timing if not. FSH and oestradiol are normal in PCOS. LH may be raised but an elevated FSH ratio is not required to make the diagnosis.
- Testosterone or androstenedione should be measured but not both. In most laboratories, testosterone is an automated assay and therefore cheaper. There is no benefit in measuring Sex hormone-binding globulin (SHBG) to calculate the free androgen index since SHBG falls as central adiposity increases. This can be assessed visually or by recording the waist circumference.
- Assess thyroid function if there is oligo- or amenorrhoea. Measure prolactin if menstrual cycle is disturbed. Prolactin may be mildly elevated (≤1000) in PCOS with irregular cycles and is of no clinical significance.
- Measure fasting lipids if BMI ≥30 kg/m^2.
- Perform oral glucose tolerance test (OGTT) if BMI ≥30/m^2, BMI of 26–30 kg/m^2 and first-degree relative with Type 2 diabetes; all Asian women with BMI ≥26 kg/m^2. Preconception OGTT is informative for the above groups.
- Serum insulin is of no clinical benefit.

Ultrasound scan
- Ovarian morphology is best assessed with transvaginal ultrasound, especially if the BMI is raised.
- An ovary can be described as polycystic if there are 12 or more antral follicles measuring 2–9 mm and/or the ovarian volume is increased above 10 mL (volume = 0.5 × length × width × thickness) (PCOS Workgroup 2004). Although both ovaries usually share the same appearance, the morphology can be described as PCO if only one meets these criteria (but see differential diagnosis below).
- Endometrial thickness should be assessed, particularly if there is oligo- or amenorrhoea.

Differential diagnosis
These only need to be formally excluded if clinically indicated.
- Congenital adrenal hyperplasia can usually be excluded by measuring serum 17-hydroxyprogesterone. If that is elevated, a short Synacthen test should be performed measuring 17-hydroxyprogesterone, cortisol, and androstenedione at 0, 30, and 60 minutes.
- Cushing's syndrome can be excluded measuring urinary cortisol in two 24-hour collections.
- An androgen-secreting tumour should be suspected if there is a short history of androgenic symptoms and/or a high serum testosterone (>5 nmol/L). Rarely, unilateral PCO appearance can be due to an ovarian tumour. Detailed ultrasound examination of the ovaries should be performed together with a magnetic resonance imaging of the adrenal glands.

Management
The treatment of PCOS remains symptomatic and some treatments are mutually exclusive, e.g. antitestosterone treatment and conception.

- Weight loss should be advised in all cases where the BMI is greater than ideal. All symptoms of PCOS are exacerbated by obesity and will improve with weight loss, including androgenic symptoms. Patients should be counselled that it will be difficult and realistic targets should be agreed. Ovulation and conception rates increase with a reduction only 5–10% of the starting weight. Although there is some limited evidence that low carbohydrate diets may be beneficial, it is much more important that a sustainable change in lifestyle is achieved than any particular type of diet is followed. Exercise is vital to success. Referral to an appropriate dietician may help as can weight management groups. Consideration should be given to pharmacotherapy and bariatric surgery if appropriate.
- Acne and hirsutism can be treated with anti-androgens: daily spironolactone in the dose range 50–150 mg orally or cyproterone acetate 25–50 mg orally for the first 10 days of the menstrual cycle are the commonest. Flutamide 250 mg is an alternative but has no advantage and may be more likely to cause abnormal liver function tests. Reliable contraception must be used during treatment with any anti-androgen due to the potential detrimental effect on the development of a male fetus. The main disadvantage of any anti-androgen is that they often cause further menstrual cycle disturbance. Cycle control is best in combination with an oestrogen, such as Dianette (which contains cyproterone acetate) or Yasmin (which contains drospirenone, a derivative of spironolactone). This combination also provides the required contraception and raises serum SHBG levels, thereby reducing the effective concentration of active androgen. When treating acne, results may be seen in 3–6 months but an improvement in hirsutism may take 9–12 months. Hair removal may still be required but treatments intervals will be prolonged. Suppression of hirsutism may be more rapid with the addition of cyproterone acetate to Dianette (for the first 10 days of each packet), although the end result is the same as with Dianette alone. However, additional cyproterone acetate may be required in the treatment of acne.
- Eflornithine cream (Vaniqa) blocks the action of the enzyme required to make hair and so reduces or stops its growth. It is useful for small areas such as on the face. It can be used in combination with an anti-androgen and like these drugs is only effective during regular use.
- Finasteride blocks the peripheral conversion of testosterone to its active counterpart dihydrotestosterone. Addition of 5 mg daily to anti-androgen treatment may be beneficial in extreme cases of hirsutism although, like flutamide, it is unlicensed for this treatment and should probably be reserved for use within specialist clinics.
- Alopecia may be stabilized with an anti-androgen although new hair growth may not occur. Serum ferritin should be kept above 70 ng/L to optimize hair growth.
- Menstrual disturbance can be treated with the contraceptive pill or with a cyclical progesterone, medroxyprogesterone acetate 10 mg for 10 days per calendar month being the most usual choice as it has few androgenic side-effects. If the woman has no androgenic symptoms, she can be treated with any contraceptive pill, although those containing norethisterone are generally best avoided. The Mirena intrauterine system can also be used. Endometrial protection should be advised using any of these methods if episodes of amenorrhoea repeatedly last longer than 3 or 4 months.

Otherwise ultrasonographic measurement of endometrial thickness with sampling if required should probably be done annually.

- Induction of ovulation is covered in Chapter 12 p. 578.

Long-term follow-up

- Those at risk of diabetes should have annual OGTT.
- Amenorrhoeic patients should have an annual ultrasound assessment of endometrial thickness with endometrial sampling if necessary. Those with irregular vaginal spotting or episodes of prolonged or heavy bleeding should be similarly assessed.
- Deranged liver function rarely occurs with spironolactone or cyproterone acetate, but annual liver function tests should be routine along with serum electrolyte measurement for those on spironolactone due to its diuretic action.
- Women should be advised not to rely on anovulatory cycles for contraception. When wanting to conceive, PCOS women with menstrual irregularity should be referred for cycle monitoring and ovulation induction 3–6 months after discontinuing contraception, depending on cycle length.

Further reading

Franks S, Webber LJ, Goh M, et al. Ovarian morphology is a marker of heritable biochemical traits in sisters with polycystic ovaries. J Clin Endocrinol Metab 2008;93:3396–402.

Gilling-Smith C, Willis D, Beard RW, Franks S. Hypersecretion of androstenedione by isolated theca cells from polycystic ovaries. Clin Endocrinol 1994;47:93–9.

PCOS Workgroup. Revised 2003 consensus on diagnostic criteria and long-term health risks related to polycystic ovary syndrome. Hum Reprod 2004;19: 41–47/Fertil Steril 81:19–25.

Polson DW, Adams J, Wadsworth J, Franks S. Polycystic ovaries: a common finding in normal women. Lancet 1988;1:870–2.

Robinson S, Kiddy D, Gelding SV, et al. The relationship of insulin insensitivity to menstrual pattern in women with hyperandrogenism and polycystic ovaries. Clin Endocrinol 1993;39:351–5.

Webber LJ, Stubbs S, Stark S, et al. Formation and early development of follicles in the polycystic ovary. Lancet 2003;362:1017–21.

Wild S, Pierpoint T, McKeigue P, Jacobs H. Cardiovascular disease in women with polycystic ovary syndrome at long-term follow up: a retrospective cohort study. Clin Endocrinol 2000;52:595–600.

Internet resources

www.pcos-uk.org.uk

Patient resources

www.verity-pcos.org.uk

Preimplantation genetic diagnosis

Definition
Preimplantation genetic diagnosis (PGD) is a recent alternative to prenatal diagnosis and termination of pregnancy (qv) (see chapter 12.37) which may be suitable for individuals or couples who carry a significant risk of transmitting a serious genetic disorder to their offspring (Lashwood 2005; Braude et al. 2002). It differs from prenatal diagnosis in that the genetic test is performed on an egg, or an early developing embryo in vitro prior to implantation into the uterus, and before pregnancy is initiated.

The procedure
PGD requires a representative sample or biopsy to be taken as a single cell from an early (day 3 or 5) embryo created in vitro by the use of IVF (qv) (see chapter 12.19) and tested for the specific disorder. IVF is undertaken, not necessarily because of infertility, but in order to gain access to early embryos for the purpose of PGD.

Indications
There are three main indications for the use of PGD.
- In autosomal single gene disorders (recessive or dominant; early or late onset).
- In sex-linked gene disorders (carried by female but expressed in males).
- For chromosome rearrangements, commonly reciprocal or Robertsonian translocations. These present with physical or mental disability or repeated miscarriage due to inheritance of unbalanced chromosomal products.

Clinical approach
In autosomal recessive gene disorders the embryo must inherit a copy of both the mutated maternal and paternal recessive genes for the disorder to manifest. Carrier embryos, which will have only one copy of the mutated gene and will usually be symptom free, may thus also be considered for replacement after PGD. This is not the case in autosomal dominant gene disorders where carriage of a single copy of the mutated gene (either matermal or paternal) is sufficient to result in the disease. Some genetic diseases manifest immediately or shortly after birth and may be lethal (e.g. spinal muscular atrophy), whereas others may result in chronic disease (e.g. cystic fibrosis). Others may not manifest until well into adult life and are thus considered late onset (e.g. Huntington's disease). Each of these examples presents different moral judgments as to whether the conditions are appropriate grounds on which to discard mutation-carrying embryos (El-Toukhy et al. 2008).

The process
- The woman's ovaries are stimulated to produce multiple Graafian follicles from which the oocytes are retrieved transvaginally using ultrasound guided needle aspiration.
- The oocytes are exposed to the partners sperm in vitro (IVF qv) (see chapter 12.19) or are individually injected with single sperm (ICSI qv) (see chapter 12.17). ICSI is preferable where a molecular rather than a FISH-based test is to be performed on the biopsy in order to minimize DNA contamination by extraneous sperm.
- Only those embryos that have reached 6–10 cells on day 3 and of sufficient morphological calibre are suitable for biopsy.

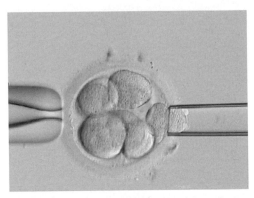

Fig. 12.32.1 Single cell being removed as a biopsy from a day 3 human preimplantation morula for genetic testing. See also colour plate section.

- A hole is made in the zona pellucida of embryo using acid or a laser, and one, sometimes two, cell is removed (Fig. 12.32.1) and is subjected to the genetic test. For a molecular based test, the DNA is amplified using a PCR to provide sufficient material for assay; or for a FISH based test, the cell is spread and stained for cytogenetic analysis (Fig. 12.32.2).
- Only those embryos found free of the mutation or chromosomally normal are considered for replacement into the uterus in order to generate a pregnancy.

Variations
- Polar body biopsy: the first and second polar bodies can be removed from the oocyte retrieved from the follicle on which a genetic test can be performed (Verlinsky 1990). This has the advantage of assessing the genetic status of the egg before any postzygotic changes during cleavage may have occurred. However, it is less reliable, more difficult to perform, and is only useful in recessive conditions or maternally inherited dominant conditions, and for some aneuploidies and chromosomal rearrangements (Fig. 12.32.3).
- Blastocyst biopsy: the embryo is biopsied on day 5 when it has formed the immediate preimplantation stage and contains many more cells. It thus has the advantage that more cells can be removed safely, providing a more reliable test (McArthuret et al. 2008). The disadvantage is that the result is needed within 24 hours so that an

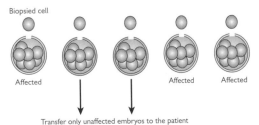

Biopsied cell

Affected   Affected   Affected

Transfer only unaffected embryos to the patient

Fig. 12.32.2 Principle of preimplantation genetic testing. See also colour plate section.

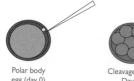

| Polar body | Cleavage stage | Blastocyst |
| egg (day 0) | Day 3 | Day 5 |

Fig. 12.32.3 Stages at which biopsy can be undertaken for PGD. See also colour plate section.

unaffected blastocyst can be transferred within the implantation window (by day 6).

Estimate of use

Although it is estimated that some 10 000 cases of PGD for serious genetic disorders have been performed worldwide since its first use in 1990 (Handyside *et al.* 1990; Verlinsky *et al.* 2004), its use is trivial compared with the number of IVF cycles performed for infertility each year (33 000 per year in the UK alone, see Table 3.19.1). PGD should be distinguished from screening for sporadic age-related aneuploidies (aneuploidy screening, preimplantation genetic screening; PGS), which also uses embryo biopsy as an adjunctive fertility enhancing procedure. Chromosome analysis by FISH or CGH of biopsies is used in order to try and improve outcome of IVF in those older infertile patients with repeated implantation failure, or repeated miscarriage (Gianaroli *et al.* 2005). Despite its ubiquitous use, it is the most common reason given for embryo biopsy internationally, randomized trials have cast significant doubt over its efficacy and safety (Jansen *et al.* 2008; Mastenbroek *et al.* 2008,10).

Further reading

Braude P, Flinter F. Use and misuse of preimplantation genetic testing. BMJ 2007;335:752–4.

Braude P, Pickering S, Flinter F, Ogilvie CM. Preimplantation genetic diagnosis. Nat Rev Genet 2002;3:941–53.

Braude P. Preimplantation diagnosis for genetic susceptibility. N Engl J Med 2006;355:541–3.

Edwards RG. Ethics of PGD: thoughts on the consequences of typing HLA in embryos. Reprod Biomed Online 2004;9:222–4.

El-Toukhy T, Williams C, Braude P. The ethics of preimplantation genetic diagnosis. Obstet Gynaecol 2008;10:49–54.

Gianaroli L, Magli MC, Ferraretti AP, *et al.* The beneficial effects of preimplantation genetic diagnosis for aneuploidy support extensive clinical application. Reprod Biomed Online 2005;10:633–40.

Goossens V, Harton G, Moutou C, *et al.* ESHRE PGD Consortium data collection IX: cycles from January to December 2006 with pregnancy follow-up to October 2007. Hum Reprod 2009 24:1786–1810.

Handyside AH, Kontogianni EH, Hardy K, Winston RM. Pregnancies from biopsied human preimplantation embryos sexed by Y-specific DNA amplification. Nature 1990;344:768–70.

Jansen RP, Bowman MC, de Boer KA, *et al.* What next for preimplantation genetic screening (PGS)? Experience with blastocyst biopsy and testing for aneuploidy. Hum Reprod 2008;23:1476–8.

Lashwood A. Preimplantation genetic diagnosis to prevent disorders in children. Br J Nurs 2005;14:64–70.

Mastenbroek S, Scriven P, Twisk M, *et al.* What next for preimplantation genetic screening? More randomized controlled trials needed? Hum Reprod 2008;23:2626–8.

McArthur SJ, Leigh D, Marshall JT, *et al.* Blastocyst trophectoderm biopsy and preimplantation genetic diagnosis for familial monogenic disorders and chromosomal translocations. Prenat Diagn 2008;28:434–42.

Verlinsky Y, Cohen J, Munne S, *et al.* Over a decade of experience with preimplantation genetic diagnosis: a multicenter report. Fertil Steril 2004;82:292–4.

Verlinsky Y, Ginsberg N, Lifchez A, *et al.* Analysis of the first polar body: preconception genetic diagnosis. Hum Reprod 1990;5:826–9.

Internet resources

ESHRE PGD consortium: www.eshre.com/ESHRE/English/SIG/Reproductive-Genetics/PGD-Consortium/page.aspx/201

Preimplantation Genetics Diagnosis International Society: www.pgdis.org/

Sex Selection and PGD: ASRM statement: www.asrm.org/Media/Ethics/Sex_Selection.pdf

HFEA information on Genetic Testing of Embryos: www.hfea.gov.uk/172.html

Premature ovarian failure

Definition

Premature ovarian failure (POF) is an ovarian defect characterized by primary or secondary amenorrhea before the age of 40 years. Approximately 1% of women under 40 years of age, 0.1% of women under 30 years of age, and 0.01% of women under 20 years of age suffer from POF. The cessation of ovarian function after puberty and before the age of 40 years strongly interferes with fertility and family planning. In most instances the aetiology is unknown but several specific causes have been identified so far. POF can be primary (spontaneous POF) or secondary (induced by radiation, chemotherapy, or surgery). Although the aetiology is very heterogeneous, the treatment and principles remain the same.

Cure rates for cancers in young women continue to improve, and therefore it is likely that the incidence of POF patients will rise rapidly.

Aetiology

The causes of POF are highly heterogeneous. There are two ways that ovarian failure can occur prematurely: failure to attain the appropriate peak follicle number; and accelerated loss of oocytes and follicles.

Many cases follow treatment for neoplastic diseases such as leukaemia, non-Hodgkin lymphoma, and ovarian/cervical carcinoma. Different chemotherapeutic agents, alkylating cytotoxics in particular, have the potential to cause progressive and irreversible damage to the ovaries. The age of the woman and the dose of chemotherapy and/or radiation are the major predictive factors in the development of ovarian dysfunction. When ovarian failure presents with primary amenorrhoea, approximately 50% will be associated with an abnormal karyotype. Two genes (POF1, POF2) have been localized on the basis of deletions in various patients and families. The most common X chromosome abnormality is Turner's syndrome, which accounts for 1 in 2000 female live births.

Of the women with POF, 10–30% have a concurrent autoimmune disease. The most common is hypothyroidism. There is also an association with Crohn's disease, rheumatoid arthritis, myasthenia gravis, and systemic lupus erythematosis. However, most cases present with secondary amenorrhea and are classified as spontaneous POF. It is not uncommon to have a positive family history but there are still few epidemiological data.

Clinical presentation

The main symptom in patients with premature ovarian failure is the cessation of menses before the age of 40 years. The symptoms vary from patient to patient and they may occur abruptly or spontaneously or develop gradually over several years. There appears to be no characteristic antecedent menstrual history. Some women develop amenorrhoea acutely after having established regular menses; some women report failure of menstruation after discontinuation of contraceptives or after completion of a pregnancy. Some women present with an irregular bleeding pattern before becoming amenorrheic. Hot flushes can be a prodromal symptom before the development of ovarian dysfunction and vasomotor symptoms, sleep disturbances, vaginal dryness, decreased libido, mood changes, and fatigue can be a result of hypo- oestrogenism. Young women who have not received oestrogen treatment are at high risk for osteoporosis of the trabecular bone of the spine with associated fractures and height loss.

Infertility is an obvious and mostly irreversible consequence of POF. There are few cases of temporary premature ovarian failure reported in the literature but the chance of subsequent spontaneous conception is 5%. There are no therapies to improve ovarian function and the only method of achieving a pregnancy is fertilization of a donor oocyte.

Diagnosis

The definition of premature ovarian failure is cessation of ovarian function in women less then 40 years of age with primary or secondary amenorrhea and high follicle-stimulating hormone (FSH) levels. The first challenge is to make the diagnosis of premature ovarian failure in a timely manner. It is a difficult diagnosis for women to accept and a carefully planned and sensitive approach is required when informing women of their diagnosis. Alzubaidi et al. (2002) quoted in their paper that 50% of women with secondary amenorrhea saw three or more clinicians before any laboratory testing was performed; 25% of women presenting with secondary amenorrhea in a general gynaecology clinic have premature ovarian failure. As a guide, it is recommended that women younger then 40 years of age suffering 3 or more months without periods should have appropriate evaluation in their first clinic appointment after excluding pregnancy.

Initial evaluation

- At the initial visit a thorough history should be taken focusing on the positive family history and concurrent autoimmune disorders.
- Hormone levels (LH/FSH, oestradiol, prolactin, TSH/T4) should be performed at least 2 occassions, and 6 weeks apart.
- Peptide factors (inhibin B and anti-Müllerian Hormone) of ovarian origin may be useful to determine the follicular reserve especially if fertility is an issue
- Karyotyping is only of interest for women with primary amenorrhoea to exclude any chromosome defects.
- Antibody screening for ovarian antibodies shows positive immunofluorescence in a few women.
- Pelvic scanning to exclude any pathology in the uterus and ovaries and to measure ovarian volume.
- Bone mineral density (BMD): estimation of BMD through DEXA.

Treatment

POF is a devastating diagnosis and many young women undergo a reactive depression in association with their diagnosis. The associated infertility is a major life change that often generates a series of symptoms similar to grief reaction. The clinician is confronted with communicating information about a sudden and unexpected diagnosis. Fogarty et al. (1999) demonstrated in their controlled study that simple statements of concern, which take very little time, can go a long way to helping women see their clinician as being more caring, sensitive, and compassionate.

The management of women with POF should be multidisciplinary with professionals from the various specialities providing the appropriate care to meet the different needs of these women.

The initial concern of women with premature ovarian failure is the need to replace oestrogen to relieve symptoms of oestrogen deficiency, maintain bone density, and reduce the risk of cardiovascular disease. Many types and route of administration of oestrogen are available and the pros and cons should be discussed. The choice of oestrogen and route of administration must be made on an individual basis. There are no controlled studies regarding the ideal hormone replacement strategy for women with premature ovarian failure. In our own database of women with premature ovarian failure, 70% of women are on oral treatment. This seems to be the most convenient way for these young women as it is easier to administer than the transdermal route in the form of a patch. On the other hand, the latter is a more physiological route of administration. Women on oestrogen treatment still need progestogen for the prevention of endometrial hyperplasia. Progestogen can be taken cyclically or continuously from an intrauterine system (Mirena IUS).

It is important to counsel women taking HRT about the possibility of a return of ovarian function and the 5% risk of pregnancy. Contraception should therefore be mentioned for women who do not want to get pregnant.

Future objectives

A multidisciplinary working group should be established to

- identify clinics with premature ovarian failure patients
- develop a national register of premature ovarian failure patients
- establish national guidelines for the treatment of premature ovarian failure patients
- propose future research to determine optimum therapeutic regimens.

Summary points

- Young women who develop premature ovarian failure have unique needs that require special care. A dedicated multidisciplinary clinic will provide ample time and the appropriate professionals to meet the needs of these emotionally traumatized women.
- The menstrual cycle is a reliable biological marker of hypothalamo-pituitary-gonadal function; disruption of regular cycles should be investigated with proper endocrine testing.
- The delay in diagnosis contributes to reduced bone density by delaying appropriate oestrogen therapy.
- HRT in POF women simply replaces ovarian hormones that should normally be produced at this age and it is of paramount importance that the women understand this in view of the general risks on HRT over the age of 50 years.
- Approximately 50% of young women with premature ovarian failure have intermittent and unpredictable ovarian function and 5% may even conceive spontaneously and unexpectedly.

- Learning the diagnosis of premature ovarian failure can be emotionally traumatic and difficult for women, therefore clinicians should spent more time with them and provide more information about their condition.
- Counselling should include explanation that remission and spontaneous pregnancy could still occur and the difference between POF and menopause should be emphasized.

Further reading

Alzubaidi NH, Chapin HL, Vanderhoof VH, et al. Meeting the needs of young women with secondary amenorrhea and spontaneous premature ovarian failure. Obstet Gynecol 2002;99:720–5.

Bondy CA, Bakalov VK. Investigation of cardiac status and bone mineral density in turner syndrome. Growth Horm IGF Res 2006;16(Suppl A):S103–8.

Coulam CB. Premature gonadal failure. Fertil Steril 1982;38:645–55.

Falsetti L, Scalchi S, Villani MT, Bugari G, Premature ovarian failure. Gynecol Endocrinol 1999;13:189–95.

Fogarty LA, Curbow BA, Wingard JR, et al. Can 40 seconds of compassion reduce patient anxiety? J Clin Oncol 1999;17:371–9.

Horner F, Kay A, Mohan E, Panay N. Management of women with premature ovarian failure at a main teaching hospital. Maturitas 2006;54S:50.

Lobo RA, Benefits and risks of oestrogen replacement therapy. Am J Obstet Gynecol 1995;173:982–9.

Massin N, Czernichow C, Thibaud E, et al. Idiopathic premature ovarian failure in 63 young women. Horm Res 2006;65:89–95.

Mishell DRJ, Stenchever MA, Droegemueller W, Herbst AL, Emotional aspects of gynecology. In: Comprehensive gynecology. St Louis: Mosby 1997:171–95.

Nelson LM, Covington SN, Rebar RW. An update: spontaneous premature ovarian failure is not an early menopause. Fertil Steril 2005;83:1327–32.

Panay N, Fenton A, Premature Ovarian Failure: a growing concern, Climacteric. 2008,11:1–3

Panay N, Kalu E. Mangement of premature ovarian failure. In: Best practice and research clinical obstetrics and gynaecology. 2008 1–12.

Portnoi MF, Aboura A, Tachdjian G, et al. Molecular cytogenetic studies of Xq critical regions in premature ovarian failure patients. Hum Reprod 2006;21:2329–34.

Singer, Hunter. Premature Menopause: a multidisciplinary approach 2000.

Sybert PV, McCauley E, Turner's syndrome. N Engl J Med 2004;351:1227–38.

Van Kasteren YM, Schoemaker J. Premature ovarian failure: a systematic review on therapeutic interventions to restore ovarian function and achieve pregnancy. Hum Reprod Up Date 1999;5:483–92.

Internet resources

Royal College of Obstetricians and Gynaecologists: www.rcog.co.uk

The British Menopause Society: www.thebms.org.uk

The Daisy Network: www.daisynetwork.org.uk

Early Menopause UK: www.earlymenopause.org

International Menopause Society: www.imsociety.org

Premenstrual syndrome

Definition

Premenstrual syndrome (PMS) has been defined as distressing physical, behavioural, and psychological symptoms not due to organic disease, which regularly occur during the same phase of each menstrual cycle and which significantly regress or disappear during the remainder of the cycle. The typical psychological symptoms can include anxiety, anger, depression, and irritability. Physical symptoms consist of bloating, weight gain, headaches, breast tenderness, and joint or muscle pain. The symptoms of PMS markedly interfere with work, regular activities, and/or relationships with others.

Epidemiology

Recent studies suggest that severe PMS affects 12–30% of menstruating women, with prevalence estimates depending on the diagnostic criteria employed.

Most women have one or more mild emotional or physical symptom in the premenstrual phase of their cycle; 5–8% have moderate to severe symptoms in association with substantial distress and interference with normal activities to an extent that interpersonal relationships can breakdown (Freeman 2007). Some studies even suggest that up to 20% of all women in their reproductive years have premenstrual complaints that could be regarded as clinically relevant (BorensteinJ et al. 2003).

Retrospectively, many adult women have noted the onset of their premenstrual symptoms as teenagers (Keye 1983). However, the peak age of presentation with severe PMS symptoms is mostly in the late 20s, but many women state they have been symptomatic for as long as 10 years before seeking advice or receiving treatment (Robinson and Swindle 2000).

Pathophysiology and aetiology

Approximately 50% of women experience a few mild symptoms for several days in the luteal phase and probably should not be diagnosed as suffering from PMS (Johnson 2004).

The exact cause of the condition is unknown, although it is almost certainly due to hormonal changes which follow ovulation or even anovulatory mid-cycle ovarian activity.

The symptoms are mostly triggered by the rise and fall of ovarian hormones after ovulation in predisposed women. The levels of sex steroids, oestrogen, progesterone, and testosterone are normal but women with PMS may be more vulnerable to normal fluctuations. Women with PMS show an alteration in their GABA receptor complex response. Studies have demonstrated reduced GABA receptor sensitivity and reduced plasma GABA levels in the luteal phase. Serotonin dysregulation with reduced serotonergic function in the luteal phase offers some plausible explanation for many cases of PMS.

There is a clear picture of 'reproductive depression' in women due to hormonal fluctuations that should be more frequently recognized (Studd and Panay 2004). There are women vulnerable to changes of ovarian hormones whose psychological symptoms start at puberty, are worse before a period, improve markedly during pregnancy, and are worse after delivery. The symptoms are worse as their periods return and in the few years before the cessation of periods. They exhibit the 'triad of hormone responsive mood disorders': premenstrual depression, postnatal depression, and perimenopausal depression.

The importance of ovulation in the aetiology of PMS is clear from the observation that women with PMS do not have symptoms before puberty, after the menopause, or during pregnancy, when they have no cyclical fluctuation of their hormone levels. They are also asymptomatic following hysterectomy and oophorectomy, many choosing to go without oestrogen replacement because they prefer to have the climacteric symptoms of hot flushes and night sweats instead of PMS symptoms. However, if the uterus is removed with conservation of ovaries, the cyclical symptoms remain in the form of PMS symptoms or menstrual migraine (without periods).

Clinical manifestations and diagnosis

More than 150 symptoms of PMS have been described in the literature, ranging from mild symptoms to those severe enough to interfere with normal life (Cronje and Studd 1989).

The physical symptoms consist of breast discomfort, headaches, bloating, and weight gain. Even more distressing are the psychological symptoms of irritability, irrational, aggressive, sometimes violent behaviour, depression, loss of self-confidence, loss of energy, and loss of libido. These may occur for up to 10–20 days per month following ovulation usually ceasing 'like flicking a switch' on the first day of menstruation. However, they may well have menstrual headaches or, like any women, heavy painful periods during this time, so they may have only about 7 good days a month. This question of 'how many good days a month do you have?' is important as it gives a measure of the severity of the condition and a baseline when assessing any improvement with therapy.

Correct diagnosis is crucial in the management of PMS. This cannot be accurately established by retrospective evaluation but needs to be made with daily prospective documentation of relevant symptoms for at least two cycles (symptom questionnaire). The initial completed questionnaires should be kept to give an objective indication of response to therapy.

Treatment

There is no single treatment universally acceptable as effective. Many treatment options have been touted as effective for PMS but only a few are supported by clinical evidence.

Lifestyle changes

Prior to any medical treatment a healthy lifestyle of reduced alcohol, caffeine, and nicotine intake, regular exercise and low fat and high-fibre diet should be the first step. Social and environmental factors can aggravate PMS symptoms. During holidays PMS symptoms seem to be less severe than during daily life. Diet plays a crucial role in the treatment of PMS and it is believed that many women experience exacerbated symptoms of PMS when their blood sugar is not under control.

Herbal preparations and other treatments

In addition to dietary changes adding specific supplements such as vitamin B6, calcium, magnesium and evening primrose oil can improve PMS symptoms. Regular exercise increases the neurotransmitter endorphin that is associated with mood changes. Complementary and alternative therapies (CAM) are widely used but in fact there is very little scientific data to support the use of CAM in PMS

(Watson *et al.* 1989). These remedies are all commonly used in the treatment of mild PMS where medicalization of the condition is not wanted.

If symptoms of stress are more significant, psychological counselling including cognitive behavioural therapy can be beneficial (Blake *et al.* 1998).

Ovulation suppression

It follows that the logical hormonal treatment of severe PMS is to suppress ovulation. This can be done by transdermal oestrogens either patches or gel (Cronje *et al.* 2004). Occasionally hormonal implantation every 6 months can be used. Monthly injections of gonadotropin-releasing hormone (GnRH) analogues such as Gonapeptyl or Zoladex act as a medical oophorectomy and certainly eradicate all symptom clusters of PMS although 'add-back' HRT is required to prevent vasomotor symptoms and osteoporosis (Leather *et al.* 1999).

Oestradiol patches are the most frequently used hormonal therapy and doses of 100 µg or 200 µg, being more than the usual dose for the menopause, are recommended producing plasma oestradiol levels of about 600–800 pmol, which will usually stop ovulation and ablate the hormonal changes that follow ovulation.

These women have a uterus and it is necessary for them to have protection by progestogen usually by the oral route. However, as they have progestogen intolerance they often have a recurrence of their PMS symptoms with the orthodox 14-day course. Thus it is justifiable and indeed correct to shorten the duration to 7 days a month, which is adequate to prevent hyperplasia in 97% of women. If there are still unacceptable PMS symptoms then a Mirena IUS should be considered for many of these patients.

The combined oral contraceptive pill is not usually effective in spite of stopping ovulation. Although it ablates the cycle, the daily progestogen component produces PMS-like symptoms for most days of the month in these women ultra-sensitive to all gestagens. However, a new type of combined contraceptive pill contains an anti-mineral corticoid and anti-androgenic progestogen drospirenone. There are no progestogenic side-effects but has a mild diuretic and anti-androgenic effect. The hormone free interval should also be less then 7 days or even being used back to back (Pearlstein *et al.* 2005).

In spite of the efficacy of these therapies there are still women who may have cyclical symptoms or may have bleeding. The ultimate form of ovulation suppression and possibly the only true cure for PMS is a hysterectomy and bilateral salpingo-oophorectomy (Domoney and Studd 2003). Clearly this procedure is only rarely performed as an alternative can usually be found. A hysterectomy with ovarian conservation will continue to have cyclical symptoms in the absence of cyclical bleeding.

Selective serotonin reuptake inhibitors

Placebo controlled studies have shown that selective serotonin reuptake inhibitors (SSRIs) are effective for severe PMS and improve both mood and physical symptoms (Wyatt *et al.* 2005). Fluoexetine, citalopram, sertraline, and paroxetine can all be implemented and are all effective. Randomized studies have also shown that half-cycle treatment is as efficacious as continuous administration

(Freeman *et al.* 1999). Unlike treating women for depression, symptoms improve within 24–48 hours of initiating therapy and there are no reports of discontinuation symptoms. The dose of fluoexetine or citalopram is 20 mg od for the continuous or cyclical treatment.

Further reading

Blake F, Salkovskis P, Gath D, et al. Cognitive therapy for premenstrual syndrome: A controlled trial. J Psychosomatic Res 1998;45:307.

Borenstein J, Dean B, Endicott J, et al. Heath and economic impact of the premenstrual syndrome. J Reprod Med 2003;48:515–24.

Cronje W, Studd J. Premenstrual syndrome and premenstrual dysphoric disorder. Prim Care 2002;29:1–12.

Cronje WH, Vashist A, Studd JWW. Hysterectomy and bilateral oophorectomy for severe premenstrual syndrome. Hum Reprod 2004;19:2152–5.

Domoney Vashist A, Studd JWW. Premenstrual syndrome and the use of alternative therapies. Ann N Acad Sci 2003;997:330–40.

Freeman E, Rickels K, Arredondo F, et al. Full-half-cycle treatment of severe premenstrual syndrome with serotonergic antidepressant. J Clin Psychopharmacol 1999;19:3 18.

Freeman E. The clinical presentation and course of premenstrual symptoms. In: O'Brien PMS, Rapkin AJ, Schmidt PJ (eds) *The premenstrual syndromes: PMS and PMDD*. Bocca Raton: Taylor&Francis 2007: 55–61.

Johnson SR. Premenstrual syndrome, premenstrual dysphoric disorder, and beyond: A clinical primer for practitioners. Obstet Gynecol 2004;104:845.

Keye W. Premenstrual syndrome. In: *Proceedings of a conference on PMS and related behavioural disorders*. Provo: BYU Division of conferences 1983: 1–10.

Leather AT, Studd JWW, Watson NR, Holland NF. The treatment of severe premenstrual syndrome with goserelin with and without 'add-back' estrogen therapy: a placebo-controlled study. Gynecol Endocrinol 1999;13:48–55.

Pearlstein T, Bachmann G, Zacur H, Yonkers K. Treatment of premenstrual dysphoric disorder with a new drospirenone-containing oral contraceptive formulation. Contraception 2005;72:414–21.

Robinson RL, Swindle RW. Premenstrual symptom severity: impact on social functioning and treatment-seeking behaviours. J Womens Health Gend Based Med 2000;9:757–68.

Royal College of Obstetricians and Gynaecologists. *Management of premenstrual syndrome*. Green-top guideline No 48, RCOG: London 2007.

Studd J, Panay N. Hormones and depression in women. Climacteric 2004;7:338–46.

Watson NR, Studd JWW, Savaas M, et al. Treatment with severe premenstrual syndrome with oestradiol patches and cyclical oral norethisterone. Lancet ii:1989;730–4.

Wyatt KM, Dimmock PW, O'Brien PM. Selective serotonin reuptake inhibitors for premenstrual syndrome. Cochrane Database Syst Rev 2005;3.

Internet resources

National Association for Premenstrual Syndrome (NAPS): www.pms.org.uk.

Womens Health Concerns: www.womens-health-concern.org.

Royal College of Obstetricians and Gynaecologists: www.rcog.co.uk.

FPA: www.fpa.org.uk

Society for endocrinology: www.endocrinology.org.

Patient UK; www.patient.co.uk.

Psychosexual problems

Psychosexual problems are common in both men and women, their prevalence depending on the definition of a dysfunction. This is a contentious issue currently but the most important factor is whether the individual is distressed by their symptoms (Table 12.35.1). The rate of female sexual dysfunction (FSD) may be up to 43% and in men up to 31% in a North American population. The International Consensus conference panel modified the framework of the International Classification of Diseases-10 and DSM-IV (Diagnostic and Statistical Manual of Mental Disorders of the American Psychiatric Association) to categorize clinical sexual disorders and thereby improve diagnosis and treatment. The improvements in physical treatment of male sexual disorders (erectile and ejaculatory disorders in particular) have led to a search for the equivalent treatments of FSD. Yet female sexual function is less easily quantifiable, as satisfaction is qualitative rather than the more quantitative measurements of male sexual function. The use of questionnaires may be helpful in a research setting but have a more limited role in clinical practice. A list of questionnaires for specific patient groups is available in the Further reading section. Asking patients about sexual activity is an important part of a gynaecological consultation. Opening questions within a consultation may be as follows and adapted to individual needs. Assumptions regarding sexual activity and orientation are likely to cause major difficulties within the doctor–patient relationship; therefore, great care should be taken to avoid them.

- Do you have a partner? Are you in a sexual relationship?
- Do you have any difficulties? Do you have pain during intercourse?
- Are these difficulties a problem for you?

Female sexual function models

It is important to have an understanding of current thinking with respect to normal functioning and when the female sexual cycle is affected to understand the categorization of FSD and its treatment. The model of Masters and Johnson has been developed over the decades into a less linear model that incorporates the multifactorial influences on female sexual activity and its modifiers. Relationship issues and the need for intimacy as expressed by physicality may be more important for women within relationships than men.

Table 12.35.1 Common presentation of sexual problems in gynaecological consultations

Overt presentation	Covert presentation
Loss of libido	Pelvic pain
Anorgasmia	Recurrent vaginal discharge
Loss of sensation	Prolapse symptoms
Non-consummation	Vulval pain
Vaginismus	Vaginismus
Coital urinary leak	Difficulty with smear taking
Vaginal dryness	Requests for labial reduction
Dyspareunia	Dyspareunia

Classification of female sexual function disorders

Desire disorders
Hypoactive desire disorder (HSDD): persistent or recurrent deficiency or absence of sexual desire/sexual fantasies/thoughts, and/or the desire for or receptivity to sexual activity that causes distress. The focus on sexual thoughts allows flexibility of definition to include those who are not in a relationship or have lost their relationships secondary to their HSDD.

Sexual aversion disorder is the persistence of phobic aversion to and avoidance of sexual activity that causes personal distress.

Sexual arousal disorder
Low sexual arousal disorder is defined as the persistent or recurrent inability to attain or maintain sexual excitement causing personal distress, which may be described as subjective feelings and/or lack of physical changes.

Persistent arousal disorder is rare but distressing and may be physical and/or psychological.

Orgasmic disorder
The persistence or recurrent difficulty or absence of achieving orgasm following sufficient stimulation and arousal. It may follow from both desire or arousal disorders or be truly independent.

Sexual pain disorders
These include dyspareunia, defined as persistent or recurrent genital pain associated with sexual intercourse. This may be physical and/or psychological, i.e. psychosomatic in origin. These origins must be explored before undertaking invasive investigations.

Vaginismus has been described by the International Consensus group as recurrent or persistent involuntary spasm of the pelvic musculature that interferes with intercourse. However, it may be situational, i.e. with only certain partners or just at speculum examination. This should be more often interpreted as a sign not a symptom of pelvic symptoms and therefore not considered a diagnosis alone.

Non-coital sexual pain disorders
Genital pain disorders induced by non-sexual stimulation, most commonly vulval pain disorders.

The prevalence of these disorders is varied depending on the population and age group. They can vary from 16–75% with desire disorder, 12–64% arousal, 16–48% orgasm, 7–68% with sexual pain, with considerable overlap. At various stages of life, sexual function and activity may change and with this an increase in sexual difficulties. An awareness of these changes may facilitate a discussion with health professionals before the behavioural changes are well established and more difficult to change.

Sexual history
It is rarely necessary to ask a comprehensive sexual history in most gynaecological settings but it is useful to be aware of the other features that may or may not be relevant to the individual patient.

- What sexual problems (primary and secondary)?
- Why is she presenting now?
- Onset? lifelong/acquired, situational/generalized, gradual/rapid onset

- Potential aetiologies: organic/psychogenic/mixed?
- Comorbidities and concurrent disease (surgery/pain/cancer/incontinence)
- Hormonal factors
- Pelvic floor dysfunction
- Psychological health
- Relationship factors.

Investigations

For most women, investigations are unnecessary as the history and examination are likely to be most revealing. However, there may be features of the consultation that invite consideration of some further tests, whether specific to gynaecological or general wellbeing. A hormone profile may or may not reveal raised pituitary hormones in a perimenopausal woman. Thyroid function tests may provide a cause for generalized lack of vitality. If a primary diagnosis presents with a secondary sexual difficulty, this needs to be explored by the appropriate physician in addition to help with the sexual problem (for instance diabetes or galactorrhoea and lack of libido with hyperprolactinaemia). Indications of generalized conditions reflected in genital complaints such as lichen planus or psoriasis may be missed if the search for both organic and psychological causes is cursory. One of the most common conditions causing sexual problems in postmenopausal women is atrophic vaginitis, even in those women using systemic hormone replacement therapy (HRT). It is simple to treat with topical oestrogens (now with an indefinite license in the UK) or non-hormonal remoisturizers.

Hormone tests may be useful in some women if there is a potential role for hormone replacement, e.g. if an individual is considering HRT or monitoring treatment to which there is no response (Table 12.35.2). It is important to remember that other medications may also modify mood and therefore libido. Synthetic progestogens can have a profound effect in susceptible individuals, whether in hormonal contraception, HRT or for management of other gynaecological conditions.

The most useful androgen measurement is the free androgen index, as this gives an indication of free, biologically active androgen. Only 1–2% of testosterone is free in the circulation: 66% is bound to sex hormone binding globulin (SHBG), 31% to albumin (which is also bioavailable. SHBG levels varies enormously in women and may contribute to poor sexual drive and arousal. In women who are using the combined contraceptive pill or oral HRT, the rise in SHBG (and therefore lowering of free testosterone) may account for a change in reported sexual activity when all other factors are stable. However, overall, population

studies have not documented correlation of hormone levels with sexual function.

The free androgen index is calculated from total testosterone and SHBG (normal range 0.4–0.8 ng/L):

$$FAI = TT \text{ (in nmol/L)}/SHBG \text{ (in nmol/L)} \times 100 \text{ (ng/L)}$$

Differing patient groups may be approached with varying techniques (Table 12.35.3). Correcting any physical problem can help but not necessarily cure FSD, as ingrained behaviours need to be addressed (e.g. avoidance/poor arousal/vaginismus). Vulval pain disorders can respond to topical treatments and systemic management of pain in addition to psychotherapeutic input. Women postpartum may need correction of atrophic vaginitis, perineal anaesthetic, and steroid injection in conjunction with debriefing and analysis of their sexual feelings (or lack thereof).

Psychosexual medicine

Sexual function is a 'mind–body' activity and therefore any sexual difficulty can have a psychological effect irrespective of its aetiology. The main tenets of psychosexual medicine use the consultation skills (see below) within the doctor–patient relationship to explore the dynamics of the sexual feelings and relationships of the patient (Table 12.35.4). The genital examination can be used as a 'moment of truth' when the underlying vulnerabilities and patterns of thinking about sexual parts are explored. Gynaecologists have privileged access to intimate examinations that can be used as more than elicitation of physical signs only. Understanding the psychological examination of the pelvis can help diagnose and provide resolution to many psychosomatic gynaecological complaints in addition to understanding the psychological impact of a physical illness.

- **L**isten
- **O**bserve
- **F**eel
- **T**hink
- **I**nterpret

Table 12.35.3 Physical conditions and treatments that may impact on male and female sexuality

Condition	Medications
Vascular disease: hypertension, atherosclerosis	Antidepressants
Dyslipidaemias	Antihypertensives
Diabetes	Antipsychotics
Chronic disease	Mood stabilisers
Depression	Diuretics
Anxiety	Anticonvulsants
Pelvic floor dysfunction: incontinence (faecal and urinary), prolapse	GnRH analogues
Pelvic surgery	H2 anatagonists
Radiotherapy	Antihistamines
Pelvic adhesions	Combined contraceptive pill
Endometriosis	Mirena IUS
Hormonal	Cyproterone
Addiction	Synthetic progestogens

Table 12.35.2 Sex hormone levels in different age groups

Hormone	Reproductive age	Natural menopause	Surgical menopause
Oestradiol	100–150	10–15	10
Testosterone	400	290	110
FSH	<10	>30 (×2, 6 weeks apart)	>30
LH	<6	>10	>10

Table 12.35.4 Psychosexual, pharmacological and physical management strategies for sexual dysfunction

Psychosexual	Pharmacological	Physical
Brief psychodynamic therapy	Oestradiol: systemic or topical	Genital self-examination: look with mirror (with doctor)
Psychotherapy	Vaginal remoisturizers	Physiotherapy: pelvic floor exercises ± biofeedback
Cognitive behavioural therapy	Testosterone: implant/gel/patch/oral	Vaginal trainers/dilators
Sex education	Tibolone	Lubricants
Couple therapy	Analgesics	Clitoral stimulators
Sensate focus	Antidepressants	Visual sexual aids
Psychoanalysis	Gabapentin	Physical sexual aids, e.g. vibrators
'Bibliotherapy'	Local anaesthetics	Vaginal trainers/dilators
	?phosphodiesterase inhibitors	Surgery
	?DHEA	?botulinum injections

The patient is central to the process: she is the 'expert'. The doctor should aim to establish the causative and maintaining factors, understanding then facilitating change and hopefully improvement. The empathic consultation may enable the exposure of subconscious feelings and fantasies, as a reflection of the physical symptoms and sexual problems. The defences and fantasies of the patient (and doctor) should be explored rather than dismissed, as their origins are important to understand. This will be part of the therapeutic pathway. Although some sex therapists follow certain theoretical disciplines, for the gynaecologist offering pragmatic care or providing treatment acceptable to the patient, a practical approach to management and referral using a combination of approaches is likely to be helpful. Understanding what other services are available locally is important to every gynaecology unit. The Internet resources section provides websites that may be able to provide this information.

Partners

Women may or may not present with their partners in gynaecological settings. Most often at the first visit, the woman will present alone. This allows her to be more open in her discussion of the sexual difficulties within her current relationship and her previous perception of her sexuality than may occur if she presents with her partner. Women are frequently protective of their partner's sexual difficulties, with development of their own secondary problems if their male partners develop erectile or ejaculatory disorders, particularly in the older age group. Yet the effectiveness of phosphodiesterase inhibitors in improving male sexual dysfunction has increased the expectations of some who may have abandoned all hope previously.

The most common male sexual problem is erectile dysfunction (ED) but desire and ejaculatory problems are frequently reported. It is important that the patient's description of impotence is clarified as it can be a general term and non-specific to laymen. ED increases with age and a careful medical and sexual history may elicit a predominantly organic problem. Although difficult to elicit, a situational ED is different from a partner who has lost his early-morning erections: the latter much more likely to indicate organic disease. New-onset erectile difficulty may pre-date the onset of cardiovascular disease. Therefore, the evaluation of men with sexual dysfunction requires blood pressure, pulse, weight, genital, and prostate examination with serum glucose, lipids, and early-morning testosterone. Although ED and, to a certain extent premature ejaculation, are compatible with pharmacological treatment, it is important to assess the psychosexual aspects of these difficulties for the couple. Treatment options for men with sexual problems are outlined below (Table 12.35.5).

Life events
Adolescence
Adolescence is a time of massive hormonal upheaval, peer group pressure, and evolving self-realization. Prior education with respect to genital function, menstrual cycles, sexual behaviour, contraception, and functional relationships are significant throughout this period as well as exposure to family attitudes. Events during this time can have a profound effect on future sexual fulfilment.

Reproductive years
Sexual function is inextricably linked with reproductive function despite the ability to control fertility and infection in the modern age.

Table 12.35.5 Treatment options for men with sexual problems

Phosphodiesterase inhibitors	
Sildenafil (Viagra)	Improves ED in 60–70%, acts in 20–60 minutes, lasts up to 8 hours
Tadalafil (Cialis)	May be useful for premature ejaculation, half-life 17 hours. May be useful for psychogenic ED
Vardenafil (Levitra)	Duration of action 8 hours
Apomorphine	Dopamine agonist, sublingual, rapid onset, shorter duration, less efficacious 50–60%
Androgens	For men with hypogonadism NB PSA measurements
Intracavernous prostaglandin	Alprostadil, most common, papaverine and phentolamine occasionally used
Intraurethral prostaglandin pellets	Alprostadil (less effective than intracavernosal)
Vacuum devices	Cost, require dexterity
Penile implants	Good success and patient satisfaction, but failure has serious implications.
Surgery	Appropriate for condition but rarely valuable

Sexually transmitted infections

Education to prevent sexually transmitted disease and treatment seeks to prevent long-term psychological consequences as well as physical. The circumstances under which an infection is introduced, its consequences and the approach to treatment has a bearing on future sexual behaviour. Management of sexually transmitted infections (STIs) should minimize adverse future behaviour: reduction of high-risk-taking sexual behaviour and normalizing sexuality in general. Advertising strategies for sex education reflect the standards and expectations of the younger age groups but may not target all communities as required.

Infertility

Counsellors, ideally with psychosexual training, are available in fertility clinics as the impact of fertility treatment is profound. It is not uncommon to encounter couples who are not having penetrative intercourse. The demands of performing to specific menstrual cycle dates and maintaining celibacy at other times takes its toll on most couples. Sex becomes goal orientated and the spontaneity may disappear. The financial, physical and psychological impact of fertility alters the relationship between the couple.

Termination of pregnancy

At the other end of the spectrum, control of fertility by termination of pregnancy is repeatedly cited by women recounting their sexual biography. This may be years after the event, often when another precipitating life event brings it to the fore.

Childbirth

Pregnancy and childbirth herald major changes for a couple, as both become different players in society with their first child. Their primary role as partner and lover changes to include mother/parent. For some pregnancy increases orgasmic potential, theoretically via an increase in oxytocin receptors, but changes may be secondary to other psychological and behavioural effects such as bonding and protection. Childbirth itself will alter sexual health. However, it is controversial whether interventions such as Caesarean section and episiotomy alter this. Overall sexual problems are common postpartum: 7–13% of women expressed a need for help, but 25% had not sought it. Advice regarding sexual function should be incorporated into routine postnatal care. Operative intervention should be very cautious in those with dyspareunia, particularly if they plan to have more children and are oestrogen deficient (still breastfeeding and no menstrual cycle). Topical oestrogen cream can safely be used in breastfeeding women.

Colposcopy

Many procedures are experienced very differently by patients when compared with healthcare professionals' perceptions. These include smear taking, speculum examination, and colposcopy. These intimate examinations may allow the patient to reveal their difficulties but clinicians can miss the opportunity to discuss them in their haste to 'console' the patient. Care must be taken to make these procedures as minimally traumatic as possible as the potential to impact on sexual functioning is marked. The potential of a diagnosis of human papillomavirus (HPV) to cause distress due to its STI nature must be recognized. Careful explanation of all aspects of colposcopy care and screening are paramount to circumvent future adverse effects.

Menopause and ageing

A number of studies have explored sexual activity and dysfunction in perimenopausal and ageing women. Overall there is a reduction in activity with age but this correlates with partner status and there is some evidence that cessation of activity is more likely to be linked to the male partner. The prevalence of desire disorders stays relatively constant through life as the younger woman is more distressed by this than the older woman. Some studies seem to indicate that sexual responsivity is related to ageing, but libido, frequency of intercourse, and dyspareunia are associated with oestrogen deficiency. Simple measures can improve the physical sequelae of hormone deficiency and tissue ageing such as topical oestrogen, non-hormonal vaginal remoisturizers and lubricants. In addition, consideration of surgery for those with medical problems such as symptomatic prolapse and stress incontinence should be complemented by a psychosexual approach.

Cancer

Aside from the physical effects of surgery, chemotherapy, and radiation the impact of a cancer diagnosis on the patient is enormous. In addition, the role of a partner as carer and provider of comfort is not always complementary to that of a sexual partner. Understanding individual feelings as experienced by the patient and their partner is key. Discussing possible problems at diagnosis and during treatment reinforces the normality of these anxieties. Training of oncology multidisciplinary teams to discuss physical interventions such as vaginal trainer use encourages continuity of care.

Sexual abuse

The possibility of sexual abuse or unwanted sexual experiences should be explored delicately. The lifetime risk of sexual assault for women worldwide is 1 in 4–6 and (in the UK 1 in 20) with a worldwide risk for men of 1 in 10. Only one in five adult rapes are reported to the police with a much lower number being pursued through the legal system. In children, it is estimated at most 1 in 20–50 are known to supervising authorities and therefore most present 'historically'. What constitutes sexual trauma will be individual and dependant on circumstance and support systems, such as the reaction of a family aware of child sexual abuse, or within the context of physical abuse. In others, over exposure to nudity and sexuality in some may constitute abuse. The British Sexual Offences Act of 2003 has responded to the change in accessibility of children and vulnerable adults via the Internet and deems them prosecutable sexual offences. It now acknowledges any penile penetration of vagina, anus, or mouth as rape, rather than sexual assault.

Conclusion

Recognition of sexual problems by the gynaecologist is mandatory. All professionals involved in women's health should have basic training and some understanding of these issues. Routine questioning regarding sexual health will determine those who need referral, but many who attend gynaecology clinics can be treated by an empathic doctor who understands the presentation of these symptoms. First-line interventions can be initiated if appropriate, including hormone therapy. Psychosexual medicine, as a branch of psychosomatic medicine pertaining to sexual problems, should be a major part of the work of gynaecologists and obstetricians, and training should focus on this area.

Further reading

American Psychiatric Association (APA). *Diagnostic and statistical manual of mental disorders*, 4th edn. Washington DC: American Psychiatric Association 2000.

Basson R, Berman J, Burnett A, *et al*. Report of the international consensus development conference on female sexual dysfunction: definitions and classifications. Urology 2000;163:888–93.

Basson R. Women's sexual dysfunction: revised and expanded definition. CMAJ 2005;172:1327–33.

Cockburn J, Pawson M (eds). *Psychological challenges in obstetrics and gynaecology*. London: Springer-Verlag 2007.

Glazener CM. Sexual function after childbirth: women's experiences, persistent morbidity and lack of professional recognition. Br J Obstet Gynaecol 1997;104:330–5.

Hayes RD, Bennett CM, Fairley CK, Dennerstein L. What can prevalence studies tell us about female sexual difficulty and dysfunction? J Sex Med 2006;3;589–95.

Laumann E, Paik A, Rosen R. Sexual dysfunction in the United States: prevalence and predictors JAMA 1999;281:537–44.

Masters WH, Johnson VE. *Human sexual response*. Boston: Little Brown 1966.

Montford H, Skrine R (eds). *Psychosexual medicine: an introduction*. London: Hodder Arnold 2001.

Rees M, Mander T (eds). *Sexual health and the menopause*. London: Royal Society of Medicine Press 2005.

Trigwell P. *Helping people with sexual problems: a practical approach for clinicians*. Mosby Elsevier 2005.

Internet resources

www.ipm.org.uk Institute of Psychosexual Medicine

www.basrt.org.uk British Association of Sexual and Relationship Therapy

www.fsrh.org.uk Faculty of Sexual and Reproductive Health

www.sda.uk.net Sexual Dysfunction Association

Questionnaires

Female sexual function index (FSFI): general population (19 items)

Profile Female Sexual Function: HSDD diagnosis in postmenopausal women (37 items)

Brief Profile Female Sexual Function: screening for HSDD (7 items)

Golombok Rust Inventory Sexual Satisfaction (GRISS): sexual relationships (28 items)

Changes in Sexual Functioning Questionnaire (CSFQ): intervention related change (14/35 items)

Prolapse and Incontinence Sexual Function questionnaire (PISQ): women with pelvic floor disorders (9/12/31 items)

Macoy Sexual Function Questionnaire (MSFQ): women with hormonal factors (19 items)

Recurrent miscarriage

Definition

Recurrent miscarriage (RM) has traditionally been defined as the loss of three or more consecutive pregnancies under 24 completed weeks' gestation. However, a recent analysis of a Scottish population-based database has suggested that after adjusting for age and smoking, the risk of a further miscarriage increased sequentially in women who had one and two miscarriages and that three miscarriages did not increase the odds any further. In the face of declining birth rates, an increasing number of clinicians now define RM as two or more consecutive pregnancy losses.

Primary RM refers to consecutive pregnancy losses with no prior successful pregnancy.

Secondary RM refers to consecutive pregnancy losses following a live birth.

Epidemiology

The statistical prediction for three consecutive miscarriages is 0.34%. However, the condition is seen to affect 1% of women. If defined as two consecutive miscarriages, the incidence is 5%.

Pathology

RM is a heterogeneous condition that has many possible causes. The pathology is therefore varied.

Aetiology

- Unexplained: the cause remains unknown in 50% of the cases.
- Maternal age and previous reproductive outcome: these are two independent risk factors for a further miscarriage. The risk of fetal loss increases steeply after the age of 35 years, rising to 75% at 45 years. Similarly, the risk of a further miscarriage increases after each consecutive miscarriage, reaching 45% after three consecutive miscarriages (RCOG 2003).
- Chromosomal and single gene disorders: 4–5% of couples with RM show changes in the karyotypes compared with 0.2% in the general population. These include balanced reciprocal translocations, Robertsonian translocations, gonosomal check with Rohan mosaic, and inversions.

Anatomical factors

- Congenital uterine malformations: 1.8%–37.6% of patients with RM have congenital uterine malformations such as septate, bicornuate, and didelphic uteri. However, the 'true impact' of these malformations on RM is questionable.
- Uterine fibroids: in addition to a mechanical effect of uterine fibroids that impedes embryonic implantation, uteri with fibroids have now been shown to have a lower expression of HOX10, a gene involved in implantation. The effect of uterine fibroids on reproductive outcome however, remains controversial.
- Acquired anatomical problems: Asherman's syndrome and cervical abnormalities resulting from trauma or surgical treatment are associated with RM.

Immunological factors

- Antiphospholipid antibody syndrome (APS): this has been reported in 15% of RM patients and in untreated pregnancies, a miscarriage rate of 90% has been reported.

- Alloimmune factors: it has been suggested that defects in the immunosuppressive factors, cytokines, and growth factors at the local maternofetal interface may be implicated in the pathogenesis of implantation failure and RM, but there is still no clear evidence to support the hypothesis that HLA incompatibility between couples, the absence of maternal leucocytotoxic antibodies or the absence of maternal blocking antibodies are related to RM.
- Natural killer (NK) cells: women with RM have higher levels of NK cells in the uterine mucosa than controls and those with the highest levels have a correspondingly high rate of miscarriage in subsequent pregnancies without treatment.
- Other immunological conditions: there might be a correlation between coeliac disease and RM but not between the presence of circulating thyroid antibodies and pregnancy outcome in euthyroid women.
- Inherited thrombophilic defects: hereditary thrombophilias due to mutations in factor V and prothrombin gene as well as deficiencies of protein C, protein S, and antithrombin are established causes of systemic thrombosis and are more prevalent in patients with disturbed pregnancy (RM, pre-eclampsia, and late fetal loss) than in patients with normal pregnancy.

Infectious causes

- Bacterial vaginosis (BV): although the association of BV with first trimester miscarriage is inconsistent, the presence of BV in the first trimester is associated with an increased risk of second trimester miscarriage and preterm delivery.
- TORCH infections: although a recognized cause of sporadic miscarriages, the role of these agents in RM is unclear and screening is not advocated.
- Endocrinological factors: RM is associated with thyroid dysfunction, polycystic ovarian syndrome (PCOS), diabetes mellitus especially type I and hyperprolactinaemia.
- Enzyme deficiencies: Some cases of RM are associated with deficiencies in either glucose-6-phosphate dehydrogenase or nitric oxide synthase which are enzymes involved in the metabolism of reactive oxygen species.
- Psychological factors: RM is associated with early pregnancy-related fear and baseline depressive symptoms

Recently identified risk factors

- Circulating microparticles: fibrin deposits have been found in the placental intervillous space of women with RM, suggesting a 'permanent, acquired procoagulatory state'. In some of these patients, there is an increased concentration of microparticles from circulating blood cells. They are believed to induce coagulation that becomes clinically manifest during pregnancy.
- Glycoproteins: the glycoprotein glycodelin, secreted in high amounts by the trophoblast seems to be downregulated in RM patients. Reduced glycodelin expression in miscarriage could lead to increased activation of the maternal immune system, thus causing rejection of the developing fetus.
- Nuclear hormone receptors and leptin: the nuclear hormonal receptor peroxisome proliferator-activated receptor (PPAR)γ seems to play a major role in facilitating

the invasion of the placental trophoblast. Leptin is connected to PPARγ by a negative feedback loop and decreased leptin levels seem to be associated with miscarriage.

Clinical approach

Investigations

Investigations for genetic factors
- Peripheral blood karyotyping of both parents has been recommended for all couples with a history of RM as the incidence of an abnormal karyotype can be as high as 3–5% in this group.
- Cytogenetic analysis of the products of conception, although an expensive tool, provides useful information for counselling and future management. If the karyotype of the miscarried pregnancy is abnormal, there is a better prognosis in the next pregnancy.

Investigations for uterine anatomical defects
- Routine two-dimensional pelvic ultrasound with or without sonohysterography is at least as sensitive in detecting uterine anomalies than the more invasive and uncomfortable procedure of hysterosalpingography and is currently recommended in all patients with RM.
- Three-dimensional ultrasound offers both diagnosis and classification of uterine malformation and its use may obviate the need for diagnostic hysteroscopy and laparoscopy in the future.
- There is currently no satisfactory objective test that can identify women with cervical weakness in the non-pregnant state.

Investigations for immunological factors
- Antiphospholipid antibody syndrome: diagnosis requires fulfilment of the criteria outlined in the updated international consensus statement. This includes the presence of at least one clinical and one laboratory-based criterion detected on two separate occasions at least 12 weeks apart.
- Alloimmune factors: testing for alloimmune factors is currently not recommended outside a research setting.
- NK cells in peripheral blood: there is poor correlation between levels of NK cells in uterine mucosa and peripheral blood and levels in peripheral blood are not representative of an individual's risk of RM. Testing is therefore not warranted.
- Testing for thyroid antibodies in women with RM is not recommended.

Investigations for inherited thrombophilias
In the absence of a randomized trial, the poor pregnancy outcome associated with inherited thrombophilias, coupled with the maternal risks during pregnancy, may justify routine screening for these conditions and offering thromboprophylaxis to those affected.

Investigations for infective causes
- Screening for bacterial vaginosis: screening low-risk women for bacterial vaginosis during the first trimester of pregnancy and treating them with oral clindamycin may reduce the risk of late miscarriage and preterm birth.
- Screening for TORCH infections is currently not recommended.

Investigations for endocrinological factors
- Hyperprolactinaemia: treatment with bromocriptine significantly reduces the rate of miscarriage.
- Other endocrinological factors: routine screening for occult diabetes and thyroid disease with oral glucose tolerance and thyroid function tests in asymptomatic women presenting with RM is uninformative. Ovarian morphology in PCOS is not predictive of pregnancy outcome. These tests are therefore not recommended.

Management

Counselling and adjuvant therapy
- Genetic counselling: the finding of an abnormal parental karyotype should prompt referral to a clinical geneticist. Genetic counselling offers the couple prognosis for future pregnancy, familial chromosomal studies and appropriate prenatal diagnosis in future pregnancies.
- General counselling: RM patients may profit not only from general supportive counselling but also from interventions like psychotherapy.

Medical management
- Progesterone: progesterone induces secretory changes in the endometrium that are essential for implantation of the embryo. Its use in the first trimester might be of benefit to women with RM.
- Metformin: the use of insulin-sensitizing agents such as metformin is associated with a reduction in miscarriage rate in women with PCOS.
- Antithrombotic treatment
  - For antiphospholipid syndrome (APS): aspirin combined with low molecular weight heparin (LMWH) significantly increases live birth rate in RM patients with APS.
  - For inherited thrombophilias: although several trials emphasize the benefit of LMWH in treatment of patients with known hereditary thrombophilia, the heparin/aspirin (HepASA) trial in Canada showed that 80% of RM patients had a successful pregnancy regardless of treatment given (heparin + aspirin versus aspirin alone) raising questions on the efficacy of LMWH treatment in this cohort of patients. However, as there is some evidence for benefit, and since the potential for harm is so small, LMWH is still considered acceptable for use in cases of inherited thrombophilia.
  - For unexplained RM: neither aspirin alone nor aspirin combined with LMWH is shown to be of any benefit in women with unexplained RM. The Scottish Pregnancy Intervention Trial has shown no reduction in pregnancy loss rate with antithrombotic agents in women with ≥2 consecutive previous pregnancy losses.
- Immunotherapy: this is of two types
  - active immunotherapy: an injection of paternal leucocytes is used to boost the subsequent maternal immune recognition of the developing conceptus. Whereas meta-analysis showed no significant benefit on pregnancy outcome in RM patients when compared with placebo, paternal immunization has recently been shown to be associated with significantly lower levels of tumour necrosis factor (TNF)-α and interferon (IFN)-γ; higher levels of CD4+ CD25+ (bright) T cells and significantly higher successful pregnancy rates in cases of unexplained RM

- passive immunotherapy: an intravenous infusion of immunoglobulins is used in the hope of neutralizing circulating maternal autoantiboidies, inhibiting complement-mediated cytotoxicity and modulating cytokine release. It may be beneficial in a subpopulation of RM patients >37 years with ≥4 miscarriages or secondary RM and in patients with high numbers of CD56+ CD3+ NK cells; this expensive treatment is not without side-effects and should only be used under controlled study conditions.
- Newer treatments
  - TNF-α inhibitors and granulocyte colony-stimulating factor (G-CSF) are promising new drugs and their use in recent studies has shown increased live birth rates when compared with placebos. They still are not recommended outside a research setting.
  - PPAR and leptin are potential targets for new treatment strategies concerning miscarriage.
  - RM patients with coeliac disease might benefit from a gluten-free diet.

Surgical management
- Surgery for anatomical factors
  - Congenital uterine anomalies: there is a suggestion that RM patients with septate uteri may profit from hysteroscopic metroplasty, but no randomized trial has assessed the benefits of this procedure on pregnancy outcome. Open uterine surgery is not recommended as it is associated with postoperative infertility and carries a significant risk of uterine scar rupture during pregnancy.
  - Fibroids: surgical treatment of uterine fibroids is controversial and depends on their size and location.
- Cervical cerclage: a Cochrane review identified no conclusive evidence that prophylactic cervical cerclage reduces the risk of recurrent midtrimester miscarriage and the insertion of a rescue cerclage for cervical shortening identified on serial ultrasound scans is questionable. Abdominal cerclage has been advocated for selected women with known cervical incompetence and failed vaginal cerclage. Although this might reduce perinatal death, it is associated with a higher risk of serious operative morbidity.
- Preimplantation genetic diagnosis and *in vitro* fertilization: this is a treatment option being explored for translocation carriers, but is a technically demanding procedure and the experience is still limited.

Complications/side-effects/sequelae
Recurrent miscarriage is being increasingly recognized as part of a spectrum of disorders resulting from faulty placentation and is found to be associated with late pregnancy complications, including intrauterine growth restriction, preterm labour, and pre-eclampsia.

Prognosis/follow-up/recurrence/future pregnancy planning
Despite a thorough evaluation, a significant proportion of cases of RM remain unexplained. The prognosis for successful future pregnancy in these cases, with supportive care alone is in the region of 75%. Attendance at a dedicated early pregnancy clinic has been shown to have a beneficial effect, although the mechanism remains unclear.

Further reading
Greer IA. Antithrombotic therapy for recurrent miscarriage? N Engl J Med 2010;362:1630–1

Rai R, Regan L. Recurrent miscarriage. Lancet 2006;368:601–611

RCOG *The investigation and treatment of couples with recurrent miscarriage.* Greentop guideline no. 17. London: RCOG 2003. www.rcog.org.uk

Toth B, Jeschke U, Rogenhofer N, *et al.* Recurrent miscarriage: current concepts in diagnosis and treatment. J Reproduct Immunol 2010;85:25–32

Patient resources
Couples with recurrent miscarriage: what the RCOG guideline means for you? www.rcog.org.uk/womens-health/clinical-guidance/couples-recurrent-miscarriage-what-rcog-guideline-means-you

The Miscarriage Association, Clayton Hospital, Northgate, Wakefield WF1 3JS: www.miscarriageassociation.org.uk

Women's Health, 52 Featherstone Street, London EC1Y 8RT: www.womenshealthlondon.org.uk

Termination of pregnancy

Introduction

Termination of pregnancy (TOP) is one of the most commonly performed gynaecological procedures in Great Britain. At least one-third of British women will have had an abortion by the time they reach the age of 45 years, with approximately 192 000 pregnancy terminations being performed each year. The UK also has the highest TOP rates among 15–19-year-old girls in Western Europe.

In 2008, for women resident in England and Wales

- the total number of abortions was 195 296, compared with 198 499 in 2007, a fall of 1.6%
- the age-standardized abortion rate was 18.2 per 1000 resident women aged 15–44, compared with 18.6 in 2007
- the abortion rate was highest at 36 per 1000, for women age 19, the same as in 2007
- the under-16 abortion rate was 4.2 and the under-18 rate was 18.9 per 1000 women, both lower than in 2007
- 90% of abortions were carried out at under 13 weeks' gestation; 73% were at under 10 weeks
- medical abortions accounted for 38% of the total
- 91% of abortions were funded by the NHS; of these, just over half (58%) took place in the independent sector under NHS contract.

Induced abortion is a healthcare need. In 1999, the International Federation of Gynaecology and Obstetrics (FIGO) recommended that 'after appropriate counselling, a woman has the right to have access to medical or surgical induced abortion, and that healthcare services have an obligation to provide such services as safely as possible'.

In 2004, the Royal College of Obstetricians and Gynaecologists (RCOG) published National evidence based guidelines on 'The Care of Women Requesting Abortion', which sets quality standards for abortion services

The aim of a termination of pregnancy service is to provide high-quality, efficient, effective, legal and comprehensive care, which respects the dignity, individuality and rights of women to exercise personal choice over their treatment. Ideally, an abortion service should be an integral component of a broader service for reproductive and sexual health, encompassing contraception and management of sexually transmitted infections.

Termination of pregnancy services should be able to offer impartial support and advice to all women with unintended pregnancy who an abortion requests regardless of age, ethnicity, language, religious or personal circumstances.

Statutory grounds for TOP

TOP or abortion is legal in Great Britain if two doctors decide in good faith that a particular pregnancy is associated with factors that satisfy one or more of five grounds specified in the Regulations of the Abortion Act and Section 37 of the Human Fertilisation and Embryology Act 1990.

A. The continuance of the pregnancy would involve risk to the life of the pregnant woman greater than if pregnancy were terminated.

B. The termination is necessary to prevent grave permanent injury to the physical or mental health of the pregnant woman.

C. The pregnancy has not exceeded its 24th week and the continuance of pregnancy would involve risk, greater than if pregnancy were terminated, of injury to physical or mental health of the pregnant woman

D. The pregnancy has not exceeded its 24th week and continuance of pregnancy would involve risk, greater than if the pregnancy were terminated, of injury to physical or mental health of the existing child(ren) of the family of pregnant women.

E. There is substantial risk if the child were born it would suffer from such physical or mental abnormality as to be seriously handicapped.

The Regulations also permit abortion to be performed in an emergency on the basis of signature of the doctor performing the procedure, which may be provided up to 24 hours after the termination. The grounds are

F. To save the life of the pregnant woman.

G. To prevent grave permanent injury to the physical or mental health of the pregnant woman at risk.

A pregnancy may only be terminated if two registered medical practitioners are of the opinion, formed in good faith, that TOP is justified within the terms of the Act. The Abortion Act has a conscientious objection clause which permits doctors to decline participating in pregnancy terminations. However, doctors are obliged to provide emergency treatment when a woman's life is at risk. Most abortions are undertaken on grounds C or D.

Access and referral to TOP services

Some 90% of abortions are performed in the NHS, with the majority being referred by GPs. Rapid access to abortion care is important to reduce the distress and complications associated with procedures undertaken at higher gestations. Services should therefore offer arrangements to minimize delay. Appointments for assessment prior to TOP can be made via a common telephone booking service that can be accessed by clients either directly, or via GPs, family planning clinics, young people's clinic, Brook clinics, and genitourinary medicine clinics. Fast track referral guidelines should also be put in place for GPs and family planning services, and attempts should be made to treat women having abortions separately from other gynaecological patients.

The Government's sexual health strategy states that no woman should wait longer than 3 weeks from the first appointment with the referring doctor to the procedure, a standard supported by professional guidelines.

RCOG recommendations on referral procedure

- All women requesting TOP should ideally be offered an assessment appointment within 5 days of referral.
- As a minimum standard, all women requesting TOP should ideally be offered an assessment appointment within 2 weeks of referral.
- Ideally all women can undergo TOP within 7 days of the procedure being agreed upon.
- As a minimum standard, all women should undergo TOP within 2 weeks of the decision being agreed upon.
- Women with urgent medical reasons requiring TOP should be seen as soon as possible.

- As a minimum standard, no woman should wait for more than 3 weeks from her initial referral to the time of abortion.

Management

A TOP service should provide counselling, contraceptive advice, gestational age assessment by ultrasound, a specialist nurse, and a clinician for clinical assessment and management.

Counselling

Counselling enables the person concerned to understand the implications of the proposed course of action for themselves and for their family. Counselling also aims at giving emotional support at times of particular stress and helps people with consequences of their decision and to help them resolve problems that may arise as a result.

Contraceptive advice following termination

- It is important to ask the patient about previous contraception and to offer contraceptive advice post termination. Before the patient is discharged following abortion, future contraception should have been discussed with each woman and contraceptive supplies should have been offered if required. The chosen method of contraception should be initiated immediately following abortion.
- Intrauterine contraception can be inserted immediately following first or second trimester abortion.
- Sterilization can be safely performed at the time of induced abortion. However, combined procedures are associated with high rates of failure and of regret on the part of the woman

Investigations

- A detailed clinical history and thorough examination to determine patient fitness for the procedure.
- Screening for chlamydia.
- Screening for HIV, hepatitis B and C is indicated in the light of clinical features, individual risk factors or prevalence.
- Preprocedure blood testing: full blood count, ABO and Rhesus blood groups, screening for red cell antibodies.
- Women who have not had a cervical smear within the recommended interval in their programme can be offered one within the TOP service.
- Ultrasound scanning of all patients prior to TOP is not considered to be an essential prerequisite.
- All services, however, must have access to scanning, as it can be a part of pre-abortion assessment, particularly where gestation is in doubt or where extrauterine pregnancy is suspected.

Consent

- Any competent young person, regardless of age, may independently seek medical advice and give valid consent to medical treatment.
- Following the Gillick case, Lord Fraser provided the Fraser Criteria for young girls under 16. Although parental involvement is ideal, girls under 16 may sign consent for TOP if they decline parental involvement and doctors feel they are 'mature' (Gillick competent) to comprehend their circumstances.

Surgical procedure

- Appropriate at gestations of 7–15 weeks

- If performed at less than 7 weeks' gestation, it is three times more likely to fail to remove products of conception than that performed at 7–12 weeks
- For first trimester suction termination either electric or manual aspiration devices may be used, as both are effective and acceptable to women and clinicians. In this process, a plastic aspiration cannula is used with a vacuum device to empty the uterus.
- Suction termination is performed as a day case procedure, usually under general anaesthesia.
- Suction termination is safer under local anaesthesia than under general anaesthesia. Consideration should be given to making this option available, particularly at low gestational ages.
- Cervical priming prior to surgical abortion reduces the risks of cervical injury by making the cervix softer and easier to dilate.
- Based on available evidence, misoprostol given in a regimen 400 μg (2 × 200 μg tablets) administered vaginally, either by the woman or a clinician, 3 hours prior to surgery remains the most widely used prostaglandin for cervical priming although it is unlicensed.
- Gemeprost 1 mg vaginally, 3 hours prior to surgery or mifepristone 600 mg orally 36–48 hours prior to surgery is licensed for use.
- During suction termination, the uterus should be emptied using the suction curette and blunt forceps (if required) only. Sharp curette should not be used.
- An ultrasound-guided procedure should be performed if there is any difficulty encountered during the procedure.
- Suction termination can be done from 12 to 15 weeks' gestation, varying according to the skills and experience of local clinicians
- For gestations above 15 weeks, surgical abortion by dilatation and evacuation (D&E), preceded by cervical preparation, is safe and effective
- The risk of cervical incompetence is increased as a result of the degree of dilatation necessary and there is a higher risk of major complications, e.g. uterine perforation and visceral damage
- Routine histopathological examination of tissue obtained at TOP is not necessary.

Medical procedure

- There has been an increase in the last few years: 30% (2006), 35% (2007), 38% (2008)
- It is a safe and effective alternative to surgery.
- Ninety per cent of women state that they would choose medical treatment for subsequent termination
- There are few contraindications to medical termination; these include:
  - ectopic pregnancy
  - chronic adrenal failure
  - long-term corticosteroid therapy
  - haemorrhagic disorders and anticoagulant therapy
  - cardiac disease
  - porphyria.

Early medical TOP

- Gestations up to 9 weeks.
- Medical abortion using Mifepristone plus prostaglandin is the most effective method of abortion at gestations of less than 7 weeks.

- Medical abortion using Mifepristone plus prostaglandin continues to be an appropriate method for women in the 7–9 week gestation band.
- Early medical TOP (up to 49 days), based on the evidence of published, but unlicensed regimes: day 1 Mifepristone 200 mg given orally, followed by 1–3 days later by misoprostol 800 µg vaginally.
- For women between 49 and 63 days, the above regimen is given, followed by a second dose of 400 µg of misoprostol if the first dose has not caused abortion. The route of the second dose of misoprostol depends on the amount of vaginal bleeding and preference.
- The following regime is licensed: mifepristone 600 mg orally followed 36–48 hours later by gemeprost 1 mg vaginally.
- If women are well informed, offered sufficient pain relief, and have a well functioning follow-up programme, this procedure can be done at home
- Early medical TOP service can be run by a nurse-led clinic without compromising on safety and effectiveness.
- The involvement of nurses in medical abortion should be encouraged, if future legislation permits, as recommended in the report from the House of Commons Science and Technology Committee.

Late medical TOP

- Gestations from 13–24 weeks.
- Mifepristone followed by prostaglandin is an appropriate method and has been shown to be safe and effective at these gestations.
- Based on the available evidence, mifepristone 600 mg orally, followed 36–48 hours later by gemeprost 1 mg vaginally every 3 hours to a maximum of five pessaries.
- Also based on evidence, but unlicensed regime includes mifepristone 200 mg orally, followed 36–48 hours later by misoprostol 800 µg vaginally, then misoprostol 400 mg orally, 3-hourly, to a maximum of four oral doses.

Other methods of TOP
Extra-amniotic route medication

- For second trimester abortions.
- A self-retaining catheter is passed through the cervix into the extra-amniotic space and a continuous infusion of PGE2 is given until the cervix is sufficiently dilated to allow catheter balloon to be expelled, followed by oxytocin infusion.

Intra-amniotic route medication

- Recommended after 20 weeks.
- Amniocentesis is performed, 100–200 mL of liquor removed, and replaced with 80–120 g of 20% urea and up to 5 µg of PGE2. This usually causes fetal demise before expulsion. Continuous ultrasound scanning is essential for the procedure, to prevent intravascular injection, leading to coagulopathy, and cardiogenic collapse.

Hysterotomy

- Nowadays, rarely performed for TOP.
- May be considered for midtrimester TOP for conjoint twins, where vaginal delivery may not be feasible

Complications

Complication rates depend on stage of gestation, method of termination, skill and experience of the operator, and coexisting factors, e.g. uterine malformation.

Haemorrhage

Haemorrhage complicates approximately 1.5 per 1000 procedures, under 13 weeks of gestation and 8.5 per 1000 over 20 weeks. Significant haemorrhage is more common in the second trimester, and if not treated promptly, can lead to significant blood loss. Oxytocics are effective in reducing intraoperative blood loss; however, its routine use is not recommended.

Uterine perforation

Uterine perforation can occur in 1–4 per 1000 procedures. When suspected at the time of TOP, laparoscopy is indicated to confirm the diagnosis. If the bleeding from the perforation is significant, it needs to be sutured. Visceral perforation may also occur at the time of TOP, the appropriate team must be involved in repair. At times, a perforation can go undiagnosed at the time of TOP and present later with abdominal pain or shock. Continuous traction of the vulsellum during cervical dilatation may be helpful in straightening the angle between the cervix and uterine cavity and reduce the risk of perforation in a markedly anteverted or retroverted uterus.

Retained products

Incidence is 1–2%. Sometimes, a repeat evacuation may be required. Ultrasound may reveal blood clots, which makes the diagnosis difficult.

Failure to abort

The incidence in surgical TOP is around 2.3 per 1000 procedures, and for medical TOP around 6 per 1000.

Cervical trauma

Incidence is 1%. Cervical priming with prostaglandin reduces the risk of cervical trauma. Dilatation above 10 mm may cause cervical incompetence.

Infection

Infection, including pelvic inflammatory disease, occurs in up to 10% of cases, although this rate is lower if bacteriological screening is performed and prophylactic antibiotics are given.

Long-term sequelae

Only a minority of women experience any long-term psychological sequelae. There are no proven associations with infertility, future pregnancy loss, breast cancer or adverse outcome in subsequent pregnancies such as low birthweight, preterm labour.

Prevention of infection

RCOG recommendations on antibiotic prophylaxis:
- metronidazole 1 g rectally at the time of abortion plus
- doxycycline 100 mg orally twice daily for 7 days, commencing on the day of abortion
  or
- metronidazole 1 g rectally at the time of abortion plus
- azithromycin 1 g orally on the day of abortion.
  Compliance is better with Azithromycin as it is a single dose regime.

Anti-D prophylaxis

According to the RCOG recommendation May 2002, anti-D immunoglobulin G (250 IU before 20 weeks of gestation and 500 IU thereafter) should be given, by injection into the deltoid muscle, to all not sensitized Rh D-negative women within 72 hours following abortion, whether by surgical or medical methods.

Sharing information and patient confidentiality

The GP, referring doctor/nurse, and doctor providing follow-up care should be informed in writing of the date of termination, method used, antibiotic treatment, other medical problems, any complications or referral to other services, and arrangements for contraception and follow-up. The woman's consent to passing on of information to professional carers should first be obtained, although the importance of the GP being informed in case of emergency should be emphasized to the woman. In order to maintain confidentiality, no information should be sent to the woman's home address unless the woman expressly wishes this.

Further reading

Abortion Act 1967. London: HMSO 1967.

Allsop JR. Termination of pregnancy. Curr Obstet Gynaecol 2004;14:285–90.

Buehler JW, Schulz KF, Grimes DA, Hogue CJ. The risk of serious complications from induced abortion: do personal characteristics make a difference? Am J Obstet Gynecol 1985;153.14–20.

Department of Health. *Abortion statistics, England & Wales: 2008.* www.dh.gov.uk

Department of Health. *The national strategy for sexual health and HIV. Implementation Action Plan.* London: DH 2002.

Ferris LE, McMain-Klein M, Colodny N, *et al.* Factors associated with immediate abortion complication. Can Med Assoc J 1996;154:1677–85.

Lipp A. A review of developments in medical termination of pregnancy. J Clin Nursing 2008;17:1411–18.

Niinimäki M, Pouta A, Bloigu A, *et al.* Immediate complications after medical compared with surgical termination of pregnancy. Obstet Gynecol 2009;114:795–80.

Peyron R, Aubeny E, Targosz V, *et al.* Early termination of pregnancy with mifepristone (RU 486) and the orally active prostaglandin misoprostol. N Engl J Med 1993;328:1560–13.

Premila S, Arulkumaran S. Termination of pregnancy. Obstet Gynaecol Reproduct Med 2007;10:301–4.

Royal College of Obstetricians and Gynaecologists (RCOG). Rh prophylaxis, anti-D immunoglobulin. Green Top Guideline No.22. London: RCOG 2002.

Royal College of Obstetricians and Gynaecologists (RCOG). *The care of women requesting induced abortion.* National Guidance-Based Clinical Guideline No. 7. London: RCOG Press 2004.

Soulat C, Gelly M. Immediate complications of surgical abortion. J Gynecol Obstet Biol Reprod (Paris) 2006;35:157–62.

Internet resources

www.dh.gov.uk/en/Publicationsandstatistics/Publications/Publications PolicyAnd Guidance/DH_080925

Benign and urogynaecology

Endometrial polyps 600
Female genital cutting 602
Fibroids 606
Ovarian cysts 610
Pelvic inflammatory disease 612
Female urinary incontinence 614
Urinary frequency and urgency 618
Urinary retention (voiding diffiulty) 620
Urinary tract injury 622
Uterovaginal prolapse 626
Urodynamic investigation 630
Vaginal discharge 632
Vesicovaginal fistulae 634
Vulval pain and pruritus 636

Endometrial polyps

Endometrial polyps are focal overgrowths of the endometrium that protrude into the uterine cavity.

Endometrial polyps are thought to arise from small areas of the endometrium that do not cycle with the rest of the endometrium. They grow but do not slough during menstruating, eventually forming a polyp which projects into the endometrial cavity.

Such polyps are common. They are detected by outpatient hysteroscopy in about 11% of women referred for the investigation of menstrual symptoms (Alexopoulos et al. 1999). They typically occur in women aged over 40 years. After the menopause, the endometrium is normally atrophic, but hormone replacement therapy does provide endometrial stimulation, leading to polyp formation.

Tamoxifen (a partial oestrogen agonist with inhibitory effects on breast tissue) treatment for breast cancer, causes endometrial stimulation, sometimes leading to polyp formation or even endometrial hyperplasia and malignancy. With tamoxifen, the incidence of polyps rises to 27%.

Pathology

- Polyps are multiple in 20% of cases.
- Smooth surfaced sessile or pedunculated with thick or slender stalk.
- Histologically, a polyp is a focal overgrowth of endometrial glands and stroma with intact overlying endometrium on three sides.

Clinical issues

Although polyps can be asymptomatic, the tip of the polyp often ulcerates and bleeds, resulting in intermenstrual bleeding in younger women or postmenopausal bleeding in older women. Other clinical presentations include menorrhagia, menometrorrhagia, or vaginal discharge.

Endometrial polyps are benign lesions with low potential for malignant transformation. The reported incidence of malignancy is about 0.5%.

Diagnosis

- Ultrasound, where transvaginal sonography (TVS) is the modality of choice with 56–96% sensitivity and 82% specificity.
- Sonohysterography (SHG) can be considered when TVS is suboptimal.
- Hysteroscopy is the most accurate diagnostic tool (Alexopoulos et al. 1999; Goldstein 2002).

Management

The first priority is to exclude endometrial malignancy in case of abnormal bleeding. Hysteroscopy and Polypectomy can be performed in cases of benign polyps.

Further reading

Alexopoulos ED, Fay TN, et al. A review of 2581 out-patient diagnostic hysteroscopies in the management of abnormal uterine bleeding. Gynaecol Endoscopy 1999;8:105–10.

Goldstein SR, Monteagudo A, et al. Evaluation of endometrial polyps. Am J Obstet Gynecol 2002;186:669–74.

Female genital cutting

Definition

Female genital mutilation (FGM) also called female genital cutting (FGC) is defined by the World Health Organization as comprising all procedures that involve partial or total removal of the external female genitalia, or other injury to the female genital organs for non-medical reasons (WHO 1997).

In communities where the practice still occurs, the term 'mutilation' is considered negative and a hindrance to social change towards elimination of the practice. The less judgemental term, female genital mutilation/cutting (FGM/C) is used by some authorities.

Classification

Female genital mutilation is classified into four main types with subdivisions (WHO 2008).

- Type I: partial or total removal of the clitoris and/or the prepuce (clitoridectomy)
  - Type Ia—removal of the clitoral hood or prepuce only
  - Type Ib—removal of the clitoris with the prepuce
- Type II: partial or total removal of the clitoris and the labia minora, with or without excision of the labia majora
  - Type IIa—removal of the labia minora only
  - Type IIb—partial or total removal of the clitoris and the labia minora
  - Type IIc—partial or total removal of the of the clitoris, the labia minora, and the labia majora
- Type III: narrowing of the vaginal orifice with the creation of a covering seal by cutting and appositioning the labia minora and/or the labia majora, with or without excision of the clitoris (infibulation)
  - Type IIIa—removal and apposition of the labia minora
  - Type IIIb—removal and apposition of the labia majora.
- Type IV: unclassified; all other harmful procedures to the female genitalia for non-medical purposes, for example pricking, piercing, incising, scraping, and cauterizing.

Prevalence

Prevalence is defined as the percentage of women aged 15–49 who have undergone any form of FGM/C. Data provided by the Demographic and Health Surveys (DHS) and Multiple Indicator Cluster Surveys (MICS) reveal a prevalence rate of 1% in Cameroon to as high as 98% in Somalia (Table 13.2.1).

The World Health Organization estimates between 100 and 140 million females worldwide have been subjected to female genital mutilation, and a further 3 million females in Africa are at risk of the procedure every year (WHO 2008).

The practice of female genital mutilation is common in some parts of Africa (mainly sub-Saharan Africa), the Middle East, and some parts of Asia. It has also been reported among the immigrant population in European countries such as the UK, France, Switzerland, Canada, America, and Australia.

In societies where FGM/C is common, it is mainly carried on young girls between infancy and age 15, and occasionally on adult women. In Nigeria, 85% of genital mutilation was carried out in infancy (www.measureddhs.com/pubs/pdf/FR148/13chapter13.pdf), in Egypt 90% of girls are cut between ages 4 and 14years (Demographic and Health survey, Egypt, 1995 and 2000). The procedure is carried out by traditional circumcisers, traditional birth attenders, nurses, and midwives and in some cases by medical doctors.

Causes

The practice of FMG/C is perpetuated by a combination of cultural, religious, and social factors within families and communities.

- Social convention: there is pressure to conform to the society norm. Failure to do so may lead to condemnation, harassment and ostracization.
- FMG/C is considered necessary for proper raising of girls in preparation for adulthood and marriage (Yoder et al., 1999).
- It is enshrined by belief of what is considered appropriate sexual behaviour. It is linked to reduction in premarital sex and marital fidelity. It is also believed to reduce female libido (Gruenbaum 2005).
- Cultural belief of femininity and modesty also contribute to continuation of FGM/C The idea that girls are beautiful and more feminine after genital mutilation persist in some society (Talle 1993).
- Religious beliefs may be associated with the practice. None of the major religious script supports the practice. The attitude of community religious leaders towards FGM/C plays a significant role in eradicating the practice.
- New groups may start the practice after migration into area where the practice is common. Women and their children may be subject to FGM/C when they marry into communities where it is widely practised.

Legal issues

FGM/C is recognized as a violation of the human rights of girls and women. Two important legally binding international human rights instruments address this issue:

- The 1979 Convention on the Elimination of All forms of Discrimination Against Women (CEDAW)
- The 1989 Convention on the Rights of the Child (CRC).

In Africa, where the majority of FGM/C occurs, the Maputo protocol (www.achr.org/english/women/protocolwomen.pdf) was adopted in 2003, and ratified by 27 member states of the African Union; it promotes women right and calls for an end to female genital mutilation. Some African countries have passed legislation abolishing the practice of female genital mutilation.

In the UK the 1985 Prohibition of Female Circumcision Act and the 2003 Female Genital Mutilation Act prohibits FGM/C in England, Scotland, and Wales. Similar legislation has been passed in countries such as Australia, Canada, Italy, New Zealand, Sweden, and the USA.

Consequences of female genital mutilation

Female genital mutilation is associated with a series of health risks and consequences. In general, the risk associated with types I, II and III are similar, but the risks tend to be more common and severe the larger the amount of genital tissue excised. The procedure is commonly carried out in unhygienic conditions, without anaesthesia, using rudimentary and crude instruments such as knives, razor blades, etc.

The acute complications include
- severe pain
- haemorrhage
- acute urinary retention
- localized infection and abscess formation
- septicaemia
- tetanus
- hepatitis and HIV infection
- death.

Late gynaecological complications include
- apareunia
- superficial dyspareunia
- sexual dysfunction with anorgasmia
- chronic pain
- Keloid formation
- dysmenorrhoea (including haematocolpos)
- urinary flow obstruction
- recurrent urinary tract infection
- HIV and hepatitis infection
- implantation dermoid cyst
- pelvic infection
- labial fusion.

The gynaecological complications results in
- difficulty conceiving
- difficulty in gynaecological examination
- difficulty in cervical cytology screening
- Psychological sequelae including post-traumatic stress disorder with associated memory loss, anxiety, depression, and increased likelihood of fear of intercourse are common (Whitehorn 2002).

Obstetric complications associated with female genital mutilation are well documented (Lovel et al. 2000; Banks et al. 2006), and include
- fear of childbirth
- increased risk of postpartum haemorrhage, Caesarean section, episiotomies, and extensive vaginal tears
- difficulty in performing vaginal examination, applying fetal scalp electrodes, or performing fetal scalp blood sampling in labour.

Female genital mutilation is also associated with increased perinatal mortality (Banks et al. 2006).

In recognition of the increased maternal and perinatal morbidity and mortality, the Royal College of Obstetricians and Gynaecologists (RCOG) issued guideline on the management of women with female genital mutilation (RCOG 2009). It recommends the identification of pregnant women that have undergone FMG/C and provision of specialist care for these women.

In women who require defibulation before childbirth, this can be done during the antenatal period or in labour. Female genital mutilation is not a contraindication to vaginal delivery, and in fact most women who have suffered female genital mutilation prefer vaginal delivery, but recourse to Caesarean section may be necessary if the woman has a fear of childbirth.

Eradication of female genital mutilation

In the last decade, the practice of FGM/C is showing a downward trend in some communities, but in others the prevalence has remained static (www.prb.org/pdf08/fgm-wallchart.pdf).

The eradication of FGM/C requires concerted effort at community, national, and global levels.
- Community level: successful community-based projects such as the Tostan project in Senegal, Guinea, Gambia, Burkina Faso, and Somalia (www.tostan.org/web/page/586/sectionid/547/pagelevel/3/interior.asp) has made a significant impact on the prevalence of FGM/C in these communities. This project is based on the promotion of human rights and emphasizes community participation. It guides the communities to define the problem and provide solutions themselves. It incorporates key elements necessary to a change social convention at the community level, including collective action, public declaration, and organized diffusion.
- National level: activity at the national level should promote a process of social change that leads to abandonment of FGM/C. These activities should involve traditional, religious, and government leaders, parliamentarians and civil society organizations. Media involvement is important for the dissemination of information about positive social change. Enactment of legislation on FGM/C at the national level serves the purpose of showing government disapproval, providing support to those who have or wish to abandon the practice and act as a deterrent. Improvements in the health, education, and the social and legal protection systems is also necessary to bring about lasting change in social conventions that perpetuate female genital mutilation/cutting.
- Regional level: the Maputo protocol adopted by members states of the African Union calls upon individual countries to create public awareness of the issue of female genital mutilation, introduce legislation to prohibit and sanction the practice of FGM/C, provide support for victims and protect women at risk of this and other harmful practices.

The Parliamentary Assembly of the council of Europe passed a resolution in 2001 calling for the introduction of national legislation, the promotion of awareness, the prosecution of those who perpetrate FGM/C, and the adoption of a more flexible approach in granting asylum to mothers and their children at risk of FGM/C.

FGM/C is a harmful practice that violates the fundamental human rights of women and children. The perpetuation of the practice in certain communities is borne out of deeply engrained sociocultural conventions. In the past decade the prevalence of FGM/C has declined, but more concerted efforts at community, national, regional, and global levels are necessary to eliminate the practice.

Further reading

Banks E, Meirrik O, Farley T, et al. WHO study group on female genital mutilation and obstetrics outcome: WHO collaborative prospective study in six African countries. Lancet 2006; 367:1835–41.

Demographic and Health survey, Egypt, 1995 and 2000.

Gruenbaum E. Socio-cultural dynamics of female genital cutting: research finding, gaps and directions. Culture Health Sexuality 2005;7:429–41.

Lovel H, McGettingan C, Mohammed Z. A systematic review of the health complication of female genital mutilation including sequelae in childbirth. Geneva: WHO 2000: www.who.int/reproductive-health/docsa/systematic_review_health_complication_fgm.pdf

RCOG. Green-top guideline no. 53. May 2009.

Talle A. Transforming women into 'pure' agnate: aspects of female infibulation in Somalia. In: Broch-Due V, Rudie I, Bleie T (eds)

Carved flesh, cast selves: gender symbols and social practices. Oxford: Berg 1993:83–106.

Whitehorn J. Female genital mutilation: cultural and psychological implications. Sexual Relationship Therapy 2002;17:161–70.

WHO. *Female genital mutilation.* Fact Sheet no. 241. Geneva: WHO 2008.

WHO/UNFPA/UNICEF *Female genital mutilation.* A joint WHO/UNFPA/UNICEF statement. Geneva: WHO 1997.

World Health Organization (WHO). *Eliminating female genital mutilation.* An interagency statement UNAIDS, UNDP, UNECA, UNESCO, UNFPA, UNHCHR, UNHCR, UNICEF, UNIFEM, WHO. Geneva: WHO 2008.

Yoder PS, Camar PO, Soumaoro B, *Female genital cutting and coming of age in Guinea.* Calverton: Macro International 1999.

Internet resources

www.measureddhs.com/pubs/pdf/FR148/13chapter13.pdf-accessed 1/11/09

www.prb.org/pdf08/fgm-wallchart.pdf

www.tostan.org/web/page/586/sectionid/547/pagelevel/3/interior.asp

www.achr.org/english/women/protocolwomen.pdf

Prohibition of Female Circumcision Act, 1985 United Kingdom.

Female Genital mutilation Act 2003: www.hmso.gov.uk/acts/act2003/2003003.htm

Fibroids

Introduction
Fibroids are well-circumscribed, benign tumours arising from myometrium and are the most common tumours of the female genital tract during the reproductive years.

Aetiology
The incidence increases with age and fibroids may in present in 25–30% women between 35 and 50 years. Risk factors include nulliparity, obesity, family history, Afro-Caribbean race (develops at early age), and hypertension. Long-term use of oral contraceptive pills, Depo-provera injections for contraception and smoking are associated with reduced risk.

Pathophysiology
Fibroid growth is related to genetic predisposition, hormonal influences, and various growth factors. Fibroids have been shown to have increased levels of both oestrogen and progesterone receptors than normal myometrium. They may enlarge in pregnancy or following treatment with tamoxifen. Fibroids shrink in size after the menopause due to reduced oestrogen exposure. Fibroids very rarely have malignant potential (0.2%), which can develop in the form of leiomyosarcoma, but most cases arise de novo.

They are composed of concentric whorls of mainly smooth muscle but may contain fibrous as well as connective tissue elements. There is a false capsule of compressed uterine muscle which allows easy enucleation of fibroids while performing myomectomy. As they enlarge they tend to outgrow the blood supply forming areas of cystic necrosis and central degeneration.

Classification
Fibroids can be classified according to the site of development
- Subserosal (1%): originating from the serosal surface of the uterus. They may become pedunculated and lose their uterine attachment and gain a secondary blood supply (parasitic fibroid)
- Intramural (91–93%): within the uterine muscle
- Intraligamentry: in the broad ligament (<1%)
- Submucous: indenting the uterine cavity (5%), classified further by the European society of Gynaecological Endoscopy into:
  - G0: where the fibroid (pedunculated) is completely within the uterine cavity
  - G1: the larger part is in the uterine cavity (intramural portion <50%) and the smaller part in the myometrium
  - G2: the larger part is in the myometrium (intramural portion >50%)
- Cervical (3%).

Clinical approach
The presentation depends upon patient's age, number of fibroids, site, and type of lesion. Most of the women are asymptomatic. Women may present with the following symptoms:
- heavy menstrual bleeding, which may lead to iron deficiency anaemia
- intermenstrual bleeding (associated with submucous fibroid)
- bladder symptoms such as increased frequency of micturition, urgency, retention of urine due to pressure effects
- abdominal fullness/swelling
- pain and discomfort
- infertility (associated with submucous fibroids)
- rare association with polycythaemia.

Examination
- Abdominal examination: palpation of pelvic mass and/or tenderness
- Speculum examination: cervical fibroid/pedunculated submucous fibroids may be visualized
- Per vaginal examination: enlarged uterus, fullness/± tenderness in adnexae.

Investigations
- History and examination are supplemented by full blood count (NICE 2007)
- Transabdominal and transvaginal ultrasound scan should be the preliminary investigation. It is important to document uterine dimensions, size, number, and position and grading (submucous) of fibroids with endometrial thickness and visualization of ovaries. Colour Doppler may reveal pedicle, absent or reduced flow within the pedicle and/or adnexal mass.
- If submucous fibroids are suspected, sonohysterography (saline infusion sonography) should be undertaken depending upon the local facilities available in the hospital.
- Inpatient or outpatient hysteroscopy.
- MRI should be used if there in any doubt about the nature of fibroid mass.
- Intravenous or CT urography may be indicated in women presenting with large fibroids and retention of urine.
- Endometrial biopsy should be carried out if there is any history of irregular bleeding/intermenstrual bleeding/abnormal endometrial thickness.

Differential diagnosis
- Adenomyosis
- Solid ovarian tumour
- Pedunculated fibroid
- All causes of pelvic mass.

Complications of fibroids
- Torsion of pedicle causing acute abdomen
- Hyaline degeneration
- Red degeneration of fibroid in pregnancy
- Malignant change: leiomyosarcoma (0.2%)
- *Infection.*

Management
Factors which should be considered are age, symptom severity, child-bearing aspirations, associated medical diseases, size and number of fibroids, desire of uterine preservation, tumour characteristics, proximity to menopause, and possibility of malignancy (rapid progression). Treatment choices are wide and include pharmacological, surgical, and radiographically directed intervention.

Pharmacological options

Non-hormonal therapies

- NSAIDs reduce the high level of prostaglandin in the uterine lining that seems to contribute to heavy periods but they are not effective in reduction of heavy bleeding secondary to fibroids.
- Tranexamic acid (antifibrinolytic) has been shown to reduce heavy menstrual loss in a Cochrane systematic review.

Hormonal therapies

- Progestogens: these compounds produce a hypo-oestrogenic effect by inhibiting gonadotrophin secretion, thus suppressing ovarian functions. Their use in fibroid-associated menorrhagia is only symptomatic control. The levonorgestrel intrauterine system (LNG-IUS) reduces blood loss and dysmenorrhoea; however, expulsion rates are higher.
- Gonadotrophin-releasing hormone (GnRH) analogues: hypo-oestrogenism reduces uterine volume and fibroid size. Cochrane review suggests it reduces the blood loss, renders surgery easier and facilitates correction of iron deficiency anaemia before surgery. There are potential short- and long-term side-effects of GnRH agonists such as postmenopausal symptoms and osteoporosis. Hormonal add-back therapy can be given to negate the symptoms.
- Antisteroid therapy: the antiprogestin RU 486, which directly inhibits the biological actions of progesterone, has been shown to decrease the uterine blood flow.

Uterine artery embolization

This is a minimally invasive procedure with a short stay in hospital. Selective arteries are occluded by the embolization of material (polyvinyl alcohol particlesvia a fluoroscopy-guided catheter inserted into the common femoral artery). The occlusion of blood supply leads to reduction in uterine and fibroid volume and menstrual loss. It is usually recommended for women with large symptomatic myomas, or women unsuitable for major surgery. The complications include pain, post-embolization syndrome, fever, pyometra, failure of regression, sepsis, and hysterectomy.

Focused ultrasound

This is a thermo-ablative technique for the treatment of uterine myomas under magnetic resonance guidance. The ultrasound waves cause marked heating, thus decreasing the uterine volume.

Indications for surgical treatment of fibroids

- Abnormal uterine bleeding not responding to medical management.
- Subfertility due to submucous fibroids; distortion of cavity or blockage of fallopian tubes by fibroids.
- Urinary symptoms such as frequency, urgency, retention, and obstruction due to fibroids.
- Pressure and or pain symptoms.
- Iron deficiency anaemia secondary to heavy menstrual bleeding due to fibroids.
- Rapid growth of fibroids with suspicion of malignancy.
- Refusal of medical management by women.
- Side-effects of medical management.

Hysteroscopic myomectomy

This is hysteroscopic resection of submucous fibroid (grades 0 and 1). The indications include abnormal uterine bleeding, history of pregnancy loss, subfertility problems, and pain. Submucous fibroids of less than 3 cm have better outcome. A single dose of GnRH agonist if given 4 weeks before the procedure decreases the size of myoma, reduces endometrial thickness, and causes less fluid absorption during the procedure.

Abdominal myomectomy

Indicated when uterine preservation for childbearing is needed, but women should be counselled regarding the risk of requiring further intervention. It is also the procedure of choice for large solitary pedunculated subserous fibroids. Pretreatment with GnRH agonist can be used to shrink the size of fibroids and minimize the blood loss. Vasocontricting agents like vasopressin can be used at the time of surgery.

Laparoscopic myomectomy

This procedure can be performed in cases of pedunculated fibroids or with intramural fibroids. Laparoscopic-assisted myomectomy involves laparoscopic dissection of fibroids and can be removed through morcellator or mini-laparotomy incision. Multilayer uterine closure should be performed.

Hysterectomy

The definitive treatment for heavy menstrual loss due to fibroids in women who have completed their family and uterine preservation is not an issue. The usual route is abdominal, but vaginal hysterectomy can be performed. Hysterectomy is not recommended for routine management of treatment of asymptomatic fibroids. The complications include technical difficulty; bowel, ureteric, and bladder injury; infection; bleeding; risk of transfusion; and deep vein thrombosis.

Hormone replacement therapy and fibroids

Oestrogen may stimulate fibroid growth and there is some evidence that Tibilone may be a better choice and may be associated with reduced fibroid growth.

Fibroids and pregnancy

Seventy-eight per cent of fibroids are unchanged or may decrease in size in pregnancy. As there is an increased uterine blood supply in pregnancy, fibroids may undergo acute ischaemic necrosis and cystic degeneration. The potential effects of fibroids on pregnancy are

- subfertility due to either blockage of tubal ostia, distortion of uterine cavity, prevention of implantation of embryo
- miscarriage
- pain due to acute ischaemic necrosis (red degeneration)
- malpresentation
- cavity distortion, which can lead to increased incidence of placental abruption, retained placenta, premature rupture of membranes, and preterm labour.
- obstructed labour, cephalopelvic disproportion
- postpartum haemorrhage.

In conclusion, there is a wide range of treatment modalities for uterine fibroids but it is paramount to select an appropriate method of treatment to suit to the need of woman.

Further reading

Becker E Jr, Lev-Toaff AS, Kaufman EP, *et al.* The added value of transvaginal sonohysterography over transvaginal sonography alone in women with known or suspected leiomyoma. J Ultrasound Med 2002;21:237–47.

Falcone T Falcone T, Gustilo-Ashby AM. Minimally invasive surgery for mass lesions. Clin Obstet Gynecol 2005;48:353–60.

Farquhar C, Arroll B, Ekeroma A, et al. Fibroids. Working Party of the New Zealand Guidelines Group. Aust NZ J Obstet Gynaecol 2001;41:125–40.

Gupta JK, Sinha AS, Lumsden MA, Hickey M. Uterine artery embolization for symptomatic uterine fibroids. Cochrane Database Syst Rev 2006;25:CD005073.

Hricak H, Tscholakoff D, Heinrichs L, Fisher MR, et al. Uterine leiomyomas: correlation of MR, histopathologic findings, and symptoms. Radiology 1986;158:385–91.

Kaunitz. Progestin-releasing intrauterine systems and leiomyoma. Contraception. 2007;75(6 Suppl):S130–3.

Lethaby A, Farquhar C, Cooke I. Antifibrinolytics for heavy menstrual bleeding. Cochrane.

Lethaby A, Vollenhoven B, Sowter M. Pre-operative GnRH analogue therapy before hysterectomy or myomectomy for uterine fibroids. Cochrane Database Syst Rev. 2000;(2):CD000547.

Lev-Toaff AS, Coleman BG, Arger PH, et al. Leiomyomas in pregnancy: sonographic study. Radiology 1987;164:375–80.

Monga AK, Woodhouse CR, Stanton SL. Pregnancy and fibroids causing simultaneous urinary retention and ureteric obstruction. Br J Urol 1996;77:606–7.

NICE. NICE guidance IPG094. Uterine artery embolisation for the treatment of fibroids. 2004.

NICE. NICE guidelines. CG44 Heavy menstrual bleeding: investigation and treatment. 2007.

Nowak RA. Fibroids: pathophysiology and current medical treatment. Baillieres Best Pract Res Clin Obstet Gynaecol 199913:223–38.

Reinsch RC, Murphy AA, Morales AJ, Yen SS. The effects of RU 486 and leuprolide acetate on uterine artery blood flow in the fibroid uterus: a prospective, randomized study. Am J Obstet Gynecol 1994;170:1623–7.

Stewart EA, et al. Clinical outcome of focused ultrasound surgery for the treatment of uterine fibroids. Fertil Steril 2006;85:22–9.

Vollenhoven B. Introduction: the epidemiology of uterine leiomyomas. Baillieres Clin Obstet Gynaecol 1998;12:169–76.

Wallach E, et al. Uterine myomas: an overview of development clinical features, and management. Obstet Gynaecol 2004;104:393–406.

Wamsteker K, Emanuel MH, de Kruif JH Transcervical hysteroscopic resection of submucous fibroids for abnormal uterine bleeding: results regarding the degree of intramural extension. Obstet Gynecol 1993;82:736–40.

Internet resources

NICE: www.nice.org.uk

Patient resources

www.fibroids.co.uk

Ovarian cysts

Ovarian cysts are a common reason for gynaecology referral.

The incidence has increased with the use of transvaginal ultrasound and computed tomography.

Pathophysiology

Cysts can occur at any age but differ in type. Germ cell tumours predominate in children. Functional cysts are more common in premenopausal women and the risk of malignancy increases after the menopause. Ninety per cent of ovarian cysts are benign, but this does vary with age.

Ovarian cysts are classified into non-neoplastic functional cysts (such as follicular and corpus luteal cysts) and neoplastic cysts.

Clinical presentation

Many ovarian cysts are asymptomatic but some will present with abdominal/pelvic pain due to torsion, rupture, or haemorrhage.

The diagnosis is made from presenting symptoms, the clinical history, and examination findings. Pain can be described as radiating down the inner thigh to the knee (referred along the cutaneous branch of the obturator nerve).

Differential diagnosis

Pain may originate from the gastrointestinal tract or urinary tract. Pelvic inflammatory disease and ectopic pregnancy should be excluded.

Ovarian cyst accidents

- Torsion: this mainly occurs in premenopausal women with cysts >6 cm in size; benign teratomas are prone to torsion but polycystic ovaries can also tort. The enlarged ovary lifts out of the pelvis because of mobility of the supporting ligaments. Torsion is more common on the right. This is thought to be due to the presence of the rectosigmoid colon on the left. Complete arterial obstruction does not usually occur and the ischaemic–haemorrhagic appearance of the adnexa is due to venous and lymphatic stasis rather than gangrene.
- Rupture: the symptoms depend on the size of the cyst and its contents that are released into the abdominal cavity. Rupture of a small cyst may be asymptomatic or have localized pain. A larger cyst may present with peritonism, especially if the contents are irritant, such as dermoid or endometriotic cysts. *Pseudomyxoma peritonei* can result from rupture of a mucinous cystadenoma.
- Haemorrhage: The theca interna is prone to haemorrhage as is the corpus luteum during formation. Haemorrhage causes pain as the cyst capsule is stretched. If the cyst ruptures intraperitoneal bleeding can occur. Cyst rupture occurs more commonly on the right.

Investigations

The aim of investigation is to exclude malignancy and triage women to the most appropriate place for them to be managed.

- Transvaginal sonography (TVS) is better than transabdominal sonography, giving better quality images of the ovaries. Dermoids and endometriomas have typical ultrasound appearances. Cysts are more likely to be malignant if there are solid components, papillary projections, and ascites, or if they are multilocular or bilateral. The specificity of TVS is not good enough for it to be used alone for screening for ovarian malignancy (NIH consensus). Colour flow Doppler studies can help to make a diagnosis of malignancy but have limited clinical application in isolation
- Magnetic resonance imaging (MRI): this is very useful to investigate further the nature of ovarian cysts suspected to be malignant. Vegetations in cystic tumours and necrosis in solid tumours can be identified. Contrast can be used to enhance images. Endometriotic cysts have a homogenous high signal intensity on T1-weighted images and low signal intensity on T2-weighted images. Dermoid cysts also have a typical appearance on MRI.

Tumour markers

- CA125 is a glycoprotein antigen; levels usually rise with epithelial ovarian malignancies but it is not specific for ovarian cancer and can be raised in other benign intra-abdominal conditions such as endometriosis, during menstruation, pelvic inflammatory disease, and non-malignant ascites.
- α-Fetoprotein (AFP) and human chorionic gonadotrophin (hCG) levels are raised in germ cell tumours but also in pregnancy.
- Inhibin levels are raised in granulosa cell tumours.
- Risk of malignancy index (RMI) is a scoring system that combines menopausal status, ultrasound findings, and CA125 levels to give an estimate of the risk of malignancy. A score of >200 is considered high risk. There are two scoring systems, the RMI 2 score gives more weight to ultrasound findings and menopausal status than RMI 1 (Table 13.4.1).
- Ovarian crescent sign is the presence of normal ovarian tissue adjacent to a cyst on detailed TVS and may help to exclude invasive malignancy.

Management

Conservative management is appropriate for many women with a simple cyst, few symptoms, and a low RMI. Expectant management is particularly appropriate for

Table 13.4.1 Risk of malignancy index scoring system

Feature	RMI 1 score	RMI 2 score
Ultrasound features	0 = none	0 = none
	1 = one abnormality	1 = one abnormality
Multilocular cyst	3 = two or more abnormalities	4 = two or more abnormalities
Solid areas		
Bilateral		
Ascites		
Intra-abdominal metastasis		
Premenopausal	1	1
Postmenopausal	3	4
CA125	U/mL	U/mL

RMI score = ultrasound score × menopausal score × CA125 level in U/mL. RMI 2 score is more sensitive than RMI 1 at predicting malignancy.

haemorrhagic cysts. A TVS can be repeated 3 months later when a high proportion of these cysts will have resolved spontaneously. Recurrent functional cysts can be suppressed by the use of the combined oral contraceptive pill.

- Suspected ovarian torsion: the diagnosis is often delayed and surgery should take place as soon as possible and should be as conservative as possible if retention of fertility is required.
- Place of surgery: as the risk of malignancy increases, the appropriate location for management changes. Cysts with a high RMI >200 should be managed in a cancer centre.
- Transvaginal cyst aspiration: this leaves the cyst capsule intact and it usually reforms and is therefore not recommended except in selected cases, for example during infertility treatment, or if a patient is not medically fit for an anaesthetic.
- Laparoscopic management: many cysts can be managed laparoscopically, resulting in reduced postoperative pain, shorter hospital stay, better cosmetic result, and quicker return to normal. This is the treatment of choice for young women wishing to retain their fertility.
- Laparoscopic cystotomy and drainage of the cyst is not recommended because the capsule is left intact, the high recurrence rates, and spillage of the contents of the cyst.
- Laparoscopic cystectomy with removal of the cyst intact is the ideal treatment. The specimen is removed in an endobag to avoid spilling the contents into the peritoneal cavity. The risk of malignancy is low. After cystectomy the defect can be left open to heal, cauterized, or sutured. None of these techniques is superior for healing or the risk of postoperative adhesions.

Ovarian cysts in pregnancy

The diagnosis of ovarian cysts has increased in pregnancy, especially in the first trimester. Most of these cysts will resolve spontaneously during the pregnancy and persistent cysts >6 cm are rare, reported in 0.07%. Ovarian cancer is very rare in women of reproductive age, and has been reported in 0.004–0.4% of pregnancies. Tumour markers are not as useful during pregnancy, α-fetoprotein, hCG, and inhibin levels are raised because of placental production. CA125 levels also rise in pregnancy and a level of 112 U/mL has been suggested as the upper limit of normal.

MRI can be used to help differentiate benign from malignant cysts and avoids the need for radiation, associated with CT. Management is dependent on the clinical symptoms, size, and features of the cyst. Most cysts <5 cm will resolve. Complex cysts should be assessed regularly by rescanning. The risk of torsion increases in the first trimester and up to 14 days after delivery and is more common on the right. Surgery should only be considered if symptomatic or if there is a risk of malignancy. If surgery is required it should be delayed until after 14 weeks to reduce the risk of miscarriage, as the pregnancy is not reliant on the corpus luteum at this stage. Laparoscopic surgery can be performed and is usually done via the open (Hassan) technique to avoid injury to the uterus. If a cyst is discovered at Caesarean section, cystectomy should be performed if it is larger than 5 cm or complex in nature.

Further reading

Antonic J, Rakar S. Colour and pulsed Doppler US and tumour marker CA 125 in differentiation between benign and malignant ovarian masses. Anticancer Res 1995;15:1527–32.

Aslam N, Ong C, Woelfer B, et al. Serum CA125 at 11-14 weeks of gestation in women with morphologically normal ovaries. Br J Obstet Gynaecol 2000;107:689–90.

Aslam N, Tailor A, Lawton F, et al. Prospective evaluation of three different models for the pre-operative diagnosis of ovarian cancer. Br J Obstet Gynaecol 2000;107:1347–53.

NIH consensus conference. Ovarian cancer. Screening, treatment, and follow-up. NIH Consensus Development Panel on Ovarian Cancer. JAMA 1995;273:491–7.

Oelsner G, Cohen SB, Soriano D, et al. Minimal surgery for the twisted ischaemic adnexa can preserve ovarian function. Hum Reprod 2003;18:2599–602.

Oyal College of Gynaecologists and Obstetricians (RCOG). Ovarian cysts in postmenopausal women. Guideline 34. London: RCOG 2003.

Platek DN, Henderson CF, Golberg GL. The management of persistent adnexal mass in pregnancy. Am J Obstet Gynecol 1996;173:1236–40.

Spencer C, Robarts P. Management of adnexal masses in pregnancy. Obstet Gynaecol 2006;8:14–19.

Yazbek J, Aslam N, Tailor K, et al. A comparative study of the risk of malignancy index and the ovarian crescent sign for the diagnosis of invasive ovarian cancer. Ultrasound Obstet Gynecol 2006;28:320–4.

Zanetta G, Lissoni A, Torri V, et al. Role of puncture and aspiration in expectant management of simple ovarian cysts: a randomised study. BMJ 1996;313:1110–3.

Pelvic inflammatory disease

Pelvic inflammatory disease (PID) is infection of the upper genital tract or reproductive organs. It is one of most common causes of morbidity in young women, with serious long-term implications if left untreated. It can cause salpingitis, oophoritis, tubo-ovarian abscess, parametritis, endometritis, peritonitis, or a combination of these. The incidence is 1.7% per annum in the UK (GUM clinics and GP practice) affecting sexually active women between 16 and 45 years with a peak incidence in 16–25 year old women.

Aetiology

The aetiology is polymicrobial, with *Chlamydia trachomatis* (20–40%) and *Neisseria gonorrhoea* (14%) being the most common causative agents. The other organisms include bacteroides, gardnerella, peptococcus, *H. influenzae*, enterococci and mycoplasma (70%) (Baveja 2001).

Risk factors

The risk factors are important in both clinical diagnosis and prevention of PID. The factors associated with PID include:
- women <25 years
- multiple sexual partners
- previous history of acute PID
- A recent new sexual partner (within the previous 3 months)
- past history of sexually transmitted disease in woman or her partner
- insertion of intrauterine device within 6 weeks
- surgical procedures such as hysteroscopy, hysterosalpingography, dilatation and curettage, *in vitro* fertilization procedure, surgical termination of pregnancy.

Sequelae

PID may cause serious long-term complications:
- infertility (10%) (Hillis SD *et al.,* 1993)
- ectopic pregnancy (1–5%)
- chronic pelvic pain (30%)
- recurrent PID
- Fitz–Hugh–Curtis syndrome (10–20%).

Clinical diagnosis

The patient with PID may be asymptomatic, or may present with non-specific symptoms. The most common symptoms and signs (positive predictive value 65–90%) are:
- lower abdominal pain usually bilateral (<1 week)
- abnormal vaginal discharge
- deep dyspareunia
- abnormal bleeding (intermenstrual, postcoital, breakthrough bleeding)
- feeling unwell with nausea and vomiting
- fever (38°C or above)
- lower abdominal/adnexal/cervical motion excitation tenderness
- palpable tender adnexal mass
- Minimum criteria for diagnosis (Centre of disease control and prevention, 2006) uterine/adnexal tenderness, cervical motion tenderness and no other cause of above signs noted.

Differential diagnosis

- ectopic pregnancy
- acute appendicitis
- endometriosis
- irritable bowel syndrome
- complications of an ovarian cyst, such as rupture or torsion
- urinary tract infection
- functional pain (pain of unknown physical origin)
- constipation.

Investigations

- High vaginal, endocervical, and urethral swabs. *N. gonorrhoea* and chlamydia infection should be confirmed using the nucleic acid amplification test. The absence of confirmed infection in the lower genital tract site does not exclude PID (Bevan *et al.,* 1995).
- Raised white cell count, leucocytosis (sensitivity 86–88%).
- Elevated C-reactive protein (74–93%).
- Elevated erythrocyte sedimentation rate (64–81%).
- Laparoscopy (specificity 100%, 15–30% no PID).
- Pelvic ultrasound scan showing thickened, fluid-filled tubes with or without free pelvic fluid or tubo-ovarian complex or Doppler studies suggesting pelvic infection (e.g. tubal hyperaemia).
- CT/MRI scan.
- Endometrial biopsy: histological evidence of endometritis (50–87%).

Management

It is recommended that clinicians should have a low threshold for treating PID empirically as delay in treatment may result in serious long-term sequelae. However, it is important to make an accurate diagnosis before informing the patient as it may have psychosocial implications for the individual. If a positive diagnosis is made then it is important to investigate and treat the sexual partner.

General measures

- Mild to moderate PID (with no tubo-ovarian abscess) can be managed on outpatient basis.
- Rule out pregnancy.
- Appropriate analgesics should be given.
- Information on current and recent medication should be obtained.
- Interactions between antibiotic therapy and hormonal contraception and other medications should be assessed and appropriate action taken must be taken.
- Outpatient antibiotic treatment should be commenced as soon as the diagnosis is suspected.
- Clear and written information (leaflets) must be provided especially regarding long-term consequences.

Hospital admission and inpatient management is advised in following conditions:
- surgical emergency cannot be excluded
- clinically severe disease
- tubo-ovarian abscess
- PID in pregnancy
- lack of response to oral therapy.

613

Intolerance to oral therapy
Antimicrobial treatment
The following are evidence-based antibiotic regimes recommended by the RCOG (2008). The women who are immune-compromised and pregnant should have inpatient treatment.

Out patient treatment regimes (Ross 2001)
- Oral ofloxacin 400 mg twice daily plus oral metronidazole 400 mg twice daily for 14 days.
- Intramuscular ceftriaxone 250 mg single dose* followed by oral doxycycline 100 mg twice daily plus metronidazole 400 mg twice daily for 14 days.
- Cefoxitin has a better evidence base for the treatment of PID than ceftriaxone but is not easily available in the UK. Ceftriaxone is therefore recommended.

Inpatient treatment regimes (Ness et al., 2002)
Intravenous antibiotic therapy should be continued for a minimum of 24 hours after clinical improvement and it should be followed by oral therapy.
- Ceftriaxone 2 g by intravenous infusion daily plus intravenous doxycycline 100 mg twice daily,* followed by oral doxycycline 100 mg twice daily plus oral metronidazole 400 mg twice daily for a total of 14 days. Oral doxycycline may be used if tolerated. An alternative third generation cephalosporin would also be acceptable.
- Intravenous clindamycin 900 mg three times daily plus intravenous gentamicin,* followed by either oral clindamycin 450 mg four times daily to complete 14 days OR oral doxycycline 100 mg twice daily plus oral metronidazole 400 mg twice daily to complete 14 days.
- Gentamicin should be given as a 2 mg/kg loading dose followed by 1.5 mg/kg three times daily or a single daily dose of 7 mg/kg may be substituted. The drug levels should be monitored.
- Intravenous ofloxacin 400 mg twice daily plus intravenous metronidazole 500 mg three times daily for 14 days.

Other treatments
- Surgical treatment: this should be considered in severe cases or where there is clear evidence of a pelvic abscess diagnosed by ultrasound. The abscess should be drained laparoscopically or by laparotomy (Lareau SM et al., 2008).
- Ultrasound-guided aspiration: pelvic fluid collection can be aspirated under ultrasonic guidance. It is less invasive and is equally effective (Corsi 1999).
- Treatment of sexual partner(s) of women with PID: The partners should be ideally tested and treated in GUM clinic but, empirical treatment should be given if testing is not possible. Patient should avoid sexual intercourse until they and their partners are fully treated and contact traced.

Special circumstances
- Pregnancy and young women: pregnant women should receive intravenous therapy. Drugs known to be toxic in pregnancy, such as tetracyclines and ofloxacin, should be avoided.
- Women with intrauterine contraceptive device (IUD): If the clinical situation is not resolved within 72 hours of starting antibiotics, then consideration should be given to remove IUD. Women wanting repeat IUD after treatment should be offered, intrauterine system (IUS).
- Women using hormonal contraception: breakthrough bleeding on hormonal contraception should be investigated for PID.

- Women with history of HIV: women treated for PID with HIV should have the same regime but drug interactions should be checked. The women should be managed in conjunction with HIV physician.

Follow up of patients with PID
- Follow up in 3 days (72 hours) is advisable if the patient is managed in the outpatient setting in order to check for further parenteral therapy or surgical intervention is required or not.
- 4–6 weeks' follow up should be organized on an outpatient basis to ensure compliance with antibiotics, adequate clinical response to treatment, contact tracing, and treatment of sexual partners and awareness of significance and sequelae of PID.

Counselling for women with confirmed PID
Women and or partners should be counselled in detail, discussing the long-term sequelae. They should be made aware that an increase in the number of episodes of PID increases the risk of infertility and ectopic pregnancy. As most PIDs are sexually transmitted, every effort should be made to reduce the patient's sexual exposure by reducing the number of sexual partners, using barrier methods of contraception, etc. HIV testing and counselling should be offered.

Further reading
Baveja G, Saini S, Sangwan K, Arora DR. A study of bacterial pathogens in acute pelvic inflammatory disease, Commun Dis 2001;33:121–5.

Bevan CD, Johal BJ, Mumtaz G, et al. Clinical laparoscopic and microbiological findings in acute salpingitis: report on a United Kingdom cohort. Br J Obstet Gynaecol 1995;102:407–14

Centers for Disease Control and Prevention sexually transmitted disease treatment guidelines.

Corsi PJ, Johnson SC, Gonik B, et al. Transvaginal ultrasound-guided aspiration of pelvic abscesses. Infect Dis Obstet Gynecol 1999;7:216–21.

Hillis SD, Joesoef R, Marchbanks PA, et al. Delayed care of pelvic inflammatory disease as a risk factor for impaired fertility. Am J Obstet Gynecol 1993;168:1503–9.

Lareau SM, Beigi RH. Pelvic inflammatory disease and tubo-ovarian abscess. Infect Dis Clin North Am. 2008;22:693–708

Ness RB, Soper DE, Holley RL, et al. Effectiveness of inpatient and outpatient treatment strategies for women with pelvic inflammatory disease: results from the Pelvic Inflammatory Disease Evaluation and Clinical Health (PEACH) Randomized Trial. Am J Obstet Gynecol 2002;186:929–37.

Pelvic inflammatory disease. NHS Library for Health. Clinical Knowledge Summaries: http://cks.library.nhs.uk

Ross JD. Outpatient antibiotics for pelvic inflammatory disease. BMJ 2001;322:251–2.

Royal College of Obstetricians and Gynaecologists (RCOG). Management of acute pelvic inflammatory disease. London: RCOG 2008: www.rcog.org.uk

Workowski KA, Berman SM. Centers for Disease Control and Prevention sexually transmitted diseases treatment guidelines. Clin Infect Dis 2007;44(Suppl 3):S73–6.

Patient resources
www.rcog.org.uk/resources/public/pdf/Acute_PID_2004.pdf

RCOG Green Top guidelines No. 32. Management of Acute pelvic inflammatory disease. Nov 2008.

Sexually transmitted infections. Family Planning Association. www.fpa.org.uk

Female urinary incontinence

Urinary incontinence (UI) is defined by the International Continence Society (ICS) as 'any involuntary loss of urine'. (Abrams 2002).

UI affects both men and women of all ages; however, it is substantially more common in women. It is often detrimental to the social, psychological, and physical wellbeing of the sufferer, as well as impacting on their families and the health service (Brocklehurst 1993). The cost of UI in Sweden and the USA accounts for 2% of the healthcare budget (Milsom 2001). Assuming the current UK healthcare budget is £90 billion, this equates to approximately £1.2 billion. This does not account for patients' own expenditure on support devices such as incontinence pads.

Considerable variation exists in the estimated prevalence of any UI with estimates from 8% to 69%, studies since 2000 are shown in Table 13.6.1. In a personal, population based, cross-sectional survey of 2500 women over the age of 21 in an English general practice in 2008, with a 60% response rate, there was a prevalence of any incontinence of 55%, with 10% of those women leaking 'a lot', or 'a flood'. Women with an overactive bladder were more than three times more likely to seek help (42%) than those with stress urinary incontinence (SUI) (12.9%), perhaps indicating that it is a more disabling condition. Social isolation is demonstrated by 25% of patients who, due to embarrassment, delay seeking advice for 5 years (Norton 1988).

Types of urinary incontinence
Urethral Conditions
- Urodynamic stress incontinence (USI) in which there is urethral sphincter incompetence diagnosed by urodynamics. SUI is the complaint of involuntary leakage on effort or exertion, or on sneezing or coughing (Abrams 2002).
- Detrusor overactivity (DO) is a urodynamic observation characterized by involuntary detrusor contractions during the filling phase which may be spontaneous or provoked (Abrams 2002). This is usually idiopathic. If associated with a neurological condition (e.g. Parkinson's disease, multiple sclerosis), it is termed neurogenic detrusor activity. DO is associated with involuntary detrusor contractions leading to urgency, frequency, nocturia, with or without leakage (urge leakage). Urge urinary incontinence (UUI) is the complaint of involuntary leakage accompanied by or immediately preceded by urgency (Abrams 2002).

- Mixed incontinence is associated with an overactive bladder with an incompetent sphincter, with the patient complaining of both stress and urge incontinence. Mixed urinary incontinence (MUI) is the complaint of involuntary leakage associated with urgency and also with exertion, effort, sneezing or coughing (Abrams 2002).
- Urinary retention with overflow. There is often no obvious cause. Chronic retention is often insidious especially in elderly people or those with neurological disease. This condition may be caused by either obstruction or more commonly in the female bladder atony. Dysfunctional voiding is characterized by an intermittent and/or fluctuating flow rate due to involuntary intermittent contractions of the peri-urethral striated muscle during voiding in neurologically normal individuals (Abrams 2002) and may coexist with or precede retention. A non-relaxing urethral sphincter obstruction usually occurs in individuals with a neurological lesion and is characterized by a reduced urine flow (Abrams 2002).
- Other causes include urinary tract infections, faecal impaction, urethral diverticulae, psychological disorders, drugs (α-adrenergic blockers), restricted mobility, dementia, and rare congenital disorders (epispadias).

Non-urethral conditions
- These are associated with continuous UI. Causes include urinary fistulae (usually secondary to surgery in the Western world and obstructed childbirth in the developing world), pelvic radiotherapy, carcinoma, and congenital anomalies (ectopic ureter and bladder exstrophy).

Risk factors for urinary incontinence
- Childbirth: parity has long been associated with UI. The Term Breech Trial noted that less UI occurred in the planned Caesarean section group (4.5%) than the planned vaginal delivery group (7.3%) at 3 months postpartum (Hannah 2002). Vaginal delivery does not appear to be associated with UUI.
- Age: the prevalence of UI increases with age. Younger women having a higher prevalence of SUI and older women more UUI and MUI. One study showing that women between the ages of 50 and 54 had more than twice the risk of severe UI than in women below 40 years (Danforth 2006).

Table 13.6.1 Summary table of prevalence studies published since 2000

Author	Irwin et al	Hunksaar et al	McGrother et al	Perry et al	Cooper and Quigley
Year	2006	2004	2004	2000	2008
Prevalence (%)	13	42	34	20	55
Method	Phone interview	Postal questionnaire	Postal questionnaire	Postal questionnaire	Postal questionnaire
Sample size	1675	2931	50 002	10 116	1463
Age range (years)	39+	18–97	40 to >80	40 to >80	21 to >75
Mean or median age	18 to 29	47.1	57	40–49	55–64
Timing	Ever	Last 30days	Last year	Ever	Ever

- Race: being of Black, Hispanic, Japanese, and Chinese races appears to offer protection (Danforth 2006).
- Oestrogen deficiency. Oestrogen receptors are found in the urethra and bladder trigone. Urogenital atrophy because of oestrogen lack is at least partly responsible for sensory urinary symptoms, and lack of urethral coaptation.
- Smoking. The relationship between smoking and UI is unclear with some studies showing a positive correlation (Danforth 2006), and others no relationship (Parazzinia 2003).
- Body mass index (BMI). A raised BMI has been identified as an independent risk factor for incontinence of all types. It has been shown that a BMI of >30 kg/m^2 increases the odds of developing UI (Parazzinia 2003; Danforth 2006). In fact, of those complaining of incontinence 65–75% were overweight or obese (BMI> 25) (Brown 1999). One explanation suggests that an increased intra-abdominal pressure with an increased BMI constantly stresses the pelvic floor muscles and weakens them. One study found that massive weight loss in morbidly obese people led to a decrease in the prevalence rate of SUI (from 61.2% to 11.6%) (Deitel 1988), another that a decrease in BMI by 5 resulted in a reduction in incontinence frequency of ≥50% (Subak 2002, 2005).
- Diabetes. There is some evidence that diabetes increases the incidence of UI by about 50% (Sampselle 2002; Hsieh 2008).
- Hysterectomy. There is evidence that women who have undergone hysterectomy are at a greater risk of developing UI (Parazzinia 2003; Hsieh 2008). A meta analysis found that the increased risk of developing UI after hysterectomy was only significant in the over 60s, suggesting the risk is a long-term not an immediate risk (Brown 2000).

History: key points

- An adequate history will allow targeting of initial therapy. Points raised should determine the duration and type of leakage (e.g. stress, urge), the amount leaked, urinary frequency, nocturia, nocturnal enuresis, leaking with intercourse. Attention to the impact on quality of life is crucial.
- Symptoms of a urinary tract infection should be sought and antibiotic treatment initiated as appropriate.
- Attention should be paid to the patient's medical history especially conditions impacting on the urinary system, e.g. diabetes, congestive heart failure, previous pelvic radiotherapy, multiple sclerosis, Parkinson's disease, chronic obstructive pulmonary disease. Drug history should be sort, e.g. diuretics, antihypertensive drugs, sedatives, antidepressants. Caffeine and alcohol intake should be recorded.
- Past surgical history, especially previous gynaecological and urological procedures, should be obtained.
- Past obstetric history should be reviewed. This should include the number, type, and difficulty of deliveries, and perineal tears.
- It is crucial to rule out any urinary tract pathology. A history of haematuria should lead to an immediate referral to a urologist. Of concern would be a sudden onset of frequency and urgency, with or without leakage, in a smoker of over 50 years of age.

Examination: key points

- Attention should be paid to abdominal, pelvic, genital, and neurological examinations, as well as general status (e.g. mobility).
- Abdominal: masses, scars, distended bladder, renal tenderness.
- Pelvic and genital: hypo-oestrogenism, pelvic organ prolapse, cough test, pelvic floor squeeze.
- Neurological: mental and general neurological status, back for asymmetry, dimples and scars, evaluate the S2–S4 nerve roots by the bulbocaverosus reflex (contraction of the external anal sphincter and perineal muscles when pressure is applied to the clitoris), sensory status of the genital area, sensory, motor and tendon reflexes of the lower limbs (sensory loss may indicate diabetes, alcoholism; ankle clonus may indicate supras-acral cord lesions).

Investigation: key points

- Urinalysis. to exclude nitrites, pyuria, bacteriuria, glycocuria, and haematuria.
- Urine culture for infection.
- Voiding diary. This quantifies fluid intake, frequency of micturition and incontinence, frequency of nocturia and volume of urine passed. A 3-day diary appears to be adequate and is associated with improved compliance than those of longer duration diaries. The aim is to limit recall bias by collecting patients' symptoms prospectively. It may also be useful in concentrating the patients mind on their symptoms.
- Assessment of post-void residual volume. This can be performed with a simple in–out catheter. However, newer ultrasound machines can accurately assess the bladder volume, avoiding the risks of catheterization.
- Perineal pad test. The 1-hour pad test has been standardized by the ICS. It is useful to grade the severity of incontinence and demonstrate leakage when other tests have failed to demonstrate incontinence.
- Pessary test. In patients with prolapse or voiding difficulties with prolapse, insertion of a pessary will mimic the post-surgical effect. This may reveal occult incontinence and will reveal the effect on urinary flow with correction of the prolapse.
- Imaging. Ultrasound of the urinary tract can be useful in detecting tumours and stones in the urinary tract as well as hydronephrosis, diverticulae, and bladder neck mobility. It is not required in the investigation of uncomplicated incontinence.
- Urodynamic evaluation. The ICS has recommended urodynamic testing prior to invasive procedures, after failed treatment, in surveillance of certain neurological dysfunctions and in complicated incontinence (Abrams 2002). This test measures bladder filling, storage, compliance, capacity, sensation during filling, and contractility. In combination with uroflowmery and residual testing, it will often allow an accurate diagnosis to be made. This is discussed in detail in Chapter xxxx.

In summary, diagnosis is made on the basis of an accurate history, detailed examination, augmented by investigations as required. Non-surgical therapy can usually be initiated on the basis of a presumptive diagnosis without the need for invasive urodynamic testing.

Treatment of urinary incontinence

Surgical procedures for UI are described in Section 15.5, Continence procedures and will not be covered here.

Conservative treatment

Patients with uncomplicated UI should be offered a trial of conservative management prior to considering surgical remedies.

Lifestyle changes

Fluid intake: a normal intake should be encouraged, generally between 1.5 and 2.0 L per 24 hours. Excessive intake will contribute to frequency and urgency. Patients will often decrease their intake to try to decrease their risk of incontinence; however, this can lead to an excessively concentrated urine that can itself be an irritant, leading to a reduced functional bladder capacity, and encourage urinary tract infections. In elderly people with nocturnal symptoms, chronic medical conditions may be present, e.g. congestive cardiac failure with ankle oedema; in these patients elevation of the legs in the afternoon or even a small dose of furosemide in the early evening may encourage diuresis of dependent fluid prior to bedtime.

Dietary intake: drinks containing caffeine (direct bladder irritant and diuretic), alcohol, and carbonated drinks should be discouraged.

Weight: as obesity is a strong risk factor for both stress and MUI, weight loss should be encouraged. This is often a difficult subject to broach with patients as a strong element of denial of any weight problem may be present. It is important to discuss this in a non-judgmental and objective manner offering appropriate support to aid compliance.

Smoking: women who smoke should be educated about the possible role of smoking in all forms of incontinence.

Constipation: constipation and faecal impaction have been implicated as factors in both stress and urge incontinence. Instructions on fluid intake, fibre, laxatives, and enemas should be given aiming for a regular daily bowel habit.

Behavioural interventions

- Scheduled toileting: planned voiding by the clock whether or not a sensation is present. This may be particularly helpful in women with cognitive impairment.
- Bladder re-education: frequent urination in UUI can lead to a reduced bladder capacity, detrusor overactivity, and leakage. The patient voids at scheduled interval, gradually increasing the time between voids and hence bladder capacity. This is very helpful in detrusor overactivity and can help SUI.
- Pelvic floor muscle retraining: an increase in urethral pressure occurs with a pelvic floor contraction; the bladder base and urethra are approximated more closely to the symphysis pubis. Long-term training increases muscle bulk and may provide urethral support. Biofeedback can aid patients who have difficulty performing pelvic floor exercises (PFE), although cones have no additional benefit to PFE alone (Cooper 1999). Functional electrical stimulation offers some benefit, but only in those who are unable to locate and contract their pelvic floor. A trial of at least 3 months of PFE is recommended before considering surgical intervention in SUI, MUI, and UUI (NICE 2006).
- Catheterization: there is a role for catheterization for short-term relief of severe uncontrollable incontinence and also for those suffering from overflow incontinence. Ideally, this is performed as clean intermittent

catheterization; occasionally an indwelling catheter is required. In the latter situation a suprapubic catheter is preferred.

Drug therapy

- SUI: Duloxetine, a combined serotonergic and noradrenaergic reuptake inhibitor, is often offered as an adjunct to PFE, or as an alternative to surgical treatment (Ghoniem 2005).
- UUI: if bladder training is ineffective then antimuscarinic drugs can be utilized. There are many available, most having similar efficacy with varying anticholinergic side-effects. Immediate-release oxybutynin is inexpensive and may be used as a first-line therapy, although the incidence of its adverse effects often lead to discontinuation. Alternatives include twice daily trospium, or once daily preparations such as extended-release oxybutynin tablets or patches, darifenacin, fesoterodine, solifenacin, or tolterodine. These drugs may be combined and will often require dose adjustment for maximal effect. Desmopressin has an important role in patients with troublesome nocturia (NICE 2006).
- MUI: drug treatment should be tailored to the most bothersome symptom. Antimuscarinic medication can be combined with duloxetine.

Surgery

This is discussed in Chapter 15.5, Continence procedures.

Further reading

Abrams P, Cardozo L, Fall M, et al. The standardisation of terminology of lower urinary tract function: report from th estandardisation sub-commitee of the International Continence Society. Neurourol Urodyn 2002;21:167–8.

Brocklehurst JC. Urinary incontinence in the community: analysis of a MORI poll. BMJ 1993;306:832–4.

Brown J, Grady D, Ouslander JG, et al. Prevalence of urinary incontinence and associated risk factors in postmenopausal women. Heart and Estrogen/Progestin Repalcement Study (HERS) Research Group. Obstet Gynecol 1999;94:66.

Brown JS, Sawaya G, Thom DH, Grady D. Hysterectomy and urinary incontinence: a systematic review. Lancet 2000;356:535–9.

Cooper JC, Monga AK. Issues 1, 2, 3, 4, 5, 6 & 7. Stress incontinence. Clinical evidence. London: BMJ Publishing Group & American College of Physicians—American Society of Internal Medicine.

Danforth KN, Townsend, MK, Lifford K, et al. Risk factors of urinary incontinence among middle aged women. Am J Obstet Gynecol 2006;194:339–45.

Deitel M, Stone E, Kassam HA, et al. Gynecologic-obstetric changes after loss of massive excess weight following bariatric surgery. J Am Coll Nutr 1988;7:147–53.

Ghoniem GM, Van Leeuwen JS, Elser DM, et al. A randomized controlled trial of duloxetine alone, pelvic floor muscle training alone, combined treatmet and no active treatment in women with stress urinary incontinence. J Urol 2005;173:1647–53.

Hannah ME, Pannuh HK, Hodnett ED, et al. Outcomes at 3 months after planned cesarean section vs planned vaginal delivery for breech presentation at term: The International Randomized Term Breech Trial. JAMA 2002;287:1822–31.

Hannested YS, Rortveit G, et al. Are smoking and other lifestyle factors associated with female urinary incontinence? The Norwegian EPINCOT Study. BMJ 2003;110:247–54.

Hsieh CH, Lee, MS, Lee MC, et al. Risk factor for urinary incontinence in Taiwanese women aged 20–59 years. Taiwan J Obstet Gynecol 2008;47:197–202.

Hunskaar S, Lose G, Sykes D, Voss S. The prevalence of urinary incontinence in women in four european countries. BJU Int 2004;93;324–30.

Irwin DE, Milsom I, Hunskar S, et al. Population based survey on urinary incontinence, overactive bladder and other lower urinary tract symptoms in five countries. Results of the EPIC study. Eur Urol 2006;50:1306–15.

McGrother CW, Donaldson MMK, Shaw C, et al. Storage symptoms of the bladder: prevalence, incidence and need for services in the UK. BJU Int 2004;93:763–9.

Milsom I, Abrams, P, Cardozo L, et al. How widespread are the symptoms of overactive bladder and how are they managed? A population based prevalence survey. BJU Int 2001:87;760–6.

National Institute of Clinical Excellence (NICE). Urinary Incontinence. The management of urinary incontinence in the female. Clinical Guideline 40. 2006: www.nice.org.uk/cg040

Norton P, McDonald, Sedgwick PM, Stanton SL. Distress and delay associated with urinary incontinence, frequency and urgency in women. BMJ 1988;297:1187–9.

Parazzinia, F, Chiaffarinoa, M, Lavezzaric V, Giambanco D and the VIVA Study Group. Risk factors for stress, urge or mixed urinary incontinence in Italy. Br J Obstet Gynaecol 2003;110:927–33.

Perry S. An epidemiological study to establish prevalence iof urinary symptoms and felt need in the community: the leicestershire MRC incontinencce study. J Public Health Med 1994;22:427–34.

Sampselle CM, Harlow SD, Skurnick J, et al. Urinary incontinence predictors and life impact in ethnically diverse perimenopausal women. Obstet Gynecol 2002;100:1230–8.

Subak LL, Johnson C, Whitcomb E, et al. Does weight loss improve incontinence in moderatley obese women? Int Urogynecol J 2002;13:40–3.

Subak LL, Whitcombe E, Shen H, et al. Weight loss: a novela and effective treatment for urinary incontinence. J Urol 2005;174:190–5.

Urinary frequency and urgency

Definition
Urinary frequency is defined as voiding more than eight times per 24 hours. Urgency is defined as a sudden and compelling desire to void that is difficult to defer. The overactive bladder syndrome (OAB) is the combination of frequency and urgency with or without urge incontinence (incontinence preceded by urgency) and nocturia (Abrams and Cardozo 2002).

Aetiology
A number of conditions can cause frequency and urgency, from within and outside the lower urinary tract.

Causes within the lower urinary tract
- Detrusor over activity
- Urinary tract infection
- Radiation cystitis
- High urinary residual
- Bladder calculus
- Bladder tumour
- Interstitial and chemical cystitis
- Sensory urgency
- Renal disease
- Urethral mucosal prolapse and caruncle
- Urethral tumour
- Urethral diverticulum.

Causes outside the lower urinary tract
- Excessive fluid intake
- Oestrogen deficiency
- Neurogenic bladder
- Uterovaginal prolapse
- Diabetes mellitus
- Diabetes insipidus
- Diuretic medication
- Pregnancy
- Pelvic mass.

Epidemiology
Frequency and urgency are common symptoms, with up to 20% women reporting frequency and 15% reporting urgency. The symptoms have significant effects on quality of life. The incidence of OAB increases with age, reported as 5% in those 18–44 years old, increasing to 20% over the age of 44 years.

Management
A number of conditions can result in frequency and urgency and it is essential that all patients have a stepwise evaluation to exclude any underlying cause.

History
A full urinary history should be taken to define any symptoms associated with the causes listed above. This will help assess the severity and how often symptoms occur. Other symptoms to consider include:
- urge incontinence
- stress-related incontinence: involuntary loss during physical examination such as coughing, running etc.
- nocturia/nocturnal enuresis
- coital incontinence

- continuous incontinence, which may be associated with a fistula or urinary retention
- drug history, including diuretic use
- neurological illness
- medical conditions such as diabetes mellitus/insipidus
- chronic/excessive drinking habits
- symptoms of prolapse

If pain or haematuria are present this needs further urgent investigation to exclude underlying urinary tract infection, bladder calculus, or tumour and any upper urinary tract lesion.

Examination
- Abdominal percussion to exclude urinary retention.
- A bimanual examination to exclude any pelvic masses such as fibroids, pregnancy or ovarian tumours.
- Perineal/vulval inspection to identify atrophic vaginitis and demonstrate any stress incontinence.
- A pelvic examination to assess any uterovaginal prolapse.
- The bladder base and urethra should be palpated to assess for tenderness which may be found in interstitial cystitis.
- Urethral examination to exclude any local lesions.
- Neurological examination to exclude any upper or lower motor neurone lesions particularly affecting the S2, S3, S4 nerve roots. This includes dorsiflexion of the toes (S3) and sensory innervations of the perineum (L1–2), lateral aspect of foot (S1), and thigh (S2).

Investigations
All patients should have the following investigations performed (as long as there is no strong suspicion of underlying malignancy).
- A midstream urine sample should be taken for an initial dipstick urinalysis to detect haematuria, glycosuria, pyuria, and bacteria. The sample should then be sent for culture and sensitivity. The presence of red cells and haematuria should be followed up with a renal ultrasound and cystoscopy.
- Urine cytology if suspicion of malignancy and in high-risk groups, e.g. smokers, patients exposed to aniline/hair dyes.
- A frequency volume chart is a useful way to evaluate abnormal fluid intake, number of voids, functional bladder capacity and leakage episodes.

More specialized investigations are required if the above investigations have not revealed the cause of symptoms. Investigations to consider include the following.
- Urodynamics: this test measures the pressure–volume relationship during filling and voiding in relation to a patient's symptoms. It should be performed when there is doubt regarding the aetiology of symptoms and in those who have had previous surgery, failed therapy and in those with voiding dysfunction. Most patients however can be treated for OAB empirically without the need for urodynamics.
- Detrusor overactivity is diagnosed on urodynamics as involuntary increases in detrusor pressure during filling or provocative manoeuvres such as coughing or running water. Low compliance may be found in the presence of a low capacity bladder. Poor voiding can be documented

- Cystoscopy: this can be performed using a rigid or flexible cystoscope. It should be performed if haematuria is present or there is a history suggestive of a urethral diverticulum or interstitial cystitis. It is also useful to measure true bladder capacity under anaesthetic.
- Imaging studies include renal ultrasound to assess for scarring, calculi, and to measure post-void urine volumes. An intravenous urogram can be performed if ultrasound suggests obstruction or a fistula. A CT scan is advocated on the presence of gross haematuria or if ultrasound has not been diagnostic,

Treatment

Treatment should be aimed at the underlying cause. For most patients with frequency urgency, treatment may be started empirically once any sinister underlying causes have been excluded and infection and high urinary residual treated (NICE 2006).

The mainstay of treatment is a combination of lifestyle changes, behavioural management, and antimuscarinic medication (Berghmans et al. 2000). Surgery is now only considered in those who have failed medical therapy.

Lifestyle changes

- Alteration in fluid intake such as avoidance of caffeine, fizzy drinks, and alcohol, which may exacerbate symptoms.
- Reduction in fluid intake to 2–2.5 L/day.
- Weight loss: this should be recommended in those with a BMI>30.

Behavioural management

This aims to teach a patient how to develop new voiding patterns by training the patient to actively increase the interval between voids and defer.

Antimuscarinic therapy

There are a number of drugs on the market that target the muscarinic receptors on the bladder wall, which are stimulated to acetylcholine released by the parasympathetic system causing bladder contraction. These drugs have been shown to have efficacy in reducing symptoms of urgency and urge incontinence (Chapple et al. 2008). Patients need to be warned about side-effects, which include dry mouth, constipation, headaches, and visual symptoms. They are contraindicated in those with a closed-angle glaucoma and myasthenia gravis.

The commonly used antimuscarinics include

- Oxybutynin: immediate release 2.5–5 mg bd/tds; extended release 5–30 mg/day
- Oxybutynin patch: 3.6 mg twice weekly
- Tolterodine: immediate release 1–2 mg/day; extended release 2–4 mg/day
- Solifenacin: extended release 5–10 mg/day
- Trospium: 20 mg bd
- Propiverine: 15 mg bd tds
- Darifenacin: 7.5–15 mg/day
- Fesoterodine: 4–8 mg/day

In those with troublesome nocturia a low dose antidepressant can be used, such as imipramine 25 mg nocte.

DDAVP (spray/tablets) can be used to reduce nocturnal urine production, although with caution in those over 65 years and with renal disease where a close review of renal function should be performed (Roxburgh et al. 2007).

Surgery

Over the last decade the surgical treatment for refractory urgency frequency has changed with newer less invasive approaches. Surgical procedures that have been used include the following.

- Augmentation cystoplasty: previously this was the procedure of choice and involved incising the bladder and inserting a portion of bowel to increase compliance. However, the procedure is associated with significant side-effects such as urinary retention, mucous production, stone formation, and malignant change within the transposed bowel.
- Detrusor myomectomy: this involves removing a portion of the detrusor from the bladder dome.

These procedures have now been superseded by the following techniques.

- Intradetrusor botulinum toxin: botulinum toxin is injected cystoscopically into the detrusor muscle or suburothelially. It is effective within a few weeks, with effects lasting on average 10 months, Side-effects include urinary retention. It is currently unlicensed for use in the bladder, although there is a large amount of research supporting its use in idiopathic and neurogenic detrusor overactivity.
- Sacroneuromodulation: this involves implantation of a pulsed generator in the S3 foramen and has 60–70% efficacy for frequency urgency (van Voskuilen et al. 2006).

Alternative therapy

A number of alternative therapies have been suggested such as acupuncture and hypnotherapy, although large good-quality studies are lacking (Emmons and Otto 2005).

Further reading

Abrams P, Cardozo L, Fall, et al. The standardisation of terminology of lower urinary tract function: report from the Standardisation Sub-committee of the International Continence Society. Neurourol Urodyn 2002;21:167–78.

Berghmans LC, Hendriks HJ Conservative treatment of urge urinary incontinence in women: a systematic review of randomized clinical trials. BJU Int 2000;85:254–63.

Chapple CR, Khullar V, Gabriel Z, et al. The effects of antimuscarinic treatments in overactive bladder: an update of a systematic review and meta-analysis. Eur Urol 2008;54:543–62.

Emmons SL, Otto L. Acupuncture for overactive bladder: a randomized controlled trial. Obstet Gynecol 2005;106:138–43.

National Institute for Health and Clinical Excellence. Urinary incontinence: the management of urinary incontinence in women. Clinical Guideline 40. London: NICE 2006: www.nice.org.uk/cg40

Roxburgh C, Cook J, et al. Anticholinergic drugs versus other medications for overactive bladder syndrome in adults. Cochrane Database Syst Rev 2007;4:CD003190.

van Voskuilen AC, Oerlemans DJ, Weil EH, et al. Long term results of neuromodulation by sacral nerve stimulation for lower urinary tract symptoms: a retrospective single center study. Eur Urol 2006;49:366–72.

Internet resources

The International Continence Society: www.icsoffice.org

Patient resources

www.bladderandbowelfoundation.org

Urinary retention (voiding difficulty)

Introduction

Normal voiding occurs when a bladder contraction is initiated and the bladder neck and the urethra are synchronously relaxed. When the falling urethral pressure and increasing intravesical pressure equate, urine flow will commence.

The act of micturition is governed by a number of contributory factors: control from higher centres, the sacral reflex arc, the innervation of the bladder muscle and sphincter mechanisms, the outflow resistance, and the speed of contraction of the detrusor muscle fibres. Abnormalities of any component of this interactive mechanism may result in voiding dysfunction.

Definitions and classification

Acute retention

Acute retention is the sudden onset of painful or painless inability to void over 12 hours, requiring catheterization with removal of a volume equal to or greater than normal bladder capacity. It is usually painful but may be painless in the presence of a neurological lesion or following an epidural anaesthetic.

Chronic retention

Chronic retention describes the insidious and painless failure of bladder emptying where catheterization yields a volume equal to at least 50% of normal bladder capacity. Chronic retention may cause urinary incontinence and occur without obvious cause.

There are usually two phases through which women pass before developing acute or chronic urinary retention. The first is asymptomatic voiding difficulty, where the woman is unaware of impaired bladder emptying. The urinary stream is reduced, and the peak flow rate is less than 15 mL/second. The maximum voiding pressure is usually normal, and there is no residual urine. The second stage is that of bladder decompensation, when symptoms of voiding difficulty appear such as hesitancy, poor stream, straining to void, and incomplete emptying, with or without urinary tract infection. The peak flow is less than 15 mL/second, the voiding pressure is reduced, and there is residual urine.

There is a paucity of data on the incidence or prevalence of voiding disorders in the absence of neuropathy. Of 600 women with symptoms of bladder dysfunction attending a urodynamic clinic, 2% had asymptomatic and 14% had symptomatic voiding difficulty. The symptomatic group tended to be older and were more likely to have had previous pelvic surgery.

Aetiology and pathophysiology

In the female, voiding can occur via one of three mechanisms: contraction of the detrusor muscle, a rise in abdominal pressure, and relaxation of the urethral sphincter and pelvic floor musculature. Therefore, voiding disorders result when these mechanisms fail, that is when the detrusor muscle is unable to maintain an effective contraction, the urethra fails to relax and lower urethral resistance, or if there is a failure in the synchronization of these two actions, resulting in detrusor sphincter dyssynergia. The latter occurs in suprasacral neurological lesions

Pharmacological causes

Obstetric epidural anaesthesia is the commonest cause of voiding dysfunction. If retention is overlooked, overdistension injury may result in long-term voiding difficulty.

Anticholinergic agents used to treat urgency and frequency are frequent causes, for example Solifenacin or Fesoterodine. It is therefore vital to exclude urinary residual before prescribing this class of agent. In women with a combination of poor voiding and detrusor instability these drugs may be used in conjunction with intermittent self-catheterization. Ganglion-blocking drugs have a similar effect to anticholinergics, and α-adrenergic agents increase urethral resistance.

Inflammatory causes

The most frequent causes of inflammation are infective, chemical, or allergic (local or systemic allergens). Voiding difficulties may result from painful stimuli and may be aggravated by urethral oedema. Primary anogenital herpetic infection may produce urinary retention by the effect of local inflammatory lesions and lumbosacral meningomyelitis

Obstructive causes

Distal urethral stenosis usually results from urogenital atrophy in the postmenopausal woman but can result from chronic fibrosis following chronic inflammation, urethral instrumentation (e.g. urethrotomy), and scarring following surgery (e.g. anterior colporrhaphy).

Acute urethral oedema may occur after bladder neck surgery or, rarely, secondary to premenstrual fluid retention.

Foreign bodies and calculi

- Bladder neck surgery (e.g. sling procedures) may cause compression.
- Extrinsic causes of obstruction include impaction of a retroverted gravid uterus, pelvic masses, and faecal impaction.
- Haematocolpos associated with cryptomenorrhoea may present with retention due to urethral obstruction.
- Urethral distortion due to genital prolapsed; 33% of women with grades 3 and 4 prolapse have evidence of urethral obstruction.

Endocrine causes

Hypothyroidism and diabetes mellitus can cause peripheral neuropathy, resulting in urinary retention.

Overdistension

Bladder overdistension as a result of mismanagement of acute or chronic retention develops insidiously and is more frequent in women than in men. It often results after failure to detect retention after pelvic surgery (e.g. hysterectomy) or epidural anaesthesia. Overdistension may occur without obvious cause and is frequently observed in elderly women with large acontractile bladders.

Urethral sphincter hypertrophy

Fowler and Kirby have described a group of women who present with voiding difficulties due to a primary defect within the striated urethral sphincter.

Detrusor myopathy

Primary changes in the detrusor muscle have been reported as a cause of retention.

Psychogenic causes

Criteria for this diagnosis are an absence of neurological and or other significant organic disease, correlation of psychological disturbance with onset of symptoms, and a response to psychotherapy or psychopharmacological agents. Psychiatric diagnoses include hysteria and depression.

Presentation

Symptoms

Impaired voiding may be asymptomatic in a few patients but the majority present with infrequent voiding, poor flow, intermittent stream, incomplete emptying, straining to void, and/or hesitancy. Others may present with overflow incontinence and frequency or urinary tract infection due to stasis. Acute retention may present with pain.

History taking should be directed towards determination of a primary cause. Neuropathy should be enquired about and a detailed drug, medical, and surgical history, including genital and urinary tract infection, should be obtained.

Signs

A careful general abdominal and pelvic examination should be performed to exclude the causes listed. A neurological examination should be performed and the lumbar region examined for stigmata of an underlying spinal disorder. The bladder may be palpable and will characteristically be dull to percussion.

Investigations

Urinary tract infection should be excluded as it may predispose to voiding difficulty. The simplest investigations are uroflowmetry and ultrasonography for residual, but cystometry and other investigations may be required to make a more accurate diagnosis.

When catheterization is performed for acute retention the residual volume should be recorded. This will confirm the diagnosis and give a guide to the severity of bladder overdistension, and may be useful in assessing prognosis.

Uroflowmetry

This is the most important initial screening procedure and is simple and non-invasive. Measurements may need to be repeated as a single measurement may be unreliable. Obstructed voiding may occur in the presence of normal uroflowmetry because the detrusor may compensate by increasing the voiding pressure. Subtracted cystometry is required to detect this.

Cystometry

The filling phase of cystometry may indicate a lower or upper motor neuron lesion. The voiding phase will confirm any disorder of bladder emptying. The following may give clues during the procedure:

- difficulty catheterizing in presence of obstruction
- residual urine greater than 50 mL
- delayed first sensation (early first sensation in upper motor neuron lesions)
- increased bladder capacity
- pressure rise during filling and compliance usually normal
- maximum voiding pressure will be raised in the presence of obstruction prior to decompensation (it will be low or non-existent when detrusor failure occurs)
- isometric pressure is usually reduced or non-existent, demonstrating poor detrusor reserve.

Radiology

A plain abdominal radiograph will disclose a full bladder, and lumbosacral film will demonstrate congenital conditions such as spina bifida occulta or acquired conditions such as intervertebral disc prolapse. Videocystourethrography can provide additional information at the time of cystometry. Trabeculation diverticula and ureteric reflux can be detected and distal urethral stenosis identified.

Ultrasonography

Abdominal ultrasonography allows non-invasive measurement of urinary residual and also assessment of the upper urinary tract.

Cystourethroscopy

Difficulty in instrumentation of the urethra will suggest stenosis. Cystoscopy will allow visualization of intravesical pathology such as trabeculation, sacculation, and diverticula.

Electromyography

May help diagnose urethral sphincter hypertrophy and multiple system atrophy.

Treatment

Prophylaxis

Prevention or early recognition of retention may avoid long-term voiding difficulty. Pre-emptive bladder drainage at radical pelvic or continence surgery or with epidural will prevent long-term problems. When there is evidence of voiding difficulty prior to continence surgery it is reasonable to counsel appropriately and teach intermittent self-catheterization.

Intermittent self-catheterization

Intermittent self-catheterization is the principal treatment for chronic urinary retention. It allows women to lead independent lives with efficient bladder emptying and low rates of urinary tract infection. There are two forms of intermittent self-catheterization: sterile and clean. The former is usually reserved for patients with neuropathic bladders in a hospital environment to prevent cross-infection.

Pharmacotherapy

Cholinergic agents, prostaglandins have been advocated but there is no real evidence that they are of any clinical benefit. Diazepam used as an anxiolytic may help with postoperative voiding problems.

In women with combined urge incontinence and retention, anticholinergic agents such as tolterodine may be used effectively in conjunction with CISC.

Surgery

If voiding difficulty is due to urethral stenosis, urethral dilatation using Hegar dilators or the Otis urethrotome are appropriate options.

Neuromodulation

This two-stage procedure involves stimulation of the S3 nerve root through the S3 foramen. The first stage is that of percutaneous nerve evaluation using a temporary stimulation wire. If this has a beneficial effect then a permanent stimulator is implanted. Early results are encouraging but the mechanism of action is not understood.

Further reading

Dwyer PL, Desmedt E. Impaired bladder emptying in women. Aust N Z J Ostet Gynaecol 1994;34:73–8.

Stanton SL, Ozsoy C, Hilton P. Voiding difficulties in the female: prevalence, clinical and urodynamic review. Ob-stet Gynecol 1983;61:144–7.

Patient resources

The Bladder and Bowel Foundation: www.bladderandbowelfoundation.org

Urinary tract injury

Definition
The close association between the lower urinary tract (LUT) and female reproductive organs predisposes the lower urinary tract to injury during gynaecological and obstetric surgery. Most LUT injuries occur during benign surgery and the majority are not recognized during the procedure.

Epidemiology
LUT injury occurs in 1–2% of all obstetric and gynaecological procedures (Dowling 1986). The true incidence is possibly higher when unreported and undiagnosed cases and those that spontaneously resolve are accounted for (Daly 1988).

Aetiology
The LUT can be injured by penetrating or blunt injury. The most common penetrating injury tends to be surgical, although external violence such as knife and gunshot or unusual sources such as migrating IUCDs, hip prosthesis surgical drains, swallowed objects and filshie clips have all been incriminated. Diathermy, particularly during laparoscopic surgery for endometriosis, accounts for a significant proportion of the injury. Predisposing factors for urinary tract injury are coexisting pelvic adhesion, an enlarged uterus, endometriosis and other causes of distorted pelvic configuration, history of previous irradiation, previous surgery, haemorrhage during surgery and the extent of surgery.

Sites of injury
LUT injury may involve the ureter, bladder, or urethra. Whereas bladder and ureteric injuries account for the majority of these, urethral injuries are becoming increasingly recognized with tape procedures for incontinence.

Classification of injury
The American Association for the Surgery of Trauma (AAST) has devised a classification for ureteric (Table 13.9.1), bladder (Table 13.9.2), and urethral injuries (Table 13.9.3). This is an anatomical classification but does not have clear prognostic implications.

Prevention
The best defence against injury to the urinary tract is knowledge of its anatomic relations and use of the avascular spaces of the pelvis to identify structures during surgery. Preoperatively, a detailed history, physical examination and evaluation of the urinary tract to rule out pre-existing urinary dysfunction should be undertaken. Imaging of the renal tract gives information on the kidneys, evidence of ureteric obstruction, and bladder for urinary residuals. Intravenous urography further defines renal function and identifies ureteral obstruction. Retrograde ureteric stenting

Table 13.9.1 AAST classification of ureteric injury

Grade I	Haematoma or contusion without devascularization
Grade II	Laceration <50% transection
Grade III	Laceration >50% transection
Grade IV	Complete transection with <2 cm of devascularization
Grade V	Avulsion with >2 cm of devascularization

Table 13.9.2 Bladder injury

Grade I	Haematoma: contusion, intramural haematoma. Laceration: partial thickness
Grade II	Laceration: extra peritoneal bladder wall laceration <2 cm
Grade III	Laceration: extraperitoneal >2 cm or intraperitoneal <2 cm
Grade IV	Laceration: intraperitoneal >2 cm
Grade V	Laceration: intra- or extraperitoneal extending to the bladder neck (trigone) or the ureteral orifice

preoperatively has not been shown to reduce the incidence of ureteric injury during surgery. When the course of the ureter is difficult to determine during surgery, ureteric catheterization or intravenous injection of methylene blue may help to delineate the ureter.

Intraoperatively, proper patient positioning, good lighting, appropriate surgical approach, adequate exposure, an early assessment of pelvic pathology, and seeking urological assistance if problems are anticipated help reduce injury. Peritoneal entry should be as high as possible to avoid a cystotomy. Following abdominal entry an attempt to restore normal anatomy and identify the ureters and bladder should be made. During vaginal surgery, downward traction on the cervix when clamping the uterine vessels and upward traction on the bladder holds the bladder and ureter out of the operative field. Blind clamping of vessels should be avoided as it is the commonest cause of urinary tract injury in obstetric practice (Neuman et al. 1991). When dissecting masses it is important to stay near the pathology and identify structures prior to ligation. The bladder should be mobilized in the downward and outward direction thus avoiding both bladder and ureteric injury. When using diathermy, particularly during laparoscopic surgery, short applications are preferable as the depth of penetration depends on both the duration and power of diathermy.

Clinical approach: diagnosis and management

Ureteric injury
Diagnosis of ureteric injury can be made intraoperatively or postoperatively, with 70% being identified postoperatively

Table 13.9.3 Urethral injury

Grade I	Contusion: blood at urethral meatus, urethrography normal
Grade II	Stretch injury: elongation without extravasation
Grade III	Partial disruption: extravasation on urethrography, contrast at injury site with contrast visualisation in bladder
Grade IV	Complete disruption: extravasation on urethrography, contrast at injury site without visualization in the bladder; <2 cm of urethral separation
Grade V	Complete disruption: complete transaction with >2 cm of urethral separation, or extension into the prostate or vagina

(Mann 1988). Intraoperatively, ureteric injury can be recognized by intravenous dye injection and extravasation of urine into the operative field. Alternatively, cystoscopy with evidence of urinary excretion, or ureteric catheterization identifies ureteric integrity.

Postoperative investigations are aimed at establishing renal function, ruling out hydronephrosis and confirming ureteric integrity and include an intravenous urogram, contrast computed tomography, retrograde ureterogram, renal ultrasound, and cystoscopy. With unilateral ureteric injury patients may have a transient rise in serum creatinine, although normal levels do not preclude ureteric injury.

Postoperative symptoms of ureteric injury tend to be variable and are shown in Table 13.9.4.

Management of ureteric injury depends largely on the site and type of injury. The general principles include achieving a tension-free anastomosis by adequate mobilization, preservation of adventitial blood supply, ureteric stenting, and passive drainage of the repair site and minimal use of sutures to avoid necrosis. Although a complete description of all repair techniques is beyond the scope of this chapter, broadly speaking when the injury is below the mid-pelvis, an ureteroneocystostomy, or ureteral reimplantation, is most commonly used. These injuries usually occur within 4–6 cm of the trigone. To ensure this is tension-free, an additional bridging procedure such as a psoas muscle hitch or Boari flap may need to be used.

When the injury occurs above mid-pelvis, there may not be enough proximal ureter left to reach the bladder for reimplantation. At this point a ureteroureterostomy, or end-to-end anastomosis of the injured ureter, becomes the best option. The ends of the ureter are spatulated to decrease the chances of stenosis occurring at the anastomotic site. An omental fat graft can be helpful to aid healing by providing an additional blood supply.

When an injury occurs such that a short proximal ureter exists, as when a substantial length of ureter has been damaged, it may no longer be possible to re-anastomose the ureter to itself. In such a case, a transureteroureterostomy, or end-to-side anastomosis of the proximal ureter to the contralateral ureter, may be required. This should be avoided if possible because stenosis at this anastomotic site could now jeopardize function in both kidneys. If the above options are not possible or the resources to execute them are not immediately available, a single J stent can be inserted into the proximal end of the cut ureter and can be brought out to the skin into a collecting device. Thus, the short ureter is able to drain but is not dissected until repair is possible. This is a temporizing measure to preserve renal function while the patient awaits definitive repair.

Bladder injury

Intraoperative bladder injury is easily identified by instilling indigo carmine in the bladder and noting for leakage of dye into the operative filed. Alternatively, cystoscopy can be used to identify the injury. Postoperatively a similar approach using a radio-opaque dye in conjunction with imaging can be used for identification of injury. Symptoms of bladder injury depend on whether the injury is intra- or extraperitoneal.

Intraperitoneal injury is associated with abdominal distension, shoulder tip pain, and if diagnosis is delayed with the development of uroascites. Peritoneal signs of tenderness and rebound will develop and if infection ensues there may be features of frank peritonitis. Extraperitoneal injury is associated with pain and an occasional rise in blood pressure. Haematuria is the hallmark of bladder injury and frank

Table 13.9.4 Symptoms and signs of ureteric injury

Fever and flank pain	Commonest symptom
Haematuria	Absent in 30%
Urinoma	Can be confirmed on USG
Abdominal distension/ ileus/peritonitis	Leakage from the wound is more common
Urinary leakage	Abdominal/vaginal
Secondary hypertension	Due to obstructive uropathy
Asymptomatic	50% have none of the above

haematuria is seen in 95% of cases with the remaining 5% having microscopic haematuria.

The management of bladder injury depends on the site, and grade of injury as well as the timing of recognition. Over half of all bladder injuries will be recognized intraoperatively and require a two-layer closure with absorbable suture to achieve an excellent result. The commonest mistake made is to miss a second rent having found one. All edges of the cystotomy must be identified and mobilized so that repair can be achieved tension free. If the injury is close to the trigone, care to avoid kinking of ureters must be taken. With intraperitoneal injury and repair, the cystotomy site should be covered by omentum or a layer of peritoneum to cushion the repair by adding bulk followed by continuous bladder drainage for at least 7 days, which promotes healing by preventing bladder distension. Isolated extraperitoneal injury can be treated by 7–10 days of continuous indwelling catheterization and expectant management. This is particularly true of injury occurring due to endoscopic procedures, i.e. laparoscopy and cystoscopy. Although prompt repair is usually desirable, with delayed recognition management may warrant delayed surgical repair after a few months to allow the oedema and inflammation to settle.

Urethral injury

Urethral injury is relatively uncommon with gynaecological surgery, and is seen more frequently with trauma to the perineum and fracture of the bony pelvis. Patients with urethral injury are usually unable to void due to extravasation of urine into the subcutaneous tissue. If they are able to void there is usual gross haematuria with swelling and ecchymosis of the perineum. In suspected urethral trauma no attempt to catheterize the urethra should be made until the site of injury has been delineated, as a partial disruption may be converted into a complete injury. Intraoperatively urethral injury is most often recognized by seeing the catheter through an incision in the wall of the urethra. The imaging of choice with suspected urethral injury is retrograde urethrogram. When undertaking urethroscopy in these patients it is best performed with a 0° scope.

Lacerations of the urethra in women should be repaired as soon as it is identified over a transurethral catheter in layers. This differs to repair in males where a delayed repair has better results. Early repair ensures that the integrity of the continence mechanism can be maintained and avoids the development of a fistula. With involvement of the proximal urethra it is important to buttress the urethrovesical junction to avoid postoperative stress incontinence. A bulbocavernosus fat pad can be used if there is a need for additional tissue depth during the repair.

Postoperative care

Following a repair, integrity of the urinary tract should be established with a cystogram or IVP to rule out extravasation or confirm ureteral patency prior to removal of catheters and stents.

Prognosis

Early recognition of urinary tract injury is associated with excellent results. Intraoperative detection and correction causes little inconvenience to the patient and is associated with minimal complications or long-term sequel. Postoperatively a high index of suspicion should be maintained and immediate investigations instituted in those with suspected injury to achieve optimal outcomes.

Further reading

Daly JW, Higgins KA. Injury to the ureter during gynecologic surgical procedures. Surg Gynecol Obstet 1988;167:19–22.

Dowling RA, Corriere JN Jr, Sandler CM. Iatrogenic ureteral injury. J Urol 1986;135:912–15.

Mann WJ, Arato M, Patsner B, Stone ML. Ureteral injuries in an obstetrics and gynecology training program: etiology and management. Obstet Gynecol 1988;72:82–5.

Neuman M, et al. Iatrogenic injuries to the ureter during gynecologic and obstetric operations. Surg Gynecol Obstet 1991;173:268–72.

Uterovaginal prolapse

Definition
The word prolapse is derived from the Latin word *prolapsus* and means a slipping forth or the falling out of place of a part or viscus. A prolapse occurs when there is a defect in the pelvic floor sufficient to allow one or more of the pelvic viscera to fall through.

Epidemiology
The incidence of genital prolapse is difficult to determine as many women do not seek medical advice. Broad estimates suggest that 50% of all parous women lose the support of the pelvic floor and have some degree of prolapse with 10–20% seeking medical aid for their problem.

Aetiology
The pathophsyiology of pelvic floor disorders is complex and multifactorial. The factors include a combination of genetic predisposition and acquired dysfunction of the muscular and connective tissue support systems due to parturition or the menopause. Damage to the pelvic diaphragm causes the levator plate to become more oblique, creating a funnel which allows the uterus, vagina, and rectum to herniated, resulting in a prolapse. In women with severe prolapse a 50% loss of motor units of the perineal muscles has been demonstrated (Sharf *et al.* 1976). There is also evidence of fascial denervation (Parks *et al.* 1977).

Normal supports of the vagina and adjacent pelvic organs are provided by the interaction between the levator ani muscle and the connective tissue supports. In adult women the pelvic floor is inherently weak, predominantly due to their upright posture. Also on account of this orthograde posture, the fascial layers of the pelvic floor are very well developed to provide support for pelvic organs. The pelvic diaphragm collectively refers to the levator ani muscles and connective tissue attachments to the pelvis (Fig. 13.10.1a). Although the levator ani muscle has two component parts, i.e. the diaphragmatic part (coccygeus and iliococcygeus muscles) and the pubovisceral part (pubococcygeus and puborectalis), it functions as a single unit. The levator ani is a skeletal muscle with a baseline resting tone and can be voluntarily contracted. The type I fibres (slow twitch) provide constant tone and the type II fibres (fast twitch) provide reflex and voluntary contractions.

Contrary to previous belief, the connective tissue fibres are just as important as the pelvic muscles in providing support to the pelvic organs, but their role is different. The fascial components consist of two types of fascia: parietal and visceral (endopelvic). Parietal fascia covers the pelvic skeletal muscles and provides attachments of the muscles to the bony pelvis. The visceral fascia exists throughout the pelvis as a meshwork of loosely arranged collagen, elastin, and adipose tissue through which blood vessels, lymphatics, and nerves travel to reach the pelvic organs. DeLancey (1992) described three levels of endopelvic fascia support for the vagina (Fig. 13.10.1b). The upper third of the vagina (level I) is suspended from the pelvic walls by vertical fibres of the paracolpium, which is a continuation of the cardinal ligament. In the middle third of the vagina (level II) the paracolpium attaches the vagina laterally to the arcus tendineus and fascia of the levator ani muscles. The vagina's lower third fuses with the perineal membrane, levator ani muscles, and perineal body (level III).

Classification
As vaginal wall prolapse is a protrusion of one or more pelvic organs (such as the bladder or the rectum) through the vaginal fascia and the displacement ('prolapse') of the associated vaginal wall from its normal location into or outside the vagina, there are different types of vaginal wall prolapse depending on the organs and sites involved. These include anterior vaginal wall prolapse (such as urethrocele and cystocele), posterior vaginal wall prolapse (such as rectocele and enterocele), and apical vaginal wall prolapse (affecting the uterus or the vault in women who have had a hysterectomy). A woman can also present with prolapse of a combination of these sites.

Many systems for staging prolapse have been described, but due to lack of subjectivity have been fraught with problems. The standard for prolapse assessment for clinical researchers is the system accepted by the International Continence Society, the Pelvic Organ Prolapse Quantification system or the POP-Q (Bump *et al.* 1996).

The POP-Q system makes measurements in centimetres in nine locations on the vagina and vulva relative to the hymen. Its advantage over previous grading systems which have included a general grading as mild, moderate, and severe to more complex classifications such as the

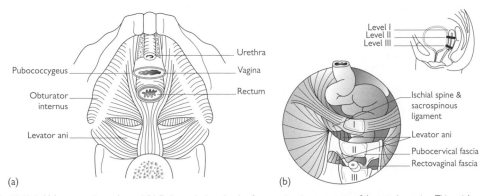

Fig. 13.10.1 (a) Levator ani complex and (b) DeLancey's three levels of connective tissue supports of the anterior vagina. This article was published in *Am J Obstet Gynecol*, Vol 166, 6, DeLancey, J.O, 'Anatomic aspects of vaginal eversion hysterectomy', pp. 1717–1724, Copyright Elsevier (1992).

Pelvic organ prolapse quantitative scoring system (POP-Q)

Aa Arbitrary point on the anterior wall, measured 3 cm from the external urethral meatus −3 to +3cm (−3 cm with no prolapse)

   Ba The most dependent portion of the anterior vagina Value is −3 with no prolapse.

   C Least supported portion of the cervix or vaginal cuff

   Ap Arbitrary point on the posterior vaginal wall, measured 3 cm from the hymen −3 to +3cm

   Bp The most dependent portion of the posterior vagina. Value is −3 with no prolapse

   D Position of the cul-de-sac. Point D ranges in value from positive to negative. It is not measured post hysterectomy.

   TVL Total vaginal length from the hymen to the posterior fornix (or vaginal apex after hysterectomy)

   GH Genital hiatus from the midpoint of the external urethral meatus to the posterior midline of hymen

   PB Perineal body from the posterior midline of hymen (GH site) to the midanal opening

Baden Walker system is that the assessment of prolapse for all sites of the vagina is done as well as a quantitative measurement of prolapse with straining relative to the hymen.

Prognosis

A large retrospective cohort study (Olsen et al. 1997) of women undergoing surgical treatment for prolapse and incontinence during 1995 which included 149 554 women age 20 or older demonstrated that the lifetime risk of undergoing a single operation for prolapse or incontinence by age 80 was 11.1%. In women undergoing surgery for prolapse, up to one-third of procedures represented recurrent operations.

Clinical approach: diagnosis

History

- Something coming down is almost universal. Women describe a vaginal lump which is usually asymptomatic when they get up in the morning and gradually gets worse as the day progresses.
- A uterine prolapse may cause protrusion of the cervix giving a feeling of pressure, and when the prolapse is protruding outside the introitus, bleeding, ulceration of the protruded lump, and discharge may be present.
- An anterior vaginal wall prolapse (cystocele) often presents with urinary symptoms. Increased frequency related to a large residual or recurrent urinary tract infection may occur. Prolapse does not cause stress incontinence (SI) and in fact the symptoms of SI may be masked by the increasing size of the prolapse. Some women may even complain of having to reduce the bulge digitally in order to pass urine, but more commonly of voiding difficulty with the need to strain, double void, or rock in order to empty their bladders. In the presence of large prolapse and vaginal eversion, back flow resulting in hydroureter and hydronephrosis may occur, although this is reversible following correction of the prolapse.
- A posterior vaginal wall prolapse (rectocele and/or enterocele) by comparison may be asymptomatic until

quite large. There may be difficulty with defaecation, with incomplete bowel emptying and passive leakage, or problems with intercourse.
- Other non-specific symptoms which may occur in patients with prolapse include pelvic pain, low back ache, and the consequences of a vaginal protrusion such as difficulty walking.

Examination

- Bimanual examination.
- Speculum examination at rest and with straining. This should be performed in the left lateral position using a Sims speculum to permit visualisation of the anterior and posterior vaginal walls separately.

Investigations

These depend on the history and examination findings and include
- urine culture
- pelvic ultrasound scan
- urodynamic studies
- proctography.

Management

Most women with prolapse are asymptomatic so may need no treatment. Current treatment options for vaginal wall prolapse include pelvic floor muscle training (physiotherapy), use of topical hormone replacement therapy, use of mechanical devices (ring or shelf pessaries), and surgery, with or without mesh reinforcement. A trial of lifestyle modification might be beneficial: weight loss, smoking cessation, treatment of constipation, electrical stimulation, or biofeedback.

Physiotherapy

There is some encouragement from the systematic review by Hagen et al. (2004) that pelvic floor muscle training, delivered by a physiotherapist to symptomatic women in an outpatient setting, may reduce severity of prolapse.

Topical hormone replacement therapy

Although there are no studies looking at the impact of oestrogen therapy in women with prolapse, oestrogen has been shown to be of benefit in women with atrophic vaginitis, thereby reducing prolapse symptoms. Taking oestrogen may also help to limit further weakness of the muscles and other connective tissues that support the uterus.

Mechanical devices

Pessaries are a good option for those who wish to remain fertile or avoid surgery. There are a variety of pessaries available, made of rubber, plastic, or silicone-based material. The commonest pessaries are the rings and shelf, but other types being increasingly used are the inflatable, the doughnut, and the Gellhorn, all of which have slightly different uses and specifications.

Surgery

Surgical correction of prolapse depends largely on the compartment which is affected. For vaginal wall prolapse it may involve an anterior colporrhaphy/anterior vaginal wall repair, posterior colporrhaphy/posterior vaginal wall repair or a vaginal hysterectomy. For a vaginal vault prolapse surgical correction may require a sacrospinous fixation, an abdominal sacrocolpopexy, or an infracoccygeal procedure which involves the use of a mesh (e.g. Apogee, Post I-Stop).

The aims of using mesh in the repair of vaginal wall prolapse are to add additional support and to reduce the risk of recurrence, particularly for women with recurrent prolapse or with congenital connective tissue disorders. The evidence for their use in routine practice and primary repairs is however lacking.

Prevention

The development of prolapse may not be completely preventable as there are a large number of factors, including genetic and familial, that contribute. Certain precautionary measures such as antenatal and postnatal exercises and avoidance of factors that increase intra-abdominal pressure (persistent heavy lifting, constipation) may however play a role.

Further reading

Bump RC, Mattiasson A, Bø K, et al. The standardization of terminology of female pelvic organ prolapse and pelvic floor dysfunction. Am J Obstet Gynecol 1996;175:10–7.

DeLancey JO. Anatomic aspects of vaginal eversion after hysterectomy. Am J Obstet Gynecol 1992;166:1717–24.

Hagen S, et al. Conservative management of pelvic organ prolapse in women. Cochrane Database Syst Rev 2004;2:CD003882.

Olsen AL, Smith VJ, Bergstrom JO, et al. Epidemiology of surgically managed pelvic organ prolapse and urinary incontinence. Obstet Gynecol 1997;89:501–6.

Parks AG, Swash M, Urich H. Sphincter denervation in anorectal incontinence and rectal prolapse. Gut 1977;18:656–65.

Sharf B, Zilberman A, Sharf M. Electromyogram of pelvic floor muscles in genital prolapse. Int J Gynecol Obstet 1976;14:2–14.

Urodynamic investigation

The term 'urodynamics' is used to describe a combination of tests that assess bladder filling and emptying.

The aim of urodynamics is to
- reproduce the patient's symptoms
- demonstrate a physiological explanation for the patient's symptoms.

Assessment of the patient with lower urinary tract dysfunction

Urodynamic assessment of a patient with lower urinary tract dysfunction includes full history, clinical examination, urinalysis, and frequency volume diary prior to embarking on laboratory tests.

History

The International Continence Society has published guidelines on the classification of lower urinary tract symptoms. The urogynaecological assessment includes specific enquiry into symptoms of
- stress urinary incontinence (SUI)
- urge urinary incontinence
- urgency, nocturia, frequency
- voiding and urinary stream
- bowel function
- sexual function and dyspareunia
- prolapse
- recurrent urinary tract infections.

Quality of life assessment

Urinary incontinence has a significant impact on a woman's quality of life. There are numerous standardized quality of life questionnaires now available.

Examination and dipstick urinalysis

Abdominal and pelvic examinations are essential to exclude a pelvic mass. Vaginal examination will help assess the degree of oestrogenization of the lower genital tract and classify and quantify any prolapse. Prolapse can be classified according to severity (mild moderate or severe) by the Baden Walker system or the International Continence Society Pelvic Organ Prolapse (ICS PoPQ) score. Neurological examination may also be necessary to determine any possible neurological cause for the patient's symptoms. Dipstick testing of urine will help detect a urinary tract infection and diabetes mellitus. Haematuria on dipstick testing confirmed on microscopy requires urgent cystoscopy to exclude a bladder tumour.

Frequency volume chart

Patients are given a frequency volume chart (FVC) prior to attending the urodynamic clinic. The patient is asked to complete a 3-day diary of the fluid intake and voiding habits. A FVC provides information about the following:
- bladder functional capacity
- daytime and night time frequency
- frequency and severity of incontinence episodes
- nature and volume of fluid intake.

Laboratory tests

Urodynamics usually involve the following:
- Uroflowmetry: plots the flow rate of urine against time. This assesses voiding function. Voiding dysfunction manifests in an interrupted, reduced or incomplete urinary stream. The patient attends with a full bladder and sits in private, on a special commode which measures the rate of micturition.
- Cystometry: once the urine has again had dipstick analysis to exclude a UTI a filling catheter and fluid-filled pressure transducer are inserted under aseptic technique into the bladder to measure the intravesical pressure. A fluid-filled pressure transducer is then inserted into the rectum or vagina. This measures intra-abdominal pressure. The bladder is then filled and provocation manoeuvres are performed by the patient. The detrusor pressure is plotted by subtracting the intra-abdominal pressure from the intravessical pressure. The bladder is filled with saline at room temperature usually at a rate of 50–100 mL/minute. Microtip solid state transducers may also be used.
- The patient is asked to inform the practitioner performing the tests when she feels the first sensation of fullness (first sensation), the first desire to void and strong desire to void. Any feelings of urgency or signs of leakage are noted on the trace.
- Mimicking the patient's symptoms of urgency with or without urinary leakage associated with a rise in detrusor pressure is called detrusor overactivty (DO). Provocation studies are then performed including coughing, jumping and laughing to provoke an involuntary leakage of urine. Urinary leakage in the absence of a rise in detrusor pressure is called urodynamic stress incontinence. At the end of provocation studies the patient is asked to void. Pressure flow analysis on voiding will again screen for a voiding disorder and differentiates between outflow obstruction (high pressure–low flow) and detrusor failure (low pressure–low flow).

Normal reference ranges:
- Flow rate:>15 mL/second
- First sensation: 150–250 mL
- First desire to void: 350–450 mL
- Strong desire to void: 400–600 mL.

Additional tests may include:
- Urethral pressure tests: urethral closure pressure and urethral leak point pressure assess the ability of the urethra to prevent leakage.
- Videourodynamics: formal cystometry performed under X-ray imaging. The filling medium is radio-opaque rather than saline. This demonstrates abnormalities in the bladder anatomy such as diverticulae. It also allows assessment of bladder anatomy in association with function. For example differentiating incontinence due to bladder neck hypermobility and urethral sphincter deficiency (ISD).
- Ambulatory urodynamics: ambulatory urodynamics are used when conventional cystometry fails to demonstrate the patient's symptoms of DO. The intravessical and rectal pressure lines are inserted but no filling catheter is used. The bladder is allowed to fill physiologically with urine. During this time the patient keeps a diary of symptoms and this is later compared with the subtracted cystometry. This test is thought to detect DO in up to 30% more women.

Further reading

Abrams P. *Urodynamics*, 2nd edn. Springer 1997.

Abrams P, Cardozo L, Fall M, *et al.* The standardization of terminology in lower urinary tract function. Neurourol Urodynam 2002;21:167–78.

Bump RC, Mattiasson A, Bø K, *et al.* The standardization of terminology of female pelvic organ prolapse and pelvic floor dysfunction. Am J Obstet Gynecol 1996;175:10–7.

Radley SC, Jones GL. Measuring quality of life in urogynaecology. Br J Obstet Gynaecol 2004;111:33–6.

Van Waalwijk van Doorn ES, Zwiers W, *et al.* A comparative study between standard and ambulant urodynamics. Neurourol Urodynam 1987;6:156.

Vaginal discharge

Vaginal discharge presents with or without irritation and has various causes.

Non-infective
- Physiological
- Cervical ectopy
- Foreign bodies
- Vulval dermatitis.

Non sexually transmitted: (caused by disturbance of normal vaginal flora)
- Bacterial vaginosis
- Candidiasis.

Sexually transmitted
- Chlamydia trachomatis
- Neisseria gonorrhoeae
- Trichomonas vaginalis.

Typical features
- Physiological: usually white, non-offensive, varies with menstrual cycle.
- Cervical ectopy: outgrowth of columnar cells from endocervix over the ectocervix causing a mucoid discharge.
- Vulval dermatitis: irritation often associated with a change in soaps, chemicals, washing powders.
- Foreign bodies: seen in children, history of retained foreign body, usually offensive smelling discharge.
- Bacterial vaginosis: 9% prevalence, profuse fishy smelling discharge, no itching or irritation. Typified by an overgrowth of anaerobic bacteria. Vagina and vulva appear normal and not inflamed.
- Candidiasis: 10% prevalence, thick white non-offensive discharge associated with vulval itching and irritation. Vagina and vulva appear red and inflamed on examination.
- *Chlamydia trachomatis*: prevalence 5–10% of women under 25 years of age. Usually asymptomatic in 80% of women but may present with a purulent vaginal discharge. Infection leads to a significant risk of developing pelvic inflammatory disease.
- *Neisseria gonorrhoeae*: prevalence is unknown, asymptomatic in 50% of women but may present with purulent vaginal discharge. May coexist in women with chlamydia and cause pelvic inflammatory disease.
- *Trichomonas vaginalis*: prevalence unknown. May be asymptomatic but often presents with a yellow offensive profuse frothy discharge associated with vaginal and vulval itching and irritation and dysuria.

Evaluation of patient with vaginal discharge

History
- Nature of discharge-colour, smell, consistency and presence or absence of vaginal irritation. If patient has pelvic pain and pyrexia, suspect pelvic inflammatory disease. Sexual history including new partners, high-risk partners, numerous partners, unprotected intercourse.

Examination
- A chaperone should be present during intimate examinations. Inspection to look at nature of discharge, vaginal and vulval inflammation. Abdominopelvic examination

to elicit pelvic tenderness or mass such as an abscess, cervical excitation indicative of pelvic inflammatory disease. Speculum examination to inspect cervix for an ectopy, cervical inflammation, purulent discharge.

Investigations
- Vaginal pH: vaginosis (pH>4.5), candidiasis (pH <4.5)
- High vaginal swab: identifies bacterial vaginosis, candidiasis and *Trichomonas vaginalis*
- Endocervical swab: *N. gonorrhoeae*
- Endocervical swab: DNA amplification test for chlamydia.
- DNA amplification techniques such as polymerase chain reaction to test for chlamydia.

Treatments
- Physiological: exclude pathological cause. Reassure patient that discharge is normal.
- Cervical ectopy: traditional treatment is cervical cautery allowing stratified squamous epithelium to grow in place of columnar epithelia.
- Vulval dermatitis: avoid using local irritants such as perfumed soaps and wipes and sprays. Vaginal douching should be avoided as this can predispose to bacterial vaginosis and candidiasis.
- Bacterial vaginosis: metronidazole 2 g single dose, then 400–500 mg twice daily for 5–7 days, intravaginal clindamycin cream (2%) once daily for 7 days or intravaginal metronidazole gel (0.75%) once daily for 5 days. Acidic gel may help reduce repeat infection.
- Candidiasis: vaginal imidazole available over the counter, or fluconazole 150 mg orally as a single dose. Recurrent candidiasis can be treated with extended regimes (not licensed) for 6 months. Regimes include fluconazole 100 mg weekly in a single dose for 6 months, clotrimazole vaginally 500 mg pessary in a single dose weekly for 6 months or itraconazole 400 mg orally in two divided doses monthly for 6 months.
- Chlamydia: doxycycline 100 mg twice daily for seven days or a single dose of azithromycin 1 g orally.
- Gonorrhoea: cefixime 400 mg as a single oral dose or a single dose of ceftriaxone 250 mg intramuscularly.
- Trichomonas vaginalis: single dose of Metronidazole 2 g orally or 400–500 mg twice daily for 5–7 days.
- A referral to genitourinary medicine and partner notification is appropriate in cases of sexually transmitted diseases.

Further reading

Bignell C. National guideline on the diagnosis and treatment of gonorrhoea in adults. Clinical Effectiveness group. British Association for Sexual Health and HIV. 2005.

British National Formulary, 56. Sept 2008.

Cook RL, Hutchison S, Ostergaard L, Braithwaite S, Ness RB. Systematic review: noninvasive testing for Chlamydia trachomatis and Neisseria gonorrhoeae. Ann Intern Med 2005;142:914–25.

Daniels D. Forster national guideline on the management of vulvovaginal candidiasis. G. Clinical Effectiveness group (British Association for Sexual Health and HIV). 2002.

FFPRHC and BASHH Guidance. The management of women of reproductive age attending non-genitourinary medicine settings complaining of vaginal discharge. J Fam Plann Reprod Health Care 2006;32:33–42.

Hay P. National guideline for the management of bacterial vaginosis. Clinical Effectiveness Group. British Association for Sexual Health and HIV. 2006.

Horner PJ, Boag F. National guideline for the management of genital tract infection with Chlamydia trachomatis. Clinical Effectiveness group. British Association for Sexual Health and HIV. 2006.

Sherrard J. National guideline on the management of Trichomonas vaginalis. Clinical Effectiveness group. British Association for Sexual Health and HIV. 2007.

Vesicovaginal fistulae

Introduction

A fistula may be defined as an abnormal communication between two or more epithelial surfaces. From a practical gynaecological point of view this means a communication between either uterus, cervix, or vagina with either the urinary tract or the bowel.

Aetiology

The true incidence of genitourinary fistulae in a given population is unknown. The aetiology may be varied but is usually in the gynaecological population is acquired rather than congenital

Obstetric

This is the commonest cause of fistulae in developing countries. These fistulae occur largely due to obstructed labour causing pressure necrosis and sloughing of the bladder, urethra, or bowel, or as a result of traumatic injury to the bladder at the time of delivery. Therefore this can happen at the time of Caesarean section, forceps delivery, craniotomy or symphisiotomy, or Gishiri. The vast majority of women who develop obstructed labour have associated fetal demise. Obstetric anal sphincter injury is associated with a 6% incidence of rectovaginal fistulae.

Surgical

The commonest cause for surgical fistulae is hysterectomy, and laparoscopic hysterectomy appears to be associated with a higher incidence than abdominal or vaginal hysterectomy. The more complicated the surgery, for example if there are adhesions, previous Caesarean section, or endometriosis or malignancy, the more likely a fistula is to arise. The experience of the surgeon is probably also a factor. Surgical fistulae may also arise after operations such as anterior or posterior repair (especially with the increasing use of mesh)or after urethral diverticulectomy or closure.

Radiation

Preoperative pelvic radiation increases the risk of postoperative fistula development. Radiation itself may be a cause of fistula.

Malignancy

Carcinoma of the cervix, vagina and rectum may present with a fistula and obviously treatment with surgery or radiotherapy can predispose to fistula.

Inflammatory bowel disease

This is the most significant cause of the intestinogenital fistulae in the UK. These usually present to the colorectal surgeons, and Crohn's disease is by far the most common cause.

Miscellaneous

This category includes infection, penetrating trauma, coital injury, infected pessary, or other foreign body or catheter-related injury.

Prevalence

It was suggested that the post-hysterectomy fistula rate is about 1 per 1300 operations in the UK. It is very difficult to give a true prevalence. In the developing world the estimated prevalence is 1–2 per 1000 deliveries. Fistula may be small or large and it is outside of the context of this article to discuss classifications.

Presentation

Fistulae between the urinary tract and the genital tract present with continuous and uncontrollable urinary leakage. This happens day and night. A small fistula may only leak intermittently and a large fistula may leak so much the woman's bladder will be constantly empty. A woman with vesicocervical or vesicouterine fistula may present with cyclical haematuria at the time of menstruation.

Classically fistulae present between 5 and 10 days after the causative injury and especially after direct surgical injury.

Urethrovaginal fistulae distal to the urethral sphincter mechanism may be asymptomatic and may not require treatment.

Rectovaginal fistulae may present with flatus passing through the vagina or faecal loss through the vagina.

Investigations

If the fistula is not obvious on clinical examination either under direct inspection with a Sims speculum, or in the case of rectovaginal on rectal examination then after excluding a urinary infection an intravesical dye test can be used. The author's preference is to use methylene blue through a catheter and to examine the vagina carefully. It is usually done in the lithotomy position. The author finds it much more useful than a 3 swab test.

IVU can be useful especially if the ureter is thought to be affected. It is also useful to know the position of the vesicovaginal fistula in relation to the ureter.

Careful examination with cystoscopy usually will allow the identification of a fistula. A small sound can be passed from the vaginal side and can be visualized in the bladder. Sometimes a fistula may be complex and have more than one opening. Again the position of the ureter, if it is close to the fistula would be noted and at the time of surgery a stent may need to be inserted.

Sigmoidoscopy and proctoscopy are used to identify fistulae especially if there is inflammatory bowel disease present.

Management

At an early stage for a urinary tract fistula not involving the ureter a urethral catheter may be inserted and a small fistula may close. A larger fistula will need time for the edges to slough off and heal before repair is attempted. Immediate repair is only appropriate if trauma is recognised within the first 24–48 hours. If infection is present then antibiotics should be used.

Preoperative care

If a woman has a large fistula, the vulval skin may be infected by ammoniacal dermatitis. Silicon barrier creams may be helpful. In developing countries it is important that the patient has appropriate nutrition to improve healing. Also in obstetric fistula there are associated with lower limb weakness, foot drop and limb contraction and physiotherapy may be useful.

Surgical management

In general principle it is best to wait till sloughing of the fistula has occurred and the edges are clean before repairing. This may take a variable length of time. Repairs which affect the urinary tract excluding ureteric fistulae can be performed either vaginally or abdominally.

Generally urologists use the abdominal route and may go directly retropubically through the bladder or trans peritoneally. The vaginal approach is associated with a far quicker recovery rate and should be the route of choice. In developing countries with larger fistulae many of the surgeons perform ureteric reimplantations through the vaginal route.

Infiltration with 1% xylocaine with 1:200000 adrenaline helps to separate the layers allowing dissection of the vagina from the underlying organ, whether it be bladder or rectum. The dissection should be such that closure is under no tension. Closure usually is undertaken in two layers with interrupted sutures usually Polyglactin 3 0 Then the vagina is closed over the repair under no tension. If the tissue is particularly poor then grafts can be interpositioned. From the vaginal side one can use either the Martius (labial fat pad) graft or bring a flap of pubococcygeus muscle across. For those using the abdominal route the omentum is often used.

Patients should be well hydrated prior to the procedure but it is the management of the bladder afterwards that is vital. Continuous bladder drainage should be ensured and the catheter should not be allowed to be blocked and therefore the catheter should be checked hourly.

In developing countries open drainage is carried out and often the patients are allowed to walk around with a bucket with the catheter draining constantly and given responsibility for their own catheter management. For surgical fistulae the author uses 14 days' catheterization whereas with obstetric fistulae in developing countries 21–42 days have been reported.

Results

For primary closure over 90% success rates are reported; however, the success rate falls if the surgery has to be repeated.

Complications include recurrence and the development of subsequent incontinence. Although this is largely thought to be stress incontinence, sometimes it is due to detrusor overactivity as the bladder has been empty for quite a long time and this may lead to a reduction in compliance and capacity. In most young women a period of bladder retraining with or without anticholinergics will resolve the overactivity and any stress incontinence may need to be treated subsequently.

Further reading

Hilton P. Fistulae. In: Shaw R, Soutter WP, Stanton SL (eds) *Gynaecology*. Elsevier science 2003: 835–56.

Vulval pain and pruritus

The vulva lies within the urogenital triangle extending to overlie the pubic symphysis and pubic bones. Embryologically it is a junctional zone derived from ectoderm, hind-gut endoderm, and mesoderm. The vulva consists of the mons pubis, the labia majora and minora, the vestibule of the vagina, the hymen, the Bartholin glands, the clitoris, and the external urethral orifice. The epidermis is a stratified squamous epithelium. Vulval pain may be acute or chronic. Idiopathic chronic vulval pain, soreness, or burning (but not itching) is called vulvodynia. Pruritus vulvae (itching of the female external genitalia) is a symptom and not a diagnosis, and when acute is often of infective aetiology but lichen sclerosis, a common non-infective condition, is a significant cause of long-term symptoms.

Vulval pain

Acute

- Infective: causes of acute pain include infected Bartholin's glands, infected sebaceous cysts, acute herpes simplex infections, occasionally other sexually transmitted diseases, candida, infected eczema, infected psoriasis, and conditions such as infected intertrigo (non-specific inflamed flexures common in the obese).
- Traumatic: these may be accidental, sexual, gynaecological, or surgical. Pain with sexual intercourse may be a feature of scarring with skin conditions including advanced lichen sclerosis (Fig.13.14.1).
- Non-infective cutaneous conditions of the vulva: several systemic conditions can lead to acute vulval pain including erosive lichen sclerosis, epidermolysis bullosa (Petersen, 1996), acrodermatitis enteropathica (Verburg, 1974), ulcerative colitis, Crohn's disease (Werlin 1992), lupus erythematosis, lichen planus, Behcet's syndrome (Wechsler and Piette 1992), fissuring of psoriatic vulval skin and neoplasia (e.g. Paget's disease and squamous cell carcinoma).
- Other causes include spinal nerve compression.

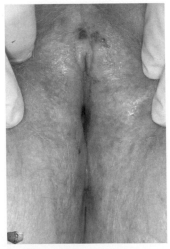

Fig. 13.14.1 Lichen sclerosis. This figure was published in Gynaecology, RW Shaw, WP Soutter and SL Stanton, Copyright Elsevier (2002) pp. 245–258.

Chronic

- Vulvodynia: the International Society for the Study of Vulvovaginal Disease (ISSVD) has defined vulvodynia as 'vulvar discomfort, most often described as burning pain, occurring in the absence of relevant visible findings or a specific, clinically identifiable, neurologic disorder'. It is not caused by infection (herpes, etc.), inflammation (lichen planus etc), neoplasia, or neurological disorders. Vulvodynia is therefore an idiopathic process. It is said to affect up to 18% of the female population and is generally regarded as an underdiagnosed difficult to treat gynaecological disorder (Gumus 2008). It is often accompanied by psychosexual problems. This is explained by two hypotheses: the presence of long-standing pain leading to the development of these problems (neuropathic hypothesis), or pre-existing distress leading to chronic vulval pain (somatic hypothesis) (Lynch 2008). It is a chronic pain lasting at least 3–6 months without an identifiable cause, i.e. a diagnosis of exclusion. However, recent work (Bowen 2008) has shown that 61% of women with a diagnosis of vulvodynia have a specific disease of the vulval skin identified by a dermatopathologist. The most common of these were lichen sclerosis, atopic dermatitis, and lichen planus. The 39% remaining had non-specific changes and hence were the true vulvodynias.
- Other causes include chronic forms of acute vulval pains listed above.

History and examination: key points

- Identify the duration of pain, past medical and surgical history, previous treatments, allergies, and sexual history, including sexually transmitted diseases.
- Examine all areas of the external genitalia ensuring that both the labia majora and labia minora are separated. Perform a vaginal examination if indicated. As vulval conditions may be manifestations of systemic disease, examine other body surfaces, scalp, nail, and oral mucosa. The diagnosis may be obvious elsewhere, e.g. lichen planus (mouth) and psoriasis (scalp).
- Demarcate the type and areas of pain with a cotton bud.
- Adequate lighting and exposure is crucial. Signs to look for include: erythema, lichenification, loss of architecture, ulceration, whiteness, discharge, and excoriation.

Special investigations

- Evaluate any vaginal discharge, e.g. with 10% potassium hydroxide for the bacterial vaginosis 'whiff test', take swabs as necessary for sexually transmitted diseases.
- Consider taking a small punch biopsy under local anaesthetic.

Treatment

Acute pain

General principles apply to most causes. Make a diagnosis and treat appropriately. Multidisciplinary working may be required with dermatologists.

Chronic pain

- Vulvodynia is a difficult condition to treat and multiple therapies have been tried all with varying degrees of success (Haefner 2005). As with all chronic pains a team of therapists including a gynaecologist, dermatologist, pain management physician, and psychologist is ideal, although expensive.

General measures
Suggestions include wearing cotton underwear during daytime and none at night, avoid vulval irritants (e.g. shampoo), clean the vulva with water alone and pat dry, apply a moisturizing emollient once clean and use adequate lubrication during intercourse.

Topical measures
Local anaesthetic preparations such as lidocaine ointment 5% or Emla cream may be used. Long-term 24-hour treatment may minimize feedback amplification of pain and allow healing. Simple petroleum jelly has been used as has topical oestrogen. One study showed low oestrogen receptor levels in women with vulvodynia (Eva 2003). Topical therapies of no proven benefit include corticosteroids, testosterone, and antifungals.

Oral therapy
Drugs used are often those utilized for any chronic pain syndrome. Oral tricyclic antidepressants are commonly used especially amitryptyline. A dose of 5–25 mg nightly increasing to a dose not exceeding150 mg daily can be used (Munday 2001). The anticonvulsant Gabapentin, starting at 300 mg orally for 3 days then increasing to 3600 mg maximum can be used as can carbamazepine (100 mg nocte increasing to a maximum of 400 mg twice daily) for refractory patients. The full therapeutic effect of oral therapies may not be apparent for weeks or months.

Other therapies
Biofeedback and physical therapy are important in vulvodynia. Physical therapy includes soft tissue mobilisation, myofascial release, trigger point pressure and electrical stimulation to alleviate pain caused by muscle spasm (Glazer 1995).

Surgery
Excision of the vulval vestibule is rarely performed and only in those who have failed other managements.

Pruritus vulvae

There are many causes of vulval itching.
- Vulval infections: these include bacterial boils, viral infections such as warts (papillomavirus), herpes simplex, molluscum contagiosum, fungal infections such as candida, tinea cruris (ringworm of the groin), pityriasis versicolor, and other infections including scabies (*Sarcoptes scabei*), pediculosis (*Phthirus pubis*, the crab louse).
- Vaginal discharge: including candidiasis, trichonomas vaginalis, and bacterial vaginosis.
- Vulval dystrophies: non-neoplastic includes lichen sclerosis, lichen planus, lichen simplex, eczema, and psoriasis. Neoplastic lesions include vulval intraepithelial neoplasia, Paget's disease of the vulva and occasional a squamous cell tumour.
- Ammoniacal dermatitis secondary to urinary incontinence
- Irritant dermatitis: reaction to detergents, perfume, bath oils, spermicides. Reactions to drugs.

- Psychological causes.
  History and examination are identical to that of vulval pain.

Differential diagnosis
This is often a challenge. One method is to make this on the basis of the vulval appearance (Black 2002).

Red rash
Tinea cruris, intertrigo, psoriasis, irritant dermatitis, allergic contact dermatitis, steroid rebound dermatitis, tinea versicolor.

White plaques
Lichen planus, lichen sclerosis, Paget's disease, vulval intraepithelial neoplasia (VIN).

Papules
VIN, condylomata acuminate, molluscum contagiosum, scabies.

Vaginitis
Bacterial vaginosis, trichomoniasis, candidiasis.
  Treatment will be guided by the diagnosis made.

Further reading.

Black M, McKay M. *Obstetric and gynecologic dermatology*, 2nd edn. 2002: 200.

Bowen AR, Vester A, Marsden L, *et al*. The role of vulvar skin biopsy in the evaluation of chronic vulvar pain. Am J Obstet Gynecol 2008;199:1–467e.6.

Eva LJ, MacLean AB, Reid WM, *et al*. Estrogen receptor expression in vulvar vestibuitis syndrome. Am J Obstet Gynecol 2003;189:458–61.

Glazer HI, Rodke G, Swencionis C, *et al*. Treatment of vulvar vestibulitis syndrome with electromyographic biofeedback of pelvic floor musculature. J Reprod Med 1995;40:283–90.

Gumus II, Sarifakiuglu E. Vulvodynia: case report and review of literature. Gyneco Obstet Invest 2008;65:155–61.

Haefner HK, Collins ME, Davis GD, *et al*. The vulvodynia guideline. J Lower Genital Tract Dis 2005;9:40–51.

Lynch PJ. Vulvodynia as a somatoform disorder. J Reprod Med 2008 53;391–6.

Munday PE. Response to treatment in dysaesthetic vulvodynia. J Obstet Gynecol 2001;40:283–90.

Petersen CS, Brooks K, Weissman K, *et al*. Pretibial epidermolysis bullosa with vulvar involvement. Acta Dermato-venerologica 1996;76:80–1.

Verburg DJ, Burd LI, Hoxtell EO, Merill LK. Acrodermatitis enteropathica in pregnancy. Obstet Gynecol 1974;44:233–7.

Wechsler B, Pietter JC. Behcets disease. BMJ 1992;304:1199–200.

Werlin SL, Esterly NB, *et al*. Crohns disease presenting as unilateral labial hypertrophy. J Acad Dermatol 1992;27:893–5.

Internet resources

International Society for the Study of Vulvovaginal Disease: www.issvd.org.

Patient resources

www.vulvalpainsociety.org/

Benign, premalignant, and malignant tumours in gynaecology

Cancer screening for women 640
Cervical cancer 644
Cervical dysplasia and human papillomavirus 648
Neoplastic conditions of the endometrium 652
Gestational trophoblastic neoplasia 658
Ovarian and fallopian tube cancer 664
Palliative care 670
Vulval cancer 676
Vulval intraepithelial neoplasia 682

Cancer screening for women

Screening for cancer in women must include both those cancers with disease presentations that are different in women and those that are unique for women. The spectrum of cancer screening and frequency are influenced by individual disease processes as well as individual risk factors. Ongoing care of women should include consideration of all cancer risk factors, modifiable behaviours, and available screening methods to reduce those risks (Ferley et al. 2004).

Wilson and Junger (1968) have outlined the criteria for the desirable characteristics of a successful screening programme. These are
- the condition should be important
- an accepted treatment must be available for the condition
- the facilities for diagnosis and treatment must be available
- a latent or early symptomatic stage must exist
- a sensitive and specific screening test must be available
- the test must be acceptable to the population
- the natural history of the condition must be understood
- an agreed treatment policy must exist
- the cost must be acceptable
- case finding must be a continuous process.

It is estimated that there will be increased incidence of gynaecological cancers over the next 5 years. The incidence of endometrial cancer will increase overall as a consequence of an ageing population, and an increasing problem of obesity. The incidence of cases of ovarian cancer, despite the use of the combined pill and hormone replacement therapy will increase due to the ageing population and more accurate assessment through the use of multidisciplinary working. Worldwide, cervical cancer remains an important disease and should be considered as the most preventable cancer through screening and in future through the use of prophylactic and therapeutic vaccines. The incidence of vulval cancer will increase due to the ageing population and due to the increased prevalence of infections with the oncogenic types of human papillomavirus (HPV). The introduction of the HPV vaccine is likely, in due course, to reduce the incidence of anogenital cancers.

Non-gynaecological cancers

Lung cancer screening
- No primary lung cancer screening is recommended, although low-dose computed tomography may benefit high-risk patients (Bach et al. 2007).
- Lung cancer remains the number one cause of cancer death overall worldwide for men and second or third for women. Primary prevention of lung cancer with smoking cessation is the ultimate goal. Women have trailed men in decreasing the rate of smoking, but are beginning to show an overall decline. In addition, women may be at risk because of secondary inhalation of smoke. At this point, routine yearly exams or computed tomography has not been shown to make a difference in early diagnosis or overall survival. Therefore, there is no screening recommendation for lung cancer in women.

Colon cancer screening
- The UK Bowel Screening Programme is currently being rolled out throughout the UK and will achieve nationwide coverage by 2009. The NHS Bowel Cancer Screening Programme offers screening every 2 years to all men and women aged 60–69.
- Colon cancer has wide geographic and ethnic variation in incidence. Family history has a major impact on the frequency of colon cancer screening. For women for whom there is a family history of familial polyposis or multiple colon cancers, with or without associated uterine and breast cancer, screening begins earlier than the recommended age of 50, and is likely to be more frequent. Screening in these patients should be full colonoscopy and managed in the context of overall screening for genetic predisposition to these cancers.
- Colonoscopy is preferred for women, given the higher incidence of right-sided lesions (Schoenfeld et al. 2005). The issues are the preparation required, the risks, and the lack of adequate access to trained health professionals. Faecal occult blood testing may have a role, but is both less sensitive and less specific than colonoscopy as a screening tool. Adequate use requires changing diet before testing to avoid false positives. It should be used with an additional evaluation. Sigmoidoscopy will miss right-sided lesions and has similar risks to colonoscopy, although technically easier.
- The use of computed tomography colonoscopy is still in the developmental stages and not appropriate at this time for standard screening.

Breast cancer screening
The NHS Breast Screening Programme provides breast screening every 3 years for all women in the UK between 50 and 70 years. Because the programme is a rolling one, every woman will receive an invitation for her first screening between her fiftieth and fifty-third birthday.

Breast cancer is the most common cause of cancer deaths for women worldwide (21% of cancer deaths for women). Access to and frequency of screening directly impact this statistic.

Family history also has a major impact on the frequency and type of breast cancer screening. In particular, women with a family history of >1 first-degree relative with breast cancer; or breast cancer in a first-degree relative before age 40; breast and ovarian cancer or independent bilateral breast cancer in the same woman; or multiple breast and ovarian cancers in the family all are at higher risk for the disease. In addition, an increased incidence of early age diagnosis of cancers in the family, such as colon cancer, may put women at higher risk. This risk requires assessment, often with genetic counselling, to determine the level of risk and the role that screening (versus other forms of cancer risk reduction such as medication or surgery) will play.

For women who are at higher risk for breast cancer, evaluation with magnetic resonance imaging (MRI), with or without concurrent mammogram, may be more sensitive and specific in the detection of early breast cancers. Ultrasound is used as an adjunct to further characterize lesions and is not used for primary screening.

Women who have had prior breast cancer should have more frequent screening depending on their overall risk for recurrence. For many of these patients, screening every 6 months may be recommended and for those at higher family risk, screening with MRI may be recommended for one of those intervals (DeMartini et al. 2008; Warner et al. 2008).

The use of clinical breast examinations has been widely promoted, but at present there is no evidence for efficacy as a sole method of screening, nor its use as an adjunct for screening. However, given the low cost and ability to pick up some lesions chronologically distant from mammographic screening, it remains generally encouraged.

Encouraging screening and assuring access to screening both make a substantial difference in early detection and overall survival with this disease. Any strategy to achieve a high participation rate is likely to result in improvements in participation and is encouraged (Bonfill et al. 2008).

Gynaecological cancers

Vulval cancer screening

In the UK there are no recommendations for vulval cancer screening for the general population.

Vulvar cancer is generally situated on the external labia majora and minora. As the most common forms of cancer in this region are squamous, close visual inspection forms the primary means of screening as with other epidermal cancers. There is no evidence that magnification of the skin with colposcopic equipment improves the overall screening outcomes.

Women at higher risk for development of these cancers, and therefore appropriate for annual screening include women with a history of cervical or vaginal dysplasia or cancer, women with high exposure to nicotine, or women with prior vulvar dysplasia or cancer. In addition, women with a history of chronic immune suppression are at higher risk. The invasive form of these cancers peaks in the 70s and 80s, therefore inspection of the vulvar areas in the 60s and beyond is warranted.

Vaginal cancer screening

There is no UK recommendation for vaginal cancer screening.

Screening may be indicated because of a past history of cervical dysplasia, cancer or prior exposure to DES (diethylstilbestrol).

Cervical cancer screening

- The NHS Cervical Screening Programme in England invites all women between the ages of 25 and 64 for a cervical screening test every 3–5 years. The new guidelines are
  - Under 25s: no screening
  - 25 years: first invitation
  - 25–49: 3 yearly
  - 50–64: 5 yearly
  - 65+: only screen those who have not been screened since aged 50 or have had recent abnormal tests.
- Cervical cancer is rare in women under the age of 25 years.
- The National Cervical Screening Programme in Scotland offers women aged 20–60 years a cervical smear every 3 years.
- In the UK, all cervical screening services have moved to liquid-based cytology (LBC) so reducing the number of inadequate smears.
- Worldwide, cervical cancer remains the number one cause of death from gynaecological cancer in underdeveloped countries with a quarter of a million deaths per year. Eighty-three per cent of the incidence and 86% of the mortality occurs in this population and the World Health Organization estimates that this will continue to rise by at least 10% if no actions are taken to prevent or screen and treat for this cancer. Given the development of both a prevention vaccine and effective screening

schemes, this is a cancer that has the potential for major reduction and virtual elimination in the future (Wright et al. 2007).
- The general recommendations for cervical cancer screening have changed based on the tight linkage to the presence of oncogenic subtypes of HPV. Recommendations for screening of women who received the HPV vaccine have not been formalized and should follow the standard guidelines until there is more clarity on the long-term success and correlates for disease with prior vaccination.
- Special efforts to recruit women from populations with limited screening and high cervical cancer incidence rates should be national concerns, as the incidence directly correlates with access to screening systems. Many alternative screening programs have been shown to have value in low resource settings and often combine rapid analysis of HPV, or visual inspection of the cervix with immediate treatment.
- HPV high risk subtype testing has become a standard component of triage of abnormal cytological results. Its use as a primary method of screening is in active research. Advantages include the rapidity of the testing, the potential for self-administration, and potentially a broader application to both resource rich and resource poor environments.

Uterine cancer screening

- There is no standard screening for uterine/endometrial cancer.
- The highest prevalence is in North America with age-standardized rates of around 15–18 per 100 000 and lowest in most of Africa and southeast Asia.
- Uterine cancer is generally a disease of women after the menopause for which less than 50% is detected on standard cervical cytology. There are potential pre-invasive forms of cancer that can be identified with endometrial sampling. An ultrasound scan and/or sampling of the endometrium is indicated in most circumstances of postmenopausal uterine bleeding as well as in select premenopausal patients with heavy, irregular bleeding to make a diagnosis of hyperplasia or cancer. Up to 25% of endometrial cancers occur in premenopausal women.
- The role of a 'screening' endometrial biopsy has been evaluated for tamoxifen, which is associated with an increased risk for endometrial cancer. To date, there is no evidence that routine screening endometrial biopsies results in greater detection or outcome differences in this population. Transvaginal uterine sonography also has a high false-positive rate and is not recommended as a screening methodology with tamoxifen.

Fallopian tube and ovarian cancer screening

- There is no evidence that screening with present modalities of ultrasound and CA125 impacts either diagnosis or outcome of ovarian or fallopian tube cancer in normal risk patients.
- The issue of whether a screening intervention might provide some protection for women at high risk for fallopian tube/ovarian/peritoneal cancer is as yet undetermined. The conventional standard of examination, ultrasound, and CA125 every 6 months for these patients who have not had risk reduction surgery has not been shown to make a difference in overall detection or outcome. The development of new serum markers, in combination with CA125 may offer an advance for the high-risk groups.

• The results of the ovarian cancer screening trial (UKCTOCS) will help to inform decisions regarding the implementation of an ovarian cancer screening programme. Public awareness of ovarian cancer is low and symptom screening may contribute to earlier diagnosis and treatment.

Further reading

Bach PB, Jett Jr, Pastorino U, *et al*. Computed tomography screening and lung cancer outcomes. JAMA 2007:279;953–61.

Bonfill X, Marzo M, Pladevall M, *et al*. Strategies for increasing the participation of women in community breast cancer screening. Cochrane Database Syst Rev 2008; 2:CD00075320.

DeMartiniW, Lehman C, Patridge S. Breast MRI for cancer detection and characterization: a review of evidence-based clinical applications. Acad Radiol 2008;15:408–16.

Ferley J, Bray F, Pisani P, Parkin DM. *GLOBOCAN 2002: cancer incidence, mortality and prevalence worldwide*. IARC CancerBAse No. 5, version 2.0. Lyon: IARC Press 2004.

Schoenfeld P, Cash B, Flood A, *et al*. Colonoscopic screening of average risk women for colorectal neoplasia. CONCCeRN Study Investigators. N Engl J Med 2005:352:2061–8.

Warner E, Messersmith H, Causer P, *et al*. Systematic Review: using magnetic resonance imaging to screen women at high risk for breast cancer. Ann Intern Med 2008;148:671–9.

Wilson JMG, Junger G. Principles and practice of screening for disease. Public Health Papers 34. Geneva: WHO 1968.

Wright TC, Massad SL, Dunton CJ, *et al*. 2006 consensus guidelines for the management of women with cervical intraepithelial neoplasia or adenocarcinoma in situ. Am J Obstet Gynecol 2007;197:340–5.

Internet resources

www.cancerscreening.nhs.uk/bowel/finalreport.pdf
www.cancerbackup.org.uk
www.isdscotland.org/isd/cancer
http://info.cancerresearchuk.org/cancerstats
www.eveappeal.org.uk/consensus

Cervical cancer

Introduction

- Carcinoma of the cervix uteri remains the second most common cancer in women under the age of 35 despite a well-established UK-wide screening programme for the detection of pre-invasive disease.
- There are over 2700 new cases of cervical cancer diagnosed per annum in the UK, and regrettably, almost 1000 women still die from this disease each year (Cancer Research UK).
- Screening will only detect 30% of women with cervical cancer with the majority of cases occurring in those outwith the current screening programme.

Risk factors

- Sexually active women are at risk of exposure to human papillomavirus (HPV). The aetiological association of HPV with genital disease is related most commonly to four subtypes which are 6, 11, 16, and 18. HPV subtypes 16 and 18 are attributed to 70% of cervical cancer cases.
- Early age at first intercourse, multiple sexual partners, oral contraceptives (some studies), cigarette smoking, low socioeconomic status, increased parity, family history, associated genital infections, and no circumcision in the male partner have also been documented as increasing the risk of developing cervical cancer.

Clinical staging

- Cervical cancer is clinically staged using the FIGO (International Federation of Gynaecology and Obstetrics) criteria and was updated in 2009. This is solely based on clinical examination and does not include findings obtained from imaging modalities such as computed tomography (CT), magnetic resonance imaging (MRI), or positron emission tomography (PET). Table 14.2.1 shows the complete FIGO staging system in detail.
- Current recommendations suggest that there is not sufficient evidence to advocate the use of sentinel node surgery in preference to pelvic lymphadenectomy to predict the tumour status of lymph nodes which are left in situ (SIGN 2008). Additionally, there is conflicting evidence regarding the average number of lymph nodes that should be attained during a surgical lymphadenectomy, and the exact relevance of this to long-term outcome in patients.

Clinical presentation

- Patients can present with common, non-specific symptoms and signs which must always be investigated appropriately (SIGN 2008). These can include intermenstrual bleeding (IMB), post-coital bleeding (PCB), postmenopausal bleeding (PMB), a clinically suspicious looking cervix, blood-stained vaginal discharge, or pelvic pain.
- Women with symptoms or signs such as those above are more likely to be diagnosed with an advanced stage cervical tumour.
- Premenopausal women with abnormal vaginal bleeding, and some postmenopausal women, when considered appropriate by clinicians, should be tested for *Chlamydia trachomatis* infection (SIGN 2008).
- There is no evidence that performing an unscheduled cervical screening smear outwith the programme is of any use (SIGN 2008).

Table 14.2.1 FIGO staging criteria

FIGO	Staging of the cervix uteri (2009)
Stage I	The carcinoma is strictly confined to the cervix (extension to the corpus would be disregarded)
IA	Invasive carcinoma which can be diagnosed only by microscopy, with deepest invasion ≤5 mm and largest extension ≥7 mm
IA1	Measured stromal invasion of ≤3.0 mm in depth and extension of ≤7 mm
IA2	Measured stromal invasion of >3.0 mm and not >5 mm with an extension of not >7 mm
IB	Clinically visible lesions limited to the cervix uteri or pre-clinical cancers greater than stage IA*
IB1	Clinically visible lesion ≤4.0 cm in greatest dimension
IB2	Clinically visible lesion >4.0 cm in greatest dimension
Stage II	Tumour invades beyond uterus, not to pelvic side wall or lower third vagina
IIA	No parametrial invasion
IIB	Parametrial invasion
Stage III	The tumour extends to the pelvic wall and/or involves lower third of the vagina and/or causes hydronephrosis or non-functioning kidney
IIIA	Tumour involves lower third of the vagina, with no extension to the pelvic wall
IIIB	Extension to the pelvic wall and/or hydronephrosis or non-functioning kidney[†]
Stage IV	The carcinoma has extended beyond the true pelvis or has involved (biopsy proven) the mucosa of the bladder or rectum. A bullous oedema, as such, does not permit a case to be allotted to Stage IV
IVA	Spread of the growth to adjacent organs
IVB	Spread to distant organs

*All macroscopically visible lesions, even with superficial invasion, are allotted to stage IB carcinomas. Invasion is limited to a measured stromal invasion with a maximal depth of 5.00 mm and a horizontal extension of not >7.00 mm. Depth of invasion should not be >5.00 mm taken from the base of the epithelium of the original tissue, superficial or glandular. The depth of the invasion should always be reported in mm, even in those cases with 'early (minimal) stromal invasion' (~1°mm). The involvement of vascular/lymphatic spaces should not change the stage allotment.
[†]On rectal examination, there is no cancer-free space between the tumour and the pelvic wall. All cases with hydronephrosis or non-functioning kidney are included, unless they are known to be due to another cause.

Pathological classification

- Cervical cancer is diagnosed by detailed histopathological examination of tumour biopsies. The World Health Organization (WHO) histological classification system is summarized in Table 14.2.2.
- Histopathology reports should feature essential criteria that can be used by multidisciplinary teams to categorize women into higher risk groups for metastatic disease which will require adjuvant treatment (Van de Putte et al. 2005). These criteria should include tumour type, size, extent of disease, which includes involvement of

Table 14.2.2 WHO histological classification, subtypes and examples of tumours of the cervix uteri

WHO classification	Subtype	Example
Epithelial	Squamous tumours and precursors	Squamous cell cancer
	Glandular tumours and precursors	Adenocarcinoma
	Other epithelial tumours	Adenosquamous
Mesenchymal/ tumour-like conditions		Leiomyosarcoma
Mixed epithelial and mesenchymal		Carcinosarcoma
Melanocytic		Malignant melanoma
Miscellaneous		Germ cell type
Lymphoid and haematopoetic		Lymphoma/leukaemia
Secondary		Various

vaginal wall or parametrium, depth of invasion, pattern of invasion (infiltrative or cohesive invasive front), lymphovascular space invasion (LVSI), status of resected margins (presence of tumour and distance from margin), status of lymph nodes (including site and number of nodes involved), and presence of pre-invasive disease if present (SIGN 2008).

Radiological staging

- It is essential that all patients with clinically visible, histologically proven cervical cancer undergo accurate radiological imaging. This is essential in planning further management of patients at time of initial diagnosis, relapse, and in the event of treatment complications. It has been reliably shown that MRI is more exact in this context than computed tomography imaging (accuracies 40–97%) (Hricak et al. 2005). MRI (including urinary tract and para-aortic nodes) is therefore the first choice of imaging modality in most patients. If MRI is contraindicated or in clinically evident FIGO Stage IV disease, a post-contrast spiral or multislice CT scan of chest, abdomen and pelvis is indicated (SIGN 2008).
- Patients who are considered inoperable (i.e. those more likely to have nodal/metastatic disease) should undergo a PET scan (SIGN 2008), as they may still be curable with chemoradiotherapy. There is evidence that PET scanning can accurately detect metastatic pelvic/para-aortic lymphadenopathy (sensitivities 75–100%) (Loft et al. 2007), which can importantly alter management and survival of patients.
- Investigation of bladder and bowel using cystoscopy and sigmoidoscopy is used if clinical staging or radiological imaging (CT/MRI) cannot omit metastatic spread to these organs.

Surgical management (non-fertility sparing)

- Surgical management of cervical cancer is becoming increasingly managed on an individual basis and should

be performed by an appropriately trained gynaecological surgeon.

- Surgery for early stage disease can allow preservation of ovarian function, avoiding early menopause. In addition less radical surgery will avoid shortening/fibrosis of the vagina which conserves sexual function in women.
- Standard treatment for FIGO IA1 disease has been simple hysterectomy, although fertility-sparing surgery should now be considered, as discussed below.
- Radical hysterectomy (RH) is recommended for FIGO IB1 disease and involves concurrent removal of uterus, cervix, parametrial tissues, and upper vagina (SIGN 2008). This is normally combined with a pelvic lymphadenectomy.
- RH is not recommended for those patients with tumour measuring >4 cm (i.e. >FIGO IB2), where the incidence of nodal metastasis is 36% compared with 6% (<2 cm tumour) (Hricak et al. 1996). There has been no difference shown in disease-free survival (DFS) or overall survival (OS) of patients with FIGO IB and IIA disease treated by RH or radical radiotherapy (Landoni et al. 1997).
- Pelvic lymphadenectomy should be performed along with simple hysterectomy if FIGO IA2 disease is present (SIGN 2008) where the risk of nodal metastasis is 3–6%, compared with ≤1% (FIGO IA1).
- Although LVSI is a prognostic indicator (see Pathological Classification), there is currently no good quality evidence supporting or refuting lymphadenectomy in FIGO IA1 disease with LVSI.
- Laparoscopic-vaginal radical hysterectomy (LVRH) is an alternative to standard RH although there are currently no randomized controlled trials (RCTs) comparing these. This technique should not be considered in those patients with tumour diameter >2 cm.

Fertility-sparing surgery

- Over the last decade, results from fertility-sparing surgery in younger women with cervical cancer have been encouraging. However, no RCTs have compared different methods of surgery for this (Dursun et al. 2007).
- In those women with early stage disease and no LVSI (FIGO IA1, IA2 or microscopic IB1), knife cone biopsy or large loop excision of the transformation zone (LLETZ) can be offered (SIGN 2008).
- A further uterine-sparing alternative to simple hysterectomy (FIGO IA2) or RH (FIGO IB1) is radical vaginal trachelectomy (RVT). This involves vaginal resection of the cervix, the upper 1–2 cm of vaginal cuff and the medial portions of the cardinal and uterosacral ligaments. The cervix is transected at the lower uterine segment and a prophylactic cerclage is placed at the time of surgery. If the tumour diameter is <2 cm and there is no LVSI, there does not appear to be an increased risk of recurrence with this more conservative approach (Dursun et al. 2007).
- These fertility-conserving measures should be combined with pelvic lymphadenectomy in FIGO IA2 or IB1.
- It is vitally important to counsel those women undergoing fertility-sparing surgery adequately, specifically in reference to the risk of recurrence of disease and pregnancy outcomes, including pregnancy loss and preterm delivery. Several studies have suggested a link between excisional surgery and risk of preterm birth (Sadler et al.

2004; Kyrgiou et al. 2006; Bruinsma et al. 2007). With some techniques, such as LLETZ, complications have been reported less often (Kyrgiou et al. 2006). Two linked studies have recently suggested that knife cone biopsy was associated with a significantly increased risk of preterm delivery, perinatal mortality and low birth weight babies <2000 g (Albrechtsen et al. 2008; Arbyn et al. 2008). This did not apply to LLETZ in this study, although this cannot be excluded. Data on pregnancy outcomes following RVT remains limited due to the current small number of procedures done.

Non-surgical management

- Patients with FIGO IB2-IVA cervical cancer who are deemed fit enough are offered treatment with combination chemoradiotherapy, as surgery is not appropriate due to the high risk of positive margins and nodal disease. Patients with positive nodes or margins following surgery should also be offered this, although there are no RCTs.
- Combination chemoradiotherapy (platinum-based compounds) is preferable as it shows an OS benefit of 52% versus 40% in those treated with radiation alone (Green et al. 2005).
- Brachytherapy, i.e. radiotherapy delivered directly to the target tissue via insertion of vaginal applicators, is a key component of the (chemo)radiotherapy part of treatment. External beam radiotherapy covers the entire pelvis.
- FIGO IVB should be offered palliative chemotherapy.

Complications and side effects of treatment

Surgery
- General complications including haemorrhage, infection (especially wound, urinary tract, chest, pelvic), visceral damage (bowel and bladder) and thromboembolism
- Lymphoedema
- Vaginal shortening
- Fistula formation
- Bladder and bowel dysfunction.

Chemoradiotherapy
- Anaemia: correction of haemoglobin is appropriate if <12 g/dL.
- Loss of ovarian function: HRT is recommended.
- Sexual dysfunction/vaginal stenosis: a vaginal stent/dilator therapy may prevent post-radiation induced complications.
- Radiation-induced skin desquamation/necrosis.
- Radiation-induced cystitis, haematuria, fistula formation, and ureteric obstruction.
- Radiation-induced proctitis, stricture, ulceration, and fistula formation.

Reducing morbidity
- Management of patients should involve a multidisciplinary team in a tertiary referral cancer centre.
- Healthcare professionals should be educated in recognising lymphoedema in either or both lower limbs which will allow prompt referral to a practitioner qualified in lymphodema management.
- Counselling, support and follow-up of women is required to improve compliance and success rates of vaginal dilators/stents, with the aim of reducing sexual morbidity.

Recognizing and managing recurrent cervical cancer

- Patients should be followed up on a 4 monthly basis for ≥2 years following treatment (SIGN 2008).
- History taking and clinical examination is important in the follow-up of patients. PET-CT is recommended 9 months following chemoradiotherapy (SIGN 2008).
- Cervical cytology or vault smears are not included in the long term follow-up of patients. However, those undergoing fertility-sparing techniques should have cervical smears at 6 months, 12 months, and annually for 4 years before future routine cervical surveillance is undertaken.
- Radiological imaging modalities in suspected recurrent disease should involve MRI or CT in first instance.
- In those who have a detectable recurrence on CT or MRI and who may be eligible for consideration of salvage therapy, a whole body PET scan or PET-CT is required.
- Salvage therapy can involve pelvic exenteration, palliative chemotherapy or other general palliative care measures. Exenteration should be considered in those women who have recurrent disease in the central pelvis following chemoradiotherapy. To minimise post-operative morbidity (40%) and mortality (less than 50% survive 5 years), a dedicated multiprofessional team should carry out the procedure.

Further reading

Albrechtsen S, Rasmussen S, Thoresen S, et al. Pregnancy outcome in women before and after cervical conisation: a population-based cohort study. BMJ 2008;337:803–5.

Arbyn M, Kyrgiou M, Simoens C, et al. Perinatal mortality and other severe adverse pregnancy outcomes associated with treatment of cervical intraepithelial neoplasia: meta-analysis. BMJ 2008;337:798–803.

Bruinsma F, Lumley J, Tan J, Quinn M. Precancerous changes in the cervix and risk of subsequent preterm birth. Br J Obstet Gynaecol 2007;114:70–80.

Cancer Research UK. UK Cervical Cancer incidence statistics. http://info.cancerresearchuk.org/cancerstats/types/cervix/incidence

Dursun P, LeBlanc E, Noqueira MC. Radical vaginal trachelectomy (Dargent's operation): a critical review of the literature. Eur J Surg Oncol 2007;33:933–41.

Green J, Kirwan J, Tierney J, et al. Concomitant chemotherapy and radiation therapy for cancer of the uterine cervix. Cochrane Database Syst Rev 2005;3.

Hricak H, Gatsonis C, Chi DS, et al. Role of imaging in pretreatment evaluation of early invasive cervical cancer: results of the intergroup study American College of Radiology Imaging Network 6651-Gynecologic Oncology Group 183. J Clin Oncol 2005;23:9329–37.

Hricak H, Yu KK. Radiology in invasive cervical cancer. AJR Am J Roentgenol 1996;167:1101–8.

Kyrgiou M, Koliopoulos G, Martin-Hirsch P, et al. Obstetric outcomes after conservative treatment for intraepithelial or early invasive cervical lesions: systematic review and meta-analysis. Lancet 2006;367:489–98.

Landoni F, Maneo A, Colombo A, et al. Randomised study of radical surgery versus radiotherapy for stage Ib-IIa cervical cancer. Lancet 1997;350:535–40.

Loft A, Berthelsen AK, Roed H, et al. The diagnostic value of PET/CT scanning in patients with cervical cancer: a prospective study. Gynecol Oncol 2007;106:29–34.

Sadler L, Saftlas A, Wang W, et al. Treatment for cervical interepithelial neoplasia and risk of preterm delivery. JAMA 2004;291:2100–6.

Scottish Intercollegiate Guidelines Network (SIGN). Management of Cervical Cancer 2008: www.sign.ac.uk/pdf/sign99.pdf

Van de Putte G, Lie AK, Vach W, *et al.* Risk grouping in stage IB squamous cell cervical carcinoma. Gynecol Oncol 2005;99:106–12.

Patient resources

Jo's Trust, Weedon Villa, Everdon, Northamptonshire, NN11 3BQ: www.jotrust.co.uk

British Society for Colposcopy and Cervical Pathology: www.bsccp. org.uk

Cancer Research UK: www.cancerhelp.org.uk

Tell Her: An Educational Website on Cervical Cancer and HPV: www.tellher.com

Cervical dysplasia and human papillomavirus

The cervix

- The cervix is composed of stroma, ectocervix and endocervix. The stroma is a mixture of fibrous, muscular and elastic tissue. The epithelium of the cervix is varied, being composed of non-keratinizing squamous epithelium and mucin-secreting columnar epithelium lining the ectocervix and endocervix respectively.
- The transformation zone (TZ), which evolves as columnar epithelium undergoes metaplasia to form squamous epithelium, is the area which exists between the original squamocolumnar junction (SCJ) and the new SCJ. This is the most common area for dysplastic lesions to develop. The TZ undergoes physiological metaplasia at different stages of development. The location of the TZ varies depending on age. In young women, the TZ is located on the outer surface of the immature cervix, whereas in menopausal women the TZ may recede into the endocervical canal, resulting in an unsatisfactory colposcopic examination.

Human papillomavirus and precursors of invasive cervical carcinoma

- Over the last 30 years, the association between human papillomavirus (HPV) and risk of anogenital cancers has been indisputably established (zur Hausen 2002). Cervical cancer resulting from exposure to the HPV remains a principal cause of death from cervical cancer worldwide.
- Invasive cervical carcinoma is preceded by a spectrum of well-defined precursor lesions (dysplastic changes) within the squamous epithelium, described as cervical intraepithelial neoplasia (CIN).
- Precursor lesions are graded CIN I–III and reflect a continuum of change. These can be generally grouped into low grade CIN I and high grade CIN II/III. Whether or when a lesion will become an invasive cancer is unknown; however, progression is more likely with higher grade CIN, which can be considered the requisite precursor to cervical cancer. Analysis has shown that approximately 30–40% of CIN III progress to invasive carcinoma if untreated (McIndoe et al. 1984). Table 14.3.1 illustrates the pathological differences between HPV and the varying degrees of cervical dysplasia.
- HPVs infect humans principally through sexual contact and complete an infectious cycle only in a fully differentiated keratinised squamous epithelium. Infection occurs via microtrauma to the epithelium. Approximately 100 types of HPV have been isolated which are grouped into low and high risk (i.e. oncogenic) categories associated with benign lesions (warts) and precancerous/cancerous lesions, respectively.
- Ninety per cent of genital warts are due to predominantly HPV 6 and 11, which are considered low risk. Oncogenic high-risk HPVs isolated in the genital tract most commonly are HPV 16, which along with HPV 18, and close relatives including HPV 31 and HPV 33, are the cause of cervical cancer. In fact, in approximately 80% of CIN II/III biopsies and 99% of biopsies taken from invasive cervical carcinoma (Smith et al. 2007), high-risk HPV DNA sequences can be isolated.
- The natural history of CIN and HPV, in effect, mirror one another. Young sexually active people are at high

Table 14.3.1 Colposcopic and pathological features of low and high-grade lesions

Feature	Low grade (CIN I)	High grade (CINII/III)
Colposcopic features		
Surface of lesion	Smooth	Smooth, raised, peeling
Border	Irregular outer	Sharp outer
Acetowhite test	Mild, appears slowly, disappears quickly	Dense, appears quickly, disappears slowly
Punctation	Fine	Coarse
Mosaic	Fine and regular	Coarse, Irregular
Pathological features		
Nuclear enlargement	Mild enlargement	Gross enlargement
Nuclear:cytoplasmic ratio	Mild increase	Gross increase
Nuclear pleomorphism	Mild degree	Moderate (CINII)/ severe degree (CINIII)
Abnormal mitoses within epithelium	Extends to basal third only	Extends to middle third (CINII)/all levels (CINIII)

risk of acquiring HPV infection. The lifetime risk of acquiring a genital infection with HPV is approximately 80%, with most infections resolving without clinical manifestations or a serological antibody response (Walboomers et al. 1999).

- When a low-risk lesion develops, i.e. CIN I, this represents the infectious cycle of HPV. Ten per cent of women will not clear the virus and develop persistent HPV infection with a strong cell-mediated immune response. Those with high-risk HPVs will carry a risk of progression to CIN II/III, and thereafter a significant risk of development of invasive carcinoma. However, many women who acquire HPV infection will not progress to cervical cancer, and therefore other cofactors may affect the risk (Muñoz et al. 2006), as shown in Table 14.3.2.

Cervical screening

- The UK National Health Service Cervical Screening call and recall Programme (NHSCSP) was established in the late 1980s and has successfully aided prevention of cervical cancer, saving approximately 5000 lives per year in the UK (Peto et al. 2004).
- The NHSCSP permits early detection, treatment and follow-up of precancerous changes of the cervix. The success behind the programme relies on the efficient call, recall and tracking of women, the use of quality assurance tools, a multidisciplinary approach to diagnosis and treatment, accredited training of clinicians and the widespread use of national clinical guidelines.

Table 14.3.2 Definite and potential cofactors affecting risk of cervical HPV carcinogenesis

Definite cofactors	Potential cofactors
Smoking	Genetic susceptibility
Long-term use of oral contraceptives	Sexually transmitted diseases including co-infection with hsv-2 or *Chlamydia trachomatis*
Co-infection with HIV	Immune response
High parity	Poor diet, malnutrition
	Use of intrauterine device

- Limitations to the programme do exist, including the inability to prevent or treat HPV by the programme, and the fact that some women will develop a malignant lesion of the cervix despite regular screening. False-positive/negative results are foreseeable due to the subjective nature of identification of abnormal cells and potential poor quality of samples.

- Quality has however improved since the introduction of liquid-based cytology (LBC), with a clear reduction in reported inadequate smears. Other suggested advantages of LBC versus conventional Pap smear tests include a more homogeneous sample collection, increased sensitivity and specificity and more efficient laboratory handling. LBC produces an enriched cellular sample with excellent preservation which is the ideal platform for ancillary tests and future molecular profiling studies.

- Cervical screening intervals have been standardized. In England and Wales, invitations are sent on a 3 yearly basis to women aged 25–49 years and 5 yearly to those aged 50–64 years (NHS Cervical Screening Programme). The lower age for first invitation to screening in Scotland is 20 years.

- The current geographical disparity between the lower ages to commence screening has raised several issues. The advantage of not screening women <25 years is the avoidance of detecting and potentially treating low grade lesions secondary to HPV exposure which will be transient and inevitably clear spontaneously. However, there is the disadvantage of potentially delaying treatment of high grade CIN and early screen-detected cancers in younger women. Of concern, it has been shown that CIN III prevalence has increased in women aged 20–24 years (19% in 2002, compared with 10% in 1986), which may be explained by both increased sexual activity and prevalence of sexually transmitted infections which expose younger women to high-risk HPVs (Wellings et al. 2001). Additionally, approximately 16% of CIN I lesions will evolve into high grade CIN after ≤2 years follow up (Holowaty et al. 1999).

- There is a worrying declining trend in screening uptake in younger women between 25–39 years, with average coverage rates being approximately 80% (NHS Screening Programme 2006–7). This threatens to increase the incidence of cervical carcinoma in future years. This may be due to multiple factors including lack of awareness of the potential for disease itself, which may be blamed on the overall success of the screening programme. Additionally, many women now delay having a family and this may lead to embarrassment and fear of an intimate

examination. The introduction of the HPV vaccination (see below) may also threaten public perception of risk by false claims in the media that this itself will protect them from the disease without the need to continue with routine screening.

Colposcopic features and treatment of cervical dysplasia

- Colposcopy is a diagnostic tool which uses magnification and illumination to visualize the cervix. Application of acetic acid to the cervix will highlight cells with high nuclear–cytoplasmic ratios, such as high grade CIN, because the nucleus obstructs light transmission. High grade cervical dysplasia appears more opaque or 'acetowhite'. Severity of lesion is linked with distinct demarcation, increased vascularity, dense acetowhite change, and characteristic proliferation of the microvasculature (punctuation or mosaicism). Colposcopic features of low and high grade CIN are shown in Table 14.3.1.

- Cervical dysplasia should be treated when there is a reasonable expectation that, if untreated, the patient will run the risk of subsequent development of cervical carcinoma. The likelihood of resolution of that lesion and the risk associated with treating the patient must be taken into account.

- The majority of low-grade lesions (CIN I) will regress spontaneously and do not require any treatment following a period of colposcopic observation.

- High grade lesions (CIN II/III) are at risk of progression to invasive disease if untreated (McIndoe et al. 1984), and should therefore be managed with ablative or excisional methods of treatment. However, high-grade lesions diagnosed in pregnancy may be followed up conservatively until delivery. Ablative treatment is only feasible if the lesion is visualized in its entirety at colposcopy and there is biopsy-confirmed pre-invasive disease with no glandular abnormality or microinvasive element. Ablation includes the use of cryotherapy, cold coagulation, electrocautery and carbon dioxide laser vaporization. The most commonly used excisional technique is LLETZ (large loop excision of the transformation zone). These procedures can be performed in an outpatient setting under local anaesthetic.

- A policy of 'see and treat', i.e. look and LLETZ, has become more common in recent years. This is performed on those lesions considered high grade, but without actual histological confirmation of this.

- Patients should undergo cytological evaluation at 6 and 12 months following surgical treatment of CIN. Annual smears should continue thereafter for a minimum of 5 years before a return to the normal screening programme.

HPV testing: when, how and why?

- A Health Technology Assessment review has concluded that HPV testing cannot currently be recommended for primary screening without further research.

- Current evidence does, however, support limited introduction of the test in order to improve the management of women with cytological samples showing borderline nuclear abnormality (BNA) or mild dyskaryosis.

- There remains uncertainty about the negative predictive value of an HPV test in the presence of persistent mild dyskaryosis and the safety associated with reduced surveillance of patients. This aspect has been evaluated in pilot studies.

- TOMBOLA (Trial of Management of Borderline and Other Low grade Abnormal smears) is a randomized controlled trial that determines both the most effective and efficient management options for women whose cervical smear tests indicate low grade CIN, incorporating the role of HPV testing for triaging these women. Clinical, economic and psychosocial outcomes have been determined in early studies. In contrast, most previous studies had looked at high grade abnormalities. Initial results from TOMBOLA suggest that women with a negative HPV test following a BNA smear result may not require referral for colposcopy. HPV risk was increased in non-white women, smokers and those using hormonal contraceptive measures.

- ARTISTIC (A Randomised Trial of HPV Testing in Primary Cervical Screening) aims to examine whether HPV testing will add effectiveness to the current cervical screening programme. Preliminary results (Kitchener et al. 2006) suggested that HPV testing has potential as a primary screening test in future practice but this would lead to a significant increase in retesting and referral rates.

- It has recently been shown that HPV testing may be a more accurate assessment of 'test of cure' following treatment for CIN than current colposcopy and/or cytology methods (Kitchener et al. 2008). Data suggest that those women who are both cytology negative and HPV negative at 6 months after treatment for CIN can be returned to routine 3 year follow-up.

- Overall, the introduction of HPV testing to triage women could facilitate a reduction in referral to colposcopy, length of follow-up following treatment of CIN, overall cost to the NHS and, importantly, anxiety for women.

Psychological sequelae of cervical screening and HPV testing

- Screening, abnormal smears and treatment of dysplastic changes of the cervix are well documented causes of anxiety and psychosexual dysfunction amongst affected women, with no correlation shown between grade of abnormality and levels of anxiety (Gray et al. 2006).

- More recently, a number of studies using well validated psychological tools have addressed reactions to being informed of a positive HPV infection (Maissi et al. 2004). The highest level of anxiety has been shown to be amongst those women with abnormal cytology and a positive HPV test compared to those with a negative HPV result. However, women with a positive HPV test but negative cytology show similar scores.

- It is imperative to continue to increase awareness of the possibility and consequences of HPV infection through educational resources in younger people.

HPV vaccines

- Screening tests are a means of detecting abnormalities within cells at an early stage, but the solution to any viral disease is a vaccine.

- Developing an attenuated HPV vaccine has been hampered by the lack of an effective culture system, but this has been solved by the production of virus-like particles (VLPs) which are structurally like a virus but essentially harmless due to a lack of DNA (Schiller et al. 2000).

- Two VLP-based prophylactic vaccines have proven to be extremely effective in clinical trials. Gardasil is a quadrivalent vaccine containing all four HPV types and is protective against genital warts (HPV 6 and 11) as well as cervical cancer (HPV 16 and 18). Cervarix is a bivalent vaccine which contains HPV 16 and 18, targeting cervical cancer. Clinical trials have shown that Gardasil and Cervarix are 100% effective in preventing infection with HPV 16 and 18 for 5 years and 4.5 years respectively. Both vaccines result in significantly higher antibody titres than those produced by natural infection (Harper et al. 2006; Villa et al. 2006). There is also preliminary evidence of cross-protection from vaccination against HPV 31 and 45 (Harper et al. 2006).

- The UK NHS HPV vaccination programme commenced in September 2008. The bivalent vaccine (Cervarix) will be used. This involves the offer of immunisation of all girls 12–13 years in a phased programme involving schools and local NHS services, with a 2 years catch-up programme commencing in 2009 for girls up to, but not including, 18 years old. There are no plans to immunise boys against HPV.

- Future research must focus on the exact degree of cross-protection against other HPV types and the effect of this vaccine on preventing high grade CIN. It may be envisaged that eventually the vaccination programme may affect the delivery of the current screening programme. However, as the vaccination programme currently will only be protective against 70% of cervical cancers, neither will replace one another and both will remain vital for the foreseeable future.

Further reading

Gray NM, Sharp L, Cotton SC, et al. Psychological effects of a low-grade abnormal cervical smear test result: anxiety and associated factors. Br J Cancer 2006;94:1253–62.

Harper DM, Franco EL, Wheeler CM, et al. Sustained efficacy up to 4.5 years of a bivalent L1 virus-like particle vaccine against human papillomavirus types 16 and 18: follow-up from randomised control trial. Lancet 2006;367:1247–55.

Holowaty P, Miller AB, Rohan T, To T. Natural history of dysplasia of the uterine cervix. J Natl Cancer Inst 1999;91:252–8.

Kitchener HC, Almonte M, Wheeler P, et al. HPV testing in routine cervical screening: cross sectional data from the ARTISTIC trial. Br J Cancer 2006;95:56–61.

Kitchener HC, Walker PG, Nelson L, et al. HPV testing as an adjunct to cytology in the follow up of women treated for cervical intraepithelial neoplasia. Br J Obstet Gynaecol 2008;115:1001–7.

McIndoe WA, McLean MR, Jones RW, Mullins PR. The invasive potential of carcinoma in situ of the cervix. Obstet Gynecol 1984;64:451–8.

Maissi E, Marteau TM, Hankins M, et al. Psychological impact of human papillomavirus testing in women with borderline or mildly dyskaryotic cervical smear test results: cross sectional questionnaire study. BMJ 2004;328:1293.

Muñoz N, Castellsague X, Barrington de Gonzalez A, Grissmann L. HPV in the etiology of human cancer. Vaccine 2006;24(Suppl 3):S1–10.

National Health Service. Cervical screening programme, England, 2006–7. NHS Health and Social Care Information Centre, Statistical Bulletin: wwwicnhsuk/statistics-and-data-collections/screening/cervical-cancer/cervical-screening-programme-2006-07-%5Bns%5D

Peto J, Gilham C, Fletcher O, Matthews FE. The cervical cancer epidemic that screening has prevented in the UK. Lancet 2004;364:249–56.

Schiller JT, Lowy DR. Papillomavirus-like particle vaccines. J Natl Cancer Inst Monogr 2000;28:50–4.

Smith JS, Lindsay L, Hoots B, et al. Human papillomavirus type distribution in invasive cervical cancer and high-grade cervical lesions: a meta-analysis update. Int J Cancer 2007;121:621–32.

Villa LL, Costa RLR, Petta CA, Andrade RP, et al. High sustained efficacy of a prophylactic quadrivalent human papillomavirus types 6/11/16/18 L1 virus-like particle vaccine through 5 years of follow up. Br J Cancer 2006;95:1459–66.

Walboomers JMM, Jacobs MV, Manos MM, et al. Human papillomavirus is a necessary cause of invasive cervical cancer worldwide. J Pathol 1999;189:12–19.

Wellings K, Nanchahal K, Macdowell W, et al. Sexual behaviour in Britain: early heterosexual experience. Lancet 2001; 358:1843–50.

zur Hausen H. Papillomaviruses and cancer: from basic studies to clinical application. Nat Rev Cancer 2002;2:342–50.

Patient resources

www.fightcervicalcancer.org.uk

Jo's Trust, Weedon Villa, Everdon, Northamptonshire, NN11 3BQ: www.jotrust.co.uk

British Society for Colposcopy and Cervical Pathology www.bsccp.org.uk

Cancer Research UK: www.cancerhelp.org.uk

Tell Her: An Educational Website on Cervical Cancer and HPV: www.tellher.com

Neoplastic conditions of the endometrium

Endometrial cancer is rising in incidence in the developed world, in association with rising obesity levels. Oestrogens are powerful stimulants of endometrial proliferation, and a 'premalignant' condition, endometrial hyperplasia, is well described. Endometrial hyperplasia may precede, or coexist with, endometrial cancer. Endometrial hyperplasia is further subdivided by WHO classification into simple and complex hyperplasia, and the management of this condition is discussed below.

Although more common in postmenopausal women, up to 25% of cases of endometrial cancer occur in premenopausal women. The majority of cases are endometrioid adenocarcinomas, and a common presenting symptom is postmenopausal bleeding. Further investigation with ultrasound/endometrial sampling is indicated in patients with postmenopausal bleeding to exclude endometrial hyperplasia/cancer. The majority of endometrial cancers are diagnosed at an early stage following presentation and investigation.

The mainstay of treatment for endometrial cancer remains surgery in the form of total abdominal hysterectomy and bilateral salpingo-ophorectomy. FIGO staging for endometrial cancer was revised in 1988 to become a surgical staging, including pelvic lymph node status. In recent years, the value of routine lymphadenectomy has been questioned.

Overall 5 year survival for all stages of endometrial carcinoma is 86%, with 97% for disease confined to the uterus.

Following surgery, adjuvant radiotherapy may be considered for patients at high risk of local relapse.

The role of chemotherapy in endometrial cancer has yet to be adequately defined.

Epidemiology

There is considerable geographic variation in the rates of endometrial cancer (Table 14.4.1).
- Endometrial cancer occurs most commonly in postmenopausal women, with 90% of cases occurring in women over the age of 50
- Women under 50 are an important group who may present with irregular menstrual bleeding, and investigation to rule out endometrial cancer in this group should be considered.
- A further important 5% of cases occur in women under 40. In these patients polycystic ovarian syndrome and genetic cancer predisposition due to Hereditary Non Polyposis Colon Cancer (HNPCC) may result in the development of endometrial cancer.

Table 14.4.1 Age-standardized incidence rate (per 100 000) for endometrial cancer

North America	22
East Asia	2.5
South/Central Asia	2.3
Central/Eastern Europe	11.8
Northern Europe	12.6

Figures produced with permission from IARC.

A number of risk factors for endometrial cancer have been identified:
- Obesity: a body mass index of greater than 29 is associated with a threefold increased risk of endometrial cancer.
- Polycystic ovarian syndrome: the anovulatory cycles lead to unopposed oestrogen stimulation of the endometrium.
- Parity: epidemiological evidence suggests that parous women have a decreased risk of developing endometrial cancer, with the first pregnancy associated with the maximum protective effect.
- Unopposed oestrogen hormone replacement therapy (HRT): the risk of endometrial hyperplasia and endometrial cancer in patients taking unopposed oestrogen HRT is well described, with an increased relative risk of around 2.7 for unopposed oestrogen HRT compared with HRT with progestogen added for at least 10 days per month.
- Anti-oestrogens: the selective oestrogen receptor modulator Tamoxifen is widely used in the treatment of breast cancer. Tamoxifen blocks the effect of oestrogen on breast tissue but has a stimulatory effect on the endometrium. The relative risk of endometrial cancer for patients using Tamoxifen for 5 years is 2.0.
- Feminizing ovarian tumours: although very rare, oestrogen secretion from ovarian tumours such as granulosa cell tumours can cause endometrial hyperplasia and cancer.
- Family history: HNPCC is a cancer susceptibility syndrome caused by a germline mutation in one of the DNA mismatch repair genes. Those with mutations have an increased risk of endometrial and ovarian cancer in addition to their risk of nonpolyposis colon cancer (Sonada et al. 2006). Consideration should be given to this syndrome in young patients presenting with either endometrial or non-polyposis colon cancer.

Aetiology

Bohkman proposed a new classification for endometrial cancer into Types I and II in 1983.

Type I endometrial cancer:
- predominates, accounting for more than 80% of cases
- is associated with oestrogenic stimulation of the endometrium
- is often associated with endometrial hyperplasia
- histologically is usually Grade 1 to 2 endometrioid adenocarcinoma
- is associated with mutations in the PTEN tumour suppression gene

Type II endometrial cancer:
- includes serous, clear cell, carcinosarcoma, small cell and other rare subtypes
- is associated with a higher risk of metastatic disease
- is not associated with oestrogenic stimulation of the endometrium
- is associated with mutations in the p53 tumour suppression gene

The risk factors for endometrial hyperplasia, and therefore Type 1 endometrial cancer, are linked to oestrogenic stimulation of the endometrium and have been outlined above.

Pathology

The pathology of endometrial hyperplasia, endometrial carcinoma and smooth muscle tumours is considered below:

Endometrial hyperplasia

- Defined as an increase in the ratio of endometrial glands to stroma greater than one to one.
- Endometrial hyperplasia is divided into simple and complex hyperplasia.
- Hyperplasia is further subdivided depending upon the presence or absence of cellular atypia.
- Although simple hyperplasia can often be differentiated from complex in view of the gland to stroma ratio (may be up to three to one in complex hyperplasia), the distinction between complex hyperplasia with atypia and G1 endometrial cancer can be difficult.

Type 1 endometrial carcinoma (80% of cases)

- Endometrioid adenocarcinoma.
- Usually G1 or G2, arising on a background of endometrial hyperplasia.
  Characterized histologically (according to FIGO system) as
- G1: well-formed glands with less than 5% solid non-squamous areas.
- G2: well-formed glands with between 6% and 50% solid non-squamous areas.
- G3: well-formed glands with more than 50% solid non-squamous areas.
  Other features such as degree of cytological atypia and infiltrative growth pattern may increase the grading to G3 (high grade).

Type 2 endometrial carcinoma (10% of cases)

- These tumours are all designated high grade.
- Serous, clear cell, mixed (adenosquamous) and small cell carcinomas form the majority of Type 2 carcinomas.
- Serous and clear cell subtypes are the most common.
- These subtypes may be found in association with high-grade endometrioid elements in a tumour.
- Ten per cent of the volume of the tumour should consist of serous or clear cell elements to allow classification of the tumour as serous or clear cell.
- Serous tumours frequently metastasize to the omentum and/or paraaortic lymph nodes.

Smooth muscle tumours

Smooth muscle tumours of the uterus range from the very common benign leiomyoma (fibroid) to sarcomas such as leiomyosarcoma or carcinosarcoma.

- Known also as malignant mixed Müllerian tumours (MMMT), carcinosarcoma, together with leiomyosarcoma, account for the majority of malignant smooth muscle tumours.
- Malignant uterine tumours account for under 5% of the total.
- The aetiology of these malignant tumours remains controversial.
- Of all patients with fibroids, less than 1% will have a leiomyosarcoma. Clinical suspicion of the diagnosis should be raised if a patient has a rapidly enlarging fibroid.
- Also included in this group of tumours are variants with an uncertain malignant potential (smooth muscle tumour of uncertain malignant potential (STUMP)).

- Histological categorisation of these intermediate risk groups of smooth muscle tumours may require specialist histology review.
- It has been suggested that factors such as obesity, oestrogen stimulation and nulliparity increase the risk of MMMT.
- There is a risk of both local and distant recurrence with leiomyosarcoma and MMMT, with lung metastases occurring frequently.

Staging

The staging of endometrial cancer is surgical following the 1988 FIGO classification, and updated in 2009 (Tables 14.4.2 and 14.4.3).

In cases unsuitable for surgery the FIGO clinical staging system of 1971 can be used.

Clinical approach

Endometrial hyperplasia

Presentation

- Endometrial hyperplasia may be asymptomatic and be detected incidentally following either a pelvic ultrasound or cervical smear (reported as glandular neoplasia).
- Postmenopausal bleeding is associated with endometrial hyperplasia in 15% of cases.
- Premenopausal bleeding irregularities leading to a diagnosis of endometrial hyperplasia may occur in patients with risk factors such as obesity, polycystic ovarian syndrome or Tamoxifen use as discussed above.

Table 14.4.2 FIGO staging for carcinoma of the corpus uteri (2009)

Stage I*	Tumour confined to the corpus uteri
IA*	No or less than half myometrial invasion
IB*	Invasion equal to or more than half of the myometrium
Stage II*	Tumour invades cervical stroma, but does not extend beyond the uterus[†]
Stage III*	Local and/or regional spread of the tumour
IIIA*	Tumour invades the serosa of the corpus uteri and/or adnexae[‡]
IIIB*	Vaginal and/or parametrial involvement[‡]
IIIC*	Metastases to pelvic and/or para-aortic lymph nodes[‡]
IIIC1*	Positive pelvic nodes
IIIC2*	Positive para-aortic lymph nodes with or without positive pelvic lymph nodes
Stage IV*	Tumour invades bladder and/or bowel mucosa, and/or distant metastases
IVA*	Tumour invasion of bladder and/or bowel mucosa
IVB*	Distant metastases, including intra-abdominal metastases and/or inguinal lymph nodes

*Either G1, G2 or G3.
[†]Endocervical glandular involvement only should be considered as Stage I and no longer as Stage II.
[‡]Positive cytology has to be reported separately without changing the stage.

Table 14.4.3 FIGO staging for uterine sarcomas (2009)

1 Leiomyosarcomas

Stage I	Tumour limited to uterus
IA	Less than 5 cm
IB	Greater than 5 cm
Stage II	Tumour extends to the pelvis
IIA	Adnexal involvement
IIB	Tumour extends to extrauterine pelvic tissue
Stage III	Tumour invades abdominal tissues (not just protruding into the abdomen)
IIIA	One site
IIIB	More than one site
IIIC	Metastasis to pelvic and/or para-aortic lymph nodes
Stage IV	Tumour invades bladder and/or rectum
IVA	Distant metastasis
IVB	

2 Endometrial stromal sarcomas (ESS) and adenosarcomas*

Stage I	Tumour limited to uterus
IA	Tumour limited to endometrium/endocervix with no myometrial invasion
IB	Less than or equal to half myometrial invasion
IC	More than half myometrial invasion
Stage II	Tumour extends to the pelvis
IIA	Adnexal involvement
IIB	Tumour extends to extrauterine pelvic tissue
Stage III	Tumour invades abdominal tissues (not just protruding into the abdomen)
IIIA	One site
IIIB	More than one site
IIIC	Metastasis to pelvic and/or para-aortic lymph nodes
Stage IV	
IVA	Tumour invades and/or rectum
IVB	Distant metastasis

3 Carcinosarcomas

Carcinosarcomas should be staged as carcinomas of the endometrium

*Simultaneous tumours of the uterine corpus and ovary/pelvis in association with ovarian/pelvic endometriosis should be classified as independent primary tumours.

The investigation of patients with postmenopausal bleeding or irregular bleeding in patients with risk factors for endometrial hyperplasia is described below.

The management of endometrial hyperplasia is primarily determined by the histological finding of cellular atypia in the endometrial biopsy.

- Endometrial hyperplasia without cellular atypia is associated with a low risk of progression to malignancy and treatment with progestogens is appropriate.
- Following initial treatment it is recommended that histological proof of regression to normal endometrial histology is obtained at 3–6 months.
- If this has not been achieved, consideration may be given to increasing the dose of progestogen or to hysterectomy.
- There is controversy about the optimum follow up regimen for patients treated in this way, but some authors advocate an annual assessment of the endometrium.
- The risk of coexisting malignancy in patients with endometrial hyperplasia with cellular atypia is commonly quoted as 20–25%, but at least one study found the risk to be as high as 50%.
- In this group, hysterectomy is recommended. In some cases, for example young patients wishing to retain fertility, treatment with progestogen has been used. Careful assessment of response is essential in this group. Patients should be warned of:
- Low pregnancy rates in studies of conservative management of endometrial hyperplasia/early endometrial cancer (15–30%)
- the significant risk of persistence or progression of the endometrial changes (20–50%)

Endometrial cancer

Symptoms of endometrial cancer
Postmenopausal bleeding is the most common presenting symptom in patients with endometrial cancer.

The clinical approach to diagnosis is based on the fact that 90% of patients with endometrial cancer are diagnosed over the age of 50, and up to 10% of patients with postmenopausal bleeding have an underlying carcinoma.

In premenopausal women, irregular bleeding may lead to endometrial sampling resulting in the diagnosis.

Investigation of postmenopausal bleeding
Increasingly, units have established 'postmenopausal bleeding clinics' in order to exclude endometrial cancer as a cause for postmenopausal bleeding.

- Using transvaginal ultrasound measurement of the endometrium, the pretest risk of endometrial cancer can be reduced from around 10% to 1% if the endometrial thickness is less than 5 mm.
- Endometrial sampling can be performed as an outpatient procedure to further investigate patients with thickened or irregular endometrial scan findings.
- Hysteroscopy can also be performed as an outpatient procedure to obtain histological samples of the endometrium.
- Hysteroscopy is viewed as the 'gold standard' investigation, either outpatient or inpatient.

Positive peritoneal cytology following hysteroscopy
Following hysteroscopy, the significance of intraperitoneal tumour cells is controversial. According to FIGO Staging, positive peritoneal cytology upstages to Stage 3a.

In one review of 17 studies, the positive cytology rate increased with grade of tumour and depth of invasion from 8% to 16% (G1 compared with G3), 8% to 17% (superficial versus deep myometrial invasion). Although there was a strong association between positive washings and recurrence, the conclusion of the review was that other adverse features predominated over the positive washings to explain these findings (Slomovitz et al. 2005).

In the review, however, only patients with G1, inner half myometrial invasion with no LVSI had unaffected survival when the washings were positive.

New developments in diagnostic investigation of PMB

With the advent of liquid based cytology, and the addition of immunocytochemistry it is possible to obtain cytological samples from the endometrial cavity. Promising results from early studies have been published, with cytohistological concordance rates of up to 98% reported.

Assessment of patients with endometrial cancer

Once the diagnosis of endometrial cancer is established, surgery is the mainstay of treatment for apparent early stage disease.

Surgery is also the mainstay for patients with smooth muscle cell tumours of the uterus, without pelvic lymphadenectomy.

Preoperative assessment with imaging modalities such as ultrasound, CT and MRI has been used to detect metastatic disease in patients with high-grade disease, and spread to the cervix or beyond the uterus.

Chest X-ray, and thorough preoperative assessment must also be performed. Many patients with endometrial cancer have a high BMI, and are at increased risk of:
- thromboembolic complications
- wound infection/breakdown
- chest infection.

Consideration is given to performing an extended hysterectomy if there is evidence of cervical stromal involvement. MRI has been used to assess this but has limitations in terms of both false-positive and false-negative results.

Treatment planning, in the primary, adjuvant, or recurrent disease setting, takes place in formal multidisciplinary team meetings. With members drawn from gynaecological oncology, medical, and clinical oncology, histo- and cytopathology, radiology, and often palliative care services, individual treatment plans are drawn up. The treatment plans are formulated with reference to agreed treatment protocols which are based on regional guidelines.

Surgery may still be appropriate in patients with evidence of metastatic disease in order to control symptoms of bleeding.

Surgery in endometrial cancer

The recommendation for surgical staging of endometrial cancer is for a midline laparotomy to be performed to allow adequate assessment of the peritoneal cavity/contents.

Peritoneal washings should be taken prior to any other procedure, followed by extrafascial total abdominal hysterectomy and bilateral salpingoophorectomy.

In patients with cervical stromal involvement, a radical hysterectomy may be considered as above.

For patients with a preoperative diagnosis of serous carcinoma, additional staging in the form of omental and paraaortic node biopsy should be considered.

Although part of the FIGO staging, the role of routine pelvic and/or paraaortic lymphadenectomy is controversial.
- In a survey of practice, 54% of American Gynaecological Oncologists reported that they routinely performed lymphadenectomy compared to 24% in the UK.
- Some studies have suggested a therapeutic benefit of lymphadenectomy, but the recent ASTEC trial (to date

the only prospective, randomised trial to determine the answer to this question) did not demonstrate a therapeutic advantage to the lymphadenectomy group. At 3 years of follow up there were identical survival rates (89% in the lymphadenectomy group versus 88% in the no lymphadenectomy group).

In recent years the role of laparoscopic hysterectomy has been evaluated in endometrial cancer.
- In published series the recurrence rates are similar for those treated by open or laparoscopic hysterectomy.
- Hospital stay is reduced in the laparoscopic group, although the risk of complications due to injury to intra-abdominal structures was higher in the laparoscopic groups in early studies.

Radiotherapy

For patients with endometrial cancer radiotherapy is delivered as external beam radiotherapy (EBRT) or by brachytherapy.
- EBRT involves the use of radiation whose source is distant from the patient.
- brachytherapy involves the use of sealed radiotherapy sources placed in close proximity to the treated tissue (e.g. intracavitary treatment).

Radiotherapy is used in three situations in endometrial cancer: as primary treatment, adjuvant treatment following surgery, or for palliation.

As primary treatment in patients not fit for surgery

Although inferior to surgery, primary radiotherapy has a 60% 5-year survival in apparent FIGO Stage 1 disease.

As adjuvant treatment following surgery

Adjuvant radiotherapy to the vaginal vault and/or pelvis has been used extensively in patients with adverse prognostic features such as:
- high-grade disease
- deep myometrial invasion
- lymphvascular space invasion (LVSI).

In this situation many studies have shown a reduction in vault recurrence in patients treated with radiotherapy, but no increase in overall survival.

Adjuvant radiotherapy can be associated with side-effects which are described as 'early' or 'late'.
- Early side-effects of pelvic radiotherapy include diarrhoea, cystitis and skin reactions, and in some cases bone marrow suppression in the pelvis.
- Late effects include bowel obstruction/fistula formation, changes in bladder capacity, and vaginal atrophy and possible narrowing of the vagina. In order to prevent vaginal narrowing it is recommended to use vaginal dilators during and following treatment.

Recent research has tried to identify subgroups of patients who might expect a survival advantage following adjuvant radiotherapy, and in whom the risk of side effects might be more justified following adjuvant radiotherapy. The PORTEC study in patients with FIGO stage 1 disease confirmed the findings of earlier studies with lower rates of vaginal/pelvic recurrence in the radiotherapy group with no overall survival advantage.

In addition, the PORTEC study showed that salvage treatment with radiotherapy in patients who develop a vault recurrence can result in long term survival in patients who have not previously received radiotherapy (Creutzberg et al. 2003).

- Only 4% of patients who had received radiotherapy relapsed locally compared with 14% of those who did not receive radiotherapy
  but
- There was an 89% complete response rate to radiotherapy following local relapse in patients who had not received radiotherapy, with a 65% 5year survival.
- Overall 8-year survival was 71% in the group who received adjuvant radiotherapy compared to 77% in the group who did not receive adjuvant radiotherapy.
- A recent systematic review concluded that
- adjuvant EBRT should not be used for low-risk (Ia, IbG1) or intermediate-risk (1bG2) endometrial cancer
  but
- is associated with a 10% survival advantage for high-risk (1cG3) tumours.

In this review the authors suggest that these findings challenge the role of staging lymphadenectomy (Johnson et al. 2007). The review interprets the data that show the reduction in local relapse following adjuvant radiotherapy without improved overall survival, and considers the risk of severe complications following radiotherapy of 3%, and the risk of minor complications at 20%.

For palliation

In addition to radiotherapy for relapsed disease at the vaginal vault which is associated with a good long-term prognosis as discussed above, radiotherapy may also be used to control bleeding in a palliative setting. In this situation one or two fractions are given. It may even be possible to use radiotherapy in this situation in patients who have previously undergone radiotherapy treatment previously.

Follow-up

Currently, the role of routine follow-up for patients with endometrial cancer confined to the uterus is being debated. Following the publication of small studies which do not show a difference in outcome for patients followed up in clinic routinely versus telephone consultations, the results of larger studies are awaited to confirm these findings.

Treatment of advanced disease

The adjuvant treatment of Stage 2 and more advanced disease remains controversial.

As discussed, for patients identified with possible Stage 2 disease on preoperative assessment, consideration of extended hysterectomy should be given.

Endometrial cancer can be classified as FIGO stage 3a with one or more of the following features:

- positive washings (see section above)
- serosal tumour involvement
- direct extension to the adenexa.

The role of adjuvant therapy in this situation remains controversial.

Adjuvant radiotherapy may be used to try and control disease in the pelvis as described above.

Chemotherapy

Chemotherapy regimens including cisplatin, carboplatin, doxorubicin and paclitaxel have been used.

Patients considered for chemotherapy treatment for endometrial cancer are often elderly, have comorbidities and may have undergone previous radiotherapy. The risk of chemotherapy in this population may be higher than for other patient groups, and this must be taken into account when considering chemotherapy treatment in this situation.

To date there is little evidence to show an overall survival advantage following chemotherapy treatment in endometrial cancer.

Treatment of recurrent disease

A common site of recurrence following surgery alone for endometrial cancer is the pelvis, and the vaginal vault in particular.

- Salvage treatment with radiotherapy in this situation can result in 5-year survival of more than 50% in published studies.
- Any role for exenterative surgery in recurrent disease must be considered in the context of the considerable morbidity reported in such patients.
- For patients with recurrent disease systemic treatment with progestogens is often used. The response rates of 15–30% have been reported, with median overall survival times of up to 13 months. The side-effects include weight gain and an increased risk of thromboembolic events.
- Chemotherapy regimens including platinum and taxane combinations have shown activity in recurrent endometrial cancer, with response rates of up to 30–40% reported, with median overall survival times of 13 months.

Further reading

Creutzberg CL, van Putten WLJ, Koper PC, et al. Survival after relapse in patients with endometrial cancer: results from a randomised trial. Gynecol Oncol 2003;89:201–9.

Johnson N, Cornes P. Survival and recurrent disease after postoperative radiotherapy for early endometrial cancer: systematic review and meta-analysis. Br J Obstet Gynaecol 2007;114:1313–20.

Slomovitz BM, Ramondetta, LM, Lee CM, et al. Heterogeneity of Stage IIIa endometrial carcinomas: implications for adjuvant therapy. Int J Gynecol Cancer 2005;15:510–16.

Sonoda Y, Barakat RR. Screening and the prevention of gynaecologic cancer: endometrial cancer. Best Practice Res Clin Obstet Gynaecol 2006;20:363–77.

Brinton LA, Lacey Jr JA, Devesa SS, Sherman ME. Epidemiology of uterine corpus cancers. In: *Gynecologic cancer: controversies in management*. Philadelphia: Elsevier Churchill Livingstone; 2004 189–207.

Creasman WT. Adenocarcinoma of the uterus. In: *Clinical gynecologic oncology*. China: Mosby Elsevier 2007:147–84.

Internet resources

www.cancerresearchuk.org
www.cancer.gov/cancertopics/types/endometrial
www.iarc.fr/

Patient resources

www.cancerbacup.org.uk
www.cancerhelp.org.uk
www.NHS.uk/illness

Gestational trophoblastic neoplasia

Definition
Gestational trophoblastic neoplasia (GTN) encompasses a diverse group of lesions that originate from the fetal trophoblast whose behaviour may be benign or malignant. The lack of histological confirmation in its malignant form often poses much difficulty and controversy in its diagnosis, investigations, and management.

Epidemiology
- There are no reliable figures on the true incidence of GTN due to the difficulties mentioned above.
- It is considered to be a rare disease in the UK, with a calculated incidence of 1 in 714 live births (RCOG 2004). However, with the problems associated with reporting, due to lack of histological diagnosis, especially with regards to partial moles, the true incidence is considered to be higher.
- There also appears to be ethnic variations in the incidence of GTN in the UK, with women from Asia having a higher incidence compared with non-Asian women (1 in 387 versus 1 in 752 live births)
- GTN may occur at any age but appears to be more frequent in teenagers and women above 40. The risk increases with previous history of GTN.

Pathology
- GTN is a heterogeneous group of diseases that arise from one or more of the three main types of trophoblasts found in the placenta: cytotrophoblast, syncytiotrophoblast, or intermediate trophoblast. They can be benign or malignant. Histologically, it is classified into complete hydatidiform mole (CHM), partial hydatidiform mole (PHM); invasive mole (IM), choriocarcinoma (CC), and placental site trophoblast tumour (PSTT).
- In recent years, new entities, including epithelioid trophoblastic tumour, have been added to this family.
- Hydatidiform mole (both CHM and PHM) is the most common form of GTN and can behave in a malignant or benign fashion. However, IM, and CC are considered to be malignant. PSTT has uncertain biological behaviour.
- CHMs are diploid and androgenetic (paternal) in origin, with no evidence of fetal tissue. They arise either as a consequence of duplication of the haploid sperm following the fertilization of an 'empty' ovum or after dispermic fertilization of an 'empty' ovum. CHMs carry a 20% risk of malignant sequelae.
- PHMs are triploid in origin with two sets of paternal haploid genes and one set of maternal haploid genes. They occur after dispermic fertilization of an ovum. There is evidence of fetal tissue or fetal red blood cells. PHMs rarely are followed by GTN but require the same follow up for potential malignant sequelae as a CHM.

Diagnosis and management of GTN
Clinical presentation
- The classic presentation of molar pregnancy include vaginal bleeding, anaemia, excessive uterine enlargement, hyperemesis gravidarum, early pre-eclampsia and hyperthyroidism, associated with remarkably elevated human chorionic gonadotrophin (hCG) titres. However, with the availability of high-resolution vaginal ultrasound and the practice of early dating scan, currently almost all patients with molar pregnancy are diagnosed and treated before they develop the classical symptoms. In almost all cases of PHM, the initial diagnosis is one of incomplete or missed abortion and the diagnosis is only made after the histological examination of the products of conception. Hence, the importance of sending for histology the products of conception in *every* case of pregnancy failure.
- Women who present with persistent abnormal vaginal bleeding after any pregnancy (normal, abortion, ectopic, or molar) should have a pregnancy test to exclude GTN.
- A high index of suspicion is necessary in women of reproductive age who present with acute respiratory or neurological symptoms, as these may be evidence of GTN in the lungs or brain. The finding of pulmonary nodules on a chest radiograph after normal pregnancy suggests GTN. These events may occur remotely from the antecedent pregnancy. A simple pregnancy test may help clinch the diagnosis.
- A young woman with an unknown primary neoplasm or poorly explained hyperthyroidism should have her serum hCG tested.
- Approximately half the cases of GTN follow molar pregnancy, one-fourth follow normal pregnancy, and one-fourth follow abortion or ectopic pregnancy.
- The major risk factors for molar pregnancy include maternal age (older than 40 and younger than 20 years) and a history of molar pregnancy.
- The risk of developing a second molar pregnancy after a primary mole is approximately 20–40 times greater than the initial risk.

Investigations
- Ultrasound remains the most important diagnostic modality in GTN. In CHM, the uterus shows the absence of a gestational sac but the cavity is filled with cystic spaces: the typical 'snowstorm' appearance. Its value is more limited in PHM with no definite diagnostic features. More recently, high-resolution vaginal ultrasound, with colour Doppler, has been used to diagnose GTN involving the uterine myometrium (IM and CC).
- Measurement of serum levels of hCG has been the traditional method of diagnosing GTN. Although very high levels are suspicious, there is no pathognomonic value of hCG to make the diagnosis. However, it is the tumour marker par excellence in the follow-up of patients with GTN to assess response to treatment and to diagnose recurrence.
- Chest X-rays are mandatory in all cases of GTN as the lungs are the commonest site for metastases.
- CT scans and MRI may be used judiciously in metastatic survey of other organs, especially the liver and brain.

Staging and prognostic scoring
GTN is unusual in gynaecological oncology for several reasons. The most common manifestation of GTN, the hydatidiform mole remains benign in most patients. In malignant GTN, the histology is not often available and treatment is based on serum levels of hCG and radiological images. Also, the anatomic stage is *less* important than other risk factors in making treatment decisions. For several years, various staging and prognostic scoring systems have been

used by clinicians to assess the prognosis and selection of the appropriate treatment of GTN, especially, metastatic GTN. However, this did not allow a meaningful comparison of the results and assess the efficacy of the treatment between different centres. The recognition that a universally accepted, precise system of classification would be needed to standardize clinical care has led to the amalgamation of two widely used systems, namely those of the Federation Internationale Gynecologie et Obstetrique (FIGO) staging and the World Health Organization (WHO) prognostic scoring systems (Table 14.5.1). A discussion on the merits of the individual system is beyond the scope of this section (Kohorn 2001). Suffice it to say that the current FIGO classification includes both the stage and scoring, for example Stage III:8, i.e. stage III disease with a prognostic score of 8. In the scoring system, scores 0–6 are considered low risk and scores 7 and above are considered high risk. Generally, in most centres, the prognostic scoring is used more often than stage to determine the treatment: low-risk patients would be treated with single-agent chemotherapy whereas high-risk patients would be treated with multi-agent chemotherapy (see below).

Management

- Patients treated for GTN should not become pregnant for approximately 6–12 months after treatment to allow accurate assessment of hCG levels.
- Fertility rates and pregnancy outcomes are similar in patients treated for GTN compared with the general population.

Complete hydatidiform mole

- The standard of care in the treatment of CHM is surgical evacuation of the uterus by suction curettage. This can be performed in any uterus regardless of its size. It is advisable that the suction be performed with a concurrent

oxytocin drip running in, to reduce the risks of haemorrhage, perforation, and trophoblastic embolization. There is no need for a routine second curettage in the absence of persistent bleeding. In older patients (>40 years), total hysterectomy, with the mole *in situ*, may be an option.

- The use of prostaglandins for medical termination or precurettage cervical dilatation is not recommended, as it has been shown to increase the risk of trophoblastic embolization to the lungs and lung metastases (Tidy et al. 2000).
- In the rare event of a twin pregnancy with one viable fetus and a molar pregnancy, the mother needs to be counselled on the risks. These include early pre-eclampsia and pulmonary embolism. But, if the mother wishes, she may be allowed to carry on the pregnancy. The chance of delivering a viable baby is about 40%. There is no increase in the risk of malignant GTN following delivery (Sebire et al. 2002).
- After evacuation of the uterus, all patients should be followed up with weekly serum HCG till they become negative; then, monthly for 6 months. Subsequent hCG measurements are required under the following circumstances: irregular vaginal bleeding; amenorrhea; evidence of metastatic disease. In the serial monitoring of HCG, three patterns that raise suspicion of malignant GTN include: (1) persistent rise in the values; (2) plateauing of the values; and(3) a secondary rise after an initial fall.
- Reliable contraception should be advised after evacuation of the mole, mainly to avoid the confusion that a new pregnancy can cause in the serial monitoring of hCG. Although barrier contraception may be the safest, they are also the least reliable. Intrauterine devices or implantable hormone devices may cause irregular vaginal bleeding which might be mistaken for persistent GTN. Oral contraceptives are the most preferred.

Table 14.5.1 FIGO 2000 classification for GTN

A. Staging	
Stage I	Disease confined to the uterus
Stage II	GTN extends outside the uterus, but is limited to the genital structures (adnexa, vagina, broad ligament)
Stage III	GTN extends to the lungs, with or without, known genital tract involvement
Stage IV	All other metastatic sites

B. Scoring	0	1	2	4
Age (years)	<40	≥40		
Antecedent pregnancy	Mole	Abortion	Term	
Interval from index pregnancy (months)	<4	4–6	7 to <13	≥13
Pretreatment serum hCG (IU/mL)	<10^3	10^3 to <10^4	10^4 to <10^5	≥10^5
Largest tumour diameter (cm) (including uterus)	<3	3 to <5	≥5	
Site of metastases	Lung	Spleen, kidney	Gastrointestinal	Liver, brain
Number of metastases		1–4	5–8	>8
Previous failed chemotherapy			Single drug	Two or more drugs

Of note is that the classification does not take into account of molar pregnancy not turning into malignant GTN and PSTT is to be reported separately.

There seems to be differing opinion as to the timing of starting the pills. In the UK, it is recommended that the contraceptive pills be started after biochemical remission (i.e. hCG becomes negative). However, in the USA and many other centres (including Singapore), the pills are prescribed soon after evacuation.

- When the patient does get pregnant after a previous molar pregnancy, it is recommended that an early transvaginal ultrasound scan is done to ensure a normal viable pregnancy. Following one molar pregnancy, the risk of a repeat molar pregnancy in a subsequent conception is 1% (Rice et al. 1989). It increases to about 15% after 2 molar pregnancies (Bagshawe et al. 1986).

Partial hydatidiform mole
- The management of PHM is the same as for CHM.

Medical complications of hydatidiform mole
- Anaemia
- Toxaemia
- Hyperthyroidism
- Hyperemesis gravidarum
- Cardiac failure
- Pulmonary insufficient (rare).

Invasive mole
- A diagnosis of IM is seldom made clinically without surgery. Most of the non-metastatic (low risk) GTN following a molar pregnancy is believed to be IM. The presence of a vascular nodule in the myometrium, following evacuation of a mole and persistent high levels or rising levels of hCG may be suggestive of an IM.
- Chemotherapy, usually with a single agent, methotrexate (MTX) or actinomycin D (ACT-D) is the treatment of choice.
- In chemoresistant cases, resection of the nodule or hysterectomy may be indicated.

Choriocarcinoma
- CC develops in about 3–5% of the patients with CHM. Of all CC, 50% are preceded by a hydatidiform mole, 25% by an abortion, and the other 25% by a full term pregnancy. A clinical diagnosis of CC is rare. Most of the metastatic (high risk) GTN, especially those outside the lungs, are believed to be CC.
- Chemotherapy with multiple agents (see below) is the treatment of choice.
- Surgery has an important role in selected cases (see below).

Further management
A diagnosis of persistent GTN is made when any of the following criteria are fulfilled:
There is a rise of HCG on three consecutive weekly measurements.
There is plateauing of the HCG levels for 3 or more weeks.
HCG levels remain elevated for 6 months or more.
There is radiological evidence of metastatic disease in the presence of positive hCG.
There is histological diagnosis of CC.
The disease is then assessed using the FIGO classification to determine the stage and risk score. It is highly recommended that patients with persistent GTN be referred to tertiary referral centres experienced in the management of GTN, so that optimal results may be obtained.

Low-risk patients (score up to 6)
- Chemotherapy with single agent is the treatment of choice in this group. Various protocols are used (see box) but they all give equally good results with reported remission rates reaching 100% in most centres.
- The role of surgery will be discussed below

Chemotherapy protocols for low risk GTN

1. Methotrexate 100 mg/m2 i.v. over 30 minutes followed by methotrexate 200 mg/m2 i.v. over 12 hours. Further therapy withheld as long as serum hCG regression pattern is satisfactory
2. Methotrexate 0.4 mg/kg i.v. or i.m. every day × 5 days; repeat every 12–14 days (7–9-day window)
3. Methotrexate 1 mg/kg i.m. on days 1, 3, 5, 7; folinic acid 0.1 mg/kg i.m on days 2, 4, 6, 8; repeat every 15–18 days (7–10-day window)
4. Methotrexate 40 mg/m2 weekly
5. Actinomycin D 10–13 µg/kg i.v. every day × 5 days; repeat every 12–14 days (7–9-day window)
6. Actinomycin D 1.25 mg/m2 i.v. every 14 days

Cycles are repeated until hCG becomes negative and a further two or three cycles are given

---

High-risk patients (score of 7 or more)
- In this group, the mainstay of treatment is with multiagent chemotherapy. Again various regimens are used (see box), but there is no strong evidence to determine the best combination chemotherapy (Xue et al. 2006). Familiarity with a particular regime seems to be the most important factor in the choice of a regime. The most common regime is the EMA/CO (etoposide, methotrexate/folinic acid rescue, dactinomycin/cyclophosphamide and vincristine). However, in many centres, including the author's, the regime of choice is EMA (without CO). Remission rate of about 86% have been reported (Newlands 2003).
- Salvage chemotherapy with novel combination of presently used drugs and use of newer drugs such as paclitaxel and gemcitabine may be required in patients with multiple metastases, especially those with liver and brain metastases and not responding to the regular combination therapy.
- Surgery has been utilized mainly in patients with chemoresistant tumour foci (see below).
- Fertility rates following chemotherapy is not reduced compared to patients who have not had chemotherapy. Outcomes of pregnancies are comparable to normal population. It is conventional to advise patients to avoid getting pregnant for at least 6–12 months after chemotherapy.

Surgery in GTN
- The traditional role of surgery in GTN has been in a salvage setting, where despite multiple cycles of chemotherapy, resistant tumour foci exist. However, primary chemotherapy is not without danger in certain sites, especially the brain, where chemotherapy can cause necrosis and haemorrhage of the tumour, which can have serious or even fatal consequence.
- There has been a recent trend to do primary surgery, in selected patients, to avoid prolonged chemotherapy or

Chemotherapy protocols in high risk GTN

EMA/CO
Week 1, Day 1
Actinomycin D 0.5 mg i.v. bolus
Etoposide 100 mg/m2 i.v. in 500 mL N saline over 30 minutes
Methotrexate 300 mg/m2 i.v. in 1 L N saline over 12 hours
Week 1, Day 2
Actinomycin D 0.5 mg i.v. bolus
Etoposide 100 mg/m2 i.v. in 500 mL N saline over 30 minutes
Folinic acid 15 mg oral/i.m 12 hourly × 4 doses, starting 24 hours after commencing methotrexate
Week 2, Day 1
Vincristine (Oncovin) 1.4 mg/m2 i.v. bolus (maximum 2 mg)
Cyclophosphamide 600 mg/m2 i.v. in 500 mL N saline over 30 minutes
EP/EMA (regime for patients with resistance to EMA/CO)
Etoposide and cisplatin alternating weekly with methotrexate, actinomycin D and etoposide
Week 1, Day 1 (EP)
Etoposide 150 mg/m2 i.v. in 500 mL N saline over 30 minutes
Cisplatin 25 mg/m2 i.v. over 4 hours
Cisplatin 25 mg/m2 i.v. over 4 hours
Cisplatin 25 mg/m2 i.v. over 4 hours
Week 2, Day 1 (EMA)
Etoposide 100 mg/m2 i.v. over 30 minutes
Methotrexate 300 mg/m2 i.v. over 24 hours
Actinomycin D 0.5 mg i.v. bolus
Week 2, Day 2
Folinic acid 15 mg po 12 hourly × 4 doses to start 24 hours after starting methotrexate

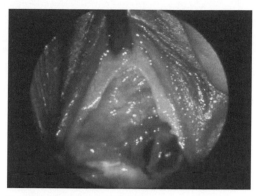

Fig.14.5.1 Vaginal metastasis in GTN.

Placental site trophopblastic tumour (PSTT)

- PSTT is among the rarest of GTN, accounting for about 1-2% of GTN. It is a very unique form of GTN, arising from the intermediate trophoblast of the placenta. It can occur after any pregnancy including molar pregnancy, abortion, term delivery, or ectopic pregnancy. It displays a wide clinical spectrum of behaviour, from benign to an extremely aggressive, metastatic tumour, often unresponsive to chemotherapy.

- Unlike other GTN, it is characterized by a *low* level of hCG. However, human placental lactogen (HPL) levels are raised in the serum and the hormone is expressed in immunostaining of the histological sections. Final diagnosis is only on histology of the curetting or hysterectomy specimen.

- Fortunately, most cases are confined to the uterus and most (85–90%) behave in a benign fashion. The most common presenting symptom is vaginal bleeding. When diagnosis is confirmed on histology, meticulous effort must be taken to identify metastatic disease. The WHO prognostic scoring is of little use in PSTT, as its behaviour is unpredictable.

- Unless child bearing is very important, current recommendation for uterus-confined PSTT is a hysterectomy with perioperative single agent chemotherapy. For metastatic disease, aggressive chemotherapy with multi-agent chemotherapy regimes like EP/EMA is preferred.

its complications. Examples of such surgery would include hysterectomy in low risk, non-metastatic disease; thoracotomy to remove large, solitary lung metastasis; and craniotomy in solitary brain metastasis at accessible sites (Ilancheran *et al.* 1980).

- Surgery may also be used when complications occur; for example, hysterectomy for a perforating invasive mole or choriocarcinoma with uncontrolled bleeding. Craniotomy may be necessary to stem cerebral haemorrhage from metastases.

- A notable exception to *avoid* surgery is vaginal metastasis. Typically, vaginal metastasis in GTN occurs in the anterior vaginal wall, just below the urethra, as a haemorrhagic nodule (Fig. 14.5.1). Any attempt to biopsy or excise the nodule can result in a torrential haemorrhage, as the nodule is often the 'tip of the iceberg' of a large vascular mass. These nodule are extremely chemosensitive and chemotherapy should be first choice; otherwise embolisation of the feeder vessels should be considered.

Radiation therapy in GTN

With the availability of effective chemotherapy, radiation always had a limited role in the treatment of GTN. It has been employed most frequently to treat patients with brain or liver metastases, in an effort to minimize haemorrhagic complications from disease at these sites (Soper 2003).

Further reading

Bagshawe KD, Dent J, Webb J. Hydatidiform mole in England and Wales, 1973-1983. Lancet 1986;673–7.

Ilancheran A, Ratnam SS. The role of surgery in gestational trophoblastic disease. Int Journal Gynecol Obstet 1980;18:237–9.

Kohorn, E. the new FIGO 2000 staging and risk factor scoring systems for gestational trophoblastic disease: description and critical assessment. Int J Gynecol Cancer 2001;11:73–7.

Newlands ES. The management of recurrent and drug-resistant gestational trophoblastic neoplasia (GTN). Best Practice Res Clin Obstet Gynaecol 2003;17:905–23.

Rice LW, Lage JM, Berkowitz RS, *et al.* Repetitive complete and partial hydatidiform moles. Obstet Gynecol 1989;74:217–9.

Royal College of Obstetricians and Gynaecologists. *The management of gestational trophoblastic neoplasia.* Clinical Green Top Guidelines 38. 2004.

Sebire NJ, Foskett M, Paradinas FJ, *et al.* Outcome of twin pregnancies with complete hydatidiform mole and healthy co-twin. Lancet 2002:359;2165–6.

Soper JT. Role of surgery and radiation therapy in GTD. Best Practice Res Obstet Gynaecol 2003;17:943–55.

Tidy J, Gillespie AM, Bright N, et al. Gestational trophoblastic disease: a study of mode of evacuation and subsequent need for chemotherapy. Gynecol Oncol 2003;78:9–12.

Xue Y, Zhang J, Wu TX, et al. Combination chemotherapy for high risk gestational trophoblastic tumour. Cochrane Database Syst Rev 2006;3:CD005196.

Ovarian and fallopian tube cancer

The incidence of ovarian cancer is low, being the fourth most common cancer in women in the UK following breast, bowel, and lung cancer. For each individual woman, the lifetime risk of ovarian cancer is estimated at 1 in 70 (1.5%). The poor 5-year survival rate in the UK of about 25% is because approximately 70% of women are diagnosed with stage 3 or stage 4 disease. Nevertheless, around 90% of patients who are found to have stage 1a and 1b ovarian cancer will have a 5-year survival.

The rates of ovarian cancer vary considerably between countries, with the highest rates in Scandinavia, North America, and the UK and are lowest in Africa, India, and the Far East. Over 6000 new cases of ovarian cancer are diagnosed each year in the UK and there are about 4500 deaths from the disease.

About 5–10% of cases are hereditary and when childbearing is complete, a hysterectomy and bilateral salpingo-oophorectomy should be considered. Although the oral contraceptive pill decreases the risk of ovarian cancer by up to 50% in women in the general population, improved diagnosis and an ageing population are likely to result in an increasing incidence of reported cases of ovarian cancer.

Over 85% of ovarian cancers are of epithelial origin. About 10% are undifferentiated and the remainder are non-epithelial cancers and are rare.

Pathology
- Ovarian tumours are classified on the basis of their cell or tissue of origin (Decruze et al. 2006).
- Neoplasms derived from coelomic epithelium (epithelial cancers)
  - serous tumour
  - mucinous tumour
  - endometroid tumour
  - mesonephroid (clear cell) tumour
  - Brenner tumour undifferentiated carcinoma
  - carcinosarcoma and mixed mesodermal tumour
  - serous cystadenomas account for approximately 50% of epithelial ovarian cancers.
- Neoplasms derived from germ cells
  - dysgerminoma
  - endodermal sinus tumour (yolk sac tumours)
  - embryonal carcinoma
  - polyembryonal
  - choriocarcinoma
  - teratoma (immature, mature or monodermal)
  - mixed forms (tumours composed of the above in any possible combination)
  - tumours composed of germ cell and sex cord stromal derivative (gonadoblastoma)
- Neoplasms derived from specialist ovarian stroma
  - granulosa-theca cell tumours (granulosa tumour and thecoma)
  - Sertoli–Leydig tumours (arrhenoblastoma and Sertoli tumour)
  - gynandroblastoma
  - lipid cell tumours
- Neoplasms derived from non-specific mesenchyme
  - fibroma, haemangioma, leiomyoma
  - lymphoma

  - sarcoma
- Metastatic ovarian tumours
  - gastrointestinal tract (Krukenberg)
  - breast
  - endometrium
  - lymphoma.

The non-epithelial cancers have an incidence of 6 per million women per year. They account for around 10–15% of all ovarian cancers and little is known about risk factors, although they do not appear to be similar to those found in patients with epithelial cancers. The malignant germ cell tumours are most common in teenagers and have been associated with the maternal use of hormones in early pregnancy. The granulosa cell tumour, which tends to occur in the older woman, is the most common malignant sex cord stromal tumour.

Aetiology
- The strongest risk factor for epithelial ovarian cancer is related to reproductive factors such as the number of lifetime ovulatory cycles. High parity, use of the combined oral contraceptive, late menarche, early menopause, and early age at first pregnancy all reduce the risk.
- 5% to 10% of all epithelial cancers are hereditary. There are three clinical genetic manifestations.
  - 'site specific' ovarian-cancer
  - hereditary breast-ovarian cancer syndromes
  Both these are associated with mutations in the BRCA1 and BRCA2 tumour suppressor genes, which are present in about 90% of hereditary cases.
  - hereditary non-polyposis colorectal cancer (HNPCC and Lynch II).
  Women with Lynch syndrome have a 40–60% of lifetime risk of endometrial cancer and a 10–12% lifetime risk of ovarian cancer. HNPCC is associated with alterations in the DNA mismatch repair genes.
  Ovarian cancers caused by BRCA mutations tend to occur in younger women. The lifetime risk of ovarian cancer is 40–50% and 20–30% for a BRCA1 and BRCA2 mutation respectively. Cancers associated with these mutations are usually poorly differentiated serous carcinomas.
- Epithelial ovarian cancers have been associated with asbestos exposure, the use of talc, endometriosis, and pelvic inflammatory disease.

Screening
Women at average risk
- An effective strategy for the early detection of ovarian cancer would significantly decrease mortality from this disease.
- To date, no screening strategies have been proven to decrease mortality from ovarian cancer and therefore screening in women at low risk of developing ovarian cancer cannot be recommended.
- CA125 and transvaginal ultrasonography to detect ovarian cancer have been used in large population-based studies as screening tools.
- Half of women with early-stage ovarian cancer will have a CA125 level within normal limits.
- Currently there is emphasis on educating women to be aware of the symptoms of ovarian cancer, such as

bloating, increasing abdominal girth, a change in bowel or bladder habit, and abdominal or pelvic discomfort.

Women with a strong family history or a proven gene mutation

- Annual screening for CA125 and transvaginal ultrasonography can be offered.
- The limitations and implications of these tests should be fully explained.
- Women with BRCA mutations should be offered prophylactic salpingo-oophorectomy once their family is complete (Griffiths et al. 2005). Those who carry the HNPCC mutation should consider prophylactic hysterectomy along with salpingo-oophorectomy.

Staging

Ovarian cancer spreads by three primary methods: direct extension to adjacent organs, exfoliation of tumour cells causing intraperitoneal dissemination, and lymphatic/vascular embolization. The omentum is the most frequent site of metastases.

The FIGO staging is based on surgical and pathological findings (Table 14.6.1). Accurate staging is essential to determine prognosis and management strategy.

Prognosis

Although staging is mainly surgical the final stage is dependent on the pathology of the surgical specimens and the cytology of peritoneal washings or ascites (Table 14.6.2).

Clinical approach

Diagnosis

Ovarian cancer generally presents with an insidious onset of vague non-specific symptoms. Many patients are referred to specialists other than a gynaecologist and clinicians need to be alert to the possibility that vague abdominal symptoms may be due to ovarian cancer.

- Main presenting symptoms in patients with primary ovarian cancer are (in order of frequency):
  - abdominal swelling
  - abdominal pain/pelvic pressure
  - gastrointestinal complaints
  - vaginal bleeding
  - dysuria
  - fatigue
  - dyspnoea
  - back pain.

Approximately 10% of women with early ovarian cancer may be asymptomatic.

- Pelvic examination will reveal a mass in 40–70% of patients and 20–30% will have clinically detectable ascites.
- Ascites, pleural effusions, enlarged inguinal, or supraclavicular lymph nodes and skin metastases suggest advanced disease.
- Where clinical examination is negative then the most valuable investigation in a woman presenting with non-specific symptoms is ultrasonography. If a pelvic mass is confirmed then a CA125 should be checked.
- A risk of malignancy index (RMI) is an effective discriminator between cancer and benign lesions (Jacob et al. 1990). The RMI is calculated using the menopausal status (M), ultrasound findings (U), and the serum CA125. The ultrasound findings are scored with 1 point for each of the following criteria.

Table 14.6.1 FIGO staging of ovarian cancer

Stage	Description
I	Growth confined to ovaries
Ia	Growth limited to one ovary, no ascites present containing malignant cells, no tumour on external surface, capsule intact
Ib	Growth limited to both ovaries, no ascites present containing malignant cells, no tumour on external surfaces, capsule intact
Ic	Tumour stage 1a or 1b but with tumour on the surface on one or both ovaries, or with capsule ruptured, or with ascites present with malignant cells, or positive peritoneal washings
II	Growth involving one or both ovaries
IIa	Extension and/or metastases to uterus and/or fallopian tubes
IIb	Extension to other pelvic tissues
IIc	Tumour stage IIa or IIb but with tumour on surface of one or both ovaries, or with capsule ruptured, or with ascites present containing malignant cells or with positive peritoneal washings
III	Tumour involving one or both ovaries with peritoneal implants outside pelvis and/or retroperitoneal or inguinal nodes, superficial liver metastases, tumour is limited to true pelvis but with histologically verified malignant extension to small bowel or omentum
IIIa	Tumour grossly limited to the true pelvis with positive nodes with microscopic seedlings of abdominal peritoneal surfaces
IIIb	Tumour one or both ovaries, peritoneal implants no greater than 2 cm in diameter, nodes negative
IIIc	Abdominal implants greater than 2 cm in diameter and/or positive retroperitoneal or inguinal nodes
IV	Growth involving one or both ovaries with distant metastasis. Includes liver parenchymal metastasis and/or pleural effusion with positive cytology

Table 14.6.2 FIGO Annual report on the results of treatment (2003)

FIGO stage	Proportion of cases (%)	5-year survival (%)
Ia	11.7	89.3
Ib	1.4	64.8
Ic	14.0	78.2
IIa	1.8	79.2
IIb	2.6	64.3
IIc	5.1	68.2
IIIa	3.0	49.2
IIIb	6.3	40.8
IIIc	41.3	28.9
IV	12.8	13.4

- multilocular cyst
- evidence of solid areas
- evidence of metastases
- presence of ascites
- bilateral lesions

RM = U × M × CA125

where U = 0 for ultrasound score 0, U = 1 for ultrasound score of 1, U = 3 for ultrasound score of 2–5, M = 1 if premenopausal, and M = 3 if postmenopausal. When an MRI cut-off level of 200 is used the sensitivity is 85% and the specificity is 97%.

- A chest X-ray and CT scan of the abdomen and pelvis will be helpful in assessing the extent of the disease and aid with the preoperative counselling of the patient and the planning of her surgery. MRI has limitations in detecting upper abdominal disease but is better than CT for the work-up of an indeterminate adnexal/ovarian mass.

Tumour markers

CA125 is a tumour-associated antigen and levels will be increased in up to 80% of women with epithelial tumours. However, increased levels can also be seen in many non-malignant conditions such as menstruation, endometriosis, pelvic inflammatory disease, acute pancreatitis, diverticulitis, and congestive cardiac failure. Other malignant tumours may also give rise to a raised CA125, including endometrial, pancreatic, breast, and lung.

Inhibin levels can be a useful marker for follow-up in patients with granulosa cell tumours, and elevated levels are also seen in postmenopausal women with mucinous tumours.

- Where investigations suggest ovarian cancer, women should be referred to a centre with a gynaecological oncology multidisciplinary team. Evidence suggests that treatment in cancer centres is associated with an improved prognosis. Women with early-stage disease may not be identified by the RMI and therefore not referred to a cancer centre.

Management

Surgery is the cornerstone for the management of patients with presumed ovarian cancer. It is diagnostic, in early-stage disease curative and most importantly allows the cancer to be staged accurately. For the majority of patients with ovarian cancer, optimizing surgery is the best way to improve survival.

Surgery

- Exploratory laparotomy is a standard approach for patients with ovarian cancer with total abdominal hysterectomy, bilateral salpingo-oophorectomy, and tumour reductive surgery.
- Optimal tumour debulking resulting in no residual tumour nodules larger than 1 cm is known to be associated with improved survival, and therefore the aim of surgery should be optimal tumour debulking wherever possible.
- Although there have been few surgical randomized controlled trials in ovarian cancer, currently only patients who are unable to tolerate surgery or who have cancer that is known preoperatively to preclude optimum tumour debulking are considered for neoadjuvant chemotherapy.
- Where neoadjuvant chemotherapy is administered, interval debulking or interval cytoreductive surgery is usually considered after three cycles, although the impact on survival is unclear.

- It is not routine to perform second-look surgery after chemotherapy outwith clinical trials as it has not been shown to be of any benefit to patients.
- Secondary tumour debulking surgery may be considered for patients with residual disease detected on second-look surgery or where an isolated late recurrence has been detected. It should not be recommended in patients who will not receive postoperative chemotherapy.
- Palliative surgery is used to alleviate symptoms and 10–40% of women with terminal ovarian cancer develop bowel obstruction. Surgery produces a rapid resolution of symptoms, although this will not be achieved in about 20% of patients. The median survival following surgery for bowel obstruction is about 2 months. The merit of surgery requires to be individualized.

Surgical technique

- In most cases a vertical incision should be used. Ascitic fluid should be drained or peritoneal washings taken for cytology. Any encapsulated tumour masses should be removed intact and all peritoneal and intestinal surfaces, liver, spleen, kidneys, lesser sac, omentum, diaphragms, and pelvic/paraortic lymph nodes examined/palpated.
- Total abdominal hysterectomy, bilateral salpingo-oophorectomy, and omentectomy should be performed and biopsies taken from any suspicious areas. An appendicectomy should be performed for mucinous tumours.
- In a patient who is medically sufficiently fit, optimal debulking (1 cm tumour diameter or less) should be attempted as this reduction in tumour load is associated with better survival by improving the effect of adjuvant chemotherapy (Bristow *et al.* 2006). Current evidence suggests that best practice for advanced ovarian cancer is cytoreductive surgery (Pomel *et al.* 2008). A recent study suggests that delay before initiating chemotherapy after major surgery is not an important factor (Aletti *et al.* 2007).
- In the UK, demonstrable benefit has been seen where a patient receives her initial surgery by a gynaecological oncologist.
- Lymphadenectomy is not routinely performed in the UK as part of maximal surgical debulking in patients who have advanced ovarian cancer, although there is some evidence that it may be associated with an improved survival. Lymphadenectomy is helpful in patients who are thought to have early stage disease.
- If a suspicious cyst is managed laparoscopically, rupture should be avoided and aspiration performed in a closed bag prior to removal of the cyst through the abdominal wall port. Laparoscopic staging is feasible but should be reserved for early stage disease because of concerns regarding port site metastases.

Management of ovarian cancer in young women

- For young nulliparous women with a stage Ia tumour, more conservative procedures should be considered.
- A unilateral oophorectomy combined with surgical staging would normally be considered optimal primary treatment for borderline or germ cell tumours. A key issue for stage Ia epithelial tumours is the histological type. Mucinous and endometroid lesions have a better prognosis than serous lesions. The tumour should be well differentiated.
- The optimal requirements for conservative management include the following: a desire to maintain fertility, a normal pelvis which is free of adhesions, no invasion of the

capsule, negative peritoneal washings, adequate evaluation of the contralateral ovary, an infracolic omentectomy, and selected lympadenectomy. Close follow-up is required with excision of the residual ovary after completion of childbearing.

Chemotherapy
- For optimally staged grade I, stage Ia, and stage 1b epithelial ovarian tumours the prognosis is excellent and chemotherapy is not usually recommended. However information from the International Collaborative Ovarian Neoplasm (ICON 1) (Colombo et al. 2003) and Adjuvant Chemotherapy in Ovarian Neoplasm (ACTION) trials confirms the benefit in terms of disease-free interval and 5-year survival of chemotherapy over observation in the population studied (Trimbos et al. 2003). The implications of these studies are unclear but patients with medium or high risk stage I ovarian cancer should be considered for chemotherapy.
- Large trials have all now confirmed that both progression-free survival and overall survival are improved in patients receiving platinum/paclitaxel chemotherapy (Piccart et al. 2000). Although survival advantages were not confirmed in the ICON 3 study, standard chemotherapy for advanced ovarian cancer in the UK is now a combination of platinum and paclitaxel.
- Chemotherapy is tailored to the individual and there remains a role for single agent carboplatin for frail or elderly patients.
- Carboplatin causes less nephrotoxicity and neurotoxicity than cisplatinum but nausea, allergic hypersensitivity reactions, gastrointestinal. and haematological side-effects can be troublesome.
- Paclitaxel commonly causes alopecia, nausea, diarrhoea, mucositis, hypersensitivity reactions, and neurological side-effects.
- There has recently been renewed interest in intraperitoneal chemotherapy and new data (GOG 172 trial) confirms that intraperitoneal chemotherapy can provide improved outcomes for patients with small volume or no visible residual disease and an intact peritoneal cavity following surgery. In this trial cisplatinum and paclitaxel were administered intraperitoneally (Armstrong et al. 2006). However, toxicity has been a significant problem with only 42% of women being able to complete all planned cycles of intraperitoneal therapy mainly because of toxicity. More studies are required to determine the place of this treatment.

Chemotherapy for relapsed disease
- Decisions about further treatment are usually made on clinical or radiological findings. A raised CA125 is seen in about 85% of cases and may predate clinical evidence of relapse by an average of 4 months.
- The choice of chemotherapy at relapse is usually based on the length of time the women has been off treatment (Ali et al. 2007).
- Women with platinum-sensitive tumours (tumours relapsing 12 months or more after initial platinum therapy) can be treated again with platinum-based chemotherapy. The ICON 4 trial using carboplatin + paclitaxel showed a 7% improvement in survival in the combined therapy group (Palmer et al. 2003). This improvement needs to be balanced against the increased toxicity of combination treatment and take into account the side-effects experienced after first line therapy.
- Women with platinum-resistant ovarian cancer (those relapsing within 6 months of completing treatment) or platinum-refractory disease (those who have progressive disease on platinum therapy) may be considered for salvage chemotherapy, which would include liposomal doxorubicin, topotecan, gemcitabine, and oral etoposide.

Other adjuvant therapies
- Radiotherapy is not currently recommended as adjuvant treatment but may have a palliative role in patients with recurrent disease.
- In view of the significant toxicity associated with chemotherapy, hormonal agents may be appropriate; 10–15% of ovarian tumours demonstrate a response. The most frequently used hormonal agents are gonadotrophin-releasing hormone agonists, tamoxifen, anti-androgens, and aromatase inhibitors such as letrozole.

Borderline malignant epithelial ovarian tumours
- Account for approximately 15% of all epithelial ovarian cancers and 95% are of the serous or mucinous type.
- The characteristics histological findings are stratification of the epithelial lining of the papillae, formation of microscopic papillary projections, pleomorphism, cellular atypia, mitotic activity, and no stromal invasion.
- Approximately 80% of women present with disease confined to the ovaries and less than 15% have advanced disease.
- There is a 10-year survival rate of approximately 95% for stage 1 disease, although recurrences may occur up to 20 years after initial treatment.
- Extra ovarian implants associated with stage III serous borderline tumours may be either invasive or non-invasive. The invasive implants are associated with a poor clinical outcome compared with the non-invasive group.
- The aim of surgery should be to completely remove the tumour. For most patients a total abdominal hysterectomy and bilateral salpingo-oophorectomy with omentectomy should be performed; however, if fertility is desired, a unilateral oophorectomy alone (provided the contralateral ovary appears healthy) does not appear to have a detrimental effect on survival.
- Women with poor prognosis borderline tumours may be prescribed chemotherapy as an adjuvant to surgery.

Non-epithelial ovarian cancers: germ cell tumours
- These tumours account for 10% of all ovarian tumours, the most common being a dysgerminoma (48%) followed by endodermal sinus (yolk sac) tumour (20%). They occur mainly in young women and a conservative approach to surgery is appropriate and radiotherapy avoided.
- Approximately 20% of patients with germ cell tumours treated with surgery alone will recur and therefore all patients except those with stage Ia dysgerminoma and stage Ia grade 1 immature teratoma should be treated with adjuvant chemotherapy.
- Bleomycin, etoposide, and cisplatin have been shown to result in a 96% sustained response rate.
- Ninety per cent of patients relapse within 2 years of initial treatment.
- Measurement of the tumour markers (hCG, AFP, and LDH) are useful as part of the preoperative evaluation and follow up monitoring.

Sex cord stromal tumours of the ovary

These constitute about 7% of ovarian malignancies.

Granulosa cell tumours

- These account for 70% of sex cord stromal tumours.
- Most tumours produce oestrogen and a few are androgenic. Serum inhibin may be a useful tumour marker.
- There are two forms: juvenile and adult. The former presents with precocious bleeding and the latter with postmenopausal bleeding. Endometrial hyperplasia or adenocarcinoma may occur as a consequence of the oestrogen production.
- The majority are diagnosed as stage I tumours and treated by hysterectomy, bilateral salpingo-oophorectomy, omentectomy, and cytoreductive surgery. In adolescent girls fertility sparing surgery should be the aim.
- Spread is similar to epithelial ovarian cancer and the stage of diagnosis seems to be the most important prognostic factor.
- The overall 5-year survival rate is around 80% however these tumours are characterised by late recurrences.
- For stage II or III tumours adjuvant chemotherapy is recommended and traditionally the combination of bleomycin, etoposide, and cisplatin has been used. Other combinations include vincristine, actinomycin, and cyclophosphamide or vinblastine, bleomycin, and cisplatin.

Sertoli–Leydig tumours

- These tumours are rare accounting for less than 0.5% of all ovarian tumours.
- The tumours may secrete oestrogen and androgen. Clinical presentation will depend on the hormones secreted, and in young women menstrual disorders are the most common symptom.
- Since over 95% of these tumours are confined to one ovary, unilateral salpingo-oophorectomy may be performed where preservation of fertility is required. In all other cases, total abdominal hysterectomy, bilateral salpingo-oophorectomy and a staging laparotomy is the appropriate management.
- Adjuvant chemotherapy (as for granulose cell tumours) is appropriate where there is a substantial risk of recurrence, although there is no evidence base to support this approach because of the rarity of the tumour.

Other uncommon ovarian tumours

- Sarcoma of the ovary (mixed Müllerian tumours (MMTs) and pure sarcomas) have a poor prognosis. After standard surgery, paclitaxel and carboplatin instead of ifosfamide and cisplatin have been used.
- Small cell carcinoma of the ovary is an aggressive tumour and following surgery the literature suggests that etoposide and cisplatin, or vincristine, actinomycin,and cyclophosphamide are the most useful combinations.

Fallopian Tube Cancer

- This is a rare malignancy.
- It is likely to have a similar aetiology and molecular pathogenesis to ovarian cancer.
- Women undergoing prophylactic bilateral oophorectomy should also have a bilateral salpingectomy performed.
- The diagnosis is rarely made preoperatively. Abnormal vaginal bleeding is the most common symptom. The classic symptoms of pain, which is often colicky, and a watery vaginal discharge are less common.

- Abnormal glandular cells on cervical smear may be seen in up to 25% of cases.
- Eight per cent will have been identified as having a pelvic mass and investigation and treatment is similar to that for ovarian cancer.
- The FIGO staging is similar to that for ovarian carcinoma using a surgical pathological staging system.
- The diagnostic pathological criteria for diagnosing a primary fallopian tube carcinoma include the following:
  The tumour should arise from the endosalpinx.
  The histology should resemble the epithelium of the tubal mucosa.
  Transition from benign to malignant epithelium should be present.
  The endometrium and ovaries should be normal or contain a tumour but by a cytological appearance, small size and distribution appear to be metastatic.
- The 5-year survival for patients with fallopian cancer is slightly higher than for ovarian cancer, perhaps reflecting the higher proportion with early stage disease. The rate of lymph node metastases is higher for fallopian tube than ovarian cancer and this will adversely affect survival.

Further reading

Aletti GD, Long HJ, Podratz KC, Cliby WA. Is time to chemotherapy a determinant of prognosis in advanced-stage ovarian cancer. Gynecol Oncol 2007;104:21–6.

Ali SN, Ledermann JA. Current practice and new developments in ovarian cancer chemotherapy. Obstet Gynaecol 2009;9:265–9.

Armstrong DK, Bundy B, Wenzel L, et al. Gynecologic Oncology Group. Intraperitoneal Cisplatinum and paclitaxel in ovarian cancer. Engl J Med 2006;354:34–43.

Bristow RE, Berek JS. Surgery for Ovarian cancer: how to improve survival. Lancet 2006;367:1558–60.

Colombo N, Guthri D, Chiari S, et al. International collaborative ovarian neoplasm trial 1: a randomised trial of adjuvant chemotherapy in women with early-stage ovarian cancer. J Natl Cancer Inst 2003;95:125–32.

Decruze SB, Kirwan JM. Ovarian cancer. Curr Obstet Gynaecol 2006;16:161–7.

FIGO (International Federation of Gynecology and Obstetrics). Annual report on the results of treatment in gynaecological cancer. Int J Gynecol Obstet 2003 83(Suppl1):IX–XXII, 1–229.

Griffiths SE, Lopes T, Edmondson RJ. The role of prolphylactic salpingo-oophorectomy in women who carry mutations of the BRCA genes. Obstet Gynaecol 2005;7:23–7.

Jacobs I, Oram D, Fairbanks J, et al. A risk of malignancy index incorporating CA125, ultrasound and menopausal status for the accurate preoperative diagnosis of ovarian cancer. Br J Obstet Gynaecol 1990;97:922–9.

Parmar MK, Ledermann JA, Colombo N, et al.; Icon and AGO Collaborators. Placlitaxel plus platinum-based chemotherapy versus conventional platinum-based chemotherapy in women with relapsed ovarian cancer: The ICON four–AGO–OVAR–2.2 Trial. Lancet 2003;361:2099–106.

Piccart MJ, Bertelsen K, James K, et al. Randomised intergroup trial of cisplatin-paclitaxel versus cisplatin-cyclophosphamide in women with advanced epithelial ovarian cancer; three year results. J Natl Cancer Inst 2000;92:699–708.

Pomel C, Barton DPJ, McNeish I, Shepherd J. A statement for extensive primary cytoreductive surgery in advanced ovarian cancer. Br J Obstet Gynaecol 2008;115:808–10.

Trimbos JB, Parmar M, Vergote I, et al. International Collaborative Ovarian Neoplasm Trial 1 and Adjuvant Chemotherapy in Ovarian Neoplasm Trial. Two parallel randomised phase iii trials of adjuvant chemotherapy in patients with early-stage ovarian carcinoma. J Natl Cancer Inst 2003;95:105–12.

Palliative care

Definition
The World Health Organization defines palliative care as improving the quality of life of patients and families who face life-threatening illness, by providing pain and symptom relief and spiritual and psychosocial support, from diagnosis through to the end of life and in to bereavement.
Palliative care
- provides relief from pain and other distressing symptoms
- affirms life and regards dying as a normal process
- intends neither to hasten or postpone death
- integrates the psychological and spiritual aspects of patient care
- offers a support system to help patients live as actively as possible until death
- offers a support system to help family cope during the patients illness and in bereavement
- uses a team approach
- aims to enhance quality of life, and may also positively influence the course of the illness
- may be valuable early in the course of the illness, in conjunction with other therapies that are intended to prolong life. These include chemotherapy or radiation therapy, and those investigations needed to better understand and manage distressing clinical complications
- puts an emphasis on open and honest communication
- respects autonomy and choice.

Knowledge of palliative care principles is encouraged as part of the practice of all health professionals caring for patients with life-limiting illness.

In the UK, the addition of gynaecological cancer nurse specialists to cancer multidisciplinary teams has greatly enhanced the care of women during diagnosis and treatment. These nurses are able to play a key role in exchange of information between hospital and community teams as well as liaising with specialist palliative care services.

For patients with complex or unresolved symptoms, or those approaching the end of life, involvement of specialist palliative care services, where available, is recommended.

Epidemiology
In the UK, about 7000 of the 17 000 women diagnosed with gynaecological cancer per annum will die from their disease. The incidence of common gynaecological cancers differs in developing and Western countries and is changing in both. The incidence of cervical cancer is falling whereas ovarian cancer is increasing. In the developed world, ovarian cancer deaths now exceed those of cervical and endometrial cancer combined. At diagnosis, two-thirds of ovarian tumours are at an advanced stage because most women with the disease are asymptomatic for a long time.

Clinical approach
Breaking bad news
Bad news can be defined as information that alters a patient's view of their future for the worse. Breaking bad news is not easy and can be daunting and demanding, but it is a skill that can be learnt, and it is an essential part of treatment and care. The following steps can assist clinicians in their approach to discussing difficult news.

- Find time and a private place.
- Try to have a relative or nurse with you.
- Know the facts before the meeting.
- Find out what the patient knows, e.g. 'What have you been told?'
- Find out what the patient wants to know, e.g. 'Are you the sort of person who likes to know everything about your illness?'
- Give a warning shot that bad news is coming, e.g. 'I'm afraid the test results were not very good'.
- Impart the news slowly, and as simply as possible, checking understanding and gauging response along the way and be prepared to stop if necessary.
- Avoid saying 'There is nothing more that can be done'. Don't lie, but offer realistic hope, e.g. controlling symptoms, treating pain, etc.
- Listen to concerns, e.g. 'What are your main concerns at the moment?'
- Encourage venting of feelings.
- Summarize concerns and give an opportunity for questions.
- Leave patients with a plan .and offer availability. Most patients need further explanation and support.

Principles of pain control in cancer
History and examination
Full assessment of the cause of the pain is integral to successful pain relief. Patients often have more than one pain, and different pains have different causes. Pain perception can be affected by psychological and emotional factors and pain can remain difficult to control if these factors are not identified and addressed.

Investigation
In the palliative care setting, investigations should be targeted at finding the cause of pain in order to plan appropriate treatment. For example, an isotope bone scan to look for bony metastases.

Unnecessary and inappropriate investigations that do not change management should be avoided.

Management
Cancer pain management may consist of drug and non-drug measures. With proper assessment and a logical step-wise approach to analgesic prescribing, at least 80% of chronic cancer pain can be controlled. Where pain is not responding to treatment, specialist advice should be sought. Consideration must also be given to treating pain by means of surgery, radiotherapy, and chemotherapy where possible and appropriate (Forbes 1998).

Common cancer-related pains
- Visceral/soft tissue
  - opioid sensitive so use 'analgesic ladder' (see below).
- Bone pain
  - sensitive to non steroidal anti-inflammatory drugs (NSAIDs)
  - partly opioid sensitive
  - radiotherapy may be helpful
  - consider intravenous bisphosphonates.
- Nerve related
  - partly opioid sensitive

- adjuvant analgesics may also be needed (see below)
- Non-drug measures such as transcutaneous electrical nerve stimulation (TENS) machine or nerve block may need to be considered in conjunction with drug therapy.

Cancer unrelated pain
1 Treatment related, e.g. constipation, radiotherapy.
2 Coincident illness or condition, e.g. diabetes, arthritis.

Principles of cancer pain control
- 'By the clock': cancer pain is continuous and therefore requires *regular* analgesia at appropriate dose intervals.
- 'By mouth': use oral route unless the patient is unable to swallow or there are concerns about absorption.
- 'By the analgesic ladder'

Analgesic ladder
- Step 1: non-opioid analgesic, e.g. paracetamol
- Step 2: weak opioid plus non-opioid, e.g. dihydrocodeine + paracetamol
- Step 3: strong opioid plus non-opioid, e.g. morphine + paracetamol

Adjuvant analgesics
Drugs primarily used for indications other than pain, but which can provide pain relief in certain situations. They can be used in combination with drugs at all steps of the analgesic ladder.
  Common adjuvant analgesics for cancer pain
1 Non steroidal anti-inflammatory drug: bone pain, pleuritic pain, hepatomegaly
2 Corticosteroid: raised intracranial pressure, hepatomegaly, and nerve compression
3 Antidepressants and anticonvulsants: neuropathic pain due to nerve damage or compression, and tenesmus.
4 Bisphosphonates: bone pain (Gralow *et al.* 2007).
  Use of strong opioids
- Gain pain control: use immediate release morphine, starting dose 5–10 mg 4 hourly (i.e. six doses daily) and titrate against pain with a 30–50% increase in dose every 2 or 3 days if pain uncontrolled. Reassess pain control each day if possible.
  1 Maintenance: change to 12 hourly modified release morphine, e.g. MST, by dividing total 24-hour morphine dose by 2. Breakthrough dose of immediate release morphine should be made available (one-sixth of 24-hour dose of morphine).
  2 Other strong opioids may be considered if the patient develops unacceptable side effects on morphine. For example, fentanyl causes less opioid induced constipation than morphine. Seek specialist advice from palliative care team if pain is unrelieved or patient has unacceptable side-effects from opioids.

Common side-effects of opioids (strong and weak)
- Constipation: must be anticipated and prevented in all patients on weak and strong opioids. A regular stimulant laxative must be commenced at the same time (see constipation section)
- Sedation: may occur with the first few doses but then usually lessens.
- Nausea: is a common problem during the first few days of treatment. If it occurs, haloperidol, domperidone, cyclizine or metoclopramide are all useful.

Principles for control of nausea and vomiting
History and examination
A logical approach to the use of antiemetics depends on knowledge of the cause of the symptom. The patient should be assessed with regard to the cause and whenever possible this cause should be addressed. Potential causes for nausea and vomiting include drugs, renal failure, deranged liver function, hypercalcaemia, ascites, bowel obstruction, constipation, brain metastases, sepsis, and humoral tumour effects.

Investigation
This may include full blood count, serum urea, and electrolytes, including corrected calcium, plain abdominal film, abdominal ultrasound scan, and head CT scan.

Management
Consider the following.
- Stop or change drugs which are causing nausea.
- Avoid drugs with anticholinergic effects if gastric stasis is present (hyoscine, antidepressants, cyclizine).
- Antiemetics may be necessary for the first few days when opioid therapy is initiated.
- Correct abnormal biochemistry, particularly malignant hypercalcaemia.

Principles of nausea and vomiting control
- Ensure chosen antiemetic is used *regularly* and to a maximum dose before changing.
- If first drug is ineffective, change to a drug from another pharmacological group.
- If first drug is partially effective, add a drug from another pharmacological group.
- Cyclizine and other anticholinergic drugs antagonize some of the effects of metoclopramide and domperidone. The combination should be avoided if possible.
- If symptoms persist for more than 24–48 hours in spite of the oral route, change to a non-oral route.
  Target antiemetic to probable cause of nausea and vomiting.
- Drug induced and biochemical: metoclopramide, haloperidol, cyclizine or levomepromazine
- Squashed stomach due to ascites or hepatomegaly, and delayed gastric emptying: metoclopramide or domperidone
- Stimulation of gastrointestinal receptors e.g. local tumour, oropharyngeal candida, bowel obstruction: cyclizine, levomepromazine
- Central causes, e.g. raised intracranial pressure, vestibular or motion related: cyclizine
- Chemotherapy induced: ondansetron, granisetron.
- Note that the place of 5HT3 antagonists in non-chemotherapy induced nausea and vomiting is not yet clear. They can cause severe constipation and should not be used first or second line.
  Medical management of malignant intestinal obstruction (Mercadante *et al.* 2007).
- About a quarter of women with advanced ovarian cancer develop bowel obstruction and medical or surgical palliative treatment can be used.
- Clinical features include abdominal pain and distension, vomiting, colic, constipation, and loud bowel sounds.
- Surgery should always be considered but may not be indicated or desired.

- It may be possible to keep a patient tolerably symptom controlled (although some vomiting may still occur) with medication given via a syringe driver, without a nasogastric tube or intravenous infusion.
- Main principles of management are to control nausea, colic, and other abdominal pain.
- Generally, when complete intestinal obstruction occurs, prokinetic agents such as metoclopramide and stimulant laxatives are to be avoided.
- In subacute obstruction, particularly if it is functional, a combination of metoclopramide and dexamethasone may be effective in restoring function.
- Patients may be able to tolerate small amounts of food and fluid if nausea is well controlled.
- If large volume vomits persist after a trial of hyoscine butylbromide (buscopan), a proton pump inhibitor can reduce gastric secretions. The somatostatin analogue octreotide may also be helpful. Seek palliative care advice.
- If thirst is severe, intravenous or subcutaneous fluids can be used, although the patient may be comfortable with good oral care and ice to suck.
- Nasogastric tube or drainage gastrostomy may be considered, in discussion with the patient, to reduce symptoms if all else fails.

Drugs in syringe driver
- Abdominal pain: morphine or diamorphine (starting dose 5–10 mg/24 hours or 50% of total oral 24-hour dose).
- Nausea: haloperidol (2.5–5 mg/24 hours) ± cyclizine (150 mg/24 hours) or levomepromazine alone (starting dose 6.25 mg/24 hours)
- Colic and to reduce secretions: hyoscine butylbromide (60–120 mg/24 hours)
- Second line to reduce secretions: octreotide (range 300–600 µg/24 hours)

Do not mix cyclizine and hyoscine butylbromide in a driver as they may precipitate.

Constipation
History and examination
Constipation (difficulty in defaecation) is common in patients with advanced cancer. Immobility, reduced oral intake, constipating drugs, and raised serum calcium are all contributory factors. Constipation should be anticipated in all patients taking opioids, 5HT3 receptor antagonists, or anticholinergic drugs (e.g. cyclizine, tricyclic antidepressants). Chronic constipation can cause anorexia, vomiting, colic, tenesmus, spurious diarrhoea, urinary retention, and mental confusion.

Abdominal palpation may reveal hard faecal material in the descending and sigmoid colon. Examination should include a rectal examination to guide management. In addition to determining the presence or absence of faeces and its consistency, it will also reveal a palpable tumour mass which may be exacerbating the problem.

Investigation
Serum urea and electrolytes will confirm any dehydration, hypokalaemia due to diuretics, or hypercalcaemia. Plain abdominal film should not be used to diagnose constipation, but may confirm dilated loops of bowel in bowel obstruction.

Management
Constipation is a common cause of distress and is better anticipated and avoided where possible. Laxatives are the main treatment of constipation in palliative care patients. They should be started as soon as strong or weak opioids are prescribed. The laxative dose should be increased if the dose of opioid is increased (Twycross et al. 1991).

A good first choice is the combination of a stimulant laxative with a softening agent, e.g. senna and docusate sodium or a combination laxative such as codanthromer.

Danthron (in codanthromer) stains urine red and should be avoided in the incontinent patient as it can cause perianal skin irritation. Its use is restricted to constipation in terminally ill patients.

Movicol is an osmotic laxative which can be effective.

In general, lactulose alone is not effective for opioid-induced constipation and should be avoided in patients with inadequate fluid intake. Lactulose can cause flatulence and abdominal cramps.

Twenty-five per cent of patients on laxatives may still need rectal measures at times. High fluid intake, fruit, and fruit juice (especially prune juice) can all help.

For patients with existing constipation, the following principles can be helpful:
- Is rectum full?
  - Hard faeces: lubricate using glycerine (glycerol) suppositories or soften with an arachis oil enema
  - When clear commence stimulant laxative with faecal softener
  - Soft faeces: start stimulant laxative
  - If no success: trial of Movicol.
- Is rectum empty?
  - Exclude obstruction or high constipation
- Is colon full?
  - If colic is present: start faecal softener
  - If colic is absent: start stimulant laxative ± softener

It is not normally necessary to use strong stimulant laxatives such as Picolax.

Fybogel is best avoided in cancer patients as many are unable to drink adequate volumes of fluid and it can lead to impaction.

Recurrent malignant ascites
History and examination
Ascites results from an imbalance between fluid influx and efflux in the peritoneal cavity.

Ascites can be asymptomatic when mild but distressing when severe. Clinical features include abdominal distension, abdominal discomfort or pain, early satiety, dyspepsia, acid reflux, nausea and vomiting, leg oedema, and breathlessness.

Ovarian cancer is the commonest primary tumour associated with ascites, present in 30% of patients at presentation and 60% in the terminal phase.

Investigation
Blood tests including urea and electrolytes, liver function tests, and INR are helpful prior to attempting an ascitic tap. Abnormal clotting may need correcting prior to drainage. Abdominal ultrasound and marking of drainage point may be advisable to confirm the presence of ascites, to avoid tumour masses, or if loculation of ascites is suspected. Ascitic fluid may be required to help with cancer diagnosis if this is the patient's presenting symptom.

Management

If appropriate and successful, chemotherapy may control ascites. However, in most cases of malignancy-related ascites, the prognosis is poor and the principle in managing these patients should be one of minimal intervention. Unnecessary investigations should be avoided and drains should be left in for only a short time.

Paracentesis is appropriate for patients with a tense distended abdomen. The aim is to remove as much fluid as possible using a suitable catheter. Individual hospitals will usually have their own protocols but the following principles apply.

- If there is substantial ascites in the form of a tense abdomen and fluid thrill, it is usually safe to proceed without diagnostic imaging. Ultrasound can be helpful to mark an area for drainage if paracentesis has been difficult in the past or if solid tumour is easily palpable. In some centres, the drain is inserted under ultrasound guidance.
- In patients with no cytological proof of malignancy, send all ascitic fluid to cytology for analysis as well as 20 mL to bacteriology for microscopy and culture
- Clamping of drains to reduce the drainage rate is usually unnecessary, particularly for volumes less than 5 L.
- There is no evidence that leaving the drain in for 24–48 hours or more is safer or more effective. Leave the catheter on free drainage for a maximum of 6 hours. and then remove (Stevenson J et al. 2002).
- The limited evidence available suggests that significant hypotension is not usually a problem, the administration of intravenous fluids is rarely needed, and intravenous albumen has no proven role.
- Diuretics: spironolactone antagonizes aldosterone and may slow down reaccumulation of ascites. The starting dose is 100–200 mg mane with a typical maintenance dose of 300 mg per day. Urea and electrolytes need to be monitored. If spironolactone alone is ineffective, frusemide 40 mg once daily can be added.
- Paracentesis may need to be repeated every 3–6 weeks if diuretics do not slow down reaccumulation.
- Peritoneovenous shunts are rarely used for malignant disease.

Breathlessness

History and examination
Cancer-related breathlessness can be caused by the cancer directly, general debility, treatment, or concurrent illness.

Potential causes include
- chest infection
- anaemia
- pleural effusion
- tense ascites
- pulmonary emboli
- lung metastases
- lymphangitis
- cancer cachexia

Investigation

Appropriate investigations to help make the diagnosis will include blood tests and a chest X-ray. Blood gases and ECG may be appropriate in the acutely unwell patient. Pulse oximetry will determine whether the patient is hypoxic.

Management

Management strategies should be targeted, where possible, at the probable cause of the breathlessness. Where this is not possible, general management principles can be applied.

- Reassurance and explanation.
- Reverse the reversible, e.g. drain pleural effusion or ascites unless the patient is in the terminal phase of their illness.
- Consider oxygen if the patient is hypoxic.
- Use of a fan, either fixed or hand held, to promote movement of air across the patients face can be helpful in the absence of hypoxia and avoids oxygen dependence.
- Occupational therapy and physiotherapy expertise can help the patient to manage their shortness of breath by adapting their environment and teaching coping strategies such as pacing and relaxation techniques.
- Pharmacological treatment includes:
  - low-dose opioids, e.g. oramorph 2.5–5 mg 6 hourly initially and titrated according to effect, duration of effect, and adverse effects
  - benzodiazepines, e.g. diazepam at a starting dose of 2 mg twice or three times daily. Use lowest effective dose as the drug can accumulate and cause memory loss and falls. Lorazepam is long acting but can be used sublingually for rapid onset in panic attacks at a dose of 0.5–1 mg.

Malignant fistulae

History and examination
The definition of a fistula is an abnormal communication between two hollow organs or between a hollow organ and the skin.

Advanced cervical cancer is the most common cause of a fistula among gynaecological malignancies. Fistulae in advanced cancer can develop as a result of postoperative infection, pelvic radiotherapy, or a combination of the two. A few are caused solely by tumour progression and necrosis. The fistula may be vesicovaginal, rectovaginal, or a combination. Patients will usually volunteer a history of pneumaturia or passage of faeces per vagina. In the case of a rectovaginal fistula, examination may reveal tumour or a palpable defect in the vaginal wall.

Investigation

Abdominal imaging such as a CT scan may be required to confirm tumour recurrence or in an attempt to identify the site of the fistula if further treatment is planned. Radiological advice will help to determine the most appropriate investigation.

Management

A multidisciplinary approach to decision-making and symptom management is recommended in these patients. This may include a gynaecological oncologist, palliative care specialist, continence nurse, and gynaecological nurse specialist.

- Patients with a poor prognosis and performance status may be best managed conservatively. Stoma may not be trouble free, and there may be psychological reasons not to want surgery. However, rectovaginal fistulae can be distressing to patients due to discomfort and odour.
- Conservative management will need to concentrate on:
  - urine collection: usually with pads, or tampons inserted in to the vagina

- faecal collection: using pads
- skin protection: use of barrier cream to prevent excoriation and soreness
- odour control (see fungating wounds).
- Surgical options will include:
  - urinary diversion: usually by formation of an ileal conduit
  - bowel diversion: the simplest possible. Widespread intra-abdominal disease can make this difficult. Increasing expertise in colonic stenting may provide new, less invasive options for management of malignant fistulae
  - fistula repair: if possible and appropriate.

Tumour fungation
History and examination
A fungating cancer is a primary or secondary tumour which has ulcerated the skin. The tumour may proliferate or cavitate and is often associated with pain, pruritis, exudate, malodour, bleeding, infection, and psychological distress to patient, carers, and family.

Investigation
Microbacterial swabs may be needed to rule out infection such as *Staphylococcus aureus* and pseudomonas as an additional cause of malodour and exudate. Serum platelet levels and clotting should be checked if heavy bleeding occurs.

Management
- If the tumour is sensitive to radiotherapy or chemotherapy, a significant reduction in tumour size and skin healing can be achieved (Forbes K 1998).
- Pain due to fungating wounds can be multifactorial. The general approach to management will be as outlined above using oral analgesia and drugs for neuropathic pain may need to be included. In addition, there is some evidence that topical morphine may reduce pain (Back et al. 1995; Krajnik et al. 1997). Nociceptive afferent nerve fibres contain peripheral opioid receptors that are silent except in the presence of local inflammation. Generally, morphine is applied as a 0.1% (1 mg/mL) gel in a water-based gel (e.g. Intrasite gel). The amount of gel varies according to the size and site of the tumour but is typically 5–10 mL applied twice to three times daily. It can be kept in place by a non-absorbable pad or dressing such as Opsite.
- Pruritis is probably caused by inflammatory agents such as prostaglandins and may respond to non-steroidal anti-inflammatory drugs.
- Exudate: specialist dressings can be chosen depending on the relative amounts of odour and infection.
- Malodour is particularly problematic. It is caused by a combination of tumour necrosis and deep anaerobic infection. Treatment includes oral or topical metronidazole, charcoal dressings, occlusive dressings such as Opsite or Granuflex, and debridement of devitalized tissue to remove the source of odour-forming bacteria using agents such as topical Manuka honey. The patient may need to be nursed in a single room. Odour in the room may be masked by aromatic oil burners. Another option is to place a cat litter tray under the bed.
- Surface bleeding may be controlled using physical measures such as application of adrenaline-soaked gauze

(1 in 1000), silver nitrate sticks, alginate dressings, and diathermy. Oral haemostatic drugs such as tranexamic acid 1 g qds may also help. Radiotherapy and embolization may be needed to control more severe recurrent spontaneous bleeding.

The syringe driver
The syringe driver is a small, portable battery-operated infusion pump, used to give medication subcutaneously over 24 hours. It can be used when other routes (e.g. oral, buccal, rectal, or transdermal) are unsuitable. Local guidelines on use will often exist. They are often used to deliver drugs at the end of life but can be useful at other stages of illness.

Indications
- Inability to swallow
- Persistent nausea and vomiting
- Interference with oral absorption
- Unconscious patient.

Mixing drugs in a syringe driver
Principles:
- Try to avoid mixing more than three drugs in a syringe at one time.
- All of the following drugs can be mixed with morphine or diamorphine in a syringe driver.
  - Antiemetic: Metoclopramide, haloperidol, cyclizine
  - Sedative and antiemetic: Levomepromazine
  - Sedative: Midazolam
  - Colic: Hyoscine butylbromide (Buscopan)
  - Terminal secretions: Hyoscine hydrobromide (crosses blood–brain barrier and sedating)
- Cyclizine and hyoscine butylbromide should not be mixed in the same syringe as they may precipitate.
- As needed (prn) doses of subcutaneous diamorphine or morphine should be prescribed for breakthrough pain, calculated to be a one-sixth of the total 24-hour dose.
- To covert from oral morphine to subcutaneous diamorphine, divide total 24-hour morphine dose by 3 to obtain total 24-hour diamorphine dose. This is based on 3 mg of oral morphine (any form) being equivalent to 1 mg of diamorphine injection.
- To convert from oral morphine to subcutaneous morphine, divide total 24-hour oral morphine dose by 2 to obtain total 24-hour subcutaneous morphine dose. This is based on 2 mg of oral morphine (any form) being equivalent to 1 mg of morphine injection.

Palliative care emergencies
Malignant hypercalcaemia
- Common in cervical cancer and is a poor prognostic sign.
- Can occur in the absence of bone metastases due to PTHrP (parathyroid hormone-related protein) produced by the tumour.
- Consider treating with intravenous fluids and intravenous bisphosphonates if the patient has a persistently raised serum corrected calcium level greater than 2.8 mmol/L and is symptomatic of hypercalcaemia, unless the patient is in the terminal phase of their illness.
- Renal function will dictate safe fluid volumes and correct dose of bisphosphonate.

Table 14.7.1 Drugs in a syringe driver for the terminal phase

Symptom	Drug	24-hour dose in syringe driver	As required subcutaneous dose (prn)
Pain	Morphine	Half of 24-hour oral dose or 10 mg in opioid naïve patient	One sixth of 24-hour dose in syringe driver or 2.5–5 mg 4 hourly
	Diamorphine	One-third of 24-hour oral dose or 10 mg in opioid naïve patient	
Nausea	Cyclizine	100–150 mg	50 mg 8 hourly
Terminal secretions	Hyoscine hydrobromide	1.2 mg	0.4 mg 4 hourly
Terminal agitation	Midazolam	10–20 mg	2.5–5 mg 4 hourly

Massive haemorrhage
- Frightening for patient, family, and staff
- If a patient is at risk of a large bleed, consider prescribing crisis medication of midazolam 2.5–5 mg subcutaneously and morphine 5–10 mg subcutaneously (or one-sixth of normal daily oral dose converted to the subcutaneous route) just in case.
  - Red or green towels or blankets should be available to soak up blood.
- Patient may become semiconscious quickly
- A reassuring presence is the most important factor; therefore, stay with the patient.
- If a second nurse or doctor is present, ask them to administer the crisis drugs.

Spinal cord compression
Consider in patients that develop problems with urinary retention, faecal incontinence, and sensory changes or loss of motor function in the lower limbs.
- Requires immediate commencement of high dose steroids (dexamethasone 4 mg qds) followed by urgent MRI scan of spine within 24 hours. Discussion with oncology team for advice regarding urgent radiotherapy or neurosurgical opinion is advised.

The terminal phase
Optimal management of the terminal phase depends on recognition that the patient is dying. Consistent communication of this fact within the medical and nursing team to the patient's family, and sometimes to the patient themselves is essential. Signs that death may be approaching include the patient becoming bed bound, only taking small amounts of food and fluid, becoming semicomatose, and no longer being able to take their tablets. This allows discontinuation of inappropriate drugs, investigations and observations, and prescription of appropriate drugs for symptom control (Ellershaw *et al.* 2003).

If the patient is unable to swallow, appropriate drugs for pain, nausea, chest secretions, and agitation can prescribed for prn (as required) administration in anticipation of symptoms, or mixed in a syringe driver if symptoms are present (Table 14.7.1).

Some centres use integrated care pathways, e.g. the Liverpool Care Pathway for the Dying Patient (LCP), as the final multiprofessional documentation. These pathways aim to standardize care for the dying patient by applying evidence-based practice and appropriate guidelines related to care of the dying.

Further reading

Back IN, Finlay I. Analgesic effect of topical opioids on painful skin ulcers. J Pain Symptom Manage 1995;10:493.

Dickman A, Schneider J, Varga J. *The syringe driver: continuous subcutaneous infusions in palliative care.* Oxford: Oxford University Press; 2005.

Ellershaw J, Ward C. Care of the dying patient: the last hours or days of life. BMJ 2003;326:30–4.

Ellershaw J, Wilkinson S. *Care of the dying: a pathway to excellence.* Oxford: Oxford University Press 2003.

Forbes K. Complications of radiotherapy for gynaecological malignancy. Eur J Palliat Care 1998;5:175–8.

Gralow J, Tripathy D. Managing metastatic bone pain: the role of bisphosphonates. J Pain Symptom Manage 2007;33 (4):462–72.

Hanks G, Cherny N, Christakis N, Fallon M (eds) *Oxford textbook of palliative medicine.* Oxford: Oxford University Press 2009.

Krajnik M, Zylicz Z. Topical morphine for cutaneous cancer pain. Palliat Med 1997;11:326.

Mercadante S, Casuccio A, Mangione S. Medical treatment for inoperable malignant bowel obstruction: a qualitative systemic review. J Pain Symptom Manage 2007;33:217–23.

Stevenson J, Gilbert J. The development of clinical guidelines on paracentesis for ascites related to malignancy. Palliat Med 2002;16:213–18.

Twycross R, Wilcox A. *Symptom management in advanced cancer.* Radcliffe Medical Press 2001.

Twycross RG, Harcourt JMV. The use of laxatives at a palliative care centre. Palliat Med 1991;13:159–60.

Internet resources

Information for professionals on drugs usage in palliative care: www.palliativedrugs.com

Website for national end of life programme containing resources, information and examples of good practice: www.endoflifecare. nhs.uk.

Scottish Intercollegiate Guidelines Network (SIGN) guidelines on control of pain in adults with cancer: www.sign.ac.uk.

Patient resources

Cancer Research UK—cancer statistics: info.cancerresearchuk.org/cancerstats/types

Macmillan Cancer Support website containing help, support and advice for those suffering from cancer and information on common cancers, treatments and side-effects: www.macmillan.org.uk

World Health Organization statements on palliative care: www. who.int/cancer/palliative/en/

Vulval cancer

Carcinoma of the vulva is a rare gynaecological cancer, accounting for 3% of gynaecological tumours, with approximately 1000 new cases registered each year in the UK, a rate of 3 per 100 000 of the population. It is the twentieth most common cancer in women and ranks as the nineteenth most common cause of cancer deaths in women. The disease commonly occurs in older women, with two-thirds of cases occurring over the age of 70 years. Approximately 15% of vulval cancers occur in women who are less than 40 years of age and are increasingly seen in younger women. Ninety per cent of cancers are squamous cell cancers and traditionally treatment has been by radical vulvectomy with groin node dissection. Over the past decade or so, the management of this condition has undergone considerable evolution with an emphasis on individualizing treatment for each case rather than a uniform surgical policy (Burke et al. 1995). These cancers are most effectively treated by a multidisciplinary team with expertise in specialized surgical and radiotherapeutic techniques.

Minimally invasive stage 1a tumours can be treated by wide local excision alone; however, all other tumours are likely to require inguinal node dissection or radiotherapy as well as definitive treatment of the vulval lesion.

Postoperative radiotherapy improves regional disease control and survival in patients with positive inguinal lymph nodes. Pelvic lymph node dissection is no longer performed. In cases of advanced vulval cancer or where there is involvement of the anus, rectovaginal septum, urethra, or vagina, complete responses have been reported using a regime of cisplatin and 5-fluorouracil (5FU) with external beam radiation to the vulva.

The physical and psychosexual impact of vulval cancer and its treatment should be managed in a proactive fashion with early involvement of nurse specialists and experts in this field (Allan 2003).

Pathology

- About 95% of malignant vulval neoplasm are squamous cell carcinomas. These tumours can be divided into subtypes. Keratinizing tumours are most common. Basaloid and warty subtypes are associated with human papillomavirus (HPV) infection and occur in younger women.
- Verrucous carcinoma is a well-differentiated squamous carcinoma that is locally invasive but does not metastasize to regional lymph nodes. Radiotherapy can lead to anaplastic change and rapid invasion.
- Malignant melanomas account for approximately 5% of vulval neoplasms. The prognosis for malignant melanomas of the vulva depends on depth of invasion as described by Breslow.
- Basal cell cancers are treated by wide local excision as this tumour rarely involves the lymphatics.
- Adenocarcinoma of the Bartholin's gland and sarcomas are extremely uncommon, each accounting for 1–2% of vulval neoplasms.

Aetiology

- There are two causes of vulval cancer, one related to HPV infection usually types 16, 18, and 31 and occurring in younger women, and the other seen in elderly patients arising in a background of differentiated vulval intraepithelial neoplasia (VIN), often after years of lichen sclerosis.
- VIN: the lifetime risk of developing vulval cancer is approximately 4–7% if a woman has VIN. However, the relationship between squamous cell carcinoma and VIN is not as well defined as in cancer of the cervix, and recent studies suggest that VIN presenting in young women carries a greater risk of recurrence with a progression to invasive cancer of 10–15%. The incidence of VIN has been reported to have increased by up to three-fold over the past two decades in women under 35 years of age.
- VIN3 can be subdivided into three types: warty, basaloid and differentiated. Basaloid and warty vulval cancer are associated with adjacent undifferentiated VIN and are often HPV positive. There is often a solitary HPV type, usually type 16.
- The more common keratinizing squamous cell carcinomas, seen in the older woman, is associated with adjacent differentiated VIN which is usually HPV negative and often associated with squamous hyperplasia and lichen sclerosis.
- Lichen sclerosis is associated with squamous cell carcinoma. About 30% of SCCs arise in women who have lichen sclerosis and the lifetime risk of developing cancer with lichen sclerosis is estimated at 3–5%. The chronic pruritus associated with this disease has been implicated in the aetiology of vulval cancer described as the 'itch scratch cycle'.
- Smoking and immunosuppression also appear to be more common in younger patients who develop vulval neoplasm. These patients are prone to multifocal, multicentric intraepithelial disease with the associated risk of carcinoma.
- P53 mutations are often seen in the HPV-negative cancers in older women.

Staging

In 1988 (updated in 2009) the FIGO (Table 14.8.1) staging for vulval cancer was changed to a surgical staging system based on the findings of the vulval excision and inguinal lymph node dissection, based on the tumour–node–metastases (TNM) classification.

Prognostic factors

- The 5-year survival for patients is related to the FIGO stage (Table 14.8.2)
- Metastatic disease in the regional lymph nodes is the most important independent prognostic factor influencing survival. Most publications have reported higher rates of recurrence and death in patients whose tumours are deeply invasive are high grade, have a high mitotic rate and/or associated with lymphovascular space invasion (Homesley et al. 1993).
- The depth of invasion is the most important factor predicting lymph node involvement. When the depth of invasion is between 1 and 2 mm the incidence of positive inguinofemoral nodes is 8%, rising to 30% when the depth of invasion is between 3 and 5 mm.
- The status of the inguinofemoral and pelvic nodes are important in predicting survival. The 5-year survival for a

Table 14.8.1 FIGO staging for vulval carcinoma (2009)

Stage I	Tumour confined to the vulva
IA IB	Lesions ≤2 cm in size, confined to the vulva or perineum and with stromal invasion ≤1.0 mm, no nodal metastasis Lesions >2 cm in size or with stromal invasions >1.0 mm, confined to the vulva or perineum, with negative nodes
Stage II	Tumour of any size with extension to adjacent perineal structures one-third lower urethra, one-third lower vagina, anus) with negative nodes
Stage III IIIA	Tumour of any size with or without extension to adjacent perineal structures (one-third lower urethra, one-third lower vagina, anus) with positive inguinofemoral lymph nodes
IIIB	(i) With one lymph node metastasis ≥5 mm) or (ii) one or two lymph node metastasis(es) (<5 mm) (i) With two or more lymph node metastases (≥5 mm) or(ii) Three or more lymph node metastases (<5 mm)
IIIC	With positive nodes with extracapsular spread
Stage IV	Tumour invades other regional (two-thirds upper urethra, two-thirds upper vagina) or distant structures
IVA	Tumour invades any of the following:(i) Upper urethra and/or vaginal mucosa, bladder mucosa, rectal mucosa, or fixed to pelvic bone, or(ii) Fixed or ulcerated inguinofemoral lymph nodes
IVB	Any distant metastasis including pelvic lymph nodes

The depth of invasion is defined as the measurement of the tumour from the epithelial stromal junction of the adjacent most superficial dermal papilla to the deepest point of invasion.

Computed tomography (CT) and magnetic resonance imaging (MRI) cannot be used to alter the FIGO stage, although they may be useful for treatment planning.

patient with negative lymph nodes is 80–90%, falling to 40–50% where there are metastases to lymph nodes. Three or more unilateral positive nodes or two or more bilateral nodes have a 30% 5-year survival.

- Both the size and the number of inguinofemoral lymph node metastases affect survival. Intracapsular metastases are associated with a better outcome than cases where there is extra capsular disease. Patients with fewer than three nodes involved have a low risk of pelvic node disease and a good prognosis.
- Patients with pelvic lymph node involvement are generally considered to have an extremely poor prognosis; however, these data were collected from patients who underwent pelvic lymph node dissections before the mid 1980s. This procedure is rarely performed nowadays

Table 14.8.2 FIGO stages

FIGO Stage	5-year survival (%)	Nodal involvement (%)
I	90	10
II	81	26
III	48	64
IV	15	89

and patients with inguinal metastases will have postoperative radiotherapy with fields that include the pelvic lymph nodes. As a consequence, the impact of current treatment on the prognosis of patients with pelvic lymph node metastases is unknown.

Clinical approach

Diagnosis

Symptoms: key points

- The vast majority of patients are symptomatic, complaining of itch, vulval pain, burning, bleeding, or swelling.
- A delay in diagnosis is not uncommon because of embarrassment both for the patient as well as the primary care physician, which may postpone examination. Topical treatments may be prescribed before a thorough examination has taken place.
- An invasive cancer may be incidental findings at the time of biopsy of presumed VIN.
- Vulval warts are uncommon in postmenopausal women and there should be a low threshold for performing a biopsy.
- Multiple biopsies may be required in patients who are immunosuppressed or exhibit evidence of HPV infection.
- A possibility of multicentric HPV-related genital intraepithelial neoplasia dictates that a thorough examination of the lower genital tract including a cervical smear and evaluation of the perianal region is required.

Investigations: key points

- Biopsy is mandatory before planning management. Increasingly photographs are used as a diagnostic aid and are particularly useful when planning primary surgical treatment.
- 'Incisional' biopsy is preferable to 'excisional' biopsy prior to a multidisciplinary team referral. A limited biopsy allows the gynaecological oncologist to fully assess the vulval lesion.
- Punch biopsy under local anaesthetic in the clinic is usually possible. A 4–6 mm punch biopsy can be taken under local anaesthetic using a *Keyes biopsy*. Ideally, the tumour should be photographed. However, a wedge biopsy may be required in larger vulval tumours or where there is discrepancy between the clinical findings and pathology. A biopsy from the edge with some normal adjacent skin is required to facilitate the diagnosis.
- Pelvic examination remains the most important tool for evaluation of the local extent of vulval tumours. The location, gross morphology, sites of involvement, and dimensions of the tumour should be carefully recorded. The proximity of the tumour to midline structures should also be noted.
- Patients with extensive disease may require examination under anaesthesia to assess the extent of involvement of structures such as the urethra and anal sphincter. Ideally these examinations should be performed by the multidisciplinary team including a gynaecological oncologist, general/urological/plastic surgeons, and radiation oncologist.
- CT and MRI can be helpful in detecting pelvic or inguinal lymphadenopathy in patients with extensive disease.
- Suspicious groin nodes should be sampled using fine needle aspiration or a similar technique, in the outpatient clinic.

Management

General: key points

- As many of the patients with a vulval cancer will be elderly with coexisting medical conditions, preoperative investigations and assessment by an anaesthetist will be required. In patients who are fit for anaesthesia, radical surgery is treatment of choice.

- The preoperative assessment should also include the likely need for occupational therapy and social services to ensure that there is a prompt supported discharge plan.

- As the treatment of vulval cancer has moved towards a more individualized, multidisciplinary approach, surgery should be undertaken in a cancer centre where there are experienced gynaecological oncology surgeons working in conjunction with other specialties.

- The treatment of vulval cancer is surgical and is carried out with curative intent. There is good evidence that patients who have inguinal metastases from vulval cancer frequently can be cured if their regional disease is addressed with appropriate treatment (radiotherapy). The vulva is richly supplied with lymphatics, and regional spread of vulval cancers is common.

- The benefit of radiotherapy in achieving local regional control and improved survival has been well demonstrated although the role of chemoradiotherapy has not yet been fully evaluated.

- There should be psychological support for patients undergoing treatment for vulval cancer at an early stage (Green 2000).

Local disease: key points

- Stage Ia tumours: many series have demonstrated that the risk of lymph metastases is less than 1% for patients with tumours that invade no more than 1 mm. These are the only cases that can safely be treated without addressing the inguinofemoral lymph nodes. Wide local excision should be performed with a 1 cm margin of normal tissue. Most gynaecologists will use a 1.5-cm margin on the fresh surgical specimen. If the surgical specimen reveals inadequate excision or deeper invasion than anticipated, then re-excision and treatment of the inguinofemoral lymph nodes is required.

- Stage Ib–II tumours: the traditional radical vulvectomy plus *en bloc* bilateral groin node dissection is rarely undertaken. Nowadays, the aim of the primary surgery is to obtain a wide excision that extends to the perineal fascia with a 2-cm margin of uninvolved tissue. In most cases, this does not require resection of the entire vulva, although it is extremely important that the primary cancer is excised with adequate margins as this directly affects the risk of local recurrence. One study suggested that the margin of clearance of tumour is the best predictor of local recurrence. All of the recurrences on the vulva occurred where the surgically free margin was less than 8 mm. Primary closure of the wound may not be possible and some form of reconstructive procedure may be required.

- When cancers are close to the urethra or anus, it may be impossible to achieve adequate tumour free margins without compromising organ function. In these circumstances collaboration with urology and colorectal surgery will be required. Chemoradiotherapy should be considered either to reduce tumour volume to allow sphincter-sparing surgery or to replace surgery completely.

- All stage Ib and stage II tumours will require treatment to the inguinofemoral lymph nodes because of the risk of regional metastases.

- Stage III–IVa tumours: radical vulvectomy with bilateral groin node dissection should be performed if it is anticipated that the tumour can be removed without compromising urethral or anal function and with negative margins.

- Fixed groin nodes should be biopsied and groin and pelvic radiation considered rather than surgery. Phase II trials of concurrent 5-fluorouracil with or without cisplatin with radiotherapy resulted in complete response rates of 53–89% for advanced disease.

- When these tumours involve the urethra, bladder, anus, rectum, or vagina, although sometimes curable with ultraradical surgical procedures, many institutions are moving towards an organ sparing approach involving radiotherapy, chemoradiotherapy with or without surgery. Multidisciplinary cooperation is required so that the best results from this approach can be achieved (Blake 2003).

- Incomplete resection of a vulva tumour should be avoided as the dose of radiotherapy required to sterilise microscopically positive surgical margins is similar to that required to control gross disease and will add morbidity without clearly improving the likelihood of local control. Dramatic responses have been seen with chemoradiotherapy, although there have been no phase III trials of chemoradiotherapy in women with vulval cancer. The results for chemoradiotherapy treatment in patients with advanced cervical and anal cancers are encouraging and are likely to be similar for vulval disease.

Vulval reconstruction: key points

- The support of the plastic surgeons can improve the cosmetic and functional result following excision of a vulval tumour. There are a wide range of surgical options which will reduce infection and breakdown particularly in the perineal area.

- There is an increasing trend towards greater use of simple rotational flaps and transposition for small and medium sized defects (e.g. lotus petal) (Yii et al. 1996). Where the defect is more extensive it may be necessary to use pedicled flaps from the thigh or abdominal wall.

Regional disease: key points

- It is essential to address the risk of spread to the inguinofemoral lymph nodes at the time of initial management of the vulval cancer. Fewer than 20% of patients survive 5 years after an inguinal recurrence of previously treated vulval cancer.

- Treatment to the regional lymph nodes applies to all vulval cancers apart from stage Ia.

- The overall incidence of positive groin nodes in early disease is about 15%. The incidence of lymph involvement increases with the depth of invasion of the tumour.

- The groin node dissection consists of removing the nodes from the superficial compartment bounded by the inguinal ligament superiorly, the border of sartorius laterally and the border of adductor longus medially. The medial deep femoral lymph nodes should also be removed, as superficial inguinal node dissection alone is associated with a higher risk of groin node recurrence. Preservation of the long saphenous vein has been advocated to reduce postoperative groin wound and subsequent lower limb problems.

- A unilateral groin node dissection is appropriate if the cancer is well lateralized, being more than 1 cm from the midline. In all other situations a bilateral dissection should be performed.
- Where a unilateral dissection has revealed positive nodes then the current practice would be to remove the contralateral nodes. The incidence of positive contralateral nodes with negative ipsilateral groin nodes where the vulval tumour is less than 2 cm in diameter, and not involving the midline, is quoted at between 0 and 0.4%.
- Where the lymph node dissection reveals inguinal metastases, postoperative radiotherapy should be considered. The standard recommendation is that postoperative radiotherapy should be given if two or more groin nodes are involved with microscopic disease or if there is evidence of extracapsular spread or complete replacement in any lymph node. Radiotherapy should be given to the lateral pelvis and inguinal regions to the side or sides with positive nodes (Thomas et al. 1989).
- Studies of patients who have positive inguinal lymph nodes after radical vulvectomy and lympadenectomy have shown that postoperative radiotherapy reduces the rate of groin recurrence and significantly improves the survival rate.
- More selective groin node surgery may be possible in the future through lymphatic mapping and sentinel node biopsy (Acheson 2007). The combination of injecting radiolabelled technetium and isosulfan blue dye looks promising for the future to reduce the morbidity from groin node dissection.

Complications/side-effects of treatment

Surgery
- General: as this disease predominantly affects elderly women between the ages of 60 and 75 years, there may be coexisting medical problems increasing the morbidity and mortality of treatment. A perioperative mortality rate of 1–2% is quoted.
  - thromboembolic disease
  - infection
  - psychological and psychosexual sequelae.
- Vulval surgery
  - wound problems, infection and breakdown
  - cystocele and rectocele
  - narrowing of the introitus
  - osteomyelitis
  - sexual dysfunction.
- Inguinofemoral lymph dissection
  - wound problems, infection and breakdown
  - groin lymphocysts
  - leg lymphoedema
  - cellulitis
  - nerve damage.

Radiotherapy
- Skin desquamation
- Skin necrosis.

Reducing morbidity: key points
- Management should involve a multidisciplinary team in a cancer centre.

- An individualized approach with separate groin incisions (triple incision approach) has replaced the classical radical surgical resection with lymphadenectomy.
- Preliminary studies indicate that sentinel nodes can be identified in most cases of vulval carcinoma which would avoid formal lymph node dissection for over 60% of patients with stage Ib/II tumours. This would help reduce the 15–20% incidence of chronic leg lymphoedema and groin wound infection and dehiscence which occurs in over 50% of cases.
- Advanced tumours and those involving bladder, urethra, rectum, or anus should be considered for chemoradiotherapy rather than ultraradical surgery with loss of organ function. Concurrent chemoradiation using cisplatin and 5FU has produced encouraging results, 'downstaging' tumours so that a surgical approach can be considered. Current chemoradiotherapeutic regimes are not well tolerated by elderly people.

Follow-up
- Although the role of routine follow up on survival has been questioned for gynaecological cancers, patients find follow up visits very reassuring and it is an opportunity to look for long-term complications of treatment and any psychosexual concerns.
- A typical follow up schedule is for all patients to be seen every 3 months for the first 2 years, every 6 months for 3 years and then discharge after 5 years.

Recurrent vulval cancer
- Management and prognosis depend on the site and extent of the recurrent disease (Piura 1993). Wide local excision of a localised recurrence provides a 56% five year survival rate when the inguinofemoral nodes are not involved. Recurrence in the regional nodes is associated a poorer prognosis and a 5-year survival of approximately 20%.
- A multidisciplinary approach involving clinical oncologists, gynaecologists and general/urological/plastic surgeons will result in the most appropriate management for this group of patients.
- Treatment options will include
  - wide local excision
  - radical vulvectomy with pelvic exenteration
  - radiotherapy or chemoradiotherapy sometimes with further surgery. Suitable chemotherapy regimes are platinum and 5FU or cisplatin, methotrexate, and bleomycin.

Bartholin's gland carcinoma
- This is a rare vulval cancer with a peak age incidence in the mid-60s.
- It has a tendency to spread into the ischiorectal fossa and to the inguinal lymph nodes.
- It may spread directly to the pelvic lymph nodes.
- Treatment is radical vulvectomy and inguinal lymphadenectomy. To achieve adequate margins the rectum and a considerable part of the vagina may need to be removed. Reconstructive surgery with support from the plastic surgeons will often be necessary.

Malignant melanoma
- This is the second most common invasive cancer in this area.

- Melanomas are usually pigmented and raised but approximately 25% may be amelanotic and resemble a squamous cell cancer.
- Prognosis is related to the size of the lesion and the depth of invasion. The Clark classification and Breslow thickness are of prognostic benefit and apply to the vulva.
- First-line treatment is radical wide local excision. Routine inguinal lymphadenectomy has little place in the management of this disease as it spreads primarily by blood born metastases. A margin of 1 cm is sufficient for lesions with a depth of less than 2 mm and a 2–3-cm margin for lesions with a depth of more than 2 mm.
- Prognosis is related to the size of the lesion and the depth of invasion, and in general it is poor because of the late stage of presentation.

Further reading

Acheson N. New developments sentinel node mapping. Obstet Gynaecol 2007;9:270–5.

Allen J. The clinical nurse specialist in gynaecological oncology–the role in vulval cancer, best practice and research. Clin Obstet Gynaecol 2003;17:591–607.

Blake P. Radiotherapy and chemoradiotherapy for carcinoma of the vulva. Best Pract Res Clin Obstet Gynaecol 2003;17:649–61.

Breslow A. Thickness, cross-sectional areas and depth of invasion in the prognosis of cutaneous melanoma. Ann Surg 1970 172:902.

Burke TW, Levenback C, Coleman RL, et al. Surgical therapy of T1 and T2 vulvar carcinoma: further experience with radical wide excision and selective inguinal lymphadenectomy Gynecol Oncol 1995; 57:215–20.

Green MS, Naumann RW, Elliot M, et al. Sexual dysfunction following vulvectomy. Gynecol Oncol 2000; 77:363–77.

Homesley HD, Bundy BN, Sealis A, et al. Prognostic factors for groin node metastasis in squamous cell carcinoma of the vulva (a Gynecologic Oncology Group Study). Gynecol Oncol 1993;49:279–83.

Thomas G, Dembo A, De Petrillo A, et al. Concurrent radiation and chemotherapy in vulvar cancer Gynecol Oncol 1989;34:263–7.

Piura B. Recurrent squamous cell carcinoma of the vulva: a study of 73 cases. Gynecol Oncol 1993;48:189–95.

Yell N. Flaps in vulval vaginal reconstruction. Br J Plastic Surg 1996;49:547–54.

Vulval intraepithelial neoplasia

Introduction

The concept of 'squamous cell carcinoma *in situ*' was first described in 1922 by French authors Hudelo *et al.* (1922). Over the years, a bewildering variety of terms, such as leucoplakia, Bowen's disease, Bowenoid papulosis, Bowenoid dysplasia, Bowenoid atypia, erythroplasia of Queyrat, carcinoma simplex, squamous cell carcinoma *in situ*, and hyperplastic dystrophy with severe atypia, have been used to describe this condition. The incidence of vulval intraepithelial neoplasia is increasing worldwide, primarily due to the increasing occurrence of this disease in young women, who account for 75% of cases (Judson *et al.* 2006).

In 1987 the International Society for the Study of Vulvovaginal Disease (ISSVD) and the International Society of Gynecological Pathologists recommended a unifying term: vulval intraepithelial neoplasia (VIN). By definition it consists of neoplastic cells confined to the boundaries of the squamous epithelium. It may regress either spontaneously or, after incomplete surgical removal, persist or progress to invasive carcinoma if untreated.

The ISSVD further recommended (ISSVD 1990) grading VIN into:
- VIN 1 mild dysplasia: only the lower third of the epithelium involved
- VIN 2 moderate dysplasia: lower half of the epithelium involved
- VIN 3 severe dysplasia/carcinoma *in situ*: lower two-thirds to full thickness involvement

This grading system was extrapolated from that applied to the non-keratinizing squamous epithelium of the cervix. However, the problems of extrapolating the grading of VIN from its cervical counterpart are that
- the vulval skin is different from its cervical counterpart in both health and disease
- cancer pathogenesis in the vulva is different from that of the cervix
- unlike the cervix, a VIN 1 to VIN 3 continuum has not been described.
- The pathological diagnosis of VIN 1 is poorly reproducible, uncommon, and generally represents reactive change or HPV effect.

Accordingly, the ISSVD in 2003 revised the terminology for squamous vulval intraepithelial neoplasia (Sideri *et al.* 2005), based on morphological manifestation, clinical characteristics, and HPV content.

VIN, usual type (VIN-u)

This is characterized by lack of cell maturation throughout the epithelium, nuclear aneuploidy, and abnormal mitotic figures and is further subdivided into
- VIN, warty type: the lesion comprises highly pleomorphic cells, keratinization, multinucleation, and verrucous surface pattern
- VIN, basaloid type: lesion comprises uniform, undifferentiated basal cell-type population
- VIN, mixed (warty/basaloid) type.

It is no longer necessary to subdivide morphologically HPV-related VIN-u into low-grade (VIN 1) and high-grade (VIN 2, 3) types. VIN 1 is a flat condyloma, and although nearly 50% contain high-risk (oncogenic) HPV types, only a minority contains HPV type 16 as opposed to high-grade VIN which carries HPV 16 in more than 90% of cases.

VIN 1 is not considered to precede high-grade VIN but may only indicate risk for developing VIN-u and thus the term VIN 1 has been discarded.

VIN, differentiated type (VIN-d)

This is HPV unrelated, with nuclear atypia and involves only the lower third or sometimes even only the basal cell layer of the squamous epithelium. The degree of nuclear atypia is similar to repair-related atypia.

Note that the occasional example of VIN which cannot be classified into either of the above VIN categories (usual type and differentiated type) may be classified as VIN, unclassified type. The rare VIN of pagetoid type may be classified as such, or placed in this category.

Abandoning the three-grade system simplifies the terminology, which better addresses the clinical need to identify vulval cancer precursors, and will also enhance diagnostic reproducibility and allow better communication among gynaecologists, pathologists, and other healthcare providers dealing with vulval disease.

Epidemiology and pathogenesis

VIN-u

- VIN-u is caused by oncogenic HPV types 16 and 18, and less frequently by other oncogenic types 33, 35, 51, 52, and 68.
- It tends to occur in younger women with a mean age of 30 years, and in most cases is associated with the same demographic, behavioural patterns and high-risk HPV-positive rates seen in women with high-grade CIN.
- There is also an associated history of smoking, multiple sex partners, and early onset of sexual activity.
- Immunosuppression and smoking may be greater risk factors for VIN than CIN.
- It is the precursor lesion of HPV-related invasive squamous cell carcinoma of the vulva, which is increasing in frequency among younger women.
- The most common symptoms of VIN-u are pruritus and a burning discomfort. VIN-u tends to be multifocal and multicentric with confluent involvement of the interlabial grooves, posterior fourchette, perineum, perianal skin, and cervical epithelium in up to two-thirds of women with VIN.
- Colposcopy is helpful in defining the limits of the lesion, in detecting foci of possible early invasion, and in the exclusion of high grade CIN with which VIN-u is often associated. The definitive diagnosis is based on biopsy of the vulva.

VIN-d

- VIN-d represents another high-grade lesion, but is of different morphology and behaviour. Comprising less than 5%, it is often recognized adjacent to an existing squamous cell carcinoma.
- It is not related to HPV and is thought to be the precursor lesion to the non-HPV-related invasive squamous cell carcinoma of the vulva observed more often in elderly women, most of whom are older than 70 years and lack the behavioural risk factors of those observed with VIN-u. It tends to be unifocal and unicentric.
- The pathogenic background may be related to chronic itch-scratch cycles that are associated with lichen simplex chronicus and lichen sclerosus (Scurry 1999).

The release of unidentified carcinogens together with the local environment of chronically irritated and inflamed skin may play a major role in the development of intraepithelial neoplasia and ultimately invasive well-differentiated keratinizing SCC of the vulva in elderly people. It is believed that this may be mediated by p53 (Yang 2000). Women with symptomatic lichen simplex chronicus or lichen sclerosus who are treated with high potency topical steroids rarely, if ever, progress to invasive squamous cell carcinoma. However, about 80% of the invasive SCC in elderly women are associated with untreated long-standing symptomatic lichen simplex chronicus or lichen sclerosus.

Natural history

VIN-u

VIN-u is now regarded as the precursor of non-keratinizing basaloid and warty SCC of the vulva skin. In a large series of 405 women with VIN 2–3 (Jones 2005), 63 women received no treatment. The lesion regressed in 47 patients and progressed to invasion before treatment in 10 patients. Seventeen women (3.8%) developed invasive vulva, perianal, or periurethral cancer more than 1 year after treatment for VIN. This is similar to a systematic review of 97 published papers involving 3322 patients by van Seters et al. (2005) in which they reported a 3.3% incidence of invasive cancer after treatment for VIN (van Seters et al. 2005). With a follow up of up to 40 years, 50% of the 405 women in Jones's series needed at least one or more treatments for persistent or new VIN. In the same series, the surgical resection margin was significantly related to the risk of requiring retreatment for persistent or recurrent disease. Positive margins were found in 47% of the women treated with excision, and they had a 50% risk of requiring retreatment in the next 5 years. On the other hand, women with negative margins had only a 15% risk of retreatment. The HPV-related invasive vulval cancers tend to be diagnosed in their early stages, and survival rates are excellent.

VIN-d

VIN-d precedes well-differentiated keratinizing SCC of the vulva skin. SCC arising from HPV-unrelated VIN tends to present with deep invasion and advanced clinical stage including lymph node metastasis (40% stage III) and 5-year survival rates of between 25–50% in women with stage III–IV disease. The risk of progression to invasion seems greater in VIN-d than in VIN-u (ISSVD 1990).

Overall the difference in prognosis of the two varieties of vulval carcinomas is due at least in part to the fact that women with VIN-u are much younger and seek medical attention much earlier than their elderly counterparts with VIN-d.

Differential diagnosis

Conditions that can mimic VIN include
- lichen sclerosus
- lichen planus
- lichen simplex chronicus
- flat or papular condylomata
- seborrhoeic keratosis
- basal cell carcinoma
- rarely, extramammary Paget's disease of the vulva.

Classically, it presents as an eczematoid, crusty, erythematous area on the vulva skin. Pruritus is present in more than 70% of patients. Histologically, it is really an intraepithelial adenocarcinoma. Diagnosis is often missed as it is treated as an eczema. It is best established by biopsy, which shows the characteristic malignant cells within the epithelium. Treatment is by wide excision, although obtaining clear margins may be difficult. These patients should also be evaluated for the possibility of synchronous neoplasms (breast, rectum, bladder, urethra, cervix, and ovary).

In most cases and where there is any doubt, or if the lesion does not respond to therapy, diagnosis must be confirmed with a biopsy.

Clinical evaluation

- There is immense variation in the clinical appearance of VIN based on colour, surface contour and topography. VIN-u, the premenopausal form, which is multifocal and multicentric is more commonly seen than VIN-d, which tends to be unicentric and occurring in the postmenopausal age group.
- About 50% of women are asymptomatic and are diagnosed either when a lesion is observed during a routine gynaecological examination or at colposcopy for abnormal cervical cytology.
- In patients with symptoms of chronic vulval irritation or pruritus, the outer genitalia must be carefully examined. The use of the colposcope to perform vulvoscopy is an important adjunct to inspection techniques. The value of performing a vulvoscopy includes:
  - defining the extent of disease
  - directing biopsies of the most severe areas
  - excluding overt invasion
  - directing laser treatment if necessary, through visualization of anatomical landmarks, thereby allowing depth of vaporization to be determined.
- The vulva must be carefully inspected for hyperkeratosis before the application of 5% acetic acid. This must be applied for a much longer period than the cervix as the vulva epithelium takes it up rather more slowly. A systematic examination must be made of the vaginal introitus, labia minora and majora, perineum, followed by the clitoris, urethral orifice, perianal area, and anal canal. During examination, the following characteristics should be documented:
  - topography: uni- or multifocal
  - surface contour: flat, raised, or micropapillary
  - colour tone: white, red, brown, grey, or dark
  - degree of acetowhite change
  - blood vessels: absent, punctuate or mosaic.
- VIN lesions are characteristically papular and over half exhibit superficial parakeratosis, which is defined as the retention of nuclear chromatin material in the usually acellular keratin layer of the epithelium.
- The Collins toluidine blue test, in which a 1% aqueous solution of dye is applied to the external genital area, and then washed off with 1% acetic acid after 2 minutes, may be useful to demonstrate this abnormal maturation of the vulva skin. Although vulvoscopy aids in localizing precancerous change, any area that looks suspicious whether it be white, grey, red, dark raised, or flat must be biopsied or excised to assess the severity of change.
- Colposcopic examination of the cervix and vagina should also be carried out.
- Biopsy of the vulva can be easily achieved with local anaesthetic in the clinic. EMLA (Eutectic Mixtures of

Local Anaesthetics) cream (lidocaine 2.5% and prilocaine 2.5%) can be applied to the area followed by local infiltration of 1% xylocaine, which will help to elevate the skin and facilitate the biopsy. A punch biopsy, a scalpel, or a proprietary Keys punch biopsy instrument may be utilized to obtain a satisfactory sample of vulva skin with 2–5 mm depth for accurate histological assessment. The small skin defect can be closed with a 3.0 suture or left to granulate after application of Monsel's (ferric subsulphate) solution, or silver nitrate.

Management of VIN

- It is important to correlate clinical symptoms and signs with histology prior to embarking on any form of therapy. Many patients are young and the emotional trauma of any procedure is considerable.
- Determining the management of patients with VIN continues to be challenging and inexperienced clinicians should refer the patient to colleagues with expertise in gynaecological dermatology.
- The rationale for treating any patient with VIN would be:
  - to relieve symptoms,
  - to avoid recurrences and the risk of invasive cancer.
- There has been a gradual trend towards individualization of treatment and conservative therapy, with preservation of normal anatomy and vulval function. Based on the new pathogenic–morphologic classification, broadly, the HPV-related VIN-u should be treated with ablative and/or excisional techniques, whereas VIN-d would be best treated with potent corticosteroid preparations or topical pro-apoptotic, non-steroidal anti-inflammatory products such as 0.1% tacrolimus.

Treatment options

Observation

This is appropriate for asymptomatic lesions and patients who will be compliant to long-term follow-up. It is essential to first rule out invasion through multiple or extended biopsies.

Surgery

- For localized lesions, CO2 laser vaporization and wide local excision are most suitable. Wide local excision is associated with recurrence rates of 12-30%, and margins of 8-10 mm are recommended. For CO2 laser vaporization, a recurrence rate of 5–40% has been described. This is as a result of treating to an insufficient depth or lateral extent. A margin of 15 mm has been found to result in lower recurrence rates than a 5 mm or less margin (Ferenczy et al. 1985). In terms of depth, laser vaporization should be carried to depths of 2–3 mm (Reid's third surgical plane) (Reid 1992) for hair-bearing areas and 1 mm for non-hair-bearing skin.
- For very extensive multifocal lesions extending into hair-bearing areas of the vulva, laser treatment would not be applicable because the necessary depth of treatment would not produce a good cosmetic result especially in young women. In such cases, skinning vulvectomy with or without skin graft would be recommended. Simple vulvectomy in a young patient is mutilating, does not significantly reduce the recurrence rate and is therefore no longer recommended. However, there may be a place for this in older patients with extensive and symptomatic VIN, to relieve symptoms and to exclude occult invasion.

- Recurrence rates range from 12% to 50% irrespective of treatment modality. Major reasons for treatment failure include failure to include all satellite lesions in the treatment field and reactivation of latent HPV DNA in vulva skin adjacent to or at a distance to the lesional epithelium. Negative surgical margins are associated with a recurrence rate of 15% whereas margin positivity is associated with a 50% recurrence rate (Yang B 2000). There appears to be two distinct groups of patients who require retreatment for VIN:
  - women diagnosed with VIN within 2 years of the original treatment who probably have persistent disease
  - another group of women who are diagnosed at 4–5 years or more who probably have new areas of VIN.
- For invasive cancer, the time intervals are a median of 2.4 years for women who progressed from their original VIN, whereas patients who were apparently originally cured but developed a new focus of disease that progressed to invasive cancer were diagnosed a median of 13.5 years after their original treatment (Yang B 2000). Multifocal lesions have a higher recurrence rate of 40% compared with 16.7% in unifocal lesions most likely due to positive resection margins.

Medical treatment

- These are used mainly in those who decline surgery or wish to preserve the cosmetic appearance of the vulva. Invasive disease must be excluded prior to medical treatment. Many of these medications are off-label use or experimental in nature.
- Imiquimod 5% cream (Aldara) is a topical immune system modulator that induces local proinflammatory cytokine production and cell-mediated immunity. Randomized trials comparing Imiquimod to placebo for treatment of VIN have demonstrated complete response in 35–80% and partial response in 10–46% in the Imiquimod arms. A skin reaction and discomfort at the treatment site is common and this affects compliance. An escalating dose regimen starting with an application once a week for 2 weeks, then twice a week for 2 weeks, then, if tolerated well, three times a week is recommended. A typical treatment course lasts 16 weeks.
- Topical 5% 5-fluorouracil (Efudex) cream is no longer used in the treatment of VIN as the chemical desquamation results in painful erosions with delayed healing and eventual scarring of the vulva and introitus.
- Experimental treatments include photodynamic therapy, ultrasonic surgical aspiration, and cidofovir, a potent antiviral agent.

Role of HPV vaccines in preventing VIN

Since HPV 16 appears to be the dominant HPV type associated with high-grade VIN, followed by HPV 18, it was anticipated that the HPV vaccine, developed primarily to reduce the incidence of cervical cancer, would also reduce the risk of VIN. This indeed was shown in the trials using the quadrivalent vaccine. Data from three placebo controlled trials showed that the immunization was 100% effective against the development of high-grade VIN caused by HPV 16/18, over a follow up period of 3 years, in the 'according-to-protocol' population.

Further reading

Ferenczy, et al. Latent papillomavirus and recurring genital warts. N Eng J Med 1985;313:784.

Hudelo M, Boulanger-Pilet M, Cailliau M. Erythrokeratodermie verruqueuse en nappes symetriques et progressives congentales. Bull Soc Fr Dermatol Syphiligr 1922;29:45.

ISSVD. Report of the Committee on Terminology of the International Society for the Study of Vulvar Diseases. New Nomenclature for Vulvar Disease J Reprod Med 1990;35:484.

Jones R. Vulvar Intraepithelial Neoplasia: Aspects of the Natural History and Outcome in 405 Women Obstet Gynecol 2005;106:1319–26.

Judson PL, Habermann EB, Baxter NN, et al. Trends in the incidence of invasive and in situ vulvar carcinoma. Obstet Gynecol 2006;107:1018.

Reid. Laser surgery in the lower genital tract. In: Coppleson M (ed.) Gynaecological oncology, vol 2, 2nd edn. Edinburgh: Churchill Livingstone 1992:1094.

Scurry J. Does lichen sclerosus play a central role in the pathogenesis of human papillomavirus negative vulvar squamous cell carcinoma? The itch-scratch-lichen clerosus hypothesis. Int J Gynecol Cancer 1999;9:89–97.

Sideri M, Jones RW, Wilkinson EJ, et al. Squamous vulvar intraepithelial neoplasia 2004 modified terminology, ISSVD Vulvar Oncology Subcommittee. J Reprod Med 2005:50:807–10.

Van Seters, et al. Is the assumed natural history of vulvar intraepithelial neoplasia iii based on enough evidence? A systematic review of 3322 published patients. Gynecol Oncol 2005;907:645.

Yang B. Vulvar intraepithelial neoplasia of the simplex (differentiated) type a clinicopathologic study including analysis of HPV and p53 expression. Am J Surg Pathol 2000:24.

Common gynaecological procedures and surgery

Colposcopy 688
Endometrial ablation techniques 690
Hysteroscopy 694
Hysterectomy 698
Continence procedures 702
Pipelle biopsy 705
Laparoscopy 706
Pelvic floor surgery 710

Colposcopy

Colposcopy is the visualization of the cervix using a magnifying lens. It is an essential part of the cervical cancer-screening programme. Colposcopy can be carried out for diagnostic or treatment purposes. Ten per cent of smears are reported to be abnormal.

Referral criteria for colposcopy based on cervical smears

Three consecutive inadequate samples:
- three tests reported as borderline nuclear change in squamous cells
- one test reported as borderline nuclear change in endocervical cells
- three tests reported as abnormal at any grade in a 10-year period
- one test reported as mild, moderate, or severe dyskaryosis
- one test showing possible invasion
- one test showing glandular neoplasia
  or
- clinically suspicious cervix.

If the patient satisfies any of the above criteria for referral to colposcopy, an invitation letter and an information leaflet are sent out to the patient.

Procedure

- Initial history is taken to enquire about periods, abnormal vaginal bleeding, contraception, etc.
- The patient is positioned in the special colposcopy couch with padded supports for the legs.
- A self-retaining speculum is inserted into the vagina to inspect the cervix.
- Any other associated pathology in the external genitalia/vagina is noted.
- The cervical smear is repeated if necessary.
- The cervix is inspected thoroughly and gently cleansed with a cotton bud moistened with saline if required.
- 3–5% acetic acid is dabbed onto the cervix and any areas acetowhite are noted after satisfactory application.

- The patient should be warned of slight stinging during this part of the procedure.
- Biopsy of any acetowhitened areas may need to be carried out.
- Lugol's iodine may need to be applied to look for lack of iodine staining in abnormal areas especially before treatment.
- A treatment procedure such as a LLETZ (large loop excision of transformation zone) may need to be carried out in a 'see and treat' setting when major grade of CIN (cervical intraepithelial neoplasia) is suspected on colposcopy examination.
- Treatment is usually carried out under local anaesthesia in an outpatient setting.
- Ensure that the patient is not dizzy as she gets off the couch.
- The findings are documented and the patient is counselled regarding the findings and time taken for the results if any.
- Patients must be warned to expect some bleeding for a week after the biopsy or 2 weeks after treatment. They should be encouraged to report heavy bleeding or abnormal discharge, which may indicate infection.

The following data should be recorded at the colposcopic examination:
- reason for referral (100%)
- grade of cytological abnormality (90%)
- whether the examination is satisfactory; this is defined as the entire squamocolumnar junction having been seen and the upper limit of any cervical lesion also being seen (100%)
- the presence or absence of vaginal and/or endocervical extension
- the colposcopic features should be recorded
- the colposcopic impression of lesion grade.

Further reading

www.bsccp.org/docs/public/pdf/nhscsp20.pdf

Patient resources

www.bsccp.org/docs/public/pdf/thecolposcopyexamination.pdf

Endometrial ablation techniques

Heavy menstrual bleeding is a very common health problem affecting quality of life and leading to anaemia. Medical treatment is frequently ineffective, although the introduction of the Mirena intrauterine system has led to a reduction in the number of surgical procedures. Hysterectomy has been the standard treatment for women with menorrhagia: it has high satisfaction rates and improved quality of life. Hysterectomy is a major operation with a relatively long recuperation period and potentially serious complications (Cooper et al. 2005) and cost implications.

Endometrial ablation (EA) is a minimally invasive alternative to hysterectomy, which can be performed as a day case procedure. The aim is to completely destroy or remove the endometrial basalis layer leading to amenorrhoea. Compared to hysterectomy, endometrial ablation offers effective treatment with high satisfaction rates, and shorter operating and recovery times. The cost is significantly lower but retreatment maybe needed in the long-term, reducing cost-effectiveness (Lethaby et al. 2004).

First-generation techniques

First-generation techniques were introduced in the early 1980s as alternatives to hysterectomy. Laser, transcervical resection of the endometrium (TCRE) and rollerball are the gold standard techniques. All these methods are performed under direct visualization with hysteroscopy, and the outcome is dependent on the skill and experience of the surgeon. They are effective techniques but have a steep learning curve during training. They are performed with the patient under general anaesthetic using glycine for distension. Glycine is non-ionic but absorption can lead to fluid overload, resulting in hyponatraemia, pulmonary and cerebral oedema leading to seizures, coma, and death (Cooper et al. 2000). The use of bipolar technology using saline distension is now a better option avoiding absorption complications. The MISTLETOE study audited complications associated with first-generation techniques and reported a total complication rate of 4.4% including two deaths. Rollerball was associated with fewer complications than laser or resection (Overton et al. 1997). Long-term complications include haematometra and pain.

Second-generation techniques

Second-generation techniques were introduced to provide safer, quicker, and more effective treatment. These techniques require less training and skill than first-generation procedures and have similar clinical outcomes. The operating time is shorter, and there is a low risk of uterine perforation. Most of the devices need a relatively normal cavity <12 cm but free fluid ablation and microwave can be performed with an irregular cavity. Patients should be counselled to ensure their family is complete and they are willing to continue contraception after the procedure. A completely septate or bicornuate uterus is a contraindication for second-generation techniques except hydro-thermablation. Each system has advantages and disadvantages and some have the potential for use in the outpatient setting. There are very few studies comparing the different techniques with each other and many use subjective improvement and amenorrhoea rates as outcome measures when quality of life should be assessed.

Microwave endometrial ablation

Microwave endometrial ablation (MEA) (Microsulis Medical) uses microwave energy to ablate the endometrium. The 7-mm probe is inserted into the uterine cavity and moved from side to side and slowly removed. The temperature is maintained at 70–80°C. The depth of ablation is 5–6 mm and the treatment takes 3–5 minutes for a normal sized uterus. Amenorrhoea rates are quoted as high as 40%. A randomized controlled trial comparing TCRE with MEA, 5-year follow up showed microwave was more satisfactory (OR 2.3, 95% CI 1.2–4.3) and acceptable (OR 3.7, 95% CI 1.3–10.1). The hysterectomy rate was 18% for MEA and 28% for TCRE (Cooper et al. 2005). The disadvantages of MEA are the size of the machine and large diameter of the probe, making it less useful in the outpatient setting. Curettage before treatment is not recommended as it increases the risk of perforation and bowel damage.

Balloon thermal ablation

There are two devices available in the UK: Cavaterm and Thermachoice. Both use the same principle of a balloon placed in the uterine cavity and hot fluid circulated within it to destroy the endometrium in contact with it. Treatment takes about 8 minutes and both systems have a good safety profile. Cavaterm can be used with cavities up to 10 cm long and Thermachoice up to 12 cm. The amenorrhoea rate is about 25%.

Free fluid endometrial ablation (hydrothermablator HTA)

Hot saline is instilled into the uterine cavity under hysteroscopic vision. Treatment takes about 10 minutes and is performed under general anaesthetic. Studies have shown similar results to rollerball ablation (Goldrath 2003). Amenorrhoea rates are 40–53%.

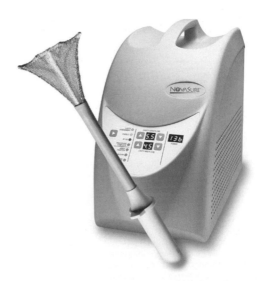

Fig. 15.2.1 Novasure device, courtesy of Hologic, Inc. and affiliates.

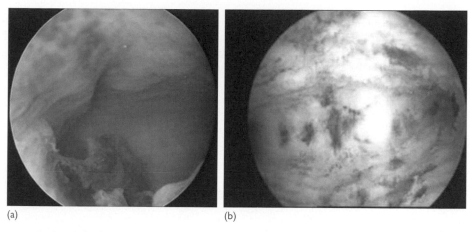

(a)   (b)

Fig. 15.2.2 (a) Endometrial cavity seen at hysteroscopy prior to Novasure ablation; (b) endometrial cavity post ablation. See also colour plate section.

Impedance bipolar radiofrequency endometrial ablation (Novasure)

A probe is inserted into the uterus containing a gold-mesh electrode, which expands to fit the shape of the cavity, the endometrium is vaporized and removed by suction. The depth of ablation is controlled by tissue impedance. Myometrium has higher impedance, and once the depth of ablation reaches it the treatment ends. Treatment takes about 90 seconds. The amenorrhoea rate is 41–59%. This is rapidly becoming the most frequently employed technology (Figs 15.2.1 and 15.2.2a,b).

Gynaclase endometrial laser intrauterine thermal therapy (ELITT)

An intrauterine diode laser emits light, which is absorbed and transformed to heat causing controlled tissue coagulation. High rates of amenorrhoea of 50–70% have been reported but limited data exist on this device (Perino 2004).

Cryoablation: Her Option

This uses cold temperature to freeze the endometrium and destroy it. The probe is cooled to −90°C and ablates to a depth of up to 12 mm. Treatment takes 10–20 minutes and requires less anaesthesia than other techniques. Its use is limited by the need for ultrasound to monitor the position of the probe and depth of ablation. This increases the cost due to the need for skilled staff and equipment. Reported efficacy is similar to rollerball ablation (Townsend 2003). Amenorrhoea rate is 28–40%.

Chemoablation

This involves instilling a chemical into the uterine cavity. Trichloroacetic acid has been used in one prospective study and the results were similar to other second-generation techniques (Kucuk 2005).

Complications of second-generation techniques

Minor postoperative complications are common, including pelvic pain, nausea, vomiting, endometritis, and urinary tract infection. Equipment failure is also more common but there is less chance of perforation than with first-generation techniques.

Endometrial preparation

Studies have shown that most second-generation techniques do not require endometrial thinning (Jack et al. 2005) except hydrothermablation and the ELITT systems.

Outpatient endometrial ablation

Most techniques can be performed on an outpatient basis under local anaesthetic, sedation, or no anaesthetic. The procedures with smaller diameter requiring less cervical dilatation and with shorter treatment times are generally better tolerated. MEA and balloon ablation have been studied on an outpatient basis and are well tolerated.

Conclusion

Endometrial ablation techniques have improved with time, becoming easier to use and safer. Rapid recovery and return to normal activities after treatment have made it a popular choice for women with menorrhagia. The outcomes for the different second-generation techniques are very similar and choice of device is personal. Cost analysis of MEA and balloon ablation concluded that these techniques were more cost-effective than first-generation techniques but further well-designed randomized controlled trials are needed.

References

Cooper JM, Bain C, et al. A randomised comparison of microwave endometrial ablation with transcervical resection of the endometrium; follow up at a minimum of five years. Br J Obstet Gynaecol 2005;112:470–5.

Cooper JM, Brady RM. Intraoperative and early postoperative complications of operative hysteroscopy. Obstet Gynaecol Clin Am 2000;27:347–66.

Garside R, Stein K, et al. A cost–utility analysis of microwave and thermal balloon endometrial ablation techniques for the treatment of heavy menstrual bleeding. Br J Obstet Gynaecol 2004; 111:1103–14.

Goldrath MH. Evaluation of HydroThermAblator and rollerball endometrial ablation for menorrhagia 3 years after treatment. J Am Assoc Gynecol Laparosc 2003;10:505–11.

Jack SA, Cooper KG, et al. A randomised controlled trial of microwave endometrial ablation without endometrial preparation in the outpatient setting: patient acceptability, treatment outcome and costs. Br J Obstet Gynaecol 2005;112:1109–16.

Kucuk M, Okman TK. Intrauterine instillation of trichloroacetic acid is effective for the treatment of dysfunctional uterine bleeding. Fertil Steril 2005;83:189–94.

Lethaby A, Shepperd S, et al. Endometrial resection and ablation versus hysterectomy for heavy menstrual bleeding. Cochrane Database Syst Rev 2004;4.

Overton C, Hargreaves J, *et al.* National survey of the complications of endometrial destruction techniques for menstrual disorders: the mistletoe study. Minimally invasive surgical techniques-laser, endothermal or endoresection. Br J Obstet Gynaecol 1997;104:1351–9.

Perino A, Castelli A, *et al.* Randomised comparison of endometrial laser intrauterine thermotherapy and hysteroscopic endometrial resection. Fertil Steril 2004;82:731–4.

Townsend DE, Duleba AJ, *et al.* Durability of treatment effects after endometrial cryoablation versus rollerball electroablation for abnormal uterine bleeding: two year results of a multicenter randomised trial. Am J Obstet Gynaecol 2003;188:699–701.

National Institute of Health and Clinical Excellence. Menstrual bleeding: fluid-filled thermal balloon and microwave endometrial ablation. Technology Appraisal 78. London: NICE 2004: www.guidance.nice.org.uk/TA78/guidance/pdf/English

Hysteroscopy

Hysteroscopy visualizes the cervical canal and uterine cavity internally with an endoscope and is used for diagnostic and operative procedures. It was first described by Pantaleoni in 1869; however, it came into routine clinical practice in the 1970s. It can be performed as an office or as an inpatient procedure. More directed biopsies can be undertaken at hysteroscopy than the traditional dilatation and curettage yielding more accurate results.

Indications for hysteroscopy
- Postmenopausal bleeding
- Menstrual irregularities
- Menorrhagia
- Dysmenorrhoea
- Intermenstrual and post-coital bleeding
- Subfertility
- Contraceptive procedure
- Misplaced intrauterine contraceptive device.

Types of hysteroscopy
1. Diagnostic: mainly performed as part of the investigation process in a patient.
2. Operative laparoscopy: aims to treat intrauterine pathology to improve the symptoms/outcome in a patient.

General make-up of a hysteroscope
The two types of hysteroscope are rigid and flexible. The rigid hysteroscope is made up of a telescope with a lens (0, 12, 30 or 70°) attached to it and an inner/outer sheath, which ranges between 5 and 10 mm. The hysteroscope come in sizes from 1.7 to 4 mm (Fig. 15.3.1). Smaller diameter hysteroscopes are used for office procedures. Some of these hysteroscopes have additional channels or operating sheaths to introduce scissors, grasping and biopsy forceps. The space between the telescope and the inner/outer sheath is necessary for the inward and outward flow of the distension medium through the telescope. A resectoscope is a special operating hysteroscope that can incorporate special instruments like an electrode (rollerball, loop, knife, or ellipsoid) or laser. These instruments allow procedures to be carried out within the uterine cavity using electric current or laser energy. The inner sheath carries the telescope, the inward flow of the medium, and the electrode. The outer sheath with perforations at the end are used for the return flow of the medium, blood, and tissue debris (Fig. 15.3.2).

The flexible hysteroscope is a soft semi-rigid telescope. It is mainly used as an outpatient/office procedure. It uses carbon dioxide gas as a distension medium.

Procedures carried out at operative hysteroscopy
- Resection/ablation of the endometrium
- Resection of a submucous myoma
- Resection of a polyp
- Resection of uterine septum
- Adhesiolysis of uterine synechiae in Ashermann's syndrome
- Removal of misplaced intrauterine contraceptive device
- Tubal sterilization (Essure procedure).

Need for distension medium
The anterior and posterior walls of the uterus are close to each other. To obtain visualization of the uterine cavity the walls need to be separated (Fig. 15.3.3). This is achieved by the distension medium. The pressure required for good

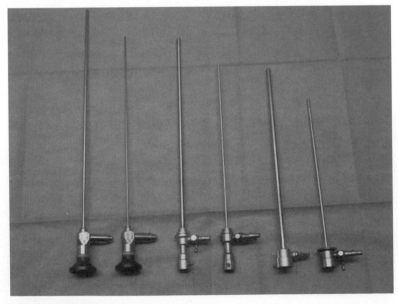

Fig. 15.3.1 2- and 4-mm hysteroscopes used for diagnostic hysteroscopy.

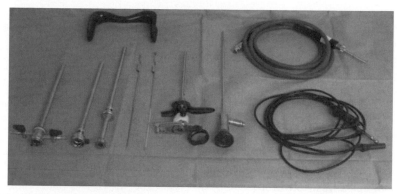

Fig. 15.3.2 Trolley set up for operative hysteroscopy.

visualization is around 75 mm of Hg with carbon dioxide gas (Valle 1998; Petrozza *et al.* 2006) and 70-100 mm of Hg with normal saline (Varol *et al.* 2002). Higher pressures will increase the risk of intravasation of the medium through the open vascular channels leading to fluid overload and pulmonary oedema. The distension medium will help to flush any blood or small tissue, which aids visualization. Over dilatation of the cervix may produce a leakage around the hysteroscope leading to lower intrauterine pressure with poor visualization.

Types of distension medium

CO_2
Used in flexible hysteroscopes, hence useful for office hysteroscopy. It has a refractory index of 1 and hence good visualization of the cavity. Absorbed into the body and removed by the lungs. Does not mix with blood and can cause poor views due to bubbling. Special insufflators are needed with maximum pressure of 100 mm of Hg and flow rates of 40–60 mL/minute (Valle 1998; Petrozza *et al.* 2006). Higher pressures can lead to cardiac arrhythmias, cardiac arrest, and gas embolism.

Normal saline
Clear isotonic low viscosity fluid. Commonly used for diagnostic procedures; however, it can be used with bipolar diathermy (Versapoint Gyne-care, SurgMaster Ethicon) and laser. Because of the presence of electrolytes,

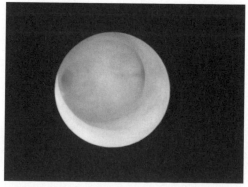

Fig. 15.3.3 Normal uterine cavity. See also colour plate section.

its conductive properties cannot be used with monopolar diathermy. It mixes with blood reducing the visibility, thus needing larger quantities during use.

Glycine 1.5%
Clear hypotonic fluid. Does not mix with blood, giving better vision if bleeding. Non-conductive and can be used with monpolar diathermy. Because of its hypotonic properties, fluid overload can lead to significant hyponatraemia with haemodilution and pulmonary oedema. Careful intraoperative working balance of the inflow and outflow needs to be maintained to prevent complications. Degraded to ammonia; hence, needs care in patients with hepatic and renal disease. Other solutions like 5% Mannitol and 3% Sorbitol can also be used and have similar properties. Dextran 70 is a high viscosity non-electrolyte and poor conductive fluid; however, because of its viscosity the instruments can get damaged. It also causes significant fluid overload and anaphylactic reaction, and can lead to disseminated intravascular coagulopathy. Hence, it is not commonly used.

Types of energy
1. Mechanical: scissors to divide adhesions, biopsy forceps to take directed biopsies.
2. Electrical: monopolar diathermy using cutting and coagulation current to resect tissues. Bipolar diathermy has similar use as monopoplar; however, can be used with isotonic solutions like Normal saline solution.
3. Laser: commonly the Nd:YAG laser is used which destroys tissue up to a depth of 5 mm. It passes easily through clear fluid.

Procedure for diagnostic hysteroscopy
• Check the indication for the procedure
• Consent and explanation of risks
• Lithotomy position.

Office hysteroscopy
Use flexible hysteroscope or small diameter rigid hysteroscope (1.7–3 mm). Cusco's speculum is used to expose the cervix. Sometimes the hysteroscope may negotiate the cervical canal without the need to grasp the cervix, otherwise use a tenaculum or littlewoods forceps to hold the anterior lip of the cervix. If dilatation is needed a paracervical block with 10 ml of 1% lignocaine would be sufficient. Introduce the scope gently under vision allowing the distension medium to fill the uterine cavity. Explain to the patient the risk of shoulder pain due to the CO_2 gas.

Evaluate the uterine cavity and cervical canal in a systematic way to avoid missing any pathology.

Inpatient hysteroscopy

Commonly performed under general anaesthetic with larger scopes of 4 mm. Expose the cervix using a Sim's speculum and hold the anterior lip of the cervix with a tenaculum or vulsellum. Dilate the cervix depending on the size and type of hysteroscope. If it is a single channel scope with no outflow sheath, then cervical dilatation up to 8 Hegar's dilator may be needed. In a dual channel hysteroscope dilatation up to 5–6 Hegar's may suffice. Beware of overdilatation as the medium will leak around the telescope, leading to poor intrauterine pressures and poor visibility.

Procedures for operative hysteroscopy

At operative hysteroscopy larger diameters scopes are used for introducing instruments, hence the cervix needs to be dilated up to No. 9–10 Hegar's dilator. In transcervical resection of the endometrium (TCRE) a rollerball electrode is used to ablate the endometrium on the fundus and cornual areas of the uterine cavity (Fig. 15.3.4). The uterine wall thickness is the thinnest at the cornual ends measuring around 5.5 mm (range 4–7 mm) (Petrozza et al. 2006); thus, precautions need to be taken during TCRE as deeper resection will perforate through the uterus. Following that the endometrium is then resected using a loop electrode which has a diameter of 4 mm. Starting on the posterior wall of the uterus the resection is done in a systematic manner either clockwise or anti-clockwise removing the endometrium all around the uterine cavity. The resection is done up to the level of the internal cervical os as further resection into the cervix can lead to significant bleeding and scarring. The medium used is usually glycine and a running balance needs to be maintained throughout the procedure. If the fluid deficit is 500–1000 mL the procedure should be rapidly completed or suspended; if the deficit is more than 1500 mL the procedure should be stopped (O'Connor and Magos 1999). It is advisable to thin the endometrium prior to the resection by GnRH analogues a month before the procedure. GnRH analogues are also useful in reducing the size and vascularity of submucosal myomas before their resection. The chips of the endometrium are removed and sent for histology. The pressure of the uterine cavity is reduced to check for any bleeding, which can be controlled using the rollerball electrode diathermy.

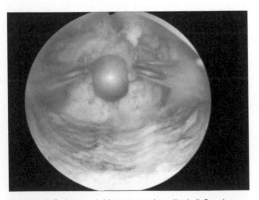

Fig. 15.3.4 Endometrial ablation using the roller ball. See also colour plate section.

Complications of hysteroscopy

Complications at diagnostic hysteroscopy are divided into (RCOG 2008).

Serious

- uterine perforation (0.76%)
- pelvic infection
- failure to visualise the uterine cavity
- damage to uterus, bladder, bowel, blood vessel

The overall serious risk at diagnostic hysteroscopy is approximately 2 in 1000 women, which is very uncommon.

Cervical stenosis, acute anteversion/retroversion, previous resection of endometrium, adhesions, and the presence of lower uterine and cervical fibroids are the common causes which lead to false passage and uterine perforation. In such cases, smaller lacrimal dilators can be used to dilate the cervix. Irrigation fluid maintained at the external os may sometimes help with hydrodilatation of the cervix and distension of the uterine cavity.

Frequent risks

- Vaginal bleeding and discharge
- Pelvic or shoulder pain

Complications at Operative hysteroscopy are more serious and can be divided as set out below.

Procedure related

- Uterine perforation leading to thermal damage of bowel, bladder, ureters and blood vessels
- Primary and secondary haemorrhage
- Cervical lacerations

Medium related

- CO_2 gas embolism
- Air embolism
- Fluid overload with hypotonic distension fluid such as glycine leading to hyponatraemia, hypokalaemia, hypo-osmolarity leading to pulmonary oedema. Electrolyte imbalances can also lead to cardiac arrythmias and cardiac arrest.
- TURS (transurethral resection syndrome) syndrome due to hyerammonaemia from the metabolism of glycine to ammonia in the body can cause coma (Hamilton and Barlow 1989; Motashaw and Dave 2001).

Delayed complications

- Dysmenorrhoea
- Haemato/pyometra
- Pregnancy
- Uterine rupture
- Delay in diagnosis in endometrial carcinoma.

Training in hysteroscopy

It is very important to be familiar with the instruments before undertaking hsyteroscopic surgery. Good hand–eye coordination needs to be developed for operative procedures. Understanding and working of the different energy sources should be mandatory. Trainees need to attend courses, lectures and need supervision when embarking on these procedures. Training on hysteroscopy trainers should be performed before carrying out procedures such as resection of the endometrium and fibroids. Training for diagnostic and minor operative hsyteroscopic procedures can be attained during the Basic and Intermediate training as outlined by the Royal College of Obstetricians and Gynaecologists (RCOG). Advanced training can be attained by completing the Advanced Training Skills Module (ATSM): 'Benign Gynaecological Surgery: Hysteroscopy' in the final years of speciality training under the supervision of RCOG preceptors.

Further reading

Valle RF. 1st edn. New York: Parthenon Publishing 1998: 22.

Petrozza J, Makai G, Sikking E. Hysteroscopy. eMedicine from WebMD. July 2006.

Varol N. Maher P, Vancaillie, *et al.* A literature review and update on the prevention and management of fluid overload in endometrial resection and hysteroscopic surgery. Gynaecol Endoscopy 2002;11:19–26.

O'Connor H, Magos A. How to avoid complications at hysteroscopic surgery. , 20. Churchill Livingstone. 1999:201–14

Diagnostic Hysteroscopy under General Anaesthesia. Royal College of Obstetricians and Gynaecologists. Consent Advice 1. December 2008.

Hamilton SA, Barlow IM. Metabolic effects of prostatectomy. J R Soc Med 1989;82:725–8.

Motashaw N, Dave S. Complications of hysteroscopy. Gynaecological Endoscopy 2001;10:203–10.

Hysterectomy

Hysterectomy is the most common major gynaecological surgery performed worldwide and in the UK (Department of Health 2007). It is the definitive treatment for many benign gynaecological disorders. It has very high satisfaction rate, improved quality of life, decreased depression and anxiety levels, and low morbidity rates.

The indications for hysterectomy with or without bilateral salpingo-opherectomy are

- fibroid uterus (34%)
- heavy menstrual bleeding not responding to medical or ablative surgical techniques (19%)
- uterine prolapse (16%)
- stage 1 endometrial cancer/cervical cancer early stages (11%)
- severe premenstrual syndrome (<1%)
- endometriosis/adenomyosis (18%)
- uncontrollable postpartum obstetric haemorrhage (<1%)

Types of hysterectomy

The approaches are abdominal, vaginal, and laparoscopic. Subtotal, total, or radical hysterectomy can be performed by the abdominal or laparoscopic approach or the routes may be combined as in laparoscopic assisted vaginal hysterectomy (LAVH).

What influences the choice of approach?

This depends on the indication for hysterectomy, history of previous abdominal surgery, or other coexisting pathology size and mobility of uterus, history of endometriosis, and the operators expertise and judgement. The surgical approach to hysterectomy should be decided by the woman in discussion with her surgeon in light of the relative benefits and hazards.

- Total abdominal hysterectomy is the removal of uterus and cervix; it can be combined with salpingo-oophorectomy. The indications include HMB, fibroid uterus >12-week size, limited vaginal access, limited uterine mobility, severe endometriosis, suspected extensive adhesions due to previous surgery, associated bilateral salpingo-oophorectomy,
- Subtotal hysterectomy is the removal of uterus with conservation of cervix. The indications include extensive adhesions and risk of complications outweighing the risk of removal of the cervix and the woman's choice to preserve the cervix.
- Vaginal hysterectomy: uterine prolapse, HMB, fibroid uterus <12-week size, ovarian conservation. The advantages are less postoperative discomfort, easy mobilization, reduced blood loss, shorter hospital stay.
- Laparoscopic hysterectomy: gynaecologist expertise, limited uterine mobility, suspected benign adnexal mass, endometriosis, and mild to moderate adhesions.

Peroperative care

Preoperative assessment is obligatory before embarking on surgery. The surgeon needs to appropriately counsel the women with regards to choice of route, removal or preservation of ovaries, removal or preservation of cervix, procedure, postoperative stay in hospital, complications of surgery, and do and don'ts after surgery. Leaflets should be provided for better understanding of the operation.

Full blood count and group and save/± cross-match should be performed.

Abdominal hysterectomy

- Asepsis
- Catherization
- Type of incision (Pfannenstiel/longitudinal)
- Open abdomen in layers with careful dissection. Cauterization of bleeding vessels for clear view.
- Head down position and abdominal cavity packed with wet large swabs to prevent bowel interference in operative field.
- Clamping and division of round and infundibulopelvic ligaments (IP ligament). Check for ureter before clamping.
- In case of salpingo-oophorectomy, the clamp is applied lateral to ovary and fallopian tube, while in ovarian conservation the clamp is applied medial to ovary and fallopian tube.
- Pedicles can be doubly clamped and IP ligament should be transfixed to achieve good haemostasis.
- Reflection of bladder along the line of uterovesical fold until cervix.
- Clamp the uterine vessels and vaginal angles.
- Opening of vagina and removing the uterus by entering the anterior fornix.
- Ligation of each of the above pedicles separately and obliteration of any dead space.
- Vaginal vault can be closed with interrupted or continuous suture.
- Check haemostasis.
- Pedicles (record numbers, suture, whether doubly ligated).
- Abdomen closed in layers.
- Type of skin closure.
- Blood loss.
- Record if drain inserted, antibiotic given intraoperatively.
- Record postoperative instructions including, trial without catheter (TWOC), thromoprophylaxis, day of removal of suture if needed.
- Any specific point of postoperative management.

Complications of hysterectomy include anaesthetic complications, thromboembolic complications, urinary retention, injury to bladder, bowel, or ureters, infection, bleeding, and febrile morbidity.

Subtotal hysterectomy

The cervix is conserved in a subtotal hysterectomy. After the ligation of uterine arteries, the uterus is incised at the level of internal os. The raw surface is sutured with interrupted sutures (vicryl 1) to secure haemostasis. The central portion (os) is diatherized in order to prevent cyclical bleeding.

The advantage of subtotal hysterectomy over total hysterectomy is fewer short-term postoperative complications, less operative time and blood loss, but there are still cases of cyclical bleeding There is no difference in long-term outcome of sexual, urinary, and bowel function between them (Lethaby et al. 2006; Thakar et al. 2008). The risks associated with subtotal hysterectomy are cancer of cervical stump, obstructive mucocele of cervix, cyclical vaginal discharge or bleeding.

Vaginal hysterectomy

There are many variations to this operation. Described here are the steps from Bonney's Gynaecological surgery.

- Positioning of patient: lithotomy position with buttocks at the end of table
- Asepsis
- Catherization of bladder
- Bimanual examination to assess the size and mobility of uterus
- Subepithelial infiltration of 20 mL of 1% lignocaine with 1 in 200 000 adrenaline to define tissue planes and reduce bleeding.
- Circumferential incision or teardrop shape made around cervix
- Reflection of bladder upwards with sharp dissection
- Dissection of posterior vaginal wall and open the pouch of Douglas.
- Three main pedicles of uterus to be secured, namely cardinal and uterosacral ligament, uterine vessels, and tubo-ovarian including round ligament.
- All pedicles are clamped, cut and the suture doubly ligated with vicryl
- The vagina is closed transversely/anteroposteriorly.
- Peritoneal closure is optional.
- Indwelling catheter and vaginal pack put in.

Record postoperative instructions including, trial without catheter (TWOC), time of removal of vaginal pack, thromoprophylaxis,

- Total blood loss, antibiotic if needed.

A recent Cochrane database review on the surgical approach to hysterectomy suggested vaginal hysterectomy should be preferred over abdominal hysterectomy and if vaginal hysterectomy is not possible, then the laparoscopic route should undertaken, but this needs more surgical expertise (Johnson et al. 2006).

The complications are similar to that of abdominal hysterectomy. In addition, there is increased risk of vaginal cuff infection, which may lead to pelvic cellulitis, septicaemia, abscesses, and vault haematoma.

Laparoscopic hysterectomy

There are various ways to perform hysterectomy by the laparoscopic route. These procedures are clearly described by Garry et al. (1994).

Hysterectomy via laparoscopic route

Laparoscopic assisted vaginal hysterectomy (LAVH)

This is vaginal hysterectomy performed after laparoscopic adhesiolysis, excision of endometriosis, or oophorectomy. The infundibulopelvic ligaments are also secured with staples or bipolar desiccation. The lower attachments of uterus such as cardinal and uterosacral ligaments and uterine vessels are approached vaginally.

Diagnostic laparoscopy with vaginal hysterectomy

Laparoscopy is performed prior and after the vaginal hysterectomy. The rational is to confirm the absence of suspected pathology before vaginal hysterectomy. Also, after vaginal hysterectomy is performed it assures complete haemostasis and allows clot evacuation if needed.

Laparoscopic hysterectomy (LH)

This procedure involves the laparoscopic ligation of uterine vessels by ligature sutures, staples, and bipolar desiccation. All surgical steps are done either vaginally or laparoscopically.

Total laparoscopic hysterectomy (TLH)

This involves the laparoscopic dissection of all vascular pedicles and all ligaments are freed from the uterus. Then, the uterus is removed vaginally or laparoscopically (morcellator). The vagina is closed with laparoscopically placed sutures.

Laparoscopic supra cervical hysterectomy

In this procedure, the uterine fundus is removed with preservation of cervix (Lyons, 1993). The uterus is removed via morcellation or by culdotomy. It is useful in women with a history of dysfunctional uterine bleeding with regular negative smears.

The advantages of laparoscopic hysterectomy are reduced blood loss, less postoperative pain, short hospital stay, quick recovery, The complications include infection, bleeding, injury to bowel, ureteric injury, bladder injury, injury to abdominal wall vessels, (2%), injury to large vessels (iliac, aorta, and inferior vena cava), subcutaneous emphysemas due to absorption of carbon dioxide in subcutaneous tissues, trocar site incisional hernias (Reich 1998).

Should the ovaries be removed or retained at the time of hysterectomy?

There is no established or acceptable standard on whether the ovaries should be retained or conserved at the time of hysterectomy. The ovaries continue to function and play an active role in secretion of oestrogen, progesterone, and androgens in a cyclical fashion until the natural menopause. Ovarian hormones influence the function of metabolic processes in liver, brain, bone, lung, skin, and other organs. Hence, absence of hormones may have an impact on these systems. Studies have revealed that bilateral oophorectomy before menopause is associated with several negative outcomes. There is an increased risk of premature death, coronary heart disease (Lobo 2007), cognitive impairment or dementia, Parkinsonism (Rocca 2008), osteoporosis and bone fractures, decline in psychological wellbeing, and decline in sexual function. There is a short-term mortality benefit following bilateral prophylactic salpingo-oophorectomy in BRCA1/2 mutation carriers and in Lynch's syndrome (Domchek 2007) and hence potential benefits for the risk of cancer reduction in women at average risk of ovarian cancer. This should be carefully weighed against the potential adverse effects of prophylactic bilateral oophorectomy on cardiovascular health, neurological health, bone health, and quality of life

Further reading

Monaghan JM, Lopes T, Naik R. . Oxford: Blackwell publishing.

Monaghan JM, et al. Total abdominal hysterectomy. In: , 10th edn. Oxford: Blackwell publishing 66–73.

Monaghan JM et al. Vaginal hysterectomy and radical vaginal hysterectomy. In: 10th edn. Blackwell publishing 95–108.

Department of health. Hospital episode statistics: 2005-2006. London (UK): Information centre, 2007: http://www.dh.gov.uk/en/Publications and statistics/Statistics/Hospital episode statistics/index.htm.

Domchek SM, Rebbeck TR. Prophylactic oophorectomy in women at increased cancer risk. Curr Opin Obstet Gynecol 2007;19:27–30.

Garry R, Reich H, Liu CY. Editorial. Laparoscopic hysterectomy-definitions and indications, Gynaecological Endoscopy 1994;3:1–3.

Johnson N, Barlow D, Lethaby A, et al. Surgical approach to hysterectomy for benign gynaecological disease. Cochrane Database Syst Re. 2006, 19;2:CD003677.

Lethaby A, Ivanova V, Johnson NP. Total versus subtotal hysterectomy for benign gynaecological conditions. Cochrane Database Syst Rev 2006 19;2:CD004993.

Lobo RA Surgical menopause and cardiovascular risks. Menopause. 2007 May-Jun;14(3 Pt 2):562-6. Review.

Reich H. Laparoscopic hysterectomy. In: Hulka JF (ed) Textbook of laparoscopy, 3rd edn. Philadelphia: Saunders 443–9.

Rocca WA, Bower JH, Maraganore DM, *et al.* Increased risk of Parkinsonism in women who underwent oophorectomy before menopause. Neurology 2008;15;70:200–9.

Thakar R, Ayers S, Srivastava R, Manyonda I. Removing the cervix at hysterectomy: an unnecessary intervention? Obstet Gynecol 2008;112:1262–9.

Patient resources

The Hysterectomy Association: www.hysterectomy-association.org.uk

Continence procedures

Definition
Stress urinary incontinence is defined as the involuntary leakage of urine on effort or exertion. Urodynamic stress incontinence is noted during urodynamics as the involuntary leakage of urine during increased abdominal pressure, in the absence of detrusor contractions.

The prevalence of stress urinary incontinence increases with age with the average age for surgical treatment around 50 years.

Treatment of stress incontinence
Treatment should be initially conservative and includes
- lifestyle advice: weight reduction, treating chronic coughs, and smoking cessation.
- pelvic floor exercises: this may include biofeedback, electrical stimulation, and use of vaginal cones
- drug therapy: duloxetine is a selective serotonin reuptake inhibitor that acts to increase urethral sphincter activity. It has 60–70% efficacy; however, its clinical use is limited by side-effects such as nausea.

Surgery may be considered for
- failed conservative treatment
- declined/unsuitable for conservative treatment
- severe symptoms.

There is some debate regarding investigations required prior to consideration for surgery. The recent NICE guidelines do not advocate that urodynamics are required in those with symptoms of pure stress incontinence. However, at present, in patients with mixed incontinence (both stress and urge incontinence), those who have had previous procedures and in those with high suspicion of voiding dysfunction, urodynamics are generally performed to confirm a diagnosis of urodynamic stress incontinence (NICE 2006).

Surgical treatment
The aims of surgery are to elevate the bladder neck and proximal urethra and/or to increase urethral outlet resistance. To date, over 100 continence procedures have been described using abdominal, vaginal, and laparoscopic routes (Jarvis 1994; Black and Downs 1996). However, over the last decade there has been a paradigm shift in continence surgery with the development of the newer minimally invasive procedures such as the midurethral and tension-free vaginal slings.

One of the difficulties in evaluation of the procedures available is that there are few good-quality studies with long-term follow-up. Previous procedures such as the anterior repair and needle suspension techniques have now been abandoned due to poor long-term results and the higher efficacy of newer procedures. The data on traditional operations such as the colposuspension and fascial slings, although greater than 10 years, have limitations as they are mainly retrospective (Alcalay et al. 1995). This is important as the choice of first procedure is important as it has much higher cure rates than subsequent repeat surgery, and there is now increasing emphasis on long-term prospective evaluation of new procedures using subjective and objective validated outcome measures.

Abdominal procedures
The Burch colposuspension was first described in 1961 and was considered the gold standard of continence surgery, with a subjective success rate of over 90%. It involves elevation of the bladder neck by placement of sutures between the lateral vaginal fornices and the ileopectineal ligament and can be performed as an open or laparoscopic procedure. Although the laparoscopic route results in less hospital stay and faster recovery, it has a longer operating time and higher complication rate and only similar efficacy if done by experienced laparoscopic surgeons. The Marshall–Marchetti–Krantz procedure is similar to this; however, it has been abandoned due to the risk of osteitis pubis, as the sutures are placed into the periosteum of the pubic bone.

Risks associated with the open colposuspension include voiding dysfunction and enterocele formation.

Sling procedures
Sling procedures were developed over 100 years ago. Slings can consist of autologous fascia or synthetic materials. They have good efficacy with continence rates of 80–90%; however, there is a high incidence of voiding dysfunction and de novo detrusor overactivity. Slings made with synthetic material are also associated with erosion.

Minimally invasive mid-urethral slings
Tension-free vaginal tape
The tension-free vaginal tape (TVT) was first described in 1996 and involves the placement of a monofilament polypropylene sling under the midurethra with the ends tunnelling retropubically. It can be performed under local, regional, or general anaesthetic and so may be performed in a day case setting. The TVT has the most robust evaluation of all of the newer invasive sling procedures with long-term cure rates of up to 90% at 10 years with little decline in efficacy over time (Nilsson et al. 2008). The UK randomized controlled trial of colposuspension compared with TVT showed similar efficacy of both procedures at 24 months (Ward et al. 2008). Although the complication rate is low, major bowel, bladder and vascular complications have been reported as well as erosion of mesh into the vagina, urethra, and bladder.

Transobturator procedures
Since the development of the TVT, there have been numerous similar slings with varying success rates. However, due to the risk of vascular and bladder complications with the TVT, the transobturator tape was proposed as an alternative technique. This has a similar placement under the midurethra; however, the ends are tunnelled through the obturator space rather than retropubically. The majority of tapes involve placement of the tape through the obturator foramen into the vaginal incision ('outside-in') versus the TVT-O ('inside-out' (Gynecare)), which places the tape via the vagina tunnelling out into the obturator space (Figs 15.5.1–15.5.3). There are a number of tapes on the market, some of which have had poor long-term evaluation. The data to date would suggest they have similar short-term efficacy to the TVT, although long-term data are still required (Latthe et al. 2007). However, although the risk of bladder injury is lower, other complications include tape erosion (~3%) and thigh pain (~15%), which is thought to be neuralgic in origin.

Recently NICE has recommended that these mid-urethral tapes should be performed in settings that allow audit of outcome and clinical governance procedures. It also

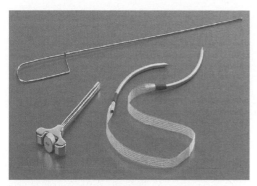

Fig. 15.5.1 Transobturator tape with needle. See also colour plate section.

recommends that to reduce the risk of erosion, a type 1 monofilament tape is used.

Minitapes
There are several tapes that are being tested which only involve a suburethral vaginal incision, but the results are awaited. The big potential advantage is these tapes can be performed as an outpatient procedure

Injection of bulking agents
There are a number of injectable agents that have been injected periurethrally or transurethrally and aim to increase urethral closure by bulking the tissue around the bladder neck. The initial agents on the market, such as Teflon, phenol, and fat, all had limited success and complications, and as such fell out of favour. More recently, new materials, such as glutaraldehye cross-linked collagen and silicone (Macroplastique), have been developed with a better long-term success rate of around 60%.

As these agents can be injected under local anaesthetic with little associated morbidity, they are an option to consider in patients
- unfit for surgery/too frail for surgery
- women deferring definitive surgery till childbearing is complete, and those who have had children
- after previous failed procedures or with fixed scarred urethras.

Artificial urinary sphincter
This is an option in those who have had previous failed surgery or after intractable stress incontinence after a radical prostatectomy. It can be placed via a transabdominal or transvaginal route. The device consists of three parts: an inflatable cuff, a pressure-regulating balloon, and a pump. The patient learns to use the sphincter by decompressing the cuff to allow voiding. Although the success rate is high, there is a high erosion rate of up to 29%, and reoperation rate for cuff problems.

Counselling
Complications of continence procedures
Because of the number of procedures in use, patients need to be counselled about the risk and benefits of each specific procedure. The benefits of newer procedures may be lower morbidity and reduced postoperative stay; however, this must be considered alongside whether there is equivalent efficacy and if there are specific potential complications.

Specific complications
Immediate
- Bleeding
- Bladder perforation: TVT ~2–18%
- Deep vein thrombosis
- Bladder perforation
- Anaesthetic complications

Short term
- Urinary tract infection
- Wound Infection
- Voiding dysfunction ~20%

Long-term
- De novo detrusor overactivity (~20%) and worsening of pre-existing detrusor overactivty in those with mixed incontinence
- Prolapse: 26% reoperation rate for prolapse post colposuspension
- Erosion (with synthetic slings/artificial sphincters)
- Leg/groin pain: ~15% post TOT/TVT-O.

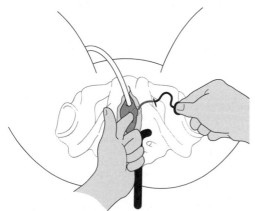

Fig. 15.5.2 Placement of tape via the obturator foramen into the vaginal incision. See also colour plate section.

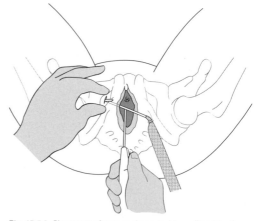

Fig. 15.5.3 Placement of tape via the vaginal tunnelling into the obturator space. See also colour plate section.

Further reading

Alcalay M, Monga A, et al. Burch colposuspension: a 10-20 year follow-up. Br J Obstet Gynecol 1995;102:740–5.

Black NA, Downs SH. The effectiveness of surgery for stress incontinence in women: a systematic review. Br J Urol 1996;78:497–510.

Jarvis GJ. Surgery for genuine stress incontinence. Br J Obstet Gynaecol 1994;101:371–4.

Latthe PM, Foon, R, et al. Transobturator and retropubic tape procedures in stress urinary incontinence: a systematic review and meta-analysis of effectiveness and complications. Br J Obstet Gynaecol 2007;114:522–331.

Nilsson CG, Palva K, et al. Eleven years prospective follow-up of tension-free vaginal tape procedure for treatment of stress urinary incontinence. Int Urogynecol J 2008;19:1043–7.

Ward KL, Hilton P, et al. Tension- free vaginal tape versus colposuspension for primary urodynamic stress incontinence: a 5 year follow up. Br J Obstet Gynaecol 2008;115:226–33.

National Institute for Health and Clinical Excellence (NICE). Urinary incontinence: the management of urinary incontinence in women. Clinical Guideline 40, London: NICE 2006: www.nice.org.uk/cg40

National Institute for Health and Clinical Excellence. Transobsturator foramen procedures for stress urinary incontinence. Clinical Guideline 40, London: NICE 2005: www.nice.org.uk/ig107

Cardozoz L, Staskin D (eds) Textbook of female urology and urogynecology, vol. 2, 2nd edn. London 2006: 801–981.

Internet resources

www.emedicine.com/checktopic

International Continence Society: www.ics.org

Patient resources

Bowel and bladder continence issues: www.bowelfoundation.org

Physiotherapy: www.womensphysio.com

Pipelle biopsy

Endometrial tissue sampling is one of the most common diagnostic procedures for the assessment of women with abnormal uterine bleeding. The main aim of the investigation is to exclude intrauterine pathology, particularly premalignant and malignant endometrial lesions. Inpatient dilatation of the cervix and curettage of the endometrium has been replaced to a large extent by the less invasive and cheaper outpatient endometrial sampling devices.

The pipelle suction aspirator was the prototype for the plastic devices that have followed. It is a flexible polypropylene cannula of 3.1 mm diameter, with a distal side port and an inner piston to generate suction. This design removed the requirement of early devices for external means of generating the necessary negative pressure for aspirating endometrial tissue into the cannula.

Procedure

The technique involves the gentle insertion of the pipelle device through the cervix into the uterus until the fundus is reached. Suction created would yield an endometrial tissue specimen into the cannula. The device is then rotated a few times around all the uterine cavity walls, with gentle back and forth movements on withdrawal to achieve a high tissue yield.

Possible difficulties

The most common reasons for failure are
- acute degrees of anteversion or retroversion of the uterus.
- narrow or stenosed cervix.

Manoeuvres to overcome this include
- adequate counselling of the patients about the procedure and what they are likely to experience to reduce failure due to poor compliance

- stabilizing the cervix with a tenaculum
- stabilizing the cannula by applying a sponge forceps to the distal end.
- applying local anaesthetic and performing gentle dilatation of the cervix
- changing to a more rigid sampling device.

Inadequate sampling, despite of good technique can be due to underlying atrophic endometrium. Pipelle biopsy has a failure rate of 3% and an inadequate specimen rate of 1.5%.

Advantages
- Rapid, less time-consuming and cheaper procedure
- Safe and less invasive procedure
- Good acceptability (less than 10% of women complain of severe pain).

Diagnostic accuracy

Meta-analysis of 7914 women has shown that pipelle biopsy is superior to other endometrial techniques in the detection of endometrial carcinoma and atypical hyperplasia. The accuracy of the pipelle in detection of endometrial carcinoma is higher in postmenopausal women (sensitivity of 99.6%) than in premenopausal women (sensitivity of 91%).

Further reading

Cornier E. The pipelle: a disposable device for endometrial biopsy. Am J Obstet Gynecol 1984;148:109–10.

Dijkhuizen FP, Mol BW, et al. The accuracy of endometrial sampling in the diagnosis of patients with endometrial carcinoma and hyperplasia. A meta-analysis. Cancer 2000;89:1765–72.

Clark TJ, Mann CJ, et al. Accuracy of outpatient endometrial biopsy in the diagnosis of endometrial hyperplasia. Acta Obstet Gynecol Scand 2001;80:784–93.

Laparoscopy

Laparoscopy is a procedure carried out through small incisions to view the inside of the abdomen and pelvis. It comes from the Greek words *La-para*, part of the body between the ribs and hips, and *Skopein*, to see. Around 250 000 women undergo laparoscopy each year (RCOG 2008). Laparoscopy is one of the most common procedures carried out in gynaecology today and classified as either

- diagnostic
  or
- operative.

However, minor procedures are now being carried out at the same time of the diagnostic laparoscopy, but appropriate consent needs to be obtained before surgery.

Indications for diagnostic laparoscopy

- Pelvic pain
- Subfertility
- Suspected ectopic pregnancy
- Malignancy.

Indications for operative laparoscopy

- Endometriosis
- Ovarian cysts
- Pelvic inflammatory disease
- Ectopic pregnancy
- Fibroid uterus
- Dysfunctional uterine bleeding
- Gynaecological malignancy.

Assessment before laparoscopic procedure

- Check indication for surgery.
- Informed consent (explain that digital images may be stored in case records).
- General and gynaecological examination. Very thin and obese patients at increased risk of complications. Pelvic examination may suggest need for operative laparoscopy.
- Check history of previous surgery and incisions on the abdomen.
- Pelvic ultrasound.
- Be familiar with the equipment.
- Have access to open surgery in case of complication
- Adequate operative time if prolonged surgery expected.

Instruments for laparoscopy

1. Laparoscope: 1.2, 5, 7, or 10 mm with 0 or 30° vision. Smaller diameters are used for diagnostic procedures. Some have an operating channel for 3-mm instruments.
2. CO_2 gas insufflators
3. Light source (usually Xenon light)
4. Camera (some laparoscopes come with integrated camera system)
5. Veress pneumoperitoneum needle
6. Trocars: 5, 10, 12 mm. There are newer trocars like the optical trocars (visual access systems), which allow visualization of the tissue being cut, radially expanding trocars and bladeless trocars, which separate the tissue rather than cutting it

7. Uterine manipulator
8. Diathermy: monopolar and bipolar
9. Operating instruments such as scissors, graspers (tooth or atraumatic), needle holders, clip applicators for sterilization, suction irrigation, etc.

Procedure for laparoscopy

Laparoscopic procedures need a lot of equipment compared with open surgery. To carry out a safe and successful procedure the operating theatre should be set up as shown in Fig. 15.7.1. All the personnel involved should be familiar with the equipment to prevent any accidents.

Positioning of the patient is very important. The patient should be placed in a dorsal lithotomy position as shown in Fig. 15.7.2, during the insertion of the veress needle and the umbilical trocar followed by a Trendelenburg position (supine position with a 45° head down tilt). This is to prevent injuries to the bifurcation of the aorta and the left iliac vein, which get pushed up by the promontory in the Trendelenburg position. The arms of the patient should be placed to her side and not perpendicular as with open surgery as this risks the chance of brachial plexus injury.

Techniques and sites of entry

The umbilicus is the preferred site for entry as the distance of the peritoneum to the abdominal skin is the shortest at the base of the umbilicus, which would avoid entry into the pre-peritoneal space (Fig. 15.7.3). A vertical incision should be taken into the base of the umbilicus rather than a subumbilical incision.

The different techniques for gaining entry into the abdominal cavity are discussed below.

Closed technique using the Veress needle

The Veress needle, preferably disposable, is first introduced perpendicular in the base of the umbilicus. Once it has traversed the abdominal wall it is then angulated at 45° aiming towards the perineum. First the Veress needle is aspirated and there should be no blood or faeculent matter aspirated. A saline test is then performed. Saline is introduced at the Veress needle and should be sucked in due to the negative intra-abdominal pressure. This is followed by reaspiration where the saline injected should not come out. Usually two clicks are felt during the insertion of the needle, the first through the rectus sheath and the second through the peritoneum. These steps may indicate a correct placement of the needle. The initial flow of CO_2 should be low, and once the correct placement of the needle is confirmed the flow rate should be increased. The initial pressure should be set between 20 and 25 mm of Hg for placement of the trocars as this helps to produce a large intra-abdominal space (bubble) between the bowel, posterior abdominal, and the anterior abdominal wall, thus reducing the risk of bowel and vascular injuries. The pressure then should be dropped to 12–15 mm of Hg for rest of the surgical procedure, which aids the anaesthetist for ventilation of the patient (Consensus document).

Open or cut down technique known as the Hasson's technique

Commonly performed by general surgeons the technique involves cutting through the layers of the abdominal wall under vision to gain entry. A blunt trocar is inserted through

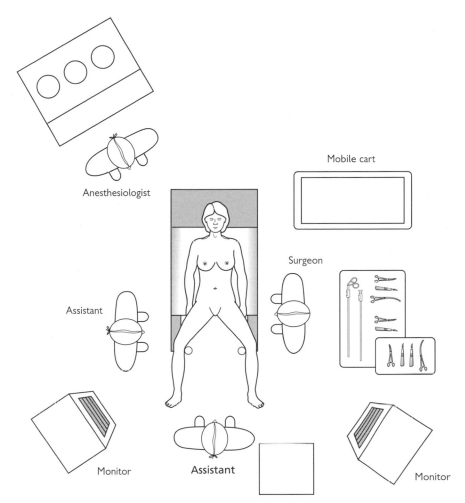

Fig. 15.7.1 Operating theatre set up (courtesy of Karl Storz and reproduced with permission).

the peritoneum. Pneumoperitoneum is established once the intra peritoneal position of the trocar is confirmed by visualization through the laparoscope. This prevents any vascular injury however the risk of bowel injury is similar to the closed technique (Hasson 1971, 1999).

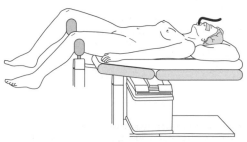

Fig. 15.7.2 Position of patient (courtesy of Karl Storz and reproduced with permission).

Direct entry technique

In this method the trocar is inserted directly into the abdomen without creating a pnuemoperitoneum. This should be carried out only in selected cases and in experienced hands. Using the newer optical trocars the different layers of the abdomen can be seen during entry with the trocar. This is useful when the port is inserted in the Palmer's point; however, the layers of the abdominal wall are not so well defined at the umbilicus and training and experience is needed to perform this technique. Several studies do not show an increased risk of major complications with this technique and some minor complications may be prevented by this method (Ahmad *et al.* 2007).

Once inside the abdomen a thorough 360° check should be performed to check for any inadvertent injuries. Additional ports under vision are usually placed in either iliac fossae lateral to the inferior epigastric vessels and the suprapubic area (Fig. 15.7.4).

In patients with laparotomy incisions, alternative sites like the Palmer's point (3 cm below the left costal margin in the midclavicular line in the left upper quadrant) should

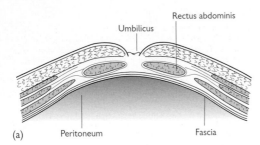

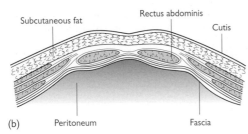

Fig. 15.7.3 Anatomy of umbilicus (courtesy of Karl Storz and reproduced with permission).

be used. There is a high rate of adhesions to the umbilicus with midline scars (50%) and with transverse scars (23%) (Audebert and Gomel 2000).

In such cases the Palmer's point should be chosen for entry with the Veress needle and primary trocar insertion. Other sites like the suprapubic and posterior vaginal fornix have been tried; however, they are associated with more complications and failures and hence not used very commonly.

Common types of gynaecological procedures carried out through laparoscopy
- Sterilization
- Salpingectomy

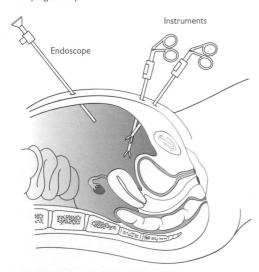

Fig. 15.7.4 Position of instruments at laparoscopy (courtesy of Karl Storz and reproduced with permission).

- Salpingostomy
- Ovarian cyst aspiration
- Ovarian cystectomy
- Oophorectomy
- Ovarian drilling in polycystic ovaries
- Adhesiolysis
- Myomectomy
- Hysterectomy
- Resection of endometriosis
- Ablation of endometriosis
- Pelvic lymphadenopathy
- Colposuspension for stress urinary incontinence
- Sacrocoplopexy for vault prolapse
- Tubal reconstructive surgery
- Oocyte retrieval in assisted conception techniques
- Misplaced intrauterine device retrieval.

Complications of laparoscopy
The risks associated with laparoscopy can be divided into serious or frequently occurring risks (RCOG 2004).

Serious risks
- Damage to bowel
- Injury to blood vessels: inferior epigastric, iliac, aorta, inferior vena cava, mesenteric
- Injury to the bladder and ureter
- Failure to gain entry to the abdominal cavity
- Uterine perforation
- Overall risk with diagnostic laparoscopy is around 2 in 1000
- In advanced laparoscopic procedures the risk of major complications can be as high as 12.5 per 1000 (Chapron et al. 1998).
- The mortality rate is between is 3 and 8 per 100 000.

Frequent risks
- Shoulder tip pain
- Bruising
- Wound infection
- Failure to identify disease
- Surgical emphysema
- Incisional hernia

During the consent procedure, these risk should be discussed with patients; the risks will vary according to the type of procedure being carried out. It is important for patients to consent for open surgery/laparotomy in case there is a complication. It is also important to remember that some patients may present with delayed complications, as thermal injuries and missed injuries can present several days later with serious consequences.

Advantages of laparoscopy
- Less analgesic requirement
- Shorter hospital stay
- Earlier mobilization
- Earlier resumption of normal activities
- Return to work earlier
- Cosmetic
- Cost saving

Training in laparoscopic surgery
Surgeons undertaking laparoscopic procedures should make themselves familiar with the equipment that is used

for the procedures. They should attend courses, lectures, and have hands-on training on pelvic trainers. Laparoscopic surgery requires good hand, foot, and eye coordination, which needs to be developed. Laparoscopic surgery requires a three-dimensional approach compared with the two dimensional views obtained at open surgery. The understanding of the different energy sources is of paramount importance and trainees need to familiarize themselves with this. Having the knowledge and using good and simple surgical principles will make laparoscopic surgery safer with good outcomes.

Training for diagnostic and minor operative laparoscopic procedures can be attained during the Basic and Intermediate training as outlined by the Royal College of Obstetricians and Gynaecologists. For further advanced training Advanced Training Skills Module (ATSM): 'Benign Gynaecological Surgery: Laparoscopy' needs to be completed.

Further reading

Consensus document concerning laparoscopic entry technique: Middlesbrough, March 19-20 1999. Gynaecol Endosc 1999; 8:403–6.

Ahmad G, Duffy J, Phillips K, Watson A. Laparoscopic entry techniques (protocol). Cochrane Database Syst Rev 2007;3:CD006583.

Audebert A J, Gomel V. Role of microlaparoscopy in the diagnosis of peritoneal and visceral adhesions and in the prevention of bowel injury associated with blind trocar insertion. Fertil Steril 2000;73:631–5.

Chapron C, Quwerleu, Bruhat MA, et al. Surgical complications of diagnostic and operative gynaecological laparoscopy: a series of 29966 cases. Hum Reproduction 1998;13:867–72.

Hasson HM. A modified instrument and method for laparoscopy. Am J Obstet Gynaecol 1971; 110:886–7.

Hasson HM. Open laparoscopy as a method of access in laparoscopic surgery. Gynaecological Endoscopy 1999; 8:353–62.

RCOG. Consent Advice 2. October 2004

RCOG. Preventing entry related gynaecological laparoscopic injuries. Green Top Guideline 49. May 2008.

Pelvic floor surgery

The management of pelvic organ prolapse is broadly divided into surgical or conservative treatment.

Conservative management includes
- lifestyle intervention such as weight loss, reducing heavy lifting and treating conditions like chronic coughing
- physical therapy, such as pelvic floor muscle training
- pessaries have been shown to be effective in the control of symptoms associated with prolapse.

Anterior vaginal prolapse

Anterior vaginal wall prolapse is thought to result from tears in or detachment of the pubocervical fascia. Lateral or paravaginal defects, midline defect or transverse defect in the pubocervical fascia are described (Karram 2001).

Symptoms

Anterior vaginal wall prolapse presents with symptoms such as vaginal bulge or mass, low back pain, pelvic pressure, or sexual difficulty. It may also be associated with stress urinary incontinence.

Surgical repair technique

The commonest method of repair of anterior vaginal wall prolapse is plication of the pubocervical fascia (anterior colporrhapy). It is carried out by making a midline longitudinal incision on the anterior vagina after infiltration with haemostatic solution containing 1% xylocaine with 1:200 000 adrenaline. The vaginal flap is dissected using the Metzenbaum scissor towards the inferior pubis ramus. This dissection is done bilaterally, thus exposing the anterior vaginal fascia. Interrupted 2-0 polyglactin stitches are used to plicate the exposed paravaginal connective tissue. The vaginal flap is trimmed and closed with absorbable interlocking stitches. Other authors use longer term absorbable sutures. This procedure can be used for recurrences; some surgeons use support meshes to enhance the repair. There appear to be complications associated with this, and further research is required.

Other methods for repair of anterior vaginal wall prolapse include carrying out a paravaginal repair; this can be done by the vaginal or abdominal route. More recently the use of synthetic material to provide support in the anterior vaginal wall has been introduced. The safety and efficacy of this latter technique is awaited.

Complications

Complications include bleeding, vaginal haematoma formation, inadvertent damage to bladder and urethra. Urinary tract infection is a common complication. Other complications include voiding difficulty and sexual dysfunction.

Posterior vaginal wall prolapse

Posterior vaginal wall prolapse commonly known as rectocele is a defect in the rectovaginal fascia. It is an out-pocketing of the anterior rectal wall and the posterior vaginal wall into the lumen of the vagina (Mellgren et al. 1995)

Symptoms

These include feeling of something falling down in the vagina, a mass in the vagina, lower abdominal or backache, difficulty passing stool, faecal incontinence, constipation. Some rectoceles are asymptomatic.

Management

Conservative measures in the management of rectocele include living an active lifestyle, eating adequate dietary fibre, adopting proper bowel training. Vaginal pessaries are also used in the non-surgical treatment of rectocele.

Surgical repair technique

The gynaecologist uses the transvaginal route for rectocele repair, whereas colorectal surgeons favour the transrectal route.

The repair of rectocele is carried out under general or local anaesthesia. An initial rectal examination is performed to assess the extent of the rectocele. Infiltration of the posterior vaginal wall using xylocaine with 1:200 000 adrenaline is performed. A longitudinal midline incision on the posterior vaginal wall is made. The vaginal flap is dissected off bilaterally exposing the rectovaginal fascia. The defect in the rectovaginal is plicated using 2-0 ployglactin suture. Excess vaginal tissue is trimmed off and the vaginal skin closed with 2-0 polyglactin suture. Perineorrhapy is carried if indicated.

Synthetic meshes or grafts are also used for repair of rectocele.

Complications

Dyspareunia is a complication that may occur after a posterior colporrhaphy.

Vaginal apical prolapse

Prolapse of the vaginal apex may occur in the presence or absence of the uterus. Traditionally, the management of uterovaginal prolapse is vaginal hysterectomy together with posterior and/or anterior compartment repair. Hysterectomy is not always considered necessary as the presence of the uterus does not affect the effectiveness of the procedure (Langer et al. 1988). This uterus-sparing approach is desirable when fertility consideration is an issue.

Symptoms

The patients with vaginal apex prolapse typically presents with symptoms such as a feeling of something coming down, vaginal pressure, sexual difficulty, difficulty emptying the bowel, urinary symptoms, such as urgency, frequency, incontinence, and voiding difficulty. Some patients are asymptomatic.

Surgical management of vaginal apical prolapse

The surgical management of vaginal apical prolapse can be carried out either by the vaginal or abdominal approach. The approach used is guided by the patient's age, presence of medical comorbidities, weight, desire for coital activity, previous abdominal surgery, and history of previous failed surgery.

Vaginal route

The advantage of the vaginal approach to management of vaginal apex prolapse include
- significant low postoperative morbidity
- can be performed either under local or regional anaesthesia
- allows for repair of other pelvic defects simultaneously

Various surgical techniques using the vaginal route have been described; these include sacrospinous vault suspension, uterosacral ligament fixation, iliococcygeus muscle fixation, McCall culdoplasty, and posterior intravaginal slingoplasty.

Sacrospinous fixation involves the attachment of the vaginal vault to the sacrospinous ligament without tension. It can be performed during vaginal hysterectomy as prophylaxis against future vaginal vault prolapse. Usually, unilateral fixation is performed when used to treat vault prolapse. Complications of the procedure include haemorrhage, nerve injury, injury to bladder and rectum, dyspareunia, postoperative stress incontinence, and voiding difficulty.

McCall culdoplasty involves suspension of the vaginal vault from the origin of the uterosacral ligament together with obliteration of the pouch of Douglas. This procedure is performed at vaginal hysterectomy to prevent occurrence of vault prolapse in the future.

The posterior intravaginal sling procedure involves the use of mesh to support the vault.

Uterus-sparing vaginal procedures are also utilized in the management of uterovaginal prolapse. These procedures include

- Manchester procedure
- sacrospinous hysteropexy
- uterosacral plication
- colpocleisis: this is carried out in elderly patients who are no longer sexually active.

Abdominal route

Sacrocolpopexy involve the using a suspensor bridge (mesh) to support the vaginal apex by attaching to the sacrum, and reperitonizing over the mesh to prevent erosion into bowel. The procedure can be done either as an open procedure or laparoscopically. Sacrocolpopexy has the advantage of allowing any concomitant intrabdominal pathology to be dealt with and it can be performed irrespective of the vaginal length.

Complications associated with sacrocolpopexy include bleeding, and injury to organs such as bowel, bladder, and ureter. Others include urinary tract infection, wound infection, postoperative ileus, and mesh erosion.

In randomized controlled trials (Benson et al. 1966; Maher et al. 2004) comparing abdominal sacrcolpopexy to vaginal sacrospinous fixation, there were more failures in the vaginal group.

Uterus-sparing abdominal procedures include

- sacrohysteropexy and sacrocervicopexy
- pectineal ligament suspension.

Further reading

Benson JT, Lucente V, McClellan E. Vaginal versus abdominal reconstructive surgery for the treatment of pelvic support defects: a prospective randomised study with long-term outcome evaluation. Am J Obstet Gynecol 1966;175:1418–22.

Bump RC, Mattiasson A, Bo K, et al. The standardisation of terminology of female pelvic organ prolapse and pelvic organ dysfunction. Am J Obstet Gynecol 1996;175:10–7.

Karram MM. Vaginal operation for prolapse. In: Baggish MS, Karram MM (eds) Atlas of pelvic anatomy and Gynaecologic surgery. Philadelphia: Saunders 2001.

Langer R, Ron-El R, Neuman M, et al. The value of simultaneous hysterectomy during burch colposuspension for urinary stress incontinence. Obstet Gynecol 1988;72:866–9.

Maher CF, Qatawneh AM, Dwyer PL, et al. Abdominal sacrocolpopexy or vaginal sacrospinous colpopexy for vaginal vault prolapse: a prospective randomised study. Am J Obstet Gynecol 2004;190:20–6.

Mellgren A, Anzen B, Nilsson BY, et al. Results of rectocoele repair. A prospective study. Dis Colon Rectum 1995;38:7–13.

Olsen AL, Smith VJ, Bergstrom VO, et al. Epidemiology of surgically managed pelvic organ prolapse and urinary incontinence. Obstet Gynecol 1997;89:501–6.

Price N, Slack A, Jwarah E, Jackson S. The incidence of reoperation for surgically treated pelvic organ prolapse: an 11-year experience. Menopause int. 2008;14:145–8.

Silva WA, Kleeman S, Segal J, et al. Effects of a full bladder and patient positioning on pelvic organ prolapse assessment. Obstet Gynecol 2004;104:37–41.

Sliskerten HMCP, Vierhout M, Bloembergen H, Schoenmaker G. Distribution of pelvic organ prolapse in the general population: prevalence, severity, aetiology and relation with function of the pelvic floor muscles. Abstract presented at the joint meeting of the ICS and IUGA, August 25–27, 2004, Paris, France.

Weber AM, Walters MD, Piedmonte MA, et al. Anterior Colporrhaphy: a randomised trial of three surgical techniques. Am J Obstet Gynecol 2001;185:1299–306

Index

N.B. 'f' following a locator indicates a figure and 't' indicates a table.

A

abdominal cysts, fetal 122
abdominal myomectomy 607
abdominal pain, in pregnancy
  aetiology 320
  clinical approach 320
  diagnosis 320–1
  epidemiology 320
  fatty liver of pregnancy 321
  inflammatory causes 321
  management 321–2
  pancreatitis 321
  placental abruption 321
  postpartum pseudo-obstruction 321
  pre-eclampsia and HELLP syndrome 321
  preterm labour 321
  surgical management 321–2
  urological causes 321
abdominal wall defects, fetal 118–20
abnormalities see fetal abnormalities
Access to Health Records Act (1990) 24
ACE inhibitors see angiotensin-converting-
  enzyme (ACE) inhibitors
achondroplasia 133
acne 198
acromegaly 284
acute fatty liver of pregnancy (AFLP)
  275–6, 321
Addison's disease 176
adenosine 232
adolescent problems see paediatric and
  adolescent problems
adrenal disorders, in pregnancy
  Addison's disease 176
  congenital adrenal hyperplasia (CAH) 176
  Conn's syndrome 177
  Cushing's syndrome 177–8
  phaeochromocytoma 176
adrenocortical steroids 210
adrenoreceptor blockers 346
Adults with Incapacity (Scotland) Act 2000 15,
  16, 26
airtravel, during pregnancy 33
albendazole 209
alcohol consumption, in pregnancy 4, 33, 61
  see also fetal alcohol syndrome (FAS)
ambiguous genitalia
  5-a-reductase deficiency 465
  aetiology 464–5
  complete androgen insensitivity syndrome
    (CAIS) 464–5, 572
  congenital adrenal hyperplasia (CAH) 464
  diagnosis 465
  gender of rearing 465–6, 483
  incidence 464
  management 465–7
  normal sexual differentiation 464
  pathophysiology of 464
  surgery for 466–7
  see also disorders of sex development
    (DSDs)
amenorrhoea 570
  see also oligomenorrhoea and amenorrhoea
aminoglycosides 209
aminosalicylates 263
amiodarone 210–11, 232
amniocentesis 351
amniotic band syndrome 126–7
amniotic fluid embolism (AFE)
  clinical approach 324
  definition 324
  diagnosis 324
  epidemiology 324
  investigations 324

  management 324–5
  pathophysiology 324
  symptoms and signs 324
amniotomy 386–7
anaemia
  causes 180
  definition 180
  diagnosis 180
  fetal 92, 146, 148, 149–50, 378
  iron-deficiency 180–1
  megaloblastic anaemias 181
  mother, effects on 180
  pregnancy and fetus, effects on 180
  prevalence 180
  screening for 33, 68
anaesthesia, in obstetrics
  anaesthesia-related mortality 367
  Caesarean sections 365
  epidural anaesthesia 365–6
  general anaesthesia 366–7
  rapid sequence induction (RSI) of
    anaesthesia 366–7
  regional anaesthesia, complications of 366t
  technique 366–7
analgesia, for labour
  definition 364
  epidemiology 364
  epidural analgesia 364–5
  pharmacological agents 364
  regional techniques 364, 365
androgen insensitivity syndrome (AIS) 482
anencephaly 98–9
aneuploidy, fetal
  antenatal screening versus prenatal
    diagnosis 168
  Down's syndrome screening 168
  Edward's syndrome 170
  first trimester tests 169
  markers 168
  model predicted DR for 5% FPR 169
  natural history 168
  neural tube defects 170
  prospective intervention studies 169
  risk calculation 168–9
  second trimester tests 169
  sequential tests 169
  strategies, possible future 169–70
  twins 170
angiotensin-converting-enzyme (ACE)
    inhibitors 211, 232, 255, 292, 345
antenatal care
  antenatal appointments 32, 35–7
  antenatal information 32
  booking appointment 32, 38–40
  care, provision and organization of 32
  clinical conditions, screening for 35
  clinical examination, of pregnant women 33
  documentation 32
  first trimester 39f
  gestational age assessment 32
  haematological conditions, screening
    for 33–5
  infections, screening for 34–5
  lifestyle considerations 32
  midwife- and GP-led models of care 32
  minor ailments, in pregnancy 33
  second trimester 35f
  third trimester 36f
antepartum haemorrhage
  causes 326
  definition 326
  examination 326
  history 326
  incidence 326
  management 326

  of indeterminate origin 326–7
  prognosis 326
anthrax 260
anti-angina drugs 210
antiarrhythmics 210–11, 232–3
antibacterials 209
antibiotic administration 351
antibodies, screening for 68
anticoagulants 233
anticonvulsants 209–11, 287
antidepressants 212, 288, 339
antiemetics 77
antihypertensives 211, 232, 254–5,
  345–6
antimuscarinic drugs 616, 619
antiphospholipid syndrome (APS)
  193, 590
antiplatelet agents 233
antiprotozoal drugs 210
antipsychotics 211–12, 288
antipyretics 208
antiretroviral drugs 246–7
antisteroid therapy 607
antithrombotics 78, 211, 213, 432
antypsychotics 343
aortic dissection/aneurysm 227–8
Apert's syndrome 112
arthrogryposis 113
asthma
  acute attack, treatment of 296–8
  definition 296
  diagnosis 296
  during pregnancy 296t
  epidemiology 296
  history 296
  management 296t
  medications 296–98
  pathology 296
  precipitants 296
  preconception 296t
  severity of 296t
  signs 296
  symptoms 296
atrial fibrillation and flutter 226
autoimmune disease
  chronic active hepatitis 183
  liver disorders 182
  multiple sclerosis 182
  myasthenia gravis 182
  primary biliary cirrhosis 183
  primary sclerosing cholangitis 183
azathioprine 210, 263
azithromycin 188

B

β-2 agonists 296
β-adrenergic antagonists 211
bacterial vaginosis 34
  aetiology 184
  clinical features 184
  complications 184
  definition 184
  diagnosis 184
  epidemiology 184
  management 184–5
  preterm delivery (PTD), prediction
    of 352
bacteriuria 34
bad news, breaking
  baby, death of 13, 14
  fertility 14
  oncology 14–15
  palliative care 670
Bakri tamponade balloon 431

balloon tamponade
  advantages of 431
  aetiology 430
  application 431–2
  clinical approach 431
  definition 430
  epidemiology 430
  pathology 430
  postoperative management 432
balloon valvuloplasty/valvotomy
  154, 233
Bartholin's gland carcinoma 679
Beckwith Wiedemann 111–12
benign and urogynaecology
  endometrial polyps 600
  female genital cutting 602–3
  female urinary incontinence 614–6
  fibroids 606–7
  ovarian cysts 610–11
  pelvic inflammatory disease (PID) 612–3
  urinary frequency and urgency 618–19
  urinary retention 620–1
  urinary tract injury 622–4
  urodynamic investigation 630
  uterovaginal prolapse 626–8
  vaginal discharge 632
  vesicovaginal fistulae 634–5
  vulval pain and pruritis 636–7
benign tumours see tumours
bereavement, and grieving process 13
beta-blockers 232
betamethazone 210
biophysical profile (BPP), fetal
  biophysical profile score 84
  clinical management protocol 84–5
  definition 84
  pathophysiology 84
biparietal diameter (BPD) 48
biscuspid aortic valve with/without coarctation
  of the aorta 228
bleeding, in early pregnancy 74
blood grouping
  cell alloantibodies 33–4
  screening for 68
blood tests, routine in pregnancy
  anaemia 68
  antibodies, screening for 68
  blood grouping 68
  Down's syndrome, screening for 69–70
  gestational diabetes (GDM), screening for 69
  haemoglobin electrophoresis 68–9
  haemoglobinopathies, and pregnancy 69
  infections, in pregnancy 70–1
  routine tests 68
  special tests 68
body mass index (BMI) 615
Bolam principle 21
Bolitho qualification 21
booking appointment (visit) 32
  aim of 38
  booking clinic, management at 38
  first trimester 39f
  lifestyle advice 38
  referrals, arrangement of 40
  risk assessment 38
  tests during 38–40
  timing of 38
bradycardia 226
brain abnormalities 112
Braxton-Hicks contractions
  51, 54–5
breast cancer screening 640–1
breastfeeding
  antidepressants 339
  baby-friendly hospital 44
  breast abscess 45
  breast, anatomy of 42
  colostrum 43–4
  contraindications to 45
  drug abuse/medications 45–6
  economic benefits 43
  engorgement 44

galactocoeles/plugged ducts 44
HIV 45
hypertension 256
immunization 258
infant benefits 43
initiation and maintenance of 43
lactation, physiology of 42
latch-on 43–4
mastitis 45
maternal benefits 42
metabolism, inborn errors of 45
nipple-related problems 45
breech delivery
  clinical approach 369
  definition 368
  epidemiology 368
  management 369–70
  medicolegal issues 22
  pathophysiology 368–9
  post 'Term Breech Trial' 370
  predisposing factors 368
  types of 368
brittle bone disease 132, 133
brow presentation
  clinical approach 371
  definition 371
  epidemiology 371
  management 371
  mechanism of labour 371

C

Caesarean myomectomy 442
Caesarean section (CS)
  adverse outcomes, factors affecting
    435–6
  aetiology 436–7
  anaesthesia 365, 438
  bladder/omentum/bowel, repair of 442
  breech delivery 370
  brow presentation 371
  cord prolapse 372–3
  decision to delivery interval 438
  definition 434
  epidemiology 434
  EXIT (ex utero intrapartum treatment)
    procedure 442
  face presentation 377
  fetal/neonatal benefits of 436–7
  general approach 438
  indications for 436
  infection, prevention of 438
  labour, managing delay 392
  lower segment 22
  maternal benefits of 436–7
  maternal morbidity 434–5
  maternal mortality 435
  multifetal pregnancy 441
  pathology 434–6
  pelvic organs, inspection of 442
  perinatal morbidity 435
  placenta praevia 403
  placenta, delivery of 441
  placental abruption 406–7
  postpartum management 442
  predictors of 436
  preparations 438–9
  prognosis 437–8
  shoulder dystocia 421
  singleton pregnancy 440–1
  skin incision 439–40
  uterine compression sutures 453
  uterine incision 440
  uterus, repair of 441–2
cancer, in pregnancy
  aetiology 328
  chemotherapy/radiotherapy, effects on
    fetus 328
  children, risks to 329
  clinical approach 328–9
  definition 328
  epidemiology 328

major considerations 328
pathology 328
screening 640–2
see also tumours, in gynaecology
carbamazepine 209
cardiac arrest 227
cardiac arrhythmias 226–7
cardiac symptoms, classification of severity
  of 224
cardiopathies 226
cardiotocography (CTG) 86–8, 354, 355,
  380–2
cardiovascular abnormalities, fetal
  aetiology and associations 94
  chromosomal defects 94
  clinical approach 95
  definition 94
  delivery, place and timing of 96
  environmental and maternal factors 94
  epidemiology 94
  family history 94
  genetic syndromes 94
  natural history, and antenatal prognosis
    94–5
  nuchal translucency 94
  perinatal management 95–6
cardiovascular system, changes in
  pregnancy 57
cardioverter defibrillators 232
Cat Cry syndrome 106
central nervous system abnormalities, fetal
  cerebral lesions, destructive 102–3
  corpus callosum, agenesis of 101–2
  Dandy-Walker complex 101–2
  microcephaly 102
  neural tube defects 98–9
  ventriculomegaly 99–100
cerebral lesions, fetal 102–3
cerebral palsy 398
cervical cancer
  clinical presentation 644
  clinical staging 644
  incidence of 644
  non-surgical management 646
  pathological classification 644–5
  radiological staging 645
  rates of in pregnancy 349
  recurrent, recognizing and managing 646
  risk factors 644
  screening 641
  surgical management 645–6
  treatment 646
cervical dysplasia
  and human papillomavirus (HPV) 648,
    649–50
  cervical screening 648–9, 650
  cervix, anatomy of 648
  colposcopic features 649
cervical glandular intraepithelial neoplasia
  (CGIN) 349
cervical intraepithelial neoplasia (CIN) 349
cervical teratomas 129
Chadwick sign, of pregnancy 50
chicken pox
  aetiology 186
  clinical approach 186
  congenital varicella syndrome 186
  epidemiology 186
  fetal outcome 187
  first trimester exposure 186
  postpartum exposure 186–7
  second trimester exposure 186
  third trimester exposure 186
  varicella screening 187
  varicella zoster virus 70, 186
chlamydia 34, 188–9
chloramphenicol 209
chloroquine 210
cholecystitis, acute 266–7
choledocal cyst 122t
chondrodysplasia punctata (CPD) 133
chorioamnionitis 400

choriocarcinoma 660
chorionic villus sampling (CVS) *versus*
    amniocentesis 152
chromosomal anomalies
  balanced translocations 106–7
  chromosome mosaicism 107
  chromosome results, abnormal 106
  confined placental mosaicism 107
  definition 106
  deletions and duplications 106
  Down's syndrome 106
  Edward's syndrome 106
  epidemiology 106
  fetal aneuploidy 106
  marker chromosomes 107
  Patau syndrome 106
  sex chromosome aneuploidies 106
  triploidy 69 106
ciprofloxacin 209
cirrhosis 277
clomiphine 504, 514
clonidine 548
clover leave 112
club foot 124
coagulation disorders
  acquired defects 191
  bleeding disorders 190
  inherited defects 190–1
colon cancer screening 640
colostrum 43–4
communication skills 12
  core clinical skill 12
  doctors-children/young people 12
  improving 16
  information transfer 12
  partnership-building 12
  patient-gynaecologist 12
  rapport-building 12
comparative genomic hybridization
    (CGH) 106
complementary therapies 32, 501, 546–7, 548,
    582–3
complete androgen insensitivity syndrome
    (CAIS) 464–5, 572
condom hydrostatic tamponade 431
confidentiality 13, 24, 485, 597
congenital adrenal hyperplasia (CAH) 176,
    464, 482
congenital cystic adenomatous malformation
    (CCAM) 136
congenital diaphragmatic hernia (CDH) 136–7
congenital heart disease 95
  see also cardiovascular abnormalities, fetal
Conn's syndrome 177
connective tissue disorder
  antiphospholipid syndrome (APS) 193
  neonatal lupus syndromes 192–3
  rheumatoid arthritis, and pregnancy 192
  scleroderma, and pregnancy 193
  systemic lupus erythematosus (SLE)
      192–3
consent
  Caesarean sections, court-ordered 21
  capacity 13, 15, 16
  children and young people 16
  decisions, reviewing 15
  emergency obstetric procedures 21
  express 13, 15
  implied 15
  informed 21, 22
  maternal immunity 21
  model for 15
  oral *versus* written 15
continence procedures
  abdominal procedures 702
  artificial urinary sphincter 703
  bulking agents, injection of 703
  counselling 703
  minimally invasive mid-urethral slings 702–3
  minitapes 703
  sling procedures 702
  stress incontinence, treatment of 702

surgical treatment 702–3
  tension-free vaginal tape 702
  transobturator procedures 702–3
contraception
  aetiology 478–9
  antiprogesterones 498
  barrier methods 478
  combined emergency 498
  contraindications 479
  copper-bearing intrauterine device 498
  counselling points 499
  definition 478
  efficacy 479, 498
  epidemiology 478
  Fraser guidelines 23–4
  hormonal methods 478
  impact 498
  indications 498
  mechanism of action 478–9, 498
  non-contraceptive benefits of 478
  non-hormonal 478
  oral 478
  pathology 478
  prevalence, by method 479
  progestogen only emergency hormonal
      contraception (PEHC) 498
  risks 478
  safety 478, 498–9
  selective oestrogen receptor modulator 498
  sterilization procedure 479
  ulipristal acetate 498
  vaccines, research on 479
  see also intrauterine devices
copper IUDs *see* intrauterine devices
cord prolapse
  definition 372
  diagnosis 372
  epidemiology 372
  management 372–3
  pathophysiology 372
  risk factors 372
cordocentesis 152
corpus callosum, agenesis of 101–2
corticosteroids 263, 351
craniosynostosis syndromes 112
Crohn's disease *see* inflammatory bowel
    disease
crown-rump length (CRL) measurement 48,
    49f
CS *see* Caesarean section (CS)
Cuscoe's speculum 9
Cushing's syndrome 177–8, 284
cyclophosphamide 209
cyclosporin 210, 263
cystic fibrosis 120–1, 300
cystic hygroma 128
cytomegalovirus (CMV) 34, 60, 196

D

Dandy-Walker complex 101–2
dating, in pregnancy
  clinical dating 48
  expected date of delivery (EDD) 48–9
  gestational age (GA) 48, 49f
deep vein thrombosis (DVT) 231, 310, 311,
    346, 432
depression 287
  see also postnatal depression
dermatology
  coincidental conditions 198
  dermatoses, pregnancy specific 198–9
  physiological changes 198
  pre-existing conditions 198
detrusor overactivity (DO) 614
diabetes, in pregnancy
  acute emergencies, management of 205
  aetiology and pathogenesis 200
  delivery, management of 205–6
  diabetes, types of 200
  diabetic ketoacidosis 205
  diagnostic criteria 200t, 201t

fetal surveillance 205
  gestational diabetes (GDM) 200–1, 203
  hypoglycaemia 205
  management of 204–5
  mortality rates 205t
  pituitary disorders 283–4
  pre-existing diabetes 203–4
  prevalence 200
  Type 1 DM 201
  Type 2 DM 201
diagnosis, of pregnancy
  Braxton-Hicks contractions 51
  breast changes 50
  breast discomfort 50
  cervical mucus, changes in 50
  cervix, changes in 50
  differential diagnosis 51f
  fatigue 50
  fetal heart sounds 51
  fetal movements 51
  fetal parts, palpation of 51
  first trimester 50
  fundal height 51
  home pregnancy test 51
  hormonal tests 50
  immunoassay 50–1
  investigations 50–1
  laboratory test kits 51
  menstruation, cessation of 50
  micturition, frequency of 50
  morning sickness 50
  objective signs 50, 51
  second trimester 51
  skin changes 50
  third trimester 51
  ultrasound 51
  uterus, changes in 50
  vagina, discolouration of 50
digoxin 232
dinoprostone (PGE2) 386
disclosure 13
  see also confidentiality
disorders of sex development (DSDs)
  46XY 572
  androgen insensitivity syndrome (AIS) 482
  clitoral surgery 483
  complete androgen insensitivity syndrome
      (CAIS) 464–5, 572
  congenital adrenal hyperplasia (CAH) 482, 572
  definition 482
  diagnosis 483
  disorders of testosterone biosynthesis 482
  gender of rearing 465–6, 483
  gonadectomy 483
  medical management 483
  Müllerian duct anomalies 572
  ovotesticular DSD 482
  presentation of 483
  Rokitansky syndrome 482–3
  surgical management 483
  Swyer's syndrome 482, 572
  Turner's syndrome 482, 572
  vagina creation 483
disseminated intravascular coagulation
    (DIC) 407
diuretics 231–2
donor insemination
  child, welfare of 485
  confidentiality 485
  counselling 484
  donor matching 485
  donor recruitment 484
  donor screening 484
  female partner, assessment of 484
  indications 484
  intracytoplasmic sperm injection (ICSI) 484
  law and regulation, UK 485
  male factor infertility 484
  rights, of parents/donor/child 485
  semen storage 484
  success rates 485
  treatment cycle, management of 485

Doppler ultrasound 5
  Doppler guidelines 93f
  fetal venous Doppler 92
  fetal vessels 90–1
  hypoxic baby 93
  middle cerebral artery (MCA) 91–2
  physics of 90
  thoracic aorta 92
  types of 90
  umbilical artery 90–1
  waveforms, assessment of 90, 91t
Down's syndrome
  chromosomal anomalies 106
  screening for 34, 69–70, 167, 168
drug use, recreational 4
drugs, in pregnancy
  ACE inhibitors 211
  adrenocortical steroids 210
  anti-angina drugs 210
  anti-arrhythmics 210–1
  anti-filarials 209
  anti-helminthic-intestinal drugs 209
  anti-hypertensives 211
  anti-schistosmals 209
  anti-trematodes 209
  antibacterials 209
  anticonvulsants/antiepileptics 209
  antiprotozoal drugs 210
  antipyretics 208
  antithrombotic drugs 211
  antithyroid drugs 211
  carbamazepine 209
  drug metabolism, in pregnancy 208–9
  fetus, effects of drugs on 208
  immunosuppressive drugs 210
  non-opioid analgesics 208
  non-steroidal anti-inflammatory drugs
    (NSAIDs) 208
  opioid analgesics 208–9
  phenobarbitone 209
  phenytoin 209
  primidone 209
  psychotherapeutic drugs 211–2
  sodium valproate 209
  US FDA pregnancy category definitions 208t
duloxetine 616
duodenal atresia 120
dysmenorrhoea
  aetiology 489
  definition 489
  epidemiology 489
  examination 489
  history 489
  investigation 489
  pathology 489
  prognosis 489
  treatment 489

E

eating disorders 287
echocardiography 95, 231
echogenic bowel
  aetiology 120–1
  cystic fibrosis 120–1
  definition 120
  diagnosis, ultrasound findings 121
  epidemiology 120
  history 121
  investigation 121
  management 121–2
eclampsia see pre-eclampsia, and eclampsia
ectopic pregnancy
  aetiology 490
  definition 490
  epidemiology 490
  examination 490
  future pregnancies 492
  history 490
  investigations 490–1
  management 491–2
ectrodactyly 124–5

eczema 198
Edward's syndrome 106, 170
Ehlers-Danlos syndrome 227–8
electrocardiogram (ECG) 230–1
electroconvulsive therapy 288
Ellis-van Creveld syndrome 133
embryo freezing
  advantages of 494
  challenges 494
  cryoprotectants, use of 494
  definition 494
  embryo development, stage of for
    freezing 494–5
  epidemiology 494
  frozen embryo replacement
    cycles 495
  legal aspects and regulation 494
  slow cooling, or vitrification 495
encephalocele 98–9
endocrine and metabolic changes, in
    pregnancy 58–9
  adrenal glands 58
  breast changes 59
  pancreas 58
  postural changes 59
  thyroid 58
endometrial ablation
  balloon thermal ablation 690
  chemoablation 691
  complications 691
  cryoablation: Her option 691
  endometrial preparation 691
  first generation techniques 690
  free fluid endometrial ablation
    (hydrothermablator HTA) 690
  gynaelase endometrial laser
    intrauterine thermal therapy
    (ELITT) 691
  impedance bipolar radiofrequency
    endometrial ablation 691
  menstrual bleeding, heavy 486–7
  microwave endometrial ablation 690
  outpatient endometrial ablation 691
  second generation techniques
    690–1
endometrial polyp
  human chorionic gonadotrophin (hCG)
    trigger 505–6
  hysteroscopic polypectomy 505
  hysteroscopy 505
  semen collection 505
  success rates 506
endometriosis
  aetiology 500
  assisted reproduction 501
  cancers, associated 500
  complementary therapies 501
  definition 500
  diagnosis 500
  endometriosis-associated infertility 501
  examination 500
  investigations 500
  pain, treatment of 500
  patient support groups 501
  quality of life, impact on 500
  symptoms 500
  treatment, empirical 500
endometrium, neoplastic conditions of
  advanced disease, treatment of 656
  aetiology 652
  clinical approach 653–5
  endometrial cancer 652, 653, 654, 655
  endometrial hyperplasia 653–4
  epidemiology 652
  pathology 653
  positive peritoneal cytology 654–5
  radiotherapy 655–6
  recurrent disease, treatment of 656
  smooth muscle tumours 653
  staging 653, 654t
epidural anaesthesia 365–6
epidural analgesia 364–5

epilepsy
  AEDs, teratogenic effects of 214
  classification of 214
  contraception 215
  genetic aspects 214
  management 214–15
  migraine 215
  post partum management 215
  preconception advice 214
  pregnancy risks 214
  seizure frequency 214
episiotomy
  definition 374
  incidence 374
  indications for 374
  perineal trauma, management and repair
    of 374–5
ergometrine 298
erythema multiform 198
erythema nodosum 198
examination
  gynaecological patient 8–9
  obstetric patient 4–5
exercise, in pregnancy 32–33
expected date of delivery (EDD) 4, 48–9
external cephalic version (ECV) 370

F

face presentation
  clinical approach 376
  definition 376
  epidemiology 376
  management 376–7
  mechanism of labour 376
  postpartum complications 377
facial abnormalities
  facial clefts 116
  micrognathia 116–7
fallopian tube cancer 641, 668
female genital mutilation (FGM) 4
  causes 602
  classification 602
  consequences of 602–3
  definition 602
  eradication of 603
  legal issues 602
  prevalence 602
female infertility see infertility, female
female pelvis see pelvis, anatomy of female
female urinary incontinence see urinary
    incontinence, female
femur length (FL) 48
fertility, in survivors of childhood malignancy
  cancer treatment effects 508
  clinical approach 509–10
  comorbidity 510
  counselling 510
  definition 508
  epidemiology 508
  Faddy-Gosden model, dose and age at
    treatment 508f
  fertility preservation 509–10, 511
  follow-up 511
  male patients 511
  management 509
  pathology 508–9
  post-treatment considerations 509
  pre-treatment considerations 509
  premature ovarian failure 508
  prognosis 509
  quick reference material 510
  radiotherapy 508–9, 511
  see also infertility, female
fetal abnormalities
  cardiovascular 94–6
  central nervous system 98–103
  chromosomal anomalies 106–7
  face 116–7
  gastrointestinal system 117–23
  genetic disorders 110–14
  head and neck 128–9

hydrops 148–50
limbs 124–7
screening for 34
skeletal abnormalities/dysplasias 132–5
thorax 136–8
urinary system 140–2
fetal alcohol spectrum disorder (FASD) 61
fetal alcohol syndrome (FAS) 61, 304
fetal aneuploidy 106
fetal blood sampling (FBS) 152
fetal goitre 128–29
fetal hydrops 113
fetal movement charts 144–5
fetal stethoscope 5
fetal surveillance, in labour
cardiotocography (CTG) 380–2
definition 378
diagnostic tests 378
epidemiology 378
fetal blood sampling 382
pathology 378–9
prognosis 379
screening tests 378
surveillance approach 379–80
fetal vesico-amniotic shunt 153
fetal pleural effusion 137–8
fetus, care of
biophysical profile (BPP) 84–5
cardiotocography (CTG) 86–9
Doppler ultrasound 90–3
fetal movement charts 144–5
fetal nuchal translucency 146–7
intrauterine growth restriction (IUGR) 156–7
invasive procedures 152–4
multiple pregnancy 158–9
oligohydramnios 160–1
placental abnormalities 162
polyhydramnios 164–5
red blood cell isoimmunization 166–7
symphyseal fundal height (SFH) 172–4
umbilical cord abnormalities 162
FGM see female genital mutilation (FGM)
fibroids
abdominal myomectomy 607
aetiology 330
antenatal care 330
Caesarean section 331
classification 606
clinical features 330
complications 606
definition 330
differential diagnosis 606
epidemiology 330
fibroid pain, management of 330–1
hormonal therapies 607
hysterectomy 607
in pregnancy 330–1
management 330–31, 606–7
miscarriage 330
myomectomy 331, 442, 553, 607
non-hormonal therapies 607
pathology 330
pathophysiology 606
pharmacological options 607
postpartum care 331
pregnancy 607
subfertility 330
surgical treatment, indications for 607
uterine artery embolization 607
fluoxetine 212
Foley catheter 431
forceps delivery
abdominal palpation 447
aetiology 446
clinical approach 447
definition 446
delivery, abandoning ('failed forceps') 450
epidemiology 446
examination, prior to forceps application 447
forceps, application of 448–9
pathology 446

preparation 447
prerequisities 447
prognosis 447
successful delivery, procedures after 449–50
traction in cephalic presentation 449
vaginal examination 447
furosemide 231–2

G
galactocoeles 44
galactopoiesis 42
galactosaemia 45
gastrointestinal abnormalities, fetal
abdominal cysts 122
anterior abdominal wall defects 118–20
exomphalos 113
gastroschisis 113
genitalia, ambiguous 113
GI tract abnormalities 120–2
pregnancies, future 122
pregnancy, termination of 122
gastroschisis 113, 400
genetic disorders, fetal
gastrointestinal abnormalities 113
inheritance patterns 110
investigations 113–14
screening 111–13
genital tract
premalignant conditions of 349
uterine anomalies 533
vaginal anomalies 532–3
genitalia, ambiguous see ambiguous genitalia
German measles see rubella
gestational diabetes (GDM) 35, 69, 200–1, 203
gestational trophoblastic neoplasia
chemotherapy 660, 661
choriocarcinoma 660
complete hydatidiform mole 659–60
definition 658
diagnosis 658–9
epidemiology 658
high-risk patients 660
invasive mole 660
low-risk patients 660
management 659–60
partial hydatidiform mole 660
pathology 658
placental site trophopblastic tumour (PSTT) 661
radiation therapy 661
surgery in 661
Gilbert's syndrome 266
Gillick competence 24
glycerine trinitrate (GTN) 351, 419
gonadectomy 467, 483
gonadotrophin-releasing hormone (GnRH) 506, 515, 525, 607
gonorrhoea
counselling 218
definition 218
diagnosis 218
epidemiology 218
examination 218
history 218
investigations 218
management 218–9
pathology 218
gynaecological cancers
incidence of 640
screening 641–2
gynaecological procedures/surgery
colposcopy 688
continence procedures 702–3
endometrial ablation techniques 690–1
hysterectomy 698–9
hysteroscopy 694–6
laparoscopy 706–9
pelvic floor surgery 710–11
pipelle biopsy 705

H
haematological changes, in pregnancy
coagulation and fibrinolysis, alterations in 58
erythrocyte, increase in 58
maternal plasma volume, increase in 58
peripheral white blood cell count, rise in 58
platelet count, fall in 58
haematological investigations, in pregnancy 38–9
haemoglobin electrophoresis 68–9
haemoglobinopathies
and pregnancy 69
clinical approach 222–3
counselling and management 223
definition 222
epidemiology 222
pathology 222
screening for 34, 39
haemolytic disease of the newborn (HDN) 68
haemophilias 190
head and neck abnormalities, fetal
cervical teratomas 129
cystic hygroma 128
fetal goitre 128–9
head circumference (HC) 48
heart disease
aetiology 228
antenatal care 230
arrhythmias 225
definition 224
epidemiology 224
fetal assessment 231
investigations 230–31
labour and delivery, management of 234–5
medical treatment 231–3
pathology 224–8
postnatal management and breastfeeding 235
pre-pregnancy/conception counseling 229–30
prognosis 228–9
pulmonary hypertension 225–6
surgical treatment 233–4
tetralogy of Fallot (TOF) 225
HELLP syndrome 344, 347
heparin 211, 233
hepatitis A 259, 260
hepatitis B 34, 60, 70, 259, 260
acute 238
antiviral drugs 240t
chronic 238–39
counselling 240
diagnosis 240
epidemiology 238
in pregnancy 240–1
management 240–1
prevention 239
hepatitis C 34
herpes simplex virus (HSV)
aetiology 242
counselling 243
definition 242
diagnosis 242
epidemiology 242
examination 242
history 242
infection, types of 242
investigations 242
management 243
maternal-fetal transmission 242
neonatal clinical manifestation 242
pathology 242
prognosis 242
risk factors 242
herpes zoster see chicken pox
HIV see human immunodeficiency virus (HIV)
holoprosencephaly 100
home birth
advantages of 384
antenatal preparation 384
complications, possible 384–5
definition 384

home birth (*Cont.*)
  eligibility criteria 384
  epidemiology 384
  future challenges 385
  maternal choice *versus* safety 385
hormone replacement therapy (HRT)
  fibroids 607
  menopause 545–47
human chorionic gonadotrophin (hCG) 52, 556–7
Human Fertilization and Embryology Act (1990) 26
human immunodeficiency virus (HIV) 34
  AIDS presenting illnesses, common 244t
  antiretroviral drugs 246–7
  breastfeeding 45
  counselling 247
  definition 244
  drug interactions 247
  epidemiology 244
  examination and investigation 246
  gynaecology, HIV in 248–9
  history 244–6
  late presentation 247
  management 246–7
  natural history 244, 245f
  prevalence 244, 245f
  prognosis 247
  screening, advantages of 71
human papillomavirus (HPV) 250–1
  cervical carcinoma, precursors of 648
  testing 649–50
  vaccines 16, 650
Human Tissue Act 2005 26
hydralazine 255, 346
hydrocortizone 210
hydrops
  aetiology 148–9
  cardiac arrhythmias 150
  chorioangiomas 150
  counselling and management 149–50
  definition 148
  diagnosis 149
  epidemiology 148
  fetal anaemia 148, 149–50
  fetal congenital infection 149
  fetal syndromes 148–9
  fetus/placenta, structural abnormalities of 148
  multiple pregnancy 148
  non-treatable causes of 150
  prognosis 149
  twin reversed arterial perfusion syndrome 149
  twin-twin transfusion syndrome 149
hypercoagulability, in pregnancy 224
hyperemesis gravidarum
  aetiology 76
  complications 78
  definition 76
  diagnosis 50
  epidemiology 76
  minor symptoms, of pregnancy 52
  prognosis 77
hyperprolactinaemia 282, 503
hypertension
  aetiology 252
  antihypertensives 254–55
  blood pressure measurement 253
  chronic 252
  clinical assessment 253
  conceptual understanding 253
  counselling 253
  definition 252
  epidemiology 252
  fetal assessment/monitoring 254
  gestational 252
  investigations 254
  labour and delivery 255–6
  pathology 252
  postnatal management 256
  prevention of 256
  prognosis 252–53

hypertrophic cardiomyopathy 226
hypopituitarism 282–83
hypoproteinaemia, fetal 146
hypothalamic/pituitary dysfunction 502–3
hypoxaemia 378
hypoxia 378–9
hysterectomy 453
  abdominal 698
  approach, choice of 698
  fibroids 607
  laparoscopic 699
  ovaries, removal of 699
  preoperative care 698
  subtotal 698
  types of 698
  vaginal 699
hystero contrast salpingography (HyCoSy) 512
hystero-salpingography (HSG) 512–3
hysteroscopic myomectomy 553, 607
hysteroscopy
  complications 696
  distension medium 694–5
  energy, types of 695
  hysteroscopes 694
  indications 694
  inpatient hysteroscopy 696
  office hysteroscopy 695–6
  procedures 694
  procedures for operative 696
  training in 696–97
  types of 694

I

imaging, in reproductive medicine
  hystero contrast salpingography (HyCoSy) 512
  hystero salpingography (HSG) 512–13
  magnetic resonance imaging 513
  selective salpingography 513
  ultrasound 512
immunization
  active, during pregnancy 259–60
  breastfeeding 258
  clinical approach 258
  definition 258
  efficacy 258
  passive, during pregnancy 260
  safety 258
  vaccination, timing of 258
  vulnerable population 258
immunoassay 50–1
immunosuppressive drugs 210
in utero shunt insertion 153
in vitro fertilization (IVF)
  adjuncts to 526
  ART 525
  blastocyst culture 506
  complications 526
  definition 524
  down-regulation, using GnRH agonist 506
  embryo transfer 506, 525–6
  endometriosis 501
  fertilization and embryo culture 506
  GnRH agonists 506
  hCG trigger 506
  infertility, incidence of 524
  intracytoplasmic sperm injection 506
  oocyte collection 525
  oocyte retrieval 506
  ovarian hyperstimulation syndrome, prevention of 567–8
  ovarian stimulation 506
  pathology 524
  prognosis 524–5
  regulation 526–7
  sperm collection 525
  success rates 506
in vitro oocyte maturation (IVM)
  definition 528
  embryo transfer 530–1
  embryology laboratory procedures 530

  epidemiology 528
  indications 528–9
  IVM cycle, monitoring and management of 530
  luteal-phase support 531
  oocyte collection procedure 530
  prognosis 529–30
  technique 528
incontinence see urinary incontinence, female
induction of labour
  clinical approach 387
  definition 386
  frequency 386
  high risk inductions 388
  indications 386
  non-pharmacological methods 387
  pharmacological methods 386–7
  risks of 386
  special indications 387
  surgical methods 386–7
induction of ovulation
  anovulation, investigation of 514
  oestrogen-deficient patients, treatment of 515
  oestrogen-replete patients, treatment of 514–15
infections
  fetal 146–47, 378
  in pregnancy 70–1
  screening for 34–5
infertility, female
  adhesions 504–5
  definition 502
  diagnosis 502
  endometrial polyp 505–6
  endometriosis 505
  fibroids 505
  in vitro fertilization (IVF) 506
  obstructive and developmental disorders 504–6
  ovulatory disorders 502–4
  sexually transmitted infections 502
  tubal occlusion 504
  see *also* male subfertility
inflammatory bowel disease
  causes 262
  clinical features 262
  complications 263–4
  contraception 264
  definition 262
  effect of pregnancy of 262
  epidemiology 262
  flare in pregnancy, medical treatment of 263
  investigations 262
  management 263
  pathology 262
  pregnancy, effect on 262–3
  rectovaginal fistulae 634
infliximab 263
influenza 259
International Federation of Gynaecologists and Obstetricians (FIGO) 20
International Planned Parenthood Federation 20
intestinal duplication cyst 122t
intracytoplasmic sperm injection (ICSI)
  clinical approach 518–19
  counselling 518
  definition 518
  epidemiology 518
  follow-up 518–19
  indications 518
  management 518
  success rates 518
intrauterine devices 498
  bleeding patterns and pain 521
  choice of 522
  clinical approach 522
  contraindications for 521
  definition 520
  duration of use 521
  ectopic pregnancy, risk of 521

efficacy 521
epidemiology 520
expulsion 521
fertility, return to 521
hormonal side-effects 521
indications for 521
insertion 522
medicated devices 520
mode of action 520
non-contraceptive benefits 522
ovarian cysts 521
pathology 520
pelvic actinomyces, and IUD 523
pelvic inflammatory disease 521
post insertion instructions 523
prognosis 521
shape 520
types of 520f, 521
intrauterine growth restriction (IUGR)
aetiology 156
definition 156
diagnosis 156–7
epidemiology 156
management 157
prognosis 156
iron deficiency 52, 180–1
ischaemic heart disease 227
IVF see in vitro fertilization (IVF)
IVM see in vitro oocyte maturation (IVM)

J

jaundice
acute and chronic viral hepatitis 266
acute cholecystitis 266–7
acute pancreatitis 267, 270
causes 266
definition 266
gall bladder disease 266
Gilbert's syndrome 266
herpes simplex hepatitis 267
history 266
investigations 266
signs 266

L

labetolol 255
labour
anaesthesia, in obstetrics 365–7
analgesia 364–5
breech 368–70
brow presentation 371
cord prolapse 372–3
definitions 390
episiotomy 374–5
face presentation 376–7
first stage 390, 392
home birth 384–5
maternal collapse 394–7
meconium-stained liquor 398–400
newborn, resuscitation of 414–17
normal physiological progress 392–3
optimizing outcomes 393
physiology 393
placenta praevia 402–4
placental abruption 406–7
postpartum haemorrhage (PPH)
    408–10
prelabour rupture of membranes at term
    (PROM) 412–13
progress, assessment of 390
retained placenta 418–19
schools of labour management 390
second stage 392
shoulder dystocia 420–2
shoulder presentation 424–5
third stage 392–3
uterine inversion 426–7
see also fetal surveillance, in labour; induction
    of labour
lactogenesis 42

laminaria tents 387
laparoscopy 321, 491
advantages of 708
assessment before 706
complications 708
indications 706
instruments for 706
procedure 706
techniques and sites of entry 706–8
theatre set up 707f
training in 708–9
umbilicus, anatomy of 708f
laparotomy 321–2
last menstrual period (LMP) 4
legal framework, for care in obstetrics and
        gynaecology
'good medicine' 20
capacity, patients lacking 25–6
children and young people 23–4
consent, in obstetrics 21–2
damage, prevention of 22
fertility treatments 26
human tissue, use of 26
medical ethics 20
medical litigation, principles of 20
medical negligence 20–1
miscellaneous legislation 25–6
sexual and reproductive rights,
    of women 20
specific obstetric conditions 22–3
standards of care 21
STIs 24–5
termination of pregnancy 23, 27
leucorrhoea, of pregnancy 55
leucotrien receptor agonists 297
lignocain 232
limb abnormalities, fetal
amniotic band syndrome 126–7
club foot 124
ectrodactly 124–5
polydactyly 126
radial aplasia 125–26
limb reduction defects 112–13
Lipkin Model, for communication 16
listeriosis
aetiology 272
definition 272
diagnosis 272
epidemiology 272
examination 272
immunocompromised states 272
investigations 272
management 272–73
neonatal infection 272
pregnancy 272
prognosis 272
lithium 211–12, 288
liver disease 274–7
acute fatty liver of pregnancy (AFLP) 275–6
cirrhosis 277
HELLP syndrome 274t, 276
hepatitis 277
liver function tests, normal pregnancy
    values 275
liver transplants 277
obstetric cholestasis (OC) 274–5
primary biliary cirrhosis 276
sclerosing cholangitis 276
Wilson's disease 277
long bones, short 112
lung cancer screening 640
lymhocytic cardiomyopathy 226
lymphatic drainage, failure of (fetal) 146
lymphocytic hypophysitis 282–3

M

macrocephaly 111
magnetic resonance imaging (MRI) 513
male subfertility
aetiology 536
chromosomal analysis 538

complications/side effects/sequelae 539
counselling 539
definition 536
diagnosis 536
DNA fragmentation 538
epidemiology 536
examination 538–9
genetic causes, of male infertility 538
history 536–7
hormone analysis 538
investigations 537–38
management 539, 540t
medications 537
prognosis 539
retrograde ejaculation 539
treatment options 539
Y chromosome gene defects 538
malignant melanoma 679–80
malignant tumours see tumours
mammogenesis 42
Marfan's syndrome 227
mastitis 44, 45
maternal collapse, in labour
aetiology 394–5
definition 394
diagnosis 395
epidemiology 394
further management 396
prevention 394
primary survey 395
prognosis 395
resuscitation 395–96
maternal medicine and infections
adrenal disorders 176–8
anaemia 180–1
autoimmune disease 182–3
bacterial vaginosis 184–5
chicken pox/herpes zoster 186–7
chlamydia 188–9
coagulation disorders 190–1
connective tissue disorder 192–3
cytomegalovirus (CMV) 196
dermatology 198–9
diabetes, in pregnancy 200–206
drugs, in pregnancy 208–12
epilepsy, and other neurological
        conditions 214–15
gonorrhoea 218–19
haemoglobinopathies 222–3
heart disease 224–5
hepatitis B (HBV) 238–41
herpes simplex virus (HSV) 242–3
HIV infection 244–9
human papillomavirus 250–1
hypertension 252–6
immunization 258–60
inflammatory bowel disease 262–4
jaundice 266–70
listeriosis 272–5
liver disease 274–7
measles: rubeola 278–9
parvovirus B19 280
perinatal group B streptococcus (GBS)
    220–1
physiological changes 282
pituitary disorders, in pregnancy
    282–4
psychiatric disorders, in
    pregnancy 286–7
renal disease 290–4
respiratory disease 296–300
rubella (German measles) 302–3
substance abuse, in pregnancy 304–5
syphilis 306–7
thromboembolic disease 310–11
thyroid and parathyroid disease 312–14
toxoplasmosis, in pregnancy 316
vulvovaginal candidiasis 318
maturity-onset diabetes of the young
    (MODY) 200
mean sac diameter (MSD) 48
measles see rubeola

measles mumps and rubella (MMR)
vaccine 302–3
mebendazole 209
meconium-stained liquor
aetiology 398
counselling 400
definition 398
depressed 400
diagnosis 398–99
epidemiology 398
fetal heart rate 399
gastroschisis, and other fetal bowel
obstruction 400
good condition 400
heavy meconium 400
home birth 400
initial management 399
light meconium 400
neonatal resuscitation 400
postnatal neonatal observation by midwifery
team 400
prematurity 399–400
prognosis 398
recurrence/future pregnancy planning 400
meningococcus 259
menopause
best practice 548–9
complementary therapies 546–7
consequences of 542–3
definitions 542
diagnosis of 543–4
epidemiology 542
hormonal changes 542
hormone replacement therapy (HRT) 545–4
hormone therapy regimes 544
lifestyle measures 544
mammography 543, 544
menstrual cycle 542
osteoporosis 543, 544
ovarian reserve, prediction of 543
pathophysiology 542–3
premature ovarian failure 542
prescribing advice, official 546
progestogens 545
testosterone preparations/regimens 546
vasomotor symptoms, management of 547–8
menorrhagia
blood tests 551
complications/side effects/sequelae 553
counselling 552
definition 550
diagnosis 550
endometrial carcinoma, risk factors 550t
epidemiology 550
examination 551
follow up 553
history 550–1
investigations 551
medical management 552
menstrual blood loss, quantification of 551
non-medical management 552
pathology 550
prognosis 550
surgical management 552–3
surgical/radiological management 552–3
uterus and endometrium, assessment
of 551–2
menstrual bleeding, heavy
aetiology 486
definition 486
diagnosis 486
epidemiology 486
pathology 486
prognosis 486
treatment 486–7
menstrual cycle, physiology of
amenorrhoea 555
clinical approach: top tips 555
cycle length, variability 555
endocrinology 554
endometrial cycle 554
follicular development 554

LH dipsticks, and polycystic ovarian
syndrome 555
menstrual cycle phases 554–5
progesterone, and body temperature 555
Mental Capacity Act (2005) 15, 16, 25–6
Mental Health Act (2007) 340
mesenteric/omental cyst 122t
metformin 205
methimazole 211
methotrexate 263
methyldopa 232, 254, 345–6
metronidazole 210, 263
microcephaly 102, 111
micrognathia 116–17
mifepristone 386
miscarriage
definition 556
diagnosis 556–7
epidemiology 556
expert adviser 558
management 557–8
nomenclature, of early pregnancy
loss 556
risk factors 556
see also recurrent miscarriage
misoprostol (PGE1) 386
mixed incontinence 614
morning sickness see hyperemesis gravidarum
multiple pregnancy
Caesarean section 441
chorionicity 158
complications 158
definition 158
delivery 158–59
dichorionic twins 158
epidemiology 158
fetal growth restriction 158
higher order 159
hydrops 148
intrapartum 159
intrauterine growth restriction
(IUGR) 156
management 158
monochorionic twins 158–9
prenatal screening 158
presentation 158
twin-twin transformation syndrome 149,
153, 158
vanishing twin 158
multiple sclerosis 182
multiple thrombosis 216
mumps 259
myasthenia gravis 182
mycophenolate mofetil (MMF) 292
myocarditis 226
myomectomy 331, 442, 553, 607

N

neck abnormalites see head and neck
abnormalities
neonatal chlamydia trachomatis 188
neonatal lupus syndromes 192–3
neonatal necrotizing enterocolitis (NEC) 43
neonatal services, optimal 351
neural tube defects, fetal 98–9
newborn, resuscitation of
congenital problems, known 415
equipment 414
incidence 414
meconium aspiration 415
newborn life support 416–17
physiology 414
preterm infants 415–16
priorities 414–15
resuscitation, stopping 416
nifedipine 255, 346
nitrofurantoin 209
nitroglycerin 210
non-opioid analgesics 208
non-steroidal anti-inflammatory drugs
(NSAIDs) 208, 607

nuchal translucency
definition 146
diagnosis 146
epidemiology 146
increased, implications of 111, 147
management 147
pathophysiology 146–7
nutritional supplements, in pregnancy 32

O

obesity 173, 435
obstetric cholestasis (OC)
aetiology 332
definition 332
diagnosis 332
endocrine factors 332
environmental factors 332
epidemiology 332
examination 332
fetal complications, aetiology of 332
genetic factors 332
history 332
investigations 333
liver disease 274–5
management 333
prognosis 332
obstetric conditions
abdominal pain, in pregnancy 320–2
amniotic fluid embolism (AFE) 324–5
antepartum haemorrhage 326–7
cancer, in pregnancy 328–9
fibroids, in pregnancy 330–1
genital tract, premalignant conditions of in
pregnancy 349
obstetric cholestasis (OC) 332–3
ovarian cysts 336–7
postnatal depression 338–40
pre-eclampsia, and eclampsia 344–4
preterm labour (preterm delivery
(PTD)) 350–2
preterm prelabour rupture of membranes
(pPROM) 354–6
prolonged pregnancy 358–9
puerperal psychosis 342–3
puerperal sepsis 360–1
obstetric techniques/procedures/surgery
balloon tamponade 430–2
Caesarean section 434–2
forceps delivery 446–50
uterine compression sutures 452–4
ventouse delivery 456–9
oesophageal atresia 120
oestrogen 52
Ogilvie syndrome 321
oligohydramnios
amnio-infusion 160–1
amniotic fluid volume, assessment
of 160
anhydramnios 160
differential diagnosis 160
epidemiology 160
fetal surveillance, in labour 379
management 160–1
pathology/aetiology 160
vesico-amniotic shunts 161
oligomenorrhoea and amenorrhoea
aetiology 562
anatomical causes 563
causes, categories of 563
clinical approach 562–4
definition 562
epidemiology 562
history 562
hypergonadotrophic
hypogonadism 564
hyperprolactinaemia 563
hypogonadotrophic hypogonadism 564
investigations 562–3
management 563
normogonadotrophic hypogonadism 564
physical examination 562

oocyte donation
  donor assessment 560
  donor management 560
  donor recruitment 560
  embryo transfer 561
  indications 560
  laboratory aspects 560–61
  law and regulation 561
  recipient management 560
  success rates 561
opioid analgesics 208–9
oral glucose tolerance test (OGTT) 200–201
Osiander's sign, of pregnancy 50
osteogenesis imperfecta 132, 133
ovarian cancer
  adjuvant therapies 667
  aetiology 664
  borderline malignant epithelial ovarian
    tumours 667
  chemotherapy 667
  clinical approach 665–8
  diagnosis 665–6
  germ cell tumours 667
  in young women 666–7
  incidence of 664
  management 666–8
  pathology 664
  prognosis 665
  sarcoma of the ovary 668
  screening 641–2, 664–5
  sex cord stromal tumours of the ovary 668
  small cell carcinoma of the ovary 668
  staging 665
  surgery 666
  tumour markers 666
ovarian cysts 122t
  acute abdominal pain 336
  aetiology 336, 610
  clinical features 336, 610
  definition 336
  differential diagnosis 610
  epidemiology 336
  in pregnancy 611
  investigations 610
  laparoscopy 611
  monitoring 336
  ovarian cyst accidents 610
  pathology 336
  pathophysiology 610
  risk of malignancy index scoring system
    610–11
  surgery, place of 611
  suspected ovarian torsion 611
  suspicious cysts, and diagnostic difficulty 337
  transvaginal cyst aspiration 611
ovarian hyperstimulation syndrome
  classification 566
  complications 568
  description of 566
  diagnosis 568
  management 568
  mechanisms 566
  pathophysiology 566
  prediction, and risk factors 566–7
  prevalence 566
  prevention 567–8
  surveillance 568
ovulation, induction of see induction of
  ovulation
oxytocin 386, 392, 408, 418–19

P

paediatric and adolescent problems
  'no vagina' 571
  adolescence, definition of 570
  amenorrhoea 570
  clinical approach 570
  delayed puberty 571
  dysmenorrhoea/pelvic pain 571
  epidemiology 570
  hypoandrogenism 571

labial adhesions 570
  menstrual dysfunction 571
  oligomenorrhoea 571
  ovarian cysts/masses 571
  polycystic ovarian syndrome (PCOS) 571
  precocious puberty 571
  premature ovarian failure 571
  thelarche/pubarche/menarche 570
  vulvovaginitis 570
  see also disorders of sex development
    (DSDs)
pain
  abdominal, in pregnancy 320–2
  cancer 670–1
  endometriosis-associated 500
  fibroids 330–1
  in early pregnancy 74
  ovarian cysts 336
  pelvic 476–7
  vulval 626
palliative care
  bad news, breaking 670
  breathlessness 673
  constipation 672
  definition 670
  emergencies 674 5
  epidemiology 670
  history and examination 670
  investigation 670
  malignant fistulae 673–4
  management 670
  nausea and vomiting, control of 671–2
  pain control, in cancer 670–1
  recurrent malignant ascites 672–3
  syringe driver, drugs in 672, 674, 675t
  tumour fungation 674
pancreatitis 267, 270, 321
parathyroid disease see thyroid and
  parathyroid disease
partogram 390, 391
parvovirus B19 60, 280
Patau syndrome 106
Pederson's hypothesis, modified 202
pelvic floor surgery
  anterior vaginal prolapse 710
  posterior vaginal wall prolapse 710
  vaginal apical prolapse 710–11
pelvic inflammatory disease (PID)
  aetiology 612
  clinical diagnosis 612
  consequences 612
  counselling 613
  description of 612
  differential diagnosis 612
  follow up 613
  investigations 612
  management 612–13
  risk factors 612
pelvic pain, chronic
  condition-specific treatment 477
  contributory factors 476
  definition 476
  empirical treatment 477
  epidemiology 476
  examination 476
  initial consultation 476
  initial history 476
  investigations 476–7
  risk factors 476
  treatment options 477
pelvis, anatomy of female
  blood supply, in pelvis 469
  bony pelvis 468
  external genitalia 470–1
  internal genitalia 471–4
  lymphatic drainage 470
  muscles 468
  nerve supply 470
  pelvic floor 468, 469f
  pelvic planes, diameter of 468t
  perineal body (central perineal
    tendon) 468–9

  soft tissues 468–9
  urogenital diaphragm 468
  veins 470
pemphigoid gestationis 198
percutaneous umbilical blood sampling
  (PUBS) 152
perinatal group B streptococcus (GBS)
  background 220
  intrapartum antibiotic prophylaxis 220
  late-onset neonatal disease 220–1
  preterm birth/low birthweight 221
  prevention of 220
  resistant organisms, emergence of 220
perineal trauma, management and
  repair of
  episiotomy 374, 375f
  postoperative care 374–5
peripartum cardiomyopathy 226
peripheral nerve compression
  syndromes 215
Pfeiffer syndrome 112
phaeochromocytoma 176
phenobarbitone 209
phenytoin 209
physiological changes, in pregnancy
  alimentary tract 56
  cardiovascular system 57–5
  endocrine and metabolic changes 58–9
  haematological changes 58
  hyperprolactinaemia 282
  respiratory tract system 56
  urinary and renal system 56–7
phytoestrogens 548
pipelle biopsy 705
pituitary disorders, in pregnancy
  acromegaly 284
  Cushing's syndrome 284
  diabetes insipidus 283–4
  hyperprolactinaemia 282
  hypopituitarism 282–3
placenta accreta 403–4
placenta praevia 35
  aetiology 402
  clinical presentation 402
  counselling 403
  definition 402
  future pregnancies 403
  incidence 402
  management 403
  placenta accreta 403–4
  risk factors 402
  screening for 402
  vasa praevia 404
placenta, retained see retained placenta
placental abnormalities
  chorioangioma 162
  circumvallate placenta 162
  placental morphology, normal variation
    in 162
placental abruption
  baby, care of 407
  Caesarean delivery 406–7
  clinical presentation 406
  complications 406, 407
  counselling 407
  definition 406
  disseminated intravascular coagulation
    (DIC) 407
  incidence 406
  management 406–7
  pathology 406
  postpartum haemorrhage 407
  renal failure 407
  risk factors for 406
  subsequent pregnancies, advice for 407
  vaginal delivery 406–7
placental site trophopblastic tumour
  (PSTT) 661
pleuro-amniotic shunt 153–4
pneumococcus 259
pneumonia 298
poliomyelitis 259

polycystic ovary syndrome (PCOS)
  acne and hirsuitism 575
  aetiology 574
  alopecia 575
  assisted reproduction 504
  clomiphine, and ovulation induction 504
  definition 574
  diagnosis 574
  eflornithine cream 575
  epidemiology 574
  examination 574–75
  finasteride 575
  follow-up, long term 576
  history 574
  investigations 575
  laparoscopic ovarian drilling (LOD) 504
  long-term consequences 574
  menstrual disturbance 575–6
  pathology 574
  weight loss 575
polydactyly 126
polyhydramnios
  aetiological treatment 165
  aetiology 164
  counselling 164
  definition of 164
  diagnosis 164
  epidemiology 164
  prognosis 164
  symptomatic treatment 165
polymorphic eruption, of pregnancy 198
postnatal depression
  and baby blues, differences between 338–9
  antidepressants 339
  clinical features 338
  counselling 339
  detection/screening/prevention 338
  electroconvulsive therapy (ECT) 339
  examination 339
  history 339
  incidence of 338
  Mother and Baby unit, admission to 339–40
  special investigations 339
  treatment 339–40
postpartum pseudo-obstruction 321
pre-eclampsia, and eclampsia 35
  abdominal pain 321
  aetiology 344
  BP, monitoring 345
  counselling 345
  definitions 344
  delivery 345, 346
  diagnosis 344–5
  epidemiology 344
  fetal monitoring 346
  future pregnancy, planning 348
  HELLP syndrome 347
  investigations 345
  magnesium sulphate 346
  management 345–7
  pathology 344
  postpartum 347–8
  pre-eclamptic toxaemia (PET) 346–4
  prognosis 344
  treatment 345–6
prednisolone 210, 297
pregnancy of unknown location (PUL)
  aetiology 80
  definition 80
  diagnosis 80–81
  ectopic pregnancy 80
  epidemiology 80
  failing PUL 80
  intrauterine pregnancy 80
  management 81
  persistent PUL 80
pregnancy, diagnosis of see diagnosis, of
    pregnancy
preimplantation genetic diagnosis
  clinical approach 578
  definition 578
  estimate of use 579

indications 578
procedure 578
process 578
variations 578–9
prelabour rupture of membranes at term
  (PROM)
  aetiology 412
  clinical questions 412
  definition 412
  diagnosis and initial assessment 412
  epidemiology 412
  feto-maternal infectious morbidity, risk
    of 412
  intrapartum antibiotic prophylaxis, advice
    against 412
  management 412–13
  neonatal infection, risk of 412
premalignant tumours see tumours
premature ovarian failure (POF)
  aetiology 581
  clinical presentation 581
  definition 580
  diagnosis 580
  future objectives 581
  hormone replacement therapy 502
  initial evaluation 580
  multidisciplinary care 581
  treatment 580–81
premenstrual syndrome (PMS)
  aetiology 582
  clinical manifestations and diagnosis 582
  complementary therapies 582–3
  definition 582
  epidemiology 582
  herbal preparations 582
  lifestyle changes 582
  ovulation suppression 583
  pathophysiology 582
  treatment 582
preparation, for pregnancy
  contraception, stopping 61
  folic acid 61
  foods to avoid 61
  healthy eating 61
  infectious disease screening 60
  lifestyle issues 61
  medicines and drugs 60
  patient information/contacts 61
  preconception care and counselling 60
  sexual health 60–1
  social assessment 60
  work environment 61
  X-rays 61
preterm delivery (PTD)
  adverse sequelae, rates of 352
  clinical assessment 350–51
  definition 350
  epidemiology and importance 350
  management 351
  prediction of 351–3
  preterm labour, as symptom 352
preterm prelabour rupture of membranes
  (pPROM)
  aetiology 354
  amniocentesis, role of 355–6
  clinical importance 354
  corticosteroid therapy 355
  definition 354
  diagnosis 354
  initial assessment 354
  management 354–5
  pathophysiology 354
  prediction of 351–2
  tocolysis 355
primary biliary cirrhosis 183
primary postpartum haemorrhage (PPH) 430
primary pulmonary hypertension 228
primary sclerosing cholangitis 183
primidone 209
probe amplification (MPLA) 106
procainamide 232
progestogens 545, 607

prolonged pregnancy
  confirmation of 358
  definition 358
  incidence of 358
  induction of labour, methods of 359
  labour abnormalities 358
  management 359
  monitoring 358–9
  perinatal morbidity 358
  perinatal mortality 358
  post-dated pregnancy, assessment of 358
  practice points 359
  recurrence, risk of 359
  risk factors for 358
  risks of 358
propylthiouracil 211
prostaglandin 298
prurigo of pregnancy 199
pruritic folliculitis of pregnancy 199
pruritis see vulval pain and pruritis
psychiatric disorders, in pregnancy
  anxiety disorders 286–7
  bipolar affective disorder 287
  clinical assessment 286
  depression 287
  eating disorders 287
  psychiatric hospital, pregnant woman
    in 288
  schizophrenia 287
  screening for 286
  subsyndromal emotional disturbances,
    prevalance of 286
  treatment principles 287
  treatments, specific 287–8
psychosexual problems
  common presentations of 584
  doctor-patient relationships 585–6
  erectile dysfunction 586
  female sexual function disorders,
    classification of 584
  investigations 585
  life events 586–7
  male and female sexuality, impact of
    conditions and treatments on 586t
  management strategies 586t
  partners 586
  psychosexual medicine 585–6
  recognition of 587
  sexual dysfunction, quantifying 584
  sexual history 584–5
psychotherapeutic drugs 211–12
puberty, delayed 571
puerperal psychosis
  aetiology 342
  clinical approach 342–3
  examination 342
  history 342
  presentation 342
  prognosis 343
  special investigations 342–3
  treatment 343
puerperal sepsis
  aetiology 360
  breast abscess 360
  definition 360
  endometriosis 360
  mastitis 360
  septic pelvic thrombophlebitis 360
  urinary tract infection 360
  wounds and episiotomy infections 360–1
puerperium
  definition of 64
  management of 65
  mother, general care of 65–6
  normal changes of 64
pulmonary embolism (PE) 310, 311
pulmonary oedema 299
pulmonary vascular disease 228

Q

quinidine 210, 232

R

rabies 259, 260
radial aplasia 125–6
ranitidine 78
recurrent miscarriage (RM)
  aetiology 590
  anatomical factors 590
  clinical approach 591
  complications/side-effects/sequelae 592
  counselling and adjuvant therapy 591
  definition 590
  epidemiology 590
  immunological factors 590
  infectious causes 590
  investigations 591
  management 591–92
  medical management 591–92
  pathology 590
  prognosis 592
  risk factors, recently identified 590–1
  surgical management 592
red blood cell isoimmunization
  definition 166
  epidemiology 166
  fetal blood transfusions 167
  prognosis 167
  red cell isoimmunized pregnancies 166–7
  Rh-negative women 166
renal disease
  acute pyelonephritis 290
  acute renal failure (ARF) 290–1
  asymptomatic bacteriuria 290
  chronic renal disease 291–3
  dialysis 293
  effect of pregnancy on 292
  fetal 113
  haemolytic uraemic syndrome 291
  management 292–3
  pregnancy, effect on 292
  renal transplant recipient 293–4
  thrombotic thrombocytopenic purpura
    (TTP) 291
  urinary tract infection 290
reproduction
  ambiguous genitalia 464–7
  chronic pelvic pain 476–7
  contraception 478–9, 498–9
  disorders of sex development (DSDs) 482–3
  donor insemination 484–6
  dysmenorrhoea 489–90
  ectopic pregnancy 490–2
  embryo freezing 494–5
  endometriosis 500–501
  female infertility 502–7
  female pelvis, anatomy of 468–74
  fertility, in survivors of childhood
    malignancy 508–11
  genital tract, malformation of 532–3
  imaging, in reproductive medicine 512–13
  in vitro fertilization 524–7
  in vitro oocyte maturation (IVM) 528–31
  induction of ovulation 514–15
  intracytoplasmic sperm injection (ICSI) 518–19
  intrauterine devices 520–3
  male subfertility 536–40
  menopause, and hormone replacement
    therapy 543–9
  menorrhagia 550–3
  menstrual bleeding, heavy 486–7
  menstrual cycle: physiology 554–5
  miscarriage, early 556–8
  oligomenorrhoea and amenorrhoea 562–4
  oocyte donation 560–1
  ovarian hyperstimulation syndrome 566–8
  paediatric and adolescent problems 570–3
  polycystic ovary syndrome (PCOS) 574–6
  preimplantation genetic diagnosis 578–9
  premenstrual syndrome (PMS) 582–3
  psychosexual problems 584–7
  recurrent miscarriage (RM) 590–2
  termination of pregnancy (TOP) 594–7

reproductive tract, anatomy of female
  anal canal 473–4
  clitoris 471
  external genitalia 470–1
  fallopian tubes 472
  hymen 471
  internal genitalia 471–4
  labia majora 470
  labia minora 471
  mons pubis 470
  ovaries 472–3
  perineum 470
  urethra 471, 473
  urinary bladder 473
  urogenital triangle 470
  uterus 471–2
  vagina 471
  vestibule 471
  vulva 470
respiratory disease
  asthma 296–8
  cystic fibrosis 300
  pneumonia 298
  pulmonary oedema 299
  restrictive lung disease 300
  sarcoidosis 299
  tuberculosis 298–9
respiratory tract system, in pregnancy 56
restrictive lung disease 300
resuscitation
  maternal 395–6, 522–3
  newborn 400, 414–17
retained placenta
  aetiology 418
  definition 418
  diagnosis 418
  epidemiology 418
  general management 418
  medical management 418
  pathology 418
  prognosis 418
  surgical management 419
reversible posterior leucoencephalopathy 215
rheumatoid arthritis, and pregnancy 192
rights 20, 485
ritonavir 247
Rokitansky syndrome 482–3, 532–3
rubella (German measles) 34, 60, 70, 259
  aetiology 302
  congenital rubella syndrome (CRS) 302
  definition 302
  diagnosis 302
  epidemiology 302
  measles mumps and rubella (MMR)
    vaccine 302–3
  pathology 302
  prognosis 302
  treatment 302–3
  vaccination 302–3
rubeola (measles)
  aetiology 278
  clinical features 278
  definition 278
  diagnosis 278
  differential diagnosis 278
  epidemiology 278
  management 278–79
  post-exposure prophylaxis 279
  pre-exposure prophylaxis 279
  prevention 279
  public health initiatives 279
Rüsch urological hydrostatic balloon 431

S

Saethre Chotzen 112
salpingectomy 491
salpingography 504, 513
salpingotomy 491
sarcoidosis 299
scleroderma, and pregnancy 193
sclerosing cholangitis 276

Sengstaken-Blakemore tube/oesophageal
  catheter 431
serum biochemistry, abnormal first
  trimester 111
sexual intercourse, in pregnancy 33
Sexual Offences Act 2003 23, 24
sexually transmitted infections (STIs) 4
  confidentiality 24
  disclosure 24–5
  genitourinary medicine (GUM) services 24–5
  gonorrhoea 218–19
  infertility, female 502
  medical colleagues with 25
  pregnant women, with HIV 25
  syphilis 35, 71, 306–7
  see also human immunodeficiency virus (HIV)
shoulder dystocia
  complications 420
  definition 420
  epidemiology 420
  fetal asphyxia, prevention of 421
  first-line manoeuvres 421
  HELPERR algorithm 422t
  management 421–22
  pathophysiology 420
  prediction and prevention 420–1
  second-line manoeuvres 421–2
  third-line manoeuvres 422
  training 422
shoulder presentation
  clinical approach 424–5
  definition 424
  epidemiology 424
  management 425
  natural history 424
  predisposing factors 424
sickle cell disease 69
  see also haemoglobinopathies
Sim's speculum examination 9
Simpson Golabi Behmel Syndrome 111
sinus venous thrombosis 215–16
skeletal abnormalities/dysplasias, fetal
  achondrogenesis types I and II 132
  achondroplasia 133
  aetiology 132
  campomelic dysplasia 133
  chondrodysplasia punctata (CPD) 133
  clinical approach 134
  counselling 134–5
  definition 132
  Ellis-van Creveld syndrome 133
  epidemiology 132
  examination 134
  investigations 134
  Jeunes asphyxiating thoracic dystrophy 133
  lethal skeletal dysplasias 132–3
  management 135
  molecular analysis 134
  non-lethal skeletal dysplasias 133
  osteogenesis imperfecta 132, 133
  pathology 132
  perinatal/infantile hypophosphatasia 133
  prognosis/recurrence risks 133–4
  short rib polydactyly 132–3
  spondyloepiphyseal dysplasia congenita
    (SEDC) 133
  thanatophoric dysplasia 132
  ultrasound findings 132
skeletal problems 112
skull shape, abnormal 112
smoking, in pregnancy 4, 33, 61, 615
sodium valproate 209
sotalol 232
Soto's syndrome 112
spina bifida 98–9
spondyloepiphyseal dysplasia congenita
    (SEDC) 133
substance abuse, in pregnancy
  aetiology 304
  clinical approach 304–5
  definition 304
  epidemiology 304

substance abuse, in pregnancy (Cont.)
  fetal alcohol syndrome 61, 304
  injecting drug use 304
  prognosis 304
sulphasalazine 209
Swyer's syndrome 482
symphyseal fundal height (SFH)
  background 172
  clinical management 173
  customized measurements 173
  definition 172
  ethnic populations, variations in 173
  future assessment of 173–4
  measurement of 172–3
  obese women, measurement in 173
  pathology 172
symptoms, of pregnancy
  aches and pains 53
  backache 53
  Braxton-Hicks contractions 54–5
  breathlessness 54
  carpal tunnel syndrome 53
  constipation and haemorrhoids 52
  heartburn 52
  insomnia 54
  nausea/vomiting 52
  palpitations 54
  pica, and ptyalism 52
  skin changes 54
  tiredness 55
  urinary problems 52–3
  vaginal discharge 55
  varicosities 53–4
syphilis 35, 71
  complications 307
  definition 306
  epidemiology 306
  management 307
  risk factors 306
  screening and diagnosis 306–7
  stages of 306
systemic lupus erythematosus (SLE) 192–3

T

tachycardia 226–7
termination of pregnancy (TOP)
  abdominal wall defects, fetal 119–20
  anti-D prophylaxis 596–7
  cervical trauma 596
  complications 596
  consent 595
  contraceptive advice following 595
  counselling 594, 595
  early medical 595–6
  failure to abort 596
  gastrointestinal abnormalities, fetal 122
  haemorrhage 596
  incidence of 594
  induced abortion, as healthcare need 594
  infection 596
  investigations 595
  late medical 596
  long-term sequelae 596
  management 595
  medical procedure 595
  medicolegal issues 23, 27
  patient confidentiality 597
  referral procedure 594–5
  retained products 596
  statutory grounds for 594
  surgical procedure 595
  uterine perforation 596
tetanus 260
tetracycline 209
thalassaemias 69
  see also haemoglobinopathies
thanatophoric dysplasia 132
theophyline 297
thorax abnormalities, fetal
  congenital cystic adenomatous malformation
    (CCAM) 136

congenital diaphragmatic hernia (CDH) 136–
  7
  fetal pleural effusion 137–8
thromboembolic disease
  definition 310
  diagnosis 310
  epidemiology 310
  examination 310
  laboratory investigations 311–12
  pathophysiology 310
thrombophilia 190–1
thrombotic thrombocytopenic purpura
  (TTP) 291
thyroid and parathyroid disease 76
  drugs 211
  hyperparathyroidism 314
  hyperthyroidism 312–13
  hypoparathyroidism 314
  hypothyroidism 312
  postpartum thyroiditis 313
  thyroid cancer 314
  thyroid function tests, normal pregnancy
    ranges 312t
  thyroid nodules 314
tocolysis 351
toxoplasmosis, in pregnancy 35, 60, 316
transcervical balloon catheter 387
transcutaneous electrical nerve stimulation
  (TENS) 364
tricyclic antidepressants 212
trimethoprim 209
triploidy 69 106
tuberculosis 298–9
tumours, in gynaecology
  cancer screening 640–2
  cervical cancer 644–6
  cervical dysplasia and human
    papillomavirus 648–50
  fallopian tube cancer 668
  gestational trophoblastic neoplasia 658–61
  gynaecological cancers 640–1
  non-gynaecological cancers 640–1
  ovarian cancer 664–8
  palliative care 670–5
  screening programme, characteristics of
    successful 640
  vulval cancer 676–80
  vulval intraepithelial neoplasia (VIN) 682–4
Turner's mosaic 106
Turner's syndrome 106, 482
twin reversed arterial perfusion syndrome 149
twin-twin transfusion syndrome (TTTS) 149,
  153, 158
twins see multiple pregnancy
typhoid 260

U

ulcerative colitis see inflammatory bowel
  disease
ultrasound 512
  see also Doppler ultrasound
umbilical artery 90–1
umbilical cord abnormalities
  abnormal length 162
  coiling 162
  marginal insertion 162
  two-vessel cord 162
  umbilical cord masses 162
  velamentous cord insertion 162
urinary and renal system, changes in pregnancy
  anatomic changes 56
  physiological changes 57
urinary frequency and urgency
  aetiology 618
  alternative therapy 619
  antimuscarinic therapy 619
  behavioural management 619
  definition 618
  epidemiology 618
  examination 618
  history 618

investigations 618–19
  lifestyle changes 619
  management 618
  surgery 619
  treatment 619
urinary incontinence, female
  antimuscarinic drugs 616
  behavioural interventions 616
  bladder re-education 616
  catheterization 616
  conservative 616
  definition of 614
  duloxetine 616
  examination 615
  history 615
  investigation 615
  lifestyle changes 616
  non-urethral conditions 614
  pelvic floor muscle restraining 616
  prevalence of 614
  risk factors 614–15
  scheduled toileting 616
  treatment 616
  types of 614
  urethral conditions 614
urinary retention
  aetiology 620
  definitions/classification 620
  detrusor myopathy 620
  endocrine causes 620
  foreign bodies and calculi 620
  inflammatory causes 620
  investigations 621
  micturition, governing factors for 620
  obstructive causes 620
  overdistension 620
  pharmacological causes 620
  presentation 621
  psychogenic causes 620
  treatment 621
  urethral sphincter hypertrophy 620
  with overflow 614
urinary system abnormalities, fetal
  aetiology 141
  definition 140
  diagnosis 142
  epidemiology 140
  management 142
  pathology 140
  prognosis 141–2
  ultrasound findings 140–1
urinary tract infections 614
  screening for 39–40
urinary tract injury 622–4
  aetiology 622
  bladder injury 623
  definition 622
  diagnosis 622
  epidemiology 622
  postoperative care 624
  prevention 622
  prognosis 624
  ureteric injury 622–3
  urethral injury 622, 623
urodynamic investigation 630
urodynamic stress incontinence (USI) 614
urogynaecology see benign and urogynaecology
ursodeoxycholic acid (UDCA) 333
uterine cancer screening 641
uterine compression sutures
  aetiology 452
  B-Lynch suture 453
  Caesarean delivery 453
  clinical approach 452–4
  efficacy, testing for 453
  epidemiology 452
  pathology 452
  postoperative management 454
  postpartum haemorrhage 452
  prognosis 452
  square suture 453
  suture material 453

transverse suture 454
U-suture 454
vaginal delivery 453
vertical suture 453
uterine inversion
    aetiology 426
    clinical presentation 426
    definition 426
    epidemiology 426
    management 426–7
    prevention 427
uterovaginal prolapse
    aetiology 626
    classification 626–37
    definition 626
    diagnosis 627
    endopelvic fascia support 626, 626f
    epidemiology 626
    management 627–8
    pelvic diaphragm, anatomy of 626, 626f
    prevention 628
    prognosis 627

V

vaginal breech delivery 369
vaginal cancer screening 641
vaginal discharge
    evaluation of patient with 632
    investigations 632
    non sexually transmitted 632
    non-infective 632
    sexually transmitted 632
    treatments 632
    typical features 632
vaginal nitric oxide donors 386
valvular diseases
    aortic valve 225
    mitral valve 224–5
    prosthetic valves 225
    pulmonary valve 225
    tricuspid valve 225
vancomycin 209
varicella zoster see chicken pox

vasodilators 232
venous congestion, fetal head and neck 146
ventouse delivery
    clinical approach 457
    contraindications for 457
    cup application, examination prior to 458
    definition 456
    epidemiology 456
    failed 459
    fetal injuries 456
    indications for 456–7
    low-risk procedure 456
    maternal injuries 456
    moderate-risk procedure 456
    prerequisites for 458
    prognosis 457
    successful delivery, procedure after 459
    traction, for cephalic presentation 458–9
    training in 459
    trial of 459
    vacuum pressure, building up 458
    ventouse cup, choice of 458
    ventouse devices 456, 457
ventriculomegaly 99–100
verapamil 232
vesicovaginal fistulae
    aetiology 634
    definition 634
    investigations 634
    malignancy 634
    management 634
    miscellaneous 634
    obstetric 634
    presentation 634
    prevalence 634
    radiation 634
    surgical management 634–5
vitamin K 333
voiding difficulty see urinary retention
von Willebrand's disease (vWD) 190
vulval cancer
    aetiology 676
    clinical approach 677–9
    diagnosis 677

incidence of 676
management 678–9
pathology 676
prognostic factors 676–7
screening 641
staging 676, 677t
treatment complications/side effects 679–80
vulval intraepithelial neoplasia (VIN)
    'squamous cell carcinoma in situ'
        concept 682
    clinical evaluation 683–4
    definition 682
    differential diagnosis 683
    epidemiology and pathogenesis 682–3
    management 684
    treatment options 684
    VIN-d (differentiated type) 682–3
    VIN-u (usual type) 682, 683
vulval pain and pruritis
    history and examination 636
    special investigations 636
    treatment 636–7
    vulval itching 637
vulvovaginal candidiasis
    clinical features 318
    definition 318
    diagnosis 318
    epidemiology 318
    risk factors 318
    treatment 318
vulvovaginitis 570

W

warfarin 211, 233
Wernicke's encephalopathy 77
Williams vaginoplasty 532–3
Wilson's disease 277
Wolff-Hirchorn syndrome 106

Y

yellow fever 259